Ernsting's Aviation Medicine

Ernsting's Aviation Medicine

Fourth edition

Air Commodore David J. Rainford
Civil Consultant in Renal Disease to the Royal Air Force,
Consultant Physician to the UK Civil Aviation Authority
and Consultant Adviser in Medicine to the Royal Air Force
of Oman

Group Captain David P. Gradwell
Royal Air Force Consultant Adviser in Aviation Medicine
and Reader in Aviation Physiology, Royal Air Force Centre
for Aviation Medicine, Royal Air Force Henlow, and Visiting
Senior Lecturer in Aviation Medicine, King's College,
London

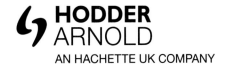

HODDER
ARNOLD

AN HACHETTE UK COMPANY

First published in Great Britain in 1978 by Tri-Med Books Ltd
Second edition 1988, paperback edition 1994, reprinted 1995
Third edition 1999 published by Butterworth-Heinemann, reprinted by
Arnold 2003
This fourth edition published in 2006 by
Hodder Arnold, an imprint of Hodder Education,
an Hachette Company UK, 338 Euston Road, London NW1 3BH

www.hoddereducation.com

Whilst the advice and information in this book are believed to be true
and accurate at the date of going to press, neither the author[s] nor the
publisher can accept any legal responsibility or liability for any errors or
omissions that may be made. In particular, (but without limiting the
generality of the preceding disclaimer) every effort has been made to
check drug dosages; however it is still possible that errors have been
missed. Furthermore, dosage schedules are constantly being revised and
new side-effects recognized. For these reasons the reader is strongly
urged to consult the drug companies' printed instructions before
administering any of the drugs recommended in this book.

British Library Cataloguing in Publication Data
A catalogue record for this book is available from the British Library

Library of Congress Cataloging-in-Publication Data
A catalog record for this book is available from the Library of Congress

ISBN 978 0 340 81319 5

4 5 6 7 8 9 10

Commissioning Editor: Joanna Koster
Project Editor: Heather Fyfe
Production Controller: Lindsay Smith
Cover Design: Sarah Rees

Typeset in 10 on 12pt Minion by Phoenix Photosetting, Chatham, Kent
Printed and bound in India by Replika Press Pvt. Ltd.

What do you think about this book? Or any other Hodder Arnold title?
Please visit our website at www.hoddereducation.com

Contents

PART II: OPERATIONAL AVIATION MEDICINE

PART III: CLINICAL AVIATION MEDICINE

Contributors

Michael Bagshaw MB BCh MRCS LRCP FFOM DAvMed DFFP FRAeS
Professor of Aviation Medicine, King's College London, London,
Army Honorary Civil Consultant in Aviation Medicine; Visiting
Professor, University of Cranfield, UK

Adrian Baker MBChB MSc MFOM DAvMed MRAeS
Surgeon Commander, Royal Navy, Principal Medical Officer, Royal
Naval Air Station Culdrose, Helston, UK

Susan M. Baker BSc PhD
Head of Human Factors, Civil Aviation Authority, Aviation House,
Gatwick Airport South, UK

Anthony J. Batchelor CBE QHS BSc MBBS FRCP DAvMed FRCP FFOM
FRAeS
Air Commodore, Royal Air Force Consultant in Medicine and
Whittingham Professor in Aviation Medicine, Royal Centre for
Defence Medicine, Birmingham, UK

Alan J. Benson BSc MSc MB ChB FRAeS
Visiting Consultant, Royal Air Force Centre of Aviation Medicine,
RAF Henlow, UK

Saliya Caldera FRCS RAF
Wing Commander, Consultant Otolaryngologist, Head and Neck
Surgeon, ENT Department, The Royal Hospital Haslar, Gosport, UK

John A. Caldwell PhD
Experimental Psychologist, Human Effectiveness Directorate, US
Air Force Research Laboratory, Wright Patterson Air Force Base,
OH, USA

J. Lynn Caldwell PhD
Diplomat, American Board of Sleep Medicine, US Air Force
Research Laboratory, Human Effectiveness Directorate, Dayton,
OH, USA

John W. Chappelow BSc CPsychol AFBPsS
Centre for Human Sciences, QinetiQ, Farnborough, UK

William J. Coker OBE QHP BSc MB ChB BA LLB FRCP DAvMed FRAeS
Air Commodore, Royal Air Force Consultant in Medicine and
Officer Commanding the Royal Air Force Centre of Aviation
Medicine, Royal Air Force Henlow, UK

John Cooke CB OBE MD FRCP FRCP(Ed) MFOM
Air Vice-Marshal RAF (retired), Retired Senior Consultant to the
Royal Air Force and Consultant Physician to the UK Civil Aviation
Authority

S. Anthony Cullen MD FRCPath FRAeS
Air Commodore (retired), Lately Royal Air Force Consultant in
Aviation Pathology, Royal Air Force Centre of Aviation Medicine,
Henlow, UK

Gary Davies MBBS MRCP(I)
Squadron Leader, Specialist Registrar in Respiratory Disease —
Royal Air Force, Prestwood, UK

Chris Elshaw BSc
QinetiQ, Farnborough, UK

John Ernsting CB OBE BSc MBBS PhD FRCP FFOM FRAeS
Air Vice-Marshal RAF (retired); Royal Air Force Honorary Civil
Consultant in Aviation Medicine; and Visiting Professor in
Applied Physiology, King's College London, London, UK

Anthony D.B. Evans BSc MSc MB ChB DAvMed MFOM
Chief, Aviation Medicine Section, International Civil Aviation
Organization, Montreal, Canada

Sally Evans MBBS DCH DRCOG DAvMed MFOM
Chief Medical Officer, UK Civil Aviation Authority, Gatwick
Airport South, UK

Eric W. Farmer BSc PhD AFBPsS
Centre for Human Sciences, QinetiQ, Farnborough, UK

Paul L.F. Giangrande BSc MD FRCP FRCPath FRCPCH
Consultant Haematologist, Oxford Haemophilia Centre and
Thrombosis Unit, Oxford Radcliffe Hospitals, Oxford

David P. Gradwell BSc PhD MB ChB FRCP DAvMed FRAeS RAF
Group Captain, Royal Air Force Consultant Adviser in Aviation
Medicine and Reader in Aviation Physiology, Royal Air Force
Centre of Aviation Medicine, Royal Air Force Henlow, Visiting
Senior Lecturer in Aviation Medicine, King's College, London, UK

Andrew D. Green MBBS FRCPath MFPH DTM&H
Wing Commander, Defence Consultant Adviser in Communicable Diseases, Defence Medical Services Department, Ministry of Defence, London; Senior Clinical Lecturer in Medicine, University of Glasgow, UK

Nicholas D.C. Green MBBS BSc DAvMed MRAeS RAF
Wing Commander, Royal Air Force Specialist in Aviation Medicine, Royal Air Force Centre of Aviation Medicine, RAF Henlow, UK

Mark Groom MB ChB MRCGP MFOM DAvMed MRAeS
Surgeon Commander, Royal Navy, Lately Principal Medical Officer, Royal Naval Air Station Yeovilton, Ilchester, UK

Alan E. Hepper BEng CEng MIMechE MRAeS ACGI
Biomedical Services Department, Defence Science and Technology Laboratory, Porton, UK

Ian R. Hill OBE MA MD PhD FRCPath LDS MRAeS
RAF Department of Aviation Pathology, RAF Centre of Aviation Medicine, Henlow, UK

Susan H. James MSc MIoA
Capability Team Leader, Defence Technology Division, QinetiQ, Farnborough, UK

Raymond V. Johnston MBA MB ChB FRCP (Glas) FFOM DAvMed
Head of the Aeromedical Centre, Civil Aviation Authority, Aviation House, Gatwick Airport South, UK

Michael Joy OBE MD FRCP FACC FESC FRAeS
Professor of Clinical Cardiology, University of Surrey and Consultant Cardiologist, Civil Aviation Authority, Aviation House, Gatwick Airport South, UK

Michael J. Kelly MBA FCIEH
Head of Food Safety & Environmental Health, British Airways, Waterside (HMAG), Harmondsworth, UK

Trevor Laundy BSc FRCP DAvMed
Group Captain, Consultant Adviser in Medicine to the Royal Air Force, Consultant Physician, MDHU Peterborough, Peterborough District Hospital, Peterborough, UK

Matthew E. Lewis MSc MBBCh DAvMed RAF
Wing Commander, Officer Commanding Accident Investigation, RAF Centre of Aviation Medicine, RAF Henlow, UK

Alistair J.F. Macmillan BSc MB ChB MFOM
Formerly Principal Medical Officer (Research), Royal Air Force Centre of Aviation Medicine, Royal Air Force Henlow, UK

Neil McGuire FRCA, RAF
Group Captain, Consultant Adviser in Anaesthetics (RAF), Adult Intensive Care, John Radcliffe Hospital, Oxford, UK

Robert T.G. Merry MBBS FRCP MRCPsych
Air Commodore (Retired), Consultant Neurologist, lately Consultant Adviser in Neurology to Royal Air Force, Consultant Neurologist and Adviser to Defence Medical Services, and Consultant Neurologist to the UK Civil Aviation Authority, UK

Helen Muir OBE
Professor of Aerospace Psychology, Cranfield University, Cranfield, UK

Denis O'Sullivan BSc PhD FInstP FRAS
Emeritus Professor, Astrophysics Section, Dublin Institute for Advanced Studies, Dublin, Ireland

David J. Rainford MBE MBBS MRCS FRCP FFOM (Hon) FRAeS RAF (Rtd)
Air Commodore, lately Commandant Royal Defence Medical College and Defence Medical Postgraduate Dean, Civil Consultant in Renal Disease to the Royal Air Force, Consultant Physician to UK Civil Aviation Authority, Consultant Adviser in Medicine to the Royal Air Force of Oman

Geoffrey E. Reid MB ChB FRCPsych DAvMed MRAeS RAF
Group Captain, Royal Air Force Consultant Adviser in Psychiatry, Royal Air Force Brize Norton, Carterton, UK

Jane Risdall MBBS MA(Cantab) DA(UK) FFARCSI
Surgeon Commander Royal Navy, Consultant in Anaesthesia and Intensive Care, lately Head of Diving and Hyperbaric Medicine, Institute of Naval Medicine, Alverstoke, Gosport, UK

Graham M. Rood PhD MSc CEng FRAES MIMechE
Consultant, QinetiQ, Farnborough, UK

Olga M. Rutherford BA MSc PhD
Lately Senior Lecturer in Physiology, King's College London, London, UK

Ian D. Sargeant MBBS FRCS FRCS(Orth) DAvMed
Wing Commander, Department of Orthopaedics, Royal Centre for Defence Medicine, Birmingham, UK; Consultant Adviser in Orthopaedics to the Royal Air Force, UK

Robert A.H. Scott MBBS FRCS(Ed) FRCOphth DM
Wing Commander, Royal Air Force Consultant Adviser in Ophthalmology, Royal Centre for Defence Medicine, Birmingham, UK; Consultant Ophthalmologist, University Hospital Birmingham NHS Trust, Birmingham, UK; Consultant Ophthalmologist, Sandwell and West Birmingham NHS Trust, Birmingham, UK; and Senior Lecturer in Ophthalmology, University of Birmingham School of Medicine, Birmingham, UK

John Skipper MB BCh FRCS RAF
Group Captain, Consultant Otolaryngologist and Consultant
Adviser in Otolaryngology to the Royal Air Force, ENT
Department, The Royal Hospital Haslar, Gosport, UK

Sheila Stork BSc(Hons) PGCE MBBS DAvMed MFOM MRAeS
Chief Medical Officer and General Manager, Safety and
Occupational Health Services, NATS, Heathrow Control Tower
Building, London Heathrow Airport, UK

J.R. Rollin Stott MA MB BChir DCH MRCP DIC DAvMed
Centre for Human Sciences, Cody Technology Park A50, QinetiQ,
Farnborough, UK

Lauren J. Thomas CPsychol
Cranfield University, Cranfield, UK

Mike Tipton MSc PhD
Professor of Human and Applied Physiology, Institute of
Biomedical and Biomolecular Sciences, Department of Sport and
Exercise Science, University of Portsmouth, Portsmouth, UK

Jane Ward BSc MB ChB PhD
Senior Lecturer in Physiology, King's College London, London,
UK

Paul Wright MB BCh MSc BAO DAvMed MRAeS
Wing Commander, RAF Centre of Aviation Medicine, Aviation
Medicine Training Wing, Royal Air Force Henlow, UK

Dazhuang Zhou BSc PhD
Astrophysics Section, Dublin Institute for Advanced Studies,
Dublin, Ireland

Foreword

When the first edition of this textbook was published nearly thirty years ago, it provided the essential material for those studying for the Diploma of Aviation Medicine at the then Royal Air Force Institute of Aviation Medicine at Farnborough; indeed I was one of those early students. Although dealing with the broader aspects of aviation and addressing physiological principle, practical and clinical issues, it was essentially a text to meet the needs of military training. Its evolution through the second and third editions was remarkable and now the fourth edition is truly an international textbook, addressing all the major issues of aviation medicine in both the military and civilian flying environments. The introduction by the editors of many new authors and topics, including important contributions from the United States of America, has brought the textbook to maturity and will undoubtedly consolidate its position as the premier textbook in the field.

Aviation medicine is not a single specialty, but brings together physiologists, clinical specialists of all disciplines and occupational physicians. All are well represented in this book. Physiological study, blue sky and operational research and their application, together with advances in clinical practice have allowed the medical world to meet the demands of the increasingly sophisticated and rapidly moving advances of the aerospace industry. The implementation of new standards by occupational physicians based on these advances, have contributed to the high levels of flight safety which both the industry and the public have a right to expect.

It gives me great pleasure to introduce the new edition of this book, now titled eponymously *Ernsting's Aviation Medicine* in tribute to the enormous contribution by Air Vice-Marshal John Ernsting to the specialty of aviation medicine and to its teaching, including through the development of this textbook. I am sure that it will be a great success and will be essential reading for all those who have an interest in this exciting and rapidly advancing field.

Air Vice-Marshal SRC Dougherty QHP MSc MBBS
FFOM DAvMed DObstRCOG FCMI FRAeS RAF
Director General Medical Services, Royal Air Force

Preface

Aviation Medicine was first published in 1978. It was followed ten years later by the second edition and in 1999 by the third. The third edition brought a change in philosophy: the text was divided into three parts, with operational aspects being added to physiology and clinical medicine. We have continued this philosophy into the fourth edition, as readers found it more user-friendly, especially when looking for data with which to answer a specific question. The format for the fourth edition follows the style of our new publisher, and we are delighted with the presentation, which is both modern and much easier to read than its predecessor. We were aware from feedback from our readers and from an international user questionnaire that there were areas of deficiency in the previous editions that had to be addressed. We hope that we have dealt with these deficiencies by the addition of new chapters in the fields of aeromedical evacuation, cosmic radiation, transport aircraft and passenger safety, passenger fitness and naval air operations. We also welcome a whole range of new authors, from research fields, the civil sector and the armed forces. It is a special pleasure to welcome our first contributors from the USA.

Originally, *Aviation Medicine* was produced primarily to meet the needs of aviation medicine training in the armed services of the UK and, in particular, to provide the reference text for students of the Diploma in Aviation Medicine of the Royal College of Physicians. The book is now aimed at a much wider audience, both civilian and military, worldwide. In the fields of fitness to fly and certification, emphasis has been placed on the principles governing decision making rather than on prescriptive regulations, which may differ from one authority to another. Knowledge of aviation medicine is pertinent to many other disciplines in the flying world, especially engineering, and we hope that this book will be a useful reference text to people in many disciplines in addition to medicine.

Professor John Ernsting was an editor for the first three editions of this book. His contributions to aviation physiology and research, and teaching and education in aviation medicine are legendary. He is known worldwide for his work and to many international readers for his supervision and support during their diploma courses. The book has been known affectionately as 'Ernsting' by successions of readers. As editors of the fourth edition, we felt it entirely appropriate that we pay tribute to Professor Ernsting by renaming the textbook *Ernsting's Aviation Medicine*. We are sure that all will approve.

Finally, we would like to thank Jo Koster, Heather Fyfe and Sarah Burrows at Edward Arnold for their help, advice and endless support in bringing the fourth edition to press.

David J. Rainford
David P. Gradwell

Acknowledgements

As with previous editions this textbook has evolved and developed. We are very grateful for and would wish to acknowledge the earlier efforts of all the authors from previous editions. In particular we would like to thank Drs JR Allan, DJ Anton, RM Harding, DH Glaister, G Maidment, GR Sharp and PJ Sowood.

PART I

Aviation physiology and aircrew systems

The Earth's atmosphere

DAVID P. GRADWELL

INTRODUCTION

This book contains chapters on the physiological, psychological and medical effects of flight. Therefore, it is appropriate to consider at the outset the nature of the environment in which all aircraft operate, i.e. the Earth's atmosphere. The form and function of the atmosphere are fundamental to the operation of all aircraft – military and civilian, fixed- and rotary-wing – influencing performance and the potential hazards faced by their occupants. An understanding of these environmental factors is thus crucial to the development of aircraft from an aerodynamic standpoint but equally important in the development of environmental control and life-support systems and essential to an appreciation of many of the principles of aviation medicine. This chapter considers the physical and chemical natures of our atmosphere and the principles of internationally accepted standards for its composition and behaviour, and provides a description of the elementary gas laws and the means of measurement adopted under differing conditions.

The development of the Earth's atmosphere has been studied extensively. The primitive atmosphere is believed not to have had the same gaseous composition as is present today. There is an interaction between the atmosphere and the land and sea masses – the *lithosphere* and *hydrosphere*, respectively – that it covers. Water from the seas is drawn into the atmosphere as water vapour, transported across sometimes great distances, and then returned to earth as freshwater precipitation. In the course of its run-off back to the sea, water modifies the Earth's surface through erosion and, importantly, provides essential support to life on Earth. The other crucial element of that capacity for life is the presence of oxygen molecules, which living organisms require for their energy and without which they cannot survive. The part of our planet in which life can naturally occur is termed the *biosphere*; this includes relatively restricted parts of the land, sea and air masses. The presence of life itself has an influence on the composition of the atmosphere, both directly and indirectly.

The atmosphere, however, is not only the source of oxygen and the medium through which the other essential requirements of life move. It also acts as a shield against the potentially harmful effects of cosmic radiation reaching the Earth and as a thermal protective layer over the Earth's surface. Depletion of the atmosphere's protective shield is already identified as a serious hazard to organisms living beneath such a defect. Human physiological processes allow life to exist in many, but not all, regions and altitudes of the Earth's surface. Unsupported exposure to environmental conditions outside this zone is hazardous and potentially fatal.

STRUCTURE OF THE ATMOSPHERE

The gases of the atmosphere are rarely, if ever, absolutely constant in position, temperature or pressure, and the rotation of the Earth and its gravitational influence have profound effects on the nature of the atmosphere. However, in practice it is possible to divide the structure of the atmosphere in a relatively simple manner, commonly described as a series of concentric 'shells' around the Earth. These shells are of varying depths and are not the same thickness at all points over the surface of the planet. Each shell or, more properly, sphere has its own distinctive qualities; the point at which one set of qualities gives way to another is termed a *pause*. One of the most valuable and widely used descriptive approaches is that based on the thermal features of each region. The successive layers of the atmosphere from the surface of the Earth outwards are the *troposphere*, the *stratosphere*, the *mesosphere*, the *thermosphere* and the *exosphere*. Thus, the level at which the thermal behaviour of the atmosphere in the troposphere changes to that of the stratosphere is termed the *tropopause*. At the outer region of the stratosphere, the *stratopause* marks the change to the mesosphere. Since the depths of the spheres vary at different points over the Earth, particularly with latitude, the altitudes at which these transitions from one part of the atmosphere to another occur also vary. These changes with latitude and thermal region, such as the Poles and the Equator, are influenced further by the effects of the seasons.

This description of the layered character of the atmosphere was established before accurate measurements were available, and it is now apparent that some of the distinctions used to delineate atmospheric regions are not as constant as thought previously. For example, temperature does not fall at a truly constant rate on ascent through the troposphere and does not remain constant in the stratosphere. Subdivisions of the stratosphere are now recognized (Figure 1.1). In a similar manner, atmospheric pressure measured at high terrestrial altitudes shows some deviation from the pattern described later. This is affected particularly by meteorological conditions and the seasons. The ascent of Mount Everest without supplemental oxygen took advantage of this effect, but the physical relationships described below are reasonably accurate and explain the physiological effects observed at altitude.

Troposphere

The troposphere is characterized by a relatively consistent fall of temperature with increasing altitude, the presence of water vapour, and the presence of large-scale air turbulence and movements, which are responsible for many of the changes in the weather. The fall of temperature with altitude is termed the *temperature lapse rate* and depends largely on local conditions. The mean lapse rate in still air is approximately 1.98 °C per 1000 feet of ascent. The decline in temperature ceases at the tropopause, the altitude of which varies with latitude and time of year. This variation arises as a consequence of the effect of solar heating of atmospheric gases. Thus, the atmosphere in Equatorial regions receives more solar energy; the air therefore is hotter and more expanded than at Polar regions. As a result, the altitude of the tropopause varies from approximately 58 000 feet at the Equator to 26 000 feet at the Poles. The temperature gradient therefore can range from an average sea-level value of 15 °C, to

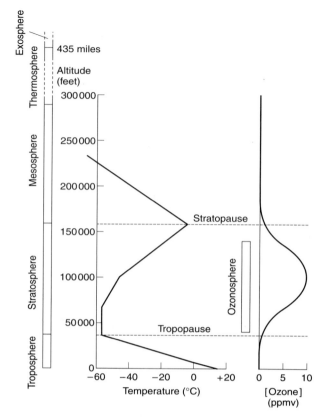

Figure 1.1   *Relationship between temperature, altitude and the layers of the atmosphere, including the ozonosphere. ppmv, parts per million by volume.*

approximately −83 °C at the tropopause over the Equator, to −53 °C over the Poles. This causes a degree of instability in the atmosphere, which contributes to the generation of the weather patterns observed.

Stratosphere

The stratosphere is the next strata of the atmosphere. It was once thought to be characterized by a fairly uniform temperature of −56 °C and an almost complete absence of water vapour. It extends from the tropopause to the stratopause at an altitude of about 158 000 feet (30 miles, 50 km) and is characterized by a high static stability. It is now known to demonstrate an overall increase in temperature, with only the lower part of the stratosphere – the isothermal layer – being at a constant temperature. Thereafter, temperature increases with altitude from about 90 000 feet to reach a maximum of −3 °C at the stratopause. The progressive rise in temperature is related to the other important feature of the stratosphere, the presence of ozone (see below). This region is termed the *ozonosphere* and extends from an altitude of about 40 000 feet to 140 000 feet. The ozonosphere is responsible for protecting the Earth from most of the ultraviolet radiation from the sun. The breakdown of ozone in this region into free ions and molecular oxygen releases heat into the atmosphere.

Mesosphere

The mesosphere, meaning 'middle region', is characterized by a rapid decline in temperature, from −3 °C at its base at the stratopause to about −110 °C at an altitude of 290 000 feet (55 miles, 85 km), making it the coldest layer of the atmosphere and at its most extreme at the Poles.

Thermosphere

The thermosphere is the uppermost region of the atmosphere. It is characterized by a continuous increase in temperature to values that depend on the activity of the sun. Temperatures can exceed 1700 °C during days of maximum solar activity but may fall to 227 °C during nights of solar calm. In air of such low density, however, temperature has no thermal significance for the air itself, although it does for any body within it. The upper limit of the thermosphere lies at an altitude of about 372 miles (600 km), i.e. at the extreme edge of the atmosphere. Since most of the particles within this layer are charged, it is also known as the *ionosphere*. The precise structure of the ionosphere varies with the energy input from the sun and is affected markedly by the 11-year cycle of solar-flare activity. The ionosphere acts as a reflector for long-wavelength electromagnetic radiation, a phenomenon that is used to facilitate radio communication between distant points on the Earth's surface.

Exosphere

At the very edge of the Earth's atmosphere, and at the beginning of true space, a final sphere, is the exosphere. There is no pause at the upper reaches of this sphere, but it becomes progressively indistinguishable from space and its composition indistinguishable from that of interplanetary gases. Within this sphere, collisions between particles are so rare as to be considered not to occur at all, and gas atoms may be regarded as having free-space trajectories. The principal components are hydrogen and helium, but even these are present at very low concentrations. The exosphere can be considered as an isothermal layer that extends into deep space.

COMPOSITION OF THE ATMOSPHERE

The composition of the atmosphere is remarkably constant between sea level and an altitude of about 300 000 feet. Air is a mixture of nitrogen, oxygen and argon, together with traces of carbon dioxide and certain rare gases such as neon and helium. Water vapour is present in variable amounts, but by convention the composition of atmospheric gases assumes it to be dry. Table 1.1 lists the constituents of dry air in percentages by volume.

The composition of air close to the surface of the Earth may be varied somewhat by a number of factors, including human activity, such as factory effluent and engine exhausts, but also natural phenomena, such as volcanic eruptions and geysers. There may be significant increases in the concentration of carbon dioxide in the air near such activity, as well as measurable levels of toxic contaminants such as carbon monoxide and methane. The lower regions of the atmosphere, up to an altitude of about 30 000 feet, i.e. the troposphere, may also contain significant quantities of water vapour. The concentration of water within a given mass of air depends largely on its location (i.e. whether it is, or has recently been, located over an area of water) and its temperature. The higher the temperature of the mass of air, the greater will be its capacity for water vapour. For many purposes, dry air may be regarded as a mixture consisting of 21 per cent oxygen and 79 per cent nitrogen, although more accurately almost one per cent is argon and the rare gases. The oxygen that is so characteristic of our atmosphere is derived from the photosynthetic processes of plants.

Ozone (O_3), the triatomic form of oxygen, is a further important constituent of the atmosphere. However, as noted above, it is present in significant concentrations only within the ozonosphere. It is a blue unstable gas formed by the irradiation of molecular oxygen in the upper atmosphere by short-wavelength (200 nm) ultraviolet light from the sun. The ultraviolet radiation is absorbed and the oxygen molecules are split into free atoms, which then either recombine with each other to reform molecular oxygen or combine with other oxygen molecules to form ozone. The amount of ozone formed at a given altitude thus depends on the concentration of oxygen molecules and the intensity of ultraviolet radiation. Above about 350 000 feet, ultraviolet radiation is so intense that all molecular oxygen is dissociated into oxygen atoms; below this altitude, molecular oxygen is more abundant and the ultraviolet

Table 1.1 *Composition of the atmosphere*

Gas	Concentration in dry air (% by volume)
Nitrogen	78.09
Oxygen	20.95
Argon	0.93
Carbon dioxide	0.03
Neon	1.82×10^{-3}
Helium	5.24×10^{-4}
Krypton	1.14×10^{-4}
Hydrogen	5.00×10^{-5}
Xenon	8.70×10^{-6}

radiation less intense, so that conditions for ozone production are created. Consequently, the concentration of ozone increases progressively as altitude is reduced below about 140 000 feet, reaching a maximum level of approximately 10 parts per million by volume (ppmv) at 100 000 feet (Figure 1.1). Below this altitude, ultraviolet radiation is much less intense, as a consequence of atmospheric absorption, and oxygen molecules are more numerous, so the concentration of ozone falls progressively to a value of less than 1 ppmv at altitudes below 40 000 feet and to about 0.03 ppmv at sea level. Furthermore, at these lower altitudes, ozone is dissociated to molecular oxygen by longer-wavelength (210–300 nm) ultraviolet light.

Ozone is a very strong oxidant and is highly toxic, exerting its clinical effects primarily upon the respiratory tract. Although in the early part of the twentieth century some clinicians believed that ozone might assist in the treatment of various diseases, acute exposure to concentrations of 0.6–0.8 ppmv for two hours is sufficient to reduce vital capacity and forced expiratory volume and to cause a fall in diffusing capacity for carbon monoxide, presumably as a consequence of alveolar oedema. Exposure to 1 ppmv is sufficient to cause lung irritation, while 10 ppmv can induce fatal pulmonary oedema. In addition, ozone has been shown to impair night vision in humans, and exposure of human cell cultures to ozone induces chromatid breakages similar to those produced by X-rays.

Some military aircraft operate within the ozonosphere, but their occupants generally will have personal oxygen systems, providing a high concentration of oxygen in the inspired breathing gas. In aircraft in which the cabin environment is pressurized to such a degree as to make it suitable as the primary means of protection against hypoxia at high altitudes, there would be a potential risk of the ozone concentration in cabin air being unacceptably high and giving rise to respiratory irritation. However, at normal engine power settings, the air entering the cabin, which will have passed through the engine compressors before reaching the cabin-conditioning system, will have been heated to high temperatures; given the thermal instability of ozone, this potentially toxic gas is thus broken down to molecular oxygen. Only at flight-idle engine power could ozone pass unaltered through the cabin-conditioning system in any significant amount, and inevitably at such power levels the aircraft will be descending out of the ozonosphere.

PHYSICS OF THE ATMOSPHERE

Density and pressure

As described above, the overall depth of the atmosphere varies with latitude and is the result of two opposing influences. The atmospheric gases are heated by the sun; the

more directly this acts, the greater the effect seen. At the outer reaches of the atmosphere, gases expand into the vacuum of space, but this effect is counteracted by the gravitational attraction exerted by the Earth, tending to draw the gases towards its surface. Air density, i.e. mass per unit volume, in the atmosphere is proportional to ambient pressure, i.e. force per unit area at a specific altitude. Atmospheric pressure falls progressively with ascent from the surface of the Earth; indeed, because gas is compressible, density and pressure both fall in an approximately exponential manner with vertical distance (altitude) from the Earth's surface, although local variations in temperature at altitude bring about modest deviations from a true exponential decline. However, the physiologically significant factor in inspired atmospheric air is its pressure; therefore, in aviation medicine, it is pressure rather than density that is used when considering the consequences of ascent to altitude.

The pressure exerted at sea level by the weight of the atmosphere is 101.3 kPa (14.7 lb/in^2). This atmospheric pressure will support a column of mercury (Hg) in an evacuated tube to a height of 760 mm. As Figure 1.2 shows, this pressure is halved to 50.7 kPa (380 mmHg) at an altitude of 18 000 feet and reduced to one-quarter (25 kPa, 190 mmHg) at an altitude of 33 700 feet. At 100 000 feet, the atmospheric pressure is one-hundredth of that at sea level.

At the upper reaches of the atmosphere, the gases are so expanded that collisions between molecules occur with decreasing frequency. By an altitude of about 262 000 feet (50 miles, 80 km) (the von Karman line), the pressure exerted by atmospheric gas has fallen to such a degree that aerodynamic forces are no longer effective and manoeuvrability of craft must be achieved by rockets or reaction jets. At even greater altitudes, the density of the atmosphere is so low that particles travel considerable distances without colliding with each other at all. In the exosphere, as described

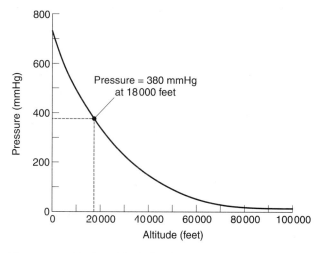

Figure 1.2 *Exponential relationship between pressure exerted by the atmosphere and altitude.*

above, some lighter particles travelling at high velocity may escape from the atmosphere completely and move into space. This characterizes the very edge of the Earth's atmosphere. Even so, the influence of the Earth's gravitational force remains strong, and only at an altitude of 1700 miles (2735 km) has it fallen to half its sea-level value.

Temperature

The temperature of the atmosphere varies markedly with altitude (Figure 1.1), but the relationship is not a simple one. For any given altitude, there are considerable geographical and temporal differences in temperature. These could be predicted from the observations on the influence of solar heating noted above, but there are several mechanisms involved in this process. Although some solar radiation is reflected away into space by the outermost layers of the atmosphere and some, particularly ultraviolet radiation, is absorbed in the upper layers, the bulk of the infrared radiation from the sun penetrates the atmosphere and reaches the Earth's surface. As the ground itself is warmed by this process, it warms the air immediately above it by radiation and conduction. The ground radiation is at a different frequency from solar radiation but still in the infrared part of the spectrum. This radiation is absorbed by carbon dioxide and water vapour in the lower atmosphere; in turn, these lower layers re-radiate part of the infrared energy. Some returns to the surface of the Earth to be radiated yet again, while the remainder passes up to be absorbed in the higher layers of the atmosphere. Thus, the atmosphere has the effect of creating a warmer environment on Earth than would occur simply as a result of solar heating in the absence of the atmosphere. This blanketing influence is termed the *greenhouse effect*.

The thermal changes that occur at or near the surface of the Earth create convection currents in the lower atmosphere and therefore contribute to the circulation of weather patterns and influence climate. Since the heating of the lower atmosphere is influenced strongly by solar infrared heating of the Earth's surface, the greater the distance above the surface, the lower the expected temperature. Thus, there is normally a progressive decline in temperature with increasing altitude, although local inversions and variations do occur. This progressive fall in temperature continues until the tropopause is reached and is then halted. The thermal patterns described previously have the effect of inhibiting further convection and thereby tend to limit weather patterns to the troposphere.

Ionizing radiation

Ionizing radiation falls on the Earth from space in a continuous stream. This high-energy subatomic particulate radiation originates either from our own sun (solar cosmic radiation) or from other stars (galactic cosmic radiation). It consists of protons (79 per cent), alpha particles (20 per cent) and the nuclei of heavier atoms (one per cent). The radiation enters the atmosphere at high velocity, in some cases approaching that of light. As the ionizing radiation enters the upper regions of the atmosphere, the primary particles collide with atoms within it at altitudes between 60 000 and 120 000 feet to produce a secondary radiation of protons, electrons, neutrons, mesons and gamma rays. Such secondary radiation has considerably less energy than its precursor, but it is capable of intense ionization. Secondary rays penetrate the lower regions of the atmosphere, but although some reach the surface of the Earth, their ionizing power diminishes rapidly at altitudes below 50 000 feet, as further collisions occur with atmospheric molecules as atmospheric density increases. At sea level, the ionizing effect of cosmic radiation is about only one-seventieth of that encountered at an altitude of 70 000 feet.

The potential to receive higher doses of ionizing radiation at high altitude has some implications for high-flying aircraft and manned spacecraft. Since these craft operate outside the protective effect of most, or all, of the Earth's atmosphere, the dose of galactic radiation increases. Manned spaceflight therefore exposes astronauts to some additional degree of radiation hazard. Although the shell of the craft provides some element of shielding in current spacecraft, it is considerably less effective than the natural shielding provided by the atmosphere. With longer endurance spaceflights being conducted in the International Space Station, and the potential for a manned mission to Mars, there is an inevitable cumulative risk arising from increased received doses of ionizing radiation. During extra-vehicular activity (spacewalks), this problem is exacerbated, since the suits worn by astronauts are far less effective than the structure of the spacecraft in providing a shield against ionizing radiation.

Standard atmospheres

The introduction of flight instrumentation that could indicate the height of an aircraft or balloon in terms of altitude and barometric pressure made it essential that a reference standard was introduced. This type of standard can be used as the basis for calibration of flight instruments, to allow accurate comparisons to be made between the performance of various aircraft and aircraft systems, and is crucially important in establishing altitude separation in busy commercial airways. In a little over 20 years of heavier-than-air flight, but coming after the rapid advances in aircraft design during the First World War and with the development of the first commercial air services, the International Committee on Air Navigation (ICAN) drew up the first internationally accepted standard atmosphere in 1924. This used simple laws to define the relationship between pressure and altitude. In the years that followed, a number of different standards were prepared and adopted both nationally and internationally. In particular, the US standard (1962), the Wright Air Development Centre (WADC) standard, the Air Research and Development Centre (ARDC; 1959) standard and the International Civil Aviation Organization (ICAO) standard (1964) were established. Even as recently as 1986, an updated standard – the Committee on Space Research international reference atmosphere – was published. Although there are differences between standards, these tend to be associated with alternative approaches to the temperature–altitude convention employed in their construction, especially with respect to the upper atmosphere, and they are very similar (and, indeed, identical in their most recent versions) for altitudes up to 65 000 feet. For the purposes of both military and civil aviation, the ICAO (1964) standard has been adopted.

INTERNATIONAL CIVIL AVIATION ORGANIZATION STANDARD ATMOSPHERE

The 1964 ICAO standard atmosphere closely represents the pressure and temperature characteristics of the real atmosphere at the temperate latitude of 45 ° North. The relationship between pressure and altitude defined by this standard, and listed in an abbreviated form in Table 1.2, is based upon the following 'ideal' assumptions:

- The air is dry and devoid of dust and has a stated composition (that given in Table 1.1).
- The atmospheric pressure at mean sea level is 760 mmHg.
- The atmospheric density at mean sea level is 1.225 kg/m³.
- The relative molecular mass of air at mean sea level is 28.9644.
- Acceleration due to gravity is 9.80665 m/s² and is constant.
- The temperature–altitude profile is as follows:

  - Temperature at mean sea level: +15 °C.
  - Mean temperature lapse rate: −1.98 °C per 1000 feet from mean sea level to 36 089 feet.
  - Height of tropopause: 36 089 feet above mean sea level.
  - Temperature of isothermal layer of stratosphere, from 36 089 to 65 616 feet: −56.5 °C.
  - Temperature rises progressively above 65 616 feet to −46 °C at 100 000 feet.

A given standard atmosphere defines the variation of pressure with altitude for a given relationship between temperature and altitude. In reality, as noted above, there are considerable variations in the temperature profile, both

with season of the year and with latitude. Table 1.3 illustrates this by comparing the ICAO standard with measured maximum and minimum temperatures at various altitudes. These temperature variations are of practical importance to both physiologists and aeronautical engineers. Thus, the physiological disturbances induced by exposure to low pressure in a hypobaric chamber are related to the pressure–altitude tables uncorrected for temperature, while the aerodynamic behaviour imparted to an airframe during its passage through the air is determined by the density altitude. Since density altitude is pressure–altitude corrected for the difference between the observed temperature and the temperature adopted by the standard atmosphere, it may therefore be regarded as a 'real' or 'true' altitude.

Gas laws and conditions of measurement

The physical laws that govern the behaviour of gases in isolation, as components of gaseous mixtures and dissolved in liquids, have a direct bearing on the understanding of the mechanisms whereby changes in altitude affect human physiology. The laws of particular relevance to physiology include Boyle's law and Charles's law, which are concerned with the relationships between pressure, temperature and volume of an ideal (hypothetical) gas, but they also extend to the behaviour of the individual components making up a mixture of gases (Dalton's law) and the behaviour of gases in solution (Henry's law and the laws of gaseous diffusion). The physical principles of gauge and absolute (abs) pressures are also pertinent, as is an understanding of the conditions of measurement applicable to atmospheric and respired gases.

BOYLE'S LAW

Boyle's law states that, measured at a constant temperature, the volume of a fixed mass of gas is inversely proportional to the pressure to which it is subjected. Expressed mathematically,

$$P \propto \frac{1}{V}$$

and therefore

$$\frac{P_1}{P_2} = \frac{V_2}{V_1}$$

where P_1 is the initial pressure, P_2 is the final pressure, V_1 is the initial volume and V_2 is the final volume.

It should be noted that the pressure here is expressed in absolute terms and not as a differential (gauge) pressure (see below). The law is modified by the presence of water vapour; therefore, since the gases in body cavities may be regarded as being saturated with water vapour at a con-

Table 1.2 *International Civil Aviation Organization (ICAO) (1964) international standard atmosphere*

Altitude ft	m	Pressure mmHg	lb/in²	Temperature (°C)	Altitude ft	m	Pressure mmHg	lb/in²	Temperature (°C)
0	0	760	14.70	+15.0	35 000	10 668	179	3.46	−54.2
1 000	305	733	14.17	+13.0	36 000	10 973	170	3.30	−56.3
2 000	610	706	13.67	+11.0	37 000	11 278	162	3.14	−56.5
3 000	914	681	13.17	+9.1	38 000	11 582	155	3.00	−56.5
4 000	1219	656	12.69	+7.1	39 000	11 887	147	2.95	−56.5
5 000	1525	632	12.23	+5.1	40 000	12 192	141	2.72	−56.5
6 000	1829	609	11.78	+3.1	41 000	12 497	134	2.59	−56.5
7 000	2134	586	11.34	+1.1	42 000	12 802	128	2.47	−56.5
8 000	2438	565	10.92	−0.9	43 000	13 107	122	2.36	−56.5
9 000	2743	543	10.50	−2.8	44 000	13 411	116	2.24	−56.5
10 000	3048	523	10.11	−4.8	45 000	13 716	111	2.14	−56.5
					46 000	14 021	106	2.04	−56.5
11 000	3353	503	9.72	−6.8	47 000	14 326	101	1.95	−56.5
12 000	3658	483	9.35	−8.8	48 000	14 630	96.0	1.85	−56.5
13 000	3962	465	8.98	−10.8	49 000	14 935	91.5	1.77	−56.5
14 000	4267	447	8.63	−12.7	50 000	15 240	87.3	1.68	−56.5
15 000	4572	429	8.29	−14.7	51 000	15 545	83.2	1.61	−56.5
16 000	4879	412	7.97	−16.7	52 000	15 850	79.3	1.53	−56.5
17 000	5182	395	7.64	−18.7	53 000	16 155	75.6	1.46	−56.5
18 000	5486	380	7.34	−20.7	54 000	16 459	72.1	1.39	−56.5
19 000	5791	364	7.04	−22.6	55 000	16 764	68.8	1.32	−56.5
20 000	6096	349	6.75	−24.6	56 000	17 069	65.5	1.27	−56.5
					57 000	17 374	62.4	1.21	−56.5
21 000	6401	335	6.48	−26.6	58 000	17 679	59.5	1.15	−56.5
22 000	6706	321	6.21	−28.6	59 000	17 983	56.8	1.10	−56.5
23 000	7010	307	5.95	−30.6	60 000	18 288	54.1	1.04	−56.5
24 000	7315	294	5.70	−32.6	65 000	19 812	42.3	0.828	−56.5
25 000	7620	282	5.45	−34.5	70 000	21 336	33.3	0.644	−55.2
26 000	7925	270	5.22	−36.5	75 000	22 860	26.2	0.507	−53.6
27 000	8230	258	4.99	−38.5	80 000	24 384	20.7	0.401	−52.1
28 000	8534	247	4.78	−40.5	85 000	25 908	16.4	0.317	−50.6
29 000	8839	236	4.57	−42.5	90 000	27 432	13.0	0.251	−49.1
30 000	9144	226	4.36	−44.4	95 000	28 956	10.3	0.199	−47.5
					100 000	30 480	8.2	0.158	−46.0
31 000	9449	215	4.17	−46.4					
32 000	9754	206	3.98	−48.4					
33 000	10 058	196	3.80	−50.6					
34 000	10 363	187	3.63	−52.4					

Table 1.3 *Worldwide maximum and minimum recorded air temperatures at various altitudes (frequency of occurrence of 10 days in 1 year)*

Altitude (ft)	ICAO (1964) standard	Temperature (°C) Maximum recorded	Minimum recorded
0	+15.0	+50	−26
10 000	−4.8	+16	−34
20 000	−25.6	−3	−48
30 000	−44.4	−21	−62
40 000	−56.5	−40	−68
50 000	−56.5	−40	−78
60 000	−56.5	−40	−86
80 000	−52.1	−40	−86
100 000	−46.0	−30	−90

ICAO, International Civil Aviation Organization.

stant (body) temperature, the equation becomes, for physiological purposes:

$$\frac{(P_1 - P_{H_2O})}{(P_2 - P_{H_2O})} = \frac{V_2}{V_1}$$

where P_{H_2O} is saturated water vapour pressure at body temperature. Since body temperature is constant, so too is P_{H_2O}.

CHARLES'S LAW

Charles's law states that the volume of a fixed mass of gas is directly proportional to its absolute temperature, measured at a constant pressure. The absolute temperature of a gas, which is measured in Kelvin, is obtained by adding 273 to its Celsius temperature, since absolute zero is −273 °C. (At absolute zero, molecular motion ceases and theoretically gases then have no volume.) Charles's law may be expressed mathematically thus:

$$V \propto T$$

and therefore

$$V = \text{constant} \times T$$

or

$$\frac{V_1}{V_2} = \frac{T_1}{T_2} = \frac{(t_1 + 273)}{(t_2 + 273)}$$

where V_1 is the initial volume, V_2 is the final volume, T_1 is the initial absolute temperature and T_2 is the final absolute temperature (absolute temperature being the sum of the temperature t_1 and t_2 in degrees Celsius plus 273).

UNIVERSAL GAS LAW

By combining Boyle's and Charles's laws, a universal or general gas law can be derived, as described by the following equation:

$$\frac{P_1 V_1}{T_1} = \frac{P_2 V_2}{T_2}$$

where P_1, V_1 and T_1 refer to the pressure, volume and temperature (in kelvins) of a mass of gas in one set of conditions and P_2, V_2 and T_2 describe them in a second set of conditions.

DALTON'S LAW

Dalton's law of partial pressures states that the pressure exerted by a mixture of gases is equal to the sum of the pressures that each would exert if it alone occupied the space filled by the mixture. The law may be expressed mathematically thus:

$$P_t = P_1 + P_2 + P_3 \dots P_n$$

where P_t is the total pressure of the mixture and P_1, P_2, $P_3 \dots P_n$ are the partial pressures of each component.

It follows that the partial pressure of any gas in a mixture is given by the relationship

$$P_x = F_x \times P_t$$

where P_x is the partial pressure of gas x, F_x is the fractional concentration of gas x in the mixture and P_t is the total pressure of the gas mixture. Thus, for example, the partial pressure of oxygen (P_{O_2}) in the dry atmosphere at mean sea-level pressure is

$$P_{O_2} = \frac{20.95}{100} \times 760 = 159.2 \text{ mmHg}$$

HENRY'S LAW

Henry's law states that the mass of gas that will dissolve in a liquid (and with which it does not combine chemically) at a given temperature is directly proportional to the partial pressure of the gas above the liquid and the solubility coefficient of the gas in the particular liquid. At equilibrium, the partial pressure of the gas in the liquid phase will be the same as that of the gas directly above the liquid. Thus, if the partial pressure of a gas in a liquid is reduced, then the amount of that gas that can be held in solution will be reduced in proportion. A simple example of the way in which Henry's law works is seen when a bottle of carbonated water is opened. The opening of the bottle causes a sudden reduction in pressure in the gas above the liquid, and gas in the liquid comes out of solution, as evidenced by the production of bubbles in the liquid. This behaviour is believed to be the basis of bubble formation (leading to decompression sickness) in body fluids on abrupt exposure to a significant reduction in environmental pressure.

LAWS OF GASEOUS DIFFUSION

Diffusion is the process whereby molecules move from regions of higher concentration to those of lower concentration. In gaseous diffusion, the molecules of one gas intermingle with those of another. The rate of diffusion of a single gas through a liquid or gaseous mixture is proportional to the difference between the partial pressures of the gas at the two points and inversely proportional to the square root of its molecular weight (Graham's law). In a liquid, the rate of diffusion is proportional to the solubility of the gas within the liquid, such that the more soluble the gas, the faster its diffusion.

Fick's law describes the diffusion of a gas through a tissue medium. When considering the effect of Fick's law in the body, the diffusion rate of a gas across a fluid membrane is proportional to the difference in partial pressure (as above), proportional to the area of the membrane and inversely proportional to the thickness of the membrane. Combined with the diffusion rate determined by Graham's law, Fick's law provides the means for calculating exchange rates of gases across membranes. The total membrane surface area of the lung alveoli (the alveolar–capillary membrane) in adults may be of the order of $100 \ m^2$ and have a thickness of less than one-millionth of 1 m, and so it is a very effective gas-exchange interface. Fick's law can be expressed mathematically thus:

$$\dot{V}_{gas} \propto \left(\frac{A}{T}\right) D(P_1 - P_2)$$

and,

$$D \propto \frac{Sol}{\sqrt{(MW)}}$$

where $\dot{V}_{gas}$ is the rate at which gas is transferred, A is the surface area of the tissue, T is the thickness of the tissue, $P_1 - P_2$ is the difference in gas partial pressure across the tissue, D is the diffusion constant, Sol is the solubility of the gas, and MW is the molecular weight of the gas.

CONDITIONS OF MEASUREMENT

Measurement of pressure

Pressure may be defined as perpendicular force per unit area. A column of liquid or gas therefore will exert a pressure that is proportional to the height of the column, the density of the material within it, and the acceleration due to gravity. Accordingly, atmospheric pressure is a reflection of the force imparted by the mass of a column of air that, at sea level, will exert a pressure on the Earth's surface of $1.033 \ kg/cm^2$ ($14.7 \ lb/in^2$, 760 mmHg, 1 atmosphere, 1 bar).

The *absolute pressure* of a gas or (confined) liquid is the total pressure it exerts and includes the effect of atmospheric pressure. Thus, an absolute pressure of zero corresponds to a complete vacuum (as is found in deep space). Pressure-measuring devices, such as pneumatic tyre pressure gauges, however, respond to the pressure present in excess of any atmospheric component. So, for example, a tyre pressure gauge may indicate a pressure of $30 \ lb/in^2$ within a tyre – which is termed the *gauge pressure* – but the absolute pressure exerted by the air within the tyre must include the local atmospheric component and thus at sea level will be $44.7 \ lb/in^2$. The gauge reading given by such an instrument therefore is the difference between two pressures, and so the instrument will register zero whenever the pressure applied to the measuring point equals that of its surroundings. The total or absolute pressure is the algebraic sum of the gauge and the local (i.e. ambient) atmospheric pressures, i.e.

absolute pressure = gauge pressure
+ local atmospheric pressure

Pressures less than atmospheric pressure will produce negative gauge pressures, and these correspond to partial vacuums. An absolute pressure, however, cannot be less than zero.

In physiology, the distinction between absolute and gauge pressures is important. In the case of a diver, for example, the diver is already under a pressure of 1 atmosphere (1 bar) at sea level before descending; a dive to a depth of 30 m will produce a gauge reading of 3 bars (3 atmospheres), but the absolute pressure will be 4 bars.

In aviation physiology, this concept is of particular relevance when considering cabin-pressurization schedules (see Chapter 6). The absolute pressure within the cabin of an aircraft equals the sum of the atmospheric pressure at its external surface (measured by static probe) and the *cabin differential pressure*; the cabin differential pressure is the difference between the absolute pressure within the aircraft and that of the atmosphere outside it. Thus:

cabin differential pressure =
internal cabin pressure (abs) – atmospheric pressure (abs)

and so,

cabin absolute pressure =
cabin differential pressure + atmospheric pressure (abs)

As an example, the atmospheric pressure surrounding an aircraft flying at 25 000 feet is 38 kPa ($5.5 \ lb/in^2$ abs). If the cabin differential pressure is 31 kPa ($4.5 \ lb/in^2$ g), then the absolute pressure within the cabin will be the sum of these, i.e. 69 kPa ($10.0 \ lb/in^2$), and the cabin altitude will be just over 10 000 feet.

Measurement of gas volumes

In physiology and medicine, the gas laws will have their greatest influence in the study of respiratory behaviour. The brief description of the laws governing the behaviour of gases implies that changes in temperature and pressure will have profound effects on the numerical values of any variables studied. Therefore, for a satisfactory appreciation of this subject, it is important that relationships between the various conditions of measurement are understood.

It is generally accepted that body temperature, including that of the lungs, is constant and that water vapour when present, as in the lungs, is at its saturation pressure. The values commonly used are a temperature of 37 °C and the saturated water vapour pressure at that temperature, which is 47 mmHg. The gas in the lungs under these conditions is stated to be at *body temperature and pressure, saturated with water vapour* (BTPS). The volumes of gases within the lungs are usually defined at BTPS conditions.

Under most circumstances, however, ambient air is at a lower temperature than gas in the lungs and, furthermore, contains less water vapour. This is not only because atmospheric air is not usually saturated with water vapour but also because, inevitably, at a lower temperature the saturated water vapour pressure is lower. If measurements are made under these conditions, then they are said to be at *ambient temperature and pressure* (ATP). If, however, respiratory measurements are made via a spirometer or if gas is collected in a bag, then the air is regarded to be saturated with water vapour and the conditions of measurement are the familiar *ambient temperature and pressure, saturated with water vapour* (ATPS).

Ambient air is heated and humidified as it passes through the upper respiratory tract, and consequently it expands in accordance with Charles's law and by virtue of water molecules evaporating within the airway. The physiological importance of this is that the volume of gas inspired (as measured by a spirometer or similar device) is less than the volume of gas taking part in respiratory exchange. The shortfall may be of the order of ten per cent in temperate climates; for the precision required by respiratory physiologists, a correction from ATPS to BTPS therefore is necessary. The correction may be expressed mathematically thus:

$$\dot{V}_{BTPS} = \dot{V}_{ATPS} \times \left[\frac{(273 + 37)}{(273 + t_a)} \right] \times \left[\frac{(P_B - P_{H_2O})}{(P_B - 47)} \right]$$

where t_a is the ambient temperature in degrees Celsius, P_B is the barometric pressure in millimetres of mercury, P_{H_2O} is the saturated water vapour pressure at t_a, and 47 is the saturated water vapour pressure at body temperature, in millimetres of mercury.

The first fraction in this equation is the term describing expansion due to heat. The second fraction is the term describing the volume increase as a consequence of added water vapour. The product therefore is the factor by which the ATPS volume must be multiplied to give the lung volume at BTPS.

When dealing with metabolic physiology, however, different requirements exist. In this case, it is the number of molecules of oxygen used and of carbon dioxide produced that are of interest, rather than the volume that they happen to be occupying at the time of measurement. It is essential, therefore, to express oxygen and carbon dioxide volumes under the precisely defined standard conditions, i.e. at *standard temperature and pressure, dry* (STPD). Standard temperature is 273 K (0 °C) and standard pressure is 760 mmHg. When defined in this way, the number of molecules contained within the STPD volume can be calculated readily, since, under STPD conditions, gases comply with Avogadro's law, i.e. 1 gram-mole of a gas will have a volume of 22.4 litres (STPD).

The correction from ATPS measurement to STPD conditions is:

$$\dot{V}_{STPD} = \dot{V}_{ATPS} \times \left[\frac{273}{(273 + t_a)} \right] \times \left[\frac{(P_b - P_{H_2O})}{760} \right]$$

Finally, in the context of breathing system definition (see Chapter 5), two further conditions of measurement are encountered that are of particular use to life-support engineers. Thus, system specifications may often quote gas volumes under *atmospheric temperature and pressure, dry* (ATPD) conditions, while consumption figures are quoted under *normal temperature and pressure* (NTP) conditions. In the UK, temperature and pressure under ATPD conditions are considered to be +15 °C and the absolute pressure of gas within the site under study (e.g. within a mask delivery hose). Similarly, the temperature and pressure under NTP conditions are +15 °C and 760 mmHg absolute, respectively.

The need to express quantities of gas under NTP conditions is a reflection of the expansile behaviour of gases on exposure to low environmental pressures; that is, once at altitude, the *volume flow* of a gas is not the same as its *mass flow*, the difference increasing with altitude. As an example, a mass flow of 4 litres (NTP)/min will provide a volume flow of about 8 litres (ATPD)/min at an altitude of 18 000 feet, where atmospheric pressure is half its sea-level value and expansion has occurred in accordance with Boyle's law. In fact, the volume flow of a gas is never the same as its mass flow, even at sea level, although the magnitude of the difference increases with altitude. This has particular relevance for respiratory physiology at altitude, since respiration is a volume flow phenomenon. This aspect is dealt with further in Chapter 2.

FURTHER READING

Andrews DG. *An Introduction to Atmospheric Physics*. Cambridge: Cambridge University Press, 2000.

Goody RM. *Principles of Atmospheric Physics and Chemistry*. Oxford: Oxford University Press, 1995.

International Civil Aviation Organization. *Manual of the ICAO Standard Atmosphere*, 2nd edn. Montreal, Canada: ICAO, 1964.

Lumb AB. *Nunn's Applied Respiratory Physiology*. Oxford: Butterworth-Heinemann, 2000.

Meteorological Office. *Handbook of Aviation Meteorology*. London: HM Stationery Office, 1971.

West JB. *Respiratory Physiology*, 7th edn. Philadelphia, PA: Lipincott, Williams & Wilkins, 2004.

2

Cardiovascular and respiratory physiology

JOHN ERNSTING, JANE WARD AND OLGA M. RUTHERFORD

INTRODUCTION

A clear understanding of the physiological disturbances induced by the stresses that occur in aviation rests on an in-depth knowledge of cardiovascular and respiratory physiology. The relevant aspects of the physiological function of these systems are described in this chapter. The material presented here is essential not only for understanding the stresses imposed on the body and the applied physiology of protective systems employed in aviation but also for a full appreciation of the functional significance of cardiovascular and respiratory diseases and their treatments in the context of aviation.

Readers who need a more comprehensive coverage of the topic than can be presented here can consult monographs on cardiovascular and respiratory physiology as given in the reference list at the end of this chapter.

CARDIOVASCULAR PHYSIOLOGY

Overview of the cardiovascular system

The human cardiovascular system consists of the systemic circulation in series with the pulmonary circulation (Figure 2.1). In the systemic circulation, blood is ejected by the left ventricle into the aorta. Nearly all this blood, having passed through the various vascular beds of the different organs and tissues, finds its way back via the systemic veins to the right side of the heart, to be pumped through the pulmonary circulation for gas exchange. This series arrangement of the systemic and pulmonary circulations means that the output of the right heart, measured in litres/minute, must be almost identical to the output of the left heart. In normal people, a small difference exists because of some anomalies in the anatomy of the normal circulation, e.g. the bronchial venous drainage as shown in Figure 2.1. Normally, the blood flow through such right-to-left-shunt pathways is less than two per cent of the cardiac output (CO).

In young people, the walls of the aorta and large arteries contain large amounts of elastin, making them very distensible. During ventricular systole, the aorta and other elastic arteries stretch, accommodating more blood and reducing systolic pressure. During diastole, they recoil, maintaining flow during ventricular relaxation and raising diastolic pressure. The difference between systolic and diastolic arterial pressure (pulse pressure) increases with age as the arteries become less elastic.

The capillary beds of most tissues and organs in the systemic circulation are in parallel with each other. The large arteries divide into smaller muscular arteries, which in turn lead to the muscular arterioles and pre-capillary sphincters, which supply the thin-walled capillaries where gas and nutrient exchange occur. The blood emerging from the capillaries passes through venules and veins, finally entering the right atrium via the inferior and superior vena cava and the coronary sinus.

In a few places in the body, two capillary beds that are functionally linked are in series with each other. In the hepatic portal system, the blood draining from gastro-intestinal capillary beds passes via the portal vein to the liver, where the products of digestion are processed. In the kidney, the blood from the glomerular capillaries drains into efferent arterioles that supply the capillaries of the renal tubules. The potential disadvantage of portal systems is reduced oxygen delivery to the downstream vascular bed. In the liver, an adequate oxygen supply is maintained

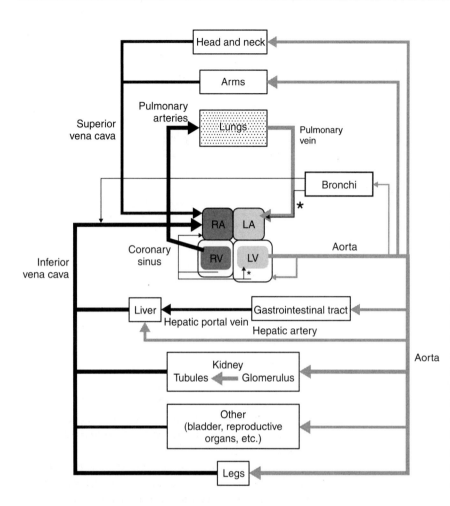

Figure 2.1   *Schematic overview of the main features of the human cardiovascular system. The white boxes represent the main organs and tissues of the systemic circulation, which are in parallel with each other and supplied by the left ventricle (LV) via the aorta. The stippled box is the pulmonary circulation, which is supplied by the right ventricle (RV) via the pulmonary arteries. The grey lines represent vessels carrying well-oxygenated blood, and the black lines represent vessels containing blood with a low oxygen content. Some deoxygenated blood from the bronchial circulation and a small amount from the left ventricular muscle join the oxygenated blood on the left side of the heart. These normal right-to-left shunts are shown by asterisks.*

via the hepatic artery. In the kidney, blood flow is normally very high relative to oxygen consumption and provides an adequate oxygen delivery to both capillary beds. However, tubular necrosis can occur when blood flow to the kidney is reduced in haemorrhage.

Typical resting blood flows to the different organs of the body are given in Table 2.1, which compares the circulation at rest and in strenuous exercise.

Measurement of cardiovascular pressures in the body

Pressures in the body are usually referred to atmospheric pressure, with pressures above atmospheric being positive and those below being negative. The International System of Units (SI) unit of pressure is the pascal (Pa) but blood pressures are still usually expressed in millimetres of mercury (mmHg), i.e. the height of a column of mercury that the pressure would support. Low pressures, such as central venous pressure, are also measured in centimetres of water (cmH$_2$O). Sometimes, especially when considering the effects of posture on blood pressure, it is helpful to know the pressure exerted by the weight of a column

Table 2.1   *Typical physiological values in a healthy 20-year-old man at rest and during maximal exercise. Actual values, especially those in maximal exercise, will vary considerably, depending on the subject's level of physical fitness and training and on environmental conditions. Blood flows for the important organs are shown both in absolute values and as a percentage of the cardiac output*

	Rest	Maximal exercise
Heart rate (bpm)	70	200
Stroke volume (ml)	75	90
CO (ml/min)	5250	18 000
(a-v) O$_2$ content (ml/ml)	0.048	0.167
O$_2$ consumption (ml/min)	250	3000
Blood flow (ml/min, % CO):		
Skeletal muscle	790 (15%)	13 000 (72%)
Skin	320 (6%)	1260 (7%)
Heart	260 (5%)	900 (5%)
Brain	790 (15%)	790 (5%)
Gastrointestinal tract	1300 (25%)	900 (5%)
Kidneys	1050 (20%)	540 (3%)

a-v, arteriovenous; bpm, beats/min; CO, cardiac output.

of blood expressed in conventional units: 1 cm blood = 1.06 cmH$_2$O = 0.78 mmHg = 0.104 kPa.

Factors affecting pressures in blood vessels

Several factors play a part in determining the pressure in any vessel in the circulation. First, blood is an incompressible liquid completely filling a system of elastic vessels. If the heart is stopped suddenly, then blood continues to flow from arteries to veins, causing arterial pressure to fall and central venous pressure to rise until, after a few seconds, pressure becomes equal throughout the circulation. This pressure – the mean circulatory filling pressure – is dependent on the blood volume contained within the circulation and the vascular capacity, which is especially affected by venous smooth muscle tone. Mean circulatory filling pressure is normally about 7 mmHg.

Second, contraction of the heart generates pressure. Left ventricular contraction generates a mean pressure in the aorta of about 90–100 mmHg. As blood flows through the systemic vessels back to the right atrium, the pressure falls progressively in a way that depends on the resistance of the vessels.

Finally, the effects of gravity modify pressures within vessels. In an open container filled with a liquid, the pressure at the surface is atmospheric or 'zero' and increases with distance below the surface because of the weight of the liquid. If the liquid has a density ρ (measured in grams per millilitre), then h metres below the surface the pressure increases by $\rho g h$ (measured in kilopascals), where g is the acceleration due to gravity (9.81 m/s^{-2}). Alternatively, h centimetres below the surface, the pressure is increased by ρh cmH$_2$O or $0.74\rho h$ mmHg.

The human circulatory system is a closed, completely liquid-filled system. In life, end-diastolic pressure in the right ventricle is close to atmospheric and is little affected by posture. Changing posture from supine to upright increases the pressure in vessels h cm below the heart and reduces the pressure h cm above it by $\rho g h$ kPa or $0.74\rho h$ mmHg or $0.78h$ mmHg, since the density of blood is about 1.06 g/cm^3.

BLOOD FLOW AND VASCULAR RESISTANCE

Fluid flows from a region of high pressure to a region of low pressure, and the flow rate is affected by the resistance to flow offered by the tube(s) or vessel(s) through which the fluid is flowing. Blood flow is usually laminar, with layers of blood moving in an orderly, streamlined fashion parallel to the walls of the vessels. Laminar flow F through a vessel or group of vessels is proportional to the pressure difference across them, i.e. arterial pressure minus venous pressure ($P_a - P_v$):

$$F = \frac{(P_a - P_v)}{R}$$

where R is the resistance to flow.

For the whole systemic circulation, flow is CO and resistance is the total peripheral resistance (TPR). The pressure difference is the mean arterial blood pressure (BP) in the ascending aorta minus the central venous pressure (CVP). CVP is the pressure in the right atrium and the great veins close to the heart.

Therefore:

$$CO = \frac{(BP - CVP)}{TPR}$$

Since in health CVP is close to atmospheric pressure, this equation is often simplified to:

$$CO \approx \frac{BP}{TPR}$$

Poiseuille studied the factors affecting laminar flow of Newtonian (constant viscosity) fluids moving along straight smooth-walled tubes and determined that:

$$R = \frac{8\eta l}{\pi r^4}$$

where R is the resistance, η is the viscosity of the fluid flowing through the tube, l is the length of the tube and r is the radius of the tube.

The human vascular system is complex and blood is non-Newtonian, as its viscosity is not constant but is reduced when flowing through vessels with diameters less than 1 mm. Nevertheless, the main principles of Poiseuille's equation apply to the human circulation. The radius of a vessel markedly affects its resistance to flow, with a halving of radius leading to a 16-fold increase in resistance. Most moment-to-moment control of blood flow through vascular beds is brought about by alterations in the radius of the smaller arteries and arterioles upstream of the vascular beds, and this vasoconstriction or vasodilation has a marked effect on the local vascular resistance and flow. Widespread vasoconstriction or vasodilation affecting many different vascular beds at the same time can markedly increase or decrease total peripheral resistance.

Red blood cells are the main blood component affecting its viscosity, which nearly doubles when haematocrit increases from its normal value of about 45 per cent to 60 per cent in polycythaemia. Polycythaemia often develops as a response to chronic hypoxia, e.g. at altitude or in chronic respiratory failure. The increased viscosity increases the work of the heart and partly offsets the beneficial effect of the increased arterial oxygen content.

In a healthy young person, a typical pressure in the ascending aorta is 120/80 mmHg, with a mean pressure of about 93 mmHg. The way in which pressure falls around the systemic circulation is determined by the distribution of resistance in the circulation. What determines this is the total resistance of all the blood vessels at each level of branching. Moving peripherally from aorta to capillaries, the resistance of individual vessels rises as the radius falls; however, at each level of branching, there are progressively more vessels in parallel with each other, which lowers their combined resistance. In the systemic circulation, the net effect of these opposing factors is such that the main resistance is located at the level of the arterioles and the largest pressure drop occurs across these vessels.

The large radius of the aorta ensures its resistance is low, as is the total resistance of vessels at the next few branching levels, so the pressure drop along the aorta and arteries is small. Mean pressure in a foot artery is only a few millimetres of mercury below that in the arch of the aorta in the supine subject.

The parallel arrangement of systemic vascular beds permits separate control of blood flow to different organs and tissues through alterations in arteriolar resistance brought about by both local and centrally integrated reflex mechanisms. As vascular beds are in parallel with each other, removing one of them, e.g. by amputating a limb, increases total peripheral resistance.

Factors affecting resistance

Vascular smooth muscle is subject to many different influences that can either increase or decrease its tone. Some of these mechanisms operate locally and change blood flow appropriately to meet the local tissue needs; others, mediated by nerves, adjust peripheral resistance and/or capacitance to meet the needs of the body as a whole, e.g. in order to maintain arterial blood pressure or core temperature. Control is hierarchical, with nervous control mechanisms able to override local mechanisms when the need arises.

AUTOREGULATION

A sudden increase in perfusion pressure increases blood flow, but in most tissues the flow falls again over the next minute or two as the arterioles constrict. This ability of a tissue to maintain a fairly constant blood flow in the face of alterations in perfusion pressure is known as autoregulation. The mechanism is partly myogenic, with the vascular smooth muscle responding to increased stretch by contracting, and partly metabolic, with increased pressure leading to increased washout of vasodilator metabolites. All vascular beds, except the pulmonary circulation, exhibit some degree of autoregulation, but the mechanism is especially well developed in the renal and cerebral circulations, where flow stays remarkably constant at perfusion pressures between about 60 and 160 mmHg in a normotensive person.

LOCAL METABOLITES

The vasodilator properties of metabolites have an important role in matching blood flow to metabolic activity in many tissues. Increased acidity, increased CO_2, increased adenosine, increased K^+, increased osmolality and increased phosphate and decreased O_2 all contribute to metabolic vasodilation, but the relative importance of these factors differs in different tissues. Metabolic hyperaemia is the main mechanism of the vasodilation in exercising skeletal muscle and probably is mediated mainly by adenosine. The cerebral circulation is especially sensitive to CO_2; when this is lowered by hyperventilation, the vasoconstriction can be severe enough to lead to visual disturbance and light-headedness.

ENDOTHELIAL FACTORS

The endothelial cells lining the blood vessels produce both vasodilator and vasoconstrictor substances. Nitric oxide (NO) is produced continuously by the enzyme endothelial nitric oxide synthase (eNOS) in normal subjects. In health, this basal NO production leads to a tonic reduction in total peripheral resistance. NO production increases when vessels are exposed to increased shear stress, causing the flow-mediated vasodilation of arteries that often follows metabolite-mediated dilation of more peripheral vessels. It allows blood flow to rise higher than would be possible otherwise. The vasodilation that accompanies inflammation also involves NO production, but in this case it follows induction of a form of NOS not normally found in the endothelium (inducible NOS, iNOS).

Other vasodilator substances produced by the endothelium include prostacyclin and endothelial-derived hyperpolarizing factor. Endothelin is a vasoconstrictor produced by the endothelium that also has an effect on basal vascular resistance in health. It is likely that alterations in the balance between endothelial vasodilator and vasoconstrictor substances are important in many common diseases, such as hypertension, pre-eclampsia and diabetes.

HORMONES

The catecholamines adrenaline (epinephrine) and noradrenaline (norepinephrine) are released into the blood from the adrenal gland when its preganglionic sympathetic fibres are stimulated. Noradrenaline is also the transmitter released by most postganglionic sympathetic nerves. Both noradrenaline and adrenaline stimulate alpha-receptors in most tissues to cause vasoconstriction and beta$_1$-receptors in the heart to increase heart rate and contractility. Circulating adrenaline can also stimulate beta$_2$-receptors in skeletal and cardiac muscle vessels to cause vasodilation. This effect dominates if adrenaline is infused, so that total peripheral resistance falls, cardiac output rises and blood pressure rises a little. In contrast, infused noradrenaline causes a marked increase in total peripheral resistance and blood pressure, which activates the arterial baroreceptor reflex. The reflex effects override the direct effects of noradrenaline on the heart, leading to bradycardia, reduced contractility and reduced cardiac output.

Antidiuretic hormone (ADH) from the posterior pituitary increases water reabsorption in the distal nephron, reducing urine output. It can also cause vasoconstriction, as indicated by its alternative name vasopressin, although higher concentrations are needed for this than for its antidiuretic action. In health, the release of ADH is controlled by plasma osmolality sensed by osmoreceptors in the hypothalamus. Vasopressin release is also stimulated by hypovolaemia, via a reduction in firing of the cardiopulmonary and arterial baroreceptors. Following haemorrhage, the antidiuretic effect of vasopressin contributes to the restoration of extracellular fluid volume, and the vasoconstriction in many tissues helps support blood pressure.

The renin–angiotensin–aldosterone system is also involved in the responses to haemorrhage, helping to restore circulating blood volume. Renin secretion from juxtaglomerular cells of the kidney is increased in hypovolaemia by several mechanisms, including increased renal sympathetic stimulation. Renin acts on plasma angiotensinogen to form angiotensin I, which is converted to angiotensin II by the action of angiotensin-converting enzyme. Angiotensin II stimulates adrenal cortical aldosterone secretion, leading to increased salt and water retention by the kidney; in addition, angiotensin II is a potent vasoconstrictor.

AUTOCOIDS (LOCAL HORMONES) AND OTHER VASOACTIVE SUBSTANCES

Many substances produced during inflammation act locally as vasodilators, including histamine, bradykinin, platelet-activating factor and prostaglandin E2. Bradykinin is also produced by sweat glands and may contribute to the skin vasodilation that occurs when core temperature rises. Serotonin and thromboxane A2 released from platelets cause local vasoconstriction.

NERVOUS CONTROL OF THE BLOOD VESSELS

At times, blood flow to a tissue needs to be adjusted to serve not its own needs but those of the body as a whole. This control is mediated mostly by nerves. Blood flow to the skin increases to many times that needed for its own metabolism as part of thermoregulatory response to heat stress. In haemorrhage, blood flow in the splanchnic, renal and cutaneous circulation is reduced below that required by local metabolic needs. The increased vascular resistance in these tissues helps to maintain blood pressure and,

hence, coronary and cerebral blood flow. The reflexes that are integrated to override local mechanisms are described later in this chapter.

The most important nerves controlling blood vessels throughout the body are sympathetic vasoconstrictor nerves. These innervate small arteries and arterioles, the constriction of which increases vascular resistance and reduces tissue blood flow and secondarily leads to a local fall in capillary and venous pressure. Veins are also innervated by sympathetic nerves. This innervation is sparse in skeletal muscle and more important in the splanchnic circulation. Sympathetic activity can reduce vascular capacitance both by reducing the flow into the veins secondary to arteriolar constriction and also by active venoconstriction.

Presympathetic nerves originate in the ventrolateral medulla. Their discharge is modulated by many cardiovascular and respiratory reflexes that are integrated in the brainstem. The bulbospinal fibres synapse with preganglionic sympathetic fibres in the intermediolateral column of the spinal cord. Preganglionic sympathetic nerves emerge from the thoracic and upper lumbar segments (T1–L3) of the spinal cord, and most synapse with the postganglionic sympathetic nerves in the ganglia of the sympathetic chain. Some preganglionic fibres pass without synapsing to the adrenal medulla, where they stimulate the release of adrenaline and, to a lesser extent, noradrenaline. The transmitter in the ganglia and adrenal medulla is acetylcholine; between postganglionic vasoconstrictor fibres and vascular smooth muscle, the transmitter is noradrenaline acting on alpha-adrenergic receptors. Sympathetic vasoconstrictor nerves have a resting tone, which means that they are discharging continuously under normal conditions. Vasodilation and venodilation are mediated by a reduction of their ongoing discharge.

OTHER NERVES INNERVATING BLOOD VESSELS

Most blood vessels are innervated only by sympathetic vasoconstrictor nerves, but some, e.g. those in the salivary glands and erectile tissue of the penis, also receive a parasympathetic vasodilator innervation. The transmitters released from the postganglionic parasympathetic nerves are acetylcholine and vasoactive intestinal peptide (VIP), substance P or NO; these are often referred to as non-adrenergic non-cholinergic (NANC) transmitters.

Vasodilation can also occur when nociceptive C-fibres are stimulated. Collaterals from these nerves release vasodilator neuropeptides such as substance P. This 'axon reflex' involves the peripheral part of the nerve rather than the central nervous system. It is responsible for the red flare surrounding a sting or injury and, together with the local redness and wheal (oedema) at the site of injury, forms part of the triple response described by Lewis.

VEINS AND CAPACITANCE VESSELS

The veins tend to be large in diameter and as a group veins offer little resistance to flow. They are much thinner-walled than the arteries and have a large internal volume. At any one time, usually about 60–70 per cent of the total blood volume is in the veins, which are, therefore, often known as capacitance vessels. The internal volume of the veins can vary greatly. When pressures within the veins are low, the veins collapse; when pressures rise, the veins become circular in cross-section, with a considerable increase in volume. If blood volume expands, veins exhibit stress relaxation, so that the initial rise in venous pressure gradually lessens. In haemorrhage, the reverse occurs, helping to lessen the fall in venous pressures. In addition, sympathetic nerves innervate many veins, permitting active control of their capacity and, thus, giving them a role in the maintenance of central venous pressures and venous return to the heart. Limb veins contain semilunar valves. Contraction of the muscles that surround the deep veins of the leg raises venous pressure, which drives the blood towards the heart. Backflow is prevented by the presence of the valves. This is known as skeletal muscle pumping. Venous return to the heart is also increased during inspiration, when the fall in intrathoracic pressure helps to suck blood back to the heart.

Fluid exchange in the capillaries: the Starling principle

Capillaries are the exchange vessels where fluids, gases, nutrients and products of metabolism move between the blood and the interstitium. The direction and magnitude of the fluid movement across the capillary at any point depends on the balance between hydrostatic and osmotic pressures across the capillary; this is the Starling principle of fluid exchange (Figure 2.2).

The main force driving fluid out of the capillaries is the hydrostatic pressure difference between the capillary and the interstitium. Capillary hydrostatic pressure falls along the capillary, with values at the arterial end depending on the vascular tone and the height above or below the heart. Interstitial fluid pressure is usually close to zero and in many tissues a few millimetres of mercury below atmospheric pressure. Hydrostatic pressure values for a typical tissue at heart level are given in Figure 2.2a (black arrows). The osmotic pressure difference opposes filtration and is due to the difference in concentration of plasma proteins across the capillary. Plasma colloid osmotic pressure is about 25 mmHg; interstitial colloid osmotic pressure is variable but about 10 mmHg (white arrows). Even this colloid osmotic pressure difference of 15 mmHg across the

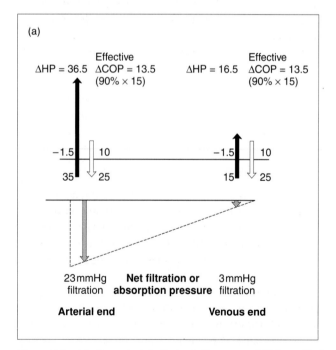

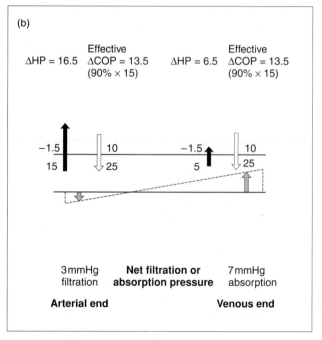

Figure 2.2 *Starling principle. Hydrostatic pressure (HP) in capillaries depends on the degree of vasoconstriction and the position of the vascular bed above or below the heart. Tissue colloid osmotic pressure (COP) and local vessel permeability to proteins also vary in different tissues. (a) Situation in a typical capillary at heart level. Hydrostatic and colloid osmotic pressures (mmHg) inside and outside the capillary are shown above, and the net filtration or absorption pressures are shown below. (b) Situation soon after the onset of vasoconstriction, which lowers the capillary hydrostatic pressures. Net reabsorption now occurs along most of the capillary, although this will not be sustained indefinitely, because the movement of fluid from interstitium to capillary will increase interstitial and reduce blood COP.*

capillary wall is only about 90 per cent exerted, because the capillary is an imperfect (slightly leaky) semipermeable membrane. It can be seen from Figure 2.2a that when all these different forces are taken into account, there is normally net filtration occurring along the entire length of the capillary in most tissues. This filtered fluid returns to the circulation via the lymphatic vessels. Oedema occurs when net filtration exceeds lymphatic drainage; this may occur if the Starling forces are altered, e.g. by a rise in capillary pressure or a fall in plasma protein concentration. Net reabsorption of fluid into capillaries may occur transiently in many tissues following haemorrhage (Figure 2.2b), because reflex vasoconstriction causes a fall in capillary pressure. This fluid movement from interstitium to blood vessel can increase circulating fluid volume by several hundred millilitres.

Pulmonary circulation

A typical pulmonary artery pressure in health is 25/8 mmHg (3.3/1.1 kPa), with a mean pressure of about 15 mmHg (2 kPa). This pressure is only about 10 mmHg above left atrial pressure, but this pressure difference is enough to drive the cardiac output through the pulmonary circulation because pulmonary vascular resistance is less than one-sixth of systemic vascular resistance.

Autoregulation does not occur in the pulmonary circulation, where holding flow constant would be unhelpful. Thus, in exercise, when increased venous return increases pulmonary artery pressure, pulmonary blood flow and, therefore, cardiac output are allowed to increase.

Nervous control of the pulmonary circulation is much less important than in the systemic circulation. Pulmonary vessels constrict in response to local hypoxia, in contrast to the vasodilation seen in systemic vascular beds. Hypoxic vasoconstriction helps to reduce ventilation/perfusion mismatching in the lungs by diverting blood flow from poorly ventilated to better-ventilated areas. When hypoxia is global, e.g. at altitude or in the presence of respiratory failure, hypoxic vasoconstriction is less helpful and simply increases pulmonary vascular resistance and can lead to right heart strain and failure.

Pulmonary capillary hydrostatic pressure at about 10 mmHg is lower than systemic capillary pressure, but there is still net filtration and lymph formation, because pulmonary interstitial protein concentration is unusually high, with an interstitial colloid osmotic pressure of 16–20 mmHg.

Control of cardiac output

Cardiac output is the product of stroke volume and heart rate. These are determined by nervous and other factors described in this section. The heart is supplied by parasympathetic nerves travelling in the vagus (X cranial nerve) and sympathetic nerves from the upper thoracic spinal cord (T1–T5). Both sympathetic and parasympathetic nerves innervate the sinoatrial (SA) node, the atrioventricular node and the atria, releasing noradrenaline and acetylcholine to act on beta$_1$-adrenergic and muscarinic receptors, respectively. The ventricular myocardium has a rich sympathetic innervation, but parasympathetic innervation is sparse.

In a healthy young person at rest, there is both tonic parasympathetic and sympathetic discharge to the SA node, but the parasympathetic discharge dominates, keeping the heart rate below its intrinsic rate of about 100 beats/min. Heart rate is also affected by temperature, rising during fever and falling in hypothermia.

Stroke volume is affected by end-diastolic volume (the preload), the contractility of the heart and the arterial blood pressure (the afterload). The Frank–Starling law of the heart states that the energy of contraction is dependent on the initial length of the cardiac muscle fibre. Venous return and heart rate both affect ventricular end-diastolic volume and, hence, the initial length of the cardiac muscle fibres at the start of ventricular systole. Increased venous return tends to increase end-diastolic volume, and increased heart rate tends to reduce it by reducing the time available for diastolic filling. The Frank–Starling mechanism helps the heart to respond to changes in preload and ensures that the outputs of the right and left heart are matched.

Changes in cardiac contractility or inotropic state refer to the changes in the energy of contraction at a given end-diastolic length. An increased contractility or positive inotropic effect means an increase in energy of contraction caused by anything other than the Frank–Starling mechanism. Sympathetic stimulation, adrenaline and drugs such as digoxin increase cardiac contractility, while myocardial ischaemia and heart failure reduce cardiac contractility. A rise in heart rate can also increase contractility (the Bowditch effect), as can an increased aortic blood pressure (the Anrep effect). Although parasympathetic vagal innervation of the ventricular myocardium is sparse, there is some evidence that vagal stimulation may reduce ventricular contractility directly as well as secondary to a fall in heart rate.

The immediate effect of a rise in mean arterial pressure is to increase the afterload on the ventricle and to reduce the stroke volume that can be achieved with a given energy of contraction. However, a rise in blood pressure can also have indirect effects on the heart that also affect stroke volume. As mentioned above, increased afterload is followed in a few beats by an increased cardiac contractility, but in the intact circulation activation of the arterial baroreceptor reflex will lead to a reflex fall in both heart rate and contractility.

Reflex control of the cardiovascular system

ARTERIAL BARORECEPTORS IN THE CAROTID SINUS AND AORTIC ARCH

The main arterial baroreceptors are located in the carotid sinus at the bifurcation of the common carotid artery and the arch of the aorta, with afferents in the glossopharyngeal and vagus nerves, respectively. These afferents synapse in the nucleus of the tractus solitarius (NTS) of the dorso-medial medulla. Individual baroreceptors respond to a relatively narrow range of pressures, with firing rising from zero to maximum as pressure increases by 20–30 mmHg from the threshold. As pressure in the carotid sinus increases, there is an increased firing of individual baro-receptors and a progressive recruitment of baroreceptors with higher thresholds, to give the sigmoid response curve of the whole nerve, where firing starts at about 50 mmHg and reaches a maximum at about 180 mmHg. Carotid baroreceptor firing is affected by pulse pressure as well as mean blood pressure. This is important in situations such as haemorrhage or standing, where a fall in stroke volume and pulse pressure reduces carotid sinus baroreceptor firing, even if mean pressure is unchanged.

A rise in mean blood pressure or pulse pressure increases arterial baroreceptor discharge and leads to increased cardiac vagal stimulation and reduced sympa-thetic stimulation to the heart and vasculature. Together, they reduce heart rate and cardiac contractility and lead to vasodilation and venodilation. Arterial baroreceptors dis-charge tonically under normal conditions, so that a fall in mean arterial blood pressure or pulse pressure reduces firing, giving a reflex tachycardia, increased cardiac con-tractility, vasoconstriction and venoconstriction.

The arterial baroreceptor control of vascular beds is variable, with strong control in the skeletal muscle and splanchnic and renal vascular beds and little effect in the coronary and cerebral circulation. Arterial baroreceptor control of the cutaneous circulation is weak, and the skin vasoconstriction and pallor in haemorrhage is probably mediated by other mechanisms, such as the rise in circu-lating vasopressin and angiotensin.

The aortic arch baroreceptors are qualitatively similar in their reflex response to the carotid sinus baroreceptors, but they are probably less sensitive to changes in pulse pres-sure. The aortic baroreceptors are close to heart level; therefore, the pressure that they are exposed to changes lit-tle as posture alters, whereas pressure in the carotid sinus falls when moving from supine to upright.

SET POINT AND GAIN OF THE ARTERIAL BARORECEPTOR REFLEX

The relationship between carotid sinus pressure and the reflex effects on blood pressure and heart rate is not fixed but can be altered by many factors acting peripherally at the carotid sinus or centrally by inputs to the brainstem. Exercise, activation of the defence response (see below) and a sustained increase in arterial blood pressure can all raise the blood pressure that the arterial baroreceptor reflex operates to maintain, whereas in sleep the operating point is lowered.

LONG-TERM CONTROL OF BLOOD PRESSURE

It is usually stated that the arterial baroreceptor reflex con-trols moment-to-moment changes in blood pressure but does not determine the mean level of blood pressure in the long term. In support of this view is the fairly rapid reset-ting of the reflex that occurs when carotid sinus pressure is maintained at a new level. Moreover, although hyperten-sion occurs immediately after arterial baroreceptor dener-vation in animals, mean blood pressure returns to near-normal values over the following weeks. Long-term blood pressure control is thought to involve the control of blood volume via the kidney, and this probably involves the cardiopulmonary baroreceptors. However, new experi-mental approaches have raised the possibility that arterial baroreceptors do have a role in long-term regulation of blood pressure in humans.

CARDIOPULMONARY RECEPTORS

In addition to the aortic baroreceptors, there are many other receptors within the thorax that have reflex effects on the cardiovascular system, including mechanoreceptors in blood vessels and the chambers of the heart, chemorecep-tors in the heart, and several groups of airway and lung receptors. The afferents from most of these receptors pass in the vagus to the brainstem, but there are also some affer-ent fibres from the heart that travel in the nerves contain-ing the cardiac sympathetic efferent fibres.

In humans, it is difficult to devise ways of stimulating these receptors discretely; consequently, those that respond to pressure or stretch are often referred to together as the cardiopulmonary baroreceptors. One technique used to study these receptors is lower-body negative pressure (LBNP), in which suction is applied around the legs and lower abdomen. This distends the veins of the lower body, producing venous pooling, reducing central venous pres-sures and mimicking the effects of gravitational stress. If low suction pressures such as 10 mmHg are used, there is a small fall in central venous pressure without a significant change in mean arterial blood pressure or pulse pressure. The forearm vasoconstriction seen with this mild LBNP is considered to be due to unloading of a subgroup of car-diopulmonary receptors often referred to as low-pressure receptors. Passively raising the legs of supine human sub-jects has the opposite effect, increasing central venous pres-sures and leading to forearm vasodilation.

Our knowledge of the effects of discretely stimulating the different groups of cardiopulmonary receptors is based largely on animal experiments, and these are outlined in the following section. It is likely that similar receptors and reflexes exist in humans and that they contribute to the responses seen when cardiopulmonary baroreceptors are stimulated or unloaded. However, it is also likely that there is considerable species difference in the strength and importance of these reflexes.

ATRIAL RECEPTORS

Receptors with large myelinated afferents are found in both the right and left atrium close to their junction with the veins; their firing increases when atrial volume increases. The reflex effects of discretely stimulating these venoatrial receptors are a tachycardia and an increased urine flow. The tachycardia is mediated largely through sympathetic efferent nerves, but there is no effect on contractility. Several mechanisms contribute to the diuresis, including reduced sympathetic discharge to the kidney and reduced renin and vasopressin secretion. The tachycardia that occurs in dogs following a rapid saline infusion (the Bainbridge reflex) probably is due to stimulation of these venoatrial receptors. This reflex is probably much less potent in humans.

Distension of the atria also produces diuresis and natriuresis by increased secretion of the hormone atrial natriuretic peptide from specialized atrial cells in response to stretch. It seems likely that by both of these mechanisms, the atria contribute to the control of blood volume.

CORONARY ARTERY BARORECEPTORS

In recent years, it has been recognized that the coronary arteries contain important baroreceptors and that these work alongside the better-known carotid sinus and aortic arch arterial baroreceptors to help control arterial blood pressure. The coronary baroreceptors appear to be as potent in their reflex vascular effects as the carotid sinus baroreceptors. They differ from the carotid sinus and aortic arch baroreceptors in that they operate over a lower range of pressures and that they have little effect on heart rate.

VENTRICULAR RECEPTORS

Ventricular receptors with vagal afferents can be stimulated by either mechanical or chemical stimuli, and many receptors respond to both. The left ventricle seems to be a more important source of these receptors than the right ventricle.

Stimulation of ventricular receptors with unmyelinated vagal afferents can produce a profound depressor reflex, with increased parasympathetic drive to the heart and reduced sympathetic drive to both the heart and the blood vessels. This reflex, known as the Bezold–Jarisch reflex, is usually provoked experimentally by coronary artery injection of either foreign substances such as veratridine or naturally occurring substances that may be produced during myocardial ischaemia, such as adenosine, bradykinin or prostaglandins.

There are also mechanosensitive and chemosensitive afferents that run with the sympathetic nerves and whose reflex effects are excitatory, i.e. they lead to tachycardia and vasoconstriction. The different types of receptors are distributed unevenly within the left ventricle, which may explain the finding that bradycardia and hypotension are more common following posterior and inferior left ventricular wall myocardial ischaemia and tachycardia and hypertension are more common with anterior wall ischaemia.

With care taken to prevent changes in coronary artery pressure, it seems that the responses (bradycardia and systemic vasodilation) to left ventricular mechanoreceptor stimulation are small and apparent only at high left ventricular distension pressures associated with large increases in left ventricular end-diastolic pressure.

In view of the fact that the stimuli needed to give reflex effects from ventricular receptors are either very high pressures or substances produced by ischaemic myocardium, it seems likely that these receptors are more concerned with responses seen in pathological situations than in normal day-to-day regulation of the circulation.

Arterial chemoreceptors, lung receptors and responses to hypoxia

Carotid body chemoreceptor stimulation increases ventilation and also has reflex effects on the cardiovascular system. The cardiovascular effects are complicated because in addition to the primary reflex effects of carotid body stimulation (i.e. bradycardia and vasoconstriction), there are secondary reflex effects of tachycardia and vasodilation, from activation of pulmonary stretch receptors as ventilation increases. In addition, carotid chemoreceptor stimulation can activate the defence areas of the brain (see below), with marked cardiovascular effects.

When the whole body is exposed to hypoxia, in addition to these direct and indirect reflex responses to peripheral chemoreceptor stimulation, there are also local effects of hypoxia on the heart and blood vessels. The local effects probably involve the release of adenosine, which in the heart leads to bradycardia and in many tissues to vasodilation. The usual cardiovascular responses to acute hypoxia observed in humans, which presumably are the net result of all these different mechanisms, are discussed in Chapter 3.

Pain and reflexes from skeletal muscle

There are numerous other afferent inputs that have reflex cardiovascular effects. Reflexes from mechanoreceptors and chemoreceptors in skeletal muscle play a part in the cardiovascular responses to exercise (see below). Stimulation of pain receptors in many locations can give rise to an increase in heart rate and blood pressure.

Reflexes contributing to the diving response

Stimulation of the face around the eyes and nose with cold water can stimulate receptors whose afferents travel in the ophthalmic and maxillary divisions of the trigeminal nerve. This can lead to reflex apnoea, bradycardia and vasoconstriction, which contribute to the diving response. The cardiovascular responses are enhanced by the direct reflex effects of peripheral chemoreceptor stimulation as the arterial partial pressure of oxygen (P_{O_2}) falls and the arterial partial pressure of carbon dioxide (P_{CO_2}) rises during the period of apnoea. These responses are especially strong in diving animals such as seals and are thought to have an oxygen-conserving role, by reducing the work of the heart and directing the reduced cardiac output to the brain.

The diving response also occurs in humans, but it is usually less intense, partly because humans usually inhale before diving into water and with stretched lungs the reflex tachycardia from stimulation of the lung airway receptors opposes the bradycardia from the facial and peripheral chemoreceptor reflexes. Occasionally, however, an excessive bradycardia occurs, particular if an unexpected immersion occurs during expiration, and this may contribute to some accidental deaths in water. A similar pattern of reflexes responses can be elicited by stimulating the inside of the nose or larynx, and this may contribute to the vagally mediated asystole that occasionally complicates laryngeal intubation during the induction of anaesthesia.

The reflex effects of cold water applied to other regions of the body are very different. Immersion of the body in cold water to the neck, excluding the face, gives rise to hyperventilation and tachycardia.

Reflexes from the urinary bladder

Distension of the urinary bladder can cause reflex tachycardia, vasoconstriction and increased blood pressure. In normal healthy humans, the rise in blood pressure is usually moderate because of the buffering action of the arterial baroreceptor reflexes. Rapid emptying of a distended bladder can cause sudden loss of this pressor reflex, which, if the depressor reflex from the arterial baroreceptors persists for a while, may cause a transient fall in blood pressure. Occasionally, this is large enough to cause fainting. This 'micturition syncope' is not uncommon in otherwise healthy young men and is especially likely when a very full bladder is emptied rapidly at night after drinking alcohol. Its main importance is that it may be confused with more serious causes of syncope, especially since, unlike the more familiar postural fainting, it often occurs suddenly with little warning that consciousness is about to be lost.

Defence or alerting response

In both humans and animals, novel or threatening stimuli can provoke behavioural responses. These can range from signs of increased alertness, such as ear-pricking in response to an unexpected sound, to full-blown rage when faced with a threatening situation. These alerting or defence responses are accompanied by a particular pattern of cardiovascular response as well as increased ventilation, piloerection and dilation of the pupils.

The cardiovascular responses include tachycardia, hypertension, vasoconstriction in the kidney and splanchnic and many other vascular beds, and vasodilation in skeletal muscle. The skeletal muscle vasodilation has several efferent mechanisms, including reduced sympathetic discharge and increased circulating adrenaline acting on beta$_2$-receptors. In some animals such as the cat, there is activation of cholinergic vasodilator nerves to skeletal muscle, but there is little evidence for the existence of such nerves in humans.

The regions of the brain that integrate these responses are known as the defence areas and include parts of the hypothalamus and amygdala. The natural stimuli that provoke these responses vary with species and individual, depending on the emotional significance of the stimulus. A telephone ringing in a quiet room may be a mild alerting stimulus to one individual or an intense stimulus to someone awaiting bad news. In experiments on humans, mental arithmetic often proves to be an effective stimulus.

Hypoxia also activates the defence areas of the brain, probably secondary to peripheral chemoreceptor stimulation. It is probably the mechanism of the repeated awakening from sleep that occurs during hypoxic episodes in patients with obstructive sleep apnoea and it may be involved in the development of the chronic hypertension that is common in these patients.

Interaction between cardiovascular and respiratory reflexes

RESPIRATORY MODULATION OF THE ARTERIAL BARORECEPTOR REFLEX AND SINUS ARRHYTHMIA

Sinus arrhythmia is the speeding up and slowing down of heart rate that occurs with inspiration and expiration, respectively, in normal individuals. In inspiration, the cardiac vagal motor neurons in the brainstem are inhibited both by central inspiratory activity and also by afferent input from the pulmonary stretch receptors; as a consequence, heart rate rises. The responses to arterial baroreceptor reflex stimulation are also inhibited during inspiration.

The inspiratory increase in heart rate can occur only if there is ongoing vagal activity to inhibit. With increasing age, cardiac vagal tone declines and sinus arrhythmia becomes less pronounced.

Cardiovascular responses to changing posture

In the upright posture, the weight of the column of blood below the heart raises both arterial and venous pressures in the feet (Figure 2.3). When standing completely still, the pressure rise in arteries and veins is similar and, hence, the pressure difference across the foot capillary bed is unchanged by the direct effect of gravity. If blood vessels were rigid, blood flow in the foot would be unaffected by changing posture. However, the pressure difference between the inside of the vessels and the outside is

increased; this is particularly important in the veins, which are easily distended by an increased transmural pressure. There is a shift of about 500 ml of blood from the thorax to the vessels below the heart, especially the lower legs, within the first minute of standing. When walking, skeletal muscle pumping reduces, but does not abolish, the postural increase in lower-leg venous pressures.

This venous pooling reduces venous return to the heart on standing, leading to a fall in stroke volume and cardiac output by the Frank–Starling mechanism. Despite this, blood pressure does not usually fall, even when skeletal muscle pumping is prevented by moving the subject passively from supine to upright on a tilt table. Several different reflexes and responses contribute to the maintenance of blood pressure following the move from supine to upright.

In the upright position, there is reduced stimulation of the carotid sinus baroreceptors, even if mean blood pressure does not fall. At the carotid sinus, about 25 cm above the heart, the effect of gravity reduces blood pressure by about 20 mmHg (2.7 kPa). In addition, the carotid sinus baroreceptors are sensitive to pulse pressure, which falls on standing, because of the reduced stroke volume. The unloading of the carotid sinus baroreceptors leads to a

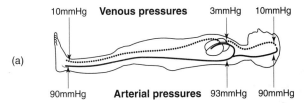

(a)

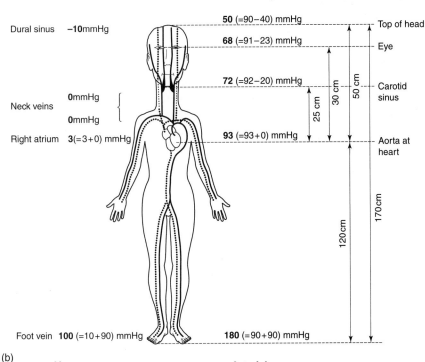

(b)

Figure 2.3 *Pressures in arteries (solid lines) and veins (dotted lines) in the supine (a) and upright (b) postures. In the supine subject, mean pressures in all arteries are close to those at heart level (in this person, 93 mmHg), falling by a few millimetres of mercury from heart to periphery. Similarly, venous pressures in peripheral veins are a few millimetres of mercury above central venous pressure. In the upright posture, the mean pressure in any artery is the mean pressure at that point in the supine position plus or minus the pressure due to the weight of the column of blood below or above the heart. Pressures in the veins below the heart are also increased when standing still by the weight of the column of blood below the heart. In veins above the heart, venous pressure also falls, but the fall is less than predicted from the height above the heart because of collapse of the neck veins, in which the fall is limited to 0 mmHg.*

reflex increase in heart rate, cardiac contractility and peripheral vasoconstriction.

The fall in central blood volume will also unload the cardiopulmonary baroreceptors, and the reflex responses, such as skeletal muscle vasoconstriction, will contribute to the rise in peripheral resistance. Reflexes from the vestibular system in response to a change in posture may also be important. Activation of the otolith organs of the vestibular system leads to reflex sympathetic activation. This vestibulosympathetic reflex may act in a feed-forward manner, causing a rapid increase in vascular resistance on standing that is then modulated by negative feedback from the arterial baroreceptor reflex.

Together, these reflexes usually maintain blood pressure during standing. The reflex tachycardia and increased contractility are not very effective in the face of a reduced venous return, and cardiac output falls by about 20 per cent on standing. A fall in mean blood pressure at heart level is prevented by matching this fall in cardiac output by a similar 20 per cent reflex increase in total peripheral resistance.

EFFECT OF POSTURE ON CAPILLARY FLUID BALANCE

The rise in foot arterial and venous pressures means that capillary hydrostatic pressure and the net filtration pressure inevitably also rise on standing. Prolonged standing makes normal feet swell, and foot and ankle oedema occurs readily in the presence of any factors increasing filtration. Increased filtration can reduce circulating blood volume and further impair venous return to the heart. Mechanisms that help to reduce the rise in capillary pressure include skeletal-muscle pumping, as this lowers venous pressure. Sympathetically mediated arteriolar vasoconstriction that occurs as part of the reflex responses to posture also reduces the rise in capillary pressure. An additional local mechanism operates that does not involve the central nervous system and causes arteriolar constriction only in vascular beds below heart level. This veni-arteriolar response is thought to be triggered by local venous distension and probably involves local sympathetic nerve networks.

EFFECT OF POSTURE ON BLOOD VESSELS ABOVE THE HEART AND ON CEREBRAL BLOOD FLOW

Each 1 cm of blood column above the heart lowers the pressure by about 0.78 mmHg (0.1 kPa). Consequently, in the arteries at the top of the head, pressure is about 40 mmHg (5.3 kPa) and at eye level about 23 mmHg (3 kPa) below that in the aorta at heart level. Venous pressures above the heart, which are low in the supine position, also are affected by gravity. The internal jugular veins in the neck are exposed to atmospheric pressure on the outside; as pressure within them falls on standing, they collapse, which limits the fall of pressure within them to 0 mmHg. Within the skull, veins do not collapse, and the pressure within the dural sinuses on top of the head is typically about −10 mmHg (−1.3 kPa).

As venous pressure in the head falls less than arterial pressure, the cerebral perfusion pressure (arterial minus venous pressure) falls on standing. As a result, cerebral blood flow falls despite autoregulation but in normal standing not enough to impair cerebral oxygen consumption.

Vasovagal fainting

Prolonged standing may cause fainting (syncope) even in healthy subjects. Blood pressure is initially maintained well on standing by the increased total peripheral resistance, but eventually, in the face of a progressively falling venous return and cardiac output, mean blood pressure begins to fall. At some point, the reflex vasoconstriction and tachycardia are suddenly replaced by a vagally mediated bradycardia and widespread vasodilation as sympathetic discharge to many vascular beds is withdrawn (Figure 2.4). At this point, blood pressure and cerebral blood flow fall precipitously and syncope occurs. Usually the subject ends up lying down and in this position venous return, cardiac output and consciousness are restored rapidly. Brain damage can occur if the subject is prevented from falling, perhaps by support from a 'helpful' bystander. Typically in the period before consciousness is lost (presyncope), the subject complains of nausea and light-headedness, looks very pale and may yawn or sigh.

The peripheral vasodilation seems to be the most important aspect of this vasovagal syncope in most people, and cardiac pacing is usually ineffective in patients with recurrent postural syncope. The mechanism that triggers the bradycardia and vasodilation is unknown. The hypothesis that reflexes from ventricular receptors might initiate it has not been supported by experimental and clinical evidence.

Vasovagal syncope may also occur in haemorrhage, heat exposure, positive-pressure breathing and hypoxia and in the presence of strong emotional stimuli; these situations are additive in their effects. A person who has lost a litre of blood may maintain a normal blood pressure lying down but faint quickly on standing.

The Valsalva manoeuvre

The Valsalva manoeuvre occurs when forced expiration is attempted but airflow is prevented by breathing against a closed glottis or, experimentally, against a manometer to measure the raised intrathoracic pressure generated (Figure 2.5).

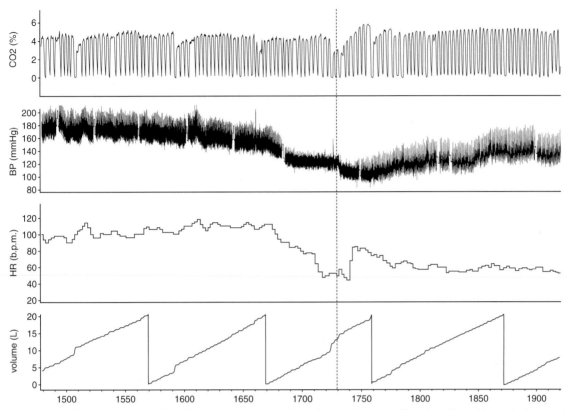

Figure 2.4   *Vasovagal faint in a healthy young volunteer subjected to combination of head-up tilt and lower-body negative pressure. Note the initial gradual fall in blood pressure (BP) and a rise in heart rate (HR), followed by a sudden marked fall in both. At the event mark, the subject was returned to the horizontal and suction switched off. Traces from above down are expired % CO_2, finger arterial blood pressure, heart rate and cumulative inspired volume.*

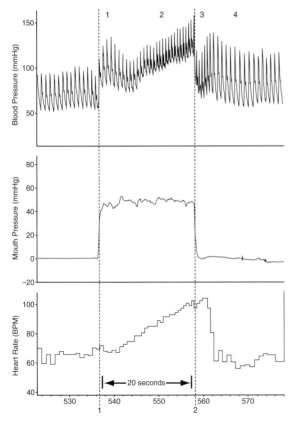

Figure 2.5   *Heart-rate and blood-pressure responses to a Valsalva manoeuvre in a healthy 20-year-old man. The subject breathed with an open glottis into a closed tube and was asked to maintain a pressure of 40 mmHg (middle trace). Finger blood pressure (top trace) was measured non-invasively using a Finapres, and the heart rate was derived beat by beat from the blood-pressure trace. The numbers represent the four phases of the Valsalva manoeuvre, as described in the text.*

A characteristic sequence of blood pressure and heart rate changes occur in normal subjects:

Phase 1: there is an immediate rise in arterial blood pressure caused by the direct effects of the raised intrathoracic pressure compressing the aorta. A brief fall in heart rate may result from activation of the arterial baroreceptor reflex.

Phase 2: the raised intrathoracic pressure impairs venous return to the thorax, which reduces cardiac output and blood pressure. The arterial baroreceptors are unloaded, leading to reflex tachycardia and peripheral vasoconstriction, which in normal people limits the fall in blood pressure.

Phase 3: at the end of the forced expiration, the sudden fall in intrathoracic pressure is transmitted to the aorta, causing aortic pressure to fall and a further reflex speeding up of heart rate.

Phase 4: the fall in intrathoracic pressure causes a sudden large increase in venous return, as the blood that has been accumulating in the abdomen, head and arms can now enter the thorax. This increases cardiac output and blood pressure and results in an arterial baroreceptor reflex bradycardia.

Cardiovascular response to exercise

In dynamic exercise such as running, the oxygen consumption increases linearly as work rate increases progressively, until a maximum is reached. Once maximum O_2 consumption ($\dot{V}O_{2\,max}$) is reached, a small further increase in work can be performed by an increase in anaerobic work, but essentially the rate of working of an individual is determined by his or her $\dot{V}O_{2\,max}$. Oxygen consumption ($\dot{V}O_2$) is equal to the product of the cardiac output (CO) and the average oxygen extraction as the blood passes through the tissues, i.e.

$$\dot{V}O_2 = CO \times (\text{arterial oxygen content} - \text{mixed venous oxygen content})$$

Both cardiac output and oxygen extraction increase as work rate increases in exercise. Arterial oxygen content remains constant at the resting value, and the maximum oxygen extraction is limited by the minimum venous oxygen content that can be achieved. This is limited by the need to maintain a capillary P_{O_2} sufficient to drive oxygen diffusion and is similar in different people. Consequently, the maximum oxygen consumption in normal people is determined largely by the maximum cardiac output that they can generate.

In health, cardiac output is increased during exercise by an increase in both heart rate and stroke volume, of which the increased heart rate is quantitatively the most important (see Table 2.1, p. 14). The maximum heart rate is reduced with age, being approximately equal to 220 minus the age in years, and the increase in stroke volume becomes proportionally larger.

In exercise, there is also some redistribution of blood flow, with vasoconstriction in non-active skeletal muscle and the splanchnic and renal circulations. Skin vasoconstriction occurs initially, but as the core temperature rises, thermoregulatory control mechanisms lead to increased cutaneous blood flow. In active skeletal muscle, there is vasodilation caused by increased local metabolite concentration. Overall, there is a fall in total peripheral resistance. The blood flow in different tissues as a proportion of cardiac output is very different from that at rest (see Table 2.1). The net effect of the rise in cardiac output and fall in total peripheral resistance is a moderate rise in blood pressure, which increases with increasing exercise intensity. Diastolic blood pressure rises less than systolic blood pressure and in some subjects may even fall a little.

The mechanisms that initiate and maintain the cardiovascular response to exercise are not resolved completely, but there is evidence that both central command and reflexes from the exercising muscles play a part. Central command refers to inputs from locomotor areas of the brain to the brainstem cardiovascular control areas, which are initiated in parallel with the motor output to the muscles. Reflexes from both chemoreceptors and mechanoreceptors in skeletal muscle can cause reflex increases in heart rate and blood pressure in response to muscle activity. All these responses are moderated by the arterial baroreceptor reflex, the operating point of which is reset to a higher pressure and heart rate in exercise.

In isometric exercise, such as weightlifting, heart rate and blood pressure also rise, but the pattern is different. With forces greater than 20 per cent of their maximum voluntary contraction, the heart rate and blood pressure increase progressively during the contraction (Figure 2.6). The rise in diastolic pressure is greater than in dynamic exercise and, relative to the oxygen consumption, the increase in mean blood pressure is larger than in dynamic exercise. In isometric exercise, the continuous contraction means that the accumulation of muscle metabolites is greater than in dynamic exercise, which may result in an increased activation of muscle chemoreceptor reflexes.

Cardiovascular aspects of temperature regulation

Alterations in skin blood flow are a very important part of the thermoregulatory responses of the body. Total skin blood flow can vary from as little as 20 ml/min during cold exposure to more than 3 l/min when the need for heat loss is great. During heat exposure, the large increase in flow to the skin and the increased volume of blood in the cutaneous veins and capillaries can have important effects

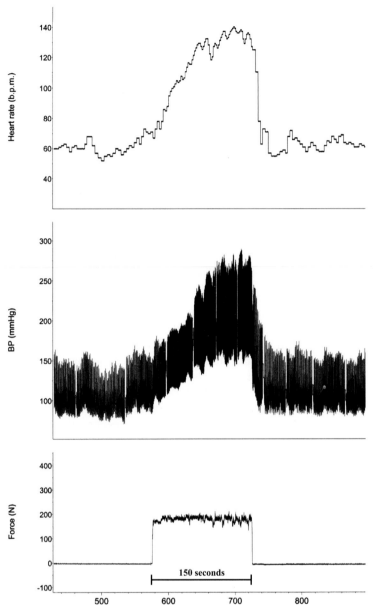

Figure 2.6 *Effects of isometric exercise on blood pressure and heart rate. A healthy 20-year-old male subject performed an isometric contraction of his left quadriceps muscle using 30 per cent of his maximum voluntary contraction force (lower trace), which he maintained for 150 seconds. Heart rate (top trace) and systolic and diastolic finger arterial blood pressure (middle trace) rose progressively during the contraction.*

on the circulation as a whole and the ability to meet the cardiovascular demands of exercise. These circulatory responses to thermal stress are discussed fully in Chapter 13.

RESPIRATORY PHYSIOLOGY

It is convenient to consider respiration as occurring in a series of steps as follows:

- Consumption of oxygen and production of carbon dioxide by the tissues.
- Exchange of gases between blood and tissues.
- Carriage of gases by blood between tissues and lungs.
- Exchange of gases between blood in the lungs and the environment.

The process underlying the exchange of gases between the blood and the environment is termed external respiration. The carriage of gases to and from the tissues, and the gas exchange in the tissues, constitute internal respiration.

Tissue respiration

CELLULAR METABOLISM

The immediate source of energy for almost all biological processes is the chemical energy held in the energy-rich bonds of adenosine triphosphate (ATP). In living material, hydrolysis of the terminal energy-rich phosphate bond of ATP is associated intimately with the performance of work. Energy-rich bonds are generated by the disruption of the chemical bonds of complex molecules, such as glucose and fatty acid, by oxidation. This process in the presence of oxygen (aerobic catabolism) results eventually in the oxidation of the complex molecules to carbon dioxide and water. One molecule of glucose, when oxidized completely, yields 38 energy-rich bonds. The breakdown of glucose can proceed part way in the absence of oxygen (anaerobic metabolism), with the formation of lactic acid. The breakdown of glucose to lactic acid, however, yields only two energy-rich bonds per molecule of glucose. Furthermore, the accumulation of lactic acid eventually limits the activity of the working tissues. Lactic acid is, however, oxidized completely by heart muscle and brain tissue and synthesized to glycogen in the liver.

The complete oxidation of the compounds produced by the breakdown of glucose, fats and proteins occurs in the mitochondria. Here, in a series of complex reactions, these compounds are oxidized to carbon dioxide and water, with the generation of many energy-rich bonds, a process termed oxidative phosphorylation. Oxidative phosphorylation requires a certain minimum molecular concentration, i.e. partial pressure, of oxygen (P_{O_2}). Above this critical value, however, the rate of oxidation is independent of the local P_{O_2}. The value of the critical P_{O_2} required at the mitochondria typically lies within the range 0.5–3.0 mmHg (0.07–0.4 kPa). Thus, if aerobic metabolism is not to be limited by the supply of oxygen, then the oxygen transport system must maintain the P_{O_2} at the mitochondria greater than 0.5–3.0 mmHg (0.07–0.4 kPa).

More than 90 per cent of the oxygen consumed by the tissues is involved in the generation of energy-rich bonds by oxidative phosphorylation. Most of the remaining consumption of oxygen also involves the removal of hydrogen from complex molecules such as amino acids and amines. Finally, a very small proportion (about one per cent) of the oxygen consumed by the tissues is involved in reactions in which oxygen is incorporated into complex organic molecules, such as biogenic amines and steroid hormones, a process known as oxygenation. The rates of certain oxygenations are reduced significantly by a fall of P_{O_2} from 100 mmHg to 60 mmHg (13.3 kPa to 8.0 kPa). Thus, although the consumption of oxygen by the tissues to generate the energy-rich bonds of ATP is almost unaffected by a reduction of the local P_{O_2} to as low as 3 mmHg (0.4 kPa), changes of cellular P_{O_2} in the range 5–100 mmHg (0.68–3.3 kPa) may have very significant effects on the rates of certain oxygenation reactions.

The major products of the complete oxidation of foodstuffs are carbon dioxide, ammonia and water. The rate at which carbon dioxide is produced is related closely to the rate at which oxygen is consumed. The ratio of the mass of carbon dioxide produced to the mass of oxygen consumed per unit time by the tissues is termed the respiratory quotient (RQ). This ratio varies with the nature of the foodstuff being oxidized. The oxidation of carbohydrates gives a RQ of 1.0; oxidation of fat or protein gives an RQ of about 0.7. The RQ of an individual on a normal mixed diet lies in the range 0.80–0.85. In contrast to the rapid gross effects when the oxygen supply is cut off, a rise in the molecular concentration of carbon dioxide in itself does not disrupt tissue function. Throughout the body, however, carbon dioxide is in equilibrium with hydrogen ions and bicarbonate ions according to the equation

$$CO_2 + H_2O \leftrightarrows H_2CO_3 \leftrightarrows H^+ + HCO_3^-$$

A rise of the concentration of carbon dioxide will, therefore, result in an increase in the concentration of hydrogen ions. This increase of acidity is tolerated by the tissues much less well than the causative rise of carbon dioxide concentration.

TISSUE OXYGEN REQUIREMENTS

The rate of oxygen consumption varies with the tissue and its activity. The oxygen consumption of cerebral tissue is 3.5 ml/min/100 g, while that of skeletal muscle varies from 0.2 ml/min/100 g at rest to 11 ml/min/100 g during hard work. The distribution of the total oxygen consumption of a resting man between the major organs of the body is summarized in Table 2.2.

The total oxygen consumption of an individual ($\dot{V}_{O_2}$) at rest in a thermally neutral environment is proportional to the surface area of the body, amounting in a healthy young man to 133 ml (standard temperature and pressure, dry, STPD)/min/m² of body surface. By far the most important determinant of $\dot{V}_{O_2}$ is the level of physical activity. Typical values of $\dot{V}_{O_2}$ for various activities are presented in Table 2.3.

BLOOD–TISSUE GAS EXCHANGE

The oxygen required for oxidation is brought to a tissue by the blood flowing through its capillaries. This flow of blood also removes the carbon dioxide produced by tissue

Table 2.2 *Partition of oxygen consumption in a normal subject (body weight 70 kg) at rest*

Organ/region	Oxygen consumption ml (STPD)/min	% total
Brain	47	19
Heart	28	11
Kidney	18	7
Splanchnic region	62	25
Skeletal muscle	75	30
Skin	5	2
Other organs	15	6
Total	250	100

The oxygen consumed by the respiratory muscles, which is included in the figure for skeletal muscles, amounts to 5 ml/min or 2% of the total.

Table 2.3 *Total oxygen consumption during various activities for an average-sized young man*

Activity	Total oxygen consumption (litres (STPD)/min)
Sleep	0.24
Lying down, fully relaxed	0.24
Lying down, moderately relaxed	0.28
Sitting at rest	0.34
Standing relaxed	0.36
Walking (5 km/h)	0.85
Running (10 km/h)	2.8
Flying an aircraft	
Level flight	0.34
Light aircraft in rough air	0.54
Taxiing	0.58
Aerobatics	0.65
Air-combat manoeuvring	1.00

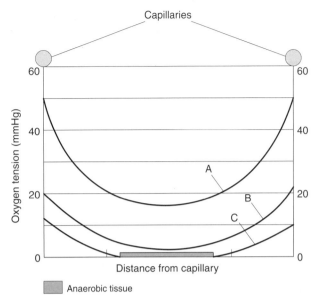

Anaerobic tissue

Figure 2.7 *Cross-section of a simple model of the distribution of tissue oxygen tension in which symmetrically arranged parallel capillaries carry blood in one direction through a tissue with uniform oxygen consumption. The solid curves (A, B, C) depict the magnitude of the oxygen tension with distance from a capillary. The tension falls to a minimum at a point midway between the two capillaries. When the oxygen tension in the capillary blood is high (A), the oxygen tension everywhere in the tissue exceeds 15 mmHg (2 kPa). When the capillary oxygen tension is reduced to about 20 mmHg (2.7 kPa) (B), the oxygen tension in the tissue midway between the capillaries falls to about 2 mmHg (0.27 kPa), whereas when the capillary oxygen tension falls to about 10 mmHg (1.33 kPa) (C), the oxygen tension of a significant part of the tissue is zero.*

respiration. The exchange of oxygen and carbon dioxide between the blood in the capillaries and the cells of a tissue occurs by simple physical diffusion. Each gas moves through the blood, the capillary wall and the cells of the tissue down the partial pressure gradient in accordance with Fick's law of diffusion. Carbon dioxide diffuses about 20 times more rapidly than oxygen. The transfer of carbon dioxide to the blood is, therefore, much less likely to be impaired than the delivery of oxygen from the blood in the capillaries to the mitochondria of the tissues.

The consumption of oxygen by the cells causes the P_{O_2} to fall progressively with distance from the blood in the capillary (Figure 2.7). As the distance from the capillary increases beyond a certain point, the oxygen supply ceases to come from that capillary and is provided by another neighbouring capillary. There are, therefore, points within a tissue where the P_{O_2} is a minimum. The condition of the local oxygen supply becomes critical when the minimum P_{O_2} falls to a level at which it limits the rate of oxidative phosphorylation, i.e. a value of 0.5–3.0 mmHg (0.07–0.4 kPa) (Figure 2.7, curve B). If the minimum P_{O_2} is reduced further, then the tissue in that region turns to anaerobic metabolism, with the formation of lactic acid (Figure 2.7, curve C). Such regions are termed lethal areas or corners.

There are two important mechanisms whereby the P_{O_2} in potential lethal corners is raised when the oxygen consumption of a tissue increases: (i) an increase in the flow of blood through the capillaries, which reduces the fall of P_{O_2} along the length of the capillary bed, and (ii) the opening up of additional capillaries, which reduces the distance over which oxygen has to diffuse. Both of these mechanisms operate in most tissues even at rest. Thus, the capillary bed normally is in a dynamic state, with new capillaries opening up as the local tissue P_{O_2} falls to a low level and other capillaries closing down. These changes in the capillaries are almost certainly mediated locally (see p. 16). The

magnitude of the changes of blood flow and capillarity that can occur in response to an increase in activity varies considerably from one tissue to another. The number of open capillaries in muscle during maximum exercise is 100–200 times greater than that at rest. There is at the same time a 20-fold increase in the blood flow. In many regions of the brain, most of the capillary bed is open even at rest, and there is only a two- to four-fold increase in the number of open capillaries during intense activity or in the face of a threat of tissue hypoxia.

The supply of oxygen to a tissue is almost always more critical than the removal of carbon dioxide, since (i) accumulation of carbon dioxide causes much less disruption of tissue function than hypoxia; (ii) carbon dioxide requires one-twentieth of the partial pressure difference needed for oxygen to diffuse at the same rate; and (iii) the tissue storage capacity for carbon dioxide is much greater than for oxygen. In most circumstances, the adjustments of the blood flow through, and the capillarity of, a tissue are set by the demand for oxygen. Paradoxically, in certain circumstances, lowering of the P_{CO_2} in the arterial blood, which increases the removal of carbon dioxide from the tissues, induces tissue hypoxia. Thus, a reduction of the arterial P_{CO_2} causes intense vasoconstriction of the cerebral arterioles so that a halving of the normal carbon dioxide tension reduces the blood flow through the brain by half and although hyperventilation on air increases the arterial P_{O_2} slightly, it induces hypoxia in brain tissue.

When the P_{O_2} in the lethal corners of a tissue is inadequate to maintain oxidative phosphorylation, energy-rich phosphate bonds can be generated only by anaerobic metabolism, with the formation of lactic acid. This situation occurs at the beginning of even light muscular exercise, since it takes time for the blood flow to the working tissue to increase to the required level. Once the blood flow has increased to raise the P_{O_2} throughout the tissue, the formation of lactic acid ceases. With very high levels of exercise, the circulation cannot meet the increase in the demand for oxygen, and lactic acid formation continues until muscular fatigue occurs.

Carriage of gases by the blood

OXYGEN

Oxygen is carried in the blood in physical solution and in chemical combination. The concentration of dissolved oxygen varies directly with the P_{O_2} of the blood. The concentration of oxygen dissolved at a P_{O_2} of 100 mmHg (13.3 kPa) is 0.3 ml (STPD)/100 ml blood, which is about 1.5 per cent of the concentration of oxygen in chemical combination with haemoglobin (Figure 2.8). Even when the arterial P_{O_2} is raised to about 650 mmHg (86.6 kPa) by

breathing 100 per cent oxygen at one atmosphere, the quantity of oxygen in physical solution (1.95 ml (STPD)/100 ml blood) is only about 40 per cent of that removed from the blood by the tissues.

Oxygen undergoes an easily reversible combination with the haemoglobin in the red cells to form oxyhaemoglobin. The maximum amount of oxygen that can combine with 1 g of haemoglobin is 1.39 ml (STPD). Therefore, the total amount of oxygen that can be carried in combination with haemoglobin in blood with a normal haemoglobin concentration of 15 g/100 ml blood (oxygen capacity of the blood) is 1.39×15, i.e. 20.8 ml (STPD)/100 ml blood. The concentration of oxygen present in the blood in combination with haemoglobin is expressed as the oxygen saturation (S_{O_2}) of haemoglobin, which is given by the relationship

$$S_{O_2} = \frac{\text{concentration of } O_2 \text{ combined with Hb}}{\text{Oxygen capacity of blood}} \times 100\%$$

The relationship between S_{O_2} and P_{O_2} is described by the oxygen dissociation curve, which is sigmoid in shape (Figure 2.8). The S_{O_2} of blood (at pH 7.4, P_{CO_2} 40 mmHg (5.3 kPa), 37 °C) is about 97.5 per cent at a P_{O_2} of 100 mmHg (13.3 kPa). For practical purposes, it can be assumed that the haemoglobin is fully saturated ($S_{O_2} = 100$ per cent) at P_{O_2} values greater than 200 mmHg (26.6 kPa). At low P_{O_2}, i.e. below about 50 mmHg (6.7 kPa), the S_{O_2} increases rapidly with P_{O_2}, whereas at higher oxygen tension the curve is much flatter. The haemoglobin is half-saturated with oxygen (P_{50}) at a P_{O_2} of 26 mmHg (3.5 kPa).

The shape of the oxygen dissociation curve of blood is of great physiological significance. The flat upper portion of

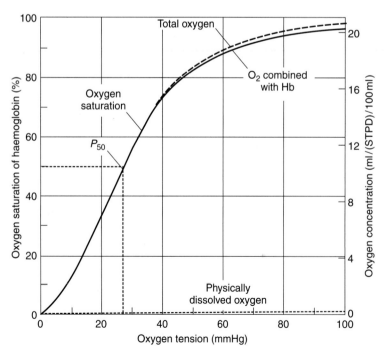

Figure 2.8 *Oxygen dissociation curve of blood. Relationship for normal blood (haemoglobin (Hb) concentration 15 g/100 mL) at pH 7.4, P_{CO_2} 40 mmHg (5.3 kPa) and 37 °C between oxygen tension and oxygen concentration (dashed curve), and oxygen saturation of haemoglobin (solid curve). The concentrations of physically dissolved and chemically combined oxygen are shown separately.*

the curve means that moderate variations of the arterial P_{O_2} about the normal value produced by breathing air at one atmosphere have relatively small effects on the concentration of oxygen in the arterial blood. Furthermore, the steep part of the curve between P_{O_2} of 40 mmHg (5.3 kPa) and 55 mmHg (7.3 kPa) ensures that during the passage of the blood through the pulmonary capillaries, the oxygen tension does not rise until much of the oxygen has been transferred to the blood. The steep portion of the curve at lower P_{O_2} greatly aids the unloading of oxygen from the blood in the tissues. The delivery of a large amount of oxygen results in only a relatively small fall in the P_{O_2} in the blood, which is an important factor in maintaining the oxygen tension in the tissue cells. Finally, the steep part of the oxygen dissociation curve tends to maintain the P_{O_2} at which oxygen is delivered to the tissues when the arterial P_{O_2} is lowered in hypoxia.

The shape of the oxygen dissociation curve is unaffected by the concentration of haemoglobin in the blood. However, a fall in pH, a rise of P_{CO_2} and a rise of temperature all shift the curve to the right. All these changes, which occur in working tissue, increase the amount of oxygen given up by the blood at a given P_{O_2}, thus facilitating oxygen delivery in the tissues. Most of the effect of carbon dioxide (the Bohr effect) can be attributed to associated changes of pH within the red cell. The Bohr effect also operates in the pulmonary capillary blood, so that the affinity of haemoglobin for oxygen increases, i.e. the oxygen dissociation curve moves to the left as carbon dioxide diffuses out of the blood into the alveolar gas.

The total concentration of oxygen in the blood is the sum of that in physical solution and that carried in combination with haemoglobin (Figure 2.8). Typical values for the concentrations of oxygen in the arterial and mixed venous blood of a normal individual at rest are given in Table 2.4.

Table 2.4 *Oxygen content of arterial and mixed venous blood of a man at rest (haemoglobin concentration 15 g/100 ml)*

	Arterial blood	Mixed venous blood
Oxygen tension		
mmHg	95.0	40.0
kPa	12.7	5.3
Oxygen concentration (mL/100 mL)		
Physically dissolved	0.29	0.12
Combined with haemoglobin	20.23	15.38
Total	20.52	15.50
Oxygen saturation (%)	97.00	74.00
Arteriovenous difference (mL/100 mL)		
Physically dissolved		0.17
Combined with haemoglobin		4.85
Total		5.02

The difference between the concentrations of oxygen $[O_2]$ in the arterial and mixed venous blood is related to the total oxygen consumption and the cardiac output by Fick's equation:

$$[O_2]\ \text{arterial} - [O_2]\ \text{mixed venous} = \frac{\text{oxygen consumption}}{\text{cardiac output}}$$

Thus, a man seated at rest with an oxygen consumption of 250 ml (SPTD)/min and a cardiac output of 5 l/min has an arteriovenous oxygen concentration difference of 5 ml/100 ml blood. Although the cardiac output increases in exercise, the increase is inadequate to meet the rise in the oxygen consumption of the tissues, so the arteriovenous oxygen difference also increases. Thus, in exercise sufficient to raise the oxygen consumption to 1 litre (SPTD)/min, the cardiac output averages 10 l/min and the arteriovenous oxygen difference becomes 10 ml/100 ml blood. Since the concentration of oxygen in the arterial blood is almost unchanged by exercise, the increased arteriovenous oxygen difference results in a reduction of the oxygen concentration in the mixed venous blood. The venous oxygen concentration falls from about 15.5 ml/100 ml ($S_{O_2} = 74$ per cent) at rest to 10.5 ml/100 ml ($S_{O_2} = 50$ per cent) in exercise, with an oxygen uptake of 1 litre (SPTD)/min.

CARBON DIOXIDE

Carbon dioxide is carried in the blood in three forms: in physical solution, as bicarbonate and in combination with protein. As with oxygen, the concentration of dissolved carbon dioxide is proportional to the tension of the gas, but carbon dioxide is some 20 times as soluble as oxygen. Thus, the concentration of dissolved carbon dioxide in blood at a P_{CO_2} of 40 mmHg (5.3 kPa) is 2.6 ml (STPD)/100 ml. Bicarbonate is formed by the dissociation of carbonic acid produced by the hydration of carbon dioxide as follows:

$$CO_2 + H_2O \leftrightarrows H_2CO_3 \leftrightarrows H^+ + HCO_3^-$$

The hydration of carbon dioxide to carbonic acid happens very slowly in the plasma, but the enzyme carbonic anhydrase in the red cells catalyses the reaction, so that significant formation of carbonic acid occurs only within the red cell. The subsequent dissociation into bicarbonate and hydrogen ions is very rapid. The bicarbonate ions formed from dissolved carbon dioxide pass back into the plasma, while the proteins within the red cell buffer the hydrogen ions. Reduced haemoglobin is a more effective buffer than oxyhaemoglobin, so that the deoxygenation of the blood that occurs in the tissue capillaries favours the formation of bicarbonate and, hence, the uptake of carbon dioxide. Conversely, oxygenation of blood in the lungs favours the conversion of bicarbonate to carbon dioxide. The concentration of carbon dioxide carried as bicarbonate in arterial blood at a P_{CO_2} of 40 mmHg (5.3 kPa) is about 44 ml (SPTD)/100 ml, which is approximately 90 per cent of the total carbon dioxide concentration. Approximately five per cent of the carbon dioxide is carried as carbamino compounds with the amine groups of proteins, especially the globin of haemoglobin:

$$HbNH_2 + CO_2 \leftrightarrows HbNHCOOH \leftrightarrows HbNHCOO^- + H^+$$

This type of reaction occurs rapidly. Since oxyhaemoglobin binds less carbon dioxide as carbamino compound than reduced haemoglobin, the reaction favours uptake of carbon dioxide in the tissues and the reverse process in the pulmonary capillaries.

The carbon dioxide dissociation curve of whole blood (Figure 2.9) is much more linear over the physiologically significant range than the oxygen dissociation curve (Figure 2.8). Since the oxygen saturation of haemoglobin affects both the bicarbonate concentration and the concentration of carbamino haemoglobin, the oxygen saturation affects the carbon dioxide dissociation curve (Figure 2.9). In vivo, the oxygen saturation of the blood falls as the carbon dioxide tension rises, so the physiological dissociation curve is of the form depicted by the dashed line in Figure 2.9. Typical values for the concentrations of carbon dioxide in the arterial and venous bloods of a normal individual at rest are given in Table 2.5. Although 90 per cent of the carbon dioxide content of blood is in the form of bicarbonate, only half of the arteriovenous carbon dioxide concentration difference is accounted for by the change in bicarbonate concentration. A third of the arteriovenous carbon dioxide difference is due to changes in the concentrations of carbamino compounds.

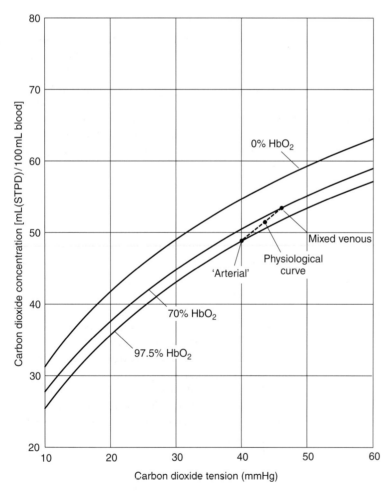

Figure 2.9 *Carbon dioxide dissociation curve of whole blood at oxyhaemoglobin (HbO$_2$) saturations of zero (fully reduced), 70 per cent (mixed venous blood at rest) and 97.5 per cent (arterial blood breathing air at rest). The dashed line depicts the relationship (the physiological curve) between carbon dioxide tension and carbon dioxide concentration, which is followed as blood takes up carbon dioxide in the tissues and gives it up in the pulmonary capillaries.*

Table 2.5 *Carbon dioxide content of arterial blood and mixed venous blood of man at rest*

	Arterial blood	Mixed venous blood
Carbon dioxide tension		
mmHg	40.0	46.0
kPa	5.3	6.1
Carbon dioxide concentration (ml/100 ml)		
Physically dissolved	2.6	3.0
As bicarbonate	43.8	46.4
As carbamino compound	2.6	3.9
Total	49.0	53.3
Arteriovenous difference (ml/100 ml)		
Physically dissolved	0.4	
As bicarbonate	2.6	
As carbamino compound	1.3	
Total	4.3	

Gas exchange in the lung

FUNCTIONAL ANATOMY

The primary function of the lung is the exchange of oxygen and carbon dioxide between the venous blood and the atmosphere. It also has other important functions, such as filtering toxic materials, e.g. blood thrombi, from the circulation, metabolism of certain biologically active agents, e.g. vasoconstrictor agents, serotonin, bradykinin and certain prostaglandins, and conversion of angiotensin I to the potent vasoconstrictor angiotensin II. It also acts as a reservoir of blood.

The structure of the lung is such that air and blood are brought into intimate contact in some 300 million air sacs or alveoli, each of which is approximately 0.3 mm in diameter. Gases are exchanged across the very thin alveolar–capillary membrane (average thickness 0.5 μm). The vast number of alveoli gives the membrane a total area of 50–100 m². Both the very large area and the thinness of the alveolar–capillary membrane serve to minimize the resistance to gas diffusion between the blood and gas phases.

The arrangement of the lung, which may be regarded as a collection of some 300 million interconnected bubbles, is inherently unstable. The forces normally generated by surface tension at the air–wall interface in bubbles of this size are relatively large. The surface tension forces tend to cause collapse of the smaller alveoli, but some of the cells lining the alveoli secrete surfactant that profoundly lowers the surface tension of the alveolar lining fluid. Surfactant promotes the stability of the lung structure. It also decreases the stiffness of the lung, reducing the effort required to ventilate it, and reduces the forces tending to draw fluid from the blood into the alveoli.

Functionally, the respiratory passages can be divided into two regions, the conducting airways and the respiratory zone. The conducting airways comprise the nose, the mouth, the pharynx, the trachea and the main, lobar, segmental and terminal bronchi. The conducting airways carry inspired air down to the gas-exchanging regions of the lungs. The gas within the conducting airways constitutes the anatomical dead space. It has a volume of about 150 ml in the average adult. The terminal bronchioles divide into respiratory bronchioles, which have alveoli attached to their walls. The final division of the airways constitutes the alveolar ducts, which are lined completely with alveoli. The respiratory bronchioles and alveolar ducts are termed the transitional and respiratory zones of the lung, since the gas contained within them (the alveolar gas) can exchange with the blood through the alveolar walls. The distance from the terminal bronchiole to the most distal alveolus is only about 5 mm. The respiratory zone has a volume of about 2500 ml and contains most of the gas held in the lung. The combined cross-sectional area of the airways increases extremely rapidly beyond the terminal bronchioles, so although inspiration causes bulk movement of gas down the conducting airways, the forward velocity of the gas becomes very low as it enters the respiratory zone. Indeed, in this zone, ventilation occurs mainly by diffusion, there being virtually no mass movement of gas. The changes in gas concentrations produced by inspiration within the airways and alveoli beyond the terminal bronchioles are abolished in less than one second.

The pulmonary arteries run into the lung tissue alongside the branching airways subdividing by way of arterioles to feed the capillary beds, which surround the alveoli. The networks of capillaries around the alveoli are very dense, and there is an almost continuous sheet of blood over the alveolar wall. The resistance to flow through the pulmonary circuit is relatively low, the mean pulmonary arterial pressure being only 15 mmHg (2 kPa).

The very large area of the alveolar–capillary membrane is vulnerable to inhaled particles. The site at which particles are removed depends on the size of the particles. Large particles are filtered out in the nose. Smaller particles, which are deposited on the walls of the conducting airways, are removed by the sheet of mucus that is continuously swept up to the epiglottis and swallowed. This mucus is secreted by the glands in the walls of the bronchi and moved by the cilia of the bronchial mucosa. Particles that are small enough to reach the alveoli are engulfed by macrophages, which pass into the circulation directly or by way of the lymphatic system.

LUNG VOLUMES

The total volume of gas held in the lungs at the end of a maximal inspiration is termed the total lung capacity and is about 6.5 litres (body temperature and pressure, saturated with water vapour, BTPS) in the average young adult male (Figure 2.10). The volume of gas in the lung at the end of a normal expiration is termed the functional residual capacity and, in our subject, would amount to about 3 litres (BTPS). At the end of a normal expiration, a further volume of gas can be expelled from the lungs. A significant amount, termed the residual volume, remains in the lungs after a maximal expiration. In our example, this would amount to about 1.5 litres (BTPS). The total volume of gas that can be expelled from the lungs after a maximum inspiration is termed the vital capacity. The vital capacity is equal to the difference between the total lung capacity and the residual volume. In our subject, it would be 5 litres (BTPS).

The tidal volume, which is the volume of gas expelled from the lungs during normal expiration, amounts to about 0.5 litres (BTPS) in a subject at rest. It should be noted that the tidal volume is only about one-sixth of the volume of gas remaining in the lungs at the end of expiration (the functional residual capacity). When the tidal volume is increased, either voluntarily or by exercise, a fraction of the increase is accommodated by a reduction of the functional residual capacity.

PULMONARY VENTILATION

Ventilation is the cyclic process of inspiration and expiration in which fresh air is drawn into the respiratory tract and pulmonary gas is expelled from it. The total volume of gas expired from the lungs per unit time is termed the pulmonary ventilation. It is generally expressed as the volume expired per minute, often called the minute volume.

The ventilation of the lungs is mainly regulated so that it provides the exchange of carbon dioxide between the blood and the atmosphere required to match the rate of production of carbon dioxide by the tissues. Over a considerable range of demands for oxygen, the pulmonary ventilation increases linearly with the oxygen uptake (Figure 2.11). Above a certain level of work, however, the pulmonary ventilation increases relatively more than the oxygen uptake. The maximum pulmonary ventilation that can be maintained for several minutes by fit young adults varies from 100 to 150 l (BTPS)/min. At low rates of physical work, pulmonary ventilation is increased mainly by an increase in tidal volume. In moderate or heavy work, the tidal volume amounts to about half the vital capacity, and there is also a progressive rise in respiratory frequency, increasing from 10–20 breaths/min at rest to 40–45 breaths/min in maximal exercise.

ALVEOLAR VENTILATION

Since exchange of gas between the inspired gas and the blood occurs only in the alveoli, it is the ventilation of alveoli rather than the total pulmonary ventilation that determines the gas exchange between the blood and the

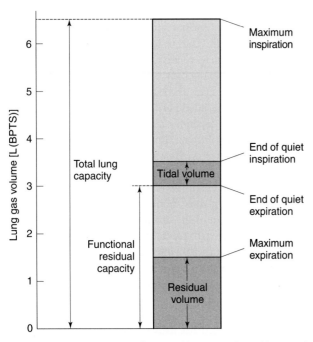

Figure 2.10 *Subdivisions of the total lung capacity, with normal values for a young male (height 1.7 m).*

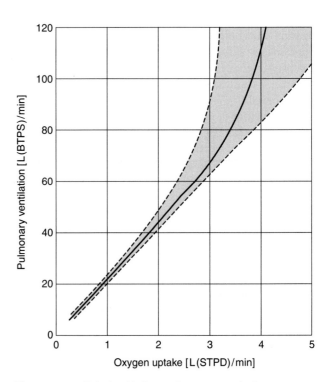

Figure 2.11 *Relationship in steady-state exercise between pulmonary ventilation and oxygen uptake (metabolic oxygen consumption). The solid curve depicts the mean and the shaded area depicts the variation (± 2 standard deviations) of this relationship for a group of 20 young healthy volunteers.*

environment. The alveolar ventilation is the volume of alveolar gas expelled per unit time. The expired gas consists of alveolar gas mixed with the volume of the previously inspired gas that had remained in the respiratory dead space. In quiet breathing, the average tidal volume of 500 ml (BTPS) will consist of 150 ml (BTPS) of inspired gas mixed with 350 ml (BTPS) of alveolar gas. Although the dead space expands with increase of tidal volume, the proportion of the tidal volume that comes from the alveoli rises as the tidal volume is increased.

There is a simple relationship between the alveolar ventilation, the rate of output of carbon dioxide, and the concentration of this gas in the alveolar gas:

$$\text{Alveolar ventilation} = K \times \frac{CO_2 \text{ output per minute}}{\text{Alveolar } P_{CO_2}}$$

Thus, with a constant rate of output of carbon dioxide, the alveolar P_{CO_2} is inversely proportional to the alveolar ventilation. This relationship is independent of environmental pressure, so with a constant metabolic production of carbon dioxide, the alveolar ventilation required to maintain a given alveolar P_{CO_2} is the same at all altitudes.

Inspired gas is not distributed evenly to the various regions of the lung. The ventilation per unit volume of lung is highest in the most dependent part and falls progressively towards the uppermost part. The weight of the lung causes a progressive increase in the pleural pressure from the upper to the lower part of the lung, so that the alveoli at the top are considerably more distended than those at the bottom. Since the stiffness of the alveoli rises progressively with increase in their volume, the expansion of the alveoli at the bottom of the lung is greater than that of those at the top. Not only do the alveoli in the lower part of the lung expand more during inspiration than those higher up, but also the initial volume of the former is less than that of the latter, so the ratio of volume of gas added to the alveoli during inspiration to their initial volume decreases progressively up the lung. These regional differences in the distribution of inspired gas are abolished in the weightless state and accentuated by exposure to increased accelerative force.

The distribution of inspired gas is also changed markedly at low lung volumes when the intrapleural pressure at the base of the lung exceeds the airway pressure. In these circumstances, the lung at the base is compressed, the small airways close and gas is trapped in the distal alveoli. The upper part of the lung, however, remains well ventilated.

DIFFUSION

The processes involved in the uptake of oxygen by the blood in the pulmonary capillaries are (i) solution of oxygen in the fluid lining the alveoli, (ii) diffusion through the alveolar–capillary membrane and through the blood plasma into the red cells, and (iii) combination with haemoglobin to form oxyhaemoglobin. Under resting

conditions, breathing air at ground level, the difference between the P_{O_2} of the mixed venous blood and the alveolar gas is about 60 mmHg (8 kPa) (Figure 2.12), and oxygen passes very rapidly into the blood. The oxygen content and, hence, the P_{O_2} of the blood increase rapidly until, after 0.2–0.25 seconds, i.e. approximately one-third of the way along the length of the capillary, the P_{O_2} of the blood and that of the alveolar gas are almost equal (Figure 2.12) and there is no difference between the P_{O_2} in the alveolar gas and that in end-capillary blood. Even in heavy exercise, when the average time for which each red cell is exposed to alveolar gas is about one-third of that at rest and oxygen

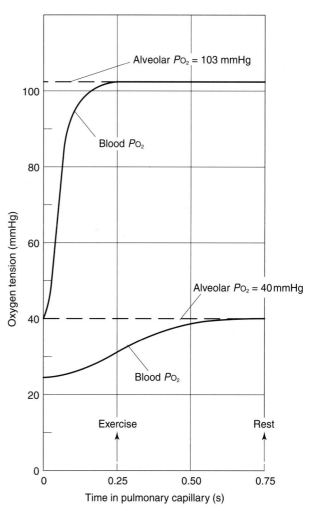

Figure 2.12 *Time course of the oxygen tension of the blood as it flows through a typical pulmonary capillary with a normal alveolar oxygen tension (103 mmHg, 13.7 kPa) and during hypoxia (alveolar oxygen tension 40 mmHg, 5.3 kPa). With the higher alveolar oxygen tension, the oxygen tension of the blood rises very rapidly, reaching that of alveolar gas before it has transversed more than one-third of the length of the capillary. Equilibration of oxygen tension between blood and alveolar gas takes longer at the lower alveolar oxygen tension. Typically, blood transverses the pulmonary capillary in 0.75 seconds at rest and 0.25 seconds in moderate exercise.*

has to cross the membrane at a greater rate, there is still no difference between the P_{O_2} of end-capillary blood and that of alveolar gas. Hypoxia reduces markedly the P_{O_2} difference between the alveolar gas and the blood entering the pulmonary capillaries, and the rate of rise of oxygen tension along the capillary is reduced, since the rate of oxygen transfer is slowed (Figure 2.12). At rest, even if the alveolar P_{O_2} is lowered to 40 mmHg (5.3 kPa), the P_{O_2} in the blood still rises to this value before it leaves the pulmonary capillary. Moderate exercise with this degree of hypoxia does, however, cause the oxygen tension of the end-capillary blood to be less than that of the alveolar gas. Thus, exercise in moderate hypoxia increases the intensity of the arterial hypoxaemia.

PULMONARY BLOOD FLOW

As noted previously, the systolic and diastolic pressures in the pulmonary artery are about 25 mmHg (3.3 kPa) and 8 mmHg (1.1 kPa), respectively, and the mean pressure is 15 mmHg (2 kPa). The pressure exerted by a column of blood equal to the height of the apex of the erect lung above the main pulmonary artery (20 cm) is 15 mmHg (2 kPa), and so the mean arterial pressure at the apex of the lung is equal to alveolar and atmospheric pressure. The mean pulmonary artery pressure increases linearly with distance below the apex to 15 mmHg (2 kPa) at the hilum of the lung and approximately 22 mmHg (2.9 kPa) at the base. Since the pulmonary veins are very thin, and the pressure in the left atrium is slightly less than alveolar pressure, the pulmonary veins above the hilum of the lung are collapsed and the pressure within them is effectively equal to alveolar pressure. Below the hilum of the lung, the pressure in the veins increases above alveolar pressure, in proportion to the weight of the column of blood from the level of the hilum. Thus, the venous pressure at the base of the lung is approximately 7 mmHg (0.9 kPa).

The pressure around the capillaries of the lung is that in the alveoli, which, during normal breathing, is within 1–2 mmHg (0.13–0.26 kPa) of atmospheric pressure. The pressure difference controlling blood flow through the capillaries above the hilum of the lung, where the veins are collapsed, is, therefore, that between pulmonary artery and alveolar pressures. Thus, the blood flow increases progressively down the upright lung from the apex to the hilum (Figure 2.13). Below the hilum, although the veins are open, so that the difference between arterial and venous pressure is constant, there is a progressive increase in the pressure in the capillaries relative to that in the alveoli, which produces a graded increase of the diameter of these vessels, so that the resistance to blood flow falls progressively with distance below the hilum (Figure 2.13). These regional differences of blood flow are reduced by the increase in the pulmonary artery pressure that occurs in exercise.

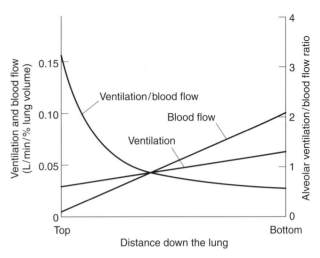

Figure 2.13 *Distribution of ventilation and blood flow in the upright lung. Both ventilation and capillary blood flow per unit volume of lung gas increase progressively with descent from the top to the bottom of the lung. The rate of increase of blood flow per unit volume, however, is considerably greater than that of ventilation per unit volume, so that the ratio of ventilation to blood flow falls progressively with distance from the top of the lung.*

VENTILATION/BLOOD FLOW RELATIONSHIPS

The relationship between the ventilation of a group of alveoli (lung unit) and the blood flow through the capillaries in their walls determines the exchange of oxygen and carbon dioxide between the gas within the alveoli and the blood and the P_{O_2} and P_{CO_2} of the alveolar gas and of end-capillary blood. The increase in flow of blood per unit distance down the lung produced by gravity is considerably greater than the corresponding rate of increase of ventilation, so that the ratio of ventilation to blood flow for each lung unit decreases with increasing distance from the top of the lung (Figure 2.13). In the erect posture, this ratio falls from 3.3 in the top seven per cent of the lung to 0.6 in the bottom ten per cent of the lung. The gradient of the ratio of ventilation to blood flow is accentuated greatly by exposure to increased acceleration.

The qualitative effects of the ratio of ventilation to blood flow upon the gas exchange and alveolar gas tension within a lung unit may be seen by considering two extreme values of the ratio. If the lung unit is ventilated but has no blood flow through its capillaries, i.e. it has a ventilation/blood flow ratio of infinity, then no oxygen will be removed from the inspired air and no carbon dioxide will be added to it. The alveolar gas tensions will, therefore, be those of inspired air. If, however, blood flows through a lung unit that is not ventilated, i.e. it has a ventilation/blood flow ratio of zero, then the P_{O_2} and P_{CO_2} in the alveolar gas will come to equal those in the blood entering the capillary and will, therefore, be equal to the tensions of these gases in the mixed venous blood. Thus, as the ventilation/blood flow ratio of a unit changes, the composition of the alveolar gas within it approaches that of inspired gas or mixed venous blood. Between these two extremes, a fall in this ratio is associated with a reduction in the P_{O_2} in the alveolar gas and, hence, in the end-capillary blood, and a rise in the P_{CO_2} of the alveolar gas and the end-capillary blood.

The progressive fall of the ratio of ventilation to blood flow from the apex to the base of the erect lung (Figure 2.13) gives rise, therefore, to a progressive reduction of the P_{O_2} in the alveolar gas from the top to the bottom of the lung, while the alveolar P_{CO_2} increases progressively down the lung. In the lung of a man sitting erect and breathing air at ground level, the alveolar P_{O_2} falls from about 130 mmHg (17.3 kPa) at the apex to about 90 mmHg (12 kPa) at the base. The corresponding values of alveolar P_{CO_2} are 28 mmHg (3.7 kPa) at the apex and 42 mmHg (5.6 kPa) at the base. The magnitude of these differences is reduced during exercise, when the regional distribution of blood flow is more even and, thus, the range of values of the ventilation/blood flow ratio is smaller.

ALVEOLAR/ARTERIAL GAS TENSIONS

The regional differences of gas exchange within the lung reduce the overall efficiency of the lungs. The P_{O_2} of the blood leaving the alveolar capillaries varies in exactly the same manner as the alveolar P_{O_2}. A lung unit with a high ventilation/blood flow ratio contributes relatively more gas to the expirate than one with a low ratio. However, a lung unit with a low ratio makes a relatively larger contribution to the total blood flow from the lung. Since lung units with a high ventilation/blood flow ratio have high alveolar P_{O_2}, and those with a low ratio have low-end capillary P_{O_2}, the P_{O_2} of the mixed expired alveolar gas is higher than that of the mixed blood leaving the lung. The P_{O_2} of the mixed pulmonary venous blood is also depressed below that of the mixed expired alveolar gas, because the additional amount of oxygen in the blood from lung units with a high P_{O_2} is less than the deficit of the oxygen content of the blood from lung units with a low P_{O_2}. This difference is a function of the sigmoid shape of the oxygen dissociation curve of blood (see p. 30). The net result of ventilation/ blood flow inequality in the normal upright lungs is that the P_{O_2} of the mixed end-alveolar capillary blood is some 4 mmHg (0.5 kPa) less than the P_{O_2} of the mixed alveolar gas. The effect is less with respect to carbon dioxide, the tension of this gas in the mixed pulmonary venous blood being only 0.5–1 mmHg (0.07–0.13 kPa) higher than the mixed alveolar P_{CO_2}. The impairment of overall gas exchange in the lungs caused by ventilation/blood flow inequality is, therefore, relatively small in healthy humans. The P_{O_2} of the blood flowing from the pulmonary capillaries is lowered by approximately a further 4 mmHg (0.5 kPa) by the admixture of venous blood from the bronchial and thebesian veins (venous shunts), so that the total alveolar/arterial P_{O_2} difference amounts to 8–10 mmHg (1.1–1.3 kPa). Exposure to raised acceleration forces and certain lung diseases that accentuate the ventilation/blood flow inequality cause larger differences between the P_{O_2} of the mixed expired alveolar gas and the arterial blood.

Control of pulmonary ventilation

NEURAL ORGANIZATION

The activity of the respiratory muscles of the chest wall, diaphragm and abdominal wall is due to the rhythmic discharge of neurons located in the medulla and pons. The primary centre, which is located in the reticular formulation of the medulla, exhibits rhythmicity even when deprived completely of afferent impulses. Stimulation of certain neurons within this medullary centre causes inspiration, while stimulation of other neurons causes expiration. The activity of this primary respiratory centre is influenced by impulses from the pontine respiratory centres, the reticular activating system and certain peripheral receptors. The important peripheral receptors are the stretch receptors in the lungs, the chemoreceptors and the arterial baroreceptors. The activity of the respiratory coordinating centres is also affected by impulses from the cerebral cortex and hypothalamus. Impulses from the hypothalamus are responsible for the increase in pulmonary ventilation produced by a rise of the temperature of the blood.

CHEMORECEPTORS

The most important factors controlling the level of pulmonary ventilation are the P_{CO_2}, the pH and the P_{O_2} of the arterial blood. The central chemoreceptors, which are situated just beneath the ventrolateral surface of the medulla, respond to the P_{CO_2} and pH of the extracellular fluid and cerebrospinal fluid, which reflect the P_{CO_2} of the arterial blood. Increases of P_{CO_2} or $[H^+]$ on the surface of this part of the medulla result in an increase in pulmonary ventilation.

The peripheral chemoreceptors are located in the carotid bodies, which lie in the bifurcations of the common carotid arteries, and the aortic bodies, which lie around the arch of the aorta. These receptors respond to change in the P_{O_2}, P_{CO_2}, pH and potassium concentration of the arterial blood. The activity of the peripheral chemoreceptors is increased markedly by a reduction of arterial P_{O_2}. The increase of pulmonary ventilation produced by arterial hypoxaemia is due solely to stimulation of the peripheral chemoreceptors, as the central effect of hypoxia is to depress pulmonary ventilation. The peripheral chemoreceptors also play a role in the matching of pulmonary ventilation to a rapid change in the arterial P_{CO_2}.

RESPONSES TO CARBON DIOXIDE

There is a very close control of the P_{CO_2} of the arterial blood. Changes in arterial P_{CO_2} give rise to immediate compensatory changes in pulmonary ventilation. Thus, a reduction of the arterial carbon dioxide tension by 5 mmHg (0.67 kPa) below the normal level removes the drive to breathe until sufficient carbon dioxide has accumulated in the blood to return the arterial P_{CO_2} to normal. Raising the arterial carbon dioxide tension by adding carbon dioxide to the inspired gas causes a rapid increase in the ventilation, until a new steady state is attained. The pulmonary ventilation is increased by about 3 litres (BTPS)/min for each 1 mmHg (0.13-kPa) increase in arterial P_{CO_2}. The sensitivity of the peripheral chemoreceptors to carbon dioxide is increased in hypoxia, so that the rise in pulmonary ventilation per 1 mmHg increase in arterial carbon dioxide tension is approximately 9 litres (BTPS)/min at an arterial oxygen tension of 30–35 mmHg (4–4.7 kPa).

The arterial P_{CO_2} of a given individual normally varies by less than 3 mmHg (0.4 kPa) throughout the waking day. There is some variation, however, of the mean arterial P_{CO_2} between individuals; it normally lies between 37 and 42 mmHg (4.9–5.6 kPa). The arterial carbon dioxide tension rises slightly above this range during sleep. The relationship between carbon dioxide tension and hydrogen ion concentration and the sensitivity of peripheral chemoreceptors to the pH of the arterial blood also results in a very close control of the latter. Thus, the pH of the arterial blood normally lies within the range 7.36–7.44.

RESPONSES TO OXYGEN

An acute reduction of the arterial P_{O_2} does not produce a significant increase in pulmonary ventilation until the tension is reduced below 45–50 mmHg (6–6.7 kPa). Below this level, there is a considerable increase in ventilation, although the latter tends to be reduced by the concomitant decrease of P_{CO_2}. If the latter is maintained at its normal resting level by adding carbon dioxide to the inspired gas as the alveolar oxygen tension is lowered, then the pulmonary ventilation is twice normal at an arterial P_{O_2} of about 38 mmHg (5.1 kPa) and four to six times greater at an arterial oxygen tension of 35 mmHg (4.7 kPa). There are large individual differences in response to arterial hypoxaemia. An increase of the arterial P_{O_2} above normal has little or no effect on pulmonary ventilation.

CORTICAL CONTROL

In the short term, there is considerable cortical control of pulmonary ventilation. It is relatively easy to reduce the arterial P_{CO_2} to half its normal value by voluntarily increas-

ing ventilation of the lungs. Hyperventilation, with a consequent reduction of the arterial P_{CO_2}, also occurs involuntarily as a result of fear or emotional disturbance. The cortical input producing the increase in ventilation in these circumstances may completely override the chemoreceptor control of respiration. The reduction in arterial P_{CO_2} can be so great that performance and even consciousness are grossly disturbed.

EXERCISE

It has been shown that exercise produces a rapid increase in ventilation, the magnitude of which is proportional to the increased oxygen uptake and carbon dioxide output. In all but heavy exercise, the increase in alveolar ventilation is matched so closely to the increased gaseous exchange in the lungs that the arterial P_{CO_2} and P_{O_2} are held very close to the values that exist at rest. The mechanism of the control of ventilation of the lungs during exercise is controversial and not understood fully. The large increases in ventilation occur without an increase in the arterial P_{CO_2} or a fall in the arterial P_{O_2}. The initial increase in ventilation at the start of exercise probably is due to nervous impulses from the motor cortex and the exercising muscles and joints.

Gas tension gradients

A valuable expression of the effectiveness of the exchange of respiratory gases between the inspired gas and the tissues is the magnitude of the tensions of each gas at various points in the transport system (Figure 2.14).

CARBON DIOXIDE

The primary factor that determines the tissue P_{CO_2} is the tension of the gas in the arterial blood. The pulmonary ventilation normally is regulated by the respiratory control mechanism, so that the arterial P_{CO_2} is held constant. The maximum P_{CO_2} in the tissues is only slightly greater than that in the blood flowing from the tissue. Typical values of the carbon dioxide tensions at various points in the carbon dioxide transport system in an individual at rest are given in Table 2.5 (p. 33).

The tissues contain relatively large stores of carbon dioxide, mainly as bicarbonate, so that a sudden sustained decrease of the arterial carbon dioxide tension, such as that produced by voluntary hyperventilation, results in a marked increase in the rate at which carbon dioxide is removed from the tissues and blood and expired from the lungs. Even when the hyperventilation reduces the arterial carbon dioxide tension by only 15 mmHg, the output of carbon dioxide in the expired gas exceeds that produced by tissue metabolism for 30–60 minutes. During this period,

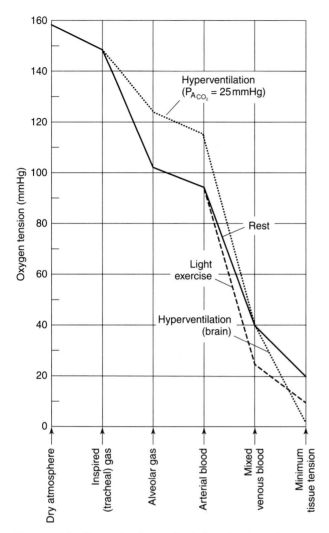

Figure 2.14 *Oxygen tension gradients from dry atmosphere to minimum tissue level in an individual breathing air at ground level at rest, during light exercise and performing hyperventilation.*

the ratio of the rate of carbon dioxide output to the rate of oxygen uptake measured at the lips – the respiratory exchange ratio – will exceed the respiratory quotient.

OXYGEN

The difference between the oxygen tensions of the inspired and alveolar gas is proportional to the ratio of oxygen consumption to alveolar ventilation. This relationship is analogous to that for carbon dioxide, the alveolar P_{CO_2} (in the absence of carbon dioxide from the inspired gas) being proportional to the ratio of carbon dioxide production to alveolar ventilation.

The alveolar P_{O_2} and P_{CO_2} are connected intimately. The relationship between the inspired P_{O_2}, the alveolar P_{O_2} and P_{CO_2} is simplest when the inspired gas is 100 per cent oxygen. Under these circumstances, the alveolar gas consists of oxygen, carbon dioxide and water vapour, and the sum of P_{O_2} and P_{CO_2} in the alveolar gas ($P_{A_{O_2}}$ and $P_{A_{CO_2}}$, respectively) equals the P_{O_2} in the inspired tracheal gas ($P_{I_{O_2}}$), i.e. inspired gas saturated with water vapour at deep body temperature (37 °C). Thus, when the inspired gas is 100 per cent oxygen,

$$P_{I_{O_2}} = P_{A_{O_2}} + P_{A_{CO_2}} \tag{1}$$

and hence

$$P_{A_{O_2}} = P_{I_{O_2}} - P_{A_{CO_2}} \tag{2}$$

This expression is a special case of the alveolar gas equation, which relates these three gas tensions. When nitrogen is present in the inspired and alveolar gas, it is necessary to introduce a correction factor into the alveolar gas equation, since the excess oxygen uptake over carbon dioxide production results in a higher concentration of nitrogen in the alveolar gas than in the inspired gas. The general form of the alveolar gas equation is:

$$P_{A_{O_2}} = P_{I_{O_2}} - P_{A_{CO_2}}(F_{IO_2} + [1 - F_{IO_2}]/R) \tag{3}$$

where F_{IO_2} is the fractional concentration of oxygen in the inspired gas (dry gas) and R is the respiratory exchange ratio.

When either $F_{IO_2} = 1$ or $R = 1$, equation 3 simplifies to equation 2. Equation 3 predicts that when breathing air and R is 0.85, the alveolar P_{O_2} rises by 0.9 mmHg (0.12 kPa) for every 1 mmHg (0.13-kPa) fall in alveolar P_{CO_2}, provided that R remains unchanged. R, however, rises towards and even exceeds 1 during hyperventilation, so that the alveolar oxygen tension rises by about 1 mmHg (0.13 kPa) for each 1 mmHg (0.13-kPa) reduction in alveolar carbon dioxide tension.

The P_{O_2} in the dry atmosphere, the inspired tracheal gas and the alveolar gas for an individual breathing air at ground level, at rest, during light exercise and while hyperventilating to reduce the alveolar P_{CO_2} to 25 mmHg (3.3 kPa) are presented in Figure 2.14. The alveolar P_{O_2} at rest is 103 mmHg (13.7 kPa), and it remains at this value during light exercise (oxygen uptake of 1 litre (STPD)/min). Hyperventilation, which reduces the alveolar P_{CO_2} to 25 mmHg (3.3 kPa) and raises R to 1, increases the alveolar P_{O_2} to 124 mmHg (15.2 kPa).

The P_{O_2} of the arterial blood is reduced below that of the mixed alveolar gas by the effects of the ventilation/blood flow inequality and the venous-to-arterial shunts. In all three conditions depicted in Figure 2.14, the fall in P_{O_2} from alveolar gas to arterial blood is 8 mmHg (1.07 kPa), so that the arterial P_{O_2} is 95 mmHg (12.7 kPa) both at rest and during light exercise. Hyperventilation, which reduces the alveolar P_{CO_2} to 25 mmHg (3.3 kPa), gives an arterial P_{O_2} of 116 mmHg (15.4 kPa).

The fall in P_{O_2} between arterial and mixed venous blood is determined by the ratio of oxygen uptake to blood flow in the tissues and the shape of the oxygen dissociation curve of the blood. These relationships are such that, in the resting state, mixed venous blood P_{O_2} is 55 mmHg (7.3 kPa) less than that of the arterial blood, i.e. 40 mmHg (5.3 kPa). In light exercise, the proportional increase in cardiac output is less than the proportional increase in the oxygen uptake by the tissues, so that the fall of P_{O_2} from arterial to mixed venous blood increases to 70 mmHg (9.3 kPa). The mixed venous blood P_{O_2}, therefore, falls to 25 mmHg (3.3 kPa). The small increase in the concentration of oxygen in the arterial blood associated with the rise of oxygen tension induced by moderate hyperventilation (alveolar P_{CO_2} 25 mmHg, 3.3 kPa) will, because of the shape of the oxygen dissociation curve, have only a very minor effect on the P_{O_2} tension of the mixed venous blood, the latter being raised by about 1 mmHg (0.13 kPa).

So far, the tissues of the body have been treated as if they were homogeneous. However, the relationship between the oxygen uptake and blood flow varies from one tissue to another, and these differences are accentuated by exercise and hyperventilation. Thus, the P_{O_2} of the blood flowing from exercising muscle is considerably lower than the P_{O_2} of the mixed venous blood during light exercise. The lowering of the arterial P_{CO_2} produced by hyperventilation reduces the blood flow to the brain, so that venous P_{O_2} of the cerebral tissues is considerably lower than that of the mixed venous blood. Thus, the P_{O_2} of jugular venous blood is reduced from 35 mmHg (4.7 kPa) at rest to 22 mmHg (2.9 kPa) by hyperventilation producing an arterial P_{CO_2} of 25 mmHg (3.3 kPa).

Oxygen tension varies from point to point within a tissue, and the concept of mean tissue P_{O_2} is of little value. A more meaningful expression of the effectiveness of the oxygen transport system is the minimum P_{O_2} in the tissues, although in reality this varies widely from one tissue to another. Estimates of the minimum tissue P_{O_2}, assuming uniform oxygen consumption, blood flow and capillary geometry throughout the body, are presented in Figure 2.14. In all three conditions considered in this figure, the minimum tissue P_{O_2} values are considerably greater than those required to maintain aerobic metabolism. The reduction in cerebral blood flow induced by hyperventilation to an arterial P_{CO_2} of 25 mmHg (3.3 kPa) does, however, reduce the minimum tissue P_{O_2} in certain areas of the brain to about 3 mmHg (0.4 kPa), which may reduce the rate of oxidative phosphorylation and, hence, impair cerebral function.

FURTHER READING

Basic cardiovascular and respiratory system textbooks

Aaronson PI, Ward JPT. *The Cardiovascular System at a Glance*, 2nd edn. Oxford: Blackwell, 2004.

Levick JR. *An Introduction to Cardiovascular Physiology*, 4th edn. London: Arnold, 2003.

Ward JPT, Ward J, Wiener CM, Leach RM. *The Respiratory System at a Glance*. Oxford: Blackwell, 2002.

West JB. *Respiratory Physiology: The Essentials*, 7th edn. Philadelphia, PA: Lippincott Williams & Wilkins, 2004.

Advanced reading

Astrand PO, Rodahl K. *Textbook of Work Physiology*, 4th edn. Champaign, IL: Human Kinetics, 2003.

Brooks VL, Sved AF. Pressure to change? Re-evaluating the role of baroreceptors in the long term control of arterial pressure. *American Journal of Physiology* 2005; **288**: R815–18.

Comroe JH, Forster RE, Dubois AB, Briscoe WA, Carlsen E. *The Lung, Clinical Physiology and Pulmonary Function Tests*, 2nd edn. Chicago: Year Book Medical Publishers, 1962.

Coote JH. Cardiovascular responses to exercise: central and reflex contributions. In: Jordan D, Marshall J (eds). *Cardiovascular Regulation*. London: Portland Press, 1995; pp. 93–111.

Cotes JE, Leathart, GL. *Lung Function: Assessment and Application in Medicine*, 5th edn. Oxford: Blackwell, 1993.

Daly M de B. Aspects of the integration of the respiratory and cardiovascular systems. In: Jordan D, Marshall J (eds). *Cardiovascular Regulation*. London: Portland Press, 1995; pp. 15–35.

Denison DM. High altitudes and hypoxia. In: Edholm OG, Weiner JS (eds). *The Principles and Practice of Human Physiology*. London: Academic Press, 1981; pp. 241–305.

Ernsting J. Respiration and anoxia. In: Gillies JA (ed.). *A Textbook of Aviation Physiology*. Oxford: Pergamon Press, 1965; pp. 214–63.

Hainsworth R. Reflexes from the heart. *Physiological Reviews* 1991; **71**: 617–58.

Hainsworth R. Syncope and fainting: classification and pathophysiological basis. In: Mathias CJ, Bannister R (eds). *Autonomic Failure: A Textbook of Disorders of the Autonomic Nervous System*. Oxford: Oxford University Press,1999; pp. 428–36.

Hughes JMB, Pride NB. *Lung Function Tests*. London: W.B. Saunders, 1999.

Jones NL. *Clinical Exercise Testing*, 4th edn. Philadelphia, PA: W.B. Saunders, 1997.

Marshall JM. Cardiovascular changes associated with behavioural alerting. In: Jordan D, Marshall J (eds). *Cardiovascular Regulation*. London: Portland Press, 1995; pp. 37–59.

Marshall JM. The integrated response to hypoxia: from circulation to cells. *Experimental Physiology* 1999; **84**: 449–70.

West JB. *Ventilation/Blood Flow and Gas Exchange*, 5th edn. Oxford: Blackwell Scientific Publications, 1990.

3

Hypoxia and hyperventilation

DAVID P. GRADWELL

INTRODUCTION

Living organisms obtain energy for their biological processes by the oxidation of complex chemical foodstuffs to simpler compounds, usually with the eventual formation of carbon dioxide, water and other waste products. Oxygen therefore is one of the most important components required for the maintenance of continued normal function by living material. The absence of an adequate supply of oxygen to the tissues, whether in quantity or molecular concentration, is termed *hypoxia* (cf. *normoxia*, which means oxygen at normal physiological levels, and *anoxia*, which means the complete absence of oxygen). Humans are extremely sensitive and vulnerable to the effects of deprivation of oxygen, and severe hypoxia nearly always results in a rapid deterioration of most bodily functions; eventually, it will lead to death. *Hypoxaemia* is a general term meaning a deficiency in the oxygenation of the blood, but it is not synonymous with the term *tissue hypoxia*, which may arise from one or more causes.

Four different types of tissue hypoxia are recognized and may be classified according to the primary mechanism involved:

- *Hypoxic hypoxia:* the result of a reduction in the oxygen tension in the arterial blood and, hence, in the capillary blood. The aetiology includes the low oxygen tension of inspired gas associated with exposure to altitude, i.e. *hypobaric hypoxia*. Other causes are hypoventilatory states, e.g. paralysis of respiratory musculature, depression of central control of respiration, airway obstruction and pulmonary atelectasis (including that due to exposure to high sustained accelerations); impairment of gas exchange across the alveolar–capillary membrane, e.g. pulmonary oedema, pulmonary fibrosis; impairment of the circulation with right-to-left shunts, as may occur with congenital or acquired communications; and ventilation–perfusion mismatches, e.g. chronic bronchitis, emphysema.
- *Anaemic hypoxia:* the consequence of a reduction in the oxygen-carrying capacity of the blood. Although the arterial oxygen tension is normal, the amount of haemoglobin available to carry oxygen is reduced and, thus, the ability to deliver oxygen molecules to the tissues is compromised. The oxygen tension of the blood falls more rapidly than normal as it flows through the capillary beds and so, at their venous ends, is inadequate to maintain the required minimum level throughout the tissue involved. Causes of anaemic hypoxia include reduced erythrocyte count, e.g. haemorrhage, increased red cell destruction, decreased red cell production; reduced haemoglobin concentration, e.g. hypochromic anaemia; synthesis of abnormal haemoglobin, e.g. sickle-cell anaemia; reduced oxygen-binding capability, e.g. carbon monoxide inhalation; and chemical alteration of haemoglobin, e.g. methaemoglobinaemia.
- *Ischaemic (stagnant or circulatory) hypoxia:* the consequence of a reduction in blood flow through the tissues. Gas exchange in the lungs and the oxygen tension and content of the arterial blood are normal, but oxygen delivery to the tissues is inadequate. This, therefore, is an example of tissue hypoxia in the absence of arterial hypoxaemia. There is increased oxygen extraction and the oxygen tension falls to a low level in the venous ends of the capillaries. Causes include local arteriolar constriction, e.g. exposure of digits to cold; obstruction of arterial supply by disease

or trauma; general circulatory failure, e.g. cardiac failure, vasovagal syncope; and the fall in cardiac output and blood pressure associated with exposure to high sustained accelerations. Oxygen therapy is of little use in such forms of hypoxia.

- *Histotoxic hypoxia:* the result of an interference with the ability of the tissues to utilize a normal oxygen supply for oxidative processes. An example is cyanide poisoning, in which the action of cytochrome oxidase of the mitochondria is completely blocked, even in the presence of adequate molecular oxygen. Certain vitamin deficiencies, for example, beriberi resulting from inadequate intake of vitamin B1, will have the effect of compromising several stages in the utilization of oxygen by the tissues. Furthermore, oxygen toxicity, a condition in which an excessive tissue pressure of oxygen occurs, itself gives rise to a failure of oxidative metabolism.

Hypoxic hypoxia as a result of a reduction in the oxygen tension in inspired gas is by far the most common form of oxygen deficiency that occurs in aviation and is considered in detail in this chapter. However, other forms of hypoxia can and do occur in aviation, e.g. anaemic hypoxia produced by carbon monoxide poisoning, the ischaemic hypoxia produced by exposure to cold, and the circulatory shunting produced by sustained accelerations, which are described in subsequent chapters. It should be remembered that one or more forms of hypoxia may occur concurrently.

Oxygen therapy is of great value in certain types of hypoxia but of little or no benefit in others. For example, increasing the partial pressure of inspired oxygen can correct the inadequacies of oxygen deficiencies in hypobaric hypoxia (up to limits addressed in the following chapter) and in hypoventilatory states. In cases of impaired diffusion, oxygen therapy can increase the molecular oxygen content of the respired gas and reduce the degree of hypoxia. However, tissue hypoxia arising from anaemia, haemoglobinopathies, circulatory deficiencies (including right-to-left shunts) and histotoxic factors may be relieved only partially or even derive no benefit at all from supplemental oxygen. Thus, in aviation, consideration must be given to the potential interaction of various forms of hypoxia, and an awareness of the limitations of oxygen therapy is required.

Hyperventilation is a state in which the level of pulmonary ventilation is in excess of that required to remove from the body an amount of carbon dioxide equal to that produced by the tissues and hence maintain equilibrium. Such overbreathing is characterized by a reduction in the alveolar and arterial tensions of carbon dioxide, a condition termed *hypocapnia*. Thus, hyperventilation may be contrasted with the conditions that arise when an increase in respiration is proportional to an increase in carbon dioxide production during, for example, exercise. Moderate hypocapnia produces a significant impairment of the ability to perform psychomotor tasks, while an acute reduction in arterial carbon dioxide to about 15 mmHg frequently causes unconsciousness. Hypocapnia is a normal concomitant of hypoxia, and indeed the two conditions produce similar symptoms, although hyperventilation can, and perhaps more commonly does, occur in its own right under certain other conditions of the flight environment, such as exposure to low-frequency vibration, emotional stress and during positive-pressure breathing.

The remainder of this chapter is concerned with a more detailed consideration of the physiological and clinical consequences of hypobaric hypoxia and hyperventilation.

ACUTE HYPOBARIC HYPOXIA: HYPOXIA IN FLIGHT

Hypobaric hypoxia is generally recognized to be the most serious single physiological hazard during flight at altitude, because on ascent, as barometric pressure falls, breathing ambient air will result in a fall of the partial pressure, and thus the molecular content, of oxygen in the lung. Even the 25 per cent reduction in the partial pressure of oxygen in the atmosphere associated with ascent to an altitude of 8000 feet produces a detectable impairment in some aspects of mental performance, while sudden exposure to 50 000 feet as a consequence of rapid decompression, which reduces the partial pressure of oxygen within the lungs to ten per cent of its sea-level value, will cause unconsciousness within 12–15 seconds and death in four to six minutes. In the past, lack of oxygen took a regular toll of both lives and aircraft: many military air personnel were killed by hypoxia in flight, while the ability of many more to perform their duties was impaired by the condition. As a result, most military air personnel receive detailed training on this topic and the opportunity to gain personal experience of hypoxia under controlled conditions in hypobaric chambers. The world of civilian flying is not exempt from this hazard, although the aircrew involved may not necessarily have had the same degree of personal experience of hypoxia in training. Tragic incidents have occurred in which the occupants of civilian aircraft have perished as a result of hypoxia at high altitudes. In one recent study of fatal general aviation accidents, in-flight hypoxia was reported to be the cause of impairment or incapacitation in more than four per cent of cases. Therefore, notwithstanding that improvements in the performance and reliability of cabin pressurization and oxygen-delivery systems have greatly reduced incidents and accidents due to hypoxia, they do still occur and constant awareness and vigilance throughout the aviation community remains essential.

Aetiology

The principal causes of hypoxia in flight are:

- ascent to altitude without supplementary oxygen
- failure of personal breathing equipment to supply oxygen at an adequate concentration and/or pressure
- decompression of the pressure cabin at high altitude.

The relative incidence of the various causes of hypoxia in flight over a 14-year period in a large military air force is presented in Table 3.1. Failure of oxygen regulators and decompression of aircraft cabins together account for more than half of the total reported incidents in this series. A further study conducted in a rather smaller air force revealed that 63 per cent of cases of hypoxia in flight in its aircraft arose from a failure of either the mask or the regulator.

The physiological consequences of hypoxia in flight can be considered in three main areas: the respiratory and cardiovascular responses to the insult, and the neurological effects of the insult itself and of the responses to it. The clinical consequences can be expected to be the result of the combination of changes in all these areas.

Respiratory responses to acute hypobaric hypoxia

The time course of the physiological changes produced by breathing air at altitude is a function of the manner in which the condition is induced. Thus, the changes usually are produced slowly by ascent at the common rate for an aircraft of 2000–3000 feet/min; more abruptly by the reversion to breathing air after failure of oxygen delivery

Table 3.1 *Relative incidence of the causes of 397 cases of hypoxia in flight in a military airforce*

Cause of hypoxia	Relative incidence (%)
Failure of oxygen supply:	
Line failure	2
Low/depleted	1
Failure of oxygen regulator	25
Regulator off	1
Inadvertent break of connection in hose between regulator and mask	9
Hose defect or failure	1
Inadequate seal of mask to face	7
Malfunction of mask valves	3
Decompression of pressure cabin	32
Toxic fumes giving rise to hypoxia	2
Other	17

NB: the demand oxygen regulators used in this air force delivered safety pressure only at altitudes over 28 000 feet.

equipment; and fastest following rapid decompression. Although breathing air during a routine steady ascent is now an uncommon cause of hypoxia in professional aircrew, it does occur in leisure flying, e.g. in people flying light aircraft, gliders and balloons, and it is convenient to begin by describing the respiratory changes induced by hypoxia produced in this manner.

ALVEOLAR GASES WHEN BREATHING AIR

The fall in partial pressure of oxygen in the inspired gas that occurs on ascent to altitude causes a progressive reduction in alveolar oxygen tension. The main determinant of the difference in oxygen tension between inspired gas and alveolar gas is the alveolar carbon dioxide tension. That this is so can be demonstrated by rearranging the alveolar air equation thus:

$$P_{I_{O_2}} - P_{A_{O_2}} = P_{A_{CO_2}} \times \left\{ F_{I_{O_2}} + \left[\frac{(1 - F_{I_{O_2}})}{R} \right] \right\}$$

where $P_{I_{O_2}}$ is the inspired (tracheal) oxygen tension, $P_{A_{O_2}}$ is the alveolar oxygen tension, $P_{A_{CO_2}}$ is the alveolar carbon dioxide tension, $F_{I_{O_2}}$ is the fractional concentration of oxygen in the (dry) inspired gas, and R is the respiratory exchange ratio.

A fall in alveolar carbon dioxide tension will reduce the difference between the oxygen tensions in the inspired and alveolar gases. But, as explained in Chapter 2, the tension of carbon dioxide in the alveolar gas is itself determined by the ratio of carbon dioxide production to alveolar ventilation, and this ratio is independent of environmental pressure. Accordingly, therefore, alveolar carbon dioxide tension remains constant on ascent to altitude, provided that the ratio of carbon dioxide production to alveolar ventilation is unchanged. In practice, however, on acute exposure to altitude, alveolar carbon dioxide tension remains constant only between sea level and an altitude of 8000–10 000 feet. Above this altitude, arterial oxygen tension falls to a level that stimulates respiration, and so alveolar carbon dioxide tension is reduced by virtue of increased alveolar ventilation. Thus, alveolar oxygen tension falls linearly with the decline in environmental pressure associated with an ascent from sea level to about 10 000 feet, but above this altitude the reduction in alveolar oxygen tension is less than would occur if there was no increase in ventilation and no consequent fall in alveolar carbon dioxide tension. The changes in alveolar gas tensions associated with ascent to altitude when breathing air are shown graphically in Figure 3.1.

The increase in pulmonary ventilation produced by exposure to an altitude above 8000–10 000 feet may be regarded as the resultant of two conflicting factors, i.e. the lowered arterial oxygen tension stimulates ventilation

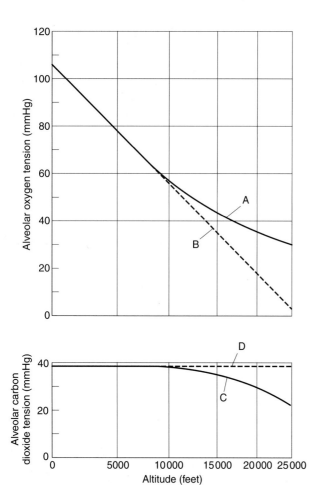

Figure 3.1 *Effect of acute exposure to various altitudes, while breathing air, on the alveolar tensions of oxygen (curve A) and carbon dioxide (curve C). The curves describe the mean values for a group of 30 subjects seated at rest. The broken lines indicate the values of alveolar tensions of oxygen (curve B) and carbon dioxide (curve D) that would be obtained if the hypoxia induced by ascent to altitude did not increase pulmonary ventilation.*

through its effect on the chemoreceptors of the carotid and aortic bodies, but the increase in ventilation is itself opposed by the respiratory depressant effect of the concomitant reduction in carbon dioxide tension. The compromise struck between these two competing influences is essentially that of the demand for an adequate oxygen supply versus the need to maintain a normal acid–base balance. The magnitude of the increase in ventilation, and hence the fall in alveolar carbon dioxide tension, exhibits considerable individual variation. During acute exposures of subjects at rest, pulmonary ventilation at 18 000 feet is 20–50 per cent greater than that observed at sea level, while at 22 000 feet it is 40–60 per cent greater.

The effect of altitude on the ventilatory response to mild and moderate exercise is a similar but slightly greater pro-portional increase in pulmonary ventilation, and such an effect can be demonstrated at altitudes as low as 3000 feet. The increase in pulmonary ventilation induced by exercise in moderate hypoxia is, however, such that alveolar carbon dioxide tension is reduced below that produced by breathing air at rest at the same altitude. There is, therefore, a corresponding rise in alveolar oxygen tension, perhaps by 3–5 mmHg.

The increase in pulmonary ventilation and cardiac output stimulated by the hypoxia arising from breathing air at altitudes of up to about 20 000 feet produces a small, almost insignificant, increase in the total oxygen consumption of the tissues and in the carbon dioxide production by them. The fall in alveolar carbon dioxide tension produced by the disproportionate rise in pulmonary ventilation, however, liberates carbon dioxide from the very substantial body stores of the gas, such that for a while the output of carbon dioxide in the expired gas actually exceeds its metabolic production by the tissues. Thus, the respiratory exchange ratio (R) is raised at the beginning of an exposure to altitude when breathing air. It returns slowly to the previous resting value as the excess carbon dioxide is removed from body stores and a steady state is regained. For example, R is raised to just over 1 on acute exposure to air at 18 000 feet, and its normal resting value of 0.85 is not regained for 30–40 minutes. Clearly, a raised value of R will produce a higher alveolar oxygen tension for a given inspired oxygen tension and alveolar carbon dioxide tension than would otherwise be the case; therefore, in the example given, with an alveolar carbon dioxide tension of 28 mmHg, alveolar oxygen tension will fall from about 41 mmHg at the beginning of the exposure to about 37 mmHg at the end.

The relationship between the alveolar tensions of oxygen and carbon dioxide therefore changes progressively throughout an exposure to a given altitude, since the alveolar oxygen tension is determined by the level of alveolar carbon dioxide and the value of R, both of which are themselves functions of the intensity of the ventilatory response to hypoxia and of the duration of exposure. The relationship between alveolar oxygen tensions and increasing altitude, with a period of 10–20 minutes spent at each, is shown graphically in Figure 3.1. The same data are presented numerically in Table 3.2, where the considerable individual variability is indicated by the values of standard deviations. In general, the alveolar oxygen tension is reduced in short-duration exposures to 45 mmHg at 15 000 feet, to 40 mmHg at 18 000 feet, to 35 mmHg at 21 000 feet and to 30 mmHg at 25 000 feet.

ALVEOLAR GASES WHEN BREATHING OXYGEN

When 100 per cent oxygen has been breathed for several hours, so that virtually all the nitrogen has been washed out of the body tissues and alveolar gas, the relationship

Table 3.2 *Mean values for alveolar gas tensions in 30 seated resting subjects after acute (10–20 minutes) exposure to breathing air at altitude*

Altitude (feet)	Inspired oxygen tension (mmHg)	Alveolar tension of oxygen (mmHg)		Alveolar tension of carbon dioxide (mmHg)	
		Mean	SD	Mean	SD
0	148	103.0	5.5	39.0	2.5
8000	108	64.0	5.0	38.5	2.6
15 000	80	44.7	5.0	30.5	2.7
18 000	69	39.5	4.2	28.0	2.5
20 000	63	36.5	4.0	26.5	2.5
22 000	57	33.2	3.0	25.0	2.6
25 000*	49	30.0		22.0	

* After 3–5 min exposure

SD, standard deviation.

between the alveolar tensions of oxygen and carbon dioxide and the environmental pressure simplifies to

$$PA_{O_2} = (P_B - P_{H_2O}) - PA_{CO_2}$$

where PA_{O_2} is the alveolar oxygen tension, P_B is the environmental pressure, P_{H_2O} is the water vapour tension at 37 °C (i.e. 47 mmHg), and PA_{CO_2} is the alveolar carbon dioxide tension.

Generally in aviation, however, the time for which 100 per cent oxygen is breathed is less than two hours, and the alveolar gas still contains a small amount of nitrogen, sufficient to exert a tension of 3–5 mmHg. Thus, in practice, the alveolar oxygen tension when breathing 100 per cent oxygen is usually some 3–5 mmHg less than that predicted by the equation, but provided that the alveolar carbon dioxide tension remains constant, alveolar oxygen tension will fall linearly with environmental pressure (as it does up to 10 000 feet when breathing air). When breathing 100 per cent oxygen, however, it is not until an altitude of 33 000–33 700 feet is reached that the alveolar partial pressure of oxygen falls to 103 mmHg, i.e. to the value observed when breathing air at sea level. When an altitude of about 39 000 feet is reached, breathing 100 per cent oxygen, the alveolar oxygen tension falls to 60–65 mmHg, i.e. to a similar value to that reached at 10 000 feet breathing air. Above 39 000 feet, the further fall in alveolar oxygen tension stimulates respiration, even though 100 per cent oxygen is being breathed, just as it does above 10 000 feet when breathing air. The alveolar oxygen tension rises by 1 mmHg for every 1 mmHg reduction in alveolar carbon dioxide tension. Thus, for example, the alveolar carbon dioxide tension at 43 000 feet is about 30 mmHg and the corresponding alveolar oxygen tension is 43–45 mmHg. Figure 3.2 is a graphical representation of the changes in alveolar gas tensions with altitude when breathing 100 per cent oxygen and should be compared with Figure 3.1.

The concept of physiologically equivalent altitudes for a person breathing air or 100 per cent oxygen is of consider-

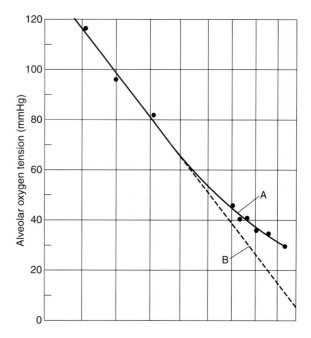
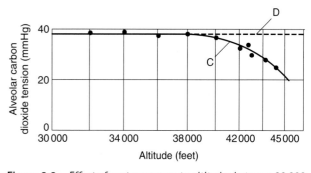

Figure 3.2 *Effect of acute exposure to altitudes between 30 000 and 45 000 feet while breathing 100 per cent oxygen on the alveolar tensions of oxygen (curve A) and carbon dioxide (curve C). The broken lines indicate the values of alveolar tensions of oxygen (curve B) and carbon dioxide (curve D) that would have occurred in the absence of any increase in pulmonary ventilation.*

able value in the design of protective equipment. However, although equivalent altitudes may be stated in terms of equality of alveolar oxygen tension, a strict interpretation of the alveolar equivalence would require steady-state conditions, the determination of the carbon dioxide tensions in both cases, and knowledge of the value of the respiratory exchange ratio. For most practical purposes, therefore, it is more satisfactory to determine equivalence on the basis of equality of inspired (tracheal) oxygen tension. Figure 3.3 describes the relationship of equivalent altitudes for both inspired gas and alveolar gas. As a simple example, the effect of the 5000-feet increase in altitude from 40 000 to 45 000 feet when breathing 100 per cent oxygen is equivalent to a 9000-feet increase in altitude from 11 000 to 20 000 feet when breathing air.

Finally, when considering the alveolar gases when breathing oxygen, it is important to consider the situation that can occur in practice as a result of a change from breathing oxygen to breathing air at altitude, such as may occur as a result of a regulator failure or disconnection of an oxygen supply hose. In such circumstances, the composition of the inspired gas changes from that containing a high concentration of oxygen to air, and the alveolar oxygen tension falls progressively as the concentration of nitrogen in the inspired and alveolar gases rises to 79–80 per cent. During the early part of this process, the oxygen tension of the inspired gas is frequently less than that of the blood returning to the alveoli, and so oxygen will pass out of the body from the returning mixed venous blood into the alveolar gas and hence into the expirate. The rate at which alveolar oxygen tension falls in these circumstances is proportional to the alveolar ventilation, but a new steady state is usually attained in the resting subject two to three minutes after the reduction in concentration of oxygen in the inspired gas.

ALVEOLAR GASES DURING RAPID DECOMPRESSION

The use of cabin-pressurization systems for aircraft flying at medium and high altitudes brings with it the possibility that the aircraft occupants could be exposed to the risks of rapid decompression should a failure occur in the structural integrity of the pressure cabin or in the pressurization system (see also Chapter 6). The sudden fall in environmental pressure that accompanies a decompression produces almost as rapid a fall in the tensions of the constituents of alveolar gas. Thus, such an emergency can produce a very profound fall in alveolar oxygen tension, the magnitude of which will depend on the gas being breathed at the moment of decompression and the ratio of the environmental pressures at the beginning and end of the event. For example, a rapid decompression from 8000 to 40 000 feet in 1.6 seconds while breathing air will cause the alveolar oxygen tension to fall from 65 mmHg to about 15 mmHg. Furthermore, since the inspired (tracheal) oxygen tension at that final altitude is only about 20 mmHg, the alveolar oxygen tension will remain below about 18 mmHg for as long as air is breathed. Under these conditions, the oxygen tension in the pulmonary capillary blood is considerably higher than that in the alveolar gas and so, as described above, oxygen passes into the alveoli from the mixed venous blood as it flows through the pulmonary capillaries. The change in alveolar tension during rapid decompression is illustrated in Figure 3.4.

Alveolar carbon dioxide tension also falls during such a decompression, since venting of the expanded alveolar gases removes carbon dioxide more quickly than it can be replaced and may reach a value of only 10 mmHg. This then partially recovers to a level of 25–30 mmHg over the ensuing 30 seconds as carbon dioxide passes rapidly from pulmonary capillary blood into the alveolar gas. The inspiration of 100 per cent oxygen during or a short time after rapid decompression will modify the changes described by causing an immediate rise in alveolar oxygen tension (Figure 3.4). The rise is rapid at first but then slows to reach a value, in this example, of about 60 mmHg some 30–40 seconds after oxygen breathing commences. Clearly, the

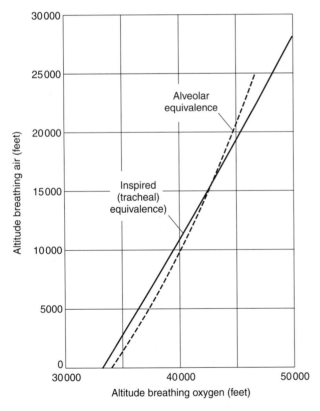

Figure 3.3 *Equivalent altitudes when breathing air and when breathing 100 per cent oxygen. The solid curve indicates equivalence based on equal tensions of oxygen in the inspired (tracheal) gas, i.e. inspired gas saturated with water vapour at 37 °C. The broken curve indicates equivalence based on equal tensions of oxygen in the alveolar gas during acute exposures of seated resting subjects for 10–15 minutes.*

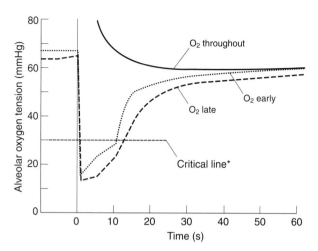

Figure 3.4 *Mean alveolar oxygen tensions of four subjects before and after rapid decompression at time 0 from 8000 feet to 40 000 feet in 1.6 seconds. Each subject was decompressed on three occasions: once breathing air before and after the decompression with 100 per cent oxygen delivered to the facemask eight seconds after time 0 (O_2 late: - - - - - - - - -), once breathing air before and after the decompression with 100 per cent oxygen delivered to the facemask two seconds after time 0 (O_2 early: ·····················), and once breathing 100 per cent oxygen throughout (O_2 throughout: ————). *Note that if the area described by the alveolar oxygen tension curve below the critical line exceeds 140 mmHg/s, then consciousness will almost certainly be lost.*

higher the final altitude and the longer the delay in administering 100 per cent oxygen, the greater will be the degree of hypoxia. The composition of the gas being breathed immediately before rapid decompression will also influence the severity of hypoxia suffered: a high alveolar oxygen tension in the inspired gas before decompression will minimize the fall in tension seen during and after decompression. Thus, for example, when 100 per cent oxygen is breathed before, during and after a rapid decompression from 8000 to 40 000 feet, alveolar oxygen tension does not fall below about 60 mmHg at any time (Figure 3.4).

The brief but profound hypoxia associated with rapid decompression has its most marked effects on the central nervous system (see below), specifically the psychomotor performance of the subject. In order to avoid the potentially catastrophic consequences of hypoxia induced by rapid decompression to a high altitude, alveolar oxygen tension must not fall below 30 mmHg. Such a fall is an inevitable consequence of a rapid decompression to a final altitude greater than 30 000 feet when breathing air, even if 100 per cent oxygen is delivered to the respiratory tract at the moment decompression occurs. The intensity of the hypoxic insult will be correspondingly greater with a higher final altitude and if delivery of 100 per cent oxygen

is delayed. These extremely rapid physiological changes have very important implications for the design of personal oxygen equipment for use at high altitudes, since they indicate that in order to avoid severe neurological disturbances after a rapid decompression, an oxygen-enriched breathing gas must be being breathed before the decompression. Indeed, the concentrations of oxygen required in the breathing gas before a rapid decompression in order to maintain an alveolar oxygen tension above 30 mmHg immediately after it and where the final altitudes are 35 000, 40 000 and 44 000 feet are 30, 40 and 60 per cent, respectively. Even then, in order to prevent significant features of hypoxia developing, 100 per cent oxygen must be delivered within two seconds of the start of rapid decompression, and therefore functional dead space in the system must be kept to a minimum to avoid delay in the delivery of oxygen to the respiratory tract.

ARTERIAL BLOOD GASES

Although the difference between the oxygen tension of the alveolar gas and that of the blood entering the pulmonary capillaries (i.e. mixed venous blood) is markedly reduced on exposure to altitude, the diffusion characteristics of the alveolar–capillary membrane are such that the tension of oxygen leaving the pulmonary capillaries still equals that of the alveolar gas when the individual is at rest. Thus, even in moderate hypoxia, the arterial oxygen tension may be only 8 mmHg less than the alveolar oxygen tension, while the carbon dioxide tension of alveolar gas is virtually equal to that of arterial blood. Typical values for the arterial blood gases of resting subjects, breathing air at various altitudes up to 20 000 feet and 100 per cent oxygen up to 45 000 feet, are presented in Table 3.3. It should be noted, however, that there are large variations in the tensions of arterial blood gases in acute hypoxia, both with time in the same individual and between individuals. For example, the oxygen saturations of the arterial blood in six resting subjects breathing air at 18 000 feet varied from 65 to 78 per cent. These large variations reflect the sensitivity of alveolar oxygen tension, and therefore arterial oxygen tension, to the level of alveolar ventilation.

The reduced transit time of blood in the pulmonary capillaries during exercise, however, results in a failure of the oxygen tension in the blood to reach equilibrium with that of the alveolar gas. The alveolar–arterial oxygen tension gradient therefore is increased by exercise in moderate hypoxia from its resting value of about 8 mmHg to 16–20 mmHg. In addition, although exercising while hypoxic does produce a small increase in alveolar oxygen tension by virtue of the alveolar hyperventilation, the large rise in the alveolar–arterial oxygen tension difference results in an overall fall in arterial oxygen tension and saturation. Thus, the symptoms and signs of hypoxia will be exacerbated by exercise.

Table 3.3 *Typical values for arterial blood gases of resting subjects acutely exposed to altitude*

Altitude (feet)	Arterial blood gases			
	Oxygen tension (mmHg)	Carbon dioxide tension (mmHg)	Oxygen concentration (mL (STPD)/100 mL blood)	Oxygen saturation of haemoglobin (%)
Breathing air				
0	95	40	20.5	97
8000	56	38	18.8	93
12 000	43	35	16.9	84
15 000	37	30	15.7	78
18 000	32	28	14.5	72
20 000	29	26	13.2	66
Breathing 100% oxygen				
33 000	95	40	20.5	97
40 000	45	38	16.9	84
43 000	36	30	15.4	76

STPD, standard temperature and pressure, dry.

Cardiovascular responses to acute hypobaric hypoxia

BLOOD FLOW

As described in Chapter 2, the rate of blood flow through a tissue bed is a cardinal determinant of the tension at which oxygen is delivered to its cells. The reverse is also the case, however, and the hypoxia produced by a reduction in oxygen tension of the inspired gas will induce both general and regional changes in the circulation. On occasion, vasovagal syncope may also complicate the picture.

GENERAL CARDIOVASCULAR CHANGES

In the resting subject, heart rate increases immediately when breathing air above 6000–8000 feet. At 15 000 feet, the increase is about 10–15 per cent above the sea-level value; it rises to a 20–25 per cent increase at 20 000 feet, and the heart rate is approximately doubled at 25 000 feet. Since stroke volume remains essentially unchanged as the heart rate increases, there is a proportional increase in cardiac output. Both heart rate and cardiac output are also elevated proportionally during exercise at altitude, although the maximum levels of each (which are the same in moderate hypoxia as when breathing air at sea level) are, however, attained at a lower degree of work under hypoxic conditions. At altitude, the maximum oxygen uptake is limited by the cardiac output and the reduced arterial oxygen saturation so that, for example, when breathing air at 15 000 feet, maximum oxygen uptake during exercise falls to about 70 per cent of the sea-level value.

Despite the increase in cardiac output, mean arterial blood pressure during moderate hypoxia usually is unchanged from that of an individual breathing air at sea level. However, the systolic pressure usually is raised, and there is an overall reduction in peripheral resistance, with a resulting increase in the pulse pressure. There is a redistribution of blood flow by local and vasomotor mechanisms. Although hypoxia causes vasodilation in most vascular beds, there are some important features of, and differences in, the responses of certain regional circulations.

REGIONAL CARDIOVASCULAR CHANGES

Acute hypoxia causes immediate increases in blood flow through the coronary and cerebral circulations, but renal blood flow is markedly reduced. Blood flow through skeletal muscle may increase by 30–100 per cent. Thus, there is a redistribution of cardiac output, with flow to essential organs such as the heart and brain increased at the expense of other less acutely essential organs, such as the viscera, skin and kidneys.

Flow through the coronary circulation increases in parallel with the rise in cardiac output, in response to the metabolic requirements of the myocardium. The increase in blood flow through the coronary vessels is such that a subject breathing air at 25 000 feet exhibits no electrocardiographic (ECG) evidence of cardiac hypoxia, even up to the point at which consciousness is lost. Cardiac reserve is reduced, however, and a profound fall in arterial oxygen tension will cause myocardial depression. In severe hypoxia, myocardial depression is reflected in the electrocardiograph by a depressed S–T segment and a reduction in the height of the T wave. Later, disorders of rhythm and conduction supervene. Occasionally, in such circumstances, there is a severe compensatory vasoconstriction of the coronary vessels that swamps all other reflex responses and causes cardiac arrest.

The response of the cerebral circulation to hypoxic hypoxia is also of considerable importance, since, not surprisingly, the changes in arterial oxygen and carbon dioxide tensions associated with that condition have profound effects. Thus, at arterial oxygen tensions above 45–50 mmHg, cerebral blood flow is determined exclusively by the arterial carbon dioxide tension to which it bears a directly linear relationship over the normal (tolerable) physiological range of 20–50 mmHg. For example, a reduction in arterial carbon dioxide tension from the normal 40 mmHg to 20 mmHg will halve cerebral blood flow. A fall in arterial oxygen tension below about 45 mmHg, however, will induce hypoxic vasodilation, so that, for example, an arterial oxygen tension of 35–40 mmHg causes a 50–100 per cent increase in blood flow through the brain. A balance therefore exists between the vasodilating effect of hypoxia on the cerebral vessels and the vasoconstricting influence of a declining arterial carbon dioxide tension caused by the hypoxic drive to ventilation. Generally, the conflict results in a reduction in cerebral blood flow when breathing air at altitudes up to about 15 000 feet, but results in an increase, modified by the degree of coexisting hypocapnia, above 16 000–18 000 feet.

Hypoxia of a degree sufficient to desaturate the blood by about 20 per cent causes a rapid reversible vasoconstriction in the pulmonary circulation, probably as a consequence of the direct action of oxygen on chemoreceptor cells in the walls of the pulmonary blood vessels. The vasoconstriction of parts of pulmonary vasculature may be the means by which local blood flow is matched to local ventilation. On acute ascent to altitude the entire pulmonary vascular bed constricts, however, which, in the presence of a raised cardiac output, increases pulmonary arterial blood pressure.

SYNCOPE

Heart rate, arterial blood pressure and cerebral blood flow are usually maintained at or above their resting values when unconsciousness occurs as the result of a gross lowering of alveolar oxygen tension (see below). In about 20 per cent of individuals, however, the immediate cause of unconsciousness in hypoxia is failure of cerebral blood flow subsequent to a precipitate fall in arterial blood pressure associated with a marked bradycardia. The mechanism underlying the fall in arterial blood pressure in this form of faint is the same as for other types of vasovagal syncope, i.e. loss of peripheral resistance in the systemic circulation brought about by profound dilation of arterioles in muscle vascular beds. Syncope is accompanied by pallor, sweating, nausea and, occasionally, vomiting.

TISSUE OXYGEN TENSION

The minimum acceptable oxygen tension in a tissue depends critically on the oxygen tension in the blood flowing through its capillaries. The major factor minimizing the fall of oxygen tension towards the venous ends of capillaries in the presence of hypoxic hypoxia is the relationship, reflected in the sigmoid shape of the oxygen dissociation curve, between oxygen tension and the saturation of haemoglobin with oxygen. A typical oxygen dissociation curve is shown in Figure 3.5.

Figure 3.5 shows that when air is breathed at sea level, producing an arterial oxygen tension of about 95 mmHg, the extraction of 5 ml of oxygen from every 100 ml of blood flowing through the tissues results in a venous oxygen tension of about 40 mmHg, i.e. a fall of 55 mmHg. The extraction of the same quantity of oxygen per unit volume of blood when the arterial oxygen tension is reduced to 32 mmHg by breathing air at 18 000 feet decreases the oxygen tension of the venous blood to 22 mmHg; thus, the fall in oxygen tension as the blood flows through the tissues is

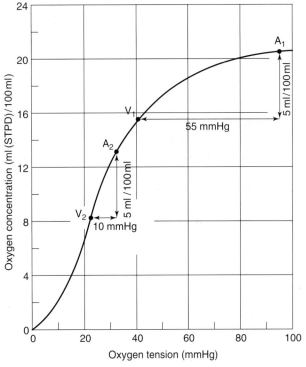

Figure 3.5 *Oxygen dissociation curve of whole blood (at a pH of 7.4 and a temperature of 37 °C), illustrating the effect of the sigmoid shape of the relationship on the fall in oxygen tension of the blood produced by the extraction of 5 ml of oxygen per 100 ml of blood by the tissues, as blood flows through them at two different levels of arterial oxygen tension. At an arterial oxygen tension of 95 mmHg (point A_1), then the extraction of 5 ml of oxygen per 100 ml of blood reduces the oxygen tension to 40 mmHg (point V_1), i.e. the fall in oxygen tension from arterial to venous blood is 55 mmHg. In moderate hypoxia, with an arterial oxygen tension of 32 mmHg (point A_2), then the extraction of the same amount of oxygen reduces the oxygen tension to 22 mmHg (point V_2), i.e. the fall in oxygen tension from arterial to venous blood is only 10 mmHg. STPD, standard temperature and pressure, dry.*

reduced to only 10 mmHg. This most important protective effect of the manner in which oxygen combines with haemoglobin results in a halving of the arteriovenous oxygen tension difference when the arterial oxygen tension is reduced from 95 to 65 mmHg, and to a reduction to a quarter when the arterial oxygen tension is 40 mmHg. Although the overall increase in cardiac output produced by acute hypoxia reduces still further the fall in arteriovenous oxygen tension difference, this effect is of much less importance than that associated with the oxygen dissociation curve. For example, the 20 per cent increase in cardiac output induced by breathing air at 18 000 feet, where the arterial oxygen tension is 32 mmHg, will raise the oxygen tension in mixed venous blood from 22 mmHg to only 24 mmHg.

Regional changes in blood flow, and especially the changes in the cerebral circulation described above, also are of importance. The marked reduction in cerebral blood flow, produced by the hypocapnia associated with the mild hypoxia induced by breathing air at 12 000 feet, can result in an appreciable further lowering of the jugular venous oxygen tension. In the more severe hypoxia associated with breathing air at 18 000 feet, the increased arteriovenous oxygen tension difference produced by hypocapnia is more than offset by the concomitant increase in alveolar and arterial oxygen tensions produced by the hyperventilation.

The combined effects of acute hypobaric hypoxia and the associated hypocapnia arising from the hypoxic drive to ventilation, induced by a reduction in the oxygen tension of inspired gas, are summarized in the gradients of oxygen tension from the dry atmosphere to the lowest tension in the tissues. Figure 3.6 illustrates oxygen tension gradients for a person breathing air at sea level and at 18 000 feet. The figure shows three oxygen tension gradients at 18 000 feet: the gradient for the body as a whole (assuming that all tissues are uniform), and two gradients for oxygen transport to the brain with mild and severe hypocapnia (alveolar carbon dioxide tensions of 35 and 20 mmHg, respectively) that would result from different degrees of increased alveolar ventilation. The curves illustrate the effect of hyperventilation on the fall in oxygen tension between inspired and alveolar gases, and the marked reduction in the fall in oxygen tension along the capillaries in hypoxia due primarily to the relationship demonstrated by the shape of the oxygen dissociation curve. The net effect in this example is that in the face of a reduction of 79 mmHg in the oxygen tension of the inspired gas, the oxygen tension of mixed venous blood is reduced by only 16 mmHg when air is breathed at 18 000 feet. The estimated minimum oxygen tension, on the simplifying assumption that the body is a single uniform tissue, is reduced only from 20 to 10 mmHg. In the absence of hyperventilation at 18 000 feet, however, the minimum oxygen tension in the brain falls to almost zero, and some decline in oxidative phosphorylation would be expected under these conditions.

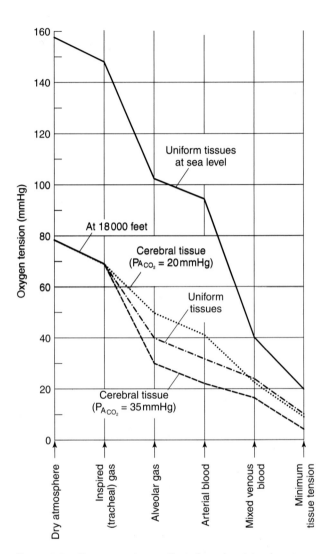

Figure 3.6 *Oxygen tension gradients from dry atmosphere to minimum tissue level in an individual breathing air at sea level and at 18 000 feet (—·—·—), assuming that body tissues are uniform and that the alveolar carbon dioxide tension is 40 mmHg at sea level and 30 mmHg at 18 000 feet. The gradients for cerebral tissue in an individual breathing air at 18 000 feet with an alveolar carbon dioxide tension of 20 mmHg (············) and 35 mmHg (-------) are also shown (see text).*

CYANOSIS

Cyanosis is a sign of clinical hypoxia and manifests itself as a bluish colouration of the skin, nail beds and mucous membranes. It is caused by the presence of an increased concentration of reduced haemoglobin in the capillaries and venules of the hypoxic tissues and is a reflection of the profound desaturation of haemoglobin at low tissue oxygen tensions. Broadly, the degree of colouration in an individual is proportional to the desaturation of the blood. There must be at least 5 g of reduced haemoglobin per 100 ml of capillary blood before cyanosis can be detected reliably, and thus it is an unreliable sign of hypoxia in the presence of significant anaemia. Conversely, an individual with polycythaemia may show signs of cyanosis in normoxia. Thus, although cyanosis is a useful sign of hypoxia, it must be treated with caution, and the central cyanosis of hypoxic hypoxia can be detected reliably only if the oxygen saturation of the arterial blood is less than 75 per cent. Normal subjects breathing air are noticeably cyanotic at altitudes above 17 000–19 000 feet.

Neurological effects of acute hypobaric hypoxia

IMPAIRMENT OF MENTAL PERFORMANCE

The impairment of psychological performance produced by lack of oxygen at altitude is of great practical significance in aviation, although there is great variability within and between individuals exposed to hypobaric hypoxia. Much of this variation is the result of differences in the respiratory response to hypoxia, with consequently very significant temporal and individual differences in the tensions of oxygen and carbon dioxide in the arterial blood when exposed to a given level of inspired oxygen tension. The hypocapnia induced by the low arterial oxygen tension affects mental performance by reducing still further cerebral tissue oxygen tension, as a consequence of the cerebral vasoconstriction it produces, and by increasing the pH of cerebral tissue.

PSYCHOMOTOR TASKS

Performance of well-learned and practised tasks generally is preserved adequately up to an altitude of at least 10 000 feet, but when alveolar oxygen falls to below 38–40 mmHg (i.e. above an altitude of 16 000–18 000 feet), simple reaction time begins to be affected, although even a reduction of the alveolar oxygen tension to 35 mmHg increases the simple reaction time by only 50 per cent on average. Performance at pursuit-meter tasks is unaffected until the altitude exceeds 12 000–14 000 feet, although the decrement of performance at this type of task does not become severe until altitudes of 16 000–17 000 feet are exceeded. More demanding tasks such as a choice-reaction time are affected, however, by much less severe degrees of hypoxia; for example, performance at such a test is usually impaired significantly at 12 000 feet. However, tasks requiring complex eye–hand coordination such as instrument flying that have been well-learned in a flight simulator before the exposure usually are unaffected until the alveolar oxygen tension is reduced below 55 mmHg (i.e. until air is breathed at altitudes above 10 000 feet). If the alveolar oxygen tension falls to less than 50 mmHg (i.e. breathing air at 12 000 ft), then there is an approximate ten per cent decrement in the ability to maintain a given air

speed, heading or vertical velocity. This decrement rises to 20–30 per cent at alveolar oxygen tensions of 40–45 mmHg (15 000 feet).

Psychomotor performance is compromised further by the impairment of muscular coordination produced by moderate and severe hypoxia. Above 15 000 feet, for example, a fine tremor of the hand develops, so the ability to hold a stylus or control lever in a fixed position in space is progressively impaired. Muscular incoordination becomes greater with increasing altitude, and the subject's writing becomes difficult to read.

COGNITIVE TASKS

Performance of previously learned coding and conceptual reasoning tasks is unaffected at altitudes up to about 10 000 feet, i.e. for as long as the alveolar oxygen tension remains greater than 55 mmHg. At alveolar tensions less than this, however, performance declines, initially slowly but then with increasing rapidity with increasing altitude. Thus, the time taken to complete a simple coding task is increased by 10–15 per cent at 15 000 feet and by 40–50 per cent at 18 000 feet. The decline in performance at conceptual reasoning tasks is even greater, although the altitude at which impairment of mental ability commences, and the severity of the decrement, varies with the difficulty and complexity of the task.

Short-term and long-term memory, as tested by paired-word association, and immediate and delayed recall of patterns and positions, are affected significantly when the alveolar oxygen tension is reduced to about 60 mmHg (breathing air at 8000–10 000 feet). Memory scores may be 25 per cent lower than at sea level at an altitude of 15 000 feet.

An individual breathing air at 8000 feet may take significantly longer to achieve optimum performance at novel tasks than is the case at sea level. For example, this degree of hypoxia has been found to double the reaction times of initial responses to a complex choice-reaction task as compared with responses at sea level. The intensity of this effect increases with altitude and complexity of the task – markedly so above 12 000 feet – and, indeed, the threshold for the detrimental effect of hypoxia on performance remains the subject of debate. Although it is recognized that there is very considerable individual variation in the threshold of effect, a number of studies have concluded that such changes can be demonstrated at altitudes as low as 5000–6000 feet.

The mechanisms responsible for the cerebral effects of mild hypoxia are not understood, although it is likely that retardation of some oxygenation processes within the brain, leading to disruption of neurotransmitter formation and decay, is involved rather than a failure of oxidative phosphorylation (see Chapter 2). This is because the oxygen tension of cerebral venous blood falls by only

2–4 mmHg on ascent from sea level to 8000 feet, and such a slight fall is unlikely to be responsible for the effects seen.

IMPAIRMENT OF THE SPECIAL SENSES

A subjective darkening of the visual field is a common symptom of hypoxia, although the individual may become aware of this only after the normal alveolar oxygen tension has been restored, when there is a marked apparent increase in the level of illumination. Even very mild hypoxia, such as that produced by lowering the alveolar oxygen tension to 75 mmHg (i.e. equivalent to breathing air at 5000 feet), can be shown in the laboratory to impair the light sensitivity of the dark-adapted eye (scotopic or rod vision). The degree of reduction in light sensitivity of scotopic vision becomes significant when the alveolar oxygen tension falls below about 50 mmHg (i.e. when air is breathed at altitudes above 12 000 feet). Retinal sensitivity in relatively bright light (photopic or cone vision) is un-affected by hypoxia until the alveolar oxygen tension is reduced below 40 mmHg. The influence of mild to moderate hypoxia on vision in the intermediate, mesopic, range between scotopic and photopic ranges is the subject of specific ongoing investigations. Finally, moderate and severe hypoxia cause restriction of the visual field, with loss of peripheral vision ('tunnelling') and the development of a central scotoma.

Auditory acuity is also reduced by moderate and severe hypoxia, but some hearing is usually retained, even after the other special senses have been lost. The effect of hypoxia on directional hearing remains under investigation and may have operational significance in the use of warning tones with a directional component given to a pilot through his headset.

LOSS OF CONSCIOUSNESS

Although the arterial oxygen tension in the cerebral tissue is of crucial importance to an individual's degree of consciousness, its effect is subject to considerable modification as a result of other influences, such as cerebral blood flow and the degree of hypocapnia present. It has been found that a much closer correlation exits between the oxygen tension of jugular venous blood and the level of consciousness under conditions of hypoxic hypoxia, provided that vasovagal syncope does not supervene. Consciousness is lost when the jugular venous oxygen tension (see Figure 3.6) is reduced to 17–19 mmHg. Unconsciousness therefore may occur with arterial oxygen tension between 20 and 35 mmHg, depending on the degree of hypocapnia. Accordingly, although consciousness usually is lost when the alveolar oxygen tension is reduced to 30 mmHg or below for a significant period of time, it is possible to lose consciousness with an alveolar oxygen tension as high as 40 mmHg if there is marked hyperventilation or to retain consciousness, at least for a time, at an alveolar oxygen ten-

sion as low as 25 mmHg if there is no hypocapnia. A subject breathing air on acute exposure to altitude therefore may become unconscious at an altitude as low as 16 000 feet or may stay conscious for some minutes as high as 24 000 feet.

EFFECTS DURING RAPID DECOMPRESSION

As described earlier, rapid decompressions to altitudes above 30 000 feet when breathing air are inevitably accompanied by a fall in alveolar oxygen tension to 30 mmHg or lower. Such severe falls will have profound neurological consequences if they are allowed to persist. Consciousness will almost certainly be lost if the duration of exposure to an alveolar oxygen tension of less than 30 mmHg, on rapid decompression, is such that on plotting the oxygen tension against time, the area of an alveolar oxygen tension curve below the 30 mmHg level is greater than 140 mmHg/s (see Figure 3.4; p. 47).

Even if air continues to be inspired at the final altitude, however, there is no decrement in the performance of a psychomotor task until 12–14 seconds after the decompression. Thereafter, at a final altitude of 40 000 feet for example, the time taken to complete the task increases to about three times its control value 20 seconds after the event. Provided that 100 per cent oxygen is inspired within eight seconds of decompression, performance at the task returns to its control level about one minute later. There is no significant decrement in performance if the severity of the decompression is such that the alveolar oxygen tension never falls below 30 mmHg and then rises rapidly as oxygen is supplied.

Thus, to ensure that the skilled performance of military aircrew is not compromised, should a loss of cabin pressurization at high altitude occur, it is essential to maintain, or rapidly restore, alveolar oxygen tension above 30 mmHg. This requirement is of obvious significance in the design of personal breathing equipment for both military and civilian aircrew, as will be discussed further in subsequent chapters.

Clinical features of acute hypobaric hypoxia

The clinical picture of acute hypobaric hypoxia is a combination of the cardiorespiratory responses and neurological effects described above; consequently, the symptoms and signs are extremely variable. The speed and order of appearance of signs, and of the severity of symptoms produced by a lowering of inspired oxygen tension, depend on the rate and the degree to which the tension is lowered and on the duration of exposure to hypoxia. Even when these factors are kept constant, however, there is considerable variation between individuals in the effects of hypoxia, although for the same individual the pattern of effects does tend to follow the same trend from one occasion to another.

The factors that may influence an individual's pattern of symptoms and signs produced by hypoxia and their personal susceptibility are as follows:

- *Intensity of hypoxia:* maximum altitude, rate of ascent and duration of exposure to altitude.
- *Physical activity:* exercise exacerbates the features of hypoxia.
- *Ambient temperature:* a cold environment will reduce tolerance to hypoxia, in part at least, by increasing metabolic workload.
- *Intercurrent illness:* similarly, the additional metabolic load imposed by ill health will increase susceptibility to hypoxia.
- *Use of certain drugs, including alcohol:* many pharmacologically active substances have effects similar to those of hypoxic hypoxia and so mimic or exacerbate the condition. Alcohol and preparations containing anti-histamines are particularly likely to cause problems.

CLINICAL PICTURE

Although in general the higher the altitude, the more marked will be the features of hypoxia, rapid rates of ascent can allow high altitudes to be reached before severe symptoms and signs occur. In such circumstances, however, unconsciousness may supervene before any or many of the classic features appear. For descriptive purposes, therefore, it is convenient to consider the influence of slow ascent to various approximate altitudes on the evolution of the clinical picture of hypoxia.

Up to 10 000 feet breathing air (up to about 39 000 feet breathing oxygen)
The resting subject has no symptoms on ascent to an altitude of 10 000 feet when breathing air, or 39 000 feet when breathing 100 per cent oxygen, but performance of novel tasks will be impaired.

From 10 000 to 15 000 feet breathing air (from about 39 000 to 42 500 feet breathing oxygen)
The warm resting subject exhibits no or few signs and has virtually no symptoms. The ability to perform skilled tasks is impaired, however, an effect of which the subject is frequently unaware. Prolonged exposure to the moderate hypoxia at about 15 000 feet frequently causes a severe generalized headache. Physical work capacity is reduced markedly, and exposure to extremes of temperature may induce symptoms and signs of hypoxia.

From 15 000 to 20 000 feet breathing air (from about 42 500 to 45 000 feet breathing oxygen)
Even in the resting subject, the symptoms and signs of hypoxia appear on acute exposure to altitudes greater than 15 000 feet when breathing air. Higher mental processes and neuromuscular control are affected; in particular, there is a loss of critical judgment and willpower. Because of the loss of self-criticism, the subject is usually unaware of any deterioration in performance or indeed of the presence of hypoxia; it is this that makes the condition such a potentially dangerous hazard in aviation. Thought processes are slowed, mental calculations become unreliable, and psychomotor performance is grossly impaired. Marked changes in emotional state are common. Thus, there may be disinhibition of basic personality traits and emotions, and the individual may become elated or euphoric or pugnacious and morose. Occasionally, the individual may become physically violent.

In parallel with this group of cerebral features, disturbances due to hypocapnia commonly occur and, indeed, may dominate the clinical picture as hyperventilation occurs. Light-headedness, visual disturbances (including tunnelling of vision) and paraesthesiae of the extremities and lips may be followed in severe cases by tetany with carpo-pedal and facial spasms. Central and peripheral cyanosis develop, and there is decreased muscular coordination with loss of the sense of touch, so that delicate or fine movements are impossible.

Physical exertion greatly increases the severity and speed of onset of all of these symptoms and signs and may lead to unconsciousness.

Above 20 000 feet breathing air (above about 45 000 feet breathing oxygen)
The resting subject exhibits a marked accentuation of the symptoms and signs described above. Comprehension and mental performance decline rapidly, and unconsciousness supervenes with little or no warning. Myoclonic jerks of the upper limbs often precede loss of consciousness, and convulsions may occur thereafter. Hypoxic convulsions are characterized by intense, maintained muscular contractions that produce opisthotonos, preceded or followed by one or more myoclonic jerks.

The early (covert) cerebral features of hypobaric hypoxia may be summarized as follows:

- *Visual function:*

  - light intensity perceived as reduced
  - visual acuity diminished in poor illumination
  - light threshold increased
  - peripheral vision narrowed.

- *Psychomotor function:*

  - learning novel tasks impaired
  - choice-reaction time impaired
  - eye–hand coordination impaired.

- *Cognitive function:* memory impaired.

The overt features of acute hypobaric hypoxia may be summarized as follows:

- personality change
- lack of insight
- loss of judgement
- loss of self-criticism
- euphoria
- loss of memory
- mental incoordination
- muscular incoordination
- sensory loss
- cyanosis
- hyperventilation:

  - dizziness
  - light-headedness
  - feelings of unreality
  - feelings of apprehension
  - neuromuscular irritability
  - paraesthesia of face and extremities
  - carpo-pedal spasm

- semi-consciousness
- unconsciousness
- death.

TIME OF USEFUL CONSCIOUSNESS

The interval that elapses between a reduction in oxygen tension of the inspired gas and the point at which there is a specified degree of impairment of performance is termed the 'time of useful consciousness' (TUC). The length of this interval is influenced by many factors, of which the most important is the accepted degree of impairment. In the laboratory, this may vary from an inability to perform complex psychomotor tasks to a failure to respond to simple spoken commands. In practice, however, the most useful concept is to regard the TUC as the period during which the affected individual retains the ability to act to correct his or her predicament.

Values for the TUC at various altitudes following hypoxia induced by changing the breathing gas from oxygen to air are presented in Table 3.4. The large standard deviations at low altitudes serve to emphasize the considerable individual variation in the TUC. The variation is a reflection of the influence of many factors, including the pulmonary ventilatory response to hypoxia and the general physical fitness, age, degree of training and previous experiences of hypoxia of the subject. It should be noted that the TUC at a given altitude is shorter when hypoxia is induced by rapid decompression rather than by slow ascent.

Consideration of the TUC when breathing 100 per cent oxygen rather than air is aided by the concept of equivalence of altitude, as described previously. This suggests that

Table 3.4 *Times of useful consciousness at various altitudes of 50 seated young men following a change from breathing oxygen to breathing air*

Altitude (feet)	Time of useful consciousness (seconds)	
	Mean	Standard deviation
25 000	270	96
26 000	220	87
27 000	201	49
28 000	181	47
30 000	145	45
32 000	106	23
34 000	84	17
36 000	71	16

an individual breathing 100 per cent oxygen at 42 000 feet would be at an alveolar equivalent of breathing air at 16 000 feet; however, at higher altitudes than this tracheal values tend to overestimate actual alveolar conditions with TUCs considerably less than might be predicted from simple equivalence.

Recovery from hypoxia and the oxygen paradox

The administration of oxygen to a hypoxic subject usually results in a rapid and complete recovery, as is also the case if environmental pressure is increased, so that alveolar oxygen tension is restored towards its normal level. A generalized headache is the only symptom that persists, and only then if the exposure to hypoxia was prolonged.

In some subjects, however, sudden restoration of the alveolar oxygen tension to normal may cause a transient (paradoxical) worsening of the severity of the symptoms and signs of hypoxia for 15–60 seconds. This oxygen paradox is usually mild and is manifest only by flushing of the face and hands and perhaps deterioration in performance of complex tasks over the immediate period following restoration of the oxygen supply. Occasionally, oxygen administration may produce a severe paradox, with the appearance of clonic spasms and even loss of consciousness. The mechanisms responsible for the phenomenon are undetermined. The paradox usually occurs in subjects who have become hypocapnic during hypoxia, and it is also accompanied by a period of arterial hypotension. It may be that there is a significant reduction in peripheral resistance on the restoration of a normal arterial oxygen tension, which induces a generalized fall in blood pressure. This hypotension, in combination with persistent and marked hypocapnia, may result in cerebral hypoperfusion and vasoconstriction that persists for some while after the restoration of the arterial oxygen tension and may intensify cerebral hypoxia for a short time. Clearly, it is important that oxygen continues to be delivered to the victim of a paradox, despite the apparent worsening of the condition on initial administration of the gas.

HYPERVENTILATION

Hyperventilation is a condition in which pulmonary ventilation is greater than that required to eliminate the carbon dioxide produced by the tissues. The consequent excessive removal of carbon dioxide from the alveolar gas, the arterial blood and the tissues results in a reduction in the tension of carbon dioxide throughout the pathway.

Furthermore, there is a close relationship between carbon dioxide tension and hydrogen ion concentration in the blood and tissues, since these substances are in equilibrium according to the equation

$$CO_2 + H_2O \leftrightarrows H_2CO_3 \leftrightarrows H^+ + HCO_3^-$$

A reduction in carbon dioxide tension will drive the equilibrium towards the left. Consequently, there is a fall in hydrogen ion concentration, i.e. a rise in pH. Thus, hyperventilation also causes an increase in the pH of blood and tissues, i.e. respiratory alkalosis.

Aetiology

As described above, hyperventilation is a normal response to hypoxia and is seen when alveolar oxygen tension is reduced to below 55–60 mmHg. It may also occur as a result of voluntary overbreathing, e.g. in preparation for a breath-hold dive into water.

More commonly, however, the condition is produced by emotional stress, particularly anxiety, apprehension and fear. Thus, a significant proportion of student pilots under instruction exhibit gross hyperventilation in flight. Indeed, it has been claimed that 20–40 per cent of student aircrew suffer from hyperventilation at some stage during flying training. The condition is also seen in experienced aircrew when, for example, they are exposed to the mental stress of a sudden in-flight emergency or when they are being trained to operate a new aircraft type. Aircraft passengers who are afraid or anxious frequently hyperventilate.

Pain sometimes induces hyperventilation, as do motion sickness and certain environmental stresses, such as high ambient temperature and whole-body vibration at 4–8 Hz as, for example, produced by clear-air turbulence when flying at low level. Finally, hyperventilation is almost invariable in aircrew during pressure breathing, and although this tendency may be reduced by training, it cannot be eliminated entirely.

Physiological features of hyperventilation

The hypocapnia of hyperventilation has no significant effect on cardiac output or arterial blood pressure, although there is a redistribution of the former. Thus, hypocapnia induces a marked vasoconstriction of the cerebral arterioles and the vessels of the skin, while blood flow through skeletal muscle is increased. Although the intense cerebral vasoconstriction tends to minimize the change in hydrogen ion concentration within cerebral tissues, it also markedly reduces the minimum tissue oxygen tension. Therefore, it is probable that many of the changes produced by gross hyperventilation, and especially deterioration in performance, appearance of slow-wave activity in the electroencephalogram and loss of consciousness, are due to a combination of hypoxia and alkalosis in the cerebral tissues.

Reduction in the arterial carbon dioxide tension to below 25 mmHg causes a significant decrement in the performance of psychomotor tasks, such as tracking and complex coordination tests. The reaction time at a two-choice task is increased by about ten per cent by such a fall and is increased by 15 per cent at an arterial carbon dioxide tension of 15 mmHg. The ability to perform complex mental tasks, such as mental arithmetic, is compromised by a reduction in carbon dioxide tension to below 25–30 mmHg. Steadiness of the hands is also impaired by a reduction in arterial carbon dioxide tension to 25 mmHg. The ability to perform manual tasks is affected markedly by the muscle spasm that occurs if arterial carbon dioxide tensions fall below 20 mmHg. Reduction of carbon dioxide tension below 10–15 mmHg produces gross clouding of consciousness and then unconsciousness.

The rise in tissue pH induced by hyperventilation increases the sensitivity of peripheral nerve fibres and reduces the threshold for their response to stimuli. The threshold is lowered by the local fall in hydrogen ion concentration and spontaneous activity occurs, giving rise to sensory disturbances, such as paraesthesiae in the face and extremities and motor disruption, in the form of reflex firing of proprioceptive fibres via the spinal cord, causing muscle spasm (tetany). Different types of nerve fibres are affected in a consistent sequence: fibres conveying information with regard to touch, position, pressure and vibration are affected first, followed by motor fibres and then cold, heat and, lastly, pain fibres.

Clinical features of hyperventilation

The earliest symptoms produced by hyperventilation become manifest when the arterial carbon dioxide tension has been reduced to 20–25 mmHg. Usually, there are feelings of light-headedness, dizziness, anxiety (which, since apprehension itself is a cause of hyperventilation, frequently establishes a vicious circle) and a superficial tingling (paraesthesiae) in the extremities and around the lips. The paraesthesiae are followed by muscle spasms, particularly of the limbs and of the face, when arterial carbon dioxide tension has fallen below 15–20 mmHg. Contraction of muscle groups in the wrist and hand and the ankle and foot give rise to carpo-pedal spasm. In this state, the thumb is flexed acutely across the palm, the hand is flexed at the wrist, the metacarpo-phalangeal joints are flexed and the inter-phalangeal joints are extended (the *main d'accoucheur*). The ankle is profoundly plantar-flexed. Spasm of the facial muscles causes stiffening of the face, and the corners of the mouth are drawn downwards (the *risus sardonicus*). In more severe hypocapnia, when arterial carbon dioxide tension is less than 15 mmHg, the whole body becomes stiff as a result of general tonic contractions of skeletal muscle (tetany).

The increased irritability of nervous tissue in moderate hypocapnia causes augmentation of tendon reflexes. An example of this lowered threshold can be demonstrated by tapping the branches of the facial nerve as they pass forward over the mandible: such tapping, in the presence of moderate alkalosis, causes twitching of the facial muscles (Chvostek's sign). Finally, as described above, moderate and severe hyperventilation produce a general deterioration in mental and physical performance, which is followed by impairment of consciousness and finally unconsciousness.

It is most important to realize that, in the uncommon event of an individual hyperventilating to the point of unconsciousness as a result of anxiety, the supervention of coma will be followed by a gradual recovery as respiration is inhibited and carbon dioxide tensions regain their normal levels. This is clearly not the case, however, if the hyperventilation has been induced by hypoxia. It will be apparent from the previous sections of this chapter that most of the early symptoms of hypoxia are very similar to those produced by hypocapnia. Indeed, the light-headedness, paraesthesiae and apprehension seen during acute hypoxia in a subject breathing air at altitudes between 15 000 and about 20 000 feet are due to the concomitant hypocapnia. Thus, hypoxia should always be suspected when symptoms or signs of hypocapnia occur at altitudes above about 12 000 feet, and the corrective procedures must be based on the assumption that the condition is caused by hypoxia until proved otherwise.

FURTHER READING

Brown EB. Physiological effects of hyperventilation. *Physiological Reviews* 1953; **33**: 445–71.

Cable GG. In-flight hypoxia incidents in military aircraft: causes and implications for training. *Aviation, Space, and Environmental Medicine* 2003; **74**: 169–72.

Crow TJ, Kelman GR. Psychological effects of mild hypoxia. *Journal of Physiology* 1969; **204**: 248.

Denison DM. High altitudes and hypoxia. In: Edholm OG, Weiner JS (eds). *Principles and Practice of Human Physiology*. London: Academic Press, 1981; pp. 241–307.

Ernsting J. The effect of brief profound hypoxia upon the arterial and venous oxygen tensions in man. *Journal of Physiology* 1963; **169**: 292–311.

Ernsting J. Prevention of hypoxia-acceptable compromises. *Aviation, Space, and Environmental Medicine* 1978; **49**: 495–502.

Ernsting J, Byford GH, Denison DM, Fryer DI. Hypoxia induced by rapid decompression from 8,000 feet to 40,000 feet: the influence of rate of decompression. Flying Personnel Research Committee Report No. 1324. London: Ministry of Defence, 1973.

Gibson TM. Hyperventilation in aircrew: a review. *Aviation, Space, and Environmental Medicine* 1979; **50**: 725–33.

Guyton AC, Hall JE. *Textbook of Medical Physiology*, 10th edn. Philadelphia, PA: W.B. Saunders, 2000.

Harding RM. The early symptoms of cerebral hypoxia. In: Amery WK, Wauquier A (eds). *The Prelude to the Migraine Attack*. London: Baillière Tindall, 1986; pp. 54–8.

Harper AM, Jennett S. *Cerebral Blood Flow and Metabolism*. Manchester: Manchester University Press, 1990.

Lambertson CJ. Respiration. In: Mountcastle VB (ed.). *Medical Physiology*. St Louis, MO: Mosby, 1980; pp. 1677–1946.

Lum LC. Hyperventilation and anxiety state. *Journal of the Royal Society of Medicine* 1981; **74**: 1–4.

National Transport Safety Board. NTSB report no. AAB-00-01. Washington, DC: National Transport Safety Board, 2000.

Taneja N, Wiegmann DA. An analysis of in-flight impairment and incapacitation in fatal general aviation accidents (1990–1998). *Proceedings of the Human Factors and Ergonomics Society*, 2002; 155–9.

Weil JV. Ventilatory control at high altitude. In: Cherniack NS, Widdicombe JG (eds). *Handbook of Physiology*, Section 3, Vol. II, Part 2. Bethesda, MD: American Physiological Society, 1986; pp. 703–27.

West JB. *Respiratory Physiology: The Essentials*, 7th edn. Philadelphia, PA: Lippincott Williams & Wilkins, 2004.

Whipp BJ. *The Control of Breathing in Man*. Manchester: Manchester University Press, 1987.

4

Prevention of hypoxia

DAVID P. GRADWELL

INTRODUCTION

Most aircraft are capable of carrying their occupants to an altitude at which hypoxia is a potential hazard. The adverse physiological effects of breathing ambient air at reduced atmospheric pressure at altitude and the associated hypoxia must be prevented during flight. For the vast majority of air travellers, this can be achieved most comfortably by the provision of an artificial pressure environment – a pressurized cabin – so that the occupants are not exposed to reduced barometric pressure (see Chapter 6). By this means, air is breathed at a sufficiently high pressure to avoid an unacceptable degree of hypoxia.

The alternative means of preventing hypoxia in flight is to increase the concentration and hence the partial pressure of oxygen in the lungs by the use of oxygen equipment. In modern commercial aircraft, the former method is used, with the latter available as an emergency system in the event of failure of the pressure cabin. In military aircraft, however, both methods of preventing hypoxia generally are employed concurrently. In this chapter, the altitudes and environmental pressures given refer to conditions surrounding the occupants of an aircraft (cabin altitude and pressure) rather than the aircraft itself.

In this chapter consideration will be given to the means by which airborne oxygen equipment can be used to protect against hypoxia by maintaining an adequate supply of oxygen to the tissues of the body despite a reduction in barometric pressure. As will have been seen in Chapter 3, the physiological ideal is for the partial pressure of oxygen in the alveolar gas to remain at the level seen when air is breathed at sea level. At altitudes up to 33 000 feet, the alveolar oxygen tension may be maintained at its ground-level value by increasing progressively the proportion of oxygen in the inspired gas. Above this altitude, however, as ambient pressure continues to diminish, the alveolar oxygen pressure falls too, even when 100 per cent oxygen is breathed. This continuing fall in the alveolar partial pressure of oxygen can be prevented only by maintaining the total alveolar gas pressure. The manoeuvre whereby the pressure in the lungs is raised above the environmental pressure is termed *positive pressure breathing* (PPB). The serious hypoxia that would otherwise occur on exposure to altitudes in excess of 40 000 feet may be prevented by this means. To be acceptable, oxygen systems must meet this primary demand in a manner that minimizes the physiological disturbance of ascent to altitude and may be required also to fulfil a secondary function, i.e. protecting the user from the additional adverse effects of inhalation of contaminated air, should it be present in the cockpit. In this chapter, the fundamental performance of oxygen systems to meet these requirements will be discussed in detail.

MINIMUM ACCEPTABLE CONCENTRATION OF OXYGEN

To prevent the fall in alveolar oxygen tension that occurs when air is breathed at reduced barometric pressures, the proportion of oxygen in the inspired gas must be increased. The fractional concentration of oxygen required in the inspired gas to maintain a desired alveolar partial pressure of oxygen (PA_{O_2}) at any particular altitude may be calculated. Figure 4.1 shows the relationship between altitude and concentration of oxygen in the inspired gas required to maintain (i) the normal PA_{O_2} (103 mmHg, 13.7 kPa), (ii) the PA_{O_2} that exists when breathing air at 5000 feet (75 mmHg, 10 kPa), and (iii) the PA_{O_2} that exists when breathing air at 8000 feet (65 mmHg, 8.7 kPa).

It might seem attractive on grounds of oxygen economy to choose a PA_{O_2} that is lower than the normal sea-level value. Thus, at 25 000 feet, the inspired gas must contain 63 per cent oxygen to maintain an alveolar oxygen tension of 103 mmHg (13.7 kPa) but only 41 per cent oxygen to provide an alveolar oxygen tension of 60 mmHg (8 kPa). However, the disadvantages of choosing a relationship between oxygen concentration and altitude that allows the alveolar oxygen tension to fall below the ground-level value are as follows:

- Even the mild degree of hypoxia associated with a lowering of the alveolar oxygen tension to 75 mmHg (10 kPa) impairs the ability to recall recently learned procedures.
- Lowering the alveolar oxygen tension to the order of

60 mmHg (8 kPa) induces a significant performance impairment, which is accentuated by physical exercise.
- There is a lower margin of safety in the event of either a partial or a complete failure of the breathing equipment to deliver oxygen to the respiratory tract.

Thus, solely on the grounds of preventing hypoxia at altitudes up to 35 000 feet, the concentration of oxygen in the inspired gas should not be allowed to fall below that required to maintain an alveolar oxygen tension of 80 mmHg (10.7 kPa). From a practical point of view, however, the third consideration in the list above is probably equally important: when an ill-fitting oxygen mask allows the oxygen delivered to the user to be diluted by the inward leakage of air, the consequent risk of hypoxia is diminished in proportion to the amount by which the concentration of oxygen in the breathing gas supply exceeds that required to prevent hypoxia. For example, at an altitude of 25 000 feet, an inward leak equal to half the pulmonary ventilation would reduce alveolar oxygen tension from 80 mmHg (10.7 kPa) to about 65 mmHg (8 kPa) (equivalent to breathing air at 8000 feet). If the oxygen system was designed to maintain an alveolar oxygen tension of 65 mmHg (8.7 kPa), then a similar leakage would reduce the alveolar oxygen tension to 40 mmHg (5.3 kPa) (equivalent to breathing air at 16 000 feet) – a very significant degree of hypoxia.

Thus, an oxygen system should be designed to deliver the concentration of oxygen, in relation to altitude, that will maintain a sea-level alveolar oxygen tension (i.e. 103 mmHg, 13.7 kPa), as indicated by the upper curve of Figure 4.1 and the minimum oxygen concentration in Table 4.1. This sea-level alveolar oxygen tension can be maintained in such a manner only up to an altitude of 33 000 feet. Above this altitude, with the continuing fall in barometric pressure, the alveolar oxygen tension falls progressively even when 100 per cent oxygen is breathed. At

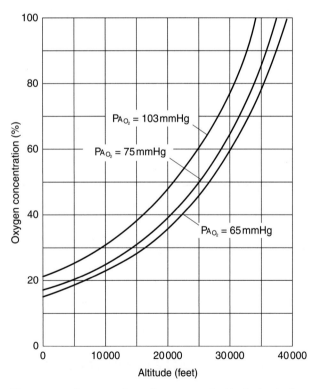

Figure 4.1 *Concentrations of oxygen required in dry inspired gas at various altitudes in order to maintain alveolar oxygen tensions of 103 mmHg (13.7 kPa) (equivalent to breathing air at ground level), 75 mmHg (10 kPa) (equivalent to breathing air at 5000 feet) and 65 mmHg (8.7 kPa) (equivalent to breathing air at 8000 feet).*

Table 4.1 *Limits for concentration of oxygen delivered to the respiratory tract by an aircraft oxygen system*

Cabin altitude (ft)	Concentration of oxygen in dry inspired gas (%)	
	Minimum	Maximum*
0	21	60
5000	25	60
10 000	31	60
15 000	38	60
20 000	49	67
25 000	63	80
30 000	81	100
33 000	95	100
35 000	100	100
40 000	100	100

*Typical values allowed by current specifications.

40 000 feet, breathing 100 per cent oxygen at ambient pressure will produce an alveolar oxygen tension of only 54 mmHg (7.2 kPa), and so above this altitude PPB (positive-pressure breathing) oxygen is required.

In certain circumstances, such as when aircrew are pressure-breathing or following loss of cabin pressurization in a military or passenger aircraft, lower alveolar oxygen tensions are acceptable for short periods. Thus, in the case of rapid decompression in a military aircraft, alveolar oxygen tensions of 30 mmHg (4 kPa) may be acceptable (although not desirable) for a very short time provided that 100 per cent oxygen is delivered within two seconds of the start of decompression; while alveolar oxygen tensions of 75 mmHg (10 kPa) are acceptable for the flight-deck crew and cabin staff of a decompressed commercial aircraft, and tensions of 50 mmHg (6.7 kPa) are acceptable for seated passengers.

MAXIMUM ACCEPTABLE CONCENTRATION OF OXYGEN

An oxygen system that provides aircrew with 100 per cent oxygen at all altitudes has the advantage of simplicity and having fewer mechanical complications and being cheaper to manufacture than a system that supplies a mixture of air and oxygen that varies appropriately with altitude. The objections to breathing 100 per cent oxygen at all altitudes in flight are as follows:

- It is uneconomical in terms of the consumption of the aircraft oxygen supply, since in order to prevent serious hypoxia, 100 per cent oxygen is required only above a cabin altitude of 33 000 feet.
- Breathing 100 per cent oxygen continuously for long periods (12–16 hours) at cabin altitudes below 18 000 feet may cause substernal discomfort due to the irritative effect of a high partial pressure of oxygen on the mucosal lining of the respiratory passages.
- Breathing 100 per cent oxygen at altitude and during return to ground level frequently gives rise, some hours later, to ear discomfort and deafness (delayed otic barotrauma). This phenomenon is due to rapid absorption of oxygen from the middle-ear cavity into the blood; the intensity of the symptoms is reduced greatly by the presence of nitrogen in the inspired gas and hence in the gas in the middle-ear cavity.
- Respiratory symptoms, such as coughing, dyspnoea and retrosternal discomfort, occurring immediately after flight in a high-performance aircraft are produced by breathing 100 per cent oxygen before and during exposure to $+G_z$ acceleration. The severity of this syndrome is increased by the use of anti-G trousers. The nature of this condition is discussed in

Chapter 8, but it should be noted that the symptoms of acceleration atelectasis may be prevented by ensuring that the concentration of nitrogen in the inspired gas is greater than 40 per cent.

For these reasons, an aircraft oxygen system should deliver a mixture of oxygen and nitrogen derived either from mixing the supply gas with air or by controlling the retention of nitrogen in molecular sieve systems (see Chapter 5). While the concentration of oxygen should vary with altitude in such a manner that the alveolar oxygen tension is maintained at or just greater than the value obtained when air is breathed at ground level (103 mmHg, 13.7 kPa), the concentration of nitrogen in the gas delivered by the system should be as high as permitted by the primary requirement to maintain the ideal oxygen tension. In practice, the concentration of oxygen delivered at a given altitude by an aircrew breathing system varies with the demand and from one regulating device to another. Thus, it is necessary to allow some deviation from the ideal oxygen concentration–altitude curve (upper curve of Figure 4.1). Typical maximum oxygen concentrations allowed by current specifications for aircrew oxygen breathing equipment are presented in Table 4.1.

At altitudes above 40 000 feet, when 100 per cent oxygen must be delivered at a pressure greater than ambient, the absolute pressure that must be contained within the lungs depends on the degree of hypoxia that is deemed acceptable; this in turn is determined by several factors, which will be discussed later in this chapter. Generally, however, most pressure breathing systems maintain an absolute pressure in the respiratory tract of between 120 and 150 mmHg (16–20 kPa). The relationship between altitude and the positive pressure at which oxygen must be delivered to the respiratory tract (breathing pressure) to maintain various absolute pressures within the lungs are shown in Figure 4.4.

PULMONARY VENTILATION IN FLIGHT

Oxygen equipment must be capable of meeting the pulmonary ventilation (respiratory minute volume) requirements of the user in a variety of situations, both on the ground and during flight. The pulmonary ventilation is determined by the metabolic rate and modified by factors such as hypoxia, excitement and anxiety. Measurements of respiratory minute volume have shown large differences in pulmonary ventilation between individuals under similar flight conditions. Typical values of respiratory minute volume obtained under various conditions of flight are shown in Table 4.2. The figures are based on data derived from many sources and relate to aircrew members who are oxygenated adequately.

Table 4.2 *Pulmonary ventilation in various conditions of flight*

Condition	Pulmonary ventilation (L (BTPS)/min)
Seated at rest	10–15
Seated active	15–50
Moving about aircraft	25–50
After running to aircraft	≤ 60

Measurements of aircrew respiratory demands have revealed that the greatest increase from resting minute volume requirements can occur when a pilot runs to the aircraft. Thus, when the pilot then connects the oxygen mask to the aircraft breathing systems, substantial minute volume demands have to be met. The mass flow of gas required from an oxygen regulator to meet a given pulmonary ventilation varies inversely with the pressure in the respiratory tract. It follows, therefore, that the sea-level requirement demands most from the delivery system in terms of mass flow. Aircrew oxygen breathing equipment should, therefore, be capable of meeting pulmonary ventilations of up to 50 litres (atmospheric temperature and pressure, dry; ATPD)/min at sea level. (It is convenient when considering breathing systems to specify flow requirements under ATPD rather than body temperature and pressure, saturated with water vapour (BTPS) conditions, the former being 84–87 per cent of the latter at normal cabin altitudes in combat aircraft.)

RESPIRATORY GAS FLOW PATTERNS IN FLIGHT

During the breathing cycle, the flow of gas in and out of the respiratory tract changes very rapidly. Oxygen equipment must be capable of responding to and meeting these changes while imposing the minimum of resistance to breathing. Respiratory gas-flow patterns related to the various conditions that occur in flight can be measured using a pneumotachograph. Typical records obtained (pneumotachograms) are shown in Figure 4.2 for:

- aircrew seated at rest (curve A)
- aircrew performing physical exercise approximating to the effort of moving about an aircraft (curve B)
- aircrew speaking aloud while seated at rest (curve C).

However, there are very wide individual variations in the airflow pattern obtained during any particular activity, and the shape of the pattern depends on the level of physical activity, the nature of the work undertaken, the degree of arm movement, posture, and the phase of flight, e.g. the level of $+G_z$ acceleration. In the resting subject (Figure 4.2,

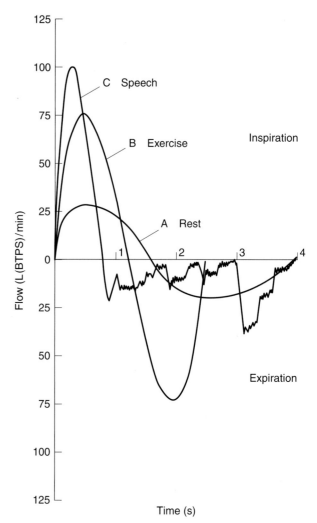

Figure 4.2 *Typical respiratory flow patterns (pneumotachograms) for aircrew seated at rest (trace A); aircrew moving about an aircraft (trace B); and aircrew speaking aloud while seated at rest (trace C). The flow throughout a single respiratory cycle is shown for each of the three conditions. BTPS, body temperature and pressure, saturated with water vapour.*

curve A), the flow of air increases rapidly at the beginning of inspiration, but then the rate of increase of flow falls progressively until the peak flow of about 25–30 litres (BTPS)/min is reached. The air velocity falls slowly and then more rapidly until it reaches zero at the end of inspiration. The whole inspiratory phase lasts for one to two seconds, and expiration follows without a pause. This lasts longer than inspiration, and the peak flow achieved is less than that occurring during inspiration. In a resting, non-speaking subject, the peak inspiratory flow is generally about three times the respiratory minute volume. During moderate exercise (Figure 4.2, curve B), the volume of gas in each phase of the breathing cycle is increased and the duration of each phase is shortened. The peak inspiratory flow also increases, but in these conditions this value amounts to only about 2.6 times the respiratory minute volume. The duration of the expiratory phase becomes shorter relative to the duration of inspiration, and at higher work rates it may be less. During speech at rest (Figure 4.2, curve C), the volume of gas breathed in each phase is similar to that during rest without speech, but the duration of inspiration is very short (0.5–0.6 seconds) and the duration of expiration is lengthened. Speech modulates the flow pattern in the expiratory phase. In inspiration during speech, the peak flow and the rate of increase and decrease of gas flow are very high. Thus, speech places one of the most severe demands on oxygen equipment in terms of the peak flow delivery and rate of change of flow.

Studies of the pressure/flow relationships, and thus the requirements placed upon a system, have allowed national and international standards for the performance of breathing systems to be defined. However, oxygen equipment must cater for the wide variety of breathing flow patterns that may occur in aircrew in flight. In addition, for any given set of circumstances, there are considerable individual variations (by as much as 100 per cent between maximum and minimum peak flow values). The mean values of gas flow, as typified in Figure 4.2, do not provide an adequate basis for the design of breathing systems. In practice, it is usual to specify the curves given by the mean values plus twice the standard deviation, which will include the gas flow requirements of 95 per cent of normal individuals. Graphs of this type show that oxygen equipment should be designed to meet inspiratory peak flows of up to 200 litres (ATPD)/min, with a maximum rate of change of 20 litres (ATPD)/s/s at these peak flows.

EXTERNAL RESISTANCE TO RESPIRATORY GAS FLOW

Most oxygen breathing equipment imposes additional flow resistance on the respiratory system. This added breathing resistance must be kept to a minimum in order to avoid undesirable physiological side effects.

There have been many experimental studies of the effects of imposed resistance to breathing, but often the results of these studies are difficult to interpret in terms of the requirements for oxygen systems, since the effects vary greatly, depending on the type and magnitude of the resistance used. Furthermore, in most studies, the external resistance has been imposed for relatively short periods (10–30 minutes).

However, the general effects of imposing external resistance to breathing in either or both of the inspiratory and expiratory phases of respiration may be stated. These effects include the following:

- Change in respiratory rhythm: moderate resistances cause slowing and deepening of respiration, while high resistances cause rapid shallow breathing.
- Decrease in pulmonary ventilation: for a given resistance, the reduction is greatest when the resistance is applied both in inspiration and in expiration.
- Reduction in alveolar ventilation: this causes an increase in alveolar carbon dioxide tension.
- Increase in functional residual capacity: this is greatest when a resistance load is applied in expiration alone.
- Reduction of maximum ventilatory capacity.
- Increase in total respiratory work per minute: this rises in an approximately linear manner with increasing resistance.
- Subjective disturbances: these range from conscious appreciation of a very slight resistance to breathing to severe resistance to breathing, with sensations of impending asphyxia.

The physiological disturbances induced by the addition of resistance to breathing show great variation of response between subjects and between the effects on the same subject on different occasions. Thus, although reduction in alveolar ventilation and hypercapnia may result from breathing against high levels of resistance, there is no doubt that susceptible subjects (e.g. aircrew untrained and inexperienced in the use of oxygen equipment) may hyperventilate and exhibit symptoms of the consequent hypocapnia. The results of one investigation into the subjective effects of applied respiratory resistance are shown in Figure 4.3. In this study, resistance was applied by means

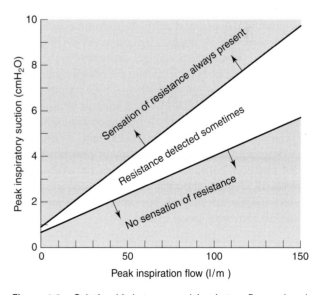

Figure 4.3 *Relationship between peak inspiratory flow and peak inspiratory suction at the nose and lips, which give rise to a sensation of resistance to breathing. The added resistance was in the form of a sharp-edged orifice. The subject's comments on the presence or absence of the sensation of resistance were recorded after exposure to it for several minutes.*

of different-size orifices. After a few minutes, the subject was asked to comment on the degree of resistance to breathing, with a view to establishing the value of resistance at which mask pressure fluctuations became perceptible. During quiet breathing (peak inspiratory flow of about 30 litres/min), an inspiratory suction of 1.6 cm water gauge (160 Pa) was not noticed by the subject. When inspiratory suction reached 2.8 cm water gauge (280 Pa), resistance was noticed on all occasions. In many aircraft oxygen systems, the ability to detect imposition of breathing resistance has been used to provide warning of either supply malfunction or inadvertent disconnection of components of the system. The sensation of resistance to breathing and the physiological disturbances produced by breathing from oxygen equipment depend not only on the total change of pressure in the mask cavity during the respiratory cycle but also on the relationship of these pressure changes to the pressure of the environment. Thus, the disturbances induced by the imposition of a given resistance to respiration are less if the mean pressure in the mask is raised slightly (2–6 cm water gauge, 200–600 Pa) above that of the environment, compared with when the mean pressure is equal to or less than the environmental pressure. Thus, in the presence of safety pressure – a small overpressure in the mask – not only would any leak be outward (rather than an inward oxygen-diluting leak) but also any small resistance to breathing is tolerated more easily.

Although it is possible to state the magnitude of resistance that will give rise to the described subjective disturbances and undesirable physiological changes, it is difficult to define the acceptable limits of resistance. In general, the aim is to keep the added breathing resistance imposed by the system to a minimum. In practical terms, the maximum acceptable limit for the resistance imposed by aircrew oxygen breathing equipment is that the total changes of pressure in the mask during the respiratory cycle should not exceed 5 cm water gauge (500 Pa) during quiet breathing (peak inspiratory and expiratory flows of 30 litres (ATPS)/min) or 11 cm water gauge (1.1 kPa) during heavy breathing (peak inspiratory and expiratory flows of 110 litres (ATPS)/min). At the maximal flows defined above, that is inspiratory peak flows of up to 200 litres (ATPS)/min, with a maximum rate of change of 20 litres (ATPS)/s/s, the total change of pressure at the mouth and nose during the respiratory cycle should not exceed 30.5 cm water gauge (3 kPa).

Added dead space

An oxygen system must either adequately and safely dispose of the expired carbon dioxide or disperse the entire expirate to ambient. To avoid significant rebreathing, the effective additional dead space imposed by the use of an oxygen mask should be no more than about 150 ml. Furthermore, following a rapid decompression, it can be essential that the gas trapped in the dead space is small, as any delay in the inspiration of a breathing gas rich in oxygen may result in severe hypoxia. These requirements for a low small added dead space are generally achievable in the closely fitting masks worn by aircrew, linked to an oxygen regulator supplying breathing gas on demand. Therapeutic oxygen masks and passenger masks used only during emergencies may utilize a rebreathing bag to economize on the supply of oxygen, and the total dead space commonly will then exceed 150 ml. However, the expirate is easily dispersed, since such masks do not fit tightly and carbon dioxide and water vapour in the expirate can be dispersed in ambient air.

PREVENTION OF HYPOXIA ABOVE 40 000 FEET

When breathing 100 per cent oxygen at 40 000 feet, where the atmospheric pressure (P_B) is 141 mmHg (18.8 kPa), the $P_{A_{O_2}}$ is 54 mmHg. A significant degree of hypoxia will occur if $P_{A_{O_2}}$ falls below 50–54 mmHg. To prevent hypoxia above 40 000 feet, therefore, an oxygen system must be capable of delivering breathing gas to the respiratory tract at pressures greater than that of the ambient environment (Figure 4.4).

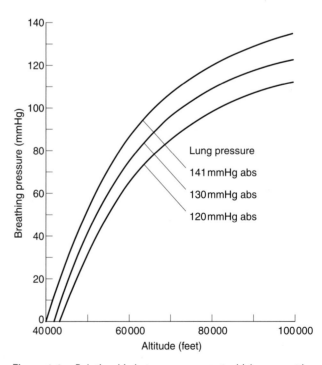

Figure 4.4   *Relationship between pressure at which gas must be delivered (relative to that of the environment) and altitude to maintain absolute pressures in the respiratory tract of 141, 130 and 120 mmHg.*

For example, at an altitude of 45 000 feet, where P_B is 111 mmHg (14.8 kPa), 100 per cent oxygen must be delivered at a positive pressure of 30 mmHg (4 kPa) to ensure that $P_{A_{O_2}}$ is elevated to the equivalent of breathing 100 per cent oxygen at 40 000 feet. It is important to remember, however, that the associated elevation of intrapulmonary pressure has significant adverse physiological consequences. These disturbances are influenced by the type of breathing system utilized. Thus, the manner in which the pressure is applied to the respiratory tract will alter the resulting respiratory and circulatory changes.

PPB was originally introduced for military flying to allow short excursions above 40 000 feet to be conducted in unpressurized aircraft without the pilot suffering an unacceptable degree of hypoxia. With the advent of pressurized cockpits, this was no longer necessary. However, pressure breathing has remained in use as an important emergency provision to enable aircrew to continue to fly their aircraft in the event of loss of cabin pressure above 40 000 feet. In recent years, it has also been adopted as a means of improving tolerance to high levels of sustained accelerations (high G_z). Therefore, an understanding of the physiological consequences of the use of pressure breathing remains of great importance. In the following sections, the physiological consequences of pressure breathing at $1\,G_z$ for altitude protection (PBA) will be considered under the following headings: respiratory effects, circulatory effects, effects on the head and neck, and the acceptable degree of hypoxia. The specific influences of the use of pressure breathing for G_z protection (PBG) will be considered in subsequent chapters.

Respiratory effects of pressure breathing

BREATHING EFFORT

Early observations on the respiratory effects of pressure breathing included comment on the reversal of the normal respiratory cycle. At breathing pressures in excess of approximately 10 mmHg (1.3 kPa), inspiration becomes a passive process, with the lungs being inflated by the breathing gas without muscular effort. Expiration, in contrast, becomes an active, tiring process, with an expiratory effort maintained continuously to support the chest and prevent overdistension of the lungs. Since elastic recoil plays little part in exhaling gas during pressure breathing, the work of breathing thereby is increased further. Furthermore, the normal inspiratory and expiratory flow patterns are markedly affected. Inspiration becomes sharper, with a more rapid rise to a peak and an abrupt end. Expiration becomes protracted because of the effort needed to breathe out against the constant positive pressure.

People experienced in pressure breathing can breathe for short periods at pressures of up to 50 mmHg (6.7 kPa),

but people unaccustomed to the procedure are unable to tolerate breathing pressures of more than about 30 mmHg (4 kPa). Trained individuals can tolerate breathing pressure of up to 30 mmHg (4 kPa) for some minutes, but inevitably this is associated with hyperventilation and fatigue. Commonly, breathing pressures greater than 30 mmHg are used only when respiratory support through the application of counter-pressure is available.

DISTENSION OF LUNGS AND CHEST

In a relaxed subject (when the distensibility of the lungs and thorax is high), the lungs are distended fully by a breathing pressure of approximately 20 mmHg (2.7 kPa). The maximum pressure that can be exerted and held in the lungs by active contraction of expiratory muscles of the chest and abdominal walls depends on the length of time for which the pressure is operative. Thus, during coughing or sneezing, the intrapulmonary pressure may reach peak values of 200–300 mmHg (27–40 kPa) for very brief periods, but these are compressive respiratory events associated with muscular activity of the chest wall and abdomen, which provides support to the lung tissue. When the pressure is held for about three seconds, the maximum expiratory pressure that can be produced is about 120 mmHg (16 kPa). If the lungs are unsupported by the chest wall, they will rupture when the intrapulmonary pressure exceeds 40–50 mmHg (5.3–6.7 kPa). However, when the lungs are supported by the walls of the thoracic cavity, intrapulmonary pressures of up to 80 mmHg (10.7 kPa) can be tolerated without damage. Intrapulmonary pressures above 80–100 mmHg (10.7–13.3 kPa) can cause tearing of the lung parenchyma when the expiratory muscles are relaxed. Gas can pass from the damaged tissue into the tissue planes, causing pneumothorax, pneumomediastinum and surgical emphysema, and into pulmonary blood vessels, causing gas embolism.

Radiographic studies of the chest while pressure breathing have shown elevation and expansion of the thoracic cage and descent of the diaphragm, despite increased muscular tone. Spirometric studies of the lung have revealed that pressure breathing gives rise to an increase in total lung capacity and, in particular, an increase in expiratory reserve volume, with a proportionate reduction in inspiratory reserve volume and an increase in residual volume, probably principally due to displacement of blood from the thorax (Figure 4.5). So, although pressure breathing at 30 mmHg (4 kPa) reduces the inspiratory reserve volume by about 2.5 litres, total lung volume is increased by 500 ml.

INCREASED PULMONARY VENTILATION

Tidal volume commonly is increased in response to pressure breathing, as is respiratory frequency, especially in people less experienced in the technique. In most subjects,

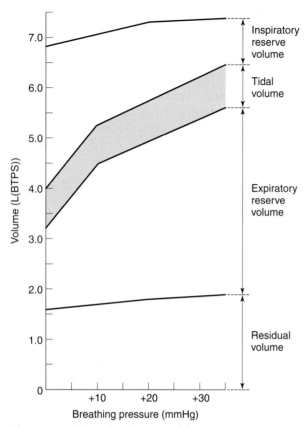

Figure 4.5 *Effect of continuous positive-pressure breathing on total lung capacity and its subdivisions. Total lung capacity, residual volume and functional residual capacity (residual volume + expiratory reserve volume) all become greater with an increase in breathing pressure. The greatest increase occurs, however, in the expiratory reserve volume, while the inspiratory reserve volume is markedly reduced.*

therefore, there is an increase in the respiratory minute volume, although there is wide individual variation in this response. Pressure breathing at 30 mmHg (4 kPa) increases the respiratory minute volume, on average, by about 50 per cent above the resting value; however, whereas some individuals double their minute volume at a breathing pressure of 30 mmHg (4 kPa), others barely respond. Although there is an increase in respiratory work, and hence carbon dioxide production, the increase in minute volume is proportionally much greater, giving rise therefore to hyperventilation, even in well-trained subjects. In untrained or inexperienced individuals, severe hyperventilation may result. Carbon dioxide tensions in the blood will then fall during pressure breathing. During pressure breathing at 30 mmHg (4 kPa), the alveolar and arterial carbon dioxide tensions are frequently as low as 25–30 mmHg (3.3–4 kPa).

RAISED INTRAPLEURAL PRESSURE

Intrapleural pressure rises as intrapulmonary pressure rises during pressure breathing. This increase in intrapleural pressure therefore is determined by the applied breathing pressure, although it is modified somewhat by the degree of lung distension that it induces. If there is no increase in lung volume, the rise in intrapleural pressure equals the applied breathing pressure. If lung distension occurs, then the rise in intrapleural pressure will be less than the applied intrapulmonary pressure by the additional elastic recoil generated in the lung tissue, which is approximately 4 mmHg (0.5 kPa) per 1 litre of distension. Thus, if lung volume is increased by 2 litre at the start of pressure breathing, then the rise in intrapleural pressure will be approximately 8 mmHg (1.1 kPa) less than the applied breathing pressure. Nonetheless, the increase in intrapleural pressure that occurs during pressure breathing is of considerable importance, since it determines the degree of pressure applied to the heart and great vessels inside the chest and thus the additional force that is applied to the circulation. It is interesting to note that chest counter-pressure (see below) will act to reduce distension of the chest wall and maintain the expiratory reserve volume closer to its normal value. Thus, for a given breathing pressure, the use of chest counter-pressure results in an increase in the intrapleural pressure relative to that which would be induced in its absence.

EFFECTS OF RESPIRATORY COUNTER-PRESSURE

The major respiratory disturbances induced by pressure breathing (i.e. lung distension, hyperventilation) may be minimized by applying counter-pressure to the surface of the trunk. Counter-pressure may be applied by a variety of methods, the most efficient of which is by gas held within a full-pressure suit, encasing the whole body in an environment at an elevated pressure, relative to ambient. Another method, which is almost as efficient, applies counter-pressure to the chest or trunk by means of a gas-filled bladder that is connected to the breathing line between the source of breathing pressure and the oronasal mask or helmet. In this way, when pressure is applied to the breathing tract, an equal gas pressure is applied in the bladder that covers the body. This is the basis of the pressure garments described in more detail in the next chapter.

Circulatory effects of pressure breathing

The most immediately significant limitation of pressure breathing as a means of extending duration of exposure to very high altitude is the profound circulatory disturbances induced by the elevation of intrathoracic pressure. Such disturbances vary with the magnitude of the pressure applied and the duration. The heart and the intrathoracic great vessels are exposed to the elevated intrapleural pressure, and it is the rise in this, rather than the intrathoracic pressure per se, that determines the stress applied to the circulation. Provided that the intrathoracic veins and the heart cavities contain blood, then the diastolic pressures within them are raised as a consequence of the rise in intrapleural pressure. The increase in intrathoracic vascular pressures gives rise to very considerable disturbance of the circulation.

POOLING OF BLOOD IN THE PERIPHERAL VASCULAR BEDS

At the start of pressure breathing, the rise in intrapleural pressure is transmitted directly to the large intrathoracic veins and the right atrium, with a consequent rise in central venous pressure. Since the pressure in the extra-thoracic veins normally is low, the flow of blood from the periphery of the body into the chest is impeded severely, and the venous outflow from the limbs ceases completely. Overall venous return to the heart does not stop altogether at the beginning of pressure breathing, since there is a maintained flow of blood from the brain and the abdominal viscera. The flow of blood from the abdomen continues, since the intra-abdominal pressure rises in parallel with that in the pleural space. Venous return and thus right atrial filling normally are aided by the reduction of intrathoracic pressure below atmospheric pressure that occurs during inspiration. Since intrathoracic pressure is above atmospheric throughout the breathing cycle during pressure breathing, this assistance to venous return and cardiac filling is impeded. The jugular venous blood flow, however, is maintained because of the indistensibility of the intracranial vascular bed.

The veins of the limbs, especially the legs, act as large capacitance vessels, and with continuing arterial outflow from the heart during pressure breathing, the veins distend with an increasing volume of blood. This increase in volume is accompanied by an increase in peripheral venous pressure, until once again peripheral venous pressure exceeds central venous (right atrial) pressure and venous return from these capacitance vessels recommences (Figure 4.6). This initial phase of very marked reduction in venous return to the heart lasts for 10–20 seconds.

The circulation through the limbs is maintained during pressure breathing by displacement of blood from within the trunk into the limbs. The amount of blood thus displaced is determined by the increase in venous pressure and the distensibility of the vessels of the limbs. One of the reflex cardiovascular changes that occur during pressure breathing is active constriction of the peripheral veins, which tends to reduce the amount of blood displaced from within the trunk. The amount of blood displaced into the limbs of a seated subject at the onset of pressure breathing at 30 mmHg (4 kPa) is of the order of 200 ml, and at 80 mmHg (10.7 kPa) it is 400 ml (Figure 4.7).

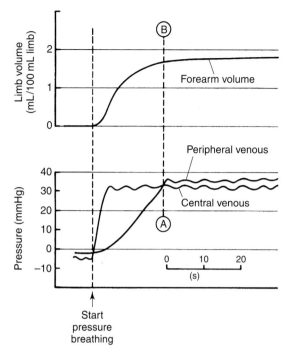

Figure 4.6 *Effect of pressure breathing at 40 mmHg with trunk counter-pressure on peripheral and central venous pressures and volume of the forearm. The central venous pressure rises rapidly to a plateau value determined by the breathing pressure. The rise of the central venous pressure raises it above the peripheral venous pressure, and the flow of blood from the limb to the heart ceases. Since arterial inflow continues, blood accumulates in the peripheral vascular bed, increasing the volume of the limb (top trace) and progressively raising the peripheral venous pressure. When the capacity vessels in the limb are distended, the peripheral venous pressure once again exceeds central venous pressure (at point A–B), so that venous outflow recommences and the volume of the limb stabilizes at a new greater value (continued increase of limb volume is due to accumulation of fluid in the tissues). For clarity, the cardiac fluctuations of venous pressure have been omitted.*

REDUCTION OF EFFECTIVE BLOOD VOLUME

The volume of blood that is available for circulatory adjustment is reduced as a consequence of the reduction in venous return, with blood pooling outside the chest. Furthermore, this gives rise to an increase in the transmural pressure within the capillary vessels of the limbs relative to the local tissue pressure. That capillary pressure rises considerably can be demonstrated by the observation of petechial haemorrhages in unsupported areas of the skin. The balance that normally exists between hydrostatic and osmotic forces at the blood–tissue fluid interface in the capillary bed is disturbed, such that fluid moves from the intravascular compartment into the tissues at a rate determined by the increase in the capillary and, hence, venous pressure. Thus, pressure breathing at 30 mmHg (4 kPa) for ten minutes will result in the loss of about 250 ml of fluid from the circulation, while pressure breathing for five minutes at 100 mmHg (13.3 kPa) will result in a loss of 500 ml of fluid into the tissues and concomitant haemoconcentration (Figure 4.7).

The total reduction in effective blood volume over time that occurs as a result of these two factors (i.e. initial pooling of blood and decrease in intravascular fluid) during pressure breathing at 30 mmHg (4 kPa) for ten minutes causes a loss in the order of 450 ml. Pressure breathing at 100 mmHg (13.3 kPa) for five minutes results in a net reduction of the effective blood volume of about 950 ml. It is not surprising, therefore, that some of the physiological responses to pressure breathing, as described below, are similar in nature to the effects of acute haemorrhage. In addition to the changes in the systemic circulation, there are also changes in the pulmonary circulation. Radiographic examinations of the chest during pressure breathing have shown a reduction in pulmonary vascular markings, due to a reduction in pulmonary blood volume, with a net shift to the systemic circulation and a reduction

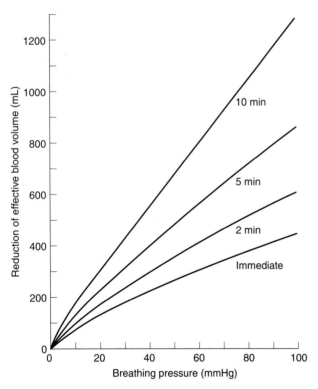

Figure 4.7 *Effects of pressure breathing with counter-pressure to the trunk on reduction of effective blood volume in seated subjects. The reduction of blood volume due to displacement of blood into the peripheral capacity vessels is indicated by the curve labelled 'Immediate'. The subsequent further reductions of effective blood volume due to loss of fluid into the tissues are indicated for pressure breathing for two, five and ten minutes.*

in heart size. Overall, the loss of circulating blood may be minimized by the application of counter-pressure, particularly over the capacitance vessels in the limbs, and this principle is used in the design of partial-pressure clothing, as described in Chaper 5.

INCREASE IN HEART RATE

Pressure breathing gives rise to a tachycardia unrelated to any effect of anxiety or anticipation. Broadly, the increase in heart rate above resting levels has been related directly to the magnitude of the applied breathing pressure, although this is mitigated to a significant extent if counter-pressure is applied to the trunk and limbs. Nonetheless, the onset of pressure breathing is associated with an immediate acceleration of the heart, often with a progressive increase in the rate throughout the period of raised breathing pressure. Hypoxia itself will, of course, cause a rise in heart rate and in combination with pressure breathing the effects can be additive. Thus, in one study, pressure breathing of 30 mmHg at ground level (with counter-pressure applied over the trunk and legs) increased heart rate, on average, by 5–10 beats/min; at 45 000 feet, the same magnitude of pressure breathing was associated with an increase in rate of 14–20 beats/min. However, in some instances, pressure breathing has been associated with heart rates in excess of 150 beats/min. The mechanism underlying the rapid change in heart rate may be mediated by receptors in the atria and great veins detecting a sharp reduction in venous return and right atrial filling.

REDUCTION IN CARDIAC OUTPUT

The pooling of blood in the periphery leads to a lowering of the effective pressure in the right atrium and, as described above, a sustained reduction in venous return. There is, therefore, a reduction in atrial filling and, consequently, in stroke volume. Even in the presence of tachycardia, cardiac output is not maintained at its normal levels. During pressure breathing at 30 mmHg (4 kPa) without trunk counter-pressure, the cardiac output is reduced by about 30 per cent compared with the resting value. If, however, trunk counter-pressure is applied, then the same degree of pressure breathing reduces the cardiac output by only 15–20 per cent. It could be expected that a greater level of counter-pressure would mitigate still further the fall in cardiac output during pressure breathing.

RISE IN ARTERIAL BLOOD PRESSURE

When a high-altitude rapid decompression initiates pressure breathing, the onset is very swift and associated with an immediate rise in arterial blood pressure. The blood pressure waveform is modified somewhat, however, becoming sharper in profile as the heart rate increases and the dicrotic notch tends to become more prominent. The immediate changes in the arterial pressure wave are similar to those observed when a subject carries out a Valsalva manoeuvre, but after the first few seconds the blood pressure will stabilize at an elevated level, although pulse pressure tends to show an exaggerated variability with respiration.

Blood pressure is raised during pressure breathing, primarily as a result of the transmission of the raised intrapleural pressure to the blood within the left ventricle. If cardiac output and peripheral vascular resistance were constant and no baroreceptor-mediated response to pressure breathing occurred, the pressure within the left ventricle would be increased by an amount equal to the rise in pleural pressure. This rise in intraventricular pressure would be reflected in the systemic arterial blood pressure. In fact, neither cardiac output nor peripheral resistance remain unchanged, and the reduction in cardiac output during pressure breathing will tend to reduce the rise in arterial blood pressure. This effect is counteracted partially by active constriction of the peripheral resistance vessels, the arterioles.

The net rise in arterial blood pressure that occurs in pressure breathing is an expression of the integrated effects of reflexes, including the compensatory circulatory adjustments that occur in this condition, i.e. the increase in heart rate and constriction of arterioles and veins. These reflex circulatory adjustments probably result from the stimulation of volume receptors in the right side of the heart, produced by the displacement of blood from the central part of the circulation into the periphery, and baroreceptor influences, which modify further the observed response. An elevation of arterial blood pressure will be detected in the carotid baroreceptors as an increase in transmural pressure, unless an equal counter-pressure is applied to prevent the walls of these vessels being stretched. This would, therefore, stimulate reflexes to lower blood pressure. Conversely, the intrathoracic baroreceptors of the aortic arch would be exposed to the increase in intrapleural pressure and unless the rise in arterial pressure was equal to that elevated intrapleural pressure, these baroreceptors would be less distended than normal and, through a reduction in their tonic discharge, in effect, signal a fall in blood pressure. This complex series of reflexes can be examined further by studying the influence of counter-pressure on the responses, as described below. It is sufficient to note in this context, however, that when pressure breathing is carried out wearing an oronasal mask (and, hence, when carotid baroreceptors are unsupported), the observed rise in blood pressure associated with a specific breathing pressure is less than when a pressure helmet is used, since with the latter, counter-pressure is applied to the anterior triangle of the neck and thus over the carotid baroreceptors.

It can be useful to consider the degree to which blood pressure rises as a result of pressure breathing as a proportion of the applied breathing pressure. Expressed as a ratio of increased blood pressure (δBP) and breathing pressure (PPB), if no attenuation of the applied pressure occurred, then the resulting arterial blood pressure would be the simple sum of the resting blood pressure and the increased breathing pressure, giving a ratio of 1. In fact, during pressure breathing at 30 mmHg (4 kPa), the rise in mean arterial blood pressure is commonly of the order of 15–20 mmHg (2–2.7 kPa), i.e. a δBP/PPB ratio of 0.5–0.7. The application of counter-pressure to the chest, abdomen, limbs and the head and neck can influence the blood pressure response to pressure breathing. Essentially, the greater the area of counter-pressure, the better the circulatory support provided. Then, the ratio as described above will more closely approach 1. The mechanisms involved are outlined below.

Although the elevation of arterial pressure by pressure breathing may be seen as a side effect of its use to improve protection against hypoxia, this response is the basis of the use of pressure breathing as a means of enhancing tolerance of $+G_z$ acceleration. The physiological mechanisms of this application of pressure breathing are discussed in Chapter 8.

PRESSURE BREATHING SYNCOPE

Cardiac output is maintained during the first 10–15 seconds following the onset of pressure breathing by the venous return from the abdomen and head, as described above. If, after that time, the breathing pressure applied to the respiratory tract remains very high (e.g. 80–100 mmHg), and if no counter-pressure is applied to the trunk, then the reduction in venous return may be so severe that the arterial blood pressure falls and consciousness may be lost within 10–15 seconds. Normally, however, the venous return to the heart is adequate to maintain a reasonable, albeit reduced, cardiac output; this, together with peripheral vasoconstriction, helps to maintain the elevated arterial blood pressure already described. Under these circumstances, there is no impairment of consciousness. If, however, pressure breathing is continued for long enough, circulatory integrity cannot be maintained and collapse occurs. The length of time that elapses before syncope occurs during pressure breathing depends primarily on the pressure that is applied to the respiratory tract and the external support of the circulation by counter-pressure assemblies. Thus, most subjects can breathe at 30 mmHg (4 kPa) for 10–20 minutes without syncope, and some may tolerate considerably longer. In one study, less than ten per cent of subjects became presyncopal after two minutes of pressure breathing at 70 mmHg (9.3 kPa) with counter-pressure applied to the trunk and lower limbs, but collapse occurred almost invariably after two minutes of breathing at a pressure of 100 mmHg (13.3 kPa) with trunk counter-pressure alone. Although studies have shown a much greater tolerance of pressure breathing in recumbent subjects, as would be expected, this is of limited value for operational aircrew following a rapid decompression of the cockpit at very high altitude. The variability of individual susceptibility may be related to a number of factors, but the likelihood of syncope during pressure breathing may be increased by hypoxia, hypocapnia, anxiety, discomfort, pain, intercurrent infection and the post-alcoholic state. In all cases, however, the symptoms and signs are very similar, and pressure-breathing collapse has the following features:

- nausea and uneasiness
- dimming of vision
- intense facial pallor
- profuse facial and palmar sweating
- loss of consciousness
- loss of postural tone
- jerky movements of limbs (occasionally major epileptiform convulsions).

The feeling of nausea and facial pallor persist for some time after consciousness returns, frequently for several hours.

Pressure-breathing syncope is accompanied by gross changes in the circulatory system. The onset of collapse is heralded by a progressive increase in heart rate and a gradual fall in the arterial blood pressure. A sudden profound bradycardia occurs, arterial blood pressure falls precipitously, and unconsciousness follows within five to ten seconds. When the pressure breathing is stopped the arterial blood pressure increases slowly over the next 30–60 seconds. The heart rate also increases, although both heart rate and arterial blood pressure may remain below resting level for as long as an hour (Figure 4.8).

Pressure-breathing collapses have many of the features of fainting of other causes, such as haemorrhage and pain. The prime cause of the sudden profound hypotension that occurs in fainting is dilation of the arterioles in muscles. The cardiac output, which usually falls in the period preceding syncope, does not decrease further when the faint occurs and thus does not contribute to the fall in arterial pressure. The disturbances of cerebral function are due to the reduction in cerebral blood flow consequent to the fall in arterial pressure. In pressure breathing syncope, the extreme peripheral arteriolar vasodilation that occurs in muscle probably is produced by vasodilator fibres of the sympathetic outflow. The nausea, abdominal discomfort, facial pallor and skin vasoconstriction are probably humoral in origin (during and following a faint, there is an increase in the secretion of antidiuretic hormone). The receptors and afferent pathways in pressure breathing syncope are, in all probability, the same as those that are responsible for syncope due to loss of blood (50 per cent of semi-reclining subjects will faint after about 1100 ml of blood has been withdrawn by venesection). The stimulus in this type of syncope may be the reduction in the intrathoracic blood volume and a sharp fall in the volume of blood in the right ventricle.

The afferent impulses responsible for initiating the cardiovascular changes (bradycardia, muscle arteriolar vasodilation, secretion of antidiuretic hormone) almost certainly arise from receptors in the walls of the right atrium and ventricle. In trained subjects, the degree by which the effective blood volume must be reduced to produce pressure-breathing syncope (about 800 ml) is similar to that which will cause fainting by venesection.

Effects of pressure breathing on the head and neck

Although the most significant physiological disturbances associated with pressure breathing may principally affect the respiratory and cardiovascular systems, the symptomatic consequences of breathing at pressures greater than ambient may be felt most clearly in the head and neck. The most common method of delivering to the respiratory

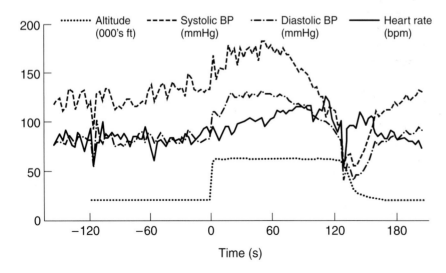

Figure 4.8 *A graph of blood pressure and heart rate during a rapid decompression which shows a PPB induced syncope. Time zero represents the moment of rapid decompression. See also colour plate 4.8.*

tract breathing gas at pressures above ambient is by means of an oronasal mask. At high breathing pressures, certain drawbacks associated with the oronasal mask may be overcome by the use of a pressure helmet. These two methods of delivering oxygen at pressures greater than ambient are discussed below.

PRESSURE BREATHING WITH AN ORONASAL MASK

Using an oronasal mask, pressure is applied to the mouth and nose, with physical support given to only a limited area of the face. There are certain mechanical limitations to the pressure that may be delivered in this manner. Most oronasal masks in current use have a specially designed reflected edge seal, which, under increased mask cavity pressures, is pressed more closely to the face. This type of mask will, when fitted correctly, hold pressures of up to 100 mmHg (13.3 kPa) without significant leakage. In order to sustain this mask cavity pressure, the tension applied to the mask by means of the harness attaching it to the helmet must be such that it counterbalances the force tending to lift the mask off the face when the delivery pressure is raised. A force of almost 60 N is necessary to seal a pressure of 40 mmHg (5.3 kPa) in the type of Royal Air Force (RAF) pressure-demand oronasal mask illustrated in Figure 4.9. Since such a high tension is neither tolerable nor necessary during routine flight, a manual or automatic means of increasing the tension when required is incorporated in the suspension harness. In the mask illustrated (Figure 4.9)

this is achieved manually by rotating a toggle over the suspension bar in order to increase the tension in the chain harness.

In practice, however, well-defined physiological effects limit the pressure that can be delivered using an oronasal mask, since no external support is applied to the floor of the mouth or the neck, eyes or ears. These effects are as follows:

Distension of the upper respiratory passages commences when the breathing pressure exceeds 10 mmHg (1.3 kPa) and progresses so that with high breathing pressures, there is distension of the mouth, the whole of the pharynx and the cervical portion of the oesophagus. It therefore makes speech difficult and impedes communication between crew members and with ground controllers. At pressures greater than about 70 mmHg (9.3 kPa), this distortion causes severe discomfort in many people, which is the main limitation to the use of oronasal masks.

Increased intravascular pressure caused by the raised intrathoracic pressure dilates the conjunctival vessels. At breathing pressures above 70–80 mmHg (9.3–10.7 kPa), the conjunctival capillaries may rupture. In contrast, the retinal vessels may constrict as a result of hypocapnia induced by the PPB. Intraocular pressure increases as breathing pressure rises. It is likely that this change in intraocular pressure provides some protection to retinal vessels during pressure breathing.

If the nasolacrimal ducts are open during pressure breathing, the gas passes directly into the conjunctival sacs, causing blepharospasm. The severity of this condition is

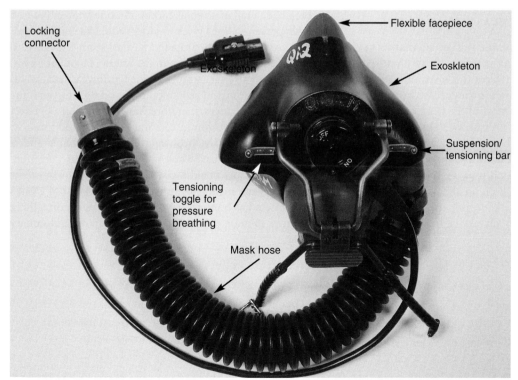

Figure 4.9 *Typical pressure-demand oronasal mask.*

related to the magnitude of the breathing pressure and, although it is uncommon below 70 mmHg, in a small proportion of people it may interfere seriously with vision.

In normal circumstances, the Eustachian tubes are occluded during pressure breathing by compression of the lower end of the tube at the pharynx. Unless the subject swallows during the exposure, the tympanic membrane remains in the normal position and auditory acuity is unchanged. Although it is difficult to swallow during pressure breathing, should it occur gas will pass up the Eustachian tube into the middle ear cavity. The ensuing rise in middle-ear pressure causes the tympanic membrane to bulge out into the external auditory canal, resulting in discomfort and reduced auditory acuity.

As pressure breathing is used as an emergency technique to provide short-duration protection against hypoxia at high altitudes, its onset coincides with rapid decompression and, hence, expansion of gas in the gastrointestinal tract. The high pressure in the oropharynx during PPB prevents the release of trapped gas from the gastric air and thus has the potential to cause upper-abdominal discomfort.

In summary, a suitable oronasal mask may be used to deliver pressures of up to 70–75 mmHg (9.3–10 kPa) to the respiratory tract, provided that the length of time for which the pressure is applied is short (i.e. about one to two minutes). Breathing for longer periods or higher pressures frequently gives rise to severe discomfort. On the other hand, a pressure of 30 mmHg (4 kPa) may be breathed for considerably longer without undue disturbance or discomfort, although even then pressure breathing is fatiguing.

PRESSURE BREATHING WITH A PRESSURE HELMET

A pressure helmet may be used as an alternative to the oronasal mask for delivering oxygen to the respiratory tract at pressures greater than that of the environment. Partial pressure helmets give support to the cheeks, the floor of the mouth and the eyes, and most of the head and the upper part of the neck are also pressurized. Thus, the pressure differentials that develop between the air passages and the skin of the head and neck when an oronasal mask is employed are eliminated and pressure breathing is symptomatically easier. In addition, no abnormal pressure differentials are applied to the vessels of the eyes. Some pressure helmets, however, do not increase the pressure in the external auditory meatus. Failure to provide counter-pressure to the outer aspect of the tympanic membrane in the presence of breathing pressures of 110–140 mmHg can be associated with rupture of the vessels in the outer layers of the membrane, giving rise to haemorrhagic bullae on its surface if a patent Eustachian tube allows the middle-ear cavity to become pressurized.

Acceptable degree of hypoxia

The pressure that must be delivered to the respiratory tract at a given altitude above 40 000 feet is determined by the degree of hypoxia that is acceptable. This is because two factors interact: from the point of view of preventing hypoxia, it is desirable to have a high breathing pressure, but from the point of view of the cardiovascular and respiratory stress imposed by pressure breathing, it is desirable to keep the breathing pressure low. Two aspects of the influence of hypoxia are of interest in the present context. The first relates to the general mental and physical performance of the individual and the second to the modifications of the cardiovascular and respiratory responses to pressure breathing that are induced by hypoxia.

A complicating feature is the fact that pressure breathing causes a certain degree of hyperventilation, even in trained subjects, and if the alveolar oxygen tension is less than 60 mmHg (8 kPa), then there is an additional stimulus to increase ventilation. The arterial carbon dioxide tension therefore is usually reduced markedly during pressure breathing at altitude. When 100 per cent oxygen is breathed, a fall in alveolar carbon dioxide tension (caused by hyperventilation) gives rise to an equal increase in alveolar oxygen tension. Initially, it may seem therefore to increase the oxygen tension in the arterial blood; however, the lowered arterial carbon dioxide tension causes cerebral vasoconstriction and reduction of blood flow through the brain. These changes, therefore, have a negligible net effect on the oxygen tension in cerebral tissue. Furthermore, as discussed previously, hypocapnia has undesirable effects on the circulation as a whole and renders the subject more liable to pressure breathing syncope.

The general mental and physical performance of groups of subjects has been determined while pressure breathing for two to four minutes with different intrapulmonary

Table 4.3 *Relationship between absolute intrapulmonary pressure and overall performance during pressure breathing*

Intrapulmonary pressure (mmHg absolute)	Equivalent altitude (ft)	Breathing pressure (mmHg)	Applied counter-pressure	Performance
141	40 000	0–141	Trunk and lower limbs	No significant impairment
130	41 600	0–70	Trunk and lower limbs	Mild impairment
120	43 300	0–60	Trunk only	Mild to moderate impairment
115	44 300	0–30	None	Moderate to severe impairment

pressures at various altitudes. The results of these studies are summarized in Table 4.3.

When significant hypoxia is present (alveolar oxygen tension < 60 mmHg, 8 kPa), the cardiovascular responses to pressure breathing are modified in that the tachycardia and increase in arterial blood pressure are greater. The most striking effect of hypoxia during pressure breathing is, however, the increased incidence of syncope. Thus, hypoxia during pressure breathing results in impaired performance and an increased risk of syncope. The effects of varying degrees of hypoxia when different degrees of body counter-pressure are applied have been investigated thoroughly. The results of these investigations have led to the development of various partial pressure systems, which are discussed in the following chapter.

FURTHER READING

Air Standardization Coordinating Committee. Minimum physiological requirements for aircrew demand breathing systems. Air Standard 61/101/06A. Air Standardization Coordinating Committee, 2000.

Ernsting J. The ideal relationship between inspired oxygen concentration and cabin altitude. *Aerospace Medicine* 1963; **34**: 991–7.

Ernsting J. Some effects of raised intrapulmonary pressure. AGARDograph 106. Maidenhead: Technivision, 1966.

Ernsting J. Prevention of hypoxia-acceptable compromises. *Aviation, Space, and Environmental Medicine* 1978; **49**: 495–502.

Ernsting J. Operational and physiological requirements for aircraft oxygen systems. In: AGARD Seventh Advanced Operational Aviation Medicine Course. AGARD report No. 697. Neuilly-sur-Seine: AGARD/NATO, 1983.

Ernsting J, Millar RL. Advanced oxygen systems for aircraft. AGARDograph 286. Neuilly-sur-Seine: AGARD/NATO, 1996.

Gradwell DP. The experimental assessment of new partial pressure assemblies. AGARD-CP-516. Neuilly-sur-Seine: AGARD/NATO, 1991.

Gradwell DP. Human physiological responses to positive pressure breathing for high altitude protection. PhD thesis, University of London, 1993.

Gradwell DP. Pressure breathing inflation schedules/ratios. Presented at Raising the Operational Ceiling AL/CF-SR-1995-0021. Armstrong Laboratory, Brooks Air Force Base, Texas, 13–15 June 1995.

Harding RM. Human respiratory responses during high performance flight. AGARDograph 312. Neuilly-sur-Seine: AGARD/NATO, 1987.

Lindelis AE, Fraser WD, Fowler B. Performance during positive pressure breathing after rapid decompression. *Human Factors* 1997; **39**: 102–10.

Morgan TR, Reid DH, Baumgardner FW. Pulmonary ventilation requirements evident in the operation of representative high performance aircraft. In: *Proceedings of 47th Annual Scientific Meeting of the Aerospace Medical Association*, 1970; p. 158.

Ryles MT, Perez-Becerra JL. The effect of positive pressure breathing for altitude protection on intraocular pressure. *Aviation, Space, and Environmental Medicine* 1996; **67**: 1179–84.

5

Oxygen equipment and pressure clothing

DAVID P. GRADWELL

INTRODUCTION

Previous chapters have described the nature of hypobaric hypoxia and physiological considerations associated with its prevention. This chapter is concerned with the way in which those physiological factors can be met in practice; it also addresses additional aspects associated with other, more general requirements of airborne oxygen systems. It is obviously essential in meeting these additional needs that no unacceptable physiological consequences occur.

The development of airborne oxygen systems in fixed-wing aircraft dates from the First World War, and over the following decades systems have evolved from crude and unreliable devices to sophisticated items of advanced technology. The differing needs of military combat and commercial passenger aircraft, and the influence of different degrees of cabin pressurization, have implications for the design of appropriate oxygen systems. Major developments commonly have been driven by the requirement to enhance the facilities and protection offered to the crew of military combat aircraft, and such improvements have thereafter been adapted for use in civil aircraft. In all cases, the primary purpose is to ensure that the user is protected adequately from hypoxia.

National military and civil aviation authorities usually set out under various regulations or statutes the minimum acceptable provision of oxygen to be carried on board aircraft registered in that state or country. In aircraft with low-differential pressure cabins (i.e. with a cabin altitude greater than 8000 feet, such as small military combat aircraft), personal oxygen equipment is worn routinely and used by the aircrew throughout flight. The definition and performance of such systems in military aircraft are addressed in relevant military documentation, e.g. Defence Standards and Military Specifications. For commercial aircraft registered in the USA, the Federal Aviation Administration (FAA) sets out the requirement for oxygen in various classes of aircraft under FAA Regulations (FARs parts 25, 121 and 135). In the UK, Schedule 4 of the Air Navigation Order (2000) requires that equipment that will deliver oxygen-enriched air or 100 per cent oxygen to the crew be installed in all commercial aircraft that fly above an altitude of 10 000 feet. Furthermore, if the aircraft is capable of maintaining its cabin altitude below 10 000 feet, then oxygen must be available in sufficient quantity to supply all crew members and passengers in the event of a failure of pressurization above 15 000 feet, and to supply all crew members and ten per cent of the passengers if pressurization fails below 13 000 feet. In all other aircraft, i.e. in those that fly unpressurized, sufficient oxygen must be carried for continuous use by all occupants whenever the aircraft is flying above 12 000 feet and for continuous use by the crew and ten per cent of the passengers for any period in excess of 30 minutes during which the aircraft flies between 10 000 and 12 000 feet. In aircraft with high-differential pressure cabins, i.e. with a cabin altitude below about 8000 feet at all times during routine flight, such as passenger aircraft and large military transport or bomber aircraft, such equipment is used only if the cabin altitude exceeds safe limits, although emergency therapeutic oxygen may be required by ill passengers at low cabin altitudes (see Chapter 54).

GENERAL CLASSES OF OXYGEN SYSTEMS

Oxygen-delivery systems may be classified into two major groups: those in which the expired gas is rebreathed (closed-circuit systems) and those in which the expired gas is dispersed to the environment (open-circuit systems). Conventional aircraft, both military and civil, employ the latter almost exclusively.

Closed-circuit oxygen systems

Oxygen is extracted from inspired gas to meet the metabolic needs of tissue oxygenation, but this demand can be met at sea level by a relatively small proportion of inspired minute ventilation. It is for this reason that the 16 per cent oxygen in expired gas (cf. 21 per cent in inspired air) is adequate to support life at sea level, as demonstrated by its use in mouth-to-mouth resuscitation techniques. Thus, considerable savings in the rate of consumption of an oxygen supply can be achieved if expired air is rebreathed from a closed circuit after removal of carbon dioxide.

This benefit, however, decreases with altitude, and there are at least four other potentially serious disadvantages of such a system. The first is the need to control the flow of oxygen into the circuit. Automation of this is difficult and complicated. The second problem is freezing: the expired and frequently the inspired gases in a closed circuit are saturated with water vapour, and so ice may occlude hoses and valves if the cabin temperature falls below 0 °C. The third problem is accumulation of nitrogen: an inboard leakage of air as a result of, for example, an ill-fitting mask will lead to a progressive increase in the concentration of nitrogen in the circuit and eventually to hypoxia. The risk of freezing may be overcome by electrical heating of critical components, and a slight overpressure in the system (safety pressure) may be imposed to ensure that any leakages are outboard; however, all of this adds to the complexity of the system. The fourth major disadvantage is the need to remove carbon dioxide. Chemical absorbers, such as barium and lithium hydroxide, can be used, but these are heavy and have to be renewed frequently. Carbon-dioxide-permeable membranes have been developed, and these could reduce considerably the bulk and inconvenience of the purification hardware, but they have not yet been seen in airborne oxygen systems.

These problems, therefore, have resulted in closed-circuit systems being used very infrequently in conventional aviation. One exception is in some forms of smoke hood for use in the event of aircraft fires. A number of systems are available that incorporate a gas cylinder containing either air or oxygen and some form of carbon dioxide absorber. Such devices are relatively simple to operate but may become hot, may be cumbersome to use and may affect vision and hearing adversely. For these reasons, they have been reserved for use by trained crew rather than passengers.

Closed-circuit oxygen systems are employed widely in anaesthetic, fire-fighting and underwater breathing equipment. They are mandatory in manned spaceflight programmes during extra-vehicular activity in which the astronauts have to carry all their consumables.

Open-circuit oxygen systems

Open-circuit oxygen systems are those in which most or all of the expired gas exhausts to the environment. These types are encountered most commonly in aviation, and the remainder of this chapter is devoted to them and the associated equipment.

Although relatively wasteful of breathing gas, an open-circuit system has the considerable merit, especially in military aviation, of simplicity. There are two main types of such systems: those in which oxygen flows from the supply source throughout the respiratory cycle (continuous flow systems) and those in which oxygen flows only during inspiration (demand flow systems). In both types, flow to the user from the source passes through a crucial component, the regulator, which essentially governs the delivery behaviour of the entire system. The major disadvantage of continuous-flow systems is that the flow of gas from the regulator has to be preset and thus cannot vary in response to the respiratory demand of the user. This disadvantage is overcome in demand systems, where the flow of gas from the regulator varies directly with inspiratory demand. Although a demand regulator is inherently more complex than a regulator providing a continuous flow, it can provide the additional automatic facilities required of oxygen equipment fitted to aircraft operating at high altitudes. Accordingly, high-performance combat aircraft are equipped with open-circuit demand oxygen systems, as are the flight decks of commercial and military transport aircraft.

OXYGEN SYSTEM REQUIREMENTS

The requirements of an adequate oxygen system can be considered under two principle interrelated categories: physiological and general.

Physiological requirements

The physiological requirements of oxygen systems were described in the previous chapter. They are:

- adequate concentration of oxygen
- adequate concentration of nitrogen
- adequate flow capacity with minimal (added external) resistance
- disposal of expirate.

General requirements

SAFETY PRESSURE

The system should maintain the desired alveolar oxygen tension even in the presence of potential inboard leakage, such as may result from an inadequate seal between the edge of the mask and the skin of the face. This requirement may be met by providing a slight but continuous overpressure in the mask (safety pressure), at least at altitudes above 12 000–15 000 feet, or by enrichment of the gas delivered to the mask, or both.

PROTECTION AGAINST TOXIC FUMES AND DECOMPRESSION SICKNESS

The user must be able to select 100 per cent oxygen manually at any cabin altitude in the event that toxic fumes or smoke contaminate the cockpit. This is especially the case when ambient cockpit air is used as the diluent of 100 per cent oxygen from the aircraft oxygen store. When decompression sickness is liable to develop or symptoms have occurred, the individual should breathe 100 per cent oxygen, and therefore it is necessary to prevent mixing of oxygen with air. The method of delivery must be such as to minimize any inboard leakage of cabin air because of an ill-fitting mask, and it is clear that the requirement for protection against toxic fumes and decompression sickness is interdependent on the provision of safety pressure.

APPROPRIATE TEMPERATURE

The inspired gas should be neither too warm nor too cold for comfort, and its temperature should therefore be within 5 °C of cockpit environmental temperature. In practice, no active method is used to achieve this requirement; reliance is placed on equilibration of temperature during passage of the breathing gas through delivery pipework within the cockpit.

CONVENIENCE

The operation of the system should, as far as possible, be automatic. Ideally, the user should be required only to don a mask (or pressure helmet) and connect it to the remainder of the system. Similarly, facilities such as safety pressure and pressure breathing should be provided automatically. The drills to cope with failures of the system should be simple.

EVALUATION OF INTEGRITY

The equipment should be designed so that it is immediately apparent to the user that there has been either a failure of the system or appropriate drills have not been carried out correctly. For example, it should not be possible for the pilot of a combat aircraft to breathe through the mask until it has been connected, correctly, to the rest of the system or for the pilot to take off without having turned on the oxygen supply. One satisfactory means of achieving such a requirement is to ensure that inspiratory resistance through the mask is high until it is connected to the system and the oxygen supply is turned on.

The user must also be able to confirm the adequacy of the seal of the mask both before and during flight. This requirement usually is met by providing a manual means of selecting some degree of positive-pressure breathing at any altitude (the press-to-test facility).

INDICATION OF SUPPLY AND FLOW

The user must have a positive indication of oxygen flow and, where appropriate, a display of the quantity of stored oxygen so that they can monitor the correct function of the oxygen system.

INDICATION OF FAILURE

In aircraft where the personal oxygen system provides the primary protection against hypoxia, any failure of the equipment that might lead to that condition must be indicated immediately and clearly to the user. Such warnings may be objective, as for example in the illumination of a low-pressure warning light, or subjective, as in an increase in inspiratory resistance on inadvertent disconnection of a supply hose.

DUPLICATION

In aircraft with low-differential pressure cabins, in which the personal oxygen system provides the primary protection against hypoxia, a degree of redundancy in the delivery system is essential. Thus, many modern oxygen regulators have a secondary regulator or a standby operating mode that can be selected if the primary regulator fails. In addition, an alternative oxygen supply should be provided in case the main supply system fails or the store becomes depleted. Such an alternative usually takes the form of a small independent source of oxygen (emergency oxygen (EO) or backup oxygen system, BOS) together with an independent delivery regulator. The volume of oxygen contained in such an emergency supply is generally based on the assumption that failure of the main supply will be followed by selection of EO and an immediate descent to below 10 000 feet. However, in systems incorporating a molecular sieve oxygen concentrator (MSOC; see below), a larger backup oxygen store may be appropriate to allow for temporary cessation of the main supply resulting, for example, from jet engine flameout.

There is no requirement for such a secondary oxygen supply in aircraft with high-differential pressure cabins, where the cabin itself provides the primary protection against hypoxia and oxygen equipment is used only if cabin pressurization fails or if toxic fumes contaminate the cabin.

PROTECTION DURING HIGH-ALTITUDE ESCAPE

In military aircraft from which abandonment at high altitude is a possibility, a separate oxygen supply is needed to protect the escapee. Clearly, the equipment must be stowed on the individual, in the parachute pack or on the seat itself in the case of assisted escape systems in which the crew member does not separate from the ejection seat until a low altitude is reached (10 000–15 000 feet). The quantity of oxygen contained in this supply must be sufficient to prevent significant hypoxia during freefall descent or until crew member–seat separation. In most military aircraft, the bail-out oxygen supply mounted on the ejection seat also serves as the secondary oxygen supply (EO or BOS) described above.

INDEPENDENCE FROM THE ENVIRONMENT

Oxygen equipment must perform satisfactorily under all the environmental extremes that may be met in flight. These inevitably include pressure changes and extremes of temperature, especially cold. With regard to the latter, the equipment must function normally after prolonged expo-

sure to temperatures as low as $-26\,^{\circ}C$ in an aircraft on the ground and to the even lower temperatures likely after a serious failure of cabin pressurization at high altitude (down to $-56\,^{\circ}C$). In combat aircraft, the mask or pressure helmet must not be displaced from the face or head by exposure to the maximum sustained accelerations (G forces) produced by the aircraft in normal flight or by exposure to the accelerations and windblast (Q forces) associated with an escape while flying at high speed. Furthermore, the mask valves must continue to function normally under such conditions.

UNDERWATER BREATHING

Aircraft that ditch in water usually sink rapidly. Therefore, oxygen equipment frequently is designed to provide breathing gas down to a certain depth (generally 30 m), and some air forces also require the bail-out oxygen supply to protect an individual who has entered water after a parachute descent.

ECONOMY OF WEIGHT, BULK AND COST

The weight and bulk (and cost) of military aircraft installations are critical logistic design features and so must be minimized within the constraints of safety. This is particularly so with regard to conventional oxygen storage systems. Clearly, therefore, physiological requirements should not be met at the expense of wastefully high flows of oxygen. For equally sound ground-logistic reasons, however, too frequent replenishment must not be necessary.

OXYGEN EQUIPMENT

Figure 5.1 lists the various general components of a typical oxygen system. This section describes each of these in turn.

Oxygen sources

Oxygen may be obtained from a store that is replenished while the aircraft is on the ground or it may be produced as required in flight by some physicochemical means. In storage, it may exist as a gas under high pressure, as a liquid at low temperature under moderate pressure, or as a solid in inert chemical combination. Both gaseous and liquid oxygen stores are in common use in military aviation, while gaseous oxygen is commonly the preferred medium for the emergency store on board commercial aircraft. Solid oxygen stores are also used in commercial aircraft, particularly as the emergency supply for passenger use in the event of loss of cabin pressurization. Finally, several methods of concentrating oxygen on board an aircraft, from an air source, have been actively investigated;

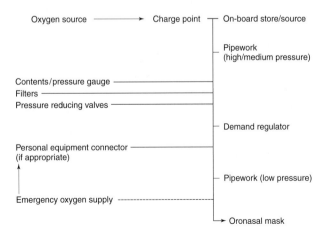

Figure 5.1 *Generic components of typical oxygen systems.*

one of these methods – the MSOC – has been installed successfully in many modern combat aircraft.

For rechargeable systems, whatever the source of breathing oxygen, the quality of the gas to be supplied must be of a high standard. It must contain at least 99.5 per cent oxygen and be odourless and virtually free of any toxic substances, e.g. the carbon monoxide concentration must be less than 0.002 per cent. The maximum allowable levels for various hydrocarbons are specified in relation to the type of storage used, since this will influence the potential contamination hazard. In order to avoid the risk of ice formation at low temperatures, the stored oxygen must also be very dry: the water content must not exceed 0.005 mg/l at 0 °C and 760 mmHg (101.3 kPa), i.e. under standard temperature and pressure (STP) conditions.

GASEOUS OXYGEN STORAGE

Gaseous oxygen usually is carried in steel cylinders at a pressure of 1800 lb/in² (12 411 kPa), although a low-pressure (450 lb/in², 3103 kPa) storage system is still employed in some aircraft and a high-pressure (5000 lb/in², 34 475 kPa) facility has been used in combat aircraft in an attempt to overcome some of the disadvantages of liquid oxygen (LOX). The capacities of cylinders commonly used in aircraft vary between 400 and 2250 litres (NTP) of oxygen when charged fully to 1800 lb/in² (12 411 kPa).

The aircraft cylinders are charged from large trolley-mounted cylinders, filled with oxygen at a maximum pressure of 3600 lb/in² (24 822 kPa), through a connection, fitted with a sealing cap and an on/off valve, mounted at or just beneath the outer skin of the aircraft. The pressure and flow of gas into the aircraft system are controlled by a regulating device on the charging trolley, while the quantity of oxygen on board is indicated by a cockpit pressure gauge connected to the main high-pressure supply pipework. A duplicate pressure gauge is often fitted at the charging point, and both gauges usually are graduated in fractions of 'full'. The pressure in a gaseous oxygen storage system normally should not be allowed to fall to ambient, thus preventing moisture from entering the system. The risk of water collecting in storage cylinders is also reduced by regular purging of the entire system, including pipework, with dry gas.

The size and number of cylinders installed, usually outside the pressure cabin, clearly will depend on the type of aircraft and its flight endurance. In military aircraft, the cylinders frequently are wire-wound to minimize shattering if hit by a projectile. The pipework connecting the cylinders to the delivery system is usually duplicated and, where two or more cylinders are installed, contains non-return valves arranged in such a way that a leak from one cylinder or junction will lead to only a partial loss of oxygen. The pressure of the oxygen is decreased by the use of reducing valves from the storage pressure to that required at the inlet to the demand valve, commonly between 70 and 200 lb/in² (483–1380 kPa).

Gaseous oxygen storage systems have several important advantages over other forms. They are relatively simple in construction and therefore inherently more reliable, gaseous oxygen is readily available worldwide, the on-board supply is available for use immediately after charging, and no gas is lost when the system is not in use. Even the gauging of the contents of a gaseous store is simpler than a liquid store. The major disadvantage, however, is that they are heavy and bulky. Table 5.1 illustrates this by comparing typical weights and overall volumes of different types of oxygen storage system.

Despite these logistic penalties, gaseous oxygen storage is the system of choice when weight and bulk are not at a great premium or when the supply is intended only for use in an emergency (and consequently is relatively small). Thus, gaseous oxygen storage commonly is used in the emergency supply to the crew and passengers on large transport aircraft and as the emergency and bail-out supplies in combat aircraft. In addition, portable and therapeutic systems generally are supplied from a small gaseous oxygen storage cylinder.

LIQUID OXYGEN STORAGE

For many years, LOX storage was the mainstay of military combat aircraft oxygen systems. This arose from its ability to yield 840 litres (NTP) of gaseous oxygen for each 1 litre of liquid oxygen, an expansion ratio almost seven times greater than that for gaseous oxygen stored at 1800 lb/in² (12 411 kPa). In addition, the low pressure at which LOX can be held in its insulated container (typically at 70–115 lb/in², 483–793 kPa) markedly reduces the overall

Table 5.1 *Comparison of typical weights and overall volumes of oxygen storage/supply systems of various types. The figures for gaseous, liquid and solid chemical sources are for systems each yielding 3000 litres (NTP) of oxygen; yield figures for molecular sieve systems are not applicable*

Storage system	Weight of charged system (kg)	Space occupied by system (L)
High-pressure cylinders containing gas at 1800 lb/in²	19	52
Liquid oxygen converter containing 3.5 litres of liquid	8	25
Solid chemical generator containing sodium chlorate	12	10
Molecular sieve oxygen concentrator	19	20

weight of liquid oxygen storage devices when compared with gaseous oxygen cylinders (see Table 5.1). However, to achieve the liquid state, oxygen must be cooled to a temperature below −183 °C at normal atmospheric pressure, i.e. its vaporization point. Much of the LOX is wasted before use; furthermore, it is a difficult and potentially hazardous material to handle. LOX production plants have been subject to a number of serious fires, both on land and on aircraft carriers at sea. Therefore, although it remains in use, most of the latest generation of combat aircraft do not have LOX systems but use MSOCs. Nonetheless, the basic principles of LOX systems and their components are outlined below.

An aircraft LOX converter consists of an insulated container, control valves and connecting pipes (Figure 5.2). The converter may be installed permanently in the aircraft, or it may be removable so that there is a choice of either replacement or recharging in situ. The LOX is contained in a double-walled stainless-steel vessel with connections through its walls at top and bottom. The capacity of the vessel varies according to the total amount of gaseous oxygen required during flight, but typically it will be 3.5, 5, 10, 25 litres. The space between the vessel walls is evacuated to reduce convective and conductive heat transfer to the LOX to a minimum. Operation of a LOX converter takes place in three distinct phases:

1. *Filling phase:* when the charging hose from the ground LOX dispenser is first connected to the vessel, LOX passes into the container and evaporates. This evaporation cools the internal walls of the system, eventually to −183 °C. Evaporation then ceases and the container fills rapidly with liquid oxygen.

2. *Build-up phase:* after disconnection of the charging hose, the top and bottom of the vessel are connected by an uninsulated pipe. LOX is now able to flow from the bottom of the container into a pressure build-up coil, where it evaporates, and thence into the top of the vessel as a gas. The heat carried in by the gas warms the surface layer of the liquid so that its vapour pressure rises. This process continues until the pressure within the container reaches the operating pressure of the converter, i.e. 70–115 lb/in^2 (483–793 kPa). The pressure closing valve then shuts, and the flow of LOX into the pressure build-up coil ceases.

3. *Delivery:* when a demand is made upon the system, gas is drawn from the top of the container, via a pressure-opening valve, to the delivery supply line and so to the user. Should the demand be so great as to cause the pressure within the container to fall below its normal level, LOX again passes into the pressure build-up coil, where it evaporates and carries gas and heat back to the top of the vessel, thus restoring the normal operating pressure.

The insulation of a LOX converter is never absolute, so that its temperature and hence the pressure of its contents rise slowly. A relief valve is fitted to limit this pressure rise, and this opens at 20–30 lb/in^2 (138–207 kPa) above normal

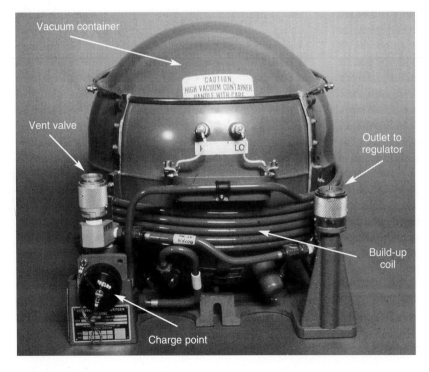

Figure 5.2 *Typical liquid oxygen converter of 10 L capacity.*

operating pressure. Such a pressure is usually attained 10–12 hours after filling, and thereafter up to ten per cent of the liquid is lost in a 24-hour period.

The amount of LOX in the vessel is monitored continuously by means of a probe immersed in the liquid and gaseous oxygen mixture, which measures the electrical capacitance between the two containing shells. The output of this capacitance probe is displayed in the cockpit and at the charging point for use during in situ refilling. The pressure at which gaseous oxygen is delivered to the main supply line is usually also displayed to the crew, or there may be a low-pressure warning device.

One major disadvantage of the simple converter described above is that any agitation of the vessel within six to eight hours of filling will produce a gross fall in delivery pressure as a result of a phenomenon termed temperature stratification. The agitation, which may be caused by the vibration of aerobatic manoeuvres or even while taxiing, disturbs the warm layer of liquid at the liquid–gas interface, so bringing colder layers of liquid into contact with the gas, which then condenses. Pressure consequently falls in the gaseous phase. This drawback may be overcome by adding sufficient heat to the contents of the container immediately after filling to raise the temperature of the liquid to that at which its vapour pressure equals its normal operating pressure; for liquid oxygen with a vapour pressure of 85 lb/in² abs (586 kPa), for example, the appropriate temperature would be −160 °C. The contents of the container are then said to be stabilized. The heat required for this stabilization is derived from the evaporation of LOX delivered to a separate, uninsulated container during the charging process. As soon as filling is complete, this liquid boils and the gas bubbles up through the liquid in the main container, condenses in so doing and heats all the liquid in the vessel to the required temperature, thus eliminating the temperature stratification. Stabilized LOX converters are installed mainly in combat aircraft.

The gaseous oxygen is warmed as it flows through the delivery pipework from the LOX converter into the pressure cabin and to the crew. This dictates that there must be either a minimum length of pipework to ensure that this warming can occur or a heat exchanger has to be incorporated in the system within the warm pressure cabin to ensure that the temperature of the gas delivery to the pilot meets the general requirement described above.

The transfer of LOX from the production plant to the aircraft is wasteful, complex and expensive. It is estimated that only 10–15 per cent of the LOX produced reaches a LOX converter in an aircraft.

A serious potential hazard of LOX is contamination by toxic materials, including the oxides of nitrogen and carbon, hydrogen sulphide and hydrocarbons. Such contamination is derived from the atmospheric air from which the LOX is produced, from plant compression and refrigeration equipment, and from storage, transport and other handling equipment. These contaminants do not evaporate at the same time as LOX, since usually they have higher boiling points, and so they can accumulate in the container. Eventually, particles or 'slugs' of contaminant may pass from the vessel into the warming coils, where they evaporate and may then be breathed by the user in relatively high concentrations. Great care must be taken therefore to eliminate the entry of contaminants during the manufacture and transfer of LOX; once in an aircraft converter, control must be exercised to ensure that the concentration of any contaminant remains very low. Routine infrared spectroscopy during ground replenishment is the preferred method used to monitor contamination.

The complexity of LOX systems results in a relatively high rate of failure of components. This and the other significant disadvantages noted above make LOX the storage method of choice only when the weight and bulk of the oxygen container must be as small as possible, and when oxygen is used routinely throughout flight, as in combat fighter aircraft. An additional benefit of the use of LOX converters in this role is that the container, essentially a vacuum flask, is unlikely to explode if punctured by enemy action.

ON-BOARD OXYGEN PRODUCTION

The need to replenish the oxygen store of an aircraft imposes considerable operational and logistic penalties on both military and civil aviation. There are also significant fire hazards associated with the production and replenishment of oxygen, especially during military operations. Because of these disadvantages, the on-board production of oxygen is obviously desirable, and several methods of so doing have been explored, with varying degrees of success. Developments towards that goal date back to the manned space programme of the 1960s. A number of different technologies have been pursued, but they may be divided conveniently into those that are dependent on a supply of compressed air and those that are not.

Air-independent systems

SOLID CHEMICAL OXYGEN GENERATION

When a mixture of sodium (or potassium) chlorate and finely divided iron is ignited, a proportion of the oxygen contained in the sodium chlorate molecule is released as gaseous oxygen, the reaction proceeding according to the equation

$$NaClO_3 + Fe = FeO + NaCl + O_2$$

The reaction is exothermic, so once the temperature of the reactants has been raised above 250 °C, it is self-generating. The proportion of iron in the mixture controls the temperature, speed of reaction and oxygen yield.

This chemical property has been used as the basis of devices that, when initiated, will produce oxygen rapidly. The sodium chlorate and iron powder are usually cast or pressed together with an inorganic binder such as fibreglass into a cylindrical mass termed a candle. The heat required to initiate the reaction is provided by a small iron-enriched zone at one end of the candle, which is activated by a percussion cap, an electric squib, a friction lighter or an electrically heated wire. The reaction proceeds at a temperature of 250–600 °C over the cross-sectional area of the candle, and oxygen is produced at a rate that is influenced by both the size of this area and the degree of insulation of the device. Thus, the desired oxygen flow–time relationship can be obtained by shaping the candle. Free chlorine, carbon monoxide and carbon dioxide may all contaminate oxygen produced in this manner, but the inclusion of a small percentage of barium peroxide neutralizes these substances, so that the purity of oxygen produced by a candle made of a sodium chlorate/iron/barium peroxide mixture approaches 99.9 per cent, with no significant concentration of toxic contaminants.

Once ignited, a sodium chlorate candle provides a continuous flow of pure oxygen and is not extinguished easily. This form of oxygen storage therefore is most appropriate for use in situations where a constant flow of oxygen is required for a specified period, such as, for example, in emergency oxygen supplies for aircraft passengers. In such cases, the cylindrical candle, with a suitable igniting mechanism fitted to one end, is enclosed in a gas-tight container within a thermally insulated shroud. A unit designed to provide oxygen for ten passengers for 30 minutes, i.e. a total oxygen supply of 1300 litres (NTP), would be 22 cm in length and 15 cm in diameter and weigh about 6 kg (see also Table 5.1).

The advantages of this form of oxygen storage include its simplicity (since oxygen can be delivered without the need for reducing valves or regulators), its almost unlimited shelf-life, its relatively small bulk, and the absence of a need for routine servicing. The sodium chlorate candle is also inert at temperatures below 250 °C, even under severe impact loads. Once initiated, oxygen delivery continues unabated. Although it is possible to devise a means whereby a solid system can be used to supply oxygen on demand (by the use of multiple candles and a reservoir), the complexity, weight and bulk of such an arrangement make it unsuitable for use as the primary supply in combat aircraft. Furthermore, although in general when handled correctly each candle is associated with a relatively low fire risk, there have been reports implicating oxygen candles in on-board fires in aircraft.

ALKALI METAL SUPEROXIDES

When treated with water, potassium superoxide liberates oxygen to form potassium hydroxide. This chemical reaction forms the basis of the use of this system in self-contained breathing escape devices. The moisture of the breath reacts with the superoxide to generate oxygen, and in a convenient co-reaction the potassium hydroxide formed reacts with expired carbon dioxide to give potassium carbonate.

REVERSED FUEL CELL AND OTHER SYSTEMS

The normal processes whereby electricity is generated as the energy released when hydrogen and oxygen combine may be reversed by supplying electrical power to a fuel cell. In this so-called reversed fuel cell, oxygen is produced at the anode and hydrogen at the cathode. Hydrogen is then oxidized to water by combination with oxygen in the air flowing over the cathode. A reversed fuel cell capable of providing 26 litres (NTP)/min of oxygen at 300–400 lb/in^2 (2068–2758 kPa) would require a supply of clean moist air at 25 lb/in^2 (172 kPa), would consume about 7 kW of electrical power, and would weigh about 30 kg. A power requirement of this magnitude makes such a system operationally impractical in the aviation environment.

The use of techniques involving the electrolysis of water have been investigated. Although it has proved possible to generate oxygen by this means, the power requirements and weight of the system mean it is currently not used.

Air-dependent systems

A number of air-dependent oxygen-generating techniques, including electrochemical oxygen concentration, praseodymium-cerium oxide systems and barium oxide (Brin process), have been investigated but not developed beyond laboratory studies. A fluomine (a chelate of cobalt) system has been developed to the stage of flight assessment, and it has been shown that fluomine could generate oxygen in dual cyclic heat-exchange beds. While one bed was absorbing oxygen, the other was desorbing it; in one development of this principle, a unit capable of delivering 26 litres (NTP)/min oxygen of 98.5 per cent purity was tested successfully in flight. The disadvantage of the system is its high cost, its relatively short lifecycle (300 operating hours) and a tendency to produce small quantities of noxious chemicals. This system therefore has been surpassed by pressure-swing adsorption systems, as described below.

PRESSURE-SWING ADSORPTION (MOLECULAR SIEVE OXYGEN CONCENTRATION SYSTEMS)

Molecular sieves are alkali-metal aluminosilicates of the crystalline zeolite family. They consist essentially of very regular tetrahedral structures of SiO_4 and AlO_4 linked by cations of sodium or calcium to form cages or cavities, which are normally filled by water molecules. These crystals can be produced synthetically and can be tailor-made in terms of the size of the cage entrances and cavities, which vary according to the precise chemical structure of the zeolite. When the sieve material is heated, the water molecules are driven off to leave an open structure with the affinity to adsorb polar molecules. The adsorption of a substance depends not only upon its degree of polarity but also upon its molecular size; clearly, then, if the molecule is too large to enter the cage, it cannot be adsorbed. The two most common types of sieve material that currently are in use are the so-called 5A and 13X. The former has some of its sodium atoms replaced by calcium, which results in a smaller cage entrance ($4.9 \times 10^{-4} \mu m$) than that of the 13X material ($1 \times 10^{-3} \mu m$).

The adsorption process is an exothermic reaction and is dependent upon both pressure and temperature. An increase in pressure generally enhances adsorption, while an increase in temperature causes a decrease. In MSOC devices, the oxygen and nitrogen are separated by virtue of the fact that nitrogen, despite its slightly larger molecular size, is held more strongly within the sieve cage than oxygen. The cage structure, especially when pressurized, induces a quadrupole moment in the nitrogen molecule, thus enhancing its adsorption energy and producing an oxygen-rich and argon-rich gas phase around the sieve. Since argon also passes through the sieve, the product gas in such a system contains a maximum of about 94 per cent oxygen, the remainder being argon. By using a pressure-swing technique, whereby the molecular sieve bed is alternately pressurized and depressurized, complete separation can be achieved. Furthermore, the adsorption of nitrogen is reversible and the bed can be purged of the gas during the depressurized phase. The adsorption of more polar molecules such as water (when in contact with the sieve material for some time) is irreversible, however, and so water contamination will deactivate a molecular sieve.

An oxygen concentrator of this type usually consists of two or more beds of molecular sieve, through each of which, in turn, conditioned compressed air from an engine bleed source is passed. Thus, in the two-bed system illustrated in Figure 5.3, one bed is depressurized and purged of its nitrogen (by means of a bleed flow of product gas from the pressurized bed) in readiness for oxygen concentration during its next pressurized phase, while the other bed is producing oxygen-enriched breathing gas. The supply of product gas therefore is continuous, and any small fluctuations in delivery pressure may be minimized by the presence of a plenum chamber.

The first operational two-bed MSOC used in the UK, capable of supplying the varying breathing requirements of a single pilot, weighed less than 19 kg, consumed about 50 W of 28 V DC electrical power, and occupied a volume of about 20 litres which is less than that of a 3.5 litre LOX converter. Such a device therefore represented an extremely attractive alternative to the LOX storage devices previously in common use, and an increasing number of combat aircraft types have now been equipped with molecular sieves. The next generation of agile fighter aircraft have molecular sieves installed, such as that illustrated in Figure 5.4, in which further savings in the weight, volume and energy requirements of the MSOC units have been achieved by arranging the sieve beds in very close proximity to one another or even, as in the unit shown, by arranging them concentrically.

The principal disadvantage of this form of oxygen production is that a failure of engine bleed air supply, as for example during an engine flameout in a single-engine aircraft, clearly will result in a failure of the molecular sieve to produce oxygen. This drawback can be overcome by the provision of a gaseous backup oxygen store that can be selected automatically if air supply to the concentrator is lost. Such a backup supply is also required to provide an immediate source of 100 per cent oxygen to prevent hypoxia following decompression of the cabin to an altitude above 30 000 feet as the speed of response of the sieve is inadequate in these circumstances. The same gaseous store, if mounted on the ejection seat, can be used to supply the crew if it becomes necessary to eject from the aircraft at high altitude.

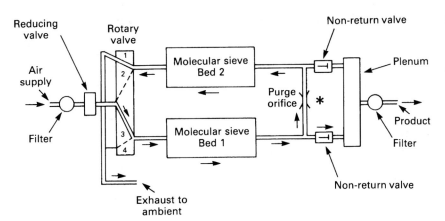

Figure 5.3 *Mode of operation of a simple two-bed molecular sieve oxygen concentrator. In this schematic molecular sieve, bed 1 is being pressurized via line 3 and delivering oxygen-rich product gas to the plenum before passing to the user. A large bleed flow of product gas is diverted to purge nitrogen from molecular sieve bed 2, via orifice * and line 1, in readiness for that bed's pressurization via line 2 when the control valve rotates. Line 4 then becomes the purge route from bed 1 via orifice *.*

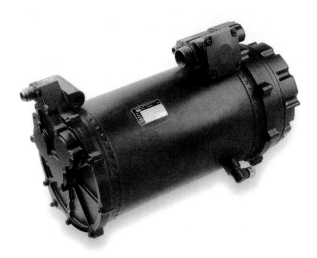

Figure 5.4 *Advanced molecular sieve oxygen concentrator, in which three beds are arranged concentrically to reduce volume. (Photograph courtesy of Honeywell International Inc.)*

In contrast to the potential lack of oxygen, an MSOC product gas concentration of 94 per cent is too rich for routine flight at normal cabin altitudes, and thus it is also necessary to provide a means of reducing the concentration of oxygen in the gas delivered to the pilot. Several generic techniques are available for the control of oxygen concentration in the product gas. The various methods used vary according to the precise design of the sieve system employed, but the techniques used have common principles and are based on the factors that may influence product gas composition. One method that has been used successfully in current aircraft exploits the characteristic of molecular sieve behaviour, whereby the concentration of oxygen in the product gas is reduced if the flow demanded through the system is increased. Artificially increasing the flow through the sieve therefore has the effect of reducing the oxygen concentration in the MSOC product gas. This technique is, however, wasteful. Another, preferred, method is to vary the bed charge and purge cycle times, either by continuous variation of cycle times or by appropriate selection of fixed fast and slow cycles. Further alternatives are to alter the purge flow, varying the control of inlet or exhaust flow and pressure control, or even to mix product gas with air as in a conventional air-mix breathing regulator. In all but the last case, the concentration of oxygen in the product gas is monitored and used in the control of operation of the sieve. Considerable effort has been expended in the development of suitable oxygen sensors for airborne use in the control of MSOC systems. These closed-loop controls have employed a number of different sensors based on a range of physical principles, including gas-fluidic properties, polarity and paramagnetism, to measure the product oxygen concentration. Sophisticated zirconia solid-state monitors using varia-

tions in the oxygen molecular occupancy of membrane vacancies have been introduced into service in some MSOC control systems. In each case, the control method and operation of the sieve unit must be robust and reliable under the wide range of environmental challenges associated with in-flight conditions.

The use of MSOC systems as the source of breathing gas for the crew of a military aircraft has implications for the mode of operation of the individual pressure-demand breathing regulator and for the selection of safety pressure (see below). Where the oxygen concentration required to meet the physiological demands of the aircrew is controlled within the MSOC system itself, it is clearly inappropriate for further dilution of the oxygen concentration to occur within the regulator. In addition, given the inexhaustible supply of breathing gas available from an MSOC, it is highly advantageous to have safety pressure applied from ground level. Both of these features allow very considerable simplification of the demand regulator used to control the flow of breathing gas to the pilot.

The logistic advantages of an MSOC clearly outweigh any disadvantages, however, and can be summarized thus:

- reduction of equipment and staffing costs by eliminating ground manufacture, transport and storage of oxygen
- further reduction of staffing costs and speedier, safer turnaround of aircraft by eliminating the need for ground replenishment of the oxygen store
- reduction in frequency of routine maintenance of the oxygen system, as a result of an increase in overall reliability
- simplification of breathing gas demand regulator and hence reduced unit cost but increased reliability.

MSOC systems are becoming the system of choice for single- and multi-crew military combat aircraft, and they are being investigated as a source of therapeutic oxygen on commercial aircraft. In the latter case, a portable unit incorporates its own compressor powered from the cabin electrical systems and uses cabin air as its gas source. Such systems have been flight-tested, and some airlines are considering either allowing their use by passengers who have such a device or providing them on request. The use of self-contained MSOC units for provision of therapeutic oxygen removes the logistic problems associated with the provision of cylinders of oxygen for a hypoxic passenger on a long flight.

CONTINUOUS FLOW DELIVERY SYSTEMS

From whatever source the breathing gas is derived, the simplest way that it can be delivered to the user is by a continuous-flow system, whether by direct flow or via some form of rebreathing or non-breathing reservoir. Although continuous-flow systems have advantages in that the accurate prediction of oxygen consumption is possible, and the resistance imposed to breathing is relatively low, direct-flow systems are extremely wasteful of breathing gas. They are also by their nature inflexible, because to meet the possible range of ventilatory demands that may be made requires a gas flow of such a volume as to potentially be distracting and inevitably this is wasteful of a limited store. Failure to meet ventilatory demands, however, would induce respiratory discomfort, as described in previous chapters. Adding a reservoir between the flow regulator and the mask decreases the rate of consumption of the aircraft oxygen store by 50–70 per cent. It is very difficult, however, to provide a continuous-flow delivery system incorporating the automatic provision of pressure breathing at very high altitudes.

Direct–flow systems

The most elementary form of continuous flow oxygen system consists of an oxygen store, a regulating device which delivers a continuous flow of oxygen, a flexible delivery hose, and a nasal or oronasal mask or via nasal cannulae. Nasal cannulae have been in use in clinical settings for some considerable time but are now used under certain conditions for the delivery of therapeutic oxygen to commercial airline passengers. With a continuous oxygen flow of 2–4 l/min clinically compromised passengers may be protected from hypoxia at normal cabin altitudes. A refinement of this system, termed pulse dose delivery (see Figure 5.5) releases a bolus of oxygen when a pressure fall induced by an inspiratory effort is detected through the

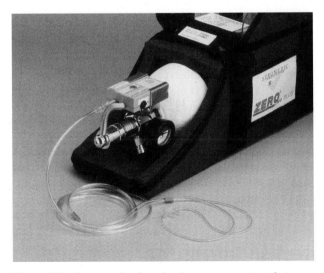

Figure 5.5 *An example of a pulse dose oxygen system that releases a bolus of oxygen when a pressure fall induced by an inspiratory effort is detected through the cannulae at the regulating device incorporated into the system. (Photograph courtesy of Aeromedic Innovations Ltd.)*

cannulae at the regulating device incorporated into the system. The balance of the ventilatory demand is met through inhalation of cabin air as is described in more detail below. Nasal cannulae systems have a number of advantages over mask systems, including being less conspicuous in their use.

When a mask system is used for therapeutic or other purposes the mask has apertures, which may be controlled by valves, through which air can be drawn into the lungs when the demanded inspiratory flow exceeds the flow of oxygen from the system. The same apertures allow expired gas to be expelled to the environment.

This form of oxygen system is very inefficient, since oxygen flowing into the mask during expiration, which occupies 50–60 per cent of the total respiratory cycle time, does not enter the respiratory tract at all. Even during inspiration, oxygen flowing into the mask will enter the lungs only when the instantaneous inspiratory flow equals or exceeds the oxygen flow. To ensure that no air is inspired, therefore, the oxygen flow must exceed the maximum inspiratory flow, which is usually about two to three times the respiratory minute volume and increases to about ten times during speech.

Despite their inefficiency, direct-flow systems are very simple and have been used widely to provide bail-out and EO in combat aircraft. A typical oxygen system of this type consists of a small cylinder containing about 55 litres (NTP) of gaseous oxygen stored at 1800 lb/in^2 (12 411 kPa), a contents gauge, an on/off valve, a metering orifice, and a delivery pipe to the inlet hose of the mask. Flow from such an EO cylinder is then triggered on ejection. More commonly, in modern ejection-seat EO systems the oxygen is delivered through a demand regulator (see below), and the pilot continues to breathe through this until pilot–seat separation occurs, at an altitude at which supplemental oxygen is no longer required.

Rebreathing reservoir systems

The efficiency of a continuous-flow oxygen system is enhanced greatly by incorporating a reservoir between the regulating device and the inlet port of the mask. In rebreathing reservoir systems, a flexible reservoir is placed in direct communication with the cavity of the mask, as shown in Figure 5.6. The addition of a reservoir ensures that all the oxygen flowing from the regulating device enters the respiratory tract during inspiration, provided that, as with direct continuous-flow systems, pulmonary ventilation equals or exceeds the flow of oxygen.

In this type of system, oxygen is delivered continuously from the regulating device into the reservoir bag. The mask usually has a single aperture, which may not be controlled by a valve and through which air may be drawn into the mask if inspiratory demand exceeds the volume of gas in

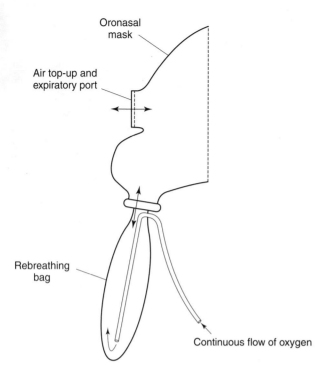

Figure 5.6 *Simple rebreathing reservoir oxygen mask. Oxygen passes at a constant flow into the distal end of the rebreathing bag. The first portion of the expirate fills the bag, while the remainder flows out through the expiratory port. The contents of the bag pass into the respiratory tract at the beginning of inspiration to be followed by the continuous flow of oxygen supplemented with air drawn in through the air inlet (top-up) port.*

the reservoir. Excess oxygen and expired gas are expelled from the mask through the same aperture, which has a resistance to flow deliberately greater than that acting against flow from the reservoir. Thus, the contents of the latter enter the respiratory tract at the beginning of each inspiration before any air is drawn in. Similarly, during expiration, the first part of the expirate passes into the reservoir, and only when this is full is expired gas expelled to the environment. In addition, oxygen flow into the reservoir bag is directed to that part that is furthest from the mask cavity, so that oxygen entering the reservoir during expiration displaces any previously expired gas. At the levels of oxygen flow employed, the volume of oxygen that enters the reservoir during expiration is less than the volume of the reservoir, so that a part of the previously expired gas is re-inspired. The gas that is rebreathed clearly includes that which was held in the respiratory dead space during the previous inspiration, and so it has a higher oxygen tension and a lower carbon dioxide tension than the alveolar gas. Rebreathing using this type of system increases oxygen economy but at the expense of an increase in the effective respiratory dead space.

Rebreathing reservoir continuous-flow oxygen equipment was used extensively in US combat aircraft during

the early 1940s, but its use had several serious disadvantages, including freezing, an inability to respond appropriately to changes in pulmonary ventilation, a lack of indication of gas flow into the mask, an inability to incorporate pressure breathing, and difficulties associated with mask leaks, which negated the value of the reservoir at all.

Because of these drawbacks, rebreathing reservoir oxygen equipment is now used mainly for the administration of therapeutic oxygen to patients in flight and to prevent hypoxia in passengers following loss of cabin pressurization in transport aircraft. The oxygen flow supplied to this type of equipment is increased from about 2 litres (NTP)/min at a cabin altitude of 20 000 feet to about 4.5 litres (NTP)/min at 40 000 feet, a volume that is adequate to prevent serious hypoxia developing in a seated passenger. Finally, it is assumed that a decompression is very unlikely to be so severe that the cabin temperature cannot be maintained above 0 °C, and the impaired performance of the system below −5 °C therefore is of no consequence.

Non-rebreathing reservoir systems

In non-rebreathing reservoir systems, a non-return valve is placed between the reservoir and the cavity of the mask so that expired gas cannot enter the reservoir. As in rebreathing systems, the mask has apertures, which may or may not be controlled by valves, through which air can be drawn into the respiratory tract to augment the oxygen supply and expired gas is expelled to the environment. To ensure that air is not drawn into the lungs until the oxygen reservoir has been emptied, the reduction in mask pressure required to draw air through the air-inlet aperture must again be greater than that required to empty the reservoir. The correct phasing of oxygen and air delivery during inspiration usually is accomplished by a combination of a very low-resistance non-return valve placed between the reservoir and the mask and a spring-loaded higher-resistance air-inlet valve placed in the mask itself.

Although used widely during the 1940s, non-rebreathing continuous-flow systems are now rare. The most successful non-rebreathing reservoir system employed in military aviation was the RAF economizer system, which was in use for almost 40 years and disappeared from service in the 1980s.

DEMAND-FLOW DELIVERY SYSTEMS

All of the disadvantages of continuous-flow delivery systems are overcome by systems in which the flow of gas from the regulator varies directly with the inspiratory demand of the user. In such systems, it is also possible to provide many of the additional automatic and manual facilities listed earlier, including air dilution, safety pressure, pressure breathing and an indication of flow. The key component in demand oxygen systems is the regulator, although the integration with it of the downstream delivery pipework and the oronasal mask is crucial. A regulator that is capable of delivering gas at increased pressure, i.e. of delivering safety pressure and pressure breathing, is termed a pressure-demand oxygen regulator.

Demand regulators

The principles underlying the design and function of demand regulators are essentially the same regardless of whether the device is panel-mounted, seat-mounted or man-mounted: all are designed to fulfil a number of automatic and manual functions, including the following:

BREATHING GAS ON DEMAND

In a demand system the flow of gas from the high-pressure source is controlled by the fluctuations in mask cavity pressure induced by respiration. To achieve this, the regulator is divided into two chambers by a flexible control diaphragm, as shown in Figure 5.7. On one side of the diaphragm, the (demand) chamber receives the high-pressure supply from the aircraft oxygen source and also communicates with the user via a delivery hose and the mask, while the (reference) chamber on the other side of the diaphragm is open to the environmental pressure of the cockpit.

The pressure changes of respiration are transmitted to the demand chamber, where they displace the flexible diaphragm. By means of a connecting lever and pivot, the position of the diaphragm controls the degree of opening of the (demand) valve through which gas from the oxygen source flows into the demand chamber and thence to the user. Thus, the reduction of pressure in the mask cavity and the demand chamber produced by the initiation of inspiration displaces the diaphragm into the chamber and opens the demand valve. The greater the inspiratory demand, the greater will be the reduction in mask cavity pressure transmitted to the demand chamber, and the further will the demand valve open, so increasing the flow of gas to the mask. When inspiration ceases, mask cavity pressure increases and so too does pressure in the demand chamber. The diaphragm is restored to its resting position, the demand valve closes and flow of gas to the mask stops. The flow of gas through the demand valve thus is equal to the instantaneous inspiratory flow.

The forces needed to open the demand valve are such that a regulator that employs a mechanical link between the control diaphragm and the valve requires the diaphragm to be relatively large if the resistance to inspiration is to be kept within acceptable limits. This type of regulator therefore has to be large enough to accommodate a diaphragm that typically is 8–10 cm in diameter. Alternatively, and especially in modern regulators, the link between the demand valve and the control diaphragm is pneumatic. In this case, the opening of a flexible demand valve is controlled by gas pressure applied to the side of the valve opposite to that exposed to the high-pressure supply line (Figure 5.8).

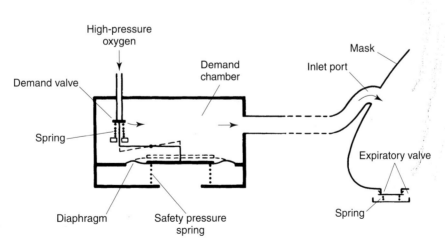

Figure 5.7 *Mode of operation of a simple demand oxygen regulator and oronasal mask system. The flow of oxygen to the mask from the high-pressure supply is controlled by the demand valve, which is held in the closed position by the demand valve spring. The reduction in pressure (produced by inspiration) within the mask, the mask hose and the regulator demand chamber displaces the control diaphragm and opens the demand valve. The rise in mask pressure when inspiration ceases allows the control diaphragm to return to its resting position and the demand valve to close. Biasing the control diaphragm by means of a safety pressure spring raises the mask pressure above that of the environment. The expiratory valve must also be biased (e.g. by spring-loading) in order to hold safety pressure in the mask.*

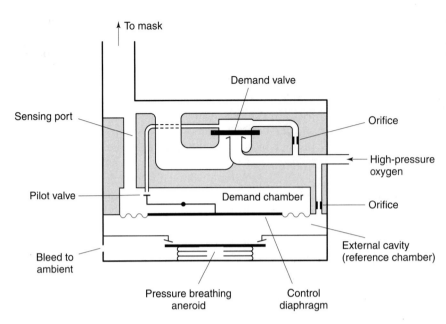

Figure 5.8 *Mode of operation of a typical servo-controlled miniature pressure-demand regulator. The flexible demand valve is held closed by the inlet pressure applied to its rear surface. The suction created by inspiration reduces the pressure within the demand chamber and opens the pilot valve. This allows the reduction in pressure to be transmitted to the back of the demand valve, which therefore opens and allows oxygen to flow through it to the mask. Pressure breathing is produced by increasing the pressure within the reference chamber, so that the control diaphragm is loaded. This is achieved by an aneroid capsule, which progressively increases the resistance to flow to the environment of a small bleed into the chamber (which itself is controlled by an orifice).*

The controlling pressure is itself determined by a second pilot valve, the opening of which is governed by a mechanical link to the control diaphragm. As before, movement of the control diaphragm is influenced by the pressure transmitted from the mask cavity to the demand chamber of the regulator. The great advantage of such servo-controlled demand regulators is the magnification of the control signal made possible by the pneumatic link. Hence, the size of the control diaphragm can be markedly reduced, and the diameter of the control diaphragm in a typical servo-controlled regulator is only 2–3 cm. Furthermore, safety pressure and pressure breathing facilities can be provided by gas-loading the control diaphragm, and all of these pneumatic control systems enable the size of the regulator to be reduced significantly.

AIR DILUTION

The physiological requirements of an oxygen system call for the dilution of oxygen in order to avoid the consequences (and waste) of breathing 100 per cent oxygen continuously and sufficient nitrogen to prevent acceleration atelectasis. Such dilution is usually achieved in conventional systems (i.e. those based on gaseous or liquid oxygen storage) by mixing cabin air with oxygen in the demand regulator. The degree of air dilution (air-mix) decreases automatically and progressively with ascent to altitude in order to maintain adequate oxygenation at all times. Two principal mechanisms are employed to draw cabin air into the regulator: suction dilution and injector dilution.

In regulators employing suction dilution, air is drawn into the demand chamber through a spring-loaded air-inlet valve (Figure 5.9a), while an aneroid capsule controls the relative resistances to flow through both this valve and

the demand valve. Thus, as altitude increases and the aneroid expands, flow through the former falls and flow through the latter rises.

Suction dilution cannot provide air-mix in the presence of safety pressure. Therefore, in systems in which that facility is provided, the suction required to induce or entrain a flow of cabin air into the demand chamber is created by passing oxygen through an injector (Venturi) as it flows from the demand valve: injector dilution. As with the suction dilution technique, the flow of cabin air is governed by another valve, the opening of which is again controlled by an aneroid capsule (Figure 5.9b). The injector dilution technique is employed widely, but it does tend to deliver a relatively high (but acceptable) concentration of oxygen during quiet breathing and at low altitudes. For example, a typical injector dilution regulator will deliver 40–50 per cent oxygen even at sea level.

In both forms of air dilution, the air-inlet port can be closed by manual operation of a shutter on the regulator, thus providing 100 per cent oxygen at any altitude in the event of toxic fumes within the cabin or if decompression sickness is suspected or is likely to develop. This manual override facility is not required in regulators used in MSOC systems, where no dilution with cabin air takes place.

A potential hazard of air dilution is that the user can continue to breathe air through the air-inlet port following a failure of the oxygen supply to the regulator. The development of hypoxia is then a distinct possibility, since the increase in resistance to inspiration associated with such a failure may well go undetected, even at cabin altitudes of 15 000–18 000 feet. In many modern regulators the risk of an undetected failure is eliminated by the incorporation of an additional valve in the air-inlet mechanism, which is

(a)

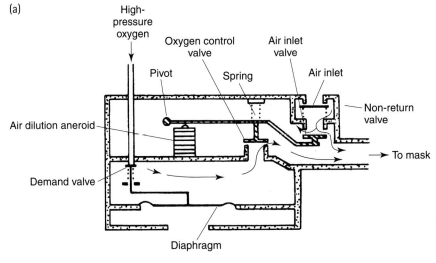

(b)

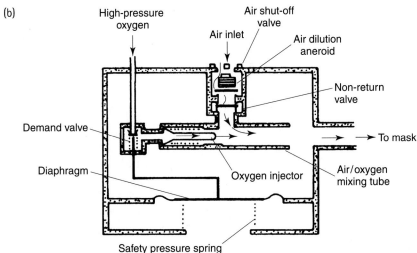

Figure 5.9 *Two techniques for diluting oxygen with cabin air, employed in demand regulator systems. (a) Mode of operation for air dilution in a suction demand regulator: suction dilution. Air is drawn into the regulator by the inspiratory effort, and the relative flows of oxygen and air are controlled by an aneroid capsule, which varies the resistances to flow through the oxygen- and air-inlet ports to the regulator outlet. (b) Mode of operation for air dilution in a pressure-demand regulator: injector dilution. In this case, air is drawn into the regulator by the suction induced by oxygen flow, from the demand valve, through an injector. The proportion of air to oxygen mixing is controlled by an aneroid capsule, which operates a throttle plate in the air-inlet port of the regulator.*

operated by oxygen pressure. This valve remains shut unless there is adequate oxygen pressure at the inlet to the regulator, and a failure of the oxygen supply pressure therefore results in the immediate occlusion of the air-inlet port, with consequent gross impedance to inspiration alerting the user.

SAFETY PRESSURE

Since the operation of the regulator demand valve depends on the transmission of pressure fluctuations produced in the mask cavity by respiration, the mask must seal well against the face and be fitted with an effective non-return expiratory valve (see Oxygen masks for aircrew, p. 89). An ill-fitting mask will induce an inboard leak of air during inspiration and thus will dilute the oxygen contained in the gas delivered by the regulator; this is a serious potential disadvantage of suction dilution demand regulators. In injector dilution demand regulators, however, this disadvantage may be prevented by creating a slight over-pressure, termed safety pressure, in the mask cavity. The

pressure in the mask then remains greater than that of the environment throughout inspiration, thus ensuring that any leak of gas as a result of an ill-fitting mask is outboard and not inboard.

Safety pressure is delivered by the demand regulator through applying an appropriate force to the control diaphragm via a spring, which displaces the diaphragm and so opens the demand valve (Figure 5.7). As soon as the pressure in the mask reaches the required level, the rise in pressure within the demand chamber overcomes the force of the spring and the diaphragm returns to its resting position and shuts the demand valve. Clearly, the mask expiratory valve must be modified so that it does not open until mask cavity pressure exceeds the nominal safety pressure. Thus, the expiratory valve may be either spring-loaded so that its opening pressure is raised at all times or compensated to the delivery pressure of the regulator, so that the raised opening pressure is present only when safety pressure is being provided. The magnitude of the safety pressure required to prevent inboard leakage around an ill-fitting mask depends on the delivery pressure-flow characteristics of the regulator and on the resistance to flow from the regulator to the mask cavity. The level of safety pressure, however, generally lies between 15 and 25 mmWg (0.15–0.25 kPa).

The disadvantage of spring-loading the control diaphragm to provide safety pressure is that gas will flow from the regulator outlet or the mask whenever they are open to the environment. Furthermore, consumption of the oxygen supply is increased at all altitudes when safety pressure is being delivered, although hypoxia arising as a consequence of an inboard mask leak is a significant risk only at altitudes above about 15 000 feet. In many demand systems, therefore, safety pressure is invoked only when it is required and is provided automatically by the expansion of a pressure-sensitive aneroid capsule, within the reference chamber, on ascent to cabin altitudes above 10 000–15 000 feet. A manual switch is also incorporated in some systems so that safety pressure can be selected at a lower cabin altitude if toxic contamination of the cockpit occurs.

PRESSURE BREATHING

The increase in regulator delivery pressure required to provide pressure breathing, and the inflation and operation of pressure garments, at cabin altitudes above 40 000 feet is achieved by progressively loading the control diaphragm with a suitable spring force, as shown in Figure 5.10 (see also Figure 5.8).

The spring force opens the demand valve, and gas flows to the mask until the pressure in the mask and in the demand chamber has built up to the required level. The diaphragm then returns to its resting position and the demand valve shuts. The load is applied to the diaphragm either by a spring, which is allowed to expand progressively under the control of an aneroid capsule within the reference chamber of the regulator, or by gas, the pressure of which is also raised by the expansion of an aneroid capsule. The required relationship between regulator delivery pressure and cabin altitude is obtained by appropriate design of the springs and controlling aneroids. As in the case of safety pressure, the pressure breathing mask must be fitted with a compensated expiratory valve. For test purposes on the ground, a means of obtaining one or two set increases in delivery pressure by manual selection is also provided: the test pressures are usually about 20 mmHg (2.7 kPa) for use with a mask alone and 40–60 mmHg (5.3–8 kPa) for use with partial pressure garments.

INDICATION OF FLOW

An indication of the passage of oxygen through the demand regulator serves as a means of confirming that oxygen flows with each inspiration and as a means of detecting outboard leakage in the presence of safety pressure or pressure breathing. Most commonly, the changes in pressure immediately downstream of the demand valve induced by flow through it are used to operate a visual indicator via some form of pressure switch. Thus, for example, pressure variations, as a consequence of flow, may deflect a small diaphragm that completes an electromagnetic circuit and operates the indicator. In the case of panel-mounted regulators, the magnetic indicator is an integral part of the device; in the case of seat- or man-mounted regulators, the indicator is located elsewhere on the instrument panel. In some systems, the flow sensor may take the form of a spring-loaded slug within the

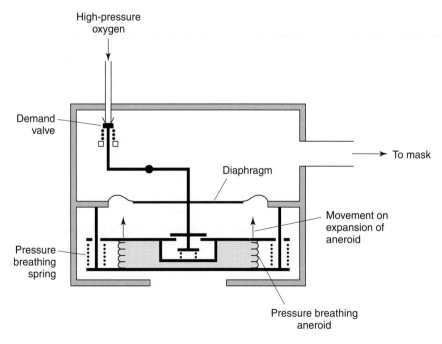

Figure 5.10 *Mode of operation for provision of pressure breathing by a demand regulator. The pressure-breathing aneroid capsule starts to expand at the altitude from which pressure breathing is to commence. This expansion allows the pressure-breathing spring to load the control diaphragm and so increase the delivery pressure from the regulator to the mask. The progressive expansion of the aneroid capsule with altitude produces concomitant increases in loading of the control diaphragm and delivery pressure from the regulator.*

lumen of the oxygen supply line to the regulator. In this case, movements of the slug produced by oxygen flow are transduced electromagnetically or by a light beam, and the indicator is again mounted in a prominent place on the instrument panel. Wherever the indicator is mounted, its regular operation is confirmed throughout flight by the user. The indicator usually displays a white bar in the presence of flow and goes black when there is no flow. The absence of oxygen flow will therefore be readily apparent, as will a continuous flow caused by an outboard leak.

INDICATION OF CONTENTS/PRESSURE

In systems supplied by gaseous or liquid oxygen, a continuous indication of the quantity of gas available is given to the user by means of gauges that display contents in fractions of 'full' or the system operating pressure. In many aircraft, both displays are provided.

Oxygen hoses and personal equipment connectors

The final routing taken by oxygen delivery pipework to the user will depend on the location within the cockpit of the demand regulator and on the presence or otherwise of an ejection seat. Furthermore, in many aircraft in which ejection seats are installed, the usual way in which the user is connected to their personal services is by means of an additional item of equipment: the personal equipment connector (PEC). The various ways in which oxygen is delivered from the source to the user are shown schematically in Figure 5.11.

In most modern UK combat aircraft, the PEC is joined to a double (duplex) seat-mounted pressure demand breathing regulator. In such cases, gas flows via the PEC to the regulator and back through the PEC to the user's oxygen hose. As well as the main oxygen supply, the PEC provides the conduits by which the EO supply, the G-trousers' supply and the electrical connections for communication can be delivered easily to the user. In some variants, an additional gas passage may be incorporated with an air supply for thermal or nuclear, biological and chemical warfare ventilation purposes. A PEC consists of

three interlocking parts – the aircraft portion, the seat portion and the man portion – which enable coupling and uncoupling of services, during routine entry and exit and during the ejection sequence, to be accomplished in a single simple action. Figure 5.12 shows a typical PEC assembly.

Wide-bore oxygen hoses are used only after the delivery pressure has been reduced by the regulator. Such hoses usually are made of vulcanized rubber, reinforced by spirally wound galvanized steel wire and covered with rubberized gauze or stockinet. They have anti-kink properties and incorporate appropriate end connectors to accommodate the fittings for different aircraft systems. The medium-pressure (70 lb/in^2, 483 kPa) hoses used in conjunction with servo-operated man-mounted pressure-demand regulators are made of narrow-bore anti-kink reinforced rubber.

Oxygen masks for aircrew

GENERAL REQUIREMENTS

A mask for aircrew use must satisfy several interrelated requirements: it must be stable and comfortable to wear for long periods, be small, fit a variety of facial sizes and shapes, and seal against the skin of the face effectively. A typical oronasal oxygen mask, such as is used by British military pilots, is illustrated in Figure 4.9 (p. 69).

Comfort demands that the facepiece of the mask should be made of a flexible material that retains that property over the whole range of temperatures in which it may be worn. Natural rubber and silicone rubber commonly are used for this purpose, but it is important that the sensitizing properties of any rubber mixture used should be as low as possible in order to reduce the potential for skin irritation and inflammation. It is also clearly desirable that body secretions should not affect the rubber adversely. The flexible facepiece generally is supported by a rigid or semi-rigid exoskeleton, which also provides the mounting for the means by which the mask is suspended from a headset or protective helmet. The mask should be as small as possible in order to reduce any restriction of the visual fields and to keep limitations on head movement to a minimum. The internal volume or dead space of the mask must be low

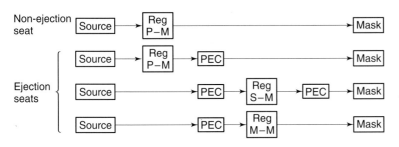

Figure 5.11 *Schematic showing the various routes by which an oxygen supply is delivered to the user in demand regulator systems. The routes depend on the location of the regulator within the cockpit and on the presence or otherwise of an ejection seat. PEC: personal equipment connector; Reg M-M, man-mounted regulator; Reg P-M, panel-mounted regulator; Reg S-M, seat-mounted regulator.*

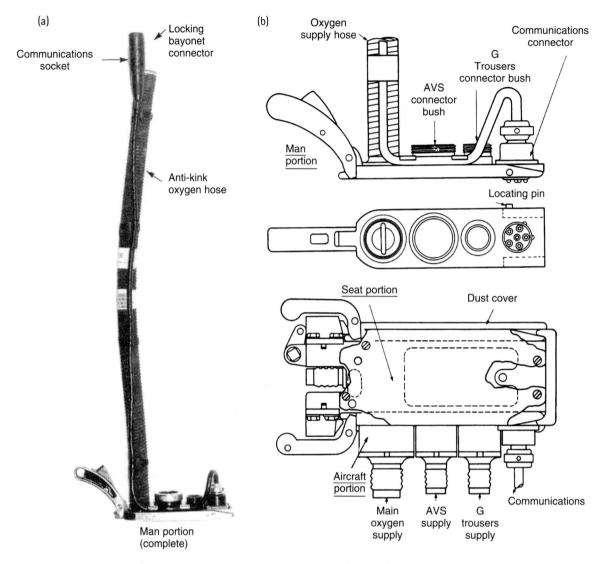

Figure 5.12 *Typical (low-pressure) personal equipment connector (PEC). AVS, air-ventilated suit.*

(typically 120–150 ml) in order to avoid significant rebreathing. Sizing is much simplified if the lower edge of the mask sits in the sulcus beneath the lower lip rather than beneath the chin itself. In the UK, until the introduction of female aircrew, only two sizes of oronasal mask were required if the line of contact with the skin was over the bridge of the nose, descending just lateral to the mouth and then passing along the sulcus below the lower lip. Because women generally have smaller faces, there is now a need for a greater size range, but it remains the case that if the chin is enclosed, even more sizes of mask are required.

The most effective and commonly used method of obtaining a seal between the mask and the face is to reflect the edge of the rubber facepiece, so that a thin flap of rubber lies on the surface of the skin within the mask cavity (Figure 5.13). A slight tension in the reflected edge causes it to lie snugly against the skin, and any increase in mask pressure, such as safety pressure or pressure breathing, will

tend to improve the seal even further. The flexibility of the mask material and of the seal must be sufficient for comfort and yet rigid enough to prevent deformation caused by accelerative forces, which tend to displace the mask. The security of the mask on the face depends primarily, however, on the suspension harness by which it is attached to the headgear and on the security of the latter on the head. A relatively rigid suspension system is required if the user is exposed to high levels of acceleration and vibration in flight, and to high levels of acceleration and windblast during an ejection sequence. The suspension system must also incorporate a means of normal adjustment of fit to the headgear and of rapid tightening for pressure breathing. One method of achieving the former is simply to place the mask comfortably on the face and lock bayonet-type connectors on the mask into one of a series of ratchet notches on the helmet. Pushing the mask further on to the face in order to engage the bayonets on a deeper notch provides

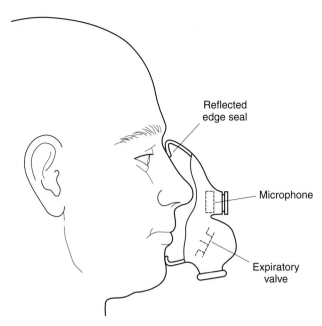

Figure 5.13 *Oronasal mask with a reflected edge seal. When gas at a raised pressure is delivered to the mask, the reflected edge of the seal is driven firmly against the skin of the face by the pressure, so preventing leakage.*

the means to enhance the seal for pressure breathing. Another, more effective, method of attaching the mask to the helmet involves engaging chains or wire cables mounted on the mask exoskeleton over adjustable hooks mounted on the helmet or headset. Tension in this case can be augmented for pressure breathing by drawing the chains or cables over a suspension/tensioning bar on the front of the mask. With the advent of routine pressure breathing for enhancement of tolerance of $+G_z$ accelerations, however, it is likely that these simple mechanical methods of mask tensioning will be superseded by automatic mechanisms. Some such systems already are in routine use by several air forces, although achieving adequate mask sealing at all breathing pressures is proving difficult.

Although the valves fitted to oxygen masks vary with the type of system in which the mask is to be used (see below), a number of general features are common to all masks. Thus, the delivery hose to the mask usually has an internal bore of 15–20 mm and has a flexible but noncrushable wall. The lower end of the hose carries a connector by which it is attached (preferably by a locking mechanism) to the supply hose from the regulator. The weight of the hose assembly is often transmitted to the personal clothing by a connecting chain attached to the mask-hose connector, in order to eliminate the downward pull by the hose on the mask. The upper end of the mask hose is attached to the inspiratory port, within which the inspiratory (inlet) valve is located. The inspiratory valve is usually placed high up in the mask to minimize the possi-

bility of its obstruction by particles of debris and to limit contact with moist expired air. An ice-guard is fitted to its internal surface to provide further protection against debris and moisture. The expiratory (outlet) valve usually is fitted in the most dependent part of the mask to allow sweat and saliva to drain effectively. Furthermore, the external surface of the expiratory valve is protected against the effects of low environmental temperatures by an extension of the rubber facepiece, which traps 10–15 ml of relatively warm expired air just beyond the valve. The walls of this extension (or snout) are flexible so that the wearer can break up and remove any ice that has accumulated within it.

The oxygen mask is also used as the carrier for the microphone component of the aircraft communication system (see Figure 5.13). The presence of a mask greatly modifies the qualities of speech, and sound-pressure levels within the mask cavity during speech may be relatively high, typically 120 dB. Furthermore, speech may be masked by noise generated during the flow of breathing gas through the regulator (particularly when man-mounted), by the flow of gas through delivery hoses and mask valves, and by the direct transmission of cabin noise through the walls of the mask or an open expiratory valve. Finally, the mask forms part of the personal protection of the head, and its stability therefore is especially vital in the event of the cockpit being breached by, for example, a bird strike or should the need arise to escape from the aircraft at high speed, with consequent exposure to high windblast (Q) forces.

PARTICULAR REQUIREMENTS OF DEMAND MASK VALVES

In demand oxygen systems in which the regulator delivers gas only when suction is created at its outlet, the associated mask requires just a single non-return valve in the outlet (expiratory) port. This valve prevents cabin air from being drawn into the lungs and also allows the creation of the suction required to open the demand valve during inspiration. Since there is no way in which gas can be discharged to the environment from the demand chamber of the regulator, expired gas cannot flow back to that chamber and so no valve is required in the inlet (inspiratory) port.

When the delivery pressure of the regulator is capable of being raised above that of the environment (i.e. when safety pressure or pressure breathing is being delivered), the non-return expiratory valve must be loaded so that it does not open under the influence of the increased mask cavity pressure. If unacceptable resistance to expiration is to be avoided, however, the setting of the expiratory valve must be such as to allow gas to be expelled from the lungs with only a small additional rise in mask cavity pressure. In those pressure demand systems in which the regulator is capable of delivering safety pressure but not pressure breathing (i.e. systems used only at cabin altitudes of less than 40 000 feet), a simple spring-loaded non-return expiratory valve may be fitted to the mask; the pressure required to open this valve is set at a slightly higher level than that of the safety pressure delivered by the regulator. When safety pressure is present, breathing when using this system is very comfortable; when safety pressure is absent, however, the spring-loading of the valve is noticeable as an increased resistance to expiration. Occasionally, therefore, the expiratory valve of the mask is fitted with a control that allows the user to raise the spring-loading manually. Such a variable resistance expiratory valve may be used to hold not only safety pressure in the mask but also low levels, e.g. 10–15 mmHg (1.3–2 kPa), of pressure breathing. This technique is not used widely because it requires manual operation and, during pressure breathing, results in excessive resistance to expiration and/or loss of oxygen.

The most satisfactory and extensively employed method of automatically varying the pressure at which the expiratory valve opens is to compensate the device (Figure 5.14). A compensated expiratory valve has a gas-loading facility, whereby the pressure in the inlet port of the mask is also transmitted, by a flexible diaphragm, piston and spring, to the valve plate on the downstream side of the expiratory valve.

The area of the flexible diaphragm/piston is equal to that of the expiratory valve port, so that any increase in the pressure at which gas is delivered to the mask is also transmitted through the compensation chamber to the underside of the valve. The expiratory valve therefore remains shut despite the increase in mask cavity pressure. The addi-

tional increase in mask cavity pressure required to open the expiratory valve is unchanged, however, so that the small increase in mask pressure induced by expiration opens the expiratory valve and allows expired gas to flow out. An additional and essential requirement of a mask fitted with a compensated expiratory valve is the need for a non-return inspiratory valve. If such a valve was not fitted in the inlet port, or if even a small leak was present around a fitted valve, then the increase in mask cavity pressure caused by expiration would be free to pass back into the mask hose and thence to the compensation chamber of the expiratory valve. The expiratory valve would then be held firmly shut by the expiratory effort, and the user would be unable to breathe out. In addition, since the inspiratory valve is prone to freezing as a result of expirate flowing over its cold surface, a deflector plate or ice-guard must be fitted to the valve to protect it against this hazard. Finally, under certain conditions, such as during excessive head movements, the mask hose may 'pump', i.e. cause an increase in pressure in the mask tube, and hence the rise in mask cavity. This rise acts to hold the expiratory valve closed, so markedly increasing the added external resistance to expiration.

Pumping can also cause the pressure in the inlet port to become less than that of the environment, although this should initiate a flow of gas from the demand breathing regulator. However, if this reduction in pressure is transmitted along the compensation tube to the expiratory valve, then this could open and allow the unacceptable possibility of inspiring air from the cabin. Equally, a failure

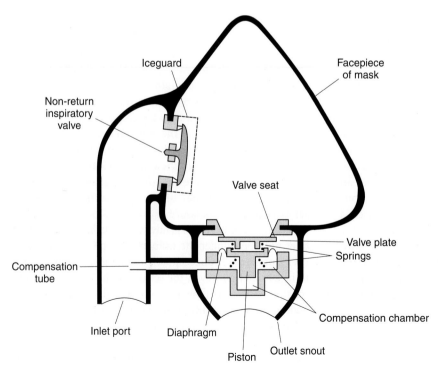

Figure 5.14 *Valve system of a pressure demand oronasal mask. The inspiratory valve is a simple non-return device, with a mesh cover that acts as an ice-guard. The expiratory valve is compensated, the pressure of gas in the inlet port also being applied along the compensation tube and through a diaphragm and piston to the external surface of the expiratory valve plate. In the resting condition, the expiratory valve is held closed by a spring in the compensation chamber. The valve plate above is separated from the diaphragm and piston below by a second spring, which ensures that any reduction in pressure within the inlet port will not open the expiratory valve.*

of gas supply through the breathing regulator would have the same effect. This sucking open of the expiratory valve may be prevented by a further refinement of the compensated expiratory valve: an additional spring interposed between the valve plate and the flexible diaphragm/piston of the compensation chamber. If pressure within the latter falls, and the diaphragm/piston moves downwards, then the expiratory valve remains sealed as a result of the valve plate being held against the valve seat by the additional spring (see Figure 5.14). A unit that incorporates such a refinement is termed a split-compensated expiratory valve.

The combination of a non-return inspiratory valve and a split-compensated expiratory valve ensures that the mask cavity pressure is controlled automatically to the datum pressure being delivered by the demand regulator, while the increase required in mask cavity pressure to open the expiratory valve during expiration remains constant at 1–2 mmHg (0.13–0.25 kPa).

In those masks used routinely throughout flight by military aircrew, and in association with a personal equipment connector, a third valve frequently is fitted to provide an anti-suffocation facility. The reason for this is that the user's portion of the personal equipment connector contains an anti-drowning, self-sealing 'prop' valve that closes the oxygen port of the connector whenever it is detached from the seat portion (see Figure 5.12). Thus, should water entry occur after an ejection escape, or should the connector release inadvertently during flight, the user is able to continue breathing through the anti-suffocation valve. In the case of water entry, the prop valve prevents the inhalation of water through the personal equipment connector. The anti-suffocation valve itself is an inward relief valve that opens when the pressure within the mask cavity falls to 9–13 mmHg (1.2–1.7 kPa) below ambient pressure, a suction sufficiently high to warn the user that the valve is operative.

Masks for passengers

Although the degree of comfort and standard of seal required of oxygen delivery masks for emergency use by passengers is considerably less than that necessary for aircrew, such masks do have some important design constraints. Thus, one size of mask must fit all shapes and sizes of face, and the mask must be easy to don and secure in place by completely untrained passengers. To this end, the mask should be circular in shape to avoid the need to orient the device on the face, and the harness is usually a simple elastic loop. Passenger masks are not usually designed for use at environmental temperatures below −5 to −10 °C.

One very common type of passenger emergency oxygen mask receives a continuous flow of oxygen and incorporates a small reservoir bag in either the rebreathing or non-rebreathing configuration (see above). At least one form of passenger mask, however, has a simple demand valve used in conjunction with a metered oxygen flow. In this case, the intervening hose between the metering orifice and the mask acts as a reservoir for oxygen during expiration.

The masks are usually stowed in overhead compartments or in the backrests of the seats. The doors of the stowage compartment are opened and the masks presented to the passengers automatically if the cabin altitude exceeds a predetermined level, commonly 13 000–15 000 feet. Flow of oxygen to the mask is not initiated, however, until the mask is actively pulled towards the face. A simple bobbin flowmeter inserted in the supply hose to the mask indicates that flow is occurring. The automatic presentation of the masks, and the magnitude of the subsequent continuous flow of oxygen, generally is controlled from the flight deck by varying the pressure in the ring main that supplies oxygen to all outlets (see also Figure 5.25; p. 99). The pressure in the ring main is itself controlled either automatically or manually by a member of the flight-deck crew.

Simple continuous-flow systems, usually of the rebreathing reservoir type, are also used to administer therapeutic oxygen to passengers in clinical need, e.g. passengers who become ill during flight and passengers for whom flight was predicted to embarrass their cardiorespiratory status. The oxygen supply is then obtained either from a direct connection to the aircraft's main oxygen store or from a portable gaseous oxygen source. An example of a simple therapeutic oxygen set is shown in Figure 5.15. National and international regulations determine the number of such therapeutic/emergency oxygen sets that are to be carried.

Smoke-hoods

Fire and toxic fumes on board an aircraft have obvious and often tragic consequences. Even if the aircraft is on the ground or manages a successful emergency landing when an emergency occurs, the occupants may succumb to smoke and fumes before escape is possible. There is, therefore, a need to provide some form of respiratory protection for crew members and passengers so threatened.

Following several such disasters in civil aircraft during the 1980s, the appropriate regulating authorities have actively pursued the possibility of providing smoke-hoods for use by passengers and crew of stricken aircraft. While the small numbers required for crew protection suggest that quite sophisticated devices could be (and, by some airlines, are) provided, the large numbers of passengers carried places severe constraints, in terms of weight, bulk and cost, on the design of suitable hoods for passenger use. Furthermore, problems of size, the ease of use by untrained subjects, compromised visibility and communication must all be addressed, as must be the all-important ability of the device to protect the user for the duration of the emergency.

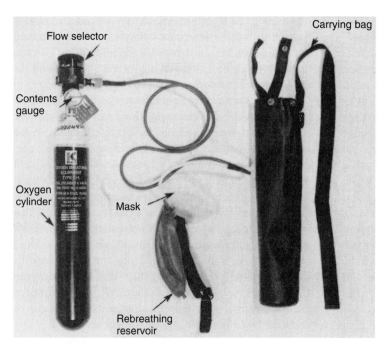

Figure 5.15   *Typical portable oxygen set for therapeutic use by passengers or walk-around use by cabin staff. Oxygen is supplied from a 120-L (NTP) capacity cylinder, at one of two preset flows, to a simple rebreathing reservoir facemask.*

Many prototype smoke-hoods, all of which envelop the head entirely, have been developed de novo or adapted from breathing devices used for other purposes. The sophistication of such equipment varies from simple hoods made of transparent plastic and equipped with a charcoal filter through which to breathe, to hoods providing an integral breathing gas supply. The source of supply may be from a chemical candle (such as in the widely used Scott (now AVOX Systems, San Antonio, TX, USA) smoke-hood for cabin staff) or from a gaseous oxygen cylinder (e.g. the Air Liquide (Paris, France) smoke-hood) combined with active or passive carbon dioxide absorption.

In military transport aircraft, where relatively few people are involved, equipment to allow a crew member to breathe in irrespirable atmospheres, e.g. when fire-fighting, can be provided with little constraint in terms of weight or bulk. A typical smoke set for such a purpose is shown in Figure 5.16. In the system illustrated, breathing gas is supplied as oxygen from two 200 litre (NTP) capacity cylinders contained in a unit carried on the chest. Oxygen is supplied on demand via a regulator assembly mounted on the side of a combined mask and visor facepiece, and expiration is through a non-return valve combined with a speech-transmitter unit. The system can provide protection in hostile environments and up to an altitude of 30 000 feet.

TYPICAL OXYGEN SYSTEMS

Examples of the various components described above are integrated to provide a complete oxygen system. The

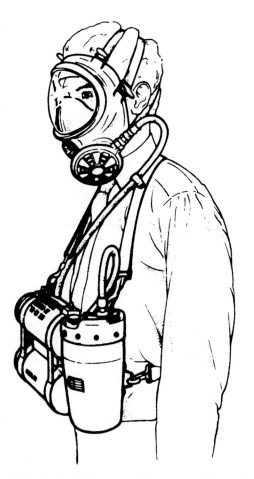

Figure 5.16   *Typical military portable oxygen set for use in irrespirable atmospheres. The weight and bulk of such equipment makes it unsuitable for use as a smoke-hood for passengers.*

choice of components and their layout clearly will depend on the type and role of the aircraft in which the system is to be installed. This section summarizes the general features of some typical oxygen systems, both in military and in civil aircraft.

Aircraft with low-differential pressure cabins: combat aircraft

Combat aircraft have low-differential pressure cabins, and so the oxygen system provides an essential element of the protection against hypoxia on ascent to cabin altitudes above 5000 feet. Consequently, those components of the oxygen system that may fail in flight are, as far as practicable, duplicated. Such an installation therefore consists of a primary or main oxygen system and a secondary or emergency oxygen system. When the aircraft is fitted with ejection seats, as is nearly always the case in modern combat aircraft, the emergency oxygen system also serves to prevent the development of serious hypoxia following escape from the aircraft at high altitude.

The main oxygen system comprises a store of oxygen or a means of production, such as an MSOC, a pressure demand oxygen regulator at each crew position, and a pressure demand oxygen mask. The emergency system comprises a small store of oxygen stowed somewhere in or on the escape equipment, so that it can also provide the bail-out supply; there is either a separate emergency oxygen regulator or the supply of emergency oxygen is delivered through a duplicated demand regulator.

The main supply in many current combat aircraft is as liquid oxygen in converters located outside the pressure cabin and that can be replaced rapidly when partially used. Single-seat aircraft are typically equipped with a 5 litre converter, while two-seat and long-range aircraft usually have 10 litre converters. Gaseous oxygen, at an appropriate operating pressure, is led from the converter by a main supply pipe through the wall of the pressure cabin to the inlet of the regulator. Similarly, in fast jet aircraft equipped with MSOC systems, the appropriately sized sieve (depending on the number of crew that it must support) is located outside the pressure cabin and supplied with compressed air drawn from the aircraft's engines. The emergency oxygen supply is carried as compressed gas in small cylinders with capacities varying from 55 to 300 litres (NTP). The contents of the emergency supply are indicated on a pressure gauge, which is checked before every flight, and the cylinder is equipped with a charging point, which allows replenishment in situ. Emergency oxygen can be selected manually in flight or automatically during the escape sequence on ejection.

The main pressure demand oxygen regulator for each crew member may be mounted in a variety of positions, and it is convenient to classify the sites used into three groups: the airframe (panel-mounted), the man (man-mounted) and the ejection seat (seat-mounted).

PANEL-MOUNTED REGULATOR SYSTEMS

When the regulator is mounted on the airframe, it is usually sited on a front or side console (panel) in such a position that its controls can be reached in flight. Wide-bore, low-pressure hose from the outlet of the regulator passes, via either single inline connectors (Figure 5.17) or a personal equipment connector (Figure 5.18), to end in a second connector in the region of the user's chest. The inlet hose of the oxygen mask then plugs directly into this connector.

In older aircraft, the associated emergency oxygen system generally is connected to the main system either at,

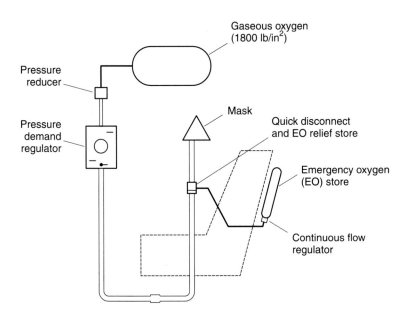

Figure 5.17 *Typical pressure demand oxygen system comprising a gaseous oxygen source, a panel-mounted demand regulator, and an oxygen mask. Breathing gas is delivered to the user via a wide-bore, low-pressure hose connected directly to the mask hose by means of a quick disconnect. The continuous flow emergency oxygen (EO) supply enters the system at the quick disconnect, which therefore also incorporates an excess-pressure relief valve.*

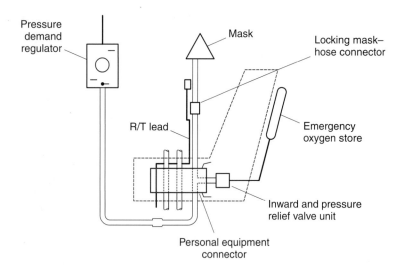

Figure 5.18 *Typical pressure demand oxygen system comprising either a gaseous or a liquid oxygen source, a panel-mounted demand regulator, and an oxygen mask. Breathing gas is delivered to the user via a wide-bore, low-pressure hose, passing via the personal equipment connector to a locking coupling at the mask hose. The emergency oxygen supply, via its own demand regulator, enters the system through the seat portion of the personal equipment connector and thence passes to the user.*

or immediately upstream of, the mask–hose coupling (see Figure 5.17), and delivery from the emergency supply is regulated by a simple orifice that provides a continuous flow. In more modern systems, however, a small pressure-demand emergency regulator may be fitted that provides 100 per cent oxygen with safety pressure from sea level, and automatic pressure breathing if necessary, delivery being via the personal equipment connector (Figure 5.18).

Panel-mounted regulators usually have large control diaphragms linked mechanically to the demand valve and are able to provide all the desirable automatic facilities described above. Figure 5.19 illustrates a typical panel-mounted oxygen regulator. The major disadvantages of panel-mounted oxygen regulator systems are that the regulator occupies valuable panel space, there is often a long unwieldy length of hose between the regulator and the mask, and the main oxygen supply cannot be routed through the emergency regulator if the main regulator fails to pass gas. The development of pneumatic servo-controlled regulators allowed miniaturization, and the consequent reduction in weight and bulk enabled other mounting sites to be utilized.

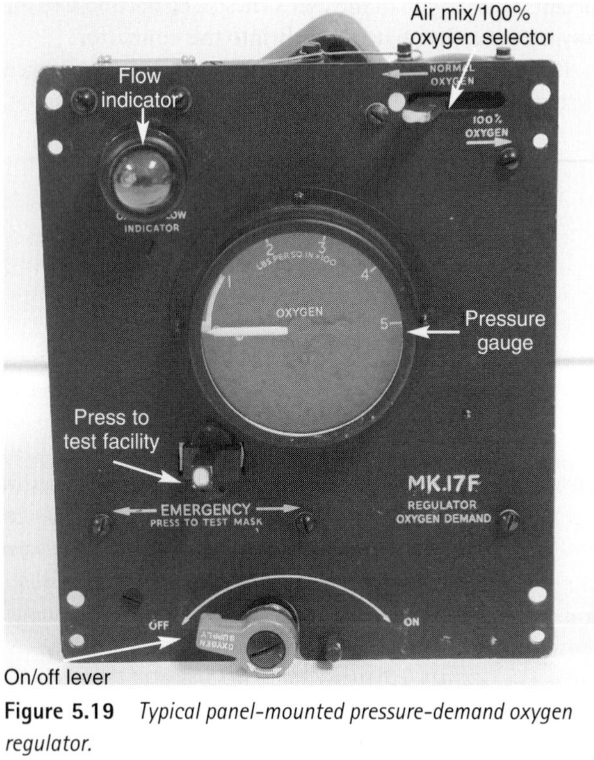

BODY–MOUNTED REGULATOR SYSTEMS

A miniaturized servo-controlled pressure demand regulator can be mounted either on the chest or on the head. The length of delivery hose from the regulator to the mask therefore is short and there is little resistance to inspiration in such systems. Oxygen at medium pressure ($70\,\text{lb/in}^2$, $483\,\text{kPa}$) is carried directly to the inlet of the regulator through narrow-bore (8 mm outside diameter) flexible hose. Routine connection/disconnection between the aircraft supply, the ejection seat and the regulator mounted on the user is accomplished via a (narrow-bore) personal equipment connector. The same device allows automatic separation of supplies during the ejection sequence. Since the main regulator travels out of the aircraft with the seat during such an event, it can be utilized by the emergency supply as well as by the main system. Consequently, the emergency oxygen supply, after passing through a reducing valve, which is usually mounted on the emergency cylinder itself, is delivered into the main supply system upstream of the main regulator (Figure 5.20).

A mask-mounted or helmet-mounted regulator can be used in association with an emergency oxygen supply carried in the personal survival pack (see below) to provide breathing gas during and immediately after a parachute descent into water and so reduce the risk of drowning. Considerations of size and weight, however, dictate that a

Figure 5.19 *Typical panel-mounted pressure-demand oxygen regulator.*

pressure-demand regulator mounted in these sites cannot provide air dilution. The additional space on the chest allows a miniaturized air-dilution device to be carried. Indeed, some chest-mounted regulators not only provide air dilution, safety pressure and pressure breathing but also incorporate a second or standby regulator that can be used in the event of failure of the main regulator. Figure 5.21 illustrates a typical chest-mounted miniature pressure-demand regulator.

Although body-mounted regulators are readily available for servicing, they are very liable to damage by handling and are required in greater numbers than panel-mounted or seat-mounted devices, since each crew member must be

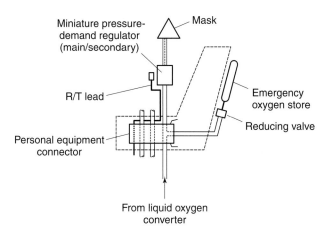

Figure 5.20 *Typical pressure-demand oxygen system comprising a liquid oxygen in source, a chest-mounted demand regulator, and an oxygen mask. Gaseous oxygen is delivered to the user via a narrow-bore, medium-pressure hose, passing via the personal equipment connector to a locked connection at the regulator. The wide-bore mask hose couples directly to the regulator. The emergency oxygen supply enters the system through the seat portion of the personal equipment connector and then passes to the regulator, which therefore is able to provide emergency oxygen on demand.*

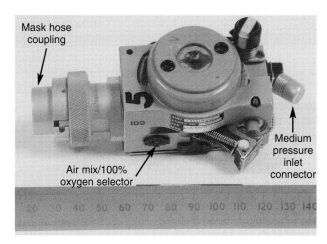

Figure 5.21 *Typical chest-mounted pressure-demand oxygen regulator.*

issued with a regulator. Furthermore, the emergency drills are relatively complicated, because separation of the regulator from direct contact with the aircraft or seat services complicates the system, increases the likelihood of problems arising, and lengthens the drills necessary to correct such problems. A final disadvantage is that miniaturization to a marked degree precludes the opportunity to incorporate additional safety features and increase system redundancy (and hence operational effectiveness). These disadvantages can be overcome, at the same time as retaining the benefits of pneumatic engineering, by mounting the regulator package on the ejection seat.

SEAT-MOUNTED REGULATOR SYSTEMS

Seat-mounted regulators may be located either on the seat structure itself or in the personal survival pack. The latter is the site of choice in which to carry the emergency/bail-out supply for the occupants of non-ejection seat aircraft, but the size and weight of emergency regulators to be carried in personal survival packs clearly must be kept as low as possible.

No such constraints apply to ejection-seat-mounted regulators, however. When used in combination with gaseous of LOX storage systems, these provide air dilution with automatic safety pressure from about 15 000 feet and pressure breathing at high altitudes. As with the other systems described, oxygen usually is delivered to the regulator via the aircraft and seat portions of a personal equipment connector. The outlet of the regulator is connected through the user portion of the personal equipment connector to a wide-bore hose that passes to the coupling by which attachment is made to the inlet hose of the oxygen mask (Figure 5.22). The emergency oxygen supply usually is controlled by a second seat-mounted (standby) pressure demand regulator that supplies 100 per cent oxygen, safety pressure from sea level, and automatic pressure breathing when required. The standby regulator can be positioned immediately adjacent to the main regulator and, indeed, may be in the same unit (such an arrangement is termed a duplex regulator); it is then possible to arrange for the main oxygen supply to be routed through either the main or the emergency regulator, thus duplicating the regulator in the main system and improving operational effectiveness. The close association of the main and standby regulators also allows the corrective drills required in the event of a failure in the system to be simplified. Figure 5.23 shows a typical seat-mounted pressure-demand oxygen regulator.

In the UK, fast jet aircraft oxygen systems that employ an MSOC also incorporate a duplex seat-mounted regulator (Figure 5.24). The technical details of such systems differ markedly from all previous oxygen systems in several fundamental areas.

Since the output pressure from a molecular sieve is usually only about 15–30 lb/in^2 (207 kPa), the regulator must

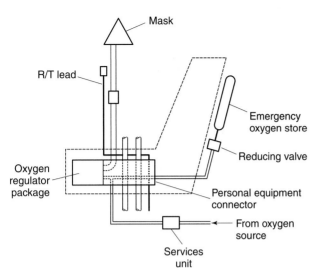

Figure 5.22 *Typical pressure demand oxygen system comprising either a gaseous oxygen or a liquid oxygen source, a seat-mounted duplex demand regulator, and an oxygen mask. Gaseous oxygen is delivered to the regulator via a narrow-bore, medium-pressure hose to the seat portion of the personal equipment connector (to which the regulator package is connected directly) and breathing gas from the regulator by way of the wide-bore, low pressure hose of the user portion of the personal equipment connector to a locking coupling with the mask hose. The emergency oxygen supply enters the system through the seat portion of the personal equipment connector and passes directly to the duplex regulator, both elements of which therefore are able to provide emergency oxygen on demand.*

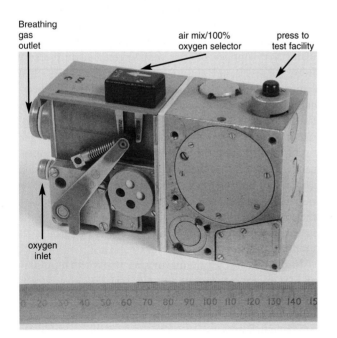

Figure 5.23 *Typical seat-mounted pressure-demand oxygen regulator.*

be engineered to function normally (i.e. to provide breathing gas on demand, safety pressure and pressure breathing) at this relatively low pressure. However, the regulator is not required to provide air dilution, since that facility is achieved by manipulation of flow through the molecular sieve (see Oxygen sources, above). In the system illustrated, control of oxygen concentration in the product gas is maintained by continuous monitoring of the partial pressure of oxygen (at the existing cabin altitude) being delivered to a new component of the system: the mixture controller. This device incorporates a sensor, which, if the product gas is too rich in oxygen, acts to reduce the concentration by altering either flow or sieve bed cycling, as described above. If the sensor detects that the oxygen content is too low, flow through the beds is slowed or the bed cycling is increased, to raise the oxygen concentration. This controlling sensor thus maintains the partial pressure of oxygen in the gas being delivered to the user at an adequate level at all altitudes. A second partial pressure sensor, set at about 160 mmHg (21.3 kPa), acts as a warning device should output from the molecular sieve fail altogether (e.g. following an engine flameout) or suddenly fall below that required for adequate oxygenation at high altitude (e.g. following a rapid decompression), or if there is a failure within the concentrator itself.

Activation of the warning sensor automatically selects the delivery of 100 per cent oxygen from a seat-mounted backup store of 200 litres (NTP) gaseous oxygen. The same store acts as the emergency oxygen supply in the event of ejection. Since the in-flight emergencies (flameout, rapid decompression) are potentially recoverable, however, a unique feature of the backup system is that it can be turned off. This is in contrast to the initiation of all other conventional emergency oxygen systems in combat aircraft, which commit the pilot to an immediate descent to below 10 000 feet, with obvious operational implications. Thus, if the pilot achieves an engine relight after a flameout, the molecular sieve will once again concentrate oxygen and the flight can proceed normally. Similarly, once the molecular sieve and mixture controller have responded to the fall in cabin pressure after rapid decompression, gaseous backup oxygen is no longer required, so the store can be conserved.

In the most advanced oxygen systems, such as those installed in the Eurofighter Typhoon and the US/UK Joint Strike Fighter, an MSOC provides the breathing gas, which is monitored by a solid-state oxygen sensor that controls the bed cycle time, as described above. As these aircraft are equipped with pressure breathing for G-protection (see Chapter 9), a close functional link is essential between the breathing regulator and the anti-G valve. To address this requirement, the two units and the PEC are combined in a single package, mounted on the side of the ejection seat. A Typhoon Aircrew Services Package (ASP) is shown in Figure 5.25.

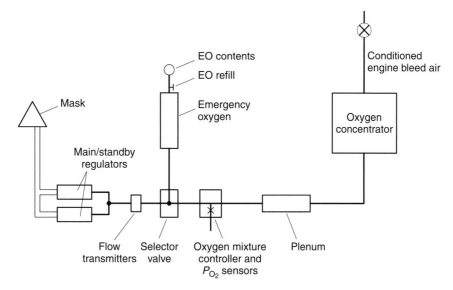

Figure 5.24 *Advanced oxygen system employing a molecular sieve oxygen concentrator and a seat-mounted duplex pressure demand regulator. Product gas is delivered from the molecular sieve to the user via the seat portion of a personal equipment connector to which the regulator is connected directly, and thence via the wide-bore, low-pressure hose of the user portion of the personal equipment connector to the locking coupling with the mask hose. In this system, the concentration of oxygen within the product gas is controlled by a sensing device, which increases flow through the concentrator if oxygen concentration is too high and decreases flow through the concentrator if oxygen concentration is too low. The emergency oxygen (EO) supply enters the system through the seat portion of the personal equipment connector and passes to the duplex regulator and thence to the user in the conventional manner. The emergency system also acts to provide a backup supply of oxygen during temporary reductions in, or failures of, adequate sieve output. Since these situations may be resolved, the emergency back-up supply may be turned off.*

ELECTRONIC

Elective breathing regulators are now becoming available which may prove to be even more reliable than current pneumatically controlled units.

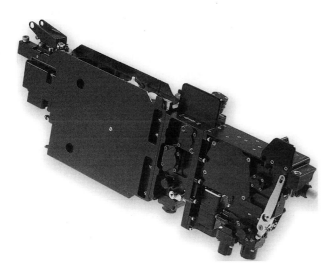

Figure 5.25 *Aircrew services package as installed in Eurofighter Typhoon contains a duplex breathing regulator, the anti-G valve and the Personal Equipment Connector in a single, seat-mounted unit. (Photo courtesy of Honeywell International Inc.)*

Aircraft with high-differential-pressure cabins: passenger aircraft

In aircraft with high-differential-pressure cabins, the oxygen system provides the second line of defence against hypoxia and is consequently used only if there is a failure of cabin pressurization or if toxic fumes contaminate the cabin atmosphere.

Because of its advantages, and especially its worldwide availability, oxygen is usually carried in passenger aircraft in gaseous form at high pressure (1800 lb/in², 12 411 kPa), although LOX is used in some aircraft and sodium chlorate candles in others. The oxygen system for the flight-deck crew is usually separate, with the exception of the oxygen store, from that for the cabin staff and passengers. The main on/off valve, the contents gauge and all the system controls are situated on the flight deck. In gaseous systems, the high-pressure supply is reduced to the working pressures of the flight-deck oxygen regulators (typically 200–400 lb/in², 1379–2758 kPa) and of the ring main for the passenger circuit (typically 70–100 lb/in², 483–690 kPa).

The flight-deck system must ensure that the crew controlling the aircraft and its subsystems are fully oxygenated at all times, since the wellbeing of the other occupants depends primarily on the crew's ability to initiate and control a rapid descent to a low and safe altitude. Therefore, the system clearly must provide oxygen for the flight-deck crew for as long as the cabin altitude exceeds 8000–10 000 feet, and so demand oxygen equipment is fitted to these crew stations. If the maximum cabin altitude on rapid decompression cannot exceed 30 000–35 000 feet, then simple suction demand regulators may be fitted, but the regulators are most commonly of the pressure demand type; these are always fitted when the cabin altitude can exceed 40 000 feet following a decompression. A regulator is mounted at each crew position and delivers oxygen via a wide-bore hose to the mask, which is placed in a purpose-designed stowage unit from which it can be extracted rapidly when required. The oxygen mask is fitted with a harness system by which it can be attached to a communications headset; a test of the adequacy of this attachment often forms part of the pre-flight checks. In the event of a rapid decompression, the crew are required to don their oxygen masks, usually within three to five seconds, and to continue to use the equipment for as long as the cabin altitude remains above 8000–10 000 feet. In certain circumstances, flying regulations require the watch-keeping members of the flight-deck crew to be wearing oxygen masks whenever the aircraft is above a specified altitude, e.g. 43 000 feet. The oxygen equipment is also used to protect the respiratory tract if toxic fumes are detected within the cabin.

The performance required of an oxygen system for passenger use is less demanding, although, as discussed earlier, oxygen must be available for all passengers when the cabin altitude exceeds 15 000 feet and for a proportion of the passengers (ten per cent) whenever the cabin altitude is between 10 000 and 15 000 feet. In practice, this means that all passenger aircraft that operate at altitudes above 25 000–35 000 feet are fitted with a passenger oxygen system. The maximum altitude at which aircraft that are not fitted with an oxygen system for passengers are allowed to operate depends on the rate of descent that can be achieved following a decompression and may vary according to national regulations; in the UK, this maximum altitude is 25 000 feet, provided that the aircraft can descend to below 12 000 feet within five minutes of loss of cabin pressure and of continuing at or below that height to its destination or other site of safe landing.

The oxygen supply for passengers is usually carried around the cabin by means of a ring main (Figure 5.26), which feeds the individual mask presentation units. Pressure in the ring main is controlled automatically, so that if the cabin altitude exceeds a predetermined level of between 10 000 and 14 000 feet, the pressure is increased to about 80 lb/in^2 (552 kPa). This rise in pressure sounds an alarm on the flight deck, opens the doors of the mask presentation units so that the masks drop in front of the passengers, and provides a high flow of oxygen when a passenger pulls the mask on to the face. The flow of oxygen after the aircraft has descended to low altitude can be reduced or turned off by the flight engineer, who can also control the pressure in the ring main manually. Portable (walk-around) oxygen sets or additional outlets from the ring main are provided in passenger aircraft for therapeutic purposes, and the cabin staff can use walk-around sets to provide assistance to passengers when the cabin altitude exceeds 10 000 feet (see Figure 5.15). Such walk-around therapeutic oxygen sets often provide two levels of oxygen flow: a 2 litre (NTP)/min level for use at altitudes below 18 000 feet and a 4 litre (NTP)/min level for use at altitudes above 18 000 feet. Finally, masks for the cabin crew are, like passenger masks, usually of the continuous flow reservoir type.

PRESSURE CLOTHING

Aircrew operating modern combat aircraft normally are protected against the hazards of high altitude by a combination of cabin pressurization and a personal oxygen system. When operating at extreme altitudes, however, additional personal protection is provided by means of pressure clothing. Such garments are normally worn un-

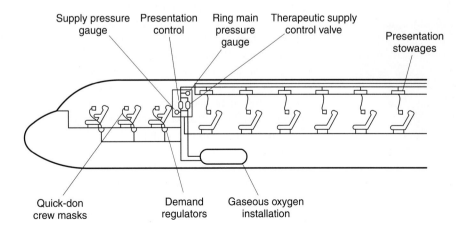

Figure 5.26 *Typical arrangement of an oxygen ring main system on board a large passenger aircraft.*

inflated and are pressurized only if the cabin altitude exceeds a certain level or if it is necessary to abandon the aircraft at high altitude (above 40 000 feet). The extent of this form of emergency equipment ranges from full-pressure suits, which apply pressure to the whole person, to partial pressure garments, which pressurize the respiratory tract together with a greater or lesser part of the external surface of the body. Pressure breathing equipment that pressurizes only the respiratory tract, via an oronasal mask, may be considered as the simplest form of partial pressure protection. Full pressure suits are also used in space flight to provide protection against exposure to the vacuum of space either as a result of a failure of the sealed cabin of the spacecraft or during extra-vehicular activity.

In most circumstances, the crew of an aircraft flying at high altitude will initiate an immediate emergency descent in the event of a failure of cabin pressurization. Operational considerations may, however, dictate that a military aircraft must remain at high altitude until the mission is completed. Thus, pressure clothing may be used either to provide the wearer with the short-term protection needed to enable a descent to be made to an altitude where such protection is no longer required, or to provide long-term protection so that the aircraft and its crew can remain safely at high altitude.

The major physiological effects of exposure to high altitude are hypoxia, decompression sickness and hypothermia, which are described in detail in Chapters 3, 7 and 13, respectively. It will be recalled that severe and unacceptable hypoxia occurs within a few seconds of exposure to altitudes above 40 000–43 000 feet, even when 100 per cent oxygen is breathed. Consequently, protection against hypoxia must be provided irrespective of whether the duration of exposure to such altitudes is short or long. The relative importance of the other effects, however, depends on the duration of exposure. Thus, a short exposure to high altitude is very unlikely to give rise to serious decompression sickness, and limited duration exposure to low environmental temperatures likewise will not cause serious impairment of performance or serious damage to subjects wearing normal aircrew clothing. However, if exposure to altitudes above 25 000 feet lasts for more than about five to ten minutes, then the risk of developing decompression sickness increases markedly. Similarly, if exposure to temperatures below approximately −34 °C lasts for more than a few minutes, uncovered skin will suffer cold thermal injury and general hypothermia may develop. Therefore, protection against hypoxia, decompression sickness and cold is essential if exposure to altitudes above about 25 000 feet is to be sustained for more than a very few minutes. Only if, by virtue of a rapid descent or an ejection, exposure will be limited to a period of less than two to five minutes can additional protection against decompression sickness and cold be omitted. These considerations lead to the following conclusions:

- Prolonged physiological protection against the effects of exposure to very high altitudes can be attained only by means of a garment that maintains a pressure equal to or greater than 282 mmHg (37.6 kPa) absolute around the body (to prevent hypoxia and decompression sickness) and to which heat can be supplied (to maintain a satisfactory thermal environment). The only form of garment that can fulfil these requirements is a full pressure suit.
- If the aircraft is able to descend rapidly, however, protection is needed only against hypoxia. In this situation, a full pressure suit once again is the ideal solution, since it applies the required pressure evenly to the respiratory tract and to the whole of the external surface of the body. Pressure differences between different parts of the body do not occur, therefore, and thus no serious physiological disturbances arise in either the cardiovascular or the respiratory system. A full pressure suit is bulky and all-enveloping, however, it impairs routine flying even when uninflated, applies a considerable heat load to the wearer, and is expensive to purchase and service. For these reasons, partial pressure garments provide a useful and attractive alternative for short-duration protection against hypoxia.

Full-pressure suits

PHYSIOLOGICAL AND GENERAL REQUIREMENTS

The distinguishing feature of a full-pressure suit is that it applies pressure evenly to the entire body surface. The magnitude of the applied pressure is determined by the need to protect against both hypoxia and decompression sickness.

Severe hypoxia can be prevented by delivering 100 per cent oxygen to the respiratory tract and maintaining an absolute pressure within the suit of at least 141 mmHg (18.8 kPa). However, since the suit is also worn in conditions where it is necessary to prevent decompression sickness, the absolute pressure within the garment ideally should not be less than 282 mmHg (37.6 kPa), i.e. equivalent to an altitude of 25 000 feet or below. However, experience has shown that an absolute pressure within the suit equivalent to an altitude of 30 000 feet (226 mmHg, 30.1 kPa) is sufficient to prevent serious decompression sickness in seated aircrew, provided that the duration of exposure is no longer than four to five hours. If the pressure within the suit is less than 226 mmHg (30.1 kPa), then serious decompression sickness may occur, the severity of which is related directly to the altitude and duration of exposure. In practice, therefore, the absolute pressure in a full pressure suit may range from as low as 141 mmHg (18.8 kPa) for short-duration protection to as high as

282 mmHg (37.6 kPa) when protection is required for several hours.

Some full pressure suits are inflated with air, oxygen being delivered to the respiratory tract via an oronasal mask mounted within the helmet (see below). Consequently, if the suit operating pressure is at the lower end of the range (i.e. 141 mmHg, 18.8 kPa), any inward leakage of air due to a poorly fitting mask will cause severe hypoxia, a risk that is clearly reduced if the pressure in the suit is higher.

Although, if necessary, heat can be delivered to a full pressure suit by various means (including ventilation with hot air, electric heating and circulation of heated liquid), its pressure-containing layer is impermeable, and the garment therefore imposes a considerable heat load. Consequently, a means of removing metabolic heat and perspiration must be provided throughout the period during which the suit is worn. It is necessary, however, to take special precautions to avoid freezing of valves by the passage through them of moist gas and to prevent misting of the inner surface of the helmet visor.

When unpressurized, a full pressure suit should not place restrictions on posture or functional movements, and it must provide an efficient oxygen and intercommunication system. It must be compatible with the aircraft escape system, and it should afford protection against any hostile ground environment that is likely to be encountered after leaving the aircraft. Finally, the pressure helmet should also provide some protection against noise and glare.

TECHNICAL CONSIDERATIONS

Full pressure suits usually consist of an impermeable inner layer of pressure-containing material with an outer retaining layer that prevents overexpansion on pressurization. It is very difficult to match the characteristics of a flexible inflated system to the shape of the human body and to match the mechanical design of the suit to the natural movement of human joints. Movement is resisted both by friction and by the force required to expel gas from the appropriate part of the suit, and delicate manipulative movements of the fingers may have to be combined with large forces at the shoulder, elbow and wrist.

Consequently, there are many problems associated with the design and construction of full pressure suits, particularly the tendency of the suit to become rigid when it is inflated, with subsequent reduction in mobility, especially at the neck, shoulder and wrist, and the marked tendency of the headpiece to rise from the trunk of the wearer. Although the movement of joints may be improved by the use of lightweight metal and gas-tight rotating bearings, the bulk, weight and additional restrictions that these impose limit the value of the full pressure suit as a flying garment in conventional aviation, even when modern fabric manufacturing techniques have been used to reduce the problems of general rigidity.

To maintain the thermal balance of a crew member wearing a full pressure suit, a large ventilating flow of gas is required beneath the impermeable layer, even when the suit is not inflated. Air is taken from the engines to provide gas for ventilation and pressurization, while an oxygen-rich supply for breathing is delivered through an oronasal mask or a helmet. Such suits therefore effectively have two separate gas compartments: one for conditioning and pressurization, and one for the breathing supply. The pressure differential between these compartments must be kept very small to avoid positive or negative pressure breathing. Furthermore, in order to prevent air being drawn into an ill-fitting mask from the remainder of the suit, the pressure within the former must not fall below that of the air inflating the latter. Expired gas from the respiratory tract may be passed either into the air compartment of the suit or directly to the exterior. There are two common methods of pressure control in full pressure suits, as illustrated in Figure 5.27.

In the first method, termed an oxygen pressure-control system (Figure 5.27a), a pressure-demand regulator is used to produce the desired absolute pressure in the oxygen compartment of the suit. This oxygen pressure is itself then used to control the air outlet valves, so that the desired pressure differential is maintained between the two compartments of the air suit. In the second method, termed an air-control system (Figure 5.27b), the pressure of the air in the suit is controlled by a barometrically operated outlet valve. A relatively simple demand valve can then be used to deliver oxygen to the breathing compartment, since the absolute pressure delivered by the oxygen regulator is determined solely by the air pressure in the suit. Finally, in space, where clearly no engine air source is available, and where the astronaut or cosmonaut may leave the spacecraft, a closed-circuit system is required. Breathing gas is circulated around the body, and a backpack unit is employed to remove carbon dioxide, water vapour, heat and odour and to add the necessary amounts of oxygen to the system. Thermal balance is maintained by a liquid-cooling garment worn under the pressure suit next to the skin.

In addition to the technical difficulties outlined above, it would be even more problematic to combine adequate protection against altitude exposure with protection against sustained acceleration, high G_z. This is achieved more easily by the combination of anti-G garments with high-altitude partial pressure assemblies (see also Chapter 9).

Partial pressure garments and assemblies

The benefits of using counter-pressure applied to regions of the body and thus to mitigate against the adverse physiological effects of pressure breathing were described in the

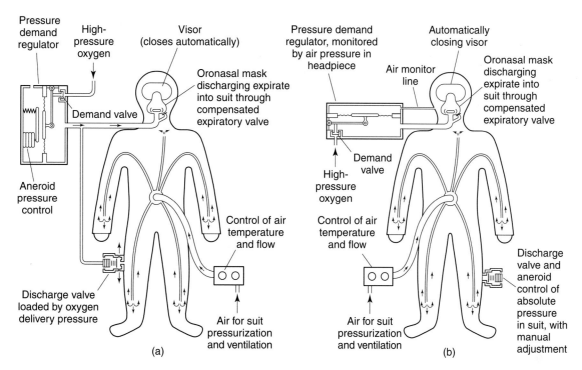

Figure 5.27 *Methods of pressure control of breathing oxygen and ventilating air in full pressure suits. (a) Oxygen pressure control system. The oxygen regulator delivers gas to the oxygen compartment of the suit (oronasal mask) at the required absolute pressure. The pressure of air in the air compartment of the suit (head, trunk and limbs) is controlled by the oxygen pressure fed to the air discharge valve. (b) Air control system. An aneroid-operated discharge valve controls the pressure of air in the air compartment, which in turn controls the pressure at which gas is delivered by the oxygen regulator to the oxygen compartment of the suit.*

previous chapter. Counter-pressure of this type is achieved by the use of partial pressure assemblies (in contrast to full-pressure suits, as described above). Partial pressure garments are less restrictive than full pressure suits and so offer considerable advantages where short-term protection against the effects of hypoxia is all that is required. From the physiological standpoint, the ideal solution is to apply counter-pressure to as much of the body as possible. The advantages of the 'partial' principle, however – i.e. low thermal load, less restriction when unpressurized, and greater mobility when pressurized – make it desirable that counter-pressure should be applied to the minimum area of the body. Thus, the proportion of the body covered by partial pressure garments represents a compromise between physiological ideal and operational expediency. Furthermore, since partial pressure assemblies for high altitude protection are used for only very short exposures, certain compromises with regard to the presence of a moderate degree of hypoxia are also acceptable. Some practical pressure breathing systems incorporating partial pressure assemblies of increasing complexity and effectiveness are described below.

MASK ALONE

The maximum breathing pressure that can be tolerated using a mask alone (i.e. without counter-pressure to

the body) is about 30 mmHg (4 kPa). If an alveolar oxygen tension of 60 mmHg (8 kPa), i.e. an absolute lung pressure (breathing pressure + environmental pressure) of 141 mmHg (18.8 kPa), is to be maintained, then this system will provide respiratory protection to an altitude of 45 000 feet. It is practical, however, to accept a greater degree of hypoxia than that associated with an alveolar oxygen tension of 60 mmHg (8 kPa). A breathing pressure of 30 mmHg (4 kPa) at 50 000 feet provides an absolute lung pressure of 117 mmHg (15.6 kPa) and an alveolar oxygen tension of 45–50 mmHg (6–6.7 kPa). Although this degree of hypoxia gives rise to very marked impairment of performance if it is experienced for any length of time, it is acceptable if a rapid descent is initiated immediately. Typically, the oxygen regulator used in this type of system delivers pressure breathing at altitudes above 40 000 feet, with the breathing pressure increasing from 0.75–7.5 mmHg (0.1–1 kPa) at 40 000 feet to about 30–34.5 mmHg (4–4.6 kPa) at 50 000 feet. Between the altitudes of 40 000 and 50 000 feet, breathing pressure increases linearly with the decrease in environmental pressure. The absolute pressure in the respiratory tract therefore falls progressively above 40 000 feet and produces a gradual increase in the intensity of the hypoxia. Above 50 000 feet, the hypoxia is very severe, and unconsciousness supervenes rapidly.

This type of pressure-breathing system is used widely throughout the world. The combination of a pressure breathing mask and a suitable oxygen regulator (capable of delivering a pressure of 30–34.5 mmHg (4–4.6 kPa) at 50 000 feet) will provide protection for one minute against the effects of loss of cabin pressurization up to cabin altitudes of 50 000 feet, provided that immediate descent at a minimum rate of 10 000 feet/min is then undertaken to below 40 000 feet. The degree of protection afforded by this system is shown diagrammatically in Figure 5.28.

CHEST AND TRUNK COUNTER-PRESSURE

Considerable physiological advantage can be gained by the application of counter-pressure to the chest or, better, the whole trunk. Furthermore, this has the added benefit of reducing the fatigue associated with pressure breathing by providing mechanical assistance to the expiratory muscles of the chest wall. An inelastic counter-pressure garment covering the chest only, commonly termed a pressure waistcoat, incorporates a pneumatic bladder in communication with the mask hose. As mask hose pressure rises, so too does the pressure in the waistcoat. There is significant benefit to using a garment with a bladder that provides full circumferential protection of the chest. This serves to reduce distension of the chest and consequently reduces

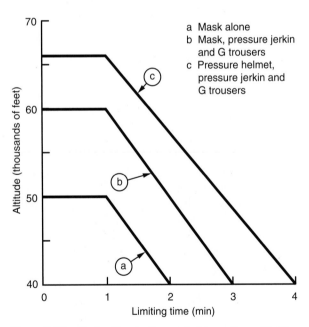

Figure 5.28 *Limits of protection against hypoxia provided by pressure breathing systems. (a) Pressure breathing mask alone (maximum breathing pressure 30–34.5 mmHg, 4–4.6 kPa). (b) Pressure breathing mask with counter-pressure to the trunk and lower limbs (maximum breathing pressure 68–72 mmHg, 9.1–9.6 kPa). (c) Partial pressure helmet with counter-pressure to the trunk and lower limbs (maximum breathing pressure 107–110 mmHg, 14.3–14.7 kPa).*

the changes in lung volumes during pressure breathing described above. Since distension of the chest is reduced, so too is the difference between the applied breathing pressure and the intrapleural pressure, i.e. there is a smaller loss of intrapulmonary pressure as a result of chest distension and the pressure breathing therefore is likely to be more effective.

However, although chest counter-pressure is helpful in providing some support to muscles of the thoracic cage, it is of little or no benefit in itself with respect to circulatory disturbances. Application of counter-pressure to the whole of the trunk, however, does contribute to circulatory support by applying compression to the abdomen. A garment covering the whole of the trunk, known as a jerkin, therefore can make higher breathing pressures tolerable and extend the allowable duration of pressure breathing. Counter-pressure jerkins are even more effective in preventing overdistension of the chest, as they offer mechanical support to the diaphragm as well as the chest wall. The abdominal element of the garment also acts to prevent visceral pooling of blood and aids venous return through the inferior vena cava.

Such mask and jerkin systems have been used in the past to provide a significant degree of protection against the adverse effects of pressure breathing and have the valuable advantage in multi-crew aircraft of allowing a considerable degree of mobility. However, counter-pressure to the trunk alone may induce syncope as a consequence of the large displacement of blood to all four limbs; therefore, to provide more effective circulatory support, limb counter-pressure is also required.

MASK WITH TRUNK AND LOWER–LIMB COUNTER-PRESSURE

A long-established partial pressure assembly used in the RAF, and copied elsewhere, incorporates both trunk and lower-limb counter-pressure and makes full use of the pressure-sealing properties of current oronasal masks to a maximum breathing pressure of 70 mmHg (9.3 kPa). Trunk counter-pressure is applied by a partial pressure jerkin (Figure 5.28), which comprises a rubber bladder restrained by an outer inextensible cover. The bladder extends not only over the whole of the trunk but also over the upper parts of the thighs, to ensure that there is adequate counter-pressure over the inguinal canals, and reduces the risk of herniation at high breathing pressures. Since the bladder is supplied from the mask hose, it is inflated to the same pressure as that delivered to the respiratory tract. In this assembly, lower-limb counter-pressure is supplied by the incorporation of anti-G trousers into the assembly, which also are inflated with gas from the breathing system.

If the absolute pressure within the lungs is maintained at 141 mmHg (18.8 kPa), then the mask/partial pressure jerkin/anti-G trousers combination will provide ideal protection to a maximum altitude of 54 000 feet. In practice, however, a certain degree of hypoxia is acceptable, and a breathing pressure of 68–72 mmHg (9.1–9.6 kPa) can be employed at 60 000 feet, where it will provide an absolute pressure in the lungs of 122–126 mmHg (16.3–16.8 kPa) and an alveolar oxygen tension of 55–60 mmHg (7.3–8 kPa). The combination of the discomfort of a high breathing pressure in the mask and a certain degree of hypoxia limits the duration of protection afforded by this ensemble. The limit, shown diagrammatically in Figure 5.28b, is an interval of 60 seconds at 60 000 feet followed immediately by descent at a rate of at least 10 000feet/min to 40 000 feet.

In this form of partial pressure assembly, both the jerkin and the anti-G trousers are inflated at the same pressure, but there are advantages to inflating the latter to a greater pressure than that being delivered to the jerkin and mask. Work carried out in a number of centres has demonstrated that if lower-body counter-pressure is provided by the inflation of anti-G trousers to a pressure considerably higher than the breathing pressure, then this serves to improve support to the diaphragm, increase venous return, resulting in the better maintenance of an appropriate blood pressure, and reduce the degree of tachycardia associated with pressure breathing. The degree to which the anti-G trousers should be inflated has been the topic of considerable research, but opinion now favours the inflation of conventional anti-G trousers to three times the

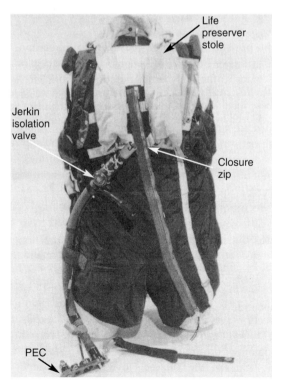

Figure 5.29 *The Royal Air Force partial pressure jerkin.*

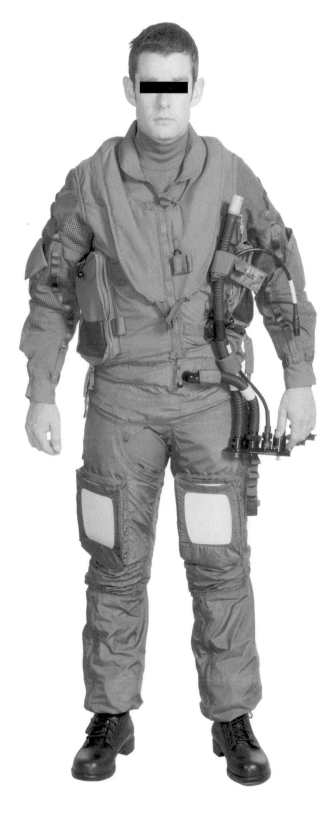

Figure 5.30 *A modern RAF counter-pressure assembly comprising a chest counter-pressure waistcoat integrated within the Flight Jacket and worn in combination with full coverage anti-G trousers which are inflated, during pressure breathing, to a pressure higher than the breathing pressure.*

breathing pressure. If the inflation of the anti-G trousers is too high, e.g. to four times a breathing pressure of 70 mmHg (9.3 kPa), this would produce a lower-body counter-pressure of some 280 mmHg (37.2 kPa), which would at least partially occlude arterial flow into the lower limbs and is uncomfortable. If anti-G trousers with enhanced body coverage are used, then the ratio of breathing pressure to trouser inflation pressure may be reduced, perhaps to just twice the mask pressure. With such assemblies, the extent of bladder coverage of the upper counter-pressure garment can be reduced drastically (and with it the bulk and weight of the garment) with few additional cardiorespiratory penalties. The abdominal portion of the anti-G trousers provides counter-pressure to the lower half of the trunk, in lieu of the abdominal portion of the jerkin as described previously. This then has considerable advantages for use in the new generation of agile combat aircraft capable of high accelerative performance at high altitude and in which bulky jerkin assemblies are less acceptable. The anti-G garments that are used therefore can be integrated into an ensemble that supports pressure breathing for both high altitude and high G (Figure 5.30).

PARTIAL PRESSURE HELMET WITH TRUNK AND LOWER-LIMB COUNTER-PRESSURE

In this system, a partial pressure helmet is the means by which pressure is delivered to the respiratory tract, a jerkin provides trunk counter-pressure, and the anti-G trousers provide lower-limb counter-pressure to reduce the circulatory disturbance induced by high breathing pressures. The disadvantages of a pressure helmet are its weight and bulk, which make it less acceptable for use in aircraft with high agility and high altitude capability.

As described therefore, a partial pressure helmet is an alternative device for applying positive pressure to the respiratory tract and to give support to the cheeks, the floor of the mouth and the eyes, so eliminating the uncomfortable pressure differentials that develop between the air passages and the skin of the head and neck when an oronasal mask is employed. In most partial pressure helmets, counter-pressure is also applied by oxygen bladders to a limited area of the upper neck, but although the extent of this coverage ensures reasonable head mobility during routine flying, severe neck discomfort may occur during pressure breathing at levels greater than 110 mmHg (14.7 kPa).

Physiologically, the pressure demand oxygen regulator used with this assembly need only provide an absolute pressure of 141 mmHg (18.8 kPa) at altitudes above 40 000 feet. In practice, however, the regulator used by the RAF in the past delivered a maximum breathing pressure of 107–110 mmHg (14.3–14.7 kPa) at 66 000 feet, so providing an absolute pressure in the lungs at that altitude of 148–151 mmHg (19.6–20.1 kPa). The partial pressure helmet/partial pressure jerkin/G-trousers ensemble there-fore could be used up to a maximum altitude of 66 000 feet, where it would provide protection for up to one minute, provided that descent to 40 000 feet follows within a further three minutes (see Figure 5.28c).

PRESSURE HELMET WITH TRUNK AND UPPER- AND LOWER-LIMB COUNTER-PRESSURE

It is clearly physiologically advantageous to include the upper limbs in the areas to which counter-pressure is applied, and a wide variety of garments have been employed to provide this extensive coverage in combination with a pressure helmet. Many garments, such as sleeved jerkins used previously in RAF systems, made use of oxygen-filled bladders that covered much of the body surface. Others, such as the United States Air Force (USAF) 'capstan' partial pressure garment, utilize a mixture of fabric tensioning by means of capstans and gas-filled bladders (see below). In these systems, an inflatable torso garment is inflated from the breathing gas, but a separate supply inflates relatively narrow tubes that run the length of the limbs to a pressure considerable greater than breathing pressure. On inflation, the capstans, which are attached to inelastic material by figure-of-eight bands around the limb, act as pneumatic levers to hold the garment encasing the limb under tension and thereby apply counter-pressure. Although this is a relatively efficient method of applying limb counter-pressure, it is restrictive, especially when inflated, since the capstans are inflated to high pressures. Such systems were in common use in the USAF in the past and remain in use in a number of Eastern European airforces to this day.

The pressure helmets employed in combination with such extensive partial pressure assemblies vary from the RAF partial pressure helmet described above (in which pressure is applied only to the face, part of the head and the upper neck) to the USAF version (in which gas is applied to the whole of the head and neck). A range of combinations have been used in the past to provide limited duration protection at very high altitudes. Most do not apply counter-pressure to the lower neck, the axillae or the hands and feet. Variants of a combined suit incorporating counter-pressure bladders, separate anti-G trousers and an air-ventilated layer have been trialled but currently are not in service. Virtually all of these systems employ oxygen regulators that maintain an absolute pressure in the respiratory tract, and over the pressurized areas of the body, of 145–150 mmHg (19.3–20 kPa). Such combinations will provide prolonged protection against the effects of hypoxia on exposure to altitudes well above 40 000 feet; for example, protection is possible for 30 minutes at 65 000–70 000 feet and for several minutes at 100 000 feet. However, protection against decompression sickness and the effects of low temperature is not provided.

Although they do not provide the same degree of physiological protection as full pressure suits, operational considerations make partial pressure assemblies an attractive alternative for short-duration protection against hypoxia at high altitude. In combination with enhanced anti-G systems, such assemblies are in relatively common use in the latest generation of fast jet combat aircraft.

FURTHER READING

Air Standardization Coordinating Committee. The minimum physiological design requirements for aircrew breathing systems. Air Standard 61/101/06A. Washington, DC: Air Standardization Coordinating Committee, 1988.

Civil Aviation Authority. CAP 393 Air Navigation: The Order and Regulations. London: Civil Aviation Authority, 2003.

Ernsting J. Operational and physiological requirements for aircraft oxygen systems. In: Seventh Advanced Operational Aviation Medicine Course. Report no. 697. Neuilly-sur-Seine: AGARD/NATO, 1984a; pp. 1—1–11.

Ernsting J. Molecular sieve on board oxygen generating systems for high performance aircraft. In: Seventh Advanced Operational Aviation Medicine Course. Report no. 697. Neuilly-sur-Seine: AGARD/NATO, 1984b; pp. 3—1–14.

Ernsting J, Miller RL. Advanced oxygen systems for aircraft. AGARDograph 286. Neuilly-sur-Seine: AGARD/NATO, 1996.

Federal Aviation Administration. FAR Code of US Federal Regulations. Parts 25, 121 and 125. Washington, DC: US Department of Transportation, 2004.

Gradwell DP. Pressure breathing inflation schedules/ratios. Presented at Raising the Operational Ceiling AL/CF-SR-1995-0021. Armstrong Laboratory, Brooks Air Force Base, Texas, 13–15 June 1995.

Macmillan AJF. The performance and deficiencies of oxygen systems fitted to current NATO interceptor aircraft. In: Seventh Advanced Operational Aviation Medicine Course. Report no. 697. Neuilly-sur-Seine: AGARD/NATO, 1984; pp. 2—1–7.

6

Principles of the pressure cabin and the effects of pressure change on body cavities containing gas

ALISTAIR J.F. MACMILLAN

INTRODUCTION

The physiological disturbances induced by exposure to the low environmental pressures encountered during flight at high altitude must be reduced to a minimum. The most effective way of providing protection against these effects is to raise artificially the pressure in the crew and passenger compartments above that of the immediate environment of the aircraft. Thus, the crew and passenger compartments of virtually all modern high-performance combat and transport aircraft are pressurized with air. At first sight, there would appear to be great advantages in maintaining the absolute pressure in the cabin at one atmosphere (760 mmHg) throughout flight. Such a requirement would, however, impose considerable penalties with regard to the weight of the pressure cabin and the pressurization equipment, the power required to pressurize the air, and, hence, the performance of the aircraft. Furthermore, the larger the pressure differential across the wall of a cabin, the greater the risk of damage to the aircraft and its occupants in the event of a failure of the structure. In practice, compromises are made between the physiological ideal of a cabin pressure of one atmosphere absolute, the weight and performance penalties of a high cabin pressure differential, and the probability of explosive failure of the cabin. The compromises that have been adopted in the design of pressure cabins can be classified into two groups. If comfort is of prime concern and the probability of structural damage to the aircraft is very remote, then the pressure in the cabin is maintained at a level at which the occupants can breathe air throughout flight. In combat aircraft, where weight is at a premium and there is a risk of failure of the integrity of the cabin due to enemy action, a much lower level of pressurization of the cabin is adopted, and the occupants breathe oxygen or an oxygen/air mixture.

There are two methods of maintaining the pressure in the cabin of aircraft above that of the immediate environment. The conventional method, used in virtually all current aircraft, is to draw air from outside the aircraft, compress it, and deliver it into the cabin. The desired pressure is maintained within the cabin by controlling the flow of compressed air out of the cabin to the atmosphere. The continuous flow of air ventilates the compartment; in most aircraft, this flow of air also controls the thermal environment within the cabin, so that the control of pressure and temperature are closely related. As modern turbofan engines were developed, the amount of fuel required to provide thrust decreased, but fuel consumption relative to extracting bleed air for control of the cabin environment increased considerably. Thus, efficient recirculation systems were developed, incorporating high-efficiency particulate air (HEPA) filters, which provided fuel savings without compromising cabin air quality. Consequently, since the mid-1980s, most passenger-carrying aircraft have been fitted with environmental control systems that recirculate 50 per cent of the air in the cabin.

At very high altitudes, the energy required to compress the low-density air to the pressure required in the cabin and the heat generated in the process of compression become excessive. It is impracticable to pressurize the cabin with external air during sustained flights at altitudes above about 80 000 feet. In these circumstances, and in the vacuum of space, the pressurizing gases must be carried within the vehicle. It then becomes uneconomical to condition the cabin with a through-flow of gas that escapes to the environment. Used gases are recycled and loss of gas is reduced to a minimum. This chapter deals only with the conventional pressure cabin.

The difference between the absolute pressure within and that of the atmosphere immediately outside an aircraft is termed the cabin differential pressure. The differential pressure is frequently controlled, so it varies with aircraft altitude. Although the pressure in the cabin generally is greater than that of the atmosphere at the aircraft altitude (i.e. a positive differential), in some circumstances, e.g. during a rapid dive, it can be less (i.e. a negative differential). The absolute pressure in an aircraft cabin is almost always stated in terms of pressure altitude (feet above mean sea level) in accordance with the International Civil Aviation Organization (ICAO) standard scale. The absolute pressure in the cabin equals the sum of the atmospheric pressure and the cabin differential pressure. Thus, the cabin pressure of an aircraft flying at an altitude of 25 000 feet (atmospheric pressure 38 kPa, 5.5 lb/in^2) and with a cabin differential pressure of 31 kPa (4.5 lb/in^2) gauge is 69 kPa (10 lb/in^2) absolute, which is equivalent to an altitude of 10 200 feet.

PHYSIOLOGICAL REQUIREMENTS

Four main groups of physiological factors must be considered when defining the requirements for a pressure cabin. The first group consists of the factors that determine the maximum acceptable cabin altitude: hypoxia, decompression sickness and expansion of gastrointestinal gas. The second group determines the maximum acceptable rate of change of cabin altitude during ascent and descent of the aircraft: the ventilation of body cavities containing gas, e.g. the middle-ear cavities and the paranasal sinuses. The third group of factors relate to the magnitude of the effects of a sudden cabin failure. The final group of factors concern the quality of the cabin air and the effect this has on comfort and well-being.

Hypoxia

The acceptable cabin altitude in an aircraft in which the occupants breathe air is set by considerations of the effects of mild hypoxia on the performance of the aircrew and on the well-being of the passengers. At altitudes greater than 10 000–12 000 feet, there is a significant impairment of ability to perform flight tasks. Indeed, individuals are detectably slower to react to a novel situation when they are breathing air at an altitude of 8000 feet; at 5000 feet, there is just detectable impairment of this type of performance. It is generally accepted that the maximum cabin altitude consistent with flight safety is 5000–7000 feet rather than the previous standard of 8000 feet. Certain people, particularly those suffering from cardiorespiratory disease, may be unable to maintain full oxygenation of tissues above 6000 feet, a matter of considerable importance in civil transport aircraft, where passengers cannot be selected for the integrity of their respiratory and cardiovascular systems. Exposure of the standard passenger population to cabin altitudes of the order of 8000 feet for several hours results in noticeable fatigue and sporadic incidents of heart failure, which are probably induced by the combination of mild hypoxia, expansion of abdominal gas, lack of movement and seated posture. Limitation of the cabin altitude to a maximum of 6000 feet has been shown to eliminate most of these incidents.

If the inspired air is progressively enriched with oxygen, then the alveolar oxygen tension ($P_{A_{O_2}}$) may be maintained at the value associated with normal air breathing at sea level up to 33 000 feet. The hypoxia induced in a person breathing 100 per cent oxygen at 40 000 feet is equivalent to that produced when he or she breathes air at 8000 feet. Since the latter was generally recognized as the maximum degree of hypoxia acceptable, it could be argued that, given 100 per cent oxygen, the cabin altitude could be allowed to rise to 40 000 feet. However, this argument ignores the effects of possible malfunction or failure of the oxygen-delivery system and the consequent rapidly increased rate at which impairment of judgement and performance develop in an individual who has to revert to breathing air above 20 000 feet. Thus, the time available to an individual to recognize that the oxygen supply has ceased and to carry out the appropriate corrective action falls from 10–12 minutes at 20 000 feet, to three to five minutes at 25 000 feet, and to 1–1.5 minutes at 33 000 feet.

Furthermore, the reduction of inspired P_{O_2} produced by a given fractional inboard leak of air due to an ill-fitting breathing mask increases with rise of altitude. In practice, the incidence and severity of hypoxia become significant at a cabin altitude of about 22 000 feet and rise markedly above that, so that 20 000–22 000 feet is now regarded as the standard limit for regular operations by crews breathing supplemental oxygen. However, some aircraft with a 25 000-feet cabin remain in service in air forces all over the world.

Decompression sickness

Although decompression sickness can occur when individuals are exposed to an altitude of 18 000 feet, it is very rare below 22 000 feet. A small but significant number of cases have occurred during exposure to altitudes between 22 000 and 25 000 feet. Since decompression sickness during routine flights is unacceptable, the maximum cabin altitude to which aircrew may be exposed should not exceed 22 000 feet. In some circumstances, it may be necessary for aircrew to operate at cabin altitudes as high as 25 000 feet; however, unless susceptible individuals are protected by pre-oxygenation, occasional cases of decompression sickness will occur.

Expansion of gastrointestinal gas

In normal healthy individuals, the stomach and intestines contain a quantity of gas, the volume of which varies between 0 and 400 ml, with an average value of 100 ml. This gas is derived from swallowed air, from the action of bacteria within the gut, and from exchange with the gases in the tissues and blood.

During ascent, the gas contained within the stomach expands and usually escapes up the oesophagus and out through the mouth. Gas bubbles within the large bowel coalesce to form large bubbles, which are vented through the anus. Some people, usually inexperienced aircrew members, have difficulty in venting gas from the mouth and anus, even with low rates of ascent. At very high rates of ascent and during rapid decompression, this difficulty increases, and even experienced aircrew members have some difficulty in expelling gas from the alimentary tract as quickly as it expands. The individual may thus develop symptoms, which vary from mild upper or lower abdominal discomfort to, in exceptional cases, very severe pain. In some sensitive individuals, the abdominal pain caused by the expanding gas may cause vasovagal syncope. Expansion of the gas in the gastrointestinal tract has never been known to produce visceral damage.

The problem of gas expansion in the alimentary tract may be aggravated if the individual is suffering from mild intestinal infection or has eaten a large quantity of foodstuffs known to be gas-forming (e.g. peas, beans, cauliflower, cabbage, high-roughage foods, carbonated drinks). With experience, aircrew members learn which foodstuffs cause excessive gas formation and adjust their diet accordingly. The incidence of abdominal discomfort or pain in healthy aircrew who are frequently exposed to high altitude is negligible when the maximum altitude does not exceed 25 000 feet. Even when such individuals are decompressed to altitudes above 40 000 feet, the incidence of abdominal pain on short-duration exposures is only two to three per cent. However, although infrequent, symptoms arising from gas expansion in the alimentary tract are the most common cause of early termination of training decompressions to high altitude.

Passengers suffering from cardiorespiratory disorders may be distressed even by a relatively small increase in the volume of gas in the abdomen produced by ascent from ground level to 8000 feet. The maximum cabin altitude of passenger and aeromedical evacuation aircraft should, therefore, be kept as low as possible, and certainly below 6000 feet.

The teeth

Expansion of gas in the teeth during ascent to altitude may cause severe toothache, known as aerodontalgia. The source of gas in the teeth may be air trapped between the tooth substance and a deep cavity filling, particularly in unlined cavities. Modern dental filling materials have reduced the incidence of trapped gas in dental fillings and aerodontalgia from this source is now rare. Aerodontalgia may, however, be experienced by aircrew with unhealthy teeth, where, for example, gas of putrefaction gathers in a small bubble at the apex of a tooth in the condition of chronic or acute apical abscess.

Rates of change of cabin altitude

High rates of ascent to altitude, e.g. 5000–20 000 feet/min, are usually tolerated very well, but descent is another matter. The difficulty of equilibration to ambient of the pressures in the gas-filled cavities of the body limits the maximum acceptable rate of increase of cabin pressure during descent. The body contains a number of gas-filled cavities that communicate with varying degrees of ease with the external environment. During ascent or descent in an aircraft or on sudden loss of cabin pressurization, the pressure of the gas within these cavities must attain equilibrium with that of the surrounding environment, otherwise the individual will suffer adverse effects.

When there is unrestricted communication between a gas-filled cavity and the outside atmosphere, gas expansion occurs with little difficulty and no discomfort. If, however, the pressure of the gas in the cavity fails to equilibrate with the outside environmental pressure, then there may be considerable discomfort, frank pain, or damage to tissues or organs of the body, which may well incapacitate the individual. The critical sites where gases can be trapped and pressures fail to equalize comprise the middle ears and paranasal sinuses.

THE MIDDLE EAR

The cavity of the middle ear is separated from the outer ear by the tympanic membrane (Figure 6.1). It communicates with the nasopharynx and, hence, the atmosphere by way of the Eustachian tube, the proximal two-thirds of which has soft walls that are normally collapsed. During ascent to altitude, the gas in the middle-ear cavity expands and

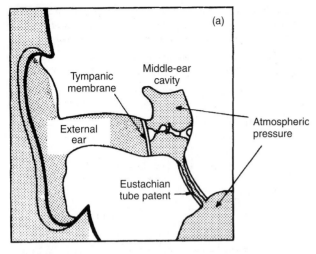

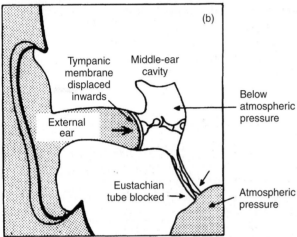

Figure 6.1 *Diagram of external and middle ear (a) at a constant altitude with a patent Eustachian tube and (b) during descent with an occluded Eustachian tube. While the Eustachian tube is patent, the pressure in the middle-ear cavity equals that in the nasopharynx, which in turn is equal to that of the atmosphere. If, however, the Eustachian tube is occluded during descent (b), the pressure in the middle-ear cavity is less than that in the nasopharynx and the atmospheric pressure, and the pressure difference across the tympanic membrane displaces it into the middle-ear cavity.*

escapes along the Eustachian tube into the nasopharynx, so that pressure remains equal on both sides of the tympanic membrane. Since the anatomical structure of the pharyngeal (or fibrous) portion of the Eustachian tube is such that it acts as a one-way valve, expanding air can escape easily to the atmosphere, and it is very unusual for passive venting of the middle ear to present difficulties during decompression. This intermittent passive ventilation of the middle ear during ascent may be appreciated as a 'popping' sensation as air escapes from the pharyngeal orifice of the Eustachian tube. On ascent, the Eustachian tube opens and

gas escapes from the middle ear into the nasopharynx approximately once every 500–1000 feet.

During descent, gas from the nasopharynx must enter the middle ear in order to maintain equilibrium between the atmospheric pressure outside and the gas pressure in the middle ear. In most individuals, the one-way valve mechanism of the Eustachian tube prevents the passive flow of gas back into the middle-ear cavity. The resultant relative increase of pressure on the outside of the tympanic membrane pushes the membrane into the middle-ear cavity. As descent continues, the membrane is pushed further into the middle-ear cavity unless gas enters through the Eustachian tube. This distortion leads to a sensation of fullness in the ear and a decrease in hearing acuity. If descent continues further without equalization of pressure between the atmosphere and the middle ear, then the differential pressure across the ear drum causes pain. In certain susceptible individuals, a rapid change of pressure in the middle-ear cavity may also affect the organs of balance in the inner ear and cause vertigo (pressure vertigo).

In order to equalize the pressure across the tympanic membrane during descent and thus prevent the development of otitic barotrauma, it is usually necessary to perform some active manoeuvre to open the Eustachian tubes. Although several simple manoeuvres, such as swallowing, yawning and jaw movements, may open the tube, these are not effective in about half the aircrew population. These individuals have to raise the pressure in the nasopharynx in order to force gas into the middle ear cavities. This rise in pressure is usually achieved by performing either a Valsalva or Frenzel manoeuvre. The Valsalva manoeuvre is carried out by attempting a forced expiration with the lips closed and the nostrils occluded by compressing the nose. This manoeuvre is used commonly in flight, but the raised intrathoracic pressure generated during the procedure may, under certain circumstances, impair cardiovascular function. The Frenzel manoeuvre raises the pressure locally in the nasopharynx. It is performed by closing the glottis and the lips while occluding the nostrils and simultaneously contracting the muscles of the floor of the mouth and pharynx. These coordinated actions are similar to those employed when blowing one's nose or stifling a sneeze and have to be learned. The Frenzel manoeuvre has the advantages of opening the Eustachian tube at lower nasopharyngeal pressures and being capable of performance during any phase of respiration.

Mention must also be made of the Toynbee manoeuvre, which consists of swallowing while the nostrils are pinched. This action also opens the Eustachian tubes at ground level but does so by generation of a reduced pressure in the nasopharynx. It is useful, therefore, for checking the patency of the tubes, but it is not recommended as a procedure for use during descent.

The frequency with which trained aircrew perform one or other of these ear-clearing manoeuvres varies considerably, from once every 1000 feet to once every 4000 feet or more. There is, however, a limit to the pressure rise that can be created within the nasopharynx, and the Eustachian tube may become locked closed when the differential pressure between the middle ear and the environment exceeds 12–16 kPa (90–120 mmHg).

Upper respiratory tract infection causes congestion and oedema of the mucosal lining of the Eustachian tube, particularly where it opens into the nasopharynx. This congestion may restrict the passage of gas into the middle-ear cavity during descent. The tympanic membrane will then be driven into the middle ear, causing deafness and pain. If descent is continued, the grossly distorted membrane may rupture, with immediate relief of the pain. The changes in the tympanic membrane and middle ear produced by failure of adequate ventilation of the latter during descent are termed otitic barotrauma. This condition commonly arises in association with upper respiratory tract infections, but it may also be caused by too rapid descent or inadequate knowledge of the correct procedures for ventilating the middle ear.

THE PARANASAL SINUSES

The paranasal sinuses are cavities located in the bones of the face and skull. The frontal sinuses communicate with the nose by relatively long ducts. Each of the other sinuses is connected to the nose by a hole in its wall. During ascent and descent, the expanding and contracting gas contained within a sinus is free to communicate with the gas in the nose, and a pressure difference does not develop between the gas in the sinus and the external atmosphere. If, however, the mucous membrane lining the passage connecting a paranasal sinus to the nose becomes inflamed and oedematous, then the normal passive ventilation of the sinus cavity may be obstructed, particularly during descent. Such a failure causes severe pain in the cheeks or forehead or deep in the head, often accompanied by watering of the eyes. Auto-inflation of the sinus cavity is not achieved easily when this condition exists, even by manoeuvres in which the pressure in the mouth and nose is raised above that of the environment. Nasal decongestants may help to re-establish auto-ventilation of the sinus cavity, but it may be necessary to limit the rate of descent. Damage to the mucosal lining may occur with subsequent haemorrhage into the sinus cavity. This condition of acute sinus barotrauma frequently recurs and eventually may require surgical treatment.

MAXIMUM ACCEPTABLE RATES OF CHANGE OF CABIN ALTITUDE

A pressure change of 14 kPa (2 lb/in^2)/min is the maximum that should be permitted for military aircraft if otitic or sinus barotrauma is to be avoided. Sudden alterations of descent rates are also undesirable. Inexperienced passengers who are not trained in the techniques of inflation of the middle ears during descent will complain of ear discomfort if the rate of increase of cabin pressure from the 6000–8000-feet maximum altitude to ground level exceeds about 1.7 kPa (0.25 lb/in^2)/min, i.e. about 500 feet/min. The maximum rate of increase of cabin pressure adopted for most civil passenger aircraft is 1 kPa (0.15 lb/in^2)/min, i.e. about 300 feet/min.

Decompression of the pressure cabin

The risk of damage to the occupants of a pressure cabin in the event of a sudden failure of its integrity increases in proportion to the ratio of the area of the defect in the wall to the volume of the cabin and to the ratio of cabin pressures before and immediately after the decompression. A more detailed account of these relationships is given later in this chapter. The cabins of transport aircraft are designed so that the ratio of the area of the maximum size of defect that could occur in the wall from the loss of a window to the volume of the cabin is as small as possible, and larger access areas such as doors and hatches are designed to open inwards. The maximum probable defect will not, therefore, produce a dangerous rate of decompression, even when the cabin pressure differential is as high as 69–83 kPa (10–12 lb/in^2) unless there is an additional major structural failure, which would possibly destroy the aircraft. In military aircraft, however, battle damage or jettison of a canopy from a small-volume cabin could lead to very rapid decompression. To limit the effects of this, the cabin differential pressure normally does not exceed 28–35 kPa (4–5 lb/in^2). However, in some combat aircraft, a dual differential pressure facility was been adopted in the past. Thus, in cruise or patrol conditions, a high differential pressure of 55–62 kPa (8–9 lb/in^2) could be selected, thereby permitting aircrew to dispense with the wearing of oxygen equipment. Reduction of the differential pressure to 28–35 kPa (4–5 lb/in^2) in danger zones minimized the effects of sudden loss of cabin pressure but enforced the use of oxygen in combat. Most aircraft with this dual pressurization capability are, however, now obsolete.

Cabin air quality

Following the introduction of recirculating environmental control systems in passenger aircraft, cabin air quality has been a subject of major interest, stimulating several studies and reviews. The elements of cabin air quality that contribute to passenger perception of comfort and well-being are ventilation, removal of contaminants, temperature, humidity and concerns regarding the spread of infections. Aircraft recirculation systems exchange the air some five to ten times more frequently than in buildings, and thus precise control of the distribution to seating zones is necessary to avoid draughts. HEPA filters ensure that contaminants such as smoke particles and microorganisms are removed. The former capability is becoming increasingly redundant, as smoking is banned by many airlines. Studies by Rydock (2004) indicate that infectious diseases are likely to be transmitted only between people sitting in close proximity to each other, and recirculation of ventilation air has a negligible effect on occupants' risk of exposure. Temperature is relatively easy to control, and flight-deck and cabin attendants should cooperate to maximize the comfort level in the cabin. However, perception of 'comfort' may vary between cabin crew and passengers, and it is not easy to provide temperature comfort for all passengers. Some areas of the aircraft are regarded by the crew as less favourable than others, e.g. the galley. Finally, without a humidifying system, low humidity is inevitable in aircraft operating at moderate and high altitudes. Typically, relative humidity levels of 12–21 per cent exist; although these low levels may cause mild symptoms of nasal dryness, no other effects are apparent. These mild effects probably can be controlled by increased fluid intake during air travel. Published data indicate that modern aircraft maintain a very high quality of ventilating air; in a study conducted for the European Commission, none of the values of the contaminants monitored were at levels of concern for the health of passengers or crew. Nevertheless, measured temperatures, relative humidities and CO_2 levels in the cabin on some flights were outside the range associated with acceptable indoor air quality and thermal comfort. Furthermore, air pollutant levels in the cabin generally were higher on the ground than at cruise altitude. An additional in-depth review of cabin air quality by the US National Research Council of the National Academy of Sciences could not identify a link between the cabin environment and reported illness (Rayman 2002). Despite the reassuring results of the studies monitoring cabin air and the literature reviews, there remains a general perception of reduction in well-being associated with air travel. Future design and technology developments should address improvements to air quality and comfort on the ground, perhaps by further improvements to filtration and better facilities for the control of ventilation and thermal comfort by both passengers and crew in the air.

PRESSURIZATION SCHEDULES

The relationship between cabin altitude and aircraft altitude is termed the cabin pressurization schedule. By convention, this is displayed graphically, with the aircraft and cabin altitudes plotted on linear pressure scales (Figure 6.2). A straight line through the origin with a slope of 1 represents the relationship between cabin and aircraft alti-

tudes when there is no pressurization. A set of straight lines parallel to the zero pressurization curve depicts various constant cabin differential pressures. It is convenient to recognize three types of relationship between cabin and aircraft altitudes. The cabin altitude may be controlled at a constant value over a range of aircraft altitudes – termed isobaric control. The cabin differential pressure may be controlled to a constant value as the aircraft altitude varies – termed differential control. There is also a form of control intermediate between isobaric and differential control, in which the differential pressure, although changing with aircraft altitude, does not do so to such an extent that the cabin altitude remains constant. In practice, these three types of control often are employed over consecutive ranges of altitudes in the same aircraft. The extent to which the pressurization schedule can be varied in flight by the crew also varies. In high-altitude combat aircraft, the cabin pressurization schedule is usually entirely under automatic control, and the pilot can only switch on or off the preset schedule. In passenger transport aircraft, the flight-deck crew can, within certain limits, vary the pressurization schedule during flight.

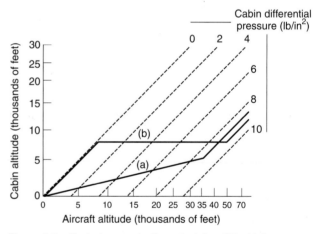

Figure 6.2 *Typical pressurization schedules of the high-differential cabins of (a) a passenger aircraft and (b) a combat aircraft. The cabin and aircraft altitudes are plotted on linear pressure scales. The zero pressurization curve (marked 0 lb/in²) passes through the origin and has a slope of 1.0. Constant differential pressures of 14, 28, 55 and 70 kPa (2, 4, 6, 8 and 10 lb/in²) are indicated by dashed lines. The cabin pressurization of the passenger aircraft (a) commences at ground level, and the maximum differential pressure (60 kPa, 8.8 lb/in², in this example) is reached at 36 000 feet. Contrastingly, in the combat aircraft (b), pressurization does not commence until an aircraft altitude of 8000 feet is reached, and the cabin altitude is held at this value until the maximum differential pressure (63 kPa, 9.2 lb/in², in this example) is reached at 50 000 feet.*

High-differential passenger cabins

The cabins of passenger-carrying aircraft operating at altitudes above 5000–8000 feet are pressurized so that the occupants can breathe air throughout flight and move freely around the cabin, and discomfort and fatigue are minimized. The structure of such aircraft is so robust and the reliability of the cabin pressurization systems so high that the risk of a serious decompression of the cabin is no greater than the risk of other forms of major structural failure. The physiological considerations require that the cabin altitude ideally does not exceed 6000 feet, and certainly not 8000 feet, and that the rate of change of cabin pressure with change of altitude of the aircraft is as small as possible: the rate of increase of pressure on descent should not exceed 1 kPa (0.15 lb/in²)/min (approximately 300 feet/min).

The maximum cabin differential pressure used during normal operation of passenger aircraft is determined by the physiological requirement and the operational ceiling of the aircraft. When the aircraft is cruising at an altitude below its operational ceiling, the flight-deck crew decides whether to select the maximum cabin differential pressure, thus maintaining a very low cabin altitude and increasing comfort, or to allow the cabin altitude to rise to the 6000–8000-feet band, thus minimizing the differential pressure but prolonging the fatigue life of the cabin structure (Table 6.1). The rate of change of cabin pressure is kept low and within the maximum for comfort of 11.7 kPa (0.15–0.25 lb/in²) (300–500 feet)/min by pressurizing the cabin from ground level and prolonging the change of cabin altitude for as long as is practicable, taking account of the rate of change of altitude of the aircraft, the pressure altitude at the airports of departure and arrival, and the cruising altitude for the flight. A typical cabin pressurization profile for the flight of subsonic jet-engined passenger aircraft is depicted by curve (a) of Figure 6.2, while the behaviour of aircraft and cabin altitudes throughout a typical flight to an aircraft altitude of 40 000 feet is shown in Figure 6.3. In such aircraft, the flight-deck crew is able to

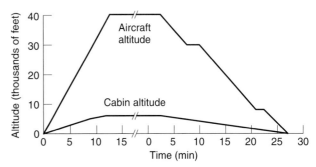

Figure 6.3 *Time course of the cabin altitude (lower curve) of a high-differential passenger aircraft during a flight (aircraft altitude, upper curve) up to 40 000 feet and back to ground level.*

select the desired aircraft altitude at which pressurization of the cabin commences or ceases, the desired rate of change of cabin altitude, and the desired maximum cabin altitude. With these variables selected, the pressurization system automatically controls the cabin differential pressure to give the required profile of cabin altitude.

High-differential combat cabins

In military aircraft, it is advantageous to be able to breathe air and so move freely within the aircraft, unencumbered by oxygen equipment. As noted previously, in the past, some bomber aircraft were provided with such a cabin pressurization schedule; however, to minimize the dangers of rapid decompression when the aircraft is liable to damage due to enemy action, a second cabin pressurization schedule similar to that for low-differential combat cabins usually was available.

Since trained combat aircrew can tolerate relatively high rates of change of cabin pressure (up to 14 kPa (2 lb/in²)/min) without discomfort, the control of the cabin pressurization system can be simplified in high-differential combat aircraft by the use of an isobaric control (curve (b) of Figure 6.2). Below a predetermined aircraft

Table 6.1 *Typical cabin pressure differentials of passenger aircraft*

Type of aircraft	Maximum operating cabin differential pressure		Maximum aircraft altitude (feet) at which cabin altitude (feet) is:	
	(kPa)	(lb/in² gauge)	6000	8000
Turbo-propeller engine	38–52	5.5–7.5	22 000	25 000
			30 500	35 000
Subsonic jet engine	59.5–62	8.6–9	37 000	44 500
			39 500	47 000
Supersonic jet engine	72.5–77	10.5–11.2	56 000	78 000
			71 000	–

altitude, e.g. 8000 feet, the cabin is unpressurized. Above the aircraft altitude at which cabin pressurization commences, the cabin altitude is held constant until the aircraft altitude at which the maximum operating differential pressure required is reached. Above this altitude, the constant maximum differential pressure is maintained, so that the cabin altitude rises.

Low-differential combat cabins

In high-performance combat aircraft, where weight and performance are primary considerations and there is often a threat to the integrity of the cabin, the crew members use oxygen equipment throughout flight and the cabin differential pressure is relatively low. The physiological requirements are that the cabin altitude should not exceed 22 000 feet, in order to minimize the effects of hypoxia due to malfunction or misuse of oxygen equipment and to reduce the incidence of decompression sickness. The maximum cabin differential pressure should not exceed 34.5 kPa gauge (5.0 lb/in^2), in order to reduce the hazard of injury on rapid decompression of the cabin. The maximum cabin differential pressures employed in practice vary between 24 and 34.5 kPa (3.5 and 5 lb/in^2). These differential pressures prevent the cabin altitude exceeding 22 000 feet at aircraft altitudes of up to 40 000 feet and 57 000 feet, respectively. The cabin altitude will not exceed 25 000 feet with differential pressures of 24 and 34.5 kPa (3.5 and 5 lb/in^2) below aircraft altitudes of 46 500 feet and 75 000 feet, respectively.

The operation of cabin pressurization control systems fitted to low-differential-cabin combat aircraft is almost always automatic. Thus, cabin pressurization commences at a fixed altitude, the value of which is kept as low as possible in order to minimize rates of change of cabin pressure with ascent and descent of the aircraft but high enough to ensure that the cabin will not be pressurized if the aircraft lands at an airfield with a high elevation. Cabin pressurization generally starts at an aircraft altitude of 5000–8000 feet. An isobaric control schedule may be used until the maximum cabin differential pressure has been achieved. At higher aircraft altitudes, this maximum differential is maintained (curve (a) of Figure 6.4). An alternative pressurization schedule (employed in some UK military aircraft) allows the cabin differential pressure to increase linearly with reduction of the absolute pressure of the aircraft environment, to the maximum differential pressure at about 40 000 feet. Above this height, the constant maximum cabin differential pressure is maintained (curve (b) of Figure 6.4). Although the use of isobaric control eliminates changes of cabin altitude over a restricted range of aircraft altitude, the UK schedule results in a significantly lower rate of increase of cabin pressure on descent from high altitude, a distinct advantage when rapid changes of aircraft altitude occur.

PRINCIPLES OF CABIN PRESSURIZATION SYSTEMS

Source of air

In piston-engined aircraft and some jet-engined aircraft (particularly multi-engined jet aircraft), air for pressurizing and conditioning the cabin is drawn from outside the aircraft and compressed by engine-driven auxiliary compressors. In most jet-engined aircraft, the air for pressurizing and conditioning the cabin is tapped off the compressor stages of the main engines, upstream of the combustion chambers. In multi-engined aircraft, generally there is one auxiliary compressor per main engine; if directly tapped air is used, it is drawn from each engine. A non-return valve in the duct from each compressed-air source prevents backflow in the event of a failure of that particular compressor. The flow of air from the engine or compressor is controlled automatically in order to give the required mass flow of air through the cabin. The total flow of air required is determined primarily by the volume of conditioned air necessary to maintain the desired thermal conditions in the cabin (for the crew, passengers and electronic equipment) and to ventilate the crew and passenger compartments (to remove carbon dioxide and odours and to replace oxygen). The inflow of air required to maintain the desired differential pressure in the cabin is generally much less than that necessary to condition the cabin. The mass flow of air into the cabin of a two-seat combat aircraft

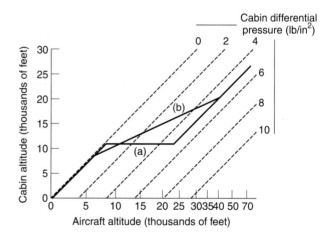

Figure 6.4 *Typical pressurization schedules for low-differential-pressure cabins of combat aircraft. The cabin is unpressurized at very low aircraft altitudes. (a) Schedule in which the differential pressure increases so that the cabin altitude remains constant with further ascent to altitude up to the maximum differential pressure (34.5 kPa, 5 lb/in^2, in this example). (b) Schedule in which the differential pressure is increased more gradually with ascent to altitude, so that the maximum is operative only at aircraft altitudes above 40 000 feet.*

is about 14–18 kg/min (30–40 lb/min) (approximately 11 000–15 000 litres (normal temperature and pressure, NTP)/min). In large passenger aircraft, a mass flow of 0.55 kg/passenger/min (1.2 lb/passenger/min; 440 litres NTP)/passenger/min) was once commonly employed. This mass flow has now been approximately halved in modern turbofan aircraft that utilize recirculating systems with HEPA filters.

The air passes from the flow controller to the conditioning equipment (heat exchangers and refrigeration system) and through a combined stop valve and non-return valve into the air distribution pipework within the cabin. The non-return valve prevents air escaping from the cabin and passing back through the air supply system in the event of a failure of the source, e.g. flameout of the engine of a single-engined aircraft or rupture of the pipework or conditioning equipment. This valve ensures that the air in the cabin is held there if there is complete failure of the supply, thus preventing catastrophic loss of cabin pressure and so minimizing the increase of cabin altitude in this type of emergency. The stop valve in the cabin air inlet can be operated from the cockpit to cut off the inflow of air if it is contaminated with smoke or oil. In many aircraft, when the airflow from the engines or compressor is shut off, a ram air inlet to the cabin opens automatically so that the cabin is ventilated with uncontaminated external air. In some aircraft, this flow of air into the cabin may be greatly increased in an emergency. This facility, which limits the rise of cabin altitude when there is a large leak, is termed 'flood flow'.

In aircraft with recirculation systems, the incoming fresh air (after conditioning) enters a mixing chamber (mix manifold), where it is combined with an equal flow of recirculated air. From the mix manifold, the air is ducted to each seating zone via an overhead ventilation distribution system. These distribution outlets run the length of the cabin; the air so distributed mixes with cabin air, which is then exhausted through metal grilles located near the cabin floor. In most aircraft, the exhaust air from the aft section of the cabin is extracted by the pressure control outflow valve and discharged overboard. The air in the forward section is continuously extracted from below the floor by recirculation fans for processing through the HEPA filters and returned to the mixing manifold.

Discharge valve and pressure controller

The air flows out of the cabin through one or more discharge valves, which impose a restriction in order to create the desired cabin differential pressure. The degree of opening of the discharge valve is controlled by either pneumatic or electric signals from the pressure controller. The pressure of the aircraft environment and the pressure of the cabin are fed to the controller, which produces an output signal to the discharge valve(s) in accordance with the pressurization schedule for the cabin. In passenger-carrying aircraft, it is possible to set the desired maximum cabin altitude and rate of change of cabin altitude on the pressure controller. If a discharge valve sticks open, the cabin loses its pressure, so in transport aircraft discharge valves and the pressure controller are duplicated. An independent method of closing a discharge valve that has failed in the open position is also desirable. The discharge valve and pressure controller are not normally duplicated in high-performance combat aircraft, where all the cabin occupants have oxygen equipment.

Safety and inward vent valves

The basic cabin pressure control system includes two further valves: safety and inward relief valves. The cabin safety valve prevents the cabin differential pressure rising above a preset maximum if the discharge valve(s) should fail to open. The setting of the safety valve is usually slightly greater (1.4–3.5 kPa gauge, 0.2–0.5 lb/in^2) than the maximum operating differential pressure. The inward relief valve is fitted to allow atmospheric air to enter the cabin if the pressure in the cabin falls below that of the atmosphere. This condition may arise during a rapid descent if the flow of air into the cabin is reduced or absent. The inward relief valve usually is set to open at a negative differential pressure of 1.4–2.0 kPa (0.2–0.3 lb/in^2).

In certain circumstances, there may be a need to decompress the cabin of an aircraft rapidly. If the cabin is filled with smoke or noxious fumes, then it may be necessary to decompress and to purge the cabin with external air through the ram air inlet. Although so drastic an action is obviously not desirable in a passenger aircraft flying at high altitude, it can be vital in aircraft carrying passengers at low altitude and in combat aircraft at any altitude. Another situation in which rapid decompression of the cabin is required is if the crew members intend to abandon the aircraft. In low-differential-pressure cabins, it is acceptable to decompress the cabin by jettisoning the cockpit canopy or door; except in dire emergencies, however, a high-differential-pressure cabin is decompressed by first fully opening all the discharge valves.

Indicators and warning systems

The performance of the cabin pressurization system is indicated to the crew of an aircraft by means of a cabin altimeter. In passenger aircraft, the rate of change of cabin altitude and the differential pressure between the cabin and the atmosphere are also displayed on the flight deck instrument panel. Failure of the pressurization control system to maintain the correct cabin altitude is normally indicated to the crew by a warning system. The warning, which may be audible or visual, or both, may be operated by the cabin altitude rising above a preset value, e.g. 10 000 feet in a high differential pressure passenger aircraft, or the cabin differential pressure falling below that which should exist at the prevailing aircraft altitude.

CAUSES OF FAILURE OF CABIN PRESSURIZATION

Although pressurization has overcome most of the physiological disturbances induced by exposure to low environmental pressure, decompression of the cabin at high altitude is associated with hazards of its own. Failure of the pressurization of aircraft cabins can be classified by cause, according to whether the fall of the cabin differential pressure is due to a reduction of the inflow of air, an excessive discharge, or failure of the cabin structure.

Reduced cabin air inflow

Marked reduction of the air supply from the engine or compressor is much more probable in single-engined aircraft than in multi-engined aircraft, since in the latter air for pressurization of the cabin commonly is tapped from all the engines or supplied by two or more engine-driven compressors. Loss of the supply of air to the cabin due to flameout of the engine of a single-engined aircraft normally results in rapid aircraft descent; if the engine fails during the climbing phase of a high-altitude ballistic manoeuvre, however, the cabin differential pressure may fall to a negligible value before the aircraft starts to descend. Other causes of inflow failure include unserviceable components in the air-conditioning system, e.g. the cabin inlet valve may stick closed. The flow of air into the cabin may be turned off by the crew because toxic material or smoke is being carried into the cabin, or as part of the escape drill. However, as long as the outflow of air through the discharge valves is prevented, failure of inflow does not cause a rapid fall of the cabin differential pressure. Pressure cabins are designed to have minimal leakage, and serviceability checks are made regularly to ensure that the leak rate remains below a specified maximum.

Failure of the pressure control system

If the pressure controller malfunctions or the cabin discharge valves stick open, then the cabin differential pressure falls. If all the discharge valves suddenly go to the fully open position, then the differential pressure will fall very rapidly to zero. Such decompressions occur more frequently in sin-gle-seated or two-seat aircraft because there is no duplication of the pressure control system. In a passenger aircraft, duplication of the components and provision of an independent facility for closing the discharge valves ensure that the cabin differential pressure does not fall significantly in the event of a failure of a discharge valve.

Structural failure

Failure of the structure can range from impaired sealing of a door, canopy or escape hatch, which may produce a small leak, to disintegration of a transparency, loss of a complete door or cockpit canopy, or even gross structural failure of the wall of the cabin. Failure of a seal or loss of a hatch, door or canopy may be caused by mechanical failure of a component such as an inflatable seal, which may not have been identified because of inadequate or faulty servicing or inadequate pre-flight/takeoff checks. Structural failure of a transparency or part of the wall of a cabin may be the result of mechanical fatigue, excessive stress, sabotage or enemy action. UK and US government regulations require that the effects of puncture of the cabin wall or a window by a bullet from a personal weapon be taken into account in the design. Gross structural failure of the wall of a cabin in the absence of enemy action or sabotage is extremely unlikely now that the significance of metal fatigue is generally appreciated. The walls may, however, be weakened by corrosion, and frequent inspections are necessary to check that the strength has not deteriorated. In military aircraft, hatches, doors and cockpit canopies may be designed to be jettisoned in flight before escape; such mechanisms may, of course, also be activated inadvertently.

Incidence

The incidence of accidental decompressions of pressure cabins is relatively low, and the incidence in commercial aircraft throughout the world is of the order of 30–40 per year. Many of these decompressions are performed voluntarily in order to cut off the flow of smoke or other toxic material into the cabin, as a precaution following cracking of a transparency, or as a planned drill following receipt of a bomb threat. Most accidental decompressions are due to failure of the compressor system, failure of the pressure control system, or opening of a hatch or door. The number of decompressions occurring in military flying even in peacetime is considerably higher than that in commercial operations. An incidence of about two to three unplanned decompressions per 100 000 flying hours has been recorded for many years. The major causes of inadvertent decompressions of military aircraft are flameout in those with single engines, malfunctions of the pressure control system, failures of transparencies and loss of canopies. In combat, there is a rise in the incidence of decompression due to enemy guns or missiles. With a few exceptions, crew and passengers survive cabin pressure failure both in commercial and in military operations. Most deaths attributable to decompression have occurred when there was massive disruption of the cabin structure due to metal fatigue. From time to time, individuals have been sucked out of a lost hatch, window or door.

PHYSICS OF RAPID DECOMPRESSION

When air can escape from a cabin, the pressure falls rapidly at first and then more slowly as the pressures inside and out approach each other and equalize (Figure 6.5). The rate at which air flows through a hole cannot exceed the local speed of sound, regardless of the size of the defect or the difference between the pressure in the cabin and that of the atmosphere. The major factors that determine the rate and time of decompression of a pressure cabin are:

- the volume of the cabin
- the size of the opening in the cabin
- the absolute pressure in the cabin at the beginning of the decompression
- the absolute pressure outside the cabin.

The larger the volume of the cabin, the slower the decompression; and the larger the defect in the wall, the faster the decompression. The ratio of the volume of the cabin to the cross-sectional area of the opening or orifice is

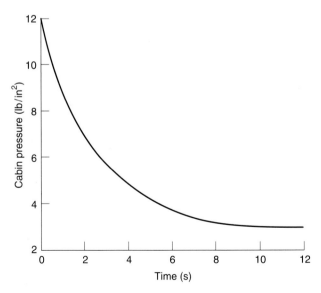

Figure 6.5 *Time course of absolute pressure of air in cabin of an aircraft during a decompression from 83 kPa (12 lb/in², 5500 feet) to 21 kPa (3 lb/in², 38 000 feet). The rate of fall of pressure, which is high at the beginning of the decompression, falls progressively as air escapes from the cabin.*

one of the main factors controlling the rate and time of decompression. Other factors being constant, the time of decompression is proportional to the ratio of cabin volume to area of the defect in the structure. The pressure ratio (cabin/ambient) is the other factor that determines the time of decompression: the larger the ratio, the longer the time of decompression. On the other hand, the actual differential pressure does not directly influence the time but does determine the severity of a decompression: the larger the pressure difference, the more severe the decompression. The absolute value of the atmospheric pressure is, of course, the primary factor that determines the physiological consequences after a rapid decompression. These often are of far greater significance than the effect of the fall of pressure itself. For any given cabin pressure differential, the higher the aircraft altitude at the instant of decompression, the greater is the ratio of cabin pressure to atmospheric pressure; and the higher the aircraft altitude, the longer the decompression time (for a constant ratio of cabin volume to area of defect).

Time of decompression

Several equations have been developed to estimate the time of decompression of a pressure cabin of given volume according to the area of the defect and the cabin and atmospheric pressures. One of the most useful and accurate is that developed by Haber and Clamann, which states that the time of decompression of a cabin is determined by the product of two factors: (i) the time constant of the cabin (t_c) and (ii) a pressure-dependent factor (P_1). t_c is calculated as follows:

$$t_c = \frac{V}{(A \times c)}$$

where V is the volume of cabin, A is the effective area of the orifice and c is the local speed of sound.

The values inserted into the equation are expressed in consistent units. The effective area of an orifice may be less than its geometric area, in that it may not behave as a sharp-edged orifice. Thus, the effective area of a defect created by sudden loss of a complete window or hatch is about 90 per cent of the geometric area. The speed of sound is related to the temperature of the air flowing through the orifice – in practice, a value of 1100 feet/s (335 m/s) is used.

P_1 is a complex function of the ratio of the cabin pressure before the decompression to the pressure in the cabin at the end of the decompression. The relationship between these two variables is depicted in Figure 6.6. The total time of decompression is given by the product

$$t_t = t_c \times P_1$$

where t_t is the total time of decompression.

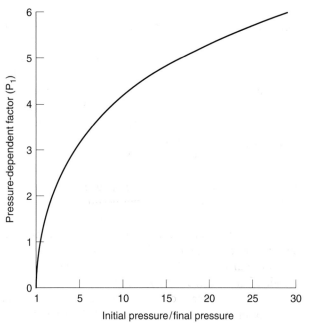

Figure 6.6 *Calculation of time of decompression of pressure cabin at a constant aircraft altitude. The curve shows the relationship between the pressure-dependent factor of the Haber–Clamann formula and the ratio of the absolute pressure in the cabin before (initial pressure) and after (final pressure) decompression.*

Examples of calculated times of decompression for the sudden disintegration of the canopy of a single-seated fighter aircraft and the loss of a window or door of a passenger aircraft are given in Table 6.2.

Effect of inflow of air

If the decompression of a cabin is due to excessive opening of discharge valves or a defect in the wall of the cabin, then the flow of air from the engine compressors into the cabin continues. The modifying effect that this inflow will have on the fall of cabin pressure is determined by the relationship between the flow and the size of the orifice in the cabin wall. If the ratio of flow to the area of the orifice is high, then this additional flow will create a significant pressure drop across the orifice, thus reducing the rate of fall of cabin pressure and raising the value to which the absolute pressure in the cabin falls at the end of the decompression. In practice, maintained inflow of air from the engine compressors is of significance only when a relatively small defect, e.g. loss of a window, occurs in a large aircraft where the inflow is high; it can maintain the cabin altitude 5000–10 000 feet lower than aircraft altitude, in spite of loss of a window at an aircraft altitude of, say, 35 000 feet. In some aircraft, the airflow into the cabin may be increased in an emergency, so limiting still further the rate of fall of cabin pressure and the final altitude reached in the cabin.

Aerodynamic suction

The pressure immediately outside a defect is seldom the static pressure exerted by the atmosphere at which the aircraft is flying. The movement of the aircraft through the air creates a fall of pressure over much of the external surface of the aircraft. The magnitude of this effect varies with the shape of the aircraft, the position of the defect, the speed and the altitude. The pressure at the external surface of the canopy of combat aircraft and at the windows and doors of transport aircraft is almost always less than the pressure altitude of the aircraft. Consequently, the fall of cabin pressure is accelerated and the final value of cabin pressure reduced below that of the atmosphere by this Venturi effect of aerodynamic suction. The aerodynamic suction at the windows of transport aircraft cruising at altitude is usually about 1.4–4 kPa gauge (0.2–0.6 lb/in^2), although this may be considerably greater at windows close to the wing roots. The aerodynamic suction over the canopy of some high-performance combat aircraft flying at speed at altitudes between 35 000 and 45 000 feet amounts to between 7 and 14 kPa gauge (1–2 lb/in^2). If the major part or the whole of the canopy of such an aircraft flying at

Table 6.2 *Calculated decompression times*

	Combat aircraft	Passenger aircraft	
Cabin volume (feet^3)	50	10 000	
Nature and area of orifice (feet^2)	Disintegration of canopy 9	Loss of window 0.5	Loss of door 12
Time constant of cabin (s)	0.005	18.2	0.76
Time of decompression (s)			
From 16 000 to 40 000 feet	0.007	–	–
From 3000 to 25 000 feet	1.3	30.9	1.3
From 5000 to 40 000 feet	–	50.0	2.1

40 000 feet is lost, then the pressure altitude in the cabin may exceed the pressure altitude of the aircraft by 8000–10 000 feet.

Cabin altitude profiles

The time course of the changes of cabin altitude following a failure of pressurization is complicated by alterations of the flight path of the aircraft during and following the incident. Usually, the pilot initiates a rapid descent and so reduces the rate of fall of cabin pressure and raises the minimum absolute pressure reached in the cabin. Thus, the cabin altitude first increases and then decreases as the aircraft descends. If the rate of decompression is very rapid, the cabin altitude rises to equal (or, if aerodynamic suction is present, to exceed) the aircraft altitude (Figure 6.7a). The cabin altitude will then fall as the aircraft descends. In large passenger aircraft, however, the decompression of the cabin is relatively slow, and descent is started well before the decompression is complete. The maximum cabin altitude attained may be very considerably less than the initial altitude of the aircraft (Figure 6.7b).

Air blast

The sudden flow of air created in a pressure cabin when a decompression occurs raises dust and debris, which may markedly reduce visibility. The mist formed by the condensation of water vapour in the expanding air adds to the problems of the crew. The velocity of the flow of air through the cabin towards a defect in its wall increases rapidly as the air approaches the hole. The air blast can blow loose articles, furnishings and even people out through the defect. Since the force of the blast is very high only close to the hole, the people at risk are those in the immediate vicinity; if there is a major structural failure, however, then many or most occupants may be severely or fatally injured by the associated air blast. The point is usually academic, since such structural failure usually leads to disintegration of the aircraft in the air.

EFFECTS ON CABIN OCCUPANTS

Provided the aircraft remains intact, the effect of failure of pressurization of a cabin on the occupants depends on three major factors: the rate of the decompression, the pressure change during the decompression, and the pressure in the cabin after the decompression. The rate and pressure range of the decompression determine the magnitude of the effects arising from the expansion of the gas within the various gas-containing cavities of the body. The intensity of the other major effects of decompression – hypoxia and decompression sickness – is determined primarily by the consequent cabin altitude, particularly the maximum cabin altitude and the subsequent pattern of change. A major deficiency in the wall of a cabin also results in a marked fall in cabin temperature, so that the occupants may suffer from cold.

Expansion of gas in body cavities

Decompression of a pressure cabin is most unlikely to give rise to symptoms in the middle ears and paranasal sinuses. However, passengers will almost certainly develop pain in the middle ear during the subsequent emergency descent, when they are exposed to a large and relatively rapid increase of cabin pressure.

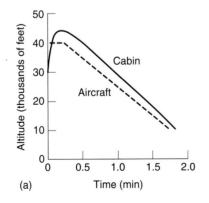 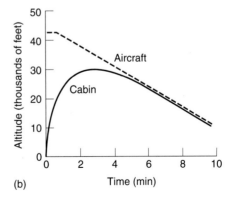

Figure 6.7 *Effects of rapid descent of aircraft and pressure of aerodynamic suction on cabin altitude after failure of cabin pressurization. (a) Behaviour of cabin altitude when the decompression is due to a large defect that allows equilibrium of pressure before descent of the aircraft has started. Aerodynamic suction at the site of the defect causes cabin altitude to exceed aircraft altitude. (b) Time course of cabin altitude when decompression occurs through a relatively small defect and descent of the aircraft is started 30 seconds after the beginning of the decompression.*

Abdominal disturbances are unlikely if the maximum cabin altitude does not exceed 25 000 feet. As the cabin altitude rises above 25 000 feet, an increasing proportion of individuals develop abdominal discomfort and pain due to expansion of gas in the stomach and intestines. The incidence of disturbances is far higher among passengers than aircrew.

The lungs

The large volume of gas in the alveoli, the relatively narrow passages that connect the alveoli to the external environment, and the susceptibility of lung tissue to damage when it is overstretched combine to make the lungs a vulnerable part of the body during the very rapid reduction of environmental pressure that occurs on sudden loss of cabin pressure. Although no serious injuries have been reported so far in human decompression with open airways, studies on experimental animals have shown that fast decompressions over large pressure ranges can cause structural damage to pulmonary tissue, with haemorrhagic, emphysematous and atelectatic changes in the lung. The ability of the human lung to withstand and adapt to sudden changes in pressure is the limiting factor in the rate or range of decompression that can be tolerated, and strict attention is paid to this factor in the design of pressurized cabins.

The decompression rate of the lungs is limited by the flow resistance offered by the pulmonary and upper airways. Thus, any environmental decompression that is faster than the maximum decompression rate of the lungs will result in a transient positive differential pressure between the gas within the lungs and the surrounding cabin environment. The faster the decompression rate of the cabin, the greater will be the transient pressure difference. The magnitude and duration of the difference between the pressure of the gas in the lungs and that of the cabin environment during a rapid decompression depend on the following factors:

- rate of decompression of the cabin in relation to the simultaneous rate of decompression of the lungs
- total change of cabin pressure during decompression
- volume of gas in the lungs at the beginning of the decompression
- ability of the lungs and thorax to expand within normal limits during decompression.

The normal expansion of the lungs and chest wall, and the flow of gas from the lungs through the airways to the environment, will reduce considerably the pressure within the lungs during a rapid decompression.

A simple model that illustrates the dynamic relationships between the pressure in the lungs and that in the cabin during a rapid decompression is depicted in Figure 6.8. The model represents the situation in which the

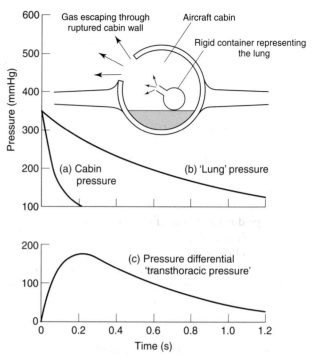

Figure 6.8 *Simple model demonstrating effects of rapid decompression of cabin of an aircraft flying at high altitude (approximately 47 000 feet) on the pressure difference between the gas within the lung and the gas surrounding the body (transthoracic pressure differential). The lung is represented by a rigid container with a relatively narrow opening into the cabin. On rupture of the cabin wall, the pressure in the cabin (a) falls to that of the environment in about 0.2 seconds. The rate at which gas escapes from the 'lung', and hence the rate at which lung pressure (b) falls, is much slower than the rate of decompression of the cabin, so there is a transient but large pressure difference between the lung and cabin gas (c).*

lungs and chest wall behave as a rigid container. The ratio of the volume of the lungs to the area of the opening from the lungs to the cabin environment (the area of an orifice equivalent to the airways) is greater in this model than the ratio of the volume of the cabin to the area of the defect in the cabin wall. Curve (a) shows the behaviour of the pressure in the cabin as it decompresses through the defect. Curve (b) depicts the time course of the pressure changes in the lungs. Curve (c) is the difference between curves (a) and (b) and represents the pressure difference between the gas in the lungs and that in the cabin – the transthoracic pressure. This pressure difference builds up rapidly to a peak and then declines gradually as the lungs progressively decompress.

Lung damage in rapid decompression is caused by stretching of the lung tissue beyond its elastic limit. As the gas within the lungs expands, the chest wall and diaphragm are displaced outwards. If the expansion of the gas within the lungs can be taken up without the final lung volume exceeding the normal total lung volume, then no damage will occur. If, however, the lung expansion induced exceeds the normal total lung volume, then the lung tissue will be overstretched. Eventually, the lung tissue will tear and blood vessels will be severed. The transthoracic pressure difference required to tear the lungs when the chest and abdominal muscles are relaxed is of the order of 80–100 mmHg. When lung tissue tears, air passes along tissue planes into the mediastinum and even up into the neck, producing surgical emphysema. Gas entering torn blood vessels passes into the systemic circulation (generalized gas embolism).

The worst case scenario is if the gas within the lung cannot escape during the fall of environmental pressure. The free flow of expanding gas to the atmosphere may be prevented by closure of the glottis, such as occurs during breath-holding, swallowing and straining, or by the characteristics of any breathing equipment being used at the time. Thus, the compensated outlet valve fitted in a typical pressure-demand oronasal mask (see Chapter 5) may well be held shut throughout and immediately after a rapid decompression. The range of decompression that is safe (i.e. the transthoracic pressure after the decompression does not exceed 50 mmHg when no gas can escape from the lungs) can be calculated if the initial volume of gas in the lungs is known. Typical limiting conditions are presented in Table 6.3. When the gas within the lungs is free to escape, it is difficult to predict whether the individual circumstances – initial and final altitudes, ratio of the volume of the cabin to the effective area of the orifice through which it is being decompressed – will produce a transthoracic pressure difference of the order of 80 mmHg and, hence, cause lung damage. Most of the information available has been obtained by animal experimentation, although there is some information with regard to 'safe' decompression for humans. The limiting conditions of the initial-to-final pressure ratio and the cabin volume-to-orifice area ratio beyond which lung damage is likely to occur in humans are presented in Figure 6.9. Although it is reasonably certain that conditions of decompression that lie to the left of the curve are 'safe' provided that the glottis is open and there is no external obstruction to the flow of gas from the lungs, decompression under conditions that lie to the right of the curve may or may not cause lung damage. In practice, lung damage due to decompression either in an aircraft or in a decompression chamber is a very rare event.

Table 6.3 *Safe limits to rapid decompression without venting of the lungs*

Initial altitude (feet)	Initial lung volume (fraction of total lung capacity)	Maximum 'safe' final altitude (feet)
8000	0.25[a]	44 000
	0.50[b]	29 700
	0.75	20 000
	1[c]	13 000
25 000	0.25[a]	61 000
	0.50[b]	46 500
	0.75	37 500
	1[c]	31 500

[a] Minimum lung volume (residual volume).
[b] Resting end-expiratory lung volume (functional residual capacity).
[c] Maximum lung volume (total lung capacity).

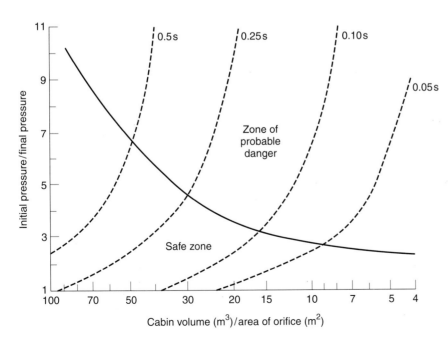

Figure 6.9 *Relationship between speed and range of a decompression and the risk of damage to the lungs as a result of the decompression. The interrupted lines depict the relationships between the ratio of the cabin volume to the area of the defect through which the decompression occurs (the ratio as expressed has the dimension of metres), the ratio of the absolute pressure in the cabin before (initial) and after (final) the decompression, and the total time of decompression, according to the Haber–Clamann equation. The solid curve separates decompressions that will not cause lung damage (provided that there is no obstruction to the flow of gas from the lungs) from those that probably will cause pulmonary damage.*

Hypoxia

By far the most important hazard of the decompression of the cabin of an aircraft flying at high altitude is hypoxia. A rapid fall of the pressure of the immediate environment produces simultaneous decreases of the oxygen tensions of the inspired and alveolar air in accordance with Dalton's law of partial pressures. There is also a concomitant decrease of the alveolar tension of carbon dioxide. The value to which the alveolar oxygen tension is reduced is determined by the composition of the gas breathed before and during the decompression, by the initial and final cabin altitudes, and by the speed of the decompression. The lower the concentration of oxygen in the inspired gas, the greater the range of decompression, the lower the final cabin pressure and the faster the speed of the decompression, the lower is the oxygen tension in the alveolar gas at the end of the decompression. Thus, a rapid decompression from 8000 feet to 40 000 feet when an individual is breathing air reduces the alveolar oxygen tension to 15–18 mmHg (2–2.4 kPa). If the final cabin altitude exceeds 30 000 feet, the alveolar oxygen tension is reduced to below the tension of oxygen in the venous blood flowing into the lungs. In these circumstances, oxygen passes out of the blood as the blood flows through the pulmonary capillaries; consequently, the blood loses oxygen to the atmosphere. The tension and concentration of oxygen in the blood leaving the lungs fall as abruptly as the alveolar oxygen tension, so that within 5–6 seconds of the start of the rapid decompression, the blood entering the capillaries of the brain and other tissues has a very low oxygen tension. Since the amount of oxygen stored in many tissues, especially the brain, is very small, the tension of oxygen in the tissues also falls rapidly. Thus, rapid decompression (one to two seconds) to a final altitude of 40 000 feet produces an impairment of performance in 12–15 seconds and leads to unconsciousness in 20 seconds.

If the aircrew members are breathing pure oxygen, then the oxygen tension of the alveolar gas is not reduced to below that of the mixed venous blood until the final altitude exceeds 48 000 feet. Rapid decompression to altitudes above 52 000 feet results in loss of useful consciousness in 10–15 seconds regardless of whether air or oxygen is breathed. The times to impairment or loss of consciousness do not change significantly with final altitudes greater than 52 000 feet because the speed of development of cerebral hypoxia is determined primarily by the lung-to-brain circulation time and the store of oxygen in the cerebral tissue, both of which are relatively constant. When the final altitude is less than 52 000 feet, the times to impairment of performance and loss of useful consciousness depend on the composition of the breathing mixture and the final altitude, as shown in Figure 6.10. Although there is always an interval of at least 12–15 seconds between the beginning of a rapid decompression to high altitude and the first

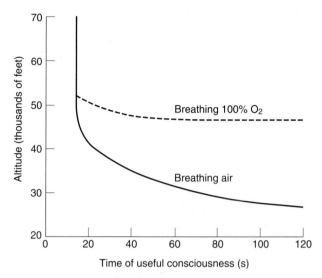

Figure 6.10 *Loss of consciousness induced by rapid decompression in 2–3 seconds to high altitude. The curves indicate the effect of the final altitude to which the decompression occurred on the time elapsing from the beginning of the decompression to the loss of useful consciousness. The solid curve shows the relationship for decompressions from 8000 feet while breathing air. The interrupted curve shows the relationship for decompression from 25 000 feet while breathing 100% oxygen.*

impairment of performance, impairment does nevertheless occur, even if the duration of the exposure to low pressure is as short as six seconds. Thus measures to restore the alveolar oxygen to a near-normal value must be well on the way to completion in less than 5–6 seconds of the beginning of a rapid, severe decompression if an adequate level of performance is to be maintained.

The interval between the beginning of a rapid decompression and loss of useful consciousness when air is breathed increases markedly as the final altitude of the decompression is reduced below 30 000 feet. Thus, useful consciousness is maintained for about 60 seconds after a rapid (three seconds) decompression to 30 000 feet and for 120–140 seconds after decompression to 25 000 feet (Figure 6.10) however. Impairment of performance occurs much earlier than loss of useful consciousness. Thus performance at psychomotor tasks is affected very significantly 45 seconds after a rapid (3 seconds) decompression to 25 000 feet.

The emergency action by the pilot of a passenger aircraft when a decompression occurs at high altitude is to initiate a rapid descent. Consequently, a plot of the cabin altitude against time assumes a triangular profile (see Figure 6.7b). The hypoxia induced by exposure to such a triangular profile with a peak altitude of 25 000 feet is very unlikely to cause seated passengers breathing air to lose consciousness, provided that the time at the peak altitude does not exceed one minute and that the total duration of the exposure to altitudes greater than 8000 feet does not exceed six minutes. Experiments on monkeys suggest that although humans are likely to lose consciousness when the peak altitude exceeds 25 000 feet, exposure to triangular profiles with peak altitudes of up to 40 000 feet should not be fatal or cause permanent brain damage, provided that the total time above 8000 feet does not exceed eight minutes. Exposure to higher peak altitudes (with approximately the same total time above 8000 feet) probably will be either immediately fatal or produce severe permanent brain damage.

Similarly, decompressions occurring in one type of transport aircraft operating at very high altitudes (above 50 000 feet) would expose the occupants to profound hypoxia. The loss of pressurization due to a small structural failure, such as loss of a window, would also expose the passengers to a decompression of triangular profile (Figure 6.11). The effects of such decompressions have also been studied in primates. As noted above, the effects of such triangular decompression profiles depend on the peak altitude and duration of the profile and may prove fatal or lead to permanent brain damage. The sequelae of various decompressions of triangular profile are illustrated in Figure 6.11, together with that of a balloonist who descended without oxygen and suffered permanent brain damage. These studies suggest that certain decompressions

of triangular profile may result in hypoxia of sufficient severity and duration to produce brain damage, but not so severe as to disrupt cardiac and respiratory function irreversibly. In animals that are impaired by decompressions of triangular profile, the brain damage is either predominantly cortical, centred on the boundary zones between the cerebral arteries and spreading from the occipital lobe across the parietal, temporal and frontal cortex, or predominantly subcortical (i.e. in the basal ganglia), with damage restricted to the neocortex. In both patterns, ischaemic necrosis is found in the hippocampus and cerebellum.

The studies carried out with decompressions of triangular profile, which essentially simulated the loss of cabin pressurization that could be expected in a supersonic transport aircraft operating around 55 000 feet and involving loss of a window together with engine failure, were of considerable practical importance during the development of supersonic transport aircraft and remain so as consideration is given to the development of the next generation of very-high-flying passenger aircraft. The studies were able to define the maximum area of the windows that would be compatible with survival without brain damage in the event of a decompression. The actual profile that could be experienced depends not only on the area of the window that may be lost but also on the altitude of the aircraft at the time of decompression and the maximum rate of descent that would be possible. Essentially, the rate of descent of a supersonic transport aircraft is limited, and the cruise altitude is determined by operational factors, and thus in this context the remaining variable that could avoid permanent brain damage, even in passengers who did not breathe oxygen during the descent, is that of the window area.

Decompression sickness

The incidence of decompression sickness becomes significant only when the cabin altitude rises above 25 000 feet and the altitude remains above this value for longer than five to ten minutes (see Figure 7.2). In practice, therefore, decompression sickness will occur only if the aircraft remains at high altitude after the decompression, so that the cabin altitude exceeds 22 000–25 000 feet for some time. Prolonged exposure to altitudes above 22 000 feet will give rise to incidents of decompression sickness unless the crew has breathed 100 per cent oxygen for some time before the decompression.

Cold

The temperature in the cabin following a failure of pressurisation is determined by the outside temperature, the

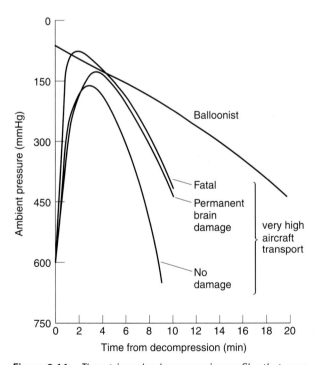

Figure 6.11 *Three triangular decompression profiles that were investigated using primates and confirmed that permanent brain damage can occur. The 'No damage' profile may be expected in the event of a small decompression in supersonic transport aircraft. Also included is the pressure–time profile of a balloonist who descended without oxygen and suffered permanent brain damage.*

nature of the cause of the decompression, and the flight path and speed of the aircraft. A large defect in the wall of the cabin of an aircraft at high altitude causes a very large fall of cabin temperature and a high flow of very cold air around the occupants. Such exposure rapidly results in cold injury of exposed skin and to a less rapid fall of body temperature (see Chapters 12 and 13). Vision may be impaired by the flow of cold air into the eyes. Outlet valves and ports of breathing equipment may be obstructed by the formation of ice. Unless the occupants are wearing special protective clothing, such as full pressure suits, it is necessary to descend quickly to increase the temperature of the air entering the cabin through the defect and, thus, reduce the severity of the cold.

Exposure to altitudes above 63 000 feet

If decompression results in exposure to an absolute pressure less than the vapour pressure of water at body temperature, i.e. 47 mmHg (6.3 kPa) (a pressure altitude of 63 000 feet), then the nature of the consequent disturbances differs from that which occurs at lower altitudes. Tissue water vaporizes as the local pressure falls below 47 mmHg (or a lower pressure, if the local temperature is below 37 °C). Thus, at altitudes between 65 000 and 70 000 feet, vaporization begins in the lungs and in the low-pressure regions of the circulation, such as the large intrathoracic veins. At higher altitudes, water vapour and other gases, such as oxygen and carbon dioxide, escape from the body fluids, a phenomenon termed ebullism. In experiments, dogs and monkeys decompressed to near-vacuum conditions (pressure 1–2 mmHg, 0.13–0.26 kPa) developed gross swelling of the soft tissues within five seconds, became unconscious in about 12 seconds, and progressed quickly to general muscle spasticity, gasping, transitory convulsions and apnoea. The products of ebullism in the veins and atria of the heart rapidly blocked the circulation. Although the electrical activity of the heart continued, the circulation ceased about ten seconds after the beginning of the exposure. As soon as the pressure increased in descent, the gases were reabsorbed into the body fluids very rapidly. Provided the duration of the exposure to near-vacuum conditions was less than two minutes, circulation and respiration in these animals recovered spontaneously. Studies on monkeys and chimpanzees suggested that exposure to a virtual vacuum for less than 1.5–2 minutes is very unlikely to be fatal or to give rise to any neurological damage.

PREVENTION OF HYPOXIA

Hypoxia is by far the most dangerous disturbance produced by failure of the pressurization of the cabin of an air-craft flying at high altitude. Oxygen delivery equipment that will prevent the otherwise inevitable impairment of performance must be available to the aircrew. A certain degree of hypoxia is acceptable in seated passengers. The primary method of alleviating this hypoxia is the rapid controlled descent of the aircraft to a safe altitude. If the cabin altitude may rise above 25 000 feet, or if recompression to below a cabin altitude of 15 000 feet in four minutes is not possible, passenger aircraft are usually fitted with an emergency system that will provide oxygen for all the passengers for the period that the cabin altitude is above 15 000 feet (see below).

Low-differential cabins

Aircrew operating low-differential-pressure cabin aircraft use their oxygen equipment throughout flight. As long as the equipment is capable of delivering 100 per cent oxygen at and above 33 000 feet and pressure breathing above 40 000 feet, serious hypoxia is unlikely if cabin pressure is suddenly lost. The design of the oxygen equipment must be such, however, that the concentration of oxygen in the mask cavity rises rapidly to the required level as soon as decompression occurs (see Chapter 5). Thus, the volume of the breathing system between the air inlet of the regulating device or the backup oxygen system changeover valve in molecular sieve oxygen concentrator (MSOC) systems and the mask cavity should be kept to a minimum (less than 600 ml). The required level of pressure breathing must be fully operative within three seconds of the time that the pressure in the respiratory tract falls below 141 mmHg (18.8 kPa) absolute.

High-differential cabins: crew

The flight-deck crew of aircraft with high-differential-pressure cabins do not need to use oxygen equipment as long as the pressure cabin is intact. A rapid decompression (decompression time less than 20 seconds) to a cabin altitude above 30 000 feet will, however, produce a significant impairment of performance in people breathing air, even if 100 per cent oxygen is delivered to the respiratory tract as soon as the decompression commences. This transient hypoxia can be avoided only by breathing 30–40 per cent oxygen (depending on the initial and final cabin altitudes) for some time before the decompression and 100 per cent oxygen as soon as the cabin pressure begins to fall. Thus, if there is a significant chance that cabin pressurization may fail, then the watch-keeping pilot should have the mask secured on his or her face and be breathing 30–40 per cent oxygen whenever the aircraft altitude exceeds 30 000 feet. If the probability of a fast decompression is very remote, as is the case in virtually all licensed passenger-carrying aircraft, then it is generally accepted that the pilot can breathe air throughout the flight, provided that he or she can don a mask and be breathing 100 per cent oxygen within three to five seconds of the cabin altitude exceeding 10 000 feet. In certain circumstances, e.g. when there is only one pilot at the controls of a passenger aircraft, UK and US government regulations require that he or she breathes an oxygen/air mixture whenever the aircraft altitude exceeds 41 000 feet. The design of the oxygen equipment for the flight-deck crew of high-differential-pressure cabin aircraft must be such that 100 per cent oxygen is delivered to the mask as soon as it is donned.

High-differential cabins: passengers

Minimizing the effects of hypoxia is best achieved by limiting the magnitude and duration of the exposure to low pressure. If decompression can result in a cabin altitude exceeding 25 000 feet, or the duration of the exposure to altitudes above 13 000 feet may be longer than 4–6 minutes, then it is current practice to fit an emergency oxygen system to supply all the passengers. Sufficient oxygen is carried to maintain the alveolar oxygen tension of all passengers above 50 mmHg (6.7 kPa) for as long as the cabin altitude exceeds 13 000 feet. UK and US government regulations also require that enough oxygen should be carried for use by a small fraction (10–15 per cent) of the passengers when the cabin altitude is between 10 000 and 15 000 feet. Although many emergency oxygen systems for passengers present oxygen masks automatically, the proportion of passengers who can be expected to use the equipment correctly is probably less than 50 per cent.

REFERENCES

Rayman RB. National Academy of Science report on cabin air quality. *Aviation, Space, and Environmental Medicine* 2002; **73**: 319.

Rydock JP. Tracer study of proximity and recirculation effects on exposure risk in an airliner cabin. *Aviation, Space, and Environmental Medicine* 2004; **75**: 168.

FURTHER READING

Brierley JB, Nicholson AN. Neurological study of simulated decompressions in supersonic transport aircraft. *Aerospace Medicine* 1969; **40**: 830–33.

Civil Aviation Authority. Air Navigation Order Aircraft Equipment, CAP 393, Schedule 4. London: Civil Aviation Authority, 1995.

Denison DM, Ledwith F, Poulton EC. Complex reaction time at simulated altitudes of 5000 feet and 8000 feet. *Aerospace Medicine* 1966; **37**: 1010–13.

Ernsting J. Prevention of hypoxia acceptable compromises. *Aviation, Space, and Environmental Medicine* 1978; **49**: 495–502.

Ernsting J, Byford GH, Denison DM, Fryer DI. Hypoxia induced by rapid decompression from 8000 feet to 40 000 feet: the influence of rate of decompression. Flying Personnel Research Committee Report No. 1324. London: Ministry of Defence (Air), 1973.

Haber E, Clamann HG. A general theory of rapid decompression. Randolph Air Force Base School of Aviation Medicine, USAF project no. 2112010008, report no. 3, 1953.

Macmillan AJF. Comfort in aircraft cabins' air quality and ventilation. *Royal Aeronautical Society Proceedings of Conference on Resting, Testing, Air Quality and Noise*, 2.12.10, 1995.

McFarland RA. *Human Factors in Air Transportation: Occupational Health and Safety*. New York: McGrawHill, 1953.

McFarland RA. Human factors in relation to the development of pressurised cabins. *Aerospace Medicine* 1971; **42**: 1303–18.

Rayman RB. Cabin air quality: an overview. *Aviation, Space, and Environmental Medicine* 2002; **73**: 211.

Thibeault C. Cabin air quality. *Aviation, Space, and Environmental Medicine* 1997; **68**: 8082.

7

Subatmospheric decompression sickness

ALISTAIR J.F. MACMILLAN

INTRODUCTION

The effects of lowered barometric pressure on the gas-containing cavities of the body are dealt with in Chapter 6. Chapter 3 deals with disturbances produced by the reduction in the partial pressure of oxygen (P_{O_2}) that occurs on ascent. There remains, however, another group of effects produced by exposure to low pressure, known collectively as decompression illness (DCI). Since the manifestations of DCI are so variable and the underlying mechanism is not well understood, this condition is usually identified by exclusion.

Subatmospheric decompression sickness is the group of effects produced by exposure to altitude that are not due to expansion of trapped or enclosed gas, arterial gas embolism following lung rupture, vaporization of tissue fluids or lowered P_{O_2}.

Although the clinical syndrome of decompression sickness was recognized in divers and compressed-air workers as caisson disease in the 1850s, the first clear description of the condition arising in men exposed to subatmospheric pressures was not made until 1930. Indeed, the production of the condition by exposure to altitude did not gain general recognition until the end of the third decade of the twentieth century. Although decompression sickness is the most generally accepted term for evolved gas disease, other terminology has been used to describe the condition, including 'the bends' (often the most common symptom, with pain in or around the joint of a limb), dysbarism, aeropathy and aeroembolism.

There are distinct differences between compressed-air and subatmospheric decompression sickness, although they share the same colloquial nomenclature for the common manifestations. Classically, the main manifestations are limb pain ('the bends'), respiratory disturbances ('the chokes'), skin irritation ('the creeps'), various disturbances of the central nervous system (CNS) ('the staggers') and cardiovascular collapse (syncope). These symptoms of subatmospheric decompression sickness virtually always subside or disappear during descent to ground level. Rarely, however, recovery does not occur after recompression to ground level, and in some cases the severity of the symptoms may increase, accompanied by a generalized deterioration in the individual's condition (post-descent collapse). This chapter addresses the features of decompression sickness and the factors that influence the incidence. Management of the condition is described in Chapter 50.

CAUSE OF DECOMPRESSION SICKNESS

Although the details of the processes underlying some of the manifestations of altitude decompression sickness remain unknown, the basic mechanism is undoubtedly the supersaturation of the tissues with nitrogen. Thus, the syndrome rarely occurs if the nitrogen normally dissolved in the body tissues and fluids is removed by breathing 100 per cent oxygen before exposure to altitude. The tissues and body fluids of an individual breathing air at ground level contain dissolved nitrogen, which exerts a partial pressure approximately equal to that of the nitrogen in the inspired air. The quantity of nitrogen contained in the body in this manner is approximately 1 litre (standard temperature and pressure, dry, STPD). As the partial pressure of nitrogen in the inspired air falls with ascent to altitude, nitrogen is carried by the blood from the tissues to the lungs, where it leaves the body in the expired gas. Since the solubility of nitrogen in blood is relatively low, and some tissues contain large amounts of nitrogen, the rate of fall of the absolute pressure of the body tissues associated with the ascent to altitude is greater than the rate of fall of the partial pressure of nitrogen in the tissues. These tissues, therefore, become supersaturated with nitrogen. Under certain circumstances, this supersaturation gives rise to the formation of bubbles of gas, the main constituent of which is initially nitrogen, in specific tissues of the body. This supersaturation concept identifies a critical component in the formation of bubbles of gas as the ratio of the tension of the inert gas in the tissues to ambient pressure (supersaturation ratio). Thus, gas exchange is the governing mechanism in the formation of the bubbles, and these bubbles subsequently grow in size by the diffusion into them of nitrogen and other gases such as oxygen and carbon dioxide from surrounding tissues. It is virtually certain that the occurrence of decompression sickness is due to this bubble formation in the tissues. Bubbles that form at one site may be carried by the circulation to another organ, where their presence may disturb the function of those tissues. Although following hyperbaric exposures bubbles may form within the interstitial spaces, there has been no unequivocal demonstration that bubbles are formed in the tissues under conditions in which altitude decompression sickness occurs in humans. However, using ultrasound technology, bubbles in the cardiovascular system can be detected, and there are many reports in the literature describing venous gas emboli (VGE). VGE are detected using a non-invasive ultrasonic echo-imaging Doppler system. The ultrasonic probe is usually placed over the precordium; although it is primarily intended to visualize the right side of the heart, a view of all four chambers is obtained. Sound recordings of the echoes from gas emboli entering the right atrium and ventricle are made and graded on a scale of 0 to 4, depending on the intensity of the visual and audible signals (Table 7.1). Correlation between the presence of the bubbles and occurrence of symptoms has not yet been established. This is perhaps not surprising, since it is likely that the growth of bubbles in the tissues that give rise to symptoms may not be related to the development of intravascular bubbles. Formation of bubbles in the lymphatic system, although identified frequently in divers and compressed-air workers, has not been described in subatmospheric exposures.

The driving pressure for bubble formation in a fluid is the difference between the partial pressure of the gas dissolved in the fluid and the absolute hydrostatic pressure. The greater the partial pressure of the gas and the lower the absolute hydrostatic pressure, the greater is the tendency for bubble formation. The increase in the partial pressure of nitrogen produced in a tissue by a given decompression depends on the solubility and the rate of diffusion of the gas in the tissue and the local blood flow. Nitrogen is highly soluble in fat; together with the low blood flow in these tissues, the rise of the partial pressure of nitrogen, and hence the magnitude of the driving pressure causing bubble formation, is greater in a tissue with a high lipid content. However, bubbles will not form in a fluid such as blood, even when the driving pressure is large, unless suitable nuclei are present. Nuclei for bubble formation consist of microscopic masses of gases attached to irregularities on the walls of a cavity, such as a blood or lymph vessel, or small particles suspended in the fluid. The distribution of such gas nuclei may account for the sites at which the disturbances occur in decompression sickness. It is very probable that bubbles have to grow to a certain critical size before the deformation that they produce is sufficient to cause symptoms or a disturbance of function. This hypothesis fits the observation that the rate of production of decompression sickness symptoms is very low immediately after ascent and that it increases to reach a peak in 20–60 minutes. Bubbles grow by a diffusion of nitrogen into the bubble, but at altitude oxygen, carbon dioxide and water vapour contribute to the establishment of nitrogen gradients. Within a bubble, oxygen and carbon dioxide partial pressures are stabilized at their tissue levels and remain the same at altitude if a sea-level alveolar P_{O_2} is maintained. However, when barometric pressure is reduced, the sum of the partial pressures of oxygen, carbon dioxide and water vapour make up an ever greater proportion of the total pressure within the bubble. Thus, the nitrogen pressure gradient between the tissues and the bubble increases as barometric pressure falls and bubble growth is faster.

Table 7.1 *Grading of venous gas emboli (VGE) detected by Doppler echo imaging systems*

Grade	Intensity of signal
0	Bubble signals absent
1	Occasional bubbles discernible
2	Fewer than half of the cardiac cycles contain bubbles
3	Most of the cardiac cycles contain bubbles
4	Bubble signals continuous throughout systole and diastole and obscure heart sounds

PRESENTATION OF DECOMPRESSION SICKNESS

Decompression sickness may arise either in flight or during exposure to reduced atmospheric pressure in an hypobaric chamber. There is considerable evidence for the existence of an altitude threshold at approximately 18 000 feet, although under certain circumstances, e.g. when decompression closely follows hyperbaric exposure in diving, the condition may occur at a much lower altitude. The incidence of decompression sickness at altitudes between 18 000 feet and 25 000 feet is low. However, work conducted with VGE monitoring has demonstrated a greater than expected incidence of both VGE and symptoms below 25 000 feet. It is probable that physical activity contributes to development of these bubbles and symptoms, since in exercising subjects asymptomatic venous bubbles have been detected at 10 250 feet and limb pain has been described at an altitude of 15 000 feet.

Clinical manifestations

The clinical manifestations of decompression sickness are extremely varied. The relative incidences of symptoms and signs during two-hour exposures to 28 000 feet and 37 000 feet are presented in Table 7.2. The clinical manifestations of decompression sickness are as follows.

JOINT AND LIMB PAINS

Often referred to as 'the bends', pain in a joint or a limb is the most common severe symptom of decompression sickness (Table 7.2). When it occurs, the pain is usually ill-localized and deep-seated. Mild aches will often develop into severe or agonizing pain if altitude is maintained or increased; ultimately, if no corrective actions are carried out, the individual may collapse. Less frequently, the pain disappears without becoming severe. More than one site may be involved. In descending order of frequency, the most commonly affected parts are the knee, shoulder, elbow, wrist or hand, ankle or foot and, rarely, hip. The pain starts as a mild ache, developing into a severe pain that spreads up and down the affected limb. Mild pain often encourages the subject to move or rub the aching part, but this action tends to increase rather than alleviate the pain. Local pressure by means of a tight bandage, a pneumatic cuff or immersion of the limb in fluid generally

Table 7.2 *Relative incidence of symptoms of altitude decompression sickness*

Symptoms	Incidence (%)	
	28 000 feet for 2 h	37 000 feet for 2 h
Joint and limb pains	74	56.5
Respiratory disturbances	4.5	6.5
Skin disturbances	7	1.6
Visual disturbances	2	4.8
Neurological disturbances	1	0
Collapse	9	25.8
Miscellaneous	2.5	4.8

relieves the pain. Symptoms almost always disappear during descent, although residual stiffness and mild aches may persist for some time. Although bubbles may be demonstrated radiologically in the synovial spaces of an affected joint, in tendon sheaths and even in fascial planes, bends pain may be present in the absence of radiological changes and, conversely, bubbles may be seen in the absence of symptoms. Similarly, VGE can be detected in approximately one-third of individuals who have no symptoms when exposed to altitude. However, VGE are detectable in almost all people with symptoms. A pain that closely resembles that of the bends can be produced by the local injection of small quantities of physiological saline into the muscles and ligaments around a joint. It is probable, therefore, that the bends is due to the formation of extravascular bubbles in these tissues.

SKIN DISTURBANCES

Itching, tingling ('the creeps') and formication of the skin often occur at altitude (Table 7.2) and are usually transient. They are of little significance; only rarely do these symptoms progress to more serious manifestations. In rare cases, the itching may be severe and accompanied by a marked hyperaesthesia. Occasionally, localized rashes, mottling and urticaria are observed, often in association with other symptoms and signs. Thus, the creeps is commonly accompanied by mottling of the skin over the chest; bluish-red patches of variable size appear and itch intensely. Discomfort associated with mottling may persist for two to three days.

The more severe skin manifestations of decompression sickness characterized by intense irritation or even pain are probably due to embolism by gas bubbles carried in the blood to the skin from other tissues of the body.

RESPIRATORY DISTURBANCES

Respiratory disturbances ('the chokes'), which are a serious manifestation of decompression sickness, occur relatively infrequently (Table 7.2). The first symptom is almost invariably a sense of constriction around the lower chest, often with a tight feeling in the epigastrium. An attempt to take a deep breath causes an inspiratory snatch that limits inspiration, and soreness develops beneath the sternum. There is frequently a general feeling of malaise and, as the condition develops, any attempt to take a deep breath causes coughing, which frequently becomes paroxysmal. If the exposure to altitude is maintained, the chokes almost invariably progresses to collapse. The symptoms of the chokes may persist for several hours after descent and may be precipitated during this period by tobacco smoke or deep inspiration. The chokes are probably part of the reflex response to irritation of the pulmonary tissues caused by the occlusion of pulmonary arterioles and capillaries by gas bubbles carried to the lungs in the circulation. Thus, the clinical picture produced by the intravenous injection of air in humans often resembles the chokes.

NEUROLOGICAL DISTURBANCES

Neurological disturbances ('the staggers') are rare in aviation decompression sickness (Table 7.2). Paralysis, paraesthesia, anaesthesia and convulsions may be present in a wide variety of clinical pictures. No disturbance of smell, taste or hearing and only one case of permanent paralysis have been reported. The focal disturbances of function in the CNS are most probably the result of gas-bubble embolism.

VISUAL DISTURBANCES

The most commonly noted visual effects are blurring of vision, scotomata, 'fortification' patterns and hemianopia. These often occur in conjunction with other symptoms such as headache and are comparable with the visual symptoms of migraine. It is not known whether these symptoms are primarily vascular or neurological, but they are probably the result of gas emboli.

COLLAPSE

A small but significant proportion of cases of decompression sickness present with a general feeling of malaise, anxiety and diminished consciousness (Table 7.2). This syndrome may occur either in the absence of any other manifestations of decompression sickness (primary collapse) or in association with the bends, the chokes or CNS disorder (secondary collapse). Typically, the individual becomes restless and pale, and the hands and face are cold and clammy with sweat. At this stage, he or she generally feels alternately hot and cold. It is followed by impairment of consciousness. The radial pulse is almost absent and there is usually bradycardia. Finally, the patient loses consciousness and may or may not jactitate. Descent is usually followed by a rapid recovery. Vomiting is quite common. Most patients develop a frontal headache.

POST-DECOMPRESSION COLLAPSE

The vast majority of individuals with decompression sickness recover either during or very shortly after descent to ground level. In a few instances, however, the symptoms may persist after return to ground level. In a small number of patients, the symptoms and signs may become worse after descent. If no preventive measures are taken, post-decompression collapse occurs in approximately one in 2500 exposures to altitudes greater than 30 000 feet. It almost never follows an altitude exposure in which no symptoms of decompression sickness occurred. Also, post-decompression collapse has never been reported when the only symptoms at altitude were mild bends at a single site or mild skin effects. The clinical picture is variable. There may be an interval of several hours between the descent to ground level and the appearance of symptoms. Typically, the patient becomes anxious, develops a frontal headache, and feels sick. He or she has facial pallor and cold sweaty extremities. There is nearly always peripheral cyanosis. General or focal signs of neurological involvement, such as weakness of the limbs, apraxia, scotomata and convulsions, may occur. Mottling of the skin across the chest and shoulders is commonly very marked. The arterial blood pressure is generally well maintained until late in the development of the illness. Finally, in the worst cases, coma supervenes. Recovery can occur at any stage, although in the past it has been very rare once coma has developed. A very consistent early finding in all cases of severe post-decompression collapse is an increase in the blood haematocrit. Typically, the haematocrit rises to 55–65 per cent. There is often also a polymorphonuclear leucocytosis, and the patient may have a high fever.

INCIDENCE OF DECOMPRESSION SICKNESS

A number of factors influence the incidence of decompression sickness. It is convenient to consider them under the headings of general and personal.

General factors

Although mild bends have been described in exercising subjects at 15 000 feet and VGE at even lower altitudes, the altitude threshold for decompression sickness in flight is generally accepted to be approximately 18 000 feet. Above this altitude (Figure 7.1), the incidence increases with altitude, although the condition occurs only very rarely below 20 000 feet and rarely below 22 500 feet.

To some extent, the threshold for the development of decompression sickness depends on the change in absolute pressure to which the individual has been exposed. Thus, breathing air at pressures greater than 1 atmosphere during the 24 hours before flight increases the susceptibility to decompression sickness, since the amount of nitrogen present in the tissues may be increased and bubbles may have been formed in the tissues asymptomatically. This effect may be avoided by not undertaking ascents to altitude for at least 12 hours after exposure to a pressure of up to 2 bar absolute (10 m of sea water) and for at least 24 hours when the pressure to which the individual has been exposed exceeds 2 bar abs. It is also possible to induce some resistance to decompression sickness by keeping the individual at reduced pressure (e.g. at a simulated altitude of 8000 feet) for at least 12 hours before ascent to above 18 000 feet. Protection acquired in this way is far from complete, and it is not practical in operational situations.

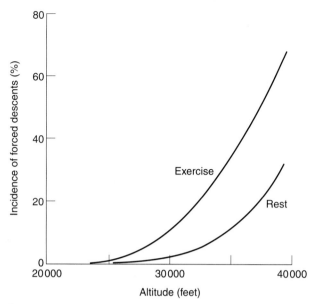

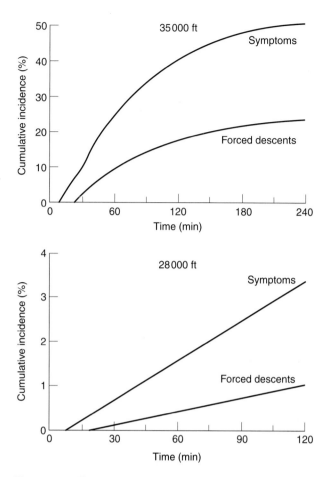

Figure 7.1   *Incidence of forced descents due to decompression sickness during two-hour exposures to various altitudes of subjects either seated at rest or carrying out moderate exercise.*

Figure 7.2   *Time course of development of symptoms and of forced descents due to decompression sickness in normal seated subjects exposed to simulated altitudes of 35 000 feet for four hours (upper graph) and 28 000 feet for two hours (lower graph).*

Decompression sickness can also be avoided if the ascent rate is very slow. Thus, mountaineers do not develop symptoms of the condition, but adoption of slow ascent rates is impracticable in aviation and, in any case, within the range normally encountered in aviation the rate of decompression per se has no significant effect on the incidence of decompression sickness.

Decompression sickness does not occur immediately on exposure to altitude (Figure 7.2). It is very rare for a case to occur before at least five minutes have passed at altitude. The rate of occurrence increases to reach a maximum at between 20 and 60 minutes exposure to altitude. The occurrence of new cases then falls, so that the total incidence approaches a plateau value, which may or may not be 100 per cent of those exposed.

Re-exposure to altitude immediately after the first exposure generally has been considered to increase susceptibility to decompression sickness. However, many of the data on which this view was generated are inconclusive, at least for early manifestations. Where a link has been claimed, symptoms generally have been more serious than current ethical standards would permit in experimental procedures. Studies comparing the incidence of VGE and decompression sickness symptoms between continuous altitude exposure of two hours at 25 000 feet with cumulative two hours of shorter exposures of 30 minutes within a four-hour period indicated that the cumulative exposures had a decreased risk (Pilmanis *et al.* 2002). It is possible that during the alternating recompressions to ground level in the cumulative exposure series, nitrogen reabsorption by the tissues was less than the desaturation that occurred

in the preceding sojourn at 25 000 feet. At the present time, however, the results of these studies are not sufficient to warrant changing the current recommendation that exposures to altitudes above 25 000 feet are separated by at least 24 hours. The interval between the two exposures should be increased to 48 hours if the currently perceived increased susceptibility is to be avoided.

As indicated earlier, exercise at altitude greatly increases the susceptibility to decompression sickness (see Figure 7.1), raises the incidence of symptoms at a given altitude and lowers the altitude at which symptoms appear. The effect of heavy exercise is roughly equivalent to an increase in the altitude of exposure of 5000 feet.

Additional factors that may play a part in the development of decompression sickness include ambient temperature and hypoxia. Some evidence exists that cold may be responsible for an increase in susceptibility. A higher incidence of decompression sickness observed in Royal Air Force (RAF) aircrew occupying inadequately heated areas of Canberra aircraft supports this view. There have been few surveys of the occurrence of decompression sickness when hypoxia is induced experimentally. However, considerable anecdotal evidence reported by experienced investigators strongly supports the opinion that the presence of hypoxia increases the incidence and severity of decompression sickness.

Personal factors

There is a true individual susceptibility to decompression sickness. Thus, on repeated exposures to the same altitude, an individual who developed decompression sickness on the first exposure is much more likely to develop the condition on a second exposure than an individual who did not have symptoms of decompression sickness on the first.

Susceptibility to decompression sickness increases with age. In the analysis of the decompression tests in which aircrew were exposed to a simulated altitude of 28 000 feet for two hours, a nine-fold increase in the likelihood of developing symptoms was demonstrated between the age bands of 17–20 years and 27–29 years. Furthermore, analysis of a US Air Force (USAF) hypobaric research database has confirmed the trend toward increased susceptibility with age, particularly in people older than 42 years.

Compared with blood and other tissues, fat tissue dissolves at least five times as much nitrogen; hence, a high body fat content possibly implies an increased susceptibility to decompression sickness. The incidence of decompression sickness is certainly greater in obese individuals. However, a reduction of the weight of an obese individual who has experienced serious symptoms of decompression sickness does not usually reduce his or her susceptibility to the condition.

Females have a higher body fat content than males, and the dissolved nitrogen in the body of a woman is greater than that in a male of the same weight. It might, therefore, be expected that females are more likely to develop decompression sickness. Many retrospective studies have supported this view, but prospective studies, stimulated by the greater role of women in the military employment, have not demonstrated the same link. One prospective programme demonstrated that although VGE occurred at significantly higher rates in men, no differences in decompression sickness were observed between the sexes (Webb et al. 2003). However, individuals of both sexes with higher body mass index and lower physical fitness developed symptoms more frequently.

There is some evidence to suggest that recent joint or limb injury sufficiently severe to cause changes in local circulation increases the incidence of bends pain at or close to the site of the lesion.

General health and other factors that affect the wellbeing of an individual can have an adverse effect on resistance to altitude exposure. Thus, the after-effects of alcohol ingestion and the presence of infection or intercurrent illness increase the susceptibility to decompression sickness. The influence of smoking on the incidence of subatmospheric decompression sickness has not been explored, but studies have been conducted in divers (Buch et al. 2003). Although data available from these studies of compressed-air decompression illness did not establish an unequivocal link between smoking and increased risk, it did appear that when symptoms occurred in divers they were more severe in heavy smokers. Thus, in addition to the myriad adverse effects attributable to smoking, the possibility of more serious detrimental effects if decompression sickness should occur must reinforce the recommendation that aircrew should not smoke.

CLASSIFICATION OF DECOMPRESSION ILLNESS

The arbitrary classification used for hyperbaric decompression illness has been widely employed to categorize manifestations of the altitude condition. This classification is as follows:

- Type I
  - pain only (the bends)
  - skin disturbances.
- Type II
  - CNS disorders
  - respiratory disorders
  - cardiovascular manifestations.

Type I DCI is generally regarded as a mild form, while type II DCI comprises the more serious conditions. However, the terms are of limited value since, type I and type II may coexist. The classification system provides no guidance to the management of the condition, and treatment must always be directed at the most serious symptoms and signs.

Other classification systems, including one that would differentiate acute manifestations and incorporate terms indicating the evolution of the presentation, have been suggested. An example of this classification would describe the creeps as 'acute, spontaneously resolving, cutaneous decompression illness'. A less complex approach identifies the major manifestations described earlier and simply categorizes them as primary or secondary manifestations. Thus, syncope may be a secondary manifestation consequent to severe bends pain.

No system currently in use is completely satisfactory, and this makes compilation of databases difficult, particularly with in-flight occurrences. Experimental studies of decompression sickness now invariably include Doppler echo imaging, and VGE can be identified and their intensity classified. However, as a diagnostic aid, even this technique is of greater value in excluding decompression sickness by the absence of bubbles than it is in confirming the diagnosis.

PREVENTION OF SUBATMOSPHERIC DECOMPRESSION SICKNESS

Decompression sickness may be prevented by limiting the reduction of environmental pressure and/or the duration of the exposure to low pressure, or by eliminating nitrogen from the tissues and body fluids before the exposure to altitude.

The threshold for the occurrence of symptoms of decompression sickness in aircraft is generally agreed to be around 18 000 feet, and thus aircrew and passengers should not be exposed to altitudes greater than this height. In practice, however, especially in military aircraft, the reduction of aircraft operating performance imposed by such a limitation may be unacceptable. The possible harmful effects of rapid decompression of the pressure cabin led in the past to the selection of a maximum cabin altitude of 25 000 feet as an acceptable compromise between the need to reduce the incidence of hypoxia and decompression sickness on the one hand and the need to avoid a high cabin pressure differential on the other. If, however, a cabin altitude of 25 000 feet is maintained for several hours, then decompression sickness will occur with sufficient frequency to be of practical importance. Since subsequent experience has shown that the incidence and harmful effects of rapid decompression of low-differential-pressure cabins was overestimated, the best practical compromise adopted in current aircraft is that the maximum cabin altitude should not exceed 22 000 feet. However, even this altitude may be too high in long flights supported by air-to-air refuelling. The need to avoid exposures to pressures greater than 1 atmosphere absolute in the 12–24-hour period before a flight has already been stated.

The removal of the nitrogen that is normally dissolved in the tissues and body fluids is accomplished by breathing 100 per cent oxygen before exposure to reduced pressure, a procedure termed 'pre-oxygenation' or 'denitrogenation' ('pre-breathe' in the USA). The removal of nitrogen from the tissues, especially those that contain a high concentration of lipid and those with a low blood flow, takes an appreciable time. The protection afforded against decompression sickness is related to the amount of nitrogen removed from the tissues and, hence, to the time for which 100 per cent oxygen is breathed. This in turn depends on the altitude and the duration of the intended exposure. Thus, pre-oxygenation for 30 minutes will ensure that the individual will not develop decompression sickness during

a short-duration exposure to an altitude of 48 000 feet if the time for which he or she is at altitudes above 25 000 feet does not exceed ten minutes. On the other hand, pre-oxygenation must be carried out at ground level for about three hours in order to prevent decompression sickness occurring during a subsequent exposure to an altitude of 40 000 feet for three hours. Pre-oxygenation is used widely to improve protection against DCI in the training of aircrew in the use of personal oxygen equipment and pressure clothing. It is current policy for aircrew in the UK who are undergoing such training in hypobaric chambers to breathe 100 per cent oxygen for 30–60 minutes (depending on the nature of the subsequent exposure) before they are exposed to altitudes in excess of 18 000 feet. Pre-oxygenation can also be used to protect experimental subjects who are to be exposed to high altitudes in hypobaric chambers and aircrew flying to high altitudes in unpressurized aircraft. It is, however, a time-consuming and complicated procedure, and although elimination of nitrogen is enhanced by exercise it is not practical in many operational situations. However, when it is possible to conduct pre-oxygenation combined with exercise, multiple short periods of exercise provide a shorter alternative to resting denitrogenation (Webb et al. 2004). Although pre-oxygenation may be most effective when carried out at ground level, it can also be of considerable value at altitude in certain operational circumstances, such as high-altitude deployment of parachutists. The parachutists breathe 100 per cent oxygen in the pressurized cabin of the dispatching aircraft (normally at a cabin altitude of 6000–8000 feet) during transit to the dropping zone and then proceed to exit the aircraft and descend using systems that deliver 100 per cent oxygen. Ideally, the duration of pre-oxygenation should be not less than one hour.

Staged decompression, which is used during ascent in diving operations, is not used in the normal aviation environment. However, staging has been adopted in the preparation for extra-vehicular activity from space shuttles. Typically, astronauts breathe 100 per cent oxygen for two hours and then the cabin pressure is reduced from sea-level equivalent to about 10 000 feet. An oxygen/nitrogen mixture is breathed during this phase for approximately 12 hours. The crew members resume breathing 100 per cent oxygen for 40 minutes before exiting the shuttle. After they have donned their full pressure suits, the cabin is depressurized and a pressure equivalent to 30 000 feet is maintained in the spacesuits.

Finally, since there is a wide variability in individual susceptibility to decompression sickness, relatively unsusceptible people may be selected by testing in a hypobaric chamber. This technique was used widely during and immediately after the Second World War in order to avoid decompression sickness in aviation. Such testing is uncommon today. However, in certain circumstances, such as the use of unpressurized training aircraft at high altitudes, selection tests are used to eliminate those aircrew members who have a high susceptibility to decompression sickness. Experience has shown that the most successful approach to the design of such tests is to simulate, in a hypobaric chamber, exposure to the most severe cabin altitude/time profile to which the aircrew member will be exposed during flight. In order to reduce the occurrence of serious cases of decompression sickness in selection testing to an absolute minimum, it is essential that the tests should be carried out by experienced medical officers and that full facilities, including a 6-atmosphere absolute hyperbaric chamber, should be available immediately for the treatment of any case that may arise.

REFERENCES

Buch DA, El Moalem H, Dovenbarger JA, Uguccioni DM, Moone RE. Cigarette smoking and decompression illness severity: a retrospective study in recreational divers. *Aviation, Space, and Environmental Medicine* 2003; **74**: 1271–4.

Pilmanis AA, Webb JT, Kannan N, Balldin U. The effect of repeated altitude exposures on the incidence of decompression sickness. *Aviation, Space, and Environmental Medicine* 2002; **73**: 525–31.

Webb JT, Kannan N, Pilmanis AA. Gender not a factor for altitude decompression sickness risk. *Aviation, Space, and Environmental Medicine* 2003; **74**: 2–10.

Webb JT, Pilmanis AA, Balldin U. Altitude decompression sickness at 7620 m following pre-breathe enhanced with exercise periods. *Aviation, Space, and Environmental Medicine* 2004; **75**: 859–64.

FURTHER READING

Buckles RG. The physics of bubble formation and growth. *Aerospace Medicine* 1968; **39**: 1062–9.

Fryer DI. Sub-atmospheric Decompression Sickness in Man. AGARDograph 129. Neuilly-sur-Seine: AGARD/NATO, 1969.

Macmillan AJF. The Management of Sub-Atmospheric Decompression Sickness. IAM report no. 489. London: Ministry of Defence, 1970 (revised 1983).

Olson RM, Krutz RW, Dixon GA. Validity of ultra-sonic monitoring at altitude for bends protection. *Aviation, Space, and Environmental Medicine* 1986; **57**: 511–20.

Pilmanis AA. *Proceedings of the 1990 Hypobaric Sickness Workshop.* Brooks Air Force Base, TX; Air Force Systems Command, 1992.

Pilmanis AA, Stegmann B. Decompression sickness and ebullism at high altitude. AGARD conference proceedings 516. Neuilly-sur-Seine: AGARD/NATO, 1991.

Rayman RB., Decompression sickness: USAF experience 1970-80. *Aviation, Space, and Environmental Medicine* 1983; **54**: 258–60.

Webb JT, Pilmanis AA. Venous gas emboli detection and endpoints for decompression sickness research. *Safe Journal* 1992; **22**: 22–5.

Effects of long-duration acceleration

NICHOLAS D.C. GREEN

INTRODUCTION

The human body is acted on continuously by the force of the Earth's gravity and is well adapted to an existence in an environment with a force of this magnitude. However, modern aircraft are capable of generating sustained acceleration resulting in much larger forces of up to nine times those due to gravity ($+9\,G_z$). This chapter is concerned with the physiological changes that are induced in humans by the inertial forces resulting from application of such sustained acceleration. Acceleration can be classified conveniently according to duration in the following manner:

- *Long duration:* long-duration acceleration acts for periods of more than two seconds. Forces of this type are typically encountered during military and civilian aerobatic aircraft manoeuvring but may also occur during launch and re-entry of space vehicles. The physiological effects of long-duration acceleration are produced by alteration in the flow and distribution of blood and body fluids, and by the distortion of tissues and organs of the body. Tolerance depends primarily on the level of plateau acceleration imposed.
- *Intermediate duration:* intermediate-duration acceleration acts for about 0.5–2 seconds. These forces are encountered in assisted escape from aircraft but may also occur during catapult launches and deck landings. Tolerance depends not only on the overall velocity change induced but also on the time taken to reach peak acceleration and the peak acceleration level attained.
- *Short duration:* short-duration acceleration acts on the body for periods of considerably less than one second.

These forces are usually encountered during ground impact and often are simply referred to as impact accelerations or impact forces. Their effects depend principally on the structural strength of the part of the body on which they act and are related to the overall velocity change induced.

The effects of short-duration, intermediate-duration and oscillating (vibration) accelerations are discussed in Chapters 10 and 14.

PHYSICAL PRINCIPLES

Knowledge of the force environment in flight is an essential prerequisite to understanding the physiological changes associated with exposure to increased acceleration. Therefore, a brief explanation of the mechanics underlying sustained acceleration is given.

Speed

Speed describes the rate of movement of a body, without specifying the direction of travel. Speed is defined as the rate of change of distance and is a scalar quantity.

Velocity

Velocity describes the rate and direction of travel of an object and thus is a vector quantity, having both magnitude and direction. The velocity of a body changes if there is a change in speed or direction of travel.

Acceleration

Acceleration describes a change of velocity of an object. It is defined as the rate of change of velocity and, like velocity, is a vector quantity having magnitude and direction. Hence, acceleration can result from a change in speed along a straight line (linear acceleration) or from a change in the direction of travel (radial acceleration). It is usually expressed in units of m/s².

In order to describe acceleration in terms that are more readily comprehensible, applied acceleration is often called G in aviation and expressed as a multiple of the acceleration due to gravity. Acceleration due to gravity is a physical constant (the gravitational constant) and is indicated by the symbol g (lower case); it has the value 9.81 m/s². Thus, the G value of an applied acceleration is given by:

$$G = \frac{\text{applied acceleration}}{g}$$

For example, if a body were exposed to 6 G, it would be accelerated at 58.86 m/s², which is six times the acceleration due to gravity (9.81 m/s²).

LINEAR ACCELERATION

A linear acceleration is an acceleration produced by a change of speed without a change in direction. In conventional aviation, prolonged linear accelerations (such as takeoff and landing) seldom reach a magnitude that will produce significant changes in human performance, as most aircraft do not exert sufficient thrust to produce extended changes in linear velocity. Linear accelerations of around 3 G to 4 G may, however, be produced during catapult-assisted takeoff, arrested landings and when reheat is engaged in certain-high performance aircraft. Prolonged linear accelerations also occur during the launch of spacecraft and when they are slowed upon re-entering the Earth's atmosphere. The magnitude of such acceleration in modern spacecraft is relatively low, the crew of the Space Shuttle generally being exposed to no more than 3 G.

RADIAL ACCELERATION

A radial acceleration is an acceleration produced by a change of direction of motion without a change of speed. The inherent design of an aircraft is such that, in order for it to fly, lift must be developed from the wings to counteract the force of gravity. Fast jet aircraft can produce far more lift than is required to counter gravity, and this can be used to change the direction of travel of the aircraft very rapidly. Considerable acceleration can be experienced in this way during banked turns and loop manoeuvres, when large radial acceleration forces are developed: accelerations of 9 G or more can be maintained for many seconds by agile military aircraft. Centrifuges used to study the effects of prolonged acceleration on humans also produce radial acceleration.

Newton's first law of motion (Box 8.1) states that a body will remain in a state of rest or in uniform motion in a straight line unless a force acts upon it. Therefore, an object constrained to move along a circular path will have the tendency to continue on a straight line that forms a tangent to the circular path. The object is prevented from moving tangentially by a force that pulls it away from the straight line towards the centre of the circle and that is responsible for the change of velocity that accompanies the change in the direction of travel. The magnitude of the radial acceleration of the object towards the centre of its circular path (centripetal acceleration) depends on the circumferential velocity of the object along its circular path and the radius of the path it follows:

$$a = \frac{v^2}{r}$$

where a is the centripetal radial acceleration, v is the circumferential velocity and r is the radius of the circular path.

Using this equation, the radial acceleration of an aircraft travelling at 500 knots (258 m/s) around a circular path with a diameter of 1 km can be calculated as 66.3 m/s² or 6.8 G. It should be noted that, due to the square term, small changes in the speed of the object will have a proportionally greater effect on the radial acceleration than small changes in radius.

ACCELERATION ONSET RATE

The rate of change of acceleration is termed acceleration onset rate or G onset rate. It is of importance when considering physiological responses to forces generated in flight and typically is expressed in units of G/s. Rate of change of acceleration is also important when considering human response to impact, where the term 'jolt' is used more commonly.

Centrifugal force

In the study of aviation physiology, it is important to consider these forces from the perspective of the human subject exposed to them. If the brakes are applied to a fast-moving car, then the occupants feel that they are being thrown forwards, although the applied force is directed backwards. The passenger's sensation is of a force in the direction opposite to that actually applied, and their body is accelerated (relative to the car) in this direction. This is explained by the action of a different force, termed inertia, which is considered in Newton's third law (Box 8.1). This

The principles relating force and motion are summarized in Newton's laws of motion.

NEWTON'S FIRST LAW

Newton's first law states that unless acted upon by a force, a body at rest will remain at rest and a body in motion will move at constant speed in a straight line. Thus, a force can produce a change in speed or in direction of motion, which is a change of velocity. Newton's first law therefore may be regarded as stating that acceleration results from the action of forces.

NEWTON'S SECOND LAW

Newton's second law states that when a force is applied to a body, the body is accelerated and the acceleration is directly proportional to the force applied and inversely proportional to the mass of the body. Expressed mathematically, the second law states:

$$F = ma$$

where F is the force, m is the mass of the body (the amount of matter in it) and a is the acceleration. This equation enables force and acceleration to be interconverted, as it may be assumed that mass is a constant. The unit of force is the newton (N), which is the force that will give a mass of 1 kg an acceleration of 1 m/s².

NEWTON'S THIRD LAW

Newton's third law states that to every action there is an equal and opposite reaction. Thus, when a force is applied to a body, it is resisted by an equal and opposite force, which is termed the force of inertia. The sensation of increased weight when being exposed to acceleration (other than gravity) is in the direction of the inertial force.

law states that every action has an equal and opposite reaction and results in human perception of an applied acceleration being a sensation of increased weight in the opposite direction. In the example given in the previous section, when an object describes a circular path, it is accelerated radially towards the centre of the circular path. By Newton's third law, the force producing the acceleration of the mass towards the centre of the circular path must be balanced by an equal force acting in the opposite direction

– the inertial force – which, since it acts outwards away from the centre of the curved path, is termed centrifugal force. The physiological effects of the radial accelerations produced by circular flight are due to centrifugal forces.

The magnitude of the centrifugal force generated by flight in a circular path is given by the equation:

$$F = \frac{mv^2}{r}$$

where F is the centrifugal inertial force, m is the mass of the body, v is the circumferential velocity and r is the radius of the curved path.

Weight

Newton's second law (see Box 8.1) enables the concept of weight to be described. Weight is the force exerted by the mass of an accelerating body and is measured in newtons (N). The force most commonly experienced by humans is weight resulting from the acceleration caused by the attraction of the Earth. This force is constant because acceleration due to gravity, g, is constant (although there is some planetary regional variation). When considering weight, the weight (W) exerted by a mass (m) when accelerated at a value of a is given by the relationship:

$$W = m \times a$$

Thus, for example, when a mass of 1 kg is acted upon by a force that produces an acceleration of 29.43 m/s² (3 G), it weighs 29.43 N. Confusion sometimes arises from the use of the term 'weight' in common parlance as a synonym for mass.

It should be noted that there is a difference between the sensation of force (weight) produced by gravity and that induced by other accelerations. Other forms of acceleration produce a sensation of force acting in a direction opposite to the change in velocity. In the case of gravity, however, both the acceleration and the sensation of weight are in the same direction, towards the centre of the Earth. Furthermore, it is only when the acceleration due to gravity is resisted fully by direct or indirect contact with the ground that normal weight is experienced, and a body has no weight if it is allowed to fall freely with an acceleration of 9.81 m/s². Thus, gravity is unique in that it can be responsible for acceleration or weight, but not for both at the same time.

Influence of gravity

The aircrew of an aircraft executing a vertical loop manoeuvre are exposed not only to the centrifugal forces induced by the radial acceleration but also to the force generated by the linear acceleration due to gravity. The relationship between the centrifugal and gravitational forces changes continuously during the manoeuvre, so that the magnitude and direction of the resultant force acting on the object vary along the flight path. The interactions of these forces may be illustrated by considering the resultant force acting on the pilot flying an aircraft in a vertical loop giving a constant radial acceleration of 1 G. The magnitude and direction of the resultant of the centrifugal inertial force (F_c) of 1 G and that due to gravity (F_g) at several stages in the loop are depicted in Figure 8.1.

When the aircraft is at the bottom of the loop, the centrifugal and gravitational forces are acting in the same direction along a line at right-angles to the longitudinal axis of the aircraft. At this point, the resultant acceleration will be 2 G and the weight of a mass will be twice its resting value. At the top of the loop, when the aircraft is inverted, the centrifugal and gravitational forces are acting along the same line but in opposition to each other, so that both the resultant acceleration and the apparent weight will be zero. At all other points in the loop, the weight lies between zero and 2 G, and the angle that the resultant makes with the longitudinal axis of the aircraft changes through 180 degrees during the loop. Thus, halfway up and halfway down the loop, the vector diagrams (Figure 8.1) show that the weight of an object will be 1.4 times its resting value. On the ascending loop, however, the resultant force is acting 45 degrees behind the normal vertical, and midway down the descending loop it acts 45 degrees forwards of the normal vertical. When the aircraft is 60 degrees from the top of the loop, the magnitude of the resultant is 1 G, and so an object will have its normal rest-

ing weight. At this position, the resultant is 60 degrees behind the normal vertical on the ascent and 60 degrees forwards of it on the descent.

Although perfect vertical loops of the type depicted in Figure 8.1 are produced in aerobatic flying, it is more usual for aircraft to fly a track made up of only part of a circular path or several different circular paths. The magnitudes and directions of the accelerative forces acting on the aircraft and its crew can be determined by treating the complex flight path as a series of sections, each with its own radius of curvature.

Acceleration terminology

In aerospace medicine, where the main interest is the effect of acceleration on humans, the direction in which an acceleration or inertial force acts is described by the use of a three-axis coordinate system (x, y, z), in which the vertical (z) axis is parallel to the long spinal axis of the body. The direction of force applied to an individual is most commonly referred to in terms of inertial reaction, rather than the applied accelerative force, as this more readily fits the human perception of the environment. Table 8.1 and Figure 8.2 show the internationally agreed standard aeromedical terminology for indicating the direction of acceleration and inertial forces acting on humans, based on terminology proposed by Gell (1961). As this terminology relates to the person and their orientation, rather than the forces acting on the aircraft, cockpit geometry is an important consideration when aircraft performance data are applied to aircrew.

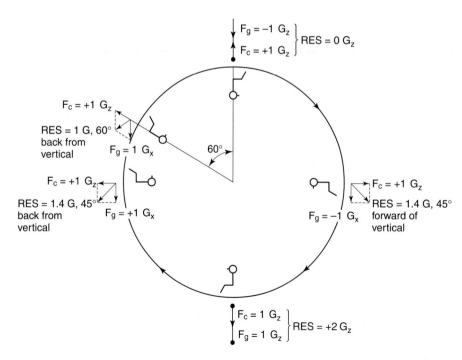

Figure 8.1 *Interaction between centrifugal inertial force (F_c) and gravitational force (F_g) on the pilot of an aircraft flown in a loop. The vector diagrams show that the resultant (RES) of the centrifugal and inertial forces varies from +2 G_z at the bottom of the loop to 0 G_z at the top. While descending, the resultant acts forward of the long axis of the body; during ascent, it acts behind the long axis.*

Table 8.1 *Three-axis coordinate system for describing direction of acceleration and inertial forces acting on a human*

Direction of acceleration	Direction of resultant inertial force	Physiological and vernacular descriptors	Standard terminology
Headwards	Head to foot	Positive G, eyeballs down	+G$_z$
Footwards	Foot to head	Negative G, eyeballs up	−G$_z$
Forwards	Chest to back	Transverse AP G, supine G, eyeballs in	+G$_x$
Backwards	Back to chest	Transverse PA G, prone G, eyeballs out	−G$_x$
To the right	Right to left side	Left lateral G, eyeballs left	+G$_y$
To the left	Left to right side	Right lateral G, eyeballs right	−G$_y$

AP, anteroposterior; PA, postero-anterior.

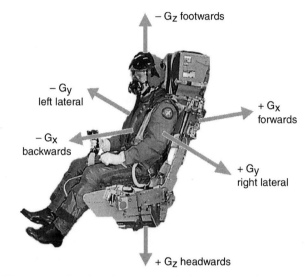

Figure 8.2 *Standard aerospace medical terminology for describing the direction of acceleration and inertial forces. The vector arrows indicate the direction of the resultant inertial forces.*

EXPOSURE TO +G$_z$ ACCELERATION

The number of aviators around the world who are exposed regularly to high sustained +G$_z$ acceleration is relatively small, being restricted almost entirely to a few hundred or more military personnel in any one country. Although civilian aerobatic flyers also experience high levels of +G$_z$ acceleration (as much as +9 to −9 G$_z$), their aircraft generally are incapable of sustaining acceleration due to limitations of thrust, and consequently their G exposure tends to be brief, limiting the physiological sequelae. In a military setting, exposure to acceleration is dependent on the aircraft type operated; however, most aircrew will be exposed to at least +6 G$_z$ during their basic flying training. Exposure to +6 G$_z$ acceleration usually results from turns, particularly during air combat manoeuvring (ACM), and ground attack flights, where dive recovery and missile avoidance may mandate abrupt changes in direction.

Within the RAF, until recently there was little exposure to high G in operational (front-line) flying duties, as many of the aircraft types operated were not designed for high-G manoeuvring, with typical acceleration exposures in front-line flying rarely exceeding +5 G$_z$. In countries that have operated aircraft such as the F15, F16 and F18 for some years, aircrew exposure to sustained high G levels is greater. Such aircraft may sustain +7 to +9 G$_z$ for five to ten seconds and accelerations above +5 G$_z$ for up to one minute. Aircrew may be expected to gain between 500 and 5000 hours' experience flying these aircraft types, and one to five per cent of this time might be under sustained high +G$_z$ conditions. The net result is a whole-career G dose measured in hours for these aircrew.

The introduction of agile aircraft such as Eurofighter Typhoon into the RAF will increase aircrew acceleration exposure. Typhoon is capable of sustaining +9 G$_z$ almost indefinitely, with an acceleration onset rate in excess of 10 G/s. Along with similar next-generation agile aircraft, such as F22, Joint Strike Fighter, Rafale and Gripen, Typhoon brings new physiological problems to the aircrew that will fly the aircraft and necessitates improvement in the G-protection provided. Furthermore, the ability to sustain high G for longer periods of time may mean that overall aircrew exposure to sustained +G$_z$ acceleration will increase, the consequences of which must yet be determined.

Musculoskeletal effects of +G$_z$ acceleration

The most readily apparent effects of exposure to increased +G$_z$ acceleration are brought about by the increased weight of the soft tissues, head, limbs and trunk. This is obvious to the pilot or centrifuge subject who tries, with difficulty, to elevate their arms at +3 G$_z$; upward movement of the arms becomes almost impossible above +7 G$_z$, although fine movement, such as that in the fingers, tends to be preserved due to their relatively low mass. More importantly, above +3 G$_z$, it is impossible for most people to stand up from the seated position, making unassisted escape (e.g. from a damaged aircraft) impossible. For this reason, among many others, assisted-escape systems such as ejection seats are employed in high-performance aircraft.

The soft tissues of the face are also seen to be affected by acceleration exposure, with a drooping or sagging appearance even at +2 G_z, which can, at higher acceleration levels, lead to involuntary closure of the eyes in inexperienced subjects. Even without the added weight of headgear, an individual cannot raise their head once the neck has been allowed to flex at accelerations above about +8 G_z. When a typical protective helmet (weighing perhaps 2 kg) is worn, this limitation occurs at +4 to +6 G_z. Of particular relevance is the position of the centre of gravity of the head, relative to the atlanto-occipital joint and cervical vertebrae. Head-mounted equipment such as helmets, sights, displays and night-vision goggles may bring the centre of gravity forward and encourage forwards flexion of the head under +G_z acceleration. For all these reasons, repetitive exposures to long-duration +G_z acceleration lead to fatigue and, in particular, neck pain and associated soft-tissue injury (see Chapter 9).

Cardiovascular effects of +G$_z$ acceleration

Exposure to increased +G_z acceleration has a profound effect on the cardiovascular system, first manifested by visual symptoms and then, at sufficiently high levels of acceleration, by loss of consciousness. These effects are not limited to the latest aircraft types and were observed at least as early as 1918 (Head 1920). The circulatory disturbance is a result of simple Newtonian physics applied to the fluid compartments within the body. Exposure to +G_z acceleration produces immediate major changes in the distribution of pressure in the arterial and venous systems, which, in turn, induce shifts of blood towards the more dependent parts. These initial disturbances evoke reflex compensatory changes, which tend to reduce the magnitude of the initial effects.

HYDROSTATIC PRESSURE

The cardiovascular changes under +G_z acceleration result from an increased hydrostatic gradient present in the arterial and venous systems under increased +G_z acceleration. The hydrostatic pressure resulting from exposure of a column of fluid to acceleration is given by

$$p = h\rho g$$

where p is the pressure exerted by a column of fluid, h is the height of that column, ρ is the density of fluid and g is the acceleration to which it is exposed. As g is increased, so the pressure exerted by the column of fluid is increased, provided the other factors remain constant. In the upright individual, the immediate effect of +G_z acceleration is therefore to accentuate the pressure gradients that normally exist due to gravity. However, the vascular pressure in the right and left sides of the heart remains essentially unchanged at the beginning of +G_z exposure, as this pressure is created with reference to the pressure in the pleural space and hence atmospheric pressure.

The acceleration increases the weight of the columns of blood above and below the heart, so that the vascular pressure above the level of the heart is decreased and the pressure below the heart is increased. Consider the column of blood in the arterial system between the heart and the head of a seated individual. In most adults, this equates to about 30 cm in height. If the density of blood is assumed to be 1.06 g/ml and g is assumed to be 9.81 m/s^2, then the pressure drop at head level caused by exposure to +1 G_z may be calculated using the formula above to be approximately 22 mmHg. This simple model assumes the vasculature to consist of inelastic tubes. Thus, the hydrostatic pressure between heart and head when seated at rest under Earth's gravity will result in a head-level blood pressure that is approximately 22 mmHg lower than that at heart level. Similarly, exposure to five times the Earth's gravity (+5 G_z) will result in a hydrostatic pressure drop of $5 \times 22 = 110$ mmHg. If heart-level systolic blood pressure is assumed to be 110 mmHg, and in the absence of any cardiovascular reflexes, it can be seen that most individuals will have little or no head-level blood pressure at this acceleration level. This principle is illustrated diagrammatically in Figure 8.3. This simple model assumes that no vertical

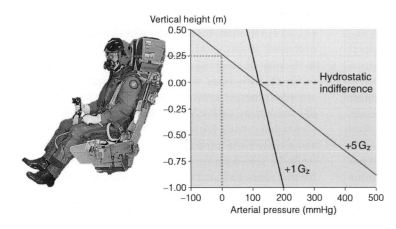

Vertical height (m)

Hydrostatic indifference

+5 G_z

+1 G_z

Arterial pressure (mmHg)

Figure 8.3 *Variation in arterial pressure in a seated individual at +1 G_z and +5 G_z at different vertical separations from the point of arterial hydrostatic indifference at heart level. The dotted line corresponds to head-level arterial pressure at +5 G_z.*

movement of the heart occurs within the thorax under +G$_z$ acceleration; in reality, subjects exposed to +G$_z$ acceleration without an anti-G suit experience descent of the heart and diaphragm. However, the magnitude of this descent is relatively small, and at +5 G$_z$, a 5 cm increase in the head-to-heart distance has been estimated, equating to a further reduction in blood pressure of only 4 mmHg per G.

Figure 8.4 shows the pressures in the arterial tree of an individual seated upright at +1 G$_z$ and +4.5 G$_z$. In this example, the mean arterial pressure at heart level both at +1 G$_z$ and at +4.5 G$_z$ is 100 mmHg. The mean pressure in the cerebral arteries at eye level, which is 30 cm vertically above the heart, is 22 mmHg less than heart-level pressure at +1 G$_z$ and 99 mmHg less at +4.5 G$_z$. Thus, the mean cerebral arterial pressure falls from 78 mmHg at +1 G$_z$ to only 1 mmHg at +4.5 G$_z$. The pressure in the femoral artery, which is approximately 60 cm below the heart, is 100 + 44 = 144 mmHg at +1 G$_z$. The pressure exerted by the 60-cm column of blood is increased to 198 mmHg at +4.5 G$_z$, so that the femoral artery pressure at this level of acceleration is approximately 300 mmHg.

The corresponding pressures in the venous part of the systemic circulation are also shown in Figure 8.4. The pressure in the right atrium of the heart is virtually atmospheric both at +1 G$_z$ and at +4.5 G$_z$. At +1 G$_z$, the pressure in the cerebral veins at eye level is of the order of −20 mmHg. On exposure to +4.5 G$_z$, the increase in the weight of the column of blood between the cerebral veins and the heart would be expected to reduce the pressure in the cerebral veins to about −100 mmHg. The high negative transmural pressure across the walls of the jugular veins in the neck reduces the lumen of the veins greatly, increasing the resistance to flow through them, so that, in practice, the pressure in the jugular bulb falls to only about −50 mmHg on exposure to +4.5 G$_z$.

BLOOD VOLUME DISTRIBUTION

The changes in intravascular pressure described above have an effect on the size of the blood vessels, since the latter is determined by the vascular transmural pressure (the difference between intravascular and extravascular pressure), the distensibility of the vessel and the amount of blood available to fill it. In turn, changes in the size of the vessels have major effects on the regional blood flow and blood content. Thus, an increase in the transmural pressure of small arteries and arterioles below the level of the heart will reduce the peripheral resistance and increase local blood flow, while a decrease in the transmural pressure of veins above the level of the heart can produce complete collapse of the vessels and cessation of blood flow through them.

Although at the onset of exposure to +G$_z$ acceleration, the arterial pressure at the level of the heart is unchanged, this pressure falls progressively over the first 6–12 seconds. This fall of mean arterial pressure is due to a fall in the

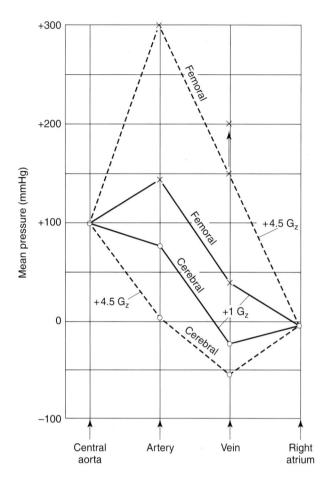

Figure 8.4 *Immediate effect of exposure to +1 and +4.5 G$_z$ on the mean pressures at the following points in the circulation of a seated individual: (a) immediately downstream of the aortic valve; (b) in the cerebral arteries and veins at the horizontal level of the eye; (c) in the femoral artery and vein; and (d) in the right atrium. Secondary changes in the circulation that occur over the first 30–60 seconds of the exposure to +G$_z$ modify the magnitude of these pressures. The pressure in the femoral vein rises progressively during the first 30–60 seconds of the exposure to +G$_z$ acceleration as blood accumulates in the capacity vessels of the lower limbs.*

peripheral resistance and a reduction in the output of the left side of the heart. The fall of peripheral resistance is caused by the large increase in the transmural pressure of the arterioles in the dependent parts of the arterial tree, while the increase in venous pressure in the regions below the heart causes dilation of the capacity vessels. The rate of distension of these vessels depends on their visco-elastic properties and the magnitude of the pressure change. During the period when distension is occurring, there is a regional redistribution of blood volume in the venous compartment. If it is assumed that the venous valves are competent at preventing backfilling into the dependent veins (which may not be true at high pressure), then filling occurs via the arterial supply. During the filling phase, inflow to the venous compartment continues, but outflow, and hence venous return back to the right side of the heart, is greatly reduced or absent.

The net result of these changes is that if acceleration is maintained, then a progressive fall of pressure occurs throughout the arterial tree for 6–12 seconds after the onset of the acceleration. At a particular transmural pressure, determined largely by the tone of the vessel wall, no further increase in venous vessel diameter occurs, venous pressure overcomes central pressure and flow is re-established, such that venous return is restored towards the initial state, tending to limit further reduction in arterial pressure.

The redistribution of blood volume produced by $+G_z$ acceleration occurs mainly towards the lower limbs. Little volume increase can occur in the capacity vessels within the abdomen, since intra-abdominal pressure rises in parallel with the venous pressure. It has been found that some 60–100 ml of blood is pooled in the lower limbs of a seated subject exposed to $+5\ G_z$ for 15 seconds, although the circulation is already compromised by gravity, as some 300–800 ml of blood is pooled in the lower limbs upon adoption of the upright posture. The relatively small blood volume shift seen during increased $+G_z$ acceleration has led some to suggest that, overall, the head–heart hydrostatic gradient has far greater influence on human acceleration tolerance than blood volume redistribution.

The rise of pressure within the capillaries in the lower limbs also causes transudation of fluid from the blood to the tissues, so that there is a progressive loss of fluid from the circulation. The rate of fluid loss into the tissues of the lower limbs during a sustained exposure to $+5\ G_z$ is about 270 ml/min (Howard 1965). In practical terms, aircrew exposure to acceleration during flight is sustained typically for periods of 15 seconds or less, and so the effects of transudation are less apparent. Repeated short exposures during a sortie do, however, sometimes lead to some noticeable swelling in dependent limbs, particularly where no counter-pressure has been applied.

High vascular transmural pressure may also be seen in the forearms if these are held significantly below the level of the heart, a posture usually demanded by low placement of an aircraft's control column and throttle. The pressure rise may be high enough to cause high-G arm pain (see Chapter 9).

BARORECEPTOR REFLEX

The blood-pressure changes and blood volume redistribution provoked by exposure to increased G_z acceleration produce reflex responses involving the arterial baroreceptors and possibly also the low-pressure cardiopulmonary receptors and arterial chemoreceptors. Additionally, exposure to acceleration may modify activity in skeletal muscle mechanoreceptors and metaboreceptors, lung-stretch receptors and vestibular receptors (Cheung and Bateman 2001), leading to modulation of cardiovascular function. Reflexes at the local level are also likely to influence the blood-pressure response to acceleration exposure.

Arterial baroreceptors are located in the adventitial layer of the carotid sinus and aortic arch. These mechanoreceptors respond to stretch, and the arterial transmural pressure governs the deformation and hence afferent output rate. They exhibit both static and dynamic properties: a fall in carotid artery pressure due to acceleration exposure may produce a cessation of output as blood pressure drops, followed by re-initiation of activity at a lower rate than the pre-acceleration baseline. Reduced activity is conveyed via the IX and X cranial nerves to the nucleus tractus solitarius in the medulla. The output of the nucleus tractus solitarius is relayed to the nucleus ambiguus, containing vagal cardiac motor neurons and to the caudal ventrolateral medulla, which influences sympathetic output (the hypothalamus also modulates these areas). Heart rate is increased by reduced vagal inhibition and vasoconstriction occurs (predominantly in muscle and the splanchnic region), leading to increased peripheral resistance. Cardiac contractility is increased, both directly and by release of adrenaline (epinephrine) from the adrenal medulla. Increase in renal sympathetic nerve activity stimulates renin secretion, activating the renin–angiotensin system to produce angiotensin II (resulting in generalized vasoconstriction) and aldosterone (resulting in salt and water retention).

Thus, the baroreceptor reflex provides a compensatory mechanism to preserve head-level blood pressure under increased acceleration, and measurement of blood pressure under acceleration demonstrates this as a characteristic recovery 6–12 seconds after the onset of acceleration exposure (Figure 8.5). Exposure to $+4\ G_z$ typically produces a maximum heart rate of around 120–140 beats/min. The venous return to the right side of the heart starts to increase by 10–15 seconds after the onset of acceleration exposure, and the output of the left side of the heart increases within a few beats. The venous return and the cardiac output continue to rise over the next 20–40 seconds: cardiac output after 30–60 seconds exposure to $+4\ G_z$ is reduced by about 20 per cent below the resting value. Overall, the compensatory changes tend to restore the heart-level arterial blood pressure, so that after 40–60 seconds of exposure to moderate levels of acceleration ($+3$ to $+5\ G_z$), the mean arterial blood pressure at heart level is similar to the pre-exposure level.

Baroreceptor sensitivity ('gain') is modified by various factors, including age and arterial wall distensibility. Additionally, the 'set point' to which blood pressure is regulated can be modified by central and peripheral factors. It is possible that exposure to acceleration and the muscular exertion of anti-G straining may invoke central (upward) resetting of the baroreceptors. Peripheral resetting of the

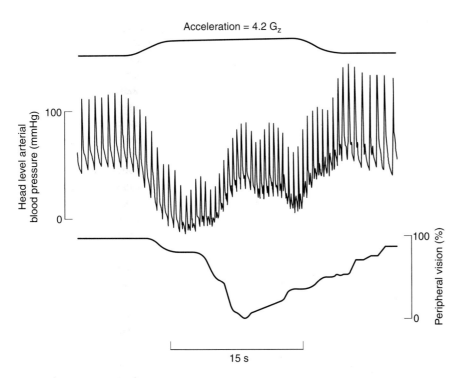

Acceleration = 4.2 G$_z$

Head level arterial blood pressure (mmHg)

100

0

Peripheral vision (%)

100

0

15 s

Figure 8.5 *Effects of a 15-second exposure to +4.2 G$_z$ on head-level arterial blood pressure and peripheral vision. Note that peripheral vision is lost progressively as arterial blood pressure falls, with blackout (zero peripheral vision) occurring some six seconds after the point of lowest pressure. Thereafter, both blood pressure and vision recover as compensatory reflexes develop.*

baroreceptors, whereby the set point is modified by baroreceptor exposure to a new pressure for 15 minutes or more, has not been thought to occur in the context of fast jet aviation. This is because exposure to acceleration in fast jet aircraft usually is brief, in the order of 5–20 seconds. In practical terms, it has long been assumed that no physiological adaptation to acceleration exposure occurs. However, this does not explain the phenomenon of 'layoff', whereby aircrew who have not flown at high G for a period of a week or more notice a reduction in their G tolerance on return to flying. Some cardiovascular adaptation to orthostatic stress has been demonstrated experimentally (Convertino 1998, 1999; Convertino *et al.* 1998; Newman *et al.* 1998, 2000; Schlegel *et al.* 2003), although the mechanism of this adaptation is unclear. One mechanism might involve central baroreceptor resetting. However, this is complicated further by the relationship between carotid and aortic baroreceptor stimulation under acceleration. Like upright tilt, the hydrostatic gradient results in more profound changes in the output of carotid baroreceptors than of those at the aortic arch, near to the heart. This is dissimilar to the situation of volume depletion (e.g. by haemorrhage) or lower-body negative pressure (LBNP), where both sets of receptors are exposed to a similar pressure change. The central integration of baroreceptor responses in the two scenarios is likely to differ.

Visual effects of +G$_z$ acceleration

To an aviator or an experimental subject on a human centrifuge, visual symptoms are the first overt manifestation of

the cardiovascular effects of acceleration exposure. The earliest recorded acknowledgement of visual changes associated with +G$_z$ exposure appears to be that by Head (1920). Head reported that a test pilot flying a Sopwith triplane in a +4.5 G$_z$ banked turn experienced 'characteristic darkening of the sky which was preliminary to fainting'. Changes in visual function have since become recognized by aircrew as an important antecedent to impending G-induced loss of consciousness, and familiarity with visual symptoms is an important part of high-G training for aircrew.

Classically, the pattern of visual loss associated with +G$_z$ exposure is described in terms of 'grey-out' and 'blackout'. Grey-out is usually described as a cone-shaped loss of vision, which starts at the periphery of vision with relative sparing of central vision, and encroaching centrally at higher levels of acceleration. The vision in the periphery is variously described as grey or black, but in practical terms subjects are unable to respond to a light stimulus presented in the affected part of the visual field.

However, not all subjects report identical visual symptoms, and there appears to be a subgroup of people who report a widespread dimming of both central and peripheral vision simultaneously, with apparent reduction in contrast sensitivity. Some subjects also report seeing lines and shapes of various colours under these conditions.

A more definite visual symptom is that of 'blackout'. In this setting, 'blackout' refers to complete loss of vision with preserved consciousness, in distinction to the colloquial term for loss of consciousness or faint. Usually it is the end result of the classical grey-out pattern described above, in which vision becomes an ever-narrowing tunnel, until finally central vision is lost while hearing and mental processes are maintained. Blackout occurs at acceleration levels higher than those that cause grey-out, and little further $+G_z$ acceleration (usually around 0.5 G) is required to cause loss of consciousness. Under certain circumstances, aircrew can use the warning symptoms of grey-out and blackout to avoid G-induced loss of consciousness (G-LOC) by taking corrective action. However, at high acceleration onset levels, these symptoms may not be present (this effect is described more fully below). The largest study to investigate the acceleration levels associated with visual symptoms was conducted using 1000 aircrew (Cochran *et al.* 1954). This revealed that blackout occurred at $+4.8 G_z$ (standard deviation 0.8 G), and loss of consciousness followed at $+5.4 G_z$ (standard deviation 0.9 G). However, there is a large variation in the level of acceleration at which a given loss of peripheral vision occurs, due to factors such as body stature, physical condition, level of illumination of the visual field and target and, in particular, the degree of muscle relaxation.

Whatever the level of acceleration, vision is not disturbed for some five seconds after the beginning of the exposure. At moderate levels of acceleration, the intensity of the visual symptoms often decreases 8–12 seconds after the onset of the acceleration. This improvement is due to compensatory cardiovascular responses restoring the flow of blood to the retina. Thus, during exposure to $+5.0 G_z$, blackout may occur after six seconds but vision is restored some six seconds later. Normal vision usually returns three to five seconds after the manoeuvre ends.

Figure 8.5 illustrates these changes as recorded in a subject seated in a Farnborough centrifuge and exposed to $+4.2 G_z$ for 15 seconds. Note the initial fall in arterial blood pressure at head level (recorded using a Finapres (OHMEDA) monitor with the finger and sensor supported at eye level) followed by an obvious tachycardia and partial recovery in pressure. Peripheral vision was monitored using a subject-operated tracking device and closely mirrors the blood pressure changes, with blackout occurring a few seconds after the point of lowest pressure.

The visual disturbances produced by $+G_z$ acceleration are caused by retinal ischaemia. The various degrees of grey-out are due to progressive reduction in the flow of blood to the retina; complete cessation of the flow causes blackout. The eye has an internal (intraocular) pressure of around 10–20 mmHg, so the pressure in the central retinal artery must exceed 20 mmHg, otherwise blood flow will cease. Blackout occurs during $+G_z$ acceleration when the systolic arterial pressure at eye level falls below 20 mmHg. Using an ophthalmoscope, the retinal arteries and arterioles can be seen to be empty when the arterial pressure is less than 20 mmHg (Duane 1954).

Figure 8.5 demonstrates that there is an interval of four to six seconds between the cessation of retinal blood flow and loss of vision. It is generally held that the time delay relates to metabolism of local oxygen in the blood and tissues. Thus, retinal function decays when local 'reserves' of oxygen have expired. Similarly, on recovery, the return of vision is delayed for a few seconds after the arterial pressure at eye level has risen above 20 mmHg. This delay is due to the time taken to regenerate the oxygen store and thereby raise the oxygen tension in the retina above the minimum required for normal function. Despite the blackout, consciousness is preserved until the cerebral arterial pressure is reduced to 0–10 mmHg.

The peripheral distribution of the loss of vision in grey-out (or coning of vision) traditionally has been ascribed to the vascular anatomy of the retina. This explanation relies on the assumption that the retina has a single blood supply from the central retinal artery, an end artery that penetrates the globe at the optic disc and forms multiple branches, becoming more numerous and smaller in diameter towards the periphery. Thus, a reduction in central retinal artery pressure will cause blood flow in peripheral retinal vessels to be overcome by intraocular pressure first, as the peripheral vessels have the lowest pressure. The explanation is probably somewhat oversimplified, as it does not address blood supply to the fovea, which is avascular and nourished by the choroidal circulation. Moreover, the hypothesis does not explain the alternative, more uniform pattern of visual loss seen in some individuals. Recently, it has been suggested that extraocular venous resistance is an important factor (Cirovic and Frazer 2003). Unfortunately, due to the technical difficulties involved, a thorough understanding of the aetiology of visual symptoms under increased acceleration has not yet been gained.

G-induced loss of consciousness

Exposure to $+G_z$ stress somewhat greater than that required to produce visual blackout results in G-LOC. As consciousness is lost, there is total loss of muscle tone, so that the head and body slump. During recovery in the few seconds following acceleration exposure, clonic muscle activity may occur, which is likely to be due to differences in cerebral activation as blood returns to the brain. This is not epileptic in nature and is of no significance, except that it may be useful in identifying a G-LOC episode. Furthermore, it is possible that an aircraft control or switch could be operated inadvertently during this activity.

Incapacitation due to G-LOC can be divided into two periods: a period of absolute incapacitation, lasting for 10–15 seconds, during which the individual is unconscious, and a period of relative incapacitation lasting for 30 seconds or more, during which the individual is conscious, but suffering from confusion and disorientation, such that he or she is unable to control the aircraft (Whinnery *et al.* 1987). The total incapacitation time, which could be a minute or longer, is sufficient for a fast-moving aircraft to impact with the ground. In the period 1982–2001, the USAF has lost 29 aircraft to G-LOC (Lyons *et al.* 2004a).

In the hours following G-LOC, G tolerance may be reduced and certain psychological effects may persist. Therefore, aircrew are recommended to terminate the sortie and not to fly for the remainder of the day following a G-LOC episode. Physiological amnesia in up to 50 per cent of cases following G-LOC may mean that aircrew may be unaware of having had an episode. Confidential surveys from various armed forces around the world suggest that 10–20 per cent of all military pilots have suffered from G-LOC at least once. However, considering that some individuals may have suffered from post G-LOC amnesia, this may be an underestimate. G-LOC occurs more commonly in training aircraft, although the resulting accident rate is higher in single-seat fighters (Lyons *et al.* 2004b).

The syndrome of 'almost loss of consciousness' (A-LOC) has also been described. This is a rather loose collection of signs and symptoms of a physiological, emotional and cognitive nature. Features include sensory abnormalities, amnesia, confusion, euphoria, paralysis and reduced auditory acuity. One particularly notable feature is the apparent disconnection between the desire and the ability to perform an action. Certain features (e.g. tremor) may persist for some time after the acceleration exposure has ceased. The aetiology is thought to be similar to that of G-LOC. The syndrome has the potential to cause significant loss of aircrew performance, but it has not received widespread publicity in the aviator community.

Effects of +G$_z$ acceleration on the cerebral circulation

The hydrostatic effect of acceleration greater than about +3.5 G$_z$ on arterial pressure reduces the arterial pressure at the level of the brain to a value that, under normal gravity, would be below that required to maintain an adequate cerebral blood flow. Similarly, exposure to +4.5 G$_z$ reduces the arterial pressure at head level to virtually zero. Furthermore, exposure to +G$_z$ acceleration sufficient to induce blackout (when the arterial pressure at eye level must be less than 20 mmHg) does not necessarily result in loss of consciousness. Although reflex compensatory changes partially restore arterial pressure at brain level 6–12 seconds after the onset of acceleration, the incidence of unconsciousness is much lower than would be expected. Several mechanisms are responsible for the continued flow of blood through the brain during exposure to +3 to +5 G$_z$, even though the arterial pressure at head level is only 0–20 mmHg.

First, the cerebral vessels and brain are enclosed in a rigid bony box and surrounded by cerebrospinal fluid. The pressure of the cerebrospinal fluid falls, owing to hydro-static effects, in parallel with the reduction of vascular pressure at head level, so that the pressure difference across the walls of the intracranial vessels remains close to normal and the vessels remain open. Second, there is active vasodilation of the arterioles of the cerebral circulation, so that the resistance to flow through them is reduced. Third, the column of blood in the upper part of the veins in the neck creates a siphon effect, which maintains the cerebral circulation for as long as the column remains unbroken. Thus, a pressure difference between the arterial and venous sides of the cerebral circulation of the order of 50–60 mmHg is maintained at an acceleration of +4 to +5 G$_z$ by a pressure in the jugular bulb of −50 mmHg.

At higher levels of acceleration, however, further lowering of the pressure within the upper part of the jugular veins causes these vessels to collapse completely, thereby breaking the siphon. Blood then ceases to flow through the brain, and unconsciousness supervenes in a few seconds. As the siphon breaks, the cerebral vessels are emptied of blood, so that only the oxygen stored as dissolved gas in the cerebral tissue is left to maintain aerobic metabolism. This store is exhausted in some three to five seconds.

Effect of +G$_z$ acceleration on skin capillaries

The high vascular transmural pressure across the walls of the capillaries in the skin of dependent parts produced by exposure to increased +G$_z$ acceleration not only gives rise to transudation of fluid but also may cause rupture of these vessels, with the formation of petechiae. Thus, it is not unusual to find showers of petechial haemorrhages on the foot, leg, buttocks and forearm after repeated or prolonged exposures to accelerations greater than about +6 G$_z$. This appearance is commonly termed 'G-measles'. Occasionally, a larger vessel (usually a small vein or venule) may rupture, leading to a subcutaneous collection of blood. This usually occurs at higher acceleration levels in unsupported areas such as the popliteal fossa; although sometimes it is painful, the condition is generally self-limiting.

Effect of +G$_z$ acceleration on cardiac rhythm

Benign cardiac dysrhythmias frequently occur during and immediately following exposures to high sustained levels of +G$_z$ acceleration. Most common are premature ventricular contractions and premature atrial contractions, which tend to occur during the acceleration exposure itself. Sinus arrhythmia, and occasionally brief atrioventricular block, is seen more commonly after acceleration exposure has ended. Premature ventricular beats with bigeminy or trigeminy may also occur under +G$_z$ acceleration; rarely, episodes of supraventricular tachycardia and ventricular tachycardia have been observed. These changes are probably related to the profound changes in heart rate induced by autonomic imbalance during and following G-exposure. Experience in the USA suggests that rhythm disturbances are more likely to occur during simulated air combat manoeuvres, which are the most physically demanding aspect of centrifuge training.

Hormone response to +G$_z$ acceleration

Acceleration stress induces a specific endocrine response with increases in serum cortisol, adrenaline and noradrenaline levels (Mills 1985). The cortisol response is too slow to have an effect on tolerance to an acute exposure to acceleration, but it may be significant in prolonged or repeated exposures. This may explain why pilots like to pull G before air-to-air combat in order to 'tone up' their physiology. The acute release of catecholamines and vasopressin (antidiuretic hormone) may also enhance G-tolerance by increasing peripheral resistance. Indeed, the first exposure to +G$_z$ acceleration of a series has been shown to produce visual symptoms at a lower acceleration level than subsequent exposures – the so-called 'first-run effect'. A rise in plasma renin has also been observed following exposure to +G$_z$ acceleration; this promotes salt and water retention via angiotensin II and hence aldosterone secretion. It is possible that increased circulating angiotensin II levels may also contribute directly to acceleration tolerance by promoting peripheral vasoconstriction. In addition, it should be noted that the psychological stress of a centrifuge run, particularly in a novice subject, may induce an anticipatory tachycardia due to catecholamine release.

Tolerance to +G$_z$ acceleration

Several problems arise in defining tolerance to acceleration. The nature of the endpoint for G-tolerance can be defined in a number of ways: grey-out, blackout or physical exhaustion can be used – the most appropriate endpoint depends on the rate of application and duration of the accelerative stress. The time from the onset of the acceleration to the appearance of grey-out, blackout or G-LOC is a function of the rate at which the acceleration is applied, particularly when this is less than 1 G/s. Thus, the level of acceleration at which blackout occurs is, on average, 1 G higher with a rate of onset of 0.1 G/s as compared with an onset rate of 1 G/s. In most fast-jet aviation, the rate of onset of acceleration for peak accelerations above +4 G$_z$ generally is much greater than 1 G/s, and the duration of exposure is usually defined as the total time for which the acceleration exceeds +1 G$_z$. During prolonged G exposure, e.g. during simulated air combat manoeuvring on the centrifuge, fatigue becomes an important factor and time to physical exhaustion is sometimes used as a measure of tol-

erance under these circumstances. A further problem with the determination of G-tolerance is the large variation between individuals, such that in one series of experiments, the acceleration required to produce blackout varied between subjects from +2.7 G$_z$ to +7.8 G$_z$ (mean value +4.7 G$_z$ with a standard deviation of ±0.8 G).

With these limitations in mind, a compilation of centrifuge data on tolerance to +G$_z$ acceleration in relaxed unprotected subjects is presented in Figure 8.6. The endpoints are unconsciousness or blackout, whichever occurred first. The increase in tolerance beyond ten seconds is due to the operation of compensatory cardiovascular responses. Figure 8.6 shows that, theoretically, a subject could be taken to +14 G$_z$ and brought back to +1 G$_z$ without any visual loss if the acceleration exposure were completed within a few seconds. However, if the subject remained at +14 G$_z$ for more than a few seconds, unconsciousness would occur without any premonitory grey-out, since the oxygen stores of both the eyes and the brain become exhausted at about the same rate. A very slow onset of acceleration allows cardiovascular reflexes to develop, and the trough seen in Figure 8.6 may then be avoided. Thus, tolerance to +G$_z$ acceleration at an onset rate of 0.1 G/s is about 1 G greater than at an onset rate of 1 G/s. The effect of G onset rate on tolerance is summarized in Figure 8.7.

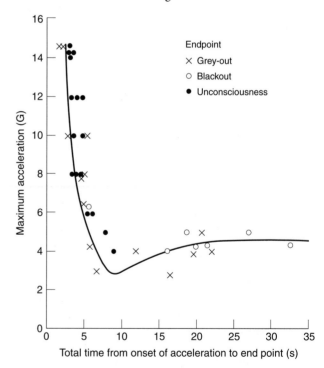

Figure 8.6 *Compilation of centrifugal data on tolerance to +G$_z$ in relaxed seated subjects (without the use of any protective device). The endpoints are blackout or unconsciousness, whichever occurred first. The results plotted in this figure were obtained with a variety of rates of onset of acceleration. The increase in tolerance beyond ten seconds is due to compensatory cardiovascular changes.*

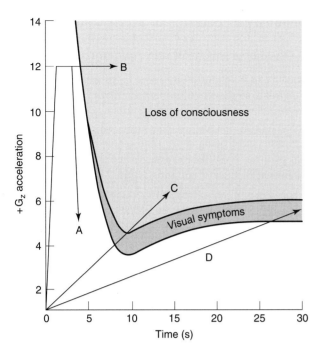

Figure 8.7   *Tolerance to +G$_z$ acceleration and effect of onset rate. A brief rapid-onset exposure to +12 G$_z$ (10 G/s) can be tolerated without visual loss (A), but this is if prolonged for more than four seconds (B), loss of consciousness may occur without visual warning. Even a moderately fast rate of onset (C) outpaces the cardiovascular reflexes, although loss of consciousness will then be preceded by symptoms of grey-out and blackout of retinal origin. A slow (0.1 G/s) rate of onset (D) allows compensatory reflexes to develop during the application of the stress, symptoms now appearing at a higher G level.*

Factors affecting tolerance to +G$_z$ acceleration

TEMPERATURE

Exposure to heat reduces tolerance to +G$_z$ acceleration. A 1 °C rise of deep body temperature reduces the level of acceleration at which blackout occurs by 30–40 per cent (Howard 1965). The reduction in tolerance is due to cutaneous vasodilation and the shift of blood to the periphery that occurs in response to a rise of body temperature. The lower peripheral resistance and reduced central blood volume then enhance the reduction of arterial pressure produced by the acceleration.

BLOOD GLUCOSE CONCENTRATION

Tolerance to positive acceleration is reduced by a falling blood glucose concentration. A 50 per cent reduction of the glucose concentration below the resting value reduces the blackout threshold by about 0.6 G (Howard 1965). However, once the fall in glucose concentration has produced a hypoglycaemic reaction, with feelings of cold and

hunger, sweating and tremor, the acceleration threshold is raised above the normal resting value by about 0.5 G. This increase in tolerance is due to arterial hypertension produced by the catecholamines secreted in the hypoglycaemic reaction.

ALCOHOL

Ingestion of alcohol reduces tolerance to +G$_z$ acceleration. A dose of 110 ml of whisky was found to reduce the grey-out threshold by 0.1–0.4 G (Howard 1965). It is likely that this effect is due, in part, to alcohol-induced vasodilation and also to depression of central responses. Dehydration associated with alcohol consumption may also have an effect on G-tolerance. Overall, however, the performance impairment from alcohol consumption is much more likely to be a contributory factor in aircraft accidents and incidents than any effect on G-tolerance.

HYPERVENTILATION AND HYPOXIA

Hyperventilation markedly reduces tolerance to +G$_z$ acceleration. Reduction of the arterial carbon dioxide tension to the order of 2.6–3.3 kPa (20–25 mmHg) by two minutes of vigorous hyperventilation reduces the grey-out threshold by about 0.6 G (Howard 1965). Moderate hyperventilation was found to precipitate unconsciousness in some individuals exposed to +3 G$_z$. The increase in cerebral vascular resistance produced by hypocapnia accentuates the reduction in blood flow through the brain caused by a fall in arterial pressure at head level under increased +G$_z$ acceleration. As would be expected, the breathing of five to ten per cent carbon dioxide in air causes a significant increase in G-tolerance, but the associated headache makes its use impractical.

Hypoxia also reduces tolerance to +G$_z$ acceleration. A reduction in blackout threshold of 0.5 G has been demonstrated when breathing air at the equivalent of 10 000 feet, which is usually regarded as an altitude below which supplementary oxygen is not required. Reduction of arterial oxygen tension to 9.3 kPa (70 mmHg) reduces the threshold for blackout by 0.6 G, and more severe degrees of hypoxia (inspired oxygen tension 7.3 kPa, 55 mmHg) have been shown to reduce the blackout threshold by 0.8–1.2 G (Howard 1965).

DISTENSION OF THE STOMACH

Distension of the stomach increases tolerance to +G$_z$ acceleration. The ingestion of 1.5 litres of water has been shown to increase the threshold for blackout by 0.6–1.3 G. This effect may be due in part to the distended stomach reducing the descent of the diaphragm and heart during the exposure, but it may also be related to a central reflex elevation of arterial blood pressure.

INTERCURRENT INFECTION

Intercurrent infection, such as an upper respiratory tract infection, reduces tolerance to $+G_z$ acceleration. This is particularly true if body temperature is raised, although it is possible that there is also some reduction in the effectiveness of central mechanisms that usually elevate arterial blood pressure under acceleration stress.

HYDRATION

The fast jet cockpit environment may lead to significant dehydration during a sortie, particularly if this involves performance of the physically demanding anti-G straining manoeuvre (see Chapter 9). The effects of heat on aviators are discussed more fully in Chapter 12. It is known that dehydration can reduce endurance to G exposure, e.g. during air combat, which is likely to be related directly to the reduction in circulating volume. It is important to emphasize to aircrew that deliberate dehydration, e.g. to avoid the potential problems of in-flight urination, may have a detrimental effect on G-tolerance.

GENDER AND BODY MORPHOLOGY

No difference has been demonstrated in G-tolerance between men and women (Wiegman *et al.* 1995). It might be expected that as average female stature is less than male stature, a smaller hydrostatic gradient between heart and head would result in improved tolerance to $+G_z$ acceleration. However, offset against this, the female resting blood pressure is often lower than that of males, and also the relationship between stature and head-to-heart distance may be different in both sexes. Indeed, it is recognized anecdotally that squat individuals tend to have better G-tolerance than tall people, but this not a reliable predictor, as a multitude of other factors, including age, blood pressure and diet, may also have influence.

TIME OFF FROM FLYING

It is recognized widely that time off from flying for more than a few days can result in reduced G-tolerance on return to the cockpit. This is sometimes termed 'layoff'. As a consequence, aircrew should be advised to take care when pulling G during their first few sorties after a break in flying. The physiological basis of this effect has been discussed above (see Baroreceptor reflex).

PRECEDING –G_z EXPOSURE

Exposure to $-G_z$ (footwards) acceleration reduces tolerance to a following $+G_z$ exposure. This is sometimes called the 'negative-to-positive G' or 'push–pull' effect. The physiological basis of this effect is explained below (see Exposure to $-G_z$ acceleration).

Pulmonary effects of +G_z acceleration

PULMONARY VENTILATION AND LUNG VOLUMES

Exposure to acceleration up to $+5\,G_z$ causes little respiratory embarrassment. Pulmonary ventilation may increase substantially in novice centrifuge subjects, but in trained subjects (and aircrew) it tends to fall, an increase in respiratory rate being more than offset by a decrease in tidal volume. This effect is exaggerated by inflation of the abdominal bladder of an anti-G suit. The total lung and vital capacities are unaffected by accelerations up to $+3\,G_z$, but exposure to $+5\,G_z$ reduces them by about 15 per cent. Exposure to $+G_z$ acceleration causes descent of the abdominal contents and diaphragm, thereby increasing the functional residual capacity (FRC). The FRC is increased by about 500 ml at $+3\,G_z$. The descent of the diaphragm produced by $+G_z$ acceleration is greatly reduced, or even reversed, by inflation of an anti-G suit (Glaister 1970).

REGIONAL LUNG VENTILATION

Exposure to $+G_z$ acceleration accentuates the regional differences in the distribution of ventilation that are present in the lungs of an upright individual at $+1\,G_z$. The increased weight of the lung magnifies the pressure gradient down the pleural cavity, which amounts to about $0.2\,cmH_2O$ per 1 cm of lung per G. Thus, at $+5\,G_z$, the pleural pressure at the base of the lung is $30\,cmH_2O$ greater than that at the apex. The larger gradient of pleural pressure induces greater differences in the distension of alveoli down the lung. Alveoli at the apices are more distended, while those at the bases are closer to their minimum volumes as compared with their sizes at $+1\,G_z$. These changes accentuate the differences in alveolar ventilation down the lung (ventilation per unit alveolar volume) (Figure 8.8). Thus, at $+3\,G_z$, the gradient of ventilation down the lung is three times that present at $+1\,G_z$.

Of greater relevance, however, is the cessation of ventilation of alveoli at the base of the lung caused by $+G_z$ acceleration. Independent of overall lung volume, relative alveolar volumes decrease down the lung to an extent such that alveoli towards the base attain their minimal volume and their associated airways close. The lung volume (on breathing out from total lung capacity) at which this closure can first be detected is termed the closing volume of the lung and increases linearly with acceleration (Figure 8.9). Closure of terminal airways in dependent lung tissue will, therefore, occur whenever the lung volume at which a subject breathes is less than the closing volume, and alveoli distal to the closed airways will contain their residual volume of trapped gas. Since inflation of the abdominal bladder of an anti-G suit raises the diaphragm and reduces the FRC, its use markedly increases the number of non-

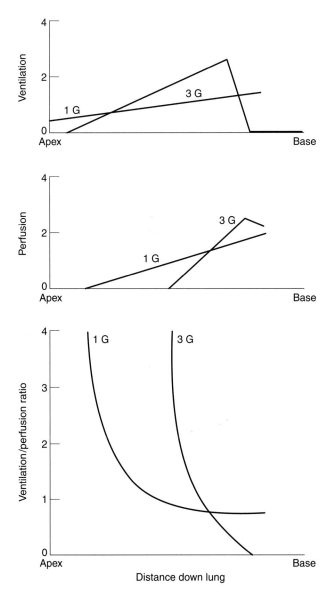

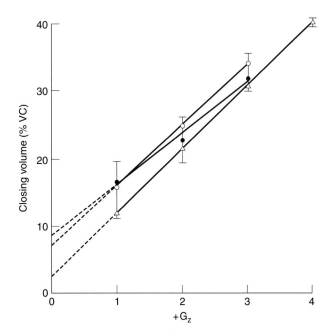

Figure 8.9 *Effect of +G$_z$ acceleration on the closing volume of the lung expressed as a percentage of the vital capacity (VC). Values are individual means and the overall range for three subjects (△, ●, ○). Closure was detected by analysing the expirate to detect a sudden increase in the concentration of a tracer gas, a bolus of which had been inhaled at residual volume during the preceding maximal inspiration.*

Figure 8.8 *Vertical distributions of alveolar ventilation, perfusion and ventilation/perfusion ratio in the upright lung of an individual exposed to +1 G$_z$ and +3 G$_z$ expressed relative to values that would exist if gas and blood were distributed uniformly. Exposure to +3 G$_z$ increases the gradient of ventilation per unit of alveolar volume down the lung three-fold over that which exists at +1 G$_z$. Blood flow to virtually all the upper half of the lung ceases at +3 G$_z$ and the gradient of flow per unit alveolar volume is tripled in the lower half. The volume of lung tissue that is ventilated but not perfused (that which has a ventilation/perfusion ratio of infinity) is increased markedly by exposure to +3 G$_z$ which also increases the spread of ventilation/perfusion ratios in the lower portion of the lung and produces a region of perfused but non-ventilated alveoli at the extreme base.*

ventilated alveoli in the lower part of the lung (Figure 8.10).

REGIONAL PULMONARY BLOOD FLOW

The distribution of blood flow through the lung is affected greatly by +G$_z$ acceleration, because the external pressure to which the vessels are exposed (i.e. alveolar gas pressure) is the same throughout the lung and is unaffected by acceleration and because the pressure in the pulmonary circulation is relatively low. The mean pulmonary artery and pulmonary venous pressures at the level of the junction of the middle and lower thirds of the lung are unaffected by +G$_z$ acceleration. Typical values for these pressures are 15 mmHg and zero, respectively. The vascular pressures above and below this level are determined by hydrostatic forces, so even at +1 G$_z$ the mean arterial pressure falls to zero 20 cm above the junction of the middle and lower thirds (just at the apex of the lung). At +4 G$_z$, the mean pulmonary artery pressure is zero only 5 cm above the junction of the middle and lower thirds, and as a consequence mean pulmonary artery pressure is zero throughout the upper half of the lung. Therefore, the proportion of the lung that is not perfused increases with increasing acceleration from the uppermost 1 or 2 cm at +1 G$_z$ to the whole

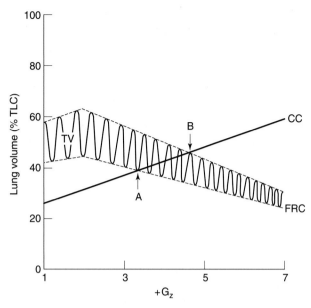

Figure 8.10 *Effect of +G$_z$ acceleration on functional residual capacity (FRC) and closing capacity (CC) expressed as a percentage of total lung capacity (TLC) for a subject wearing an anti-G suit that starts to inflate at +2 G$_z$. The combination of acceleration and anti-G suit inflation causes a reduction in FRC and tidal volume (TV). With increasing acceleration, terminal airways in the lung bases will start to close at end-expiration at point (A) but reopen in the ensuing inspiration until point (B), remaining closed thereafter. By increasing the FRC and TV, the performance of an anti-G straining manoeuvre or breathing under positive pressure will move points (A) and (B) to the right and thus increase the level of +G$_z$ at which acceleration atelectasis (absorption of alveolar gas trapped by airway closure) may develop.*

PULMONARY GAS EXCHANGE AND ARTERIAL OXYGEN SATURATION

As we have seen, exposure to +G$_z$ acceleration accentuates the increases in ventilation and blood flow with distance down the lung that occur under normal gravity. The mag-

nitude of the changes in ventilation and blood flow down the lung differ, so that +G$_z$ acceleration accentuates the ventilation–perfusion inequalities that are present in the normal erect lung (see Figure 8.8). In particular, with increasing +G$_z$ acceleration, there is a progressively larger volume of the upper lung that is ventilated but not perfused, which amounts to about one-half of the lung at +5 G$_z$. There is also a progressively larger volume of basal lung that is perfused but not ventilated, and so has a ventilation/perfusion ratio of zero. The ventilated but non-perfused region at the top of the lung simply adds to the respiratory dead space and does not, in practice, interfere with the oxygenation of the arterial blood. The considerable spread of ventilation/perfusion ratios present in that portion of the lung that is both ventilated and perfused causes only a small reduction of the oxygen tension of the arterial blood, since the blood flow is distributed preferentially to the better ventilated lower part of the lung. However, the perfused but non-ventilated alveoli in the lowermost part of the lung do significantly impair the oxygenation of the arterial blood. The oxygen tension of the gas trapped in the non-ventilated alveoli falls within a few seconds, by absorption of oxygen into the blood, to equal that of the mixed venous blood. The blood flowing through these alveoli thereafter constitutes a right-to-left shunt. The proportion of the cardiac output shunted in this manner increases with acceleration and at +5 G$_z$ may amount to 50 per cent (Glaister 1970). This right-to-left shunt reduces markedly the oxygen saturation and tension of the systemic arterial blood. Desaturation of the arterial blood becomes apparent at +3 G$_z$, and sustained exposure to +5 G$_z$ for one minute reduces the arterial oxyhaemoglobin saturation to about 85 per cent (mean arterial oxygen tension 6.9 kPa, 52 mmHg).

Breathing 100 per cent oxygen before exposure to +G$_z$ acceleration delays the onset of arterial desaturation, as the alveolar gas trapped in the non-ventilated alveoli has a very high tension and the oxygen content of the blood flowing through them will fall only to that of mixed venous blood after virtually all this alveolar gas has been absorbed. Inflation of an anti-G suit increases the fall of the oxygen saturation of the arterial blood produced by +G$_z$ acceleration, since elevation of the diaphragm and fall in FRC increases the number of alveoli that are perfused but not ventilated.

LUNG COLLAPSE

As discussed above, terminal airways serving alveoli at the base of the lung close on exposure to +G$_z$ acceleration, so that ventilation of their component alveoli ceases, although they continue to be well-perfused. The closed airways open again as soon as the exposure to acceleration ends and ventilation resumes because the alveoli have continued to contain some trapped gas. Since these non-ven-

of the upper half of the lung at +4 to +5 G$_z$. Above the level at which the pulmonary venous pressure is zero, the blood flow through the alveoli is determined by the difference between arterial and alveolar gas pressures. The progressive rise in the pulmonary artery pressure down the lung, and in pulmonary venous pressure below the junction of the middle and lower thirds, results in a corresponding increase in regional blood flow (see Figure 8.8). The rise in blood flow with distance down the lung increases with increasing acceleration. However, blood flow decreases in the most dependent part of the lung because the rise of interstitial pressure is transmitted to the alveolar gas when terminal airways close, thus increasing the local resistance to blood flow.

tilated alveoli are perfused, gaseous exchange continues between the gas trapped in them and the mixed venous blood flowing through their septa. This blood absorbs the trapped gas from the alveoli at a rate limited by the rate at which the least soluble gas, usually nitrogen, is removed. However, if little or no nitrogen is present when the acceleration is applied, as will be the case if 100 per cent oxygen has been breathed before the exposure, then the trapped gas will be absorbed very rapidly and many alveoli will be rendered gas-free. High surface-tension forces will then maintain the walls of the gas-free alveoli in contact, and the affected part of the lung will remain collapsed (atelectatic) after the acceleration exposure has ended. It then takes the relatively high pressure created in the collapsed lung by a deep inspiration or cough to separate the septal walls, reopen the alveoli and allow ventilation to resume.

Exposure to sustained acceleration above about +3 G$_z$ produces acceleration atelectasis when 100 per cent oxygen has been breathed before the exposure and an anti-G suit has been used during the exposure. The condition can arise without an anti-G suit, but the severity of lung collapse is then considerably less. There is a wide individual variation in susceptibility, both in the level and duration of acceleration required to produce atelectasis and in the magnitude of the effect. The symptoms, which usually are not apparent until after the exposure, or even after the flight in which the exposure occurred, consist of a dry cough, with or without substernal discomfort or pain, which is exacerbated by a deep inspiration. Chest radiographs reveal basal lung collapse with loss of the costophrenic and cardiophrenic angles and atelectatic shadowing at both lung bases. Radiographic signs of collapse can occur in the absence of symptoms. The symptoms and radiographic signs usually clear completely after several deep inspirations, which often provoke bouts of coughing. In the absence of deep breathing, however, basal collapse may persist for 24 hours or more. The vital capacity may be reduced by up to 60 per cent of the normal value, but the volume of lung collapsed is considerably less than this and the limitation of deep inspiration is largely reflex in origin. The lung collapse induced by several exposures to moderate levels of +G$_z$ acceleration while breathing 100 per cent oxygen produces a right-to-left shunt of the order of 20–25 per cent of the cardiac output, sufficient to reduce the arterial oxygen tension to 8 kPa (60 mmHg). The minimum concentration of nitrogen required in the gas breathed before exposure to acceleration in order to prevent significant acceleration atelectasis is approximately 40 per cent.

Any factor that alters the FRC of the lung during acceleration exposure will affect the magnitude of the induced right-to-left shunt (and hence arterial oxygen desaturation) and the development of acceleration atelectasis. Such factors include positive pressure breathing during acceleration and the anti-G straining manoeuvre (see Chapter 9). Pressure breathing causes a mechanical increase in the FRC

and so should improve arterial oxygen saturation and decrease atelectasis, although the degree of this increase may be reduced by the use of chest counter-pressure and the abdominal bladder of the anti-G suit. The anti-G straining manoeuvre includes an inspiratory gasp before the strain, so that lung volumes are likely to be greater than when relaxed. It may also be noted that obesity decreases the FRC, while smoking increases the closing capacity of the lung, and so these factors may also influence shunting and atelectasis during exposure to +G$_z$ acceleration.

EXPOSURE TO −G$_z$ ACCELERATION

Flight conditions that give rise to −G$_z$ (footwards) acceleration are outside loops and spins, simple inverted flight, recovery from such manoeuvres and 'unloading' of G to gain energy during air combat. Tolerance to −G$_z$ acceleration is much lower than that for +G$_z$ acceleration, and the symptoms produced by even −2 G$_z$ are unpleasant and alarming. Furthermore, low levels of −G$_z$ produce serious decrements of performance. Although military fast jet aircraft are often stressed to withstand up to −3 G$_z$, aircrew are not often exposed to high negative G due to the limited tactical use of such manoeuvres.

The physiological disturbances arise primarily in the cardiovascular system. The inertial forces increase the vascular pressures in the upper thorax, head and neck and reduce the pressure in the abdomen and lower limbs, so displacing blood towards the head.

Physical effects of −G$_z$ acceleration

The feeling of heaviness and the interference with movement in the limbs produced by exposure to −G$_z$ acceleration are similar to those experienced with +G$_z$ exposure. The unpleasant symptoms associated with −G$_z$ acceleration occur primarily in the head. Exposure to −1 G$_z$ produces a sense of fullness and pressure in the head; this becomes very disagreeable at −2 G$_z$ and develops to a severe throbbing headache, which may persist for some hours after the exposure. There is marked vascular congestion, and exposure for some seconds to −2.5 G$_z$ or more produces oedema of the eyelids and petechial haemorrhages in the skin of the face and neck. Congestion of the mucosal lining of the air passages may cause difficulty in breathing and epistaxis may occur. The eyes rapidly become uncomfortable, and at −2.5 to −3 G$_z$ they feel as if they are 'popping out of the head'. The conjunctivae are suffused, and descent of the lower eyelid and excessive lacrimation can cause reddening and blurring of the vision. Subconjunctival haemorrhages may also occur, although susceptibility to this is reduced by repeated exposures, presumably as the more fragile vessels are repaired. Exposure to acceleration of greater than −4 to −5 G_z for more than about six seconds can cause mental confusion and unconsciousness.

Cardiovascular effects of −G_z acceleration

The immediate hydrostatic effect of −G_z acceleration is to increase the vascular pressure in the regions above (anatomically) the heart and to decrease them below this level. The arterial pressure at head level is immediately increased by the additional pressure exerted by the column of blood between the aortic valves and the head. Thus, the mean arterial pressure at eye level increases immediately by 20–25 mmHg per G, so that it becomes 170 mmHg on exposure to −3 G_z. The venous pressure at head level takes several seconds to rise to a plateau level, as blood has to flow through the capillary bed to fill the capacity vessels before the venous pressure attains an equilibrium value. The venous pressure at eye level at −3 G_z rises to above 100 mmHg, the effective length of the venous column being from the level of the diaphragm to the head.

The rapid and large increase of arterial pressure in the neck stimulates the baroreceptors of the carotid sinus. The response to this stimulation is bradycardia and generalized arteriolar vasodilation. The intense stimulation of the carotid baroreceptors causes a large discharge of vagal efferent impulses, which, in turn, produce bradycardia and a variety of cardiac dysrhythmias, ranging from simple prolongation of the P–R interval to complete atrioventricular dissociation, with ectopic beats and asystole. Cardiac dysrhythmias almost invariably occur on exposure to acceleration more negative than −1 G_z. Periods of asystole of five to seven seconds are not uncommon at −2.5 G_z. The dysrhythmias greatly reduce cardiac output, such that mean arterial pressure at head level declines after the initial increase caused by the acceleration. The generalized arteriolar dilation also contributes to the reduction of arterial pressure.

The increase in pressure in cerebral vessels produced by −G_z acceleration exposure generally is balanced externally by similar increases in the pressure of the cerebrospinal fluid, such that there is no rise in transmural pressure and little risk of rupture of vessels within the skull. Although for the first two to three seconds there is a large increase of arterial pressure at brain level, the full development of venous engorgement and the consequent rise of venous pressure at this level, and the reduction of cardiac output produced by stimulation of the carotid sinus, combine to reduce progressively the arteriovenous pressure difference across the cerebral vascular bed. The cerebral blood flow, therefore, becomes increasingly compromised, and mental confusion and unconsciousness may result. However, the immediate cause of loss of consciousness on exposure to −G_z acceleration is generally a prolonged cardiac asystole or a slow ectopic rhythm.

Pulmonary effects of −G_z acceleration

Exposure to −G_z acceleration produces a headward displacement of the diaphragm and reduces the vital capacity and the functional residual capacity. It also reduces pulmonary ventilation. The regional distribution of ventilation and blood flow within the lung are changed by −G_z exposure in ways analogous to those produced by +G_z acceleration. In −G_z exposure, however, the apical region of the lung is better ventilated and perfused than the basal region. Since the level within the lung at which pulmonary vascular pressures are unchanged by acceleration is at the junction of the middle and basal thirds, most of the lung remains perfused under −G_z acceleration. Closure of terminal airways occurs, trapping gas in the apical regions, and the continuing flow of blood through unventilated alveoli constitutes a right-to-left shunt and arterial oxygen desaturation as with +G_z acceleration. Acceleration atelectasis produced by −G_z exposure (when breathing 100 per cent oxygen) occurs at the apices of the lungs. As the functional residual capacity is reduced by −G_z exposure, atelectasis occurs more readily than with +G_z acceleration and without the intervention of an inflated anti-G suit.

Tolerance to −G_z acceleration

−G_z acceleration is not tolerated well. The limit is set by discomfort in the head, oedema of the soft tissues of the face, petechial and subconjunctival haemorrhages and loss of consciousness. The maximum acceleration that can be tolerated is around −5 G_z for five seconds. A level of −3 G_z can be tolerated by most individuals in the seated posture for 10–15 seconds, while −2 G_z is tolerated for several minutes. A degree of adaptation may develop with repeated exposures, and experienced aerobatic display competitors may tolerate brief exposure to up to −9 G_z without immediate sequelae.

Exposure to −G_z acceleration also reduces tolerance to a following +G_z exposure, since cardiovascular reflexes and the distribution of blood volume have been reset disadvantageously. Figure 8.11, recorded in a centrifuge fitted with a three-axis gondola control, illustrates this situation. Following a period at rest, exposure to −1.8 G_z caused a pronounced bradycardia and a gradual fall in blood pressure at heart level. An immediate reversal in acceleration vector to +2.4 G_z then caused a profound fall in blood pressure, and vision was lost momentarily before tachycardia led to a recovery in blood pressure. A control exposure to +2.4 G_z produced a much smaller fall in blood pressure without visual symptoms.

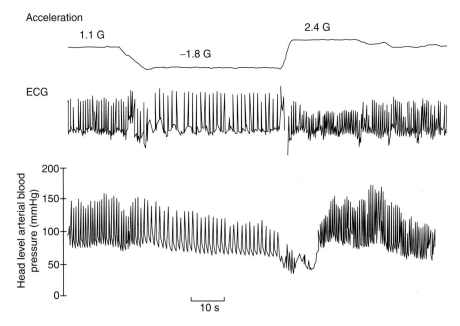

Figure 8.11 *Recording of electrocardiogram and heart-level arterial blood pressure (Portapres monitor with the height-correction unit referenced to heart level) from a subject in a human centrifuge exposed to −1.8 G_z for 30 seconds followed immediately by a +2.4 G_z exposure.*

EXPOSURE TO G_x ACCELERATION

Long-duration acceleration acting at right-angles to the long axis of the body occurs rarely in present-day conventional flight. Such acceleration is usually confined to catapult launch, rocket and jet-assisted takeoff and carrier landings, although forces in excess of −2 G_x may build up during flat spins. The forces in these manoeuvres are, however, small relative to human tolerance and do not give rise to specific problems.

In early space flights, the acceleration needed to achieve the velocities required for orbit or escape from Earth's gravitational field were such that they could be tolerated by the occupants of space vehicles only if the inertial forces were applied transversely across the long axis of the body. For current manned space vehicles such as the Space Shuttle, these accelerations act for several minutes and involve peaks of only around +3 G_x. As vision of the external world and instruments and the operation of controls are much easier when the individual lies supine rather than prone, prolonged transverse acceleration is almost always experienced with the body accelerated towards its anterior (ventral) surface (+G_x) and seldom with the body accelerated towards its posterior (dorsal) surface (−G_x). Accordingly, the effects of forwards acceleration are considered here in greater detail. Since with transverse accelerations the inertial forces act at right-angles to the long axis of the body, gross effects in the systemic circulation do not occur. The major physiological disturbances produced by transverse acceleration occur in the respiratory system, and these limit tolerance to this form of acceleration stress.

Physical effects of +G_x acceleration

Increase in the weight of the limbs becomes apparent at +2 G_x, with difficulty in breathing usually noted at +3 G_x. At and above +5 G_x, there is a consistent ache in the chest, which is generally most severe at the lower third of the sternum or epigastrium and which frequently radiates along the costal margins. The pain is aggravated by inspiration, which becomes progressively more difficult and shallow with increasing acceleration until around +9 to +12 G_x, at which point there is severe difficulty in breathing. At about +15 G_x, inspiration is extremely difficult and there is a severe vice-like pain in the chest. The limbs cannot be lifted at +8 G_x, although with the forearms supported fine controlled movements of the wrist and fingers are possible up to and above +15 G_x. Lifting the head is impossible at +7 to +9 G_x, or less when heavy headgear is worn. Petechial haemorrhages may occur in the unsupported regions of the posterior surface of the body.

Cardiovascular effects of +G_x acceleration

Since the hydrostatic pressure gradient produced by +G_x acceleration is much smaller than that produced by +G_z acceleration, there are less pronounced effects on the cardiovascular system. The pressure in the right atrium is raised by +G_x acceleration to about 20 mmHg at +5 G_x. This increase is due to blood displaced to the thorax from the lower limbs and, to some extent, the abdomen when the legs are elevated. There is a similar rise in venous pressure throughout the body at the horizontal level of the heart.

Visual disturbances do not occur when the body is truly supine, and arterial pressure in the brain usually is increased by exposure to $+G_x$ acceleration. However, it is unusual for the long axis of the body to be completely horizontal in situations in which exposure to $+G_x$ occurs. The respiratory discomfort produced by $+G_x$ is minimized when the trunk is inclined slightly (15–25 degrees) towards the acceleration vector, and the head is frequently flexed on the trunk to improve all-round vision. In these circumstances, a small but important component of $+G_z$ is created that may result in loss of vision and unconsciousness due to the vertical distance (parallel to the acceleration vector) between the heart and the head. With trunk and head elevated to 25 degrees, blackout occurs at about $+10\,G_x$ and consciousness is lost at $+14$ to $+16\,G_x$. When the angle of the back to the horizontal is only ten degrees, blackout does not occur until $+16\,G_x$, and consciousness is not lost until the acceleration exceeds $+20\,G_x$. At $+5\,G_x$ with trunk and head elevated, the increase in right atrial pressure produces a small rise in cardiac output of about 20 per cent. This in turn causes a rise of mean aortic pressure of about 20–30 mmHg over that at $+1\,G_x$.

Heart rate is usually reduced by $+G_x$ acceleration when the body is fully supine. Slight flexion of the trunk, with the associated introduction of a small $+G_z$ component, results in an increase in heart rate. Cardiac dysrhythmias, consisting mainly of premature atrial and ventricular contractions, are commonly seen on exposure to $+G_x$ acceleration above $+6$ to $+8\,G_x$. These disturbances of rhythm, which disappear on cessation of the exposure, are probably due to distension of the right atrium.

Pulmonary effects of $+G_x$ acceleration

The increase in weight of the abdominal contents under increased $+G_x$ acceleration displaces the diaphragm towards the chest. Inspiratory capacity becomes restricted and expiratory reserve volume is reduced. At $+5\,G_x$, the vital capacity is reduced by 75 per cent and the expiratory reserve volume falls to zero, so that the functional residual capacity becomes equal to the lung's residual volume. The residual volume is unaffected by $+G_x$ acceleration. The vital capacity becomes progressively smaller with increasing acceleration until, at about $+12\,G_x$, it equals the reduced tidal volume. However, the falling tidal volume is more than offset by an increase in the respiratory frequency, so that the pulmonary ventilation is actually increased. As described above, the magnitude of the disturbances to breathing and the chest discomfort can be reduced by raising the back to about 25 degrees to the horizontal. This posture markedly reduces the displacement of the abdominal contents towards the thoracic cavity. Respiratory discomfort and difficulty with breathing are also reduced by flexion of the hips

and knees to 90 degrees, with the long axis of the thighs parallel to the acceleration vector.

The distribution of inspired gas within the lung in the supine posture is controlled by the same factors as in the upright lung. Exposure to $+G_x$ progressively reduces the ventilation of the alveoli at the back of the lungs, while ventilation of the front of the lung remains fairly uniform. At $+5\,G_x$, the alveoli in the posterior third of the lungs are unventilated.

The horizontal level in the supine lung at which the pulmonary arterial and venous pressures are unaffected by transverse accelerations lies approximately one-quarter of the distance from the anterior to the posterior surface of the lung, about 5 cm deep to its anterior surface. The pulmonary artery pressure at the anterior surface of the lung is of the order of 11 mmHg (15 cm H_2O) at $+1\,G_x$ and will be reduced to zero at this point by $+4\,G_x$. With increased $+G_x$ acceleration, the regional blood flow increases progressively from the front towards the back of the lung. The blood flow falls off somewhat in the most posterior part of the lung due to the rise in interstitial pressure, which increases vascular resistance.

The absence of perfusion in the very anterior part of the lung, and the increased spread of ventilation/perfusion ratios produced by $+3$ to $+4\,G_x$ exposure produce only minor disturbances of the overall gas exchange between inspired gas and blood. The occurrence of a large number of unventilated but perfused alveoli in the posterior part of the lung forms a right-to-left shunt, which has a profound effect on overall gas exchange and produces desaturation of the oxyhaemoglobin of the systemic arterial blood. Exposure to $+6\,G_x$ when breathing air reduces the arterial saturation to 80–87 per cent, while exposure to $+8\,G_x$ reduces it to 72–82 per cent. Desaturation also occurs when 100 per cent oxygen is breathed before and during an exposure to $+G_x$ acceleration, although the fall of saturation is delayed and its extent somewhat reduced.

Acceleration atelectasis of the posterior part of the lung occurs during exposure to $+G_x$ acceleration when 100 per cent oxygen is breathed before and during the exposure. The mechanism of this collapse is the same as that responsible for the lung collapse that occurs on exposure to $+G_z$ acceleration of subjects breathing 100 per cent oxygen. Closure of terminal airways occurs at the posterior (most dependent) part of the lung during $+G_x$ exposure, with a reduction in FRC being due to the increased weight of the abdominal contents rather than to the inflation of an anti-G suit (which occurs during $+G_z$ exposure). The symptoms of lung collapse due to $+G_x$ exposure are similar to those produced by $+G_z$ acceleration. Breathing 100 per cent oxygen before and during exposure to $+6\,G_x$ for two to three minutes produces a 40 per cent reduction of the vital capacity, and the associated right-to-left shunt of blood through the collapsed lung reduces the saturation of the oxyhaemoglobin of the arterial blood to about 75 per cent.

Tolerance to +G$_x$ acceleration

Tolerance to $+G_x$ acceleration is set primarily by the increased difficulty of breathing produced by the increased weight of the anterior chest wall and abdominal contents, the latter acting on the diaphragm. The maximum voluntary tolerance for periods of exposure between 5 and 150 seconds is of the order of $+14$ to $+15\,G_x$, although above $+12\,G_x$ tolerance depends much on motivation and training. The chest pain and difficulty in breathing are reduced by elevating the trunk, but tolerance is then lowered by the occurrence of visual symptoms. Breathing under a positive pressure of 0.7 kPa/G (pressure of 4.9–5.6 kPa at $+7$ to $+8\,G_x$) balances the extra weight of the anterior chest wall and restores functional residual capacity, vital capacity and tidal volume to near-normal $+1\,G_z$ levels. Additionally, the rise in intrathoracic pressure increases arterial blood pressure to a comparable degree and enhances G-tolerance. Under these conditions, an acceleration of $+10\,G_x$ has been tolerated for 30 seconds with little decrement of vision or psychomotor performance. Even without positive pressure breathing, an acceleration of $+8\,G_x$ can be tolerated for at least six minutes with the trunk elevated by ten degrees.

Tolerance to −G$_x$ acceleration

Tolerance to $-G_x$ acceleration is influenced considerably by the support afforded to the front of the body. In a seated attitude, support comes from the restraint harness, whereas in the fully prone position, the body is usually supported by a specially contoured couch. Exposure to backwards acceleration in the seated position, using a conventional restraint harness, results in the head being forced on to the chest and the upper and lower limbs being extended forward at right-angles to the trunk. With $-G_x$ acceleration induced in a flat spin, this effect makes operation of the ejection seat handle difficult and reduces the effectiveness of the restraint harness's automatic shoulder retraction, so compromising ejection safety. The inertial force displaces blood from the trunk into the head and the limbs. The vascular pressures increase progressively towards the free ends of the limbs. The rise in pressure and distension of the vessels in the head and distal portion of the limbs causes pain (especially in the lower limbs) and petechial haemorrhages. Tolerance to sustained backwards acceleration with a conventional restraint harness is of the order of ten seconds at $-5\,G_x$ and five minutes at $-3\,G_x$. When the head and limbs are restrained so that the seated posture is maintained, the tolerance is increased to the order of 30 seconds at $-8\,G_x$.

When the whole body is supported in the prone position by a contoured couch, exposure to backwards acceleration

causes difficulty in breathing, nasal drip, salivation, sagging of the lower eyelid and petechial haemorrhages in the more dependent parts of the body.

As with $+G_x$ acceleration, the major physiological disturbances occur in the respiratory system. The reduction of vital capacity and the functional residual capacity produced by $-G_x$ acceleration is, however, markedly less than that produced by $+G_x$ acceleration, since in the former the inertial forces pull the abdominal contents and diaphragm away from the thoracic cavity. Much depends on the extent to which the weight of the thorax is supported on the anterior chest wall. If support is restricted to the shoulders and hips, respiration is facilitated and the FRC is greater than at a corresponding level of $+G_x$ acceleration. The proportion of dependent (anterior) lung alveoli that are not ventilated during $-G_x$ exposure is correspondingly less than at a comparable level of $+G_x$. This results in an arterial oxyhaemoglobin saturation of 94 per cent on exposure to $-6\,G_x$ compared with 80 per cent at $+6\,G_x$.

The head may be extended on the trunk, or the head and the chest may be raised from the horizontal position in order to improve forwards vision. Exposure to $-G_x$ acceleration (with a small $+G_z$ component) then reduces the vascular pressures in the eye and brain. However, even with the chest and head elevated to an angle of 25 degrees from the horizontal, which is a comfortable posture, vision is unimpaired on exposure to $-12\,G_x$. Tolerance to sustained $-G_x$ acceleration by a person supported by a couch in the prone or semi-prone position is in excess of five minutes at $-5\,G_x$ and two minutes at $-10\,G_x$.

EXPOSURE TO G$_y$ ACCELERATION

With the exception of some experimental aircraft concepts, significant G_y (lateral) acceleration does not occur under normal fast jet flight conditions. Forces around $\pm 2\,G_y$ may be generated by some agile aircraft during roll manoeuvres at high angles of attack. Such levels of acceleration in general have little effect, but the effect on head mobility and the risk of neck injury (see Chapter 9) should be considered, as should the potential for spatial disorientation (see Chapter 28). Greater levels of lateral acceleration (± 3 to $\pm 4\,G_y$) have profound effects on pulmonary function, as the weight of the mediastinal contents acts on the dependent (left or right) lung to induce airway closure with consequent right-to-left shunting and susceptibility to atelectasis. Indeed, the influence of the increased mediastinal weight at ± 3 to $\pm 4\,G_y$ is such that the left and right lungs inflate and deflate sequentially.

REFERENCES

Cheung B, Bateman WA. G-transition effects and their implications. *Aviation Space and Environmental Medicine* 2001; **72**: 758–62.

Cirovic S, Frazer W. A mathematical model of the eye circulation subjected to G_z acceleration (abstract). *Aviation, Space, and Environmental Medicine* 2003; **74**: 447–8.

Cochran LB, Gard PW, Norswirthy ME. Variations in human G tolerance to positive acceleration. Report no. USN/SAM/NASA/NM-001-059.020.10. Pensacola, FL: US Navy, 1954.

Convertino VA. High sustained $+G_z$ acceleration: physiological adaptation to high-G tolerance. *Journal of Gravitational Physiology* 1998; **5**: P51–4.

Convertino VA. Effects of high sustained $+G_z$ acceleration on adaptation of autonomic functions associated with blood pressure regulation (abstract). *Aviation, Space, and Environmental Medicine* 1999; **70**: 368.

Convertino VA, Tripp LD, Ludwig DA. Female exposure to high G: chronic adaptations of cardiovascular functions. *Aviation, Space, and Environmental Medicine* 1998; **69**: 875–82.

Duane TD. Observations on the fundus oculi during blackout. *Archives of Ophthalmology* 1954; **51**: 343–55.

Gell CF. Table of equivalents for acceleration terminology. *Aerospace Medicine* 1961; **32**: 1109–11.

Glaister DH. *The Effects of Gravity and Acceleration on the Lung.* London: NATO Advisory Group for Aerospace Research and Development, 1970.

Head H. The sense and stability of balance in the air. In: *Medical Research Council Report into the Medical Problems of Flying.* London: HM Stationery Office, 1920; pp. 214–56.

Howard P. The physiology of positive acceleration. In: Gillies JA (ed.). *A Textbook of Aviation Physiology.* Oxford: Pergamon Press, 1965; pp. 551–687.

Lyons T, Davenport C, Copley GB, *et al.* Preventing G-induced loss of consciousness: 20 years of operational experience. *Aviation, Space, and Environmental Medicine* 2004; **75**: 150–53.

Lyons T, Kraft N, Grayson K, *et al.* Analysis of mission and aircraft factors in G-induced loss of consciousness in the USAF: 1982–2002 (abstract). *Aviation Space and Environmental Medicine* 2004; **75 (section II)**: B56.

Mills FJ. The endocrinology of stress. *Aviation, Space, and Environmental Medicine* 1985; **56**: 642–50.

Newman DG, White SW, Callister R. Evidence of baroreflex adaptation to repetitive $+G_z$ in fighter pilots. *Aviation, Space, and Environmental Medicine* 1998; **69**: 446–51.

Newman DG, White SW, Callister R. The effect of baroreflex adaptation on the dynamic cardiovascular response to head-up tilt. *Aviation, Space, and Environmental Medicine* 2000; **71**: 255–9.

Schlegel TT, Wood SJ, Brown TE, *et al.* Effect of 30-min $+3G_z$ centrifugation on vestibular and autonomic cardiovascular function. *Aviation, Space, and Environmental Medicine* 2003; **74**: 717–24.

Whinnery JE, Burton RR, Boll PA, Eddy DR. Characterisation of the resulting incapacitation following unexpected $+G_z$-induced loss of consciousness. *Aviation, Space, and Environmental Medicine* 1987; **58**: 631–6.

Wiegman JF, Burton RR, Forster EM. The role of anaerobic power in human tolerance to simulated air combat maneuvers. *Aviation, Space, and Environmental Medicine* 1995; **66**: 938–42.

FURTHER READING

AGARD/NATO. Current concepts on G protection research and development. AGARD lecture series no. 202 Neuilly-sur-Seine: AGARD/NATO, 1995.

Burton RR, Whinnery JE. Biodynamics: sustained acceleration. In: DeHart RL, Davis JR (eds). *Fundamentals of Aerospace Medicine.* Philadelphia, PA: Lippincott Williams & Wilkins, 2002; pp. 122–53.

9

Protection against long-duration acceleration

NICHOLAS D.C. GREEN

INTRODUCTION

In civilian aerobatic aircraft and military fast jets, the object of G-protection is to minimize the fall in head-level blood pressure that would otherwise occur on exposure to increased $+G_z$ acceleration. Protection against long-duration acceleration can be divided into two areas: voluntary actions taken by the aircrew to enhance G-tolerance, and G-protective systems provided with the aircraft. Of the latter, the most widely used is the anti-G suit, which has been in regular use since the 1950s; more recently, with the advent of agile fast jet aircraft, advanced anti-G-protective systems have been introduced.

VOLUNTARY MANOEUVRES

History

Symptoms of visual disturbance and, rarely, loss of consciousness were experienced by aircrew as early as 1918 (Head 1920). Although these observations initially were regarded as a curiosity, the onset of the Second World War and the requirement for tactical superiority in air combat led to intensive efforts by both sides to improve aircrew G-tolerance. In an attempt to minimize the effects of acceleration, a number of voluntary manoeuvres were performed; some of these survive, in an altered form, to the present day. Hunching forward in the cockpit was found to improve G-

tolerance by as much as 1 G, because the heart-to-brain distance was reduced. When used in combination with elevation of the legs, by means of an accessory rudder bar to reduce venous pooling, the Germans claimed that up to 2 G improvement in tolerance could be gained. However, hunching is not useful in practice, as the harness would provide inadequate restraint in this position, and vision from the cockpit would be limited severely. Shouting and generalized muscle-tensing were successful, and at least the latter remains in use in a modified form today.

Muscle-tensing

Experiments conducted in aircraft during the Second World War demonstrated that generalized sustained contraction of skeletal muscles could increase G-tolerance by 2 G or more. The beneficial action of this manoeuvre is due to a combination of several factors:

- Increased tissue pressure applies mechanical pressure to arteries and arterioles, thus causing a reduction in vessel diameter. The associated rise in peripheral resistance leads to an increase in arterial blood pressure, because blood pressure is equal to the product of cardiac output and total peripheral resistance.
- Increased tissue pressure applies mechanical pressure to veins, limiting venous pooling and possibly causing a shift of blood to the thorax. In this way, venous return is preserved.

- Increased intra-abdominal pressure helps to prevent descent of the diaphragm under increased +G acceleration, which would otherwise increase the heart-to-head distance and so reduce head-level blood pressure.
- There is a slowly developing reflex-induced rise in blood pressure.

Valsalva manoeuvre

The Valsalva manoeuvre, or forcible exhalation against a closed glottis, improves G-tolerance in a similar manner to shouting, as described above. Both intrathoracic and intra-abdominal pressures are increased, and the pressure increase is transmitted directly to the heart and great vessels, raising systemic arterial blood pressure. Under increased +G_z acceleration, this manoeuvre helps maintain cerebral perfusion by minimizing the reduction in head-level blood pressure. However, the protective effect of this manoeuvre is short-lived. When the manoeuvre is started, blood pressure is elevated, but after only a few cardiac cycles, pulse and systolic arterial pressures begin to drop, often to lower than the resting value. This is because the elevated intrathoracic pressure leads to a reduction in venous return from the periphery and, hence, a decrease in cardiac filling and stroke volume. Therefore, if a Valsalva manoeuvre is prolonged for more than three to four seconds under increased +G_z acceleration, G-tolerance will be reduced.

Anti-G straining manoeuvre

The anti-G straining manoeuvre (AGSM) is now accepted widely as a means of combining the beneficial effects of the techniques described above and circumventing some of their shortcomings. It is a combination of muscle-tensing and the Valsalva manoeuvre performed rhythmically every three to four seconds. To gain maximum protection from the manoeuvre, muscle-tensing should be sustained throughout the acceleration exposure and not relaxed during breathing. Exhalation and subsequent inhalation should be performed as rapidly as possible, as blood pressure falls precipitously during this phase. Furthermore, there is some evidence to suggest that the negative intrathoracic pressure generated during brisk inhalation may augment venous return and so improve cardiac output.

This manoeuvre forms the mainstay of G-protection for civilian aerobatic pilots and is employed in combination with anti-G trousers by the great majority of military fast jet aircrew. It subsumes earlier straining manoeuvres such

as the L1 (similar, but with abdominal muscle-tensing only) and the M1 (in which air is exhaled through a partially closed glottis, in combination with abdominal muscle-tensing). In order to encourage rapid inhalation and expiration during the manoeuvre, the AGSM has occasionally been termed the 'hook manoeuvre' in the USA, as a description of the sound that is made if the manoeuvre is being performed correctly.

The AGSM can provide more than 4 G improvement in G-tolerance if it is performed correctly. When used in combination with standard anti-G trousers, it should enable most aircrew to tolerate +9 G_z for at least ten seconds. When performing the manoeuvre under increased +G_z acceleration, it should be emphasized that head-level arterial blood pressure is not normal; on the contrary, it is usually of just sufficient magnitude to provide adequate cerebral perfusion, which, at very high accelerations, may be as low as 30 mmHg systolic and 0 mmHg diastolic.

The AGSM has the advantage of being a simple procedure that can be used in any aircraft without the installation of special equipment and can be combined with other methods of enhancing G-tolerance (such as anti-G trousers) with additive effect. However, the manoeuvre is physically exhausting and, furthermore, distracts from the primary task of flying the aircraft and engaging in air combat. A further disadvantage of the AGSM is that distraction by the flying task may result in an inadequate strain. Under such circumstances, it is possible that G-induced loss of consciousness (G-LOC) may occur; this has been demonstrated in video evidence from aircraft mishaps in the US Air Force (USAF). Speech is difficult, if not almost impossible, while performing AGSM at high +G_z levels, and so the manoeuvre may have a profound effect on communication.

Although the AGSM is used widely, other straining manoeuvres do exist. In China, the Qigong manoeuvre has been shown to provide similar improvements in G-tolerance to the AGSM, but with less fatigue (Zhang et al. 1991). In Eastern Europe and Russia, a device called the statergometer has been used as an aid to training, on which specific exercises can be performed to improve the effectiveness of straining.

Avoidance of additive stresses

The manoeuvres described above can offer a very effective improvement in aircrew G-tolerance if performed correctly. However, other factors, described in detail in the last chapter, may coalesce to reduce G-tolerance, and so it is important that aircrew are taught to avoid these additive stresses in order to maintain their normal acceleration tolerance.

G-PROTECTIVE SYSTEMS

History

ABDOMINAL BELTS

The first attempts to produce a G-protective garment came with the development of abdominal belts in the 1930s and 1940s. It was hypothesized that use of the belt would prevent blood pooling in the abdomen under increased +G_z acceleration. Belts of various types were produced, including inelastic, elastic, water-filled and air-filled. Work was discontinued, as the G-protection afforded by these garments was poor in comparison to that of a garment that included coverage of the lower limbs.

ARTERIAL OCCLUSION

At around the same time, arterial occlusion suits were investigated, in which the flow of blood into all four limbs was prevented under increased +G_z acceleration. Although the suit gave excellent protection, the major limiting factor was ischaemic pain, which developed when acceleration was sustained over long periods. An additional disadvantage was that although arterial occlusion is effective in preventing pooling of blood in the limbs during acceleration, it has no effect on the volume of blood already present in the peripheral vessels. This method of protection was abandoned in favour of the anti-G suit.

WATER IMMERSION

The principle of a rigid suit filled with water had been suggested as a method of G-protection by the Germans in 1934. Blackout threshold could be raised by 2 G when the water level was as high as the lower ribs. The pressure exerted on the surface of the body by the water is proportional to the height of the column multiplied by the applied acceleration. Since the entire cardiovascular system is subjected to similar forces distributed in the same way, the two opposing pressures cancel out and the vascular transmural pressures remain unchanged. The tendency for blood to pool in the lower parts of the body and for blood pressure at head level to fall during applied acceleration should be prevented by total water immersion, and excellent protection has been demonstrated. However, breathing is difficult unless some method of pressure breathing is employed; furthermore, water immersion cannot protect the lungs, so ventilation perfusion inequalities still develop. At very high G levels, there is a risk of lung damage. Considering these limitations, and the cumbersome equipment required, the method has been considered impractical for aircraft application. In centrifuge experiments, however, accelerations of up to +35 G_z have been sustained for five seconds without visual symptoms developing.

Indeed, the starting point for the development of the present day pneumatic anti-G suit was the water-filled suit designed by Franks in Canada and used in the early years of the Second World War. This early form of anti-G suit consisted of a pair of trousers made of inelastic fabric, which was filled with water before flight and which provided balanced external pressure during exposure to +G_z acceleration. This suit gave excellent protection, providing blackout thresholds of +6.2 G_z and +7.7 G_z in air tests (Brook 1990). However, it had many disadvantages: not only was it bulky and cumbersome, but the weight of water limited movement. Complaints were made of loss of 'feel' because of the tendency of the body to 'float' in the water. Worst of all, there was a strong diuresis on emptying the suit. The final demise of the water-filled anti-G suit came when it was demonstrated that the protection given by the suit when inflated with air to a pressure of 6.9 kPa (1 lb/in^2) per G was equal to or greater than that of the same suit filled with water. The lightness and convenience of an anti-G suit inflated with air represented a considerable advantage over the cumbersome water-filled suit, and efforts were concentrated towards the development of the pneumatically inflated suit in its present form.

More recently, the concept of a fluid-filled suit has been resurrected with a design that uses 'fluid muscles' in the form of columns of fluid integrated into a tight-fitting garment. Under increased +G_z acceleration, an increase in hydrostatic pressure in the columns causes tensioning of the garment and, hence, mechanical counter-pressure of the limbs. This form of suit appears to offer a similar level of G-protection to that of conventional pneumatic designs, although there remains some debate about its efficacy at high G levels (Eiken et al. 2002).

PNEUMATIC SUITS

The first true operational pneumatic anti-G suit was Professor Cotton's pneumatic flying suit. This three-bladder graded pressure suit, developed in Australia in 1940, had limited use by aircrew in the Pacific Campaign during the Second World War. Graded pressure suits, in which the pressure was highest in the calves and reduced proximally, were developed by Clark, Baldes and Wood in the USA, and the same team investigated arterial occlusion suits and capstan suits. Capstan suits were designed to be less bulky and offer less thermal stress than standard suits and worked by tensioning the fabric over the limbs by inflation of a separate inflatable tube.

Anti-G suits

Ultimately, the standard five-bladder anti-G suit in service today arose as a result of the requirement for better mobility and comfort in the garment (Figure 9.1). The garment is trouser-like, cut away at the crotch and knees to permit greater mobility and to reduce heat load. It consists of an outer restraining layer made of a non-stretch material containing five interconnecting non-circumferential bladders. The bladders and their outer restraining coverings fit over the abdomen and wrap around the thighs and calves of the wearer; the girth of the outer restraining layer may be adjusted by means of lacing cords. The suit inflates to a uniform pressure throughout, through a flexible hose connected to the aircraft anti-G system. The maximum improvement in G-tolerance that has been claimed for a suit of this type is around 2 G, but in practical use, when laced to a comfortable tension, the improvement is more usually in the region of 1 to 1.5 G.

The anti-G suit increases tolerance to $+G_z$ acceleration in the following manner:

- Mechanical tissue compression maintains peripheral vascular resistance and reduces venous pooling in the lower limbs, in a similar manner to skeletal muscle-tensing. There may also be a headward shift of blood, returning blood to the thorax, such that cardiac output is maintained.
- The abdominal bladder of the suit supports the abdominal wall and thereby reduces the amount by which the diaphragm is displaced downwards. The anti-G suit tends, therefore, to prevent the increase in the vertical distance between the heart and brain that is normally caused by increased $+G_z$ acceleration.

The anti-G suit acts to reduce the magnitude of both the initial and the delayed effects of increased $+G_z$ acceleration on the cardiovascular system. The inflation of the suit at the beginning of an exposure produces an immediate increase in peripheral vascular resistance in the lower limbs and prevents the descent of the diaphragm. The anti-G suit also reduces the magnitude of the peripheral pooling of blood that occurs later in the exposure. To ensure that the initial mechanisms are fully effective, the inflation of the anti-G suit must be rapid – at most, within two to three seconds of the peak of the applied acceleration (Burton 1988).

Anti-G valve

The anti-G valve controls the flow of gas, usually air from the engine compressor, into the anti-G suit. The valve, which may be mechanical or electronic, senses the prevailing $+G_z$ acceleration and supplies the required pressure accordingly. At present, mechanical valves are more common. They typically consist of an orifice, the opening of which is controlled by a mass, supported by a spring and a diaphragm, which is exposed to the pressure in the suit. The increase in the weight of the control mass that occurs on exposure to acceleration opens the orifice and allows air to flow into the suit until the pressure in the latter, acting on the diaphragm of the valve, balances the increase in force exerted by the control mass. As the applied acceleration is decreased, the suit pressure opens the orifice and the suit deflates.

With the introduction of agile aircraft with very rapid rates of onset of G, valves have been introduced that provide higher gas flows in order to minimize inflation delays. Many of these are mechanical, but electronic anti-G valves, which anticipate gas-flow requirements by sensing both instantaneous G and the rate of onset of G, are planned to enter service in the near future. Pre-inflation of the anti-G suit to 1 kPa will hasten inflation, as the volume of gas subsequently needed to achieve maximum pressure is reduced, but many people find the pre-inflated anti-G suit cumbersome and uncomfortable in the cockpit.

Most anti-G valves supply a pressure that increases linearly with acceleration, of approximately 8.6 kPa (1.25 lb/in^2) per G, which is the UK schedule. The USA uses a slightly different schedule of 10.3 kPa (1.5 lb/in^2) per

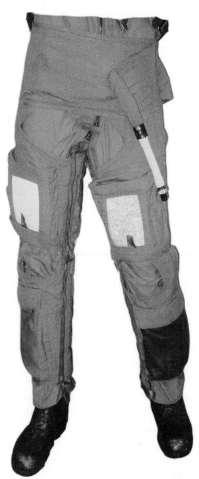

Figure 9.1 *Standard Royal Air Force externally worn anti-G suit Mark 10. The bladders over the abdomen, thighs and calves are inflated and deflated through the flexible hose attached to the abdominal bladder.*

G. Inflation pressure schedules above this tend to cause discomfort. In contrast, lower pressure schedules may become acceptable with the use of extended coverage anti-G suits (see below). Typically, the anti-G valve is designed so that garment inflation does not start until the acceleration exceeds +2 G_z in order to avoid unnecessary and distracting anti-G trouser inflation under conditions of buffet and during gentle turns.

HIGH-G TRAINING

The requirement for centrifuge-based high-G training was identified after the G-LOC surveys conducted during the 1980s. The first high-G training course was held by the USAF in 1983. Many countries around the world now conduct centrifuge training programmes for their aircrew. It is methodologically difficult to demonstrate the effect of high-G training on accident rates: in the USAF, a decrease has been shown in the G-LOC accident rate from the pre G-LOC awareness and centrifuge training era (1982–84) to the post-training era (1985–94) (Lyons *et al.* 2004), but no statistically significant reduction in G-LOC accident rates could be demonstrated over the whole period (1982–2001). However, in individual cases of low tolerance, training has been effective and has allowed such aircrew to continue flying high-performance aircraft.

Basic training consists of detailed briefings on the physiological basis for acceleration-induced visual disturbance and loss of consciousness; a demonstration of a good anti-G straining manoeuvre; and individual centrifuge experience. Centrifuge acceleration profiles may take the form of simple exposures to a single $+G_z$ level for a preset duration of time or more complex simulated air combat manoeuvres, in which the $+G_z$ level is varied in a manner akin to that of an aircraft engaged in air combat. More recently, the advent of dynamic flight simulation has offered a further improvement in centrifuge training potential. In these systems, the pilot controls the centrifuge, which is configured like a flight simulator with head-up and out-of-window displays. In this manner, aircrew can perform tail-chasing and air combat against a simulated aircraft target, which has the potential to enhance greatly the realism and aircrew acceptability of centrifuge training. This in turn may lead to a better transfer of training to the flight environment and a further reduction in G-LOC incidents.

The occasional loss of consciousness, inevitable during a centrifuge training programme, may be beneficial in drawing attention to the risks and to the slow recovery and confusion that follow. There is some evidence to suggest that prior experience of loss of consciousness may shorten subsequent recovery times (Whinnery *et al.* 1987), and it has been argued that such experience should be given to all aircrew.

The objectives of any high-G training programme should include the following:

- To promote aircrew awareness of the potential for G-LOC.
- To enhance aircrew anticipation of circumstances that might result in G-LOC and to recognize the symptoms.
- To develop an efficient and effective AGSM.
- To develop confidence in the ability to sustain high $+G_z$ acceleration.

The importance placed on high-G training is likely to grow with the introduction of agile fast jets. To this end, the latest human centrifuges match the onset rate performance of agile aircraft (up to 10 G/s). With the introduction of advanced G-protection, a certain amount of training time will be devoted to familiarization with, and correct use of, positive pressure breathing for G protection, because the correct breathing technique must be learned and practised to gain full benefit from the system.

PHYSICAL FITNESS

As described above, the AGSM is a fatiguing manoeuvre, and exhaustion is likely to limit the total time for which high $+G_z$ acceleration can be tolerated. Although there is no evidence to suggest that absolute G-tolerance can be improved by physical conditioning, some, but not all, studies have shown that whole-body strength training can significantly increase endurance at sustained high $+G_z$ acceleration. For example, a centrifuge exposure that consisted of alternating 15-second periods at +4.5 and $+7\,G_z$ could be tolerated for longer (411 seconds instead of 232 seconds) – an increase of 77 per cent – following weight-training (Epperson *et al.* 1985).

Aerobic fitness does not appear to have any great effect on G-tolerance, according to experimental findings thus far. Indeed, anecdotal evidence suggests that excessive aerobic fitness may be deleterious to G-tolerance, since it induces an imbalance between sympathetic and parasympathetic activity. Excessive vagal tone may lead to bradycardia or even asystole and subsequent loss of consciousness. Therefore, it is generally recommended that fitness training should not be pursued so far as to cause the resting heart rate to fall below 55 beats/min.

DRUGS

A number of attempts have been made to improve G-tolerance with drugs that increase vasomotor tone. In all cases, the pharmacodynamics of these agents, and their side effects, have proven to be incompatible with use in the aviation environment. Hypertensive drugs such as catecholamines, amphetamine and even inspired CO_2 have been investigated with little success, and at present there does not appear to be any drug that is suitable to improve G-tolerance. Some people have proposed that it may be possible to shorten recovery time after G-LOC with a pharmacological agent, but this has not been proven experimentally.

NECK PAIN

High $+G_z$ acceleration, particularly when sustained for long periods, combined with high G_z onset rate and heavy helmet weights are all predisposing factors for neck pain. Neck pain can be experienced even in moderately agile aircraft, such as many jet trainers, but the incidence in highly agile aircraft is likely to be greater due to the predisposing factors listed above. Instructors and non-pilot aircrew such as navigators and weapons operators may be at increased risk of experiencing neck pain, as they are less likely to be prepared for sudden manoeuvres (Green 2003). High-G-related neck pain can be divided into two categories: acute pain of sudden onset in flight and chronic degenerative disease.

Acute in-flight neck pain

Acute in-flight pain is most commonly caused by ligamentous injury or muscle strain. The neck is particularly vulnerable when at the extremes of extension and rotation, which is, unfortunately, a common position for aircrew to adopt as they pull G, e.g. during a 'check 6' manoeuvre, in which the aircrew turn to look over their shoulders for aircraft following them. In one study, 89.1 per cent of Japanese F15 pilots were found to suffer from acute pain when 'checking 6' (Kikukawa et al. 1994). More serious causes of acute in-flight pain have been revealed with magnetic resonance imaging (MRI) techniques. Cervical disc protrusion and even annular tears in the discs have been noted, particularly in the region of C3–4 (Hamalainen et al. 1994). Some of these protrusions have extended far enough to cause spinal-cord compression. At least one episode of acute cervical compression fracture has been noted in flight in an F16 pilot (Andersen 1988), and there are also reports of fractured spinous processes and facet-joint dislocation.

Degenerative disease

Degenerative cervical disease usually takes the form of disc degeneration with osteophyte formation. The lifetime incidence of neck pain has been reported in studies by the US Navy at 60 per cent (Knudson et al. 1988) and by the Finnish Air Force at 48 per cent (Hamalainen 1999). Some studies noted increased incidence with increased aircraft agility. Unfortunately, however, there is a high prevalence of spinal abnormalities on MRI and cervical radiography of asymptomatic individuals, which makes analysis of $+G_z$ acceleration-related injury difficult. However, meta-analysis of G-related spinal degeneration studies has shown conclusively that degenerative spinal disease occurs more commonly in fighter pilots than in age-matched controls (Oakley 1999). A longitudinal study of Swedish aircrew suggests that although fast-jet pilots are at increased risk of premature development of degenerative spinal lesions, with increasing age the difference between pilots and controls diminishes (Petren-Mallmin and Linder 2001).

Prevention of neck injury will become an important issue over the next few years. Unfortunately, aircrew helmets are becoming heavier rather than lighter, with the addition of night-vision equipment and helmet-mounted display systems. A number of attempts to provide support of the head and neck under $+G_z$ have failed to allow satisfactory head mobility, which is essential for air combat. The evidence that neck muscle strength-training provides protection against acute in-flight neck pain or degenerative disease is lacking. Although some authors claim that there is some reduction in acute in-flight neck pain with specific exercises (Kikukawa et al. 1994; Jones et al. 2000), this is not a universal finding. Further investigation into the aetiology of $+G_z$ associated cervical pathology and the efficacy of neck-muscle conditioning as a preventive measure is necessary.

AGILE AIRCRAFT

Aircraft with modern flight-control systems, employing 'fly-by-wire' technology and inherently unstable aerodynamics, are able to generate and sustain high $+G_z$ forces more rapidly, over a wider range of air speeds and altitudes, and for longer than ever before. The risk of G-LOC is greater because there are no premonitory visual symptoms at high G onset rates, and the ability to sustain high $+G_z$ levels for a considerable period of time may lead to aircrew fatigue if performing the AGSM. In order to address these issues, some agile aircraft have been equipped with advanced anti-G protection.

Advanced anti-G protection

The design aim of advanced anti-G protection is to enhance aircrew tolerance to high $+G_z$ acceleration with minimal fatigue. Advanced anti-G protection is automatic and requires little or no voluntary action from the aircrew. In addition to limiting fatigue, this has the advantage of freeing attention to the flying task and also greatly reduces the risk of G-LOC from inadequate performance of the AGSM. It commonly comprises one or more of extended-coverage anti-G trousers, positive pressure breathing for G-protection (PBG), and alteration of cockpit geometry and pilot position.

EXTENDED-COVERAGE ANTI-G TROUSERS

In order to provide more counter-pressure to the lower limbs, at greater mechanical efficiency, the area of cover of the anti-G suit has been extended (Figure 9.2). Extended-coverage suits utilize circumferential bladders, which improve venous return to the thorax under increased $+G_z$ acceleration. Peripheral vascular pooling is reduced, and the fall in cardiac output is minimized, resulting in an increase in relaxed G-tolerance of 2–2.5 G compared with the unprotected individual. A common problem with these garments is the reduction in mobility and increase in thermal burden that are imposed by the extended bladder coverage. Careful suit design combined with an appropriate

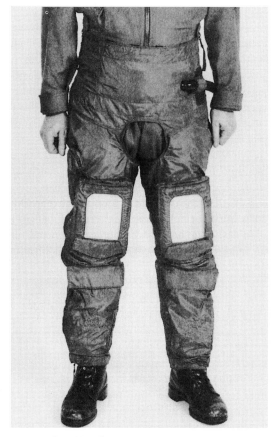

Figure 9.2 *Example of extended coverage anti-G trousers. The circumferential bladders cover over 90 per cent of the lower limbs, providing greater G protection than the standard anti-G suit.*

choice of materials are required to minimize these effects. A large range of garment sizes is required to encompass both male and female aircrew. In addition, there is some evidence to suggest that due to morphological differences, a modified garment design for females is necessary to limit discomfort.

Extended-coverage anti-G trousers provide improved G protection at minimal financial cost and without the need for major aircraft modification. Consequently, it is a relatively simple process to retrofit them into existing aircraft types. However, due to their increased inflated bulk, care must be taken to avoid cockpit interactions (e.g. with the control column or the ejection seat path). Furthermore, the performance of the anti-G valve should be considered, as the inflation rate of extended-coverage trousers may be slower because of their larger volume.

POSITIVE-PRESSURE BREATHING FOR G-PROTECTION

The effective automation of the Valsalva manoeuvre by the addition of PBG raises intrathoracic pressure and reduces fatigue. Positive pressure breathing has been used for many years as an emergency measure for high-altitude protection, but PBG takes advantage of a different physiological consequence of breathing at increased pressure. The elevation of intrathoracic pressure acts directly on the heart and great vessels to increase blood pressure on a virtually one-to-one basis but is mirrored by a rise in central venous pressure, compounding the decrease in venous return to the thorax caused by exposure to increased $+G_z$ acceleration. It is essential therefore that there is adequate support of venous return, and this can best be provided by extended-coverage anti-G trousers. The combination of PBG and extended-coverage garments enables most individuals to maintain clear vision at $+9\,G_z$ with little or no straining (some tensing is usually required). When matched for age and height, there is little evidence to show any sex difference in the G-protection provided by such systems.

In order to prevent lung over-distension by balancing forces across the chest wall, a chest counter-pressure garment is worn when pressure breathing at above 4 kPa (30 mmHg) for either altitude or G-protection. Although exhalation under PBG is assisted by the presence of a chest counter-pressure garment, the increased weight of the chest wall under G alone may be sufficient. Indeed, there is evidence to suggest that lung overdistension can be prevented by the increased weight of the chest wall and aircrew clothing alone, without the need for a chest counter-pressure garment, and some forces now use PBG operationally without chest counter-pressure.

PBG is supplied by a modified breathing regulator, driven by a control signal from the anti-G valve, to provide a schedule of pressure that increases with increasing $+G_z$ acceleration. This arrangement prevents the activation of

PBG without concomitant anti-G suit inflation, which would severely compromise the circulation. A typical pressure breathing schedule cuts in at +4 G_z and increases linearly at 1.6 kPa (12 mmHg) per G to a peak pressure of 8 kPa (60 mmHg) at +9 G_z (Figure 9.3). The peak pressure can be extended to 9.3 kPa (70 mmHg) in aircraft capable of +12 G_z.

The improvement in G-tolerance afforded by the combination of extended-coverage anti-G trousers and PBG is not without cost. Aircraft systems must be modified to deliver PBG, and the additional body-mounted equipment and clothing may decrease aircrew mobility and comfort and increase thermal stress. The system must integrate with other equipment, such as biological and chemical warfare protection. An effective oronasal mask seal must be achieved to prevent distracting mask leakage when using PBG, preferably with some means of automatic mask tensioning. The stability of helmet-mounted display images must be ensured, as PBG and mask tensioning tend to displace the helmet on the head, so moving the displayed image out of the visual field.

High +G_z-associated forearm pain

High vascular pressure may exist in the forearms if they are positioned in a dependent position under high +G_z acceleration, due to the increased hydrostatic gradient. The pressure may be increased still further by the addition of PBG. With the aircraft control column and throttle in conventional positions, forearm venous pressure may reach 250–300 mmHg at +9 G when using PBG, and this is associated with deep, poorly localized pain, which is probably

due to vascular overdistension. At the upper end of the physiological pressure range and beyond, collagen fibres become an important determinant of vessel-wall elasticity, and it is likely that vessel-wall stretch involving the collagen components is associated with the development of pain. There is evidence for vascular pain receptors (nociceptors) innervated by A-delta fibres, which are the most likely pain afferents in this case.

Arm pain may be abolished by locating the top of the aircraft's control column and throttle at or close to heart level. Attempts have been made to reduce arm discomfort with a tightly applied bandage material over the forearms, but this has not been shown to give any improvement experimentally. Many would recognize that the severity of arm pain experienced in the research environment on a human centrifuge is greater than that in the air. The distraction of the flying task and limited duration at peak +G_z acceleration during operational flying may go some way towards reconciling this discrepancy. Additionally, there is some suggestion that adaptation to high-G arm pain may occur.

POSTURE

Any measure that reduces the vertical distance between the heart and brain will provide a degree of protection against acceleration. This approach to G-protection has never been adopted in operational aircraft because a seat reclined to greater than 65 degrees is required to improve G-tolerance significantly (Glaister and Lisher 1977). In this position, it is impossible to gain a 360-degree view from the cockpit, as the head cannot be rotated adequately, and this is completely unacceptable for a fighter aircraft in a combat situation. In aircraft with reclined seats, such as F16 and Rafale, the seat-back angle is approximately 30 degrees, which adds very little (if any) improvement to G-tolerance; the principal benefit is in terms of seat comfort. Elevation of the legs helps to discourage peripheral venous pooling, and this has been employed to good effect in the cockpit of Rafale.

FUTURE G-PROTECTION

If further increases in aircraft agility and sustained +G_z acceleration level are required, then there is little alternative than to provide a solution including a reclined seat. The improvements in display technology, and the emergence of viable virtual reality systems, coupled with the increasing threat of laser weapons, have led to investigation of a 'windowless' cockpit, in which the pilot can be fully reclined. However, the expense of developing such systems

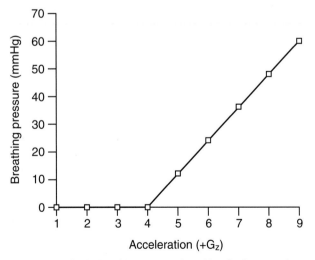

Figure 9.3 *Typical positive pressure breathing for G-protection schedule. Positive-pressure breathing is supplied above +G_z to enhance G tolerance, usually in combination with extended-coverage anti-G trousers.*

may be prohibitive, and unless a clear requirement exists for a manned aircraft capable of such high-G manoeuvring, it is likely that the emergence of unoccupied combat aircraft will meet future requirements for aircraft agility.

REFERENCES

Andersen HT. Neck injury sustained during exposure to high-G forces in the F16B. *Aviation Space and Environmental Medicine* 1988; **59**: 356–8.

Brook WH. The development of the Australian anti-G suit. *Aviation Space and Environmental Medicine* 1990; **61**: 176–82.

Burton RR. Anti-G suit inflation rate requirements. *Aviation Space and Environmental Medicine* 1988; **59**: 2–5.

Eiken O, Kolegard R, Lindborg B, *et al.* A new hydrostatic anti-G suit vs a pneumatic anti-G system: preliminary comparison. *Aviation Space and Environmental Medicine* 2002; **73**: 703–8.

Epperson WL, Burton RR, Bernauer EM. Effectiveness of specific weight training regimens on simulated aerial combat maneuvering G tolerance. *Aviation Space and Environmental Medicine* 1985; **56**: 534–9.

Glaister DH, Lisher BJ. The effect of a reclined sitting position on psychomotor performance during exposure to high sustained +G_z acceleration. Flying Personnel Research Committee report no. 1362. London: RAF Institute of Aviation Medicine; 1977.

Green NDC. Acute soft tissue neck injury from unexpected acceleration. *Aviation Space and Environmental Medicine* 2003; **74**: 1085–90.

Hamalainen O. Cervical injury and degeneration in the Finnish Air Force. In: Burton, R. (ed.). NATO RTO technical report 4, AC/323(HFM)TP/9. Neuilly-Sur-Seine: AGARD/NATO, 1999; pp. 39–43.

Hamalainen O, Visuri T, Kuronen P, Vanharanta H. Cervical disk bulges in fighter pilots. *Aviation Space and Environmental Medicine* 1994; **65**: 144–6.

Head H. The sense and stability of balance in the air. In: *Medical Research Council Report into the Medical Problems of Flying*. London: HM Stationery Office, 1920; pp. 214–56.

Jones JA, Hart SF, Baskin DS, *et al.* Human and behavioural factors contributing to spine-based neurological cockpit injuries in pilots of high performance aircraft: recommendations for management and prevention. *Military Medicine* 2000; **165**: 6–12.

Kikukawa A, Tachibana S, Yagura S. G-related musculoskeletal spine symptoms in Japan Air Self Defence Force F-15 pilots. *Aviation Space and Environmental Medicine* 1994; **65**: 269–72.

Knudson R, McMillan D, Doucette D, Seidel M. A comparative study of G-induced neck injury in pilots of the F/A-18, A-7 and A-4. *Aviation Space and Environmental Medicine* 1988; **59**: 758–60.

Lyons T, Davenport C, Copley GB, *et al.* Preventing G-induced loss of consciousness: 20 years of operational experience. *Aviation Space and Environmental Medicine* 2004; **75**: 150–53.

Oakley CJ. Meta-analysis of studies on cervical degeneration of fighter pilots. In: Burton, R. (ed.). NATO RTO technical report 4, AC/323(HFM)TP/9. Neuilly-Sur-Seine: AGARD/NATO, 1999; pp. 67–70.

Petren-Mallmin M, Linder J. Cervical spine degeneration in fighter pilots and controls: a 5-year follow-up study. *Aviation Space and Environmental Medicine* 2001; **72**: 443–6.

Whinnery JE, Burton RR, Boll PA, Eddy DR. Characterisation of the resulting incapacitation following unexpected +G_z-induced loss of consciousness. *Aviation Space and Environmental Medicine* 1987; **58**: 631–6.

Zhang SX, Guo HZ, Jing BS, *et al.* Experimental verification of effectiveness and harmlessness of the Qigong maneuver. *Aviation Space and Environmental Medicine* 1991; **62**: 46–52.

FURTHER READING

AGARD/NATO. High G physiological protection training. AGARDograph no. 322. Neuilly-sur-Seine: AGARD/NATO, 1990.

AGARD/NATO. High altitude and high acceleration protection for military aircrew. AGARD conference proceedings no. 516. Neuilly-sur-Seine: AGARD/NATO, 1991.

AGARD/NATO. Current concepts on G protection research and development. AGARD lecture series no. 202. Neuilly-sur-Seine: AGARD/NATO, 1995.

10

Short-duration acceleration

MATTHEW E. LEWIS

INTRODUCTION

Short-duration accelerations resulting in injury or death can be inflicted not only on the occupants of vehicles involved in crashes but also on pedestrians, sports people, people falling from heights and people exposed to explosions and bomb blasts. Injuries may be received when a person in motion comes into collision with a solid object or when an object or missile strikes a stationary person. Irrespective of the circumstances surrounding the accident, injury occurs when a person is exposed to forces of a critical magnitude for a brief period of time, and the degree of injury is related to the magnitude and duration of the applied forces. The study of impact injury can be summarized as what we hit, how we hit it, how long we hit it for, how many times we hit it, and which part of the body is hit. Before introducing injury-reduction programmes, it is necessary to understand how accidents cause injuries the nature of the forces contributing to the injuries, and the characteristics of the type of accident under consideration.

SHORT-DURATION VERSUS LONG-DURATION ACCELERATION

When assessing injuries incurred during aviation or automotive accidents, we encounter occupants who have been exposed to high forces for very brief periods of time. The time course of an impact event is extremely short, usually 0.1–0.5 seconds. Experiments carried out on human and animal subjects have demonstrated the essential features in the study of the effects of impact accelerations to be the magnitude of the peak acceleration, the duration of exposure, the momentum change, the jolt, the nature of the forces of inertia and the site of application to the body.

The effects of short-duration accelerations are related principally to the structural strength of the part of the body on which they act and to the overall velocity change induced in the body. In contrast, intermediate-duration accelerations are forces that persist for 0.5–2 seconds, such as during ejections from aircraft, catapult launches and deck landings. Human tolerance to intermediate-duration accelerations depends not only on the overall velocity change induced but also on the time taken to reach peak acceleration and on the peak acceleration level attained. Long-duration acceleration, which can be experienced in various aircraft manoeuvres, imposes forces that last more than two seconds and have a duration of perhaps minutes. Human tolerance to sustained acceleration depends principally on the plateau level of the acceleration imposed on the body, as the response to long-duration acceleration is due to the effects of physiological changes arising from hydrostatic pressure gradients and from alterations in the flow and distribution of blood and body fluids.

An alternative way of distinguishing long- and short-duration acceleration can be by the response of the human: with long-duration acceleration, the stresses can be considered as mainly physiological and sustained; with short-duration (or impact) acceleration, the stresses are considered as mainly mechanical and transitory. For example, events such as unconsciousness may arise in both, but the causations differ: unconsciousness following impact acceleration is caused mainly by physical trauma, while with long-duration acceleration it is usually caused by reduced cerebral perfusion.

A human tolerance curve in which peak acceleration is plotted against the length of time for which it may be tolerated has the form illustrated in Figure 10.1. For whole-body impacts, each point on the 45-degree sloping left-hand part of the graph represents a combination of acceleration (a) and time (t), which gives a constant velocity change ($v = at$), while the right-hand horizontal part indicates sensitivity to a constant plateau acceleration. The intersection of the two lines may show a dip, as indicated by the dotted line, where dynamic overshoot caused by body-resonance effects amplifies the transmitted forces and causes a reduction in tolerance.

MECHANICS OF IMPACT

The profile of acceleration forces acting on an aircraft during a crash is determined by the manner in which the aircraft decelerates as its velocity is resisted by friction with the ground or by collision with stationary objects. When an aircraft impacts the ground during an accident, the aircraft experiences an opposing force of very short duration. This force decelerates the aircraft, reducing the initial speed to a final speed, which eventually will be zero. The peak magnitude of this opposing force will depend on the length of time for which the force acts. If the time is short, then a higher peak force will result compared with when the time available is longer. The aircraft by virtue of it mass (m) and velocity (v) will have kinetic energy (KE) as follows:

$$KE = 1/2\ mv^2$$

If the structure of a crashing aircraft is crushed or deformed progressively, then much of the kinetic energy of the crash is absorbed, and the overall deceleration profile is relatively smooth. If parts of the crashing aircraft plough into the ground, however, the aircraft velocity is reduced more rapidly, and peaks of abrupt decelerations of high magnitude are produced, with the highest peak values occurring when the aircraft strikes solid objects, such as rocks or buildings. When an aircraft ditches, the forces acting on the airframe reflect not only the speed of the aircraft and its angle of incidence with the water but also the orientation of the aircraft with respect to the wave front and the sea state at the time of the accident. There is often little attenuation from airframe deformation during a planned ditching, as water tends to produce a uniform load distribution across the lower surfaces of the fuselage.

The velocity of an aircraft before a crash may be known with some accuracy from in-flight data recording, or it may be estimated from the resulting structural deformation. However, the deceleration depends on the nature of the terrain struck and, in particular, on the distance (s) over which the vehicle is brought to rest. Assuming a constant deceleration, this can be calculated from the pre-impact velocity in G units from the equation

$$G = v^2/2gs$$

In practice, the crash-deceleration pulse is more likely to approximate to a triangle or saw-tooth, in which case the peak deceleration will be twice that calculated above, but at least an approximation will be obtained of the magnitude of the forces imposed on the vehicle's occupants.

Although information on the crash pulse of the aircraft can be determined from analysis of the impact dynamics, it is the magnitude of the forces acting on the occupant that is more important. In certain circumstances, the forces reaching the occupant of a crashing aircraft may be significantly less than those occurring in the aircraft structures immediately surrounding the person. This is due to the surrounding structures collapsing and crushing, and thus absorbing part of the kinetic energy and attenuating the severity of the force before it can reach the occupant.

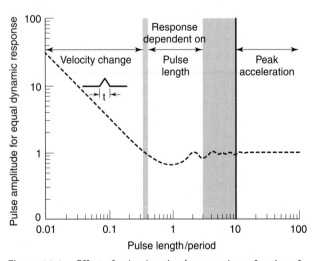

Figure 10.1 *Effect of pulse duration (expressed as a fraction of the natural period of oscillation of a simple dynamic system) on the amplitude of the triangular impact pulse needed to give an equal dynamic response. Shaded areas indicate transitions between the three zones in which the dynamic response (acceleration tolerance) depends primarily on velocity change, pulse length or peak acceleration.*

Crash-worthy design features can be used to allow the structures to collapse progressively in a controlled manner and so increase the chances of human survival. The magnitude of the forces on the occupant may also be well in excess of those occurring in the surrounding structures. In such crashes, the occupant, by virtue of inadequate restraint or poor seat design, experiences little deceleration during the early part of the impact. Inevitably, at some later point in the crash, the occupant will strike the aircraft or come to full harness extension and thereby be decelerated suddenly to the vehicle's velocity in a very short time.

As with sustained acceleration, the direction in which an impact force acts on a human being is described by a three-coordinate system in which the x axis describes forces acting in the fore and aft direction at right-angles to the longitudinal axis of the body, the y axis indicates laterally applied loads, and the z axis describes accelerations in the long axis of the body. It is important to distinguish between the applied force and the resultant inertial force, as these act in opposite directions. For example, the deceleration of a crashing car (backwards acceleration) displaces the driver's internal organs forwards; this resultant (inertial) force is called $-G_x$. The tolerance to backwards acceleration of the occupant of an aircraft or vehicle seat depends critically on the effectiveness of the support provided to the front of the body by a restraint harness. If no obstacles are present within the flail envelope, then the head will be flung down on to the chest, and the arms and legs will be thrown forwards at right-angles to the body. Without restraint, the occupant will simply continue forwards at their initial velocity until they strike a solid object such as an instrument panel or bulkhead.

Significant lateral ($\pm G_y$) accelerations do not occur under normal flight conditions. However, in crashes, significant $\pm G_y$ accelerations can occur, particularly to the seat occupants of military fixed-wing and rotary-wing aircraft fitted with sideways-facing crew positions or passenger seats. In these crashes, the severity and type of injury sustained by the occupant is dependent on the restraint provided, the nature of any contact with airframe structures, and the displacement of the body, especially the head, neck and limbs.

Significant $+G_z$ acceleration can occur in crashes associated with a high sink rate, particularly in helicopters. Tolerance to accelerations in this axis is influenced by the seat-back angle, the sitting platform and the posture of the occupant. Headwards ($+G_z$) acceleration is reacted primarily through the buttocks and spinal column, and the posture of the occupant and the effectiveness of any restraint harness provided influence the incidence of spinal column injury. Footwards ($-G_z$) accelerations are reacted through any restraint harness and may occur during inverted crashes or following a rollover.

IMPACT: THE PHYSICAL BASIS OF INJURY

Impact injury refers to structural disruption of biological tissue as a result of a short-duration physical event and causes tissue disruption by placing stress on the tissue. Tissues can be stressed in different ways. Forces that tend to compress tissues produce compression stress; the opposite of compression stress is tension, produced by forces that tend to pull tissues apart. A positive or negative single number can, therefore, be used to describe compression-tension stress. Axial compression or tension stress is not the only kind of stress that can be placed on tissues, and mathematically a total of six numerical values are required for a complete description, namely:

- compression–tension load
- fore–aft bending
- left–right bending
- fore–aft shear
- left–right shear
- clockwise–anticlockwise torsion.

Bending of a tissue structure results in a number of internal stresses and will place one side in tension and the other in compression. Shear stress is produced by a non-aligned force couple, which, if aligned, would have produced compression or tension. Since the force is non-aligned, it tends to produce slip. Torsion is produced by axial torque and can produce locally in the tissue tension, compression and shear.

Injury mechanisms are descriptions of the process by which an injury occurs. Defining the mechanism of injury ultimately involves specifying the principal stresses that produce an injury. Since injury is simply strain beyond the yield point, where strain is defined as the change in a dimension divided by the original dimension, the prevention of injury requires limiting strain to the recoverable portion of a load–deformation curve. Limiting the strain can be achieved by limiting the applied force that produces it and/or applying the force over a larger or more tolerant part of the body.

Visco-elasticity is a material property whereby a change of stress occurs under constant deformation or a change in deformation occurs under constant load. All biological tissues, including hard tissues such as bone, have the property of visco-elasticity and will break under different loads, depending on the rate of application of the load, the nature of the force and the time over which the force is applied. Human bones may sustain without breaking a higher force applied rapidly and withdrawn, but may break when a lower force is applied more slowly. As biological tissues are visco-elastic, the rate of loading and the strain rate are critical to the production of injury; the faster the load is applied, the stiffer the material behaves. At some discernible level of deformation magnitude and rate, the tissue will not be able to recover, and damage to the tissue or injury will occur. This level of response is the injury threshold and indicates the tolerance of the body organ or tissue to impact.

HUMAN TOLERANCE AND VELOCITY CHANGE

Defining human tolerance levels to short-duration accelerations is not a simple task, due to the variability of individual response and the need to state the level of injury that is considered acceptable. Short-duration acceleration forces can be separated into three broad categories: tolerable, injurious and fatal. In this classification, tolerable forces may produce minor superficial trauma, such as bruises and abrasions, which do not incapacitate; injurious forces result in moderate to severe trauma, which may or may not incapacitate; and fatal injuries result in death. These distinctions are important, since research data are often based on the results of voluntary exposures to impact, while in accidents, survival without permanent injury may be a necessary compromise in vehicle design.

In a vehicle crash, the instantaneous change in velocity, Δv, is a good predictor of injury severity. The probability of an occupant receiving injury or death increases with increasing Δv, although the relationship between Δv and injury severity is non-linear and influenced by physiological and anatomical variabilities of the vehicle occupant. This relationship is ill-defined in aircraft accidents, due to the relatively small number on which full crash analyses have been carried out, but extensive data have been derived from car-crash studies. Figure 10.2 was derived from the United States National Accident Sampling System (NASS) data for the decade 1982–91 and relates the probability of car-driver injury or fatality against Δv (Evans 1993). A database of more than 22 000 crashes in which Δv either was known or could be estimated from vehicle deformation allows a clear relationship to be seen. From such data, the influence of driver characteristics, seatbelt systems, airbags and so on can be determined, provided that numbers are adequate for statistical analysis.

FACTORS AFFECTING HUMAN TOLERANCE TO SHORT-DURATION ACCELERATION

Magnitude and duration of applied force

In general, under similar conditions, the longer the duration of the impact pulse, the lower the acceleration level that can be tolerated. This follows simply from the sensitivity of injury tolerance to the induced velocity change.

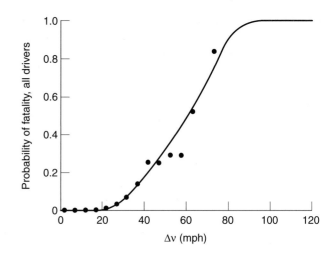

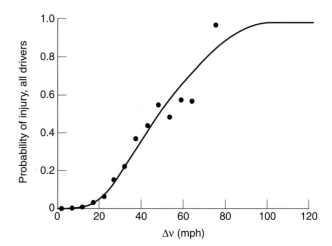

Figure 10.2   *Relationship between the probability of a car driver being killed or injured and the velocity change (Δv) incurred in the crash (from Evans 1993).*

Rate of onset of applied force

If the conditions of the impact are the same, then the slower the rate of onset of the acceleration, the better the impact will be tolerated. For example, if the rate of onset of the acceleration is 1000 G/s in a given $-G_x$ impact, then signs of injury may be evident; however, these signs could be absent if the rate of onset is slowed to 60 G/s. The effect of rate of onset of acceleration is related to the natural resonant frequency of the whole body or of individual organs and to the compliance, the ability of the mechanical system to respond to an applied force, of the visco-elastic systems of the bones, joints and ligaments.

Direction of applied force

The body can withstand much greater forces applied in the $+G_x$ axis due to the larger supported surface area of the body in this orientation. The same applies to the $-G_x$ axis given optimum support and head restraint. Accelerations in the $\pm G_z$ axis place greater strain on the organs suspended in the body cavities, and the tolerance to impact is reduced. The limited research on the effects of $\pm G_y$ impacts indicates these to have the lowest tolerance limits, especially when the head is unrestrained. In this situation, neck pain caused by this force imposes a voluntary limit of some $\pm 8\,G_y$.

Site of application of acceleration

In general, some parts of the body, such as the back and buttocks, are more able to withstand a given force than other, more vulnerable parts, such as the limbs and head. For this reason, restraint systems should be designed so as to apply loads to the body's strong points such as the pelvic bones rather than to the abdomen.

HUMAN TOLERANCE: ACCELERATION MAGNITUDE AND DIRECTION

Figures 10.3 and 10.4 are presented as an attempt to amplify Figure 10.1 and to bring in the influences of posture and restraint. The graphs underline the enormous range of accelerations that may or may not be tolerable and show the futility of trying to answer the apparently simple and frequently asked question – how much G can the body stand?

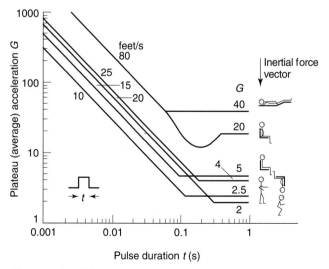

Figure 10.3 *Tolerance to whole-body impacts in the postures and restraints indicated by the stick figures and for a downward-acting inertial force vector. Inset numbers indicate tolerable velocity change (Δv) for brief impacts and tolerable G for somewhat longer impacts.*

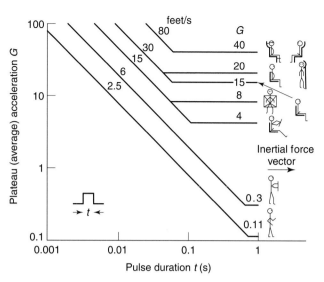

Figure 10.4 *Tolerance to whole-body impacts plotted as for Figure 10.3, but for horizontally acting force vectors.*

Since tolerance to impact forces depends on the imposed Δv and tolerance to long-duration forces depends on the plateau level of acceleration imposed, a tolerance plot should be comprised of two connected lines – one for impact having a 45-degree slope connecting points of equal Δv and the other horizontal and set at a given acceleration level (Figure 10.1, p. 170). Figure 10.3 illustrates tolerance curves for lying, seated and standing subjects exposed to a vertical force vector, with an idealized rectangular pulse form and with acceleration and timescales being plotted on logarithmic scales, a form of presentation made essential by variations in input data of several orders of magnitude. The greatest tolerance is seen when the forces are distributed most widely, i.e. when lying supine on a form-fitting couch or when falling on to a conforming surface such as soft snow. The least tolerance is seen when free-standing, as in a falling lift. Note that the two lower curves cross over, since a knees-bent posture attenuates the transmission of forces to the upper body but cannot sustain prolonged loads. The other curves in Figure 10.3 refer to impacts with the differing postures and restraints illustrated by the stick figures. The seated figure with torso restraint represents the case of ejection from an aircraft and illustrates the trough in tolerance caused by a resonance overshoot for an impulse lasting about 200 ms. The final curves illustrate the lower tolerances of unrestrained bodies, which will slump forwards, and to $-G_z$ impacts, with the forces acting through shoulder and lap restraints.

Figure 10.4 is a similar plot, but for horizontal force vectors. It illustrates the very wide range in tolerance caused by diverse postures and tolerance criteria. The upper curve is the same as the upper curve in Figure 10.3, but turned through 90 degrees, and could represent a passenger in a rear-facing aircraft seat (with lap-belt to prevent rebound) or in a forward-facing seat with full-body restraint. Note the provision of adequate head fixation and the assumption that the seat itself is capable of withstanding 40 G without failure. The tolerance criterion in these accident situations is survival without incapacitating injury. The lowest curve is for a person stepping on to a moving walkway, where the much gentler tolerance criterion is the requirement to remain upright even if aged and encumbered with luggage. The intermediate curves illustrate forward-facing aircrew with five-point harnesses, and a lateral impact with uniform body support; a forward-facing airliner or car passenger with seatbelt, and the unlikely assumption of adequate free space in front to preclude injury to the flailing head and limbs; an unbelted car driver attempting to support themselves on the steering wheel; and a passenger jumping on to a moving bus fitted with a grab handle (as in the old London double-decker buses).

ANATOMICAL AND PHYSIOLOGICAL ASPECTS OF IMPACT TOLERANCE

Injury can result from a direct blow to the body by a solid object or from an indirectly transmitted force, such as when the humerus or clavicle is fractured from an impact transmitted up the outstretched arm during a fall. Either mechanism of injury can result in damage to the skeletal framework of the body or to the soft tissues and internal organs.

Skeletal injury

Damage to the bony skeleton of the body, including the joints, is the most common injury seen in the crash environment. Injuries to the upper and lower extremities are particularly common, and these may not be reduced by the provision of effective restraint harnesses, chiefly due to the presence of solid objects within the flail envelope. The direction of the forces and the rate at which they are applied, together with an estimation of the loads involved, may be obtained from an examination of the fracture type.

Joints

Joint disruption can result in an unstable joint or a joint in which the range of movement has become either restricted or more than normally mobile. The application of a force that stresses a joint beyond its normal range of motion results in the failure of the ligaments, tendons and the joint capsule.

Abdominal cavity

The abdominal cavity reacts to an impact as would a fluid-filled or hydraulic cavity. The force of a blow to any part of the abdomen is transmitted to all organs and structures within the abdominal cavity virtually unchanged. Hence, a potentially rapidly fatal rupture of the diaphragm, liver or spleen can occur from blunt trauma to any part of the abdomen. Some damping of the pressure waves generated by an abdominal impact occurs through compression of the air and gas in the intestines and stomach, and some occurs through the action of the muscles of the abdominal wall and the muscular layers of the various viscera. Blunt trauma can result in abdominal injury by several mechanisms, such as pressure-wave transmission, compression and shear forces. The visco-elastic properties of the individual organs influence the tolerance to impact and blast. However, it would appear that intestinal injury in vehicle crashes occurs mainly in response to submarining, i.e. bending the torso, under a lap-belt.

Chest

In vehicle trauma, the chest is the most commonly injured part of the body after the head and limbs. Impact injuries to the chest are often rapidly fatal, as all the contents of the chest are vital to life. Major life-threatening injuries to the chest compromise the respiratory and circulatory systems and can result in hypoxic brain damage or death. Severe decreases in the amount of oxygen available for transport by an intact circulatory system can result from impaired breathing mechanics following damage to ribs and diaphragm as well as from the alterations associated with pneumothorax, haemothorax and lung contusions. Disruption of the circulatory system, with potentially fatal decreases in the blood volume available for oxygen transport, can be the result of blunt trauma to the chest. Non-penetrating cardiac injuries (ruptures of the myocardium, cardiac septa, pericardium and valvular apparatus) and rupture of the aorta are frequently seen at post-mortem examinations of the victims of vehicle trauma.

Head and face

The head is the most frequently injured region of the body in vehicle crashes in which the occupants have been restrained by a three-point belt. Such injury is the predominant cause of death in vehicle crashes. The definition of head-injury tolerance is fraught with difficulty and still requires clarification. In pursuing the study of head and brain injury, some researchers have equated head injury with brain injury, while others have related head injury to fracture of the skull. As it is possible to have brain injury without a skull fracture, and skull fracture without brain injury, difficulties arise in the correlation of the results of observations and experiments.

Spine

Back injuries incurred during an aircraft crash may involve the musculoskeletal structures of the vertebral column and/or the spinal cord itself. When considering the evidence for the mechanism of injury to the vertebral column, consideration must be given to the fact that post-accident appearances will not indicate the maximum deformation that occurred at the time of maximal loading. The determination of the mechanism for vertebral column injury in any one accident is complicated further by the variation in response to identical applied loads that arise from individual anatomical and physiological characteristics. The pattern of injury will depend on which of the elements in the vertebral column is the weakest link in a particular individual, such as when intervertebral disc lesions are affected by the degeneration of the disc that occurs with increasing age. Injuries from the same applied loads may be modified in different individuals by the action of the vertebral muscles, especially if pre-tensioning of the vertebral muscles has taken place before the impact.

The motion of the spine is complex and occurs as coupled motions. Lateral bending involves rotation about the horizontal and vertical axes as well as translation perpendicular to the horizontal plane; hence, lateral bending may cause any combination of transverse shear in the horizontal plane, rotational shear about the vertical axis, and tensile and compressive stresses in the vertebral bodies. Furthermore, similar injuries may be produced by a number of different mechanisms. The tolerance of the vertebral column to impact is not uniform down its length, with, in general terms, fractures of the cervical vertebrae being less stable than those of the lumbar vertebrae. Stability of the vertebral column following impact injury is paramount in determining the overall survival of the casualty. High cervical fractures with instability of the neck are likely to result in injury or transection of the spinal cord, and high spinal-cord injuries are often fatal or result in quadriplegia.

The majority of the injuries to the vertebral column arising from vehicle accidents involve the thoracolumbar spine. The response of the thoracic vertebrae to impact is modified by the presence of the ribs, whereas the increasing size of the lumbar vertebrae and the orientation of the joint facets of the lumbar vertebrae lead to increased stability of the lower vertebral column. The forces required to cause fractures or fracture dislocations of the thoracolumbar spine are very large due to the size of the vertebral bodies and supporting ligaments.

An awareness of the most likely sequence of events in a particular accident, with some assessment of the probable kinematics of the occupant, will allow the determination of the most likely mechanism of a spinal injury. Consideration must be given to the type of restraints employed as the different belt configurations are associated with characteristic injuries such as hyperflexion over a lap-belt or rotation and hyperflexion over a three-point harness.

OCCUPANT CHARACTERISTICS AND TOLERANCE TO IMPACT

The limiting factor of all methods of emergency escape and crash survival protection is the tolerance of the occupant to acceleration and applied forces. The current state of knowledge concerning human impact tolerances is incomplete. While most human volunteer studies have been conducted on young healthy male subjects under controlled conditions, they have been terminated voluntarily at levels below that of irreversible injury. Few experimental data are available for females. Due to the range of human variability, data derived from volunteer male subjects must be used with caution in other applications. Animals have been used to obtain physiological data at impact levels above those injurious to human volunteers, and cadavers offer a means of determining structural limits of tissues but cannot provide the physiological information that must be obtained on living systems.

Human beings can be grouped by gender, each with its own set of related characteristics, but also they are infinitely variable in age, race, build, fitness, genetic predisposition and freedom from disease. Attempts to quantify impact tolerance limits result only in approximations and generalizations, making it necessary in any one accident to analyse occupant injury mechanisms individually. Furthermore, individual variability must be considered, for tolerance under identical test conditions may vary in the same individual as well as from person to person. Accidental freefalls provide the means of determining human tolerances to extreme impacts beyond those to which human volunteers may be subjected. Other estimates of impact tolerances are obtained from clinical studies of impact trauma and from reconstruction of automotive and aircraft accidents.

The tolerance limits for fatality and injury have been derived from research carried out in a variety of institutions using a multiplicity of experimental devices and techniques. The limited numbers of impacts using scarce resources and the variability of the subjects themselves have allowed only an approximation of tolerance limits. The utilization of anthropomorphic test devices (ATDs), or crash-test dummies, to provide repeatable impact conditions has suffered from the employment of a number of different types of ATD, each with its own characteristic responses and limitations. The protocols, measurements and recording techniques employed in these research programmes have been many and varied, making it extremely difficult to compare the results obtained either with other ATD tests or with tests using biological subjects.

Impact testing and anthropomorphic test devices

Any attempt to standardize human tolerance limits from actual accidents where so many variables exist needs to be circumspect and confined to broad limits only. Researchers in the fields of human bioengineering and medicine have been seeking alternative sources of information on human impact tolerances. The development of increasingly sophisticated ATDs and recording devices able to withstand repeated impacts has continued to provide a tool for research into the effects of short-duration accelerations but, as with live data, the 'human tolerance limits' derived from ATD impact research must be treated with some circumspection.

ATDs have been developed for use in the automobile and aviation industry. They were manufactured to improve the biofidelity and injury-prediction measurements for human models in automotive occupant-restraint testing. The principal design attributes required of an ATD to serve as an effective human surrogate are anthropometry, biofidelity, repeatability, reproducibility, durability, measurement capability, sensitivity, simplicity and ease of use. In practice, compromises between several different requirements are made to produce the final dummy design.

One significant deficiency of most ATDs in their use for ejection testing and for vertical impact analysis is the lack of a flexible spine: the lumbar and thoracic spines of ATDs are relatively rigid. During a live ejection, the seat occupant is forcibly flexed forward within the seat harness, with the spine usually pivoting around the thoracolumbar junction. The forces appear to be maximal in this region, and this is where classically the majority of spinal injuries occur. The ATD's inability to reflect accurately the true movement of the ejection-seat occupant significantly compromises the data obtained from such tests. Modifications are being made to develop an ATD with a flexible spine, but a number of technical difficulties need to be overcome before such an ATD will become available for widespread use.

Thresholds for injury

The potential for aircrew to sustain injuries during impact or ejection can be determined by comparing the data measured from the ATD load cells and accelerometers recorded during accident simulations with the forces above which injury is likely to occur: comparisons with the accident test simulation data give an indication of the potential for injury in the test impacts.

The injury thresholds or injury assessment reference values (IARVs) refer to a human response level below which a specified significant injury is considered unlikely to occur for the given size of individual. If a response measurement is below its corresponding IARV, then the occurrence of the associated injury for that size occupant is considered unlikely for the accident environment being simulated. However, being below the specified IARV does not assure that significant injuries will not occur, since IARVs are not specified for all of the injury types that an occupant might experience; in addition, the ATD is instrumented to measure only a limited set of responses. Exceeding an IARV defined in the ATD does not necessarily imply that its human counterpart would experience that injury if exposed to the same test conditions. In many cases, the difference between an IARV and its corresponding injury threshold level is not known because the biomechanical data do not exist to define accurately the injury threshold level.

No experimental programme will be able to reproduce fully the conditions met in an accident, and data from all experimental programmes require validation against known injuries from the analysis of real accidents. Mathematical models are being developed to assist the understanding of the nature of the forces encountered during accidental impact, and although these and the new generation of ATDs are becoming more biofidelic, they are not human beings. Neither mathematical models nor ATDs break in an impact, but they lack the internal structure of the human body and are unable to mimic realistically the result of impact accelerations on organs and body tissues. In the long term, finite element mathematical models are likely to be the main tools used in impact analysis, but their use will depend on proper validation and continual updating from accident-derived data.

Finally, an accident may be considered survivable in terms of the injuries recorded as a result of accelerative forces, but death may ensue from another cause, such as a penetrating injury or internal or external haemorrhage. A survivable accident may become unsurvivable in the presence of a minor head injury causing a short period of unconsciousness and the failure to escape a post-crash fire or effect an underwater escape. Relatively minor but incapacitating limb injuries similarly can prevent survivors of the initial event surviving the post-crash sequelae. In other words, the outcome of any accident will depend not only on the nature of the injuries directly resulting from the body's response to impact but also on complicating factors arising from any injury caused by the deformation of the airframe, penetrating injuries, environmental factors such as fire or water, and the rapidity with which emergency services can respond, and the provision of expert medical care.

REFERENCES

Evans L. Driver injury and fatality risk in two-car crashes versus mass ratio inferred using Newtonian mechanics. *Accident Analysis and Prevention* 1993; **26**: 609–16.

FURTHER READING

AGARD. Anthropomorphic dummies for crash and escape system testing. AGARD-AR-330. Neuilly-sur-Seine: AGARD/NATO, 1996.

Backaitis SH. *Biomechanics of Impact Injury and Injury Tolerances of the Head–Neck Complex*. Warrendale, PA: Society of Automotive Engineers, 1993.

Backaitis SH. *Biomechanics of Impact Injury and Injury Tolerances of the Abdomen, Lumbar Spine and Pelvis Complex*. Warrendale, PA: Society of Automotive Engineers, 1995.

Backaitis SH, Hertz HJ. *Hybrid III: The First Human-like Crash Test Dummy*. Warrendale, PA: Society of Automotive Engineers, 1994.

Nahum AM, Melvin JW. *Accidental Injury: Biomechanics and Prevention*, 2nd edn. New York: Springer, 2002.

Nigg BM, Herzog W. *Biomechanics of the Musculo-Skeletal System*. Chichester: John Wiley & Sons, 1994.

11

Head injury and protection

MATTHEW E. LEWIS

INTRODUCTION

Head injury is common in all forms of accident trauma. Surveys carried out on aircraft accidents have shown that 40 per cent of injuries sustained are craniofacial, and 14–20 per cent of all fatalities resulting from aircraft crashes are due to serious head injury.

Interest in the special need for head protection in the military pilot resulted from changes in the design and role of aircraft. Heavy jet-powered aircraft, introduced in the 1950s, tended to sink rapidly when power was lost, and many aircrew perished because they were unable to escape from crashing aircraft as a result of relatively minor head injury with disturbance of consciousness. Also, as the speed of aircraft increased and operational requirements demanded flight at low level in turbulent conditions, it was feared that both aircraft and occupant might be lost if the pilot lost consciousness as a result of his or her head striking cockpit structures. Consequently, protective helmets were developed for use by aircrew. Since the introduction of such helmets into military aviation there has been a marked reduction in the incidence of head injury and in many cases the wearing of a protective helmet has proved to be life-saving.

This chapter is concerned with the mechanics of head injury, the principles of head protection, and the design and specification of aircrew protective helmets.

PRINCIPLES OF HEAD INJURY

The principles of head injury described by Cairns and Holbourn (1943) have commonly been taken as the mainstays of the descriptive papers on brain injuries. The clarification of the mechanism of head injury upon impact is crucial in trying to find appropriate measures for modifications of the impacting object to reduce the severity of injuries. The nature of head injury depends on various impact conditions, but, despite extensive work being carried out, the mechanisms have not been clarified sufficiently. It is particularly important in the aviation environment to determine what kinds of mechanisms and observations are important, what parameters are required to measure in the experimental and accident reconstruction environment, and what types of head injury occur.

From a clinical view, head injuries can be classified into three categories: skull fractures, focal injuries and diffuse brain injuries. Head injuries from these three clinical classification categories can be produced from very specific forms of mechanical input. Characteristics of the mechanical input, such as the direction, magnitude, application rate, duration and point of action of the force, contribute to the type and severity of the head injury. The complex mechanical loading experienced by the head can be either static or dynamic. Static loading implies that the force is applied to the head slowly, typically over periods greater than 200 ms. Events such as earthquakes, avalanches and slowly moving vehicles that trap the head against solid structures produce these events. In aviation, static loading is seen rarely. Dynamic loading is the more common type of mechanical loading and is characterized by an input applied rapidly to the head. Dynamic loading can be of two types: impulsive and impact. Impulsive loading occurs when the head is set in motion or the moving head is arrested without being struck or impacted. It is the inertial forces produced by the way in which the head moves that cause the resulting head injury. Impact loading is the more frequent type of dynamic loading and usually results in a combination of contact forces and inertial forces. The inertial force component can be minimal in certain impact situations, such as if the head is prevented from moving when struck. The result is that most of the energy is delivered to the head as a contact force. The force applied to any tissue results in strain, which can be considered as the amount of deformation that the tissue undergoes as a result of the applied mechanical force. Depending on the direction of the applied force, the resulting strain can be tensile, compressive or shear. Since the brain is virtually incompressible in vivo, and has lower tolerance to tensile and shear strain, the latter two types of strain are the usual mechanical causes of brain damage. Unfortunately, brain deformation or strain is almost impossible to measure in impacts, particularly in vivo, and hence input variables such as head acceleration are used as alternative parameters to characterize the injury mechanisms.

MECHANICS OF HEAD INJURY

Skull injury

A number of injuries can occur as the result of the unprotected head striking a hard object or an object striking the head. When the human head is subjected to a heavy blow, the skull bones, which break in a characteristic way, absorb much of the energy of impact. The outer table of the skull gives way over an area corresponding closely with the shape of the object striking it. It is thrust into the diploe, which is compressed and shattered. The force of the blow now spreads into surrounding bone and is borne by the inner table, which first bulges and then gives way over an area somewhat larger than that of the outer table. Secondary fissures radiate outwards into surrounding bone along lines dictated by the architecture of the skull.

Broad impacts to the vault of the skull send multiple fissures radiating away from the site of the blow. As these reach the sides of the vault, they turn downwards towards the base of the skull and are directed into channels between the thicker buttresses and the floor of the skull. A very heavy blow directed from underneath the occupant may lift the upper cervical spine with such violence that it breaks away from its ring-base attachments. With skull fractures, the brain and its covering membranes are commonly injured. The skull is also flexible enough under certain conditions of impact to be dented transiently by 10 mm or so, underlying brain damage then being produced in the absence of skull fracture. The break strength of the facial and cranial bones was determined from impacted cadaveric specimens and the resulting head accelerations were measured at the point of failure. Results depended very much on the site of impact and ranged from 30 G for the nose, 40 G for the jaw and 50 G for the zygomatic arch to 100 G for front teeth, 50–100 G for the temporoparietal bone and 100–200 G for the frontal bone.

Membrane and vascular injury

Whether or not fracture of the skull takes place, an impact to the head may tear membranes and cause intracranial haemorrhage. Blood accumulates in the epidural, subdural or subarachnoid spaces according to its source. Epidural bleeding normally follows rupture of the middle or posterior meningeal arteries by violent transmitted force. The dura is lifted locally by the haemorrhage, bulges into the interior of the skull cavity, and displaces brain tissue. After a latent period during which blood accumulates, the injured person may appear dazed or temporarily concussed but soon lapses into unconsciousness as intracranial tension increases. Subdural bleeding is often associated with subarachnoid bleeding and develops by leakage from torn perforating dural veins. Escaping blood may remain localized or may spread slowly across the brain by its own pressure and by gravity. Symptoms may be quite slow to develop.

Brain injury

Inertial loading of the head, whether from impact or from impulsive loading, causes such rapid movement of the head that resultant injuries are due only to the manner in which the head moves. Head motion results in strains within the brain tissue, which can cause either functional or structural damage by two possible mechanisms. Differential movement of the skull and brain can be produced by head acceleration. A relative movement occurs because the brain is free to move to some degree within the skull and because, due to inertia, the brain movement momentarily lags behind the skull movement. In combination, these factors allow the skull and dura to move relative to the brain surface, causing localized strain at the brain surface. The parasagittal bridging veins, which are particularly susceptible to localized strain, may tear if the vascular strain tolerance is exceeded. A relative displacement in excess of some 10 mm stretches these vessels beyond their elastic limit, with resulting rupture and haemorrhage. Furthermore, it is thought that the movement of the brain away from the skull creates regions of low pressure that may be responsible for contra-coup contusions. Head motion is also injurious, as it produces strain within the brain parenchyma, leading to classical cerebral concussion, diffuse axonal injury and associated tissue-tear injury. Data suggest that the different densities of the white and grey matter result in different velocities of propagation of the mechanical impact wave through the brain parenchyma, thereby causing stress and strain. In each type of injury, the acceleration or movement of the head causes either a functional or a structural failure of neural or vascular structures, where the severity and extent of disruption are linked to the magnitude, rate, duration, direction and types of inertial loading.

Impact acceleration can be made up of two components: translational and rotational acceleration. Translational acceleration occurs when the centre of mass of the head is moved (accelerated) in a straight line; rotational acceleration occurs when the head is rotated around its centre of mass. With the exception of horizontal plane movements, pure translational acceleration is uncommon. As the head is anchored by the neck, the usual acceleration is angular acceleration, whereby the head centre of mass angulates about a point typically in the mid or lower cervical region.

Pioneering workers in the field of head injury attributed intracranial damage to deformations and accelerations of the skull and pressure gradients caused by skull deformations and acceleration due to direct impact. Translational acceleration initially was considered to be the most important mechanism, while rotational acceleration was thought to be of minimal significance. However, later research indicated that inertial rotation alone could not produce the levels of injury caused by direct impact, and about twice the rotational velocity was required to produce cerebral concussion by indirect impact (or whiplash) (Ommaya *et al.* 1966). Furthermore, it was suggested that rotation could account for approximately half of the potential for brain injury, while the remainder was attributed to direct impact. Other researchers demonstrated that translation of the head in the horizontal plane produced only focal effects, resulting in well-circumscribed cerebral contusions and intracerebral haematomas, and diffuse injuries were seen only when a rotational component was present (Gennarelli *et al.* 1972, 1996). It is believed that the principal mechanism of pure translation appears to be pressure gradient, while that of pure rotation appears to be shear stress. Angular acceleration was proposed as the cause of gliding contusions resulting from excessive strain in cerebral vessels, and the site of maximum shear occurred at a constant distance for the surface of the brain. It has also been shown that the deeper parts of the brain could be injured while the surface was uninjured and that the zone

of maximum shear became deeper as the angular acceleration pulse duration increased. Further work investigated the role of rotational acceleration in causing brain injury in live primates and physical models (Gennarelli and Thibault 1982; Gennarelli *et al.* 1981, 1982; Thibault and Gennarelli 1986). This work established that angular acceleration is the most injurious in the production of concussive injuries, diffuse axonal injury and subdural haematomas and that virtually every known type of head injury can be produced by angular acceleration.

HEAD INJURY TOLERANCE

The impact response of the head has been studied, and the forces needed to fracture the skull are reasonably well known; however, the mechanical response of the brain is difficult to quantify. Pioneering work on linear skull fractures using cadavers and anaesthetized animals led to the development of the Wayne State tolerance curve (WSTC) (Figure 11.1). The WSTC is a plot of effective head acceleration against impact duration and is based on a mixture

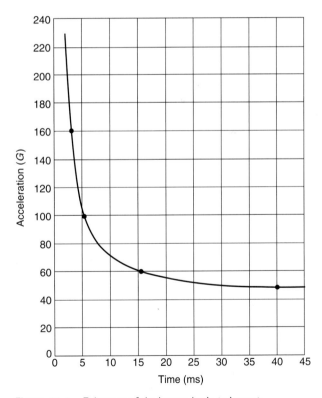

Figure 11.1 *Tolerance of the human brain to impact acceleration. The curve was developed at Wayne State University and describes the time for which a given acceleration must be applied to produce cerebral concussion. The four dots, reading from left to right, represent velocity changes of 4, 5, 9 and 20 m/s, respectively.*

of data from human cadaver drop tests, animal experimentation involving frontal hammer blows and airblasts to the exposed brain, and human volunteer sled tests. It cannot be considered definitive, as there was a considerable degree of scatter in the data, but a hyperbolic tolerance curve was drawn through the data points.

The WSTC indicates that high head accelerations are tolerable, provided that the duration is short. The WSTC utilized the peak value of the acceleration encountered, but this was subsequently changed to 'effective' acceleration, which is interpreted as average acceleration of the impact pulse. The procedure for deriving the curve exhibited a number of deficiencies, including:

- poor definition of the type of acceleration parameter to be utilized and failure to address the presence of acceleration spikes
- lack of applicability to blows other than those used in its construction
- inadequate correlation of data with living humans
- initial acceleration measurement at the contra-coup position, which may require modification due to skull resonances and vibrations.

Nevertheless, the WSTC represents one of the cornerstones for biomechanical injury criteria serving as a comparison for more recently derived models.

Gadd (1966) used the WSTC curve to derive a means of assessing the likelihood of sustaining a head injury from the acceleration–time curve of an impact. He analysed the pulse duration of an impact in its entirety rather than just the peak acceleration and determined that between 4 and 50 ms on the acceleration–time curve the WSTC is almost a straight line with a slope of −2.5 if plotted logarithmically. This he represented mathematically as the Gadd severity index (GSI), where a tolerance level of less than 1000 was stipulated as acceptable and was considered to be the median point between those occupants who survived and those who did not. A concern with the GSI is that it can give unrealistically high values for impacts that typically have much longer pulse duration. An example of such are impacts with automobile airbags or padded surfaces that are known to be less injurious, but the GSI would predict that injuries would occur despite accident and experimental evidence to the contrary.

The GSI had been developed further into the head injury criterion (HIC), which is the current standard for the Federal Motor Vehicle Safety Standard 208. The HIC is a linear head injury model developed for use in the automotive industry to assess impacts of anthropomorphic test dummy heads on to the interior structures of automobiles. The formulation of the HIC is similar to that of the GSI, but the mathematical process calculates the maximum value of the HIC over only a part of the acceleration pulse and considers only the more injurious portion of the impact pulse around the peak of the acceleration waveform.

A HIC of less than 1000 is considered to be an acceptable level, as at this value there is a 16 per cent risk of life-threatening brain injury (Figure 11.2). However, one of the difficulties with this formula is that it ascribes to the entire event a level of severity that is based on only part of the impact event. Furthermore, it contains no reference to rotational kinematics and is a poor approximation of the empirical data on which the WSTC was based. As a result, the formulation produces numbers that are too high when impacts last longer than 20 ms. Rather than correcting a fundamentally unsound equation, the current approach is to limit the time interval to the 15 ms around the peak acceleration. This has the effect of keeping the HIC artificially low in order to correspond better to reality.

Since the recognition that rotational motion may be more likely to correlate with brain injury, a number of studies have attempted to set limits for angular acceleration and angular velocity. A scaling relationship was used for the animal data to extrapolate them to adult humans. Rotational movement of the head provides far more opportunity for the brain to move relative to the skull and to distort than does linear motion. Rotational motion probably results in more significant shear strains leading to tissue disruption, but the rotational accelerations alone do not provide a complete description of events to provide a satisfactory correlation with injuries. New data may suggest that measurement of strain and strain rate, and in particular the strain/strain rate product, may be better

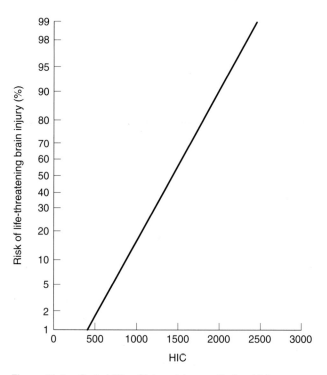

Figure 11.2 *Probability of injury risk curve for head injury criterion (HIC) for peak acceleration duration of 15 ms (after Mertz 1994).*

predictors of injury outcome. However, as yet this has limited practical significance, as strain and strain rate can be measured only on cadavers using radio-opaque markers inserted into the brain tissue.

Alternative surrogates for brain injury research are finite-element computer models. Ever increasingly sophisticated computer models are starting to provide information that is useful in the investigation of human injury due to impact. The use of such models allows the brain's response in the form of acceleration, strain, stress and pressure to be calculated. In particular, the models should be able to relate the degree and severity of the physiological changes and/or structural failure for a given mechanical input. A number of injury mechanisms have been postulated for brain injury, but more experimental confirmation of how the human brain is injured due to rotational acceleration is still needed. This would permit mathematical surrogates to become more advanced in the prediction of human response to blunt head trauma. In the case of translational acceleration, the HIC appears to be a valid tolerance criterion. However, there is no criterion for angular acceleration; this is problematic, as most head injuries result from a combination of linear and rotational acceleration. A suitable criterion combining linear and rotational acceleration therefore is required.

IMPACT ENERGY AND PROTECTION

To consider methods of head protection, a clear understanding of the human tolerance to each potential injury mechanism is essential. The relationships between velocity, acceleration and stopping distance on head impact can be made clear by means of an example. Assume that a human head weighing 5 kg and travelling at a velocity of 10 m/s strikes a solid wall. The frontal bone fractures and is depressed to a depth of 20 mm (0.02 m). Then, from the laws of motion,

$$v^2 = 2as$$

where v is the velocity (in m/s), a is the acceleration (in m/s^2) and s is the stopping distance (in m).

Then,

$$a = \frac{10^2}{(2 \times 0.02)} = 2500 \text{ m/s}^2 = 255 \text{ G}$$

The force (F) acting on the head (or wall) is given by mass multiplied by acceleration:

$$F = 5 \times 255 \text{ G, or } 1275 \text{ N}$$

The kinetic energy (KE) of the head before impact is given by $1/2mv^2$:

$$KE = 1/2 \times 5 \times 10^2 = 250 \text{ J}$$

If a constant deceleration of the head is assumed, then the duration of the impact (t) is given by the velocity divided by the acceleration:

$$t = \frac{10}{2500} = 0.004 \text{ s} = 4.0 \text{ ms}$$

It should be noted that if the skull had not fractured, then the stopping distance would have been much less (perhaps only 3 mm). In that case, the deceleration would have been 1700 G, the force 8.5 kN and the duration 0.6 ms. The input energy would still have been 250 J. This example emphasizes the profound importance of stopping distance on the forces imposed by a given head impact. It also shows how the skull and soft tissues can, as a result of a certain amount of deformation, protect the brain from excessive acceleration. The relationship between stopping distance, impact velocity and acceleration is shown in Figure 11.3.

METHODS OF PREVENTING HEAD INJURY

The problem of preventing head injury on impact may be approached in a number of ways.

Restraint harnesses can do much to prevent contact of the head with surrounding structures. However, even with acceptable harness restraint, there may be multidirectional flailing of the head, arms and legs. A more effective means of preventing contact of the head with surrounding structures during crash deceleration is by provision of a suitable head-restraint system, such as an airbag.

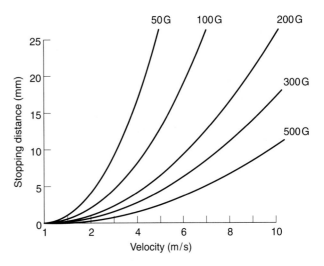

Figure 11.3 *Relationship between velocity change and stopping distance for five levels of uniform deceleration. For example, a velocity change (Δv) of 7.5 m/s requires 10 mm of theoretically perfect padding to stay within 300 G.*

The provision of adequate space in the cockpit within the occupant's immediate environment helps to reduce the injury associated with flailing of the head and contact with surrounding structures. Space is usually at a premium, however, and it is not always possible to site structural parts of the aircraft at a sufficient distance.

Where it is not possible to design the cockpit in such a way that the occupant's head is prevented from striking surrounding objects, it may be possible to treat surfaces in order to minimize injury. Injurious surfaces or projections within the head's flail envelope may be constructed from deformable material to provide a measure of energy absorption, and control knobs and switches may be made to preferentially fracture if impacted – so-called de-lethalization of the cockpit. Although many aircraft cockpits are designed following this principle, the structures and equipment used are far from ideal. However, some, for example the parachute-containing headbox on ejection seats, have been shown to be effective energy absorbers and are designed to improve head protection in high-speed ejections without any increase in helmet mass. Although the primary aim should always be to eliminate potentially lethal head impacts, in practice it is usually necessary to resort to personal head protection. Thus, the provision of a protective helmet for aircrew is now the standard method of reducing the risk of serious head injury in aircraft operations.

MECHANICS OF HELMET HEAD PROTECTION

Distribution of impact load and prevention of skull deformation

There are several possible mechanisms whereby a helmet can protect the head during impact. It can distribute the impact load so as to prevent or reduce soft-tissue injury. Similarly, it can prevent deformation of the skull and so increase tolerance to linear acceleration to the 300-G level. In either case, the requirement is for a strong inflexible shell. However, if the shell is separated from the skull by an appropriate distance, then some flexion or distortion of the shell becomes acceptable. In this case, the load has to be transmitted to a large area of cranium by a suitable suspension system or padding. A measure of the potential benefit afforded by a rigid helmet shell is given by a simple example:

A light aircraft makes a controlled wheels-up landing on a rough field and slows to rest at a modest 5 G, a level of acceleration that would be readily tolerated in terms of whole-body response. However, at 5 G, the pilot is unable to prevent his head and upper torso being thrown forwards inertially, and his head travels some 30 cm before striking the top edge of the instrument panel. In the time taken for the head to cover this distance, the aircraft velocity will have decreased by 5.4 m/s, and it is at this relative velocity that the head strike will occur (assuming no resistance to head motion from the neck musculature). Taking head mass as 5 kg, the impact energy will be 73.5 J. Without head protection, the 3 mm stopping distance offered by the soft tissues of the scalp will give an average deceleration to the head of 500 G. Acting over a small area, this greatly exceeds the strength of the frontal bone, so that a fracture will occur, with damage to the underlying brain tissue.

The same head, but wearing a well-designed protective helmet, would impact at the same velocity, but the impact energy would actually be increased by the added helmet mass to some 100 J. However, by distributing the impact over a greater area, skull distortion and fracture are prevented. In addition, the protective padding component of the helmet (see below) affords an additional 15 mm of stopping distance. The available 18 mm now allows the head to be brought to rest at an average 83 G, well below the injury threshold. Thus, not only will there be no brain damage, but also the avoidance of even transient concussion allows the pilot to extricate himself promptly in the event of a post-crash fire.

Provision of finite stopping distance

The provision of a finite stopping distance by a protective helmet can reduce the peak acceleration imposed in a given impact. Since the velocity change will be unaltered, the reduced acceleration will be applied for a longer time. In the example given above, a six-fold increase in stopping distance (from 3 to 18 mm) afforded a six-fold reduction in average deceleration (from 500 to 83 G), although the duration of the impact event was also increased by a factor of six (from 1.1 to 6.7 ms). In practice, the maximum stopping distance that can be built into a protective helmet is about 25 mm – more than this, and the device becomes unacceptably bulky. Even this theoretically available 25 mm is reduced by the relatively inefficient energy-absorbing materials that can be integrated into a practicable helmet, and only some 15 mm is actually available in which to reduce the relative velocity between head and struck object to zero before the material bottoms out and the transmitted force rises.

There are two basic energy-absorbing systems that can be used in protective helmets. Certain helmets employ a fibre-glass shell that breaks up on impact. The impact load is transmitted to the head and distributed widely by means of a suspension harness, which initially provides an air gap of about 25 mm. Each time a glass fibre ruptures or is pulled out of its resin matrix, energy is absorbed inelastically. This technique requires a strong rigid shell. A second technique makes use of a layer of rigid foam beneath the shell, which crushes on impact to about 40 per cent of its initial thickness. In this design, a lighter shell can be employed.

An important consideration of helmet design is to tune the padding material to human tolerance levels, such that the material crushes at a level of transmitted force that is just tolerable. Such padding will appear very hard and will not crush to any significant extent in a minor impact. For comfort, a double layer of padding is desirable, the inner layer of which is more yielding. In any event, all materials used should be energy-absorbing; this principle can also be applied to other helmet components such as ear cups. The hard outer shell with a crushable liner method is used widely for helmets produced in large numbers, e.g. in protective helmets for motorcyclists, as the major components can be produced cheaply and effectively by injection moulding using thermoplastics. Hybrid designs are available that use a combination of frangible shell, energy-absorbing foam and harness suspension, although the reduced air gap means that the harness is used mainly for fitting the helmet to individual heads rather than for energy absorption. Other helmets use a frangible shell and energy-absorbing padding, with additional comfort foam pads for individual sizing. This system with its reduced air space may incur a greater heat load, and its frangible shell is more liable to damage in routine use. Newer state-of-the-art helmets employ form-fit liners, which are custom-fitted to the individual aircrew member's head size and shape. In a helmet in which energy is absorbed elastically (as occurs to a certain extent with a thermoplastics shell and padding), the helmeted head will rebound on impact, and the impact energy will be increased by the addition of a post-impact head velocity. This effect is minimized with the low coefficient of restitution afforded by a frangible shell.

Protection against rotational acceleration

A very heavy helmet could reduce head angular acceleration by increasing the rotational inertia of the whole head, but only at the expense of excessive weight and an increased risk of neck injury. Hence, this mechanism has never been employed deliberately in the design of aircrew protective helmets. If a helmeted head strikes a surface at an acute angle, then the head may either slide or roll along the surface, depending on friction at the contact area. If the helmet shell is made smooth and external protuberances reduced to a minimum, then the tendency to slide is increased and rotational acceleration is reduced. For the same reason, any essential projections should be fared or designed to break away at a non-injurious force level. Novel helmet designs are being developed for motorcyclists, which incorporate multidirectional impact protection systems consisting of sliding outer shells. On impact, the shell glides over the underlying layer to reduce the rotational accelerations and velocities imparted on the brain.

Extent of helmet protection and retention

All of the mechanisms for protecting the head that have been discussed above protect only the area actually covered. Overall protection is compromised by the need to provide an adequate field of vision and head mobility. Helmets must be retained following an impact so that protection is available in the event of a repeated insult. Investigations of aircraft accidents have shown that multiple impacts are not uncommon. During the ejection sequence, the head could strike canopy fragments and the seat headbox, then strike against the separating seat, and then sustain a final ground strike on landing. Furthermore, aircraft crashes rarely impose a single axis of deceleration, and multiple head impacts are likely to occur. Despite careful fitting and the use of a chinstrap and an adjustable neck strap, helmet losses still occur, especially during high-speed ejections, as a result of high aerodynamic lift forces.

Windblast protection

In high-speed ejection, the body is suddenly thrust into an airstream that can exert a windblast pressure as great as 60 kPa at 600 knot. This pressure on the face may cause petechial and conjunctival haemorrhages and, if the mouth is open and unprotected, blast damage to the lungs. If, due to the initial posture, or as a result of the ejection forces, the head is not in contact with the headbox, then the head will be forced back by the windblast with a potentially injurious impact. Face protection in high-speed ejection is essential. The protection can be provided by an oxygen mask and visor of adequate strength to be retained during the ejection sequence.

TESTS FOR HELMET PROTECTION

No dedicated helmet standard for civilian aviation use was forthcoming until the 1990s (British Standards Institution 1996). Unlike earlier specifications, which defined helmets in terms of their materials, dimensions and production, the later performance standards defined helmets largely in terms of their function, i.e. instead of describing the helmets, the standards defined how to test the helmets. The standards served two immediate purposes: tools for the evaluation of existing helmet designs and guides for the development of new headgear.

In the UK, the military aircrew helmets currently in use are based on design standards of motorcycle helmets. In the past, there was no specific standard for military aircrew helmets. The Mk4 helmet used in rotary-wing aircraft and in fixed-wing aircraft for certain roles is tested against BS

2495, while the Mk10 or ALPHA helmet is used in aircraft fitted with ejection seats and is tested to BS 6658. Both standards were developed for the evaluation of motorcycle helmets; with the introduction of a new European standard, EN regulation 22, they will be superseded. EN regulation 22 is the result of many years of analysis of motorcycle helmet impact data, with the standard better reflecting the threat seen in motorcycle accidents. As a result, it makes its use in the procurement of aircrew helmets less tenable and makes the development of helmet test standards specifically for aircrew helmets all the more important. In the UK, a helmet standard has now been developed specifically for aircrew helmets; as with all helmet design standards it covers three major aspects: resistance to penetration, shock absorption and retention.

The standard was developed from the findings of research programmes that included assessment of existing equipment and the cockpit environment, detailed review of aircrew accident statistics including impact events and injury outcomes, impact test methodology, and evaluation techniques for damaged helmets. Two types of helmet are specified: type E for use in aircraft fitted with ejection seats and type S for aircraft fitted with static seats.

For convenience and consistency, all performance figures quoted below refer to the new UK military aircrew helmet impact standard.

Penetration resistance

To evaluate a helmet's resistance to penetration, the test helmet is mounted on a rigid headform and struck by a conical striker with a 0.5 mm radius tip. The striker weighs 1.8 kg. For a type E helmet, the striker is dropped in guided freefall from a height of 1.5 m; for a type S helmet, the striker weighs 3.0 kg and the drop height is 3 m. Test failure occurs by detecting penetration by transient electrical contact between the tip of the striker and a soft metal insert at the top of the headform.

Shock absorption

The test helmet is mounted on an instrumented headform and dropped in guided freefall on to either a flat or a hemispherical anvil. A typical helmet impact test tower is illustrated in Figure 11.4. The headform and its supporting carriage have a combined mass of 5 kg; the impact velocities, measured just before impact are given in Table 11.1. Each impact is followed by a second impact at the same site but at half the energy; on no occasion must the acceleration of the headform exceed 300 G. Helmets may be impacted at any point of the crown as well as laterally and posteriorly down to within about 40 mm of a basic plane

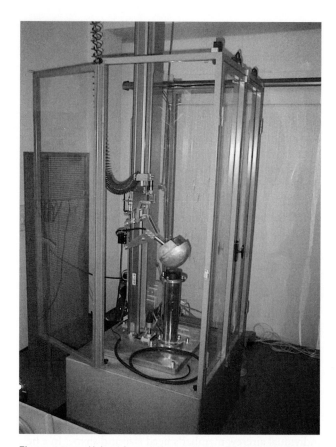

Figure 11.4 *Helmet impact drop test rig, with a monorail tower on to which the headform and helmet are attached and dropped under guided freefall on to the test anvil. The impact accelerations are measured by accelerometers mounted in the headform.*

defined as that passing through the external auditory meatus and inferior margin of the orbit.

Helmet retention

In this test, the helmet is mounted on a rigidly fixed headform and the chinstrap is preloaded through an artificial chin from which hangs a vertical bar at the lower end of which there is a stop. A magnetically released mass of 10 kg can be dropped 0.75 m down the bar, so as to impact the stop and produce a sudden jerk load. A 7 kg preload takes the slack out of the system, and maximum displacement

Table 11.1 *Representative impact velocities for shock-attenuation testing of aircrew helmets*

Impact	Anvil face	Impact velocity (m/s)	
		Type E helmet	Type S helmet
First	Flat	7.5	7.5
	Hemispherical	6.0	7.0
Second	Flat	5.3	5.3

criteria ensure that a peak force of the order of 3–4 kN must be withstood without failure or excessive stretch, either of which could result in helmet loss.

Assessment of protection

Aircrew helmets that have been involved in an ejection or crash should be examined and assessed for the protection afforded to the wearer. Close examination can reveal any impact damage, and witness marks may indicate the nature of the object struck. In suitable cases, impact tests should be conducted against a representative anvil using undamaged helmets to assess the impact forces involved in the accident; these are then compared with known human tolerance levels and the actual outcome of the accident.

OTHER FUNCTIONS OF PROTECTIVE HELMETS

Apart from providing protection against impact accelerations, protective helmets fulfil other major functions in aviation. They are mentioned here only briefly.

Helmets contribute towards achieving high levels of speech intelligibility and preventing hearing loss by reducing noise that gains access to the ear through the helmet structure. The predominant factor is the performance of the ear cup and the seal that it provides to the skin around the ear. If the ear cup is constructed from crushable materials, it can offer additional impact protection without any increase in helmet weight.

For aircrew, an antiglare filter is essential for flight. The neutral-density filter is placed as close to the eyes as possible and is adjustable so that it protects from glare but still allows the pilot to see the instruments. The antiglare visor must be as light as possible so as to stay in place during high-G manoeuvres and to keep the total mass of the helmet as low as possible.

Nuclear explosions may result in flash-blindness or retinal burns from the fireball directly or indirectly from atmospheric scatter. Protective headgear may include, or be worn with, devices that protect against nuclear flash. Similarly, headgear may also be required to integrate with chemical defence respirators or other devices worn by aircrew to protect against chemical and biological agents.

The hazard of bird-strike is always present during low-level flight. To protect the eyes from splinters of broken transparency and bird remains, the helmet must carry a visor made of polycarbonate (3 mm thick), which covers the area of the face and eyes. The lower edge of the polycarbonate visor must abut closely (gap less than 5 mm) against the oronasal mask, and it must be possible to lock down the visor in order to protect against windblast. In addition to supporting the visor, the helmet also acts as a platform from which to suspend an oxygen mask.

An extension of the head-up display principle with an aircraft-mounted collimator is to project the display information on to the inside surface of the helmet visor, where it may be viewed independently of head position. Similarly, a sight can be placed over a target by moving the head and an appropriate aim angle computed from measured head orientation. Either device requires helmet-mounted (or helmet-integrated) electronic and optical components, which will add to its mass and need to be mounted so that the centre of gravity of the helmeted head is not unduly displaced from its normal position. Heavier objects, such as night-vision goggles, which must be mounted in front of the eyes, may be counterbalanced by placing other components, such as batteries, to the rear of the helmet; provision may also be made for the goggles to separate from the helmet before ejection or impact, so as to reduce forces imposed on the neck.

HELMET COMFORT

As with other items of personal equipment, headgear should not be uncomfortable or impair the efficiency with which the wearer can perform duties inside or outside the cockpit. This is difficult to achieve, particularly if the helmet is heavy, poorly balanced, or required to keep the eye fixed in relation to helmet-mounted optics. A helmet must not impair the wearer's ability to board the aircraft, strap in securely or egress in an emergency.

When the helmet is worn in aircraft frequently exposed to sustained accelerations or vibrations, the total weight of the entire headgear ideally should not exceed 1.7 kg. The weight of the helmet and components should be well distributed over the head, and the centre of gravity of the headgear–head combination should be as close as possible to that of the head alone. The increase in the moment of inertia of the head due to the headgear should also be kept as low as possible. Since the weight of the headgear is distributed around the circumference of the head, its angular inertia (proportional to the square of the radius) increases to a greater degree than its weight. Even a simple full-face motorcyclist's helmet doubles the angular inertia of the wearer's head. The helmet should be as compact as possible to keep it away from the cockpit structure, seat, canopy and other items of aircrew personal flying equipment, to improve effective vision, and to allow free movement of the head. The outer surface of the helmet should be kept as smooth as possible in shape and texture. Any components mounted on the outer shell of the helmet should be contoured smoothly to reduce the effects of glancing blows and to avoid snagging hazards, such as with the parachute risers following ejection.

The weight of the helmet should be distributed over as large an area of the head as possible. The wearer should be able to alter the distribution and magnitude of any local pressure points and have some range of adjustment during wear (e.g. by altering tension in the chinstrap). The headgear may have to be worn for several hours at a time, and pressure points that are tolerable initially can become highly distracting, annoying and fatiguing with prolonged wear.

To be effective, the helmet must be clasped firmly to the head. It should not move when the head is moved voluntarily or involuntarily as a result of vibration or sustained accelerations; this is particularly important when the headgear includes sights and displays. A stable fit depends on good initial adjustment of the webbing harness, so that it fits snugly around the head. The chinstrap and an oxygen mask help to keep it in place, and the ear cups can provide additional sideways stability.

The user should be able to put on and take off the helmet easily and without assistance and to put on or remove parts of the assembly or the mask in the narrow confines of a cockpit.

The helmet should not impose any visual restriction. The wearer should not need to carry out excessive head movements to see above or behind in combat or to see essential cockpit instruments. The lower part of the helmet should not produce any significant restriction of head movement, either by preventing full neck mobility or by coming up against items of personal equipment worn on the upper trunk (e.g. a life preserver or other floatation device).

REFERENCES

British Standards Institution. Specification for helmets for airborne sports. BS EN 966. London: British Standards Institution, 1996.

Cairns H, Holbourn H. Head injuries in motorcyclists with special reference to crash helmets. *British Medical Journal* 1943; 1: 591–8.

Gadd CW. Use of a weighted impulse criterion for estimating injury hazard. In: *Proceedings of the 10th Stapp Car Crash Conference*. New York: Society of Automotive Engineers, 1966; pp. 164–74.

Gennarelli TA, Thibault LE. Biomechanics of acute subdural hematoma. *Journal of Trauma* 1982; **22**: 680–86.

Gennarelli TA, Ommaya AK, Thibault LE. Comparison of translational and rotational head motions in experimental cerebral concussion. In: *Proceedings of the 15th Stapp Car Crash Conference*. New York: Society of Automotive Engineers, 1972; pp. 797–803.

Gennarelli TA, Adams JH, Graham DI. Acceleration induced head injury in the monkey. I: the model, its mechanistic and physiological correlates. *Acta Neuropathology* 1981; **7** (suppl.): 23–5.

Gennarelli TA, Thibault LE, Adams JH, *et al*. Diffuse axonal injury and traumatic coma in the primate. *Annals of Neurology* 1982; **12**: 564–74.

Gennarelli TA, Thibault LE, Ommaya AK. Pathophysiologic responses to rotational and translational acceleration of the head. In: Bachaitis S (ed.). *Biomechanics of Impact Injury and Injury Tolerances of the Head-Neck Complex*. Warrendale, PA: Society of Automotive Engineers, 1996; pp. 411–23.

Mertz H. Injury assessment values used to evaluate the hybrid III response measurements. In: Bachaitis S, Mertz H, (eds). *Hybrid III: The First Human-Like Crash Test Dummy*. Warrendale, PA: Society of Automotive Engineers, 1994; pp. 407–22.

Ommaya AK, Hirsch AE, Martinez JL. The role of whiplash in cerebral concussion. In: *Proceedings of the 10th Stapp Car Crash Conference*. New York: Society of Automotive Engineers, 1966; pp. 314–24.

Thibault LE, Gennarelli TA. Biomechanics of diffuse brain injuries. In: *Proceedings of the 10th International Technical Conference on Experimental Safety*. Washington, DC: NHTSA, 1986; pp. 79–85.

FURTHER READING

AGARD. Impact head injury: responses, mechanisms, tolerance, treatment and countermeasures. Conference proceedings 597. Neuilly-sur-Seine: AGARD/NATO, 1997.

Cooper GJ, Dudley HAF, Gann DS, *et al. Scientific Foundations of Trauma*. Oxford: Butterworth-Heinemann, 1997.

Yoganandan N, Pintar F, Larson S, Sances A. *Frontiers in Head and Neck Trauma*. Amsterdam: IOS Press, 1998.

12

Human physiology and the thermal environment

MIKE TIPTON

INTRODUCTION

Ecology, from the Greek *oikos* (house), is the branch of biology concerned with the study of the relationship between an organism and the environment in which it lives. For a subtropical human, the thermal environment of Earth can represent a hostile place.

Largely due to their intellectual development, humans have been able to spread out from their Equatorial origins to explore and inhabit the rest of the planet and the space that surrounds it. In so doing, they have endeavoured, through building, engineering and clothing, to maintain the same conditions around the body as applied in their ancestral home. Thus, if one measures the mean skin temperatures of an office worker in Portsmouth, a tribesperson in the Kalahari Desert and a Laplander in the far north, they will all approximate to 33 °C. It is a measure of human ingenuity and adaptability that we can run ultramarathons in the desert, swim the English Channel, fly fast jets, climb the highest mountains and walk on the moon. While such achievements can be inspirational and receive a good deal of media attention, many occupational groups, such as military pilots and ground crew, can be presented with a combination of physical and environmental demands that push them to their physiological limits. In these cases, the challenge represented by the environment is often compounded by the heat produced by the body and the specialist clothing and equipment used.

For an aviator, the consequences of being unable to cope with a given thermal environment in a cockpit or survival situation can range from subtle decrements in perform-

ance to death. Where along that continuum an individual is placed depends on a wide range of environmental, technical and physiological factors. Over the next two chapters, we explore the impact of the thermal characteristics of the environment on aviator performance and safety, in terms of threats (thermal stress), responses (thermoregulation and pathophysiological responses) and solutions (maintaining performance, enhancing the prospect of survival and treatment).

In this chapter, the basics of thermal physiology are outlined. The physical processes involved in heat production and heat exchange with the environment are presented, and the human physiological response to thermal stress is described. Methods for quantifying both the thermal stress represented by a particular environment and the thermal strain that such environments produce within the body are reviewed briefly. An understanding of these basic principles and techniques should enable an individual to assess and prioritize the thermal threats within an environment.

In the chapter that follows, the threats associated with the thermal environment are identified, and methods to prevent and treat them are outlined.

THERMAL STRESS

Heat and temperature

In 1714, having developed the mercury-in-glass thermometer, Fahrenheit produced the scale that bears his name. In 1742, Celsius, a Swedish astronomer, proposed a scale with 100 degrees between the freezing and boiling points of water; this became known as the centigrade scale and subsequently the Celsius scale. To this day, temperature is measured using a variety of linear scales, including Celsius (°C, the Système International d'Unités (SI)-derived unit to describe temperature and temperature intervals), Fahrenheit (°F) and Kelvin (K, the SI temperature unit and the preferred unit to express thermodynamic temperature). The Celsius scale is related directly to the Kelvin scale (1 °C = 1 K), but Kelvin begins at absolute zero (−273.15 °C), the temperature below which a system achieves its lowest energy state.

The SI unit of heat energy is the joule (J), named after James Joule (1818–89), who, in addition to Julius Mayer (1814–78), demonstrated that heat is a form of energy that can be exchanged freely between inanimate objects and living organisms. Heat energy is associated with the movement of individual atoms or molecules. Rates of heat exchange (flow or flux) are usually measured in Watts (1 W = 1 J/s).

Heat and temperature are related by the specific heat capacity of a substance (c_p), i.e. the amount of heat energy required to raise the temperature of a unit mass of a material by 1 K (1 °C). The volume-specific heat capacity of a substance is obtained by multiplying the specific heat of a substance by its density (Table 12.1). Humans can be considered an open energy system into which energy can pass (influx) and from which energy escapes (efflux). The thermal energy retained is quantified in terms of tissue temperature; this changes proportionally with the average kinetic energy of its molecules. In human tissues, efflux of 3.47 kJ (0.83 kcal) of thermal energy from 1 kg of tissue results in an average tissue temperature reduction of 1 °C (mean specific heat of tissue; see Table 12.1).

Air and water: a comparison of two fluids

Although air and water are both fluids, their physical characteristics differ significantly. At 37 °C, the volume-specific heat capacity of water is 3431 times that of air; this explains the relatively greater cooling power of water compared with air. In addition, the body surface area available for heat exchange in water comes close to 100 per cent.

Table 12.1 *Physical characteristics of air, water and human tissue at 37 °C (300 K)*

	Thermal conductivity (mW/m²/K)	Specific heat (J/g/K)	Density (g/cm³)
Human tissue	–	3.47–3.56	–
Air	26.2	1.007	0.0012
Water	630.5	4.1785	0.9922

These differences between air and water have several practical consequences. In resting individuals thermo-neutral water temperature (temperature in which body temperature remains stable with only changes in skin blood flow) averages about 35 °C with a narrow range. This compares with 26 °C and a broader range in air. Skin temperature falls faster and further on immersion in water than in an air environment; upon water immersion, skin temperature is quickly 'clamped' close to water temperature. Deep body temperature cools two to five times more quickly during immersion in cold water compared with in air at the same temperature. Immersion in cold water can produce responses, such as the cold shock response (discussed in the next chapter), which, because of a slower rate of fall of skin temperature, are not seen on exposure to cold air. In addition, in comparison with air, cold water produces more profound responses earlier and at higher temperatures. For example, in lean individuals, peripheral blood flow and, as a consequence, tissue conductance are minimized when immersed in water below about 30 °C; the equivalent air temperature is 10 °C. On average, water temperature can be 11 °C higher than that of air and produce an equivalent physiological response.

A stationary upright body in air at sea level is surrounded by one atmosphere of pressure and gravity; this allows venous pooling in the lower extremities. In contrast, the greater density of water means that in a head-out upright posture, the body has a differential hydrostatic pressure over it and is in a near-weightless environment. As a consequence, a negative transthoracic pressure of about 14.7 mmHg is established, which results in negative-pressure breathing. There is a consequent cephalad redistribution of blood, which, within six heart beats of immersion, can increase central blood volume by up to 700 ml. This is associated with enhanced diastolic filling, a raised right atrial pressure and a 32–66 per cent increase in cardiac output due entirely to an increase in stroke volume, which itself is due to enhanced filling of the heart rather than alterations in afterload and contractility. Most of the renal responses seen following immersion in thermoneutral water are due to the shift in blood volume, which the body senses as hypervolaemia. These responses include diuresis, natriuresis and kaliuresis. Diuresis is usually manifest by the first or second hour of immersion, and the natriuresis peaks by the fourth or fifth hour of immersion. In fully hydrated sodium-replete individuals, head-out upright immersion can result in 200–300 per cent increases in sodium excretion and free-water clearance, with urine output reaching 350 ml/hour.

Heat (energy) balance

The first two laws of thermodynamics describe heat exchange between an object and the environment. They state that (i) energy cannot be created or destroyed but is transformed from one form to another (conservation of energy) and (ii) heat flows down a thermal gradient, i.e. from high to low temperatures. Thus, energy may be converted from one form to another (e.g. from that stored in a substance, such as food or high-energy phosphate, to heat), but in a closed system its total quantity remains unchanged.

To remain in heat balance, the heat gained by the body must match that being lost from it, i.e. there should be no net change in the amount of heat stored (S) in the body. Failure to do this can result in hyper- or hypothermia. There are four physical routes by which heat may be exchanged with the environment: conduction (K), convection (C), radiation (R) and evaporation (E). Thermal exchange by K, C and R are variously referred to as 'dry', 'sensible' (measurable) and 'non-evaporative' heat transfer. This distinguishes them from 'evaporative' heat transfer (E).

The human heat-balance equation can be expressed in different forms but always contains terms for the generation of heat within the body, heat transfer with the environment and heat storage. The equation is the basis for assessing the effects of an environment on an organism. Because it describes the relationship between heat production and exchange with the environment, it is a mathematical expression of the first law of thermodynamics (energy conservation). The basic equation is:

$$M - (\pm W) = R \pm C \pm K - E \pm S$$

To remain in heat balance, S in the following rearranged equation must equal zero:

$$S = M - (\pm W) \pm R \pm C \pm K - E$$

where the terms are expressed as a rate of energy flow (flux) per unit area. The unit for each term is Watts (Joules/second), and it is traditional to standardize for people of different sizes by expressing the rates of heat gain or loss per square metre of total body surface area (W/m^2).[1]

M is the metabolic energy utilization (metabolic rate). W is measurable external work (this is positive when performing measurable external work and negative when work is performed on the subject).

For S to remain stable in a cool environment (below body temperature), the heat produced by M must be matched by that lost by K, C, R and E. In a hot environment (above body temperature), the heat produced by metabolism (M) and that gained by K, C and R must be matched by that lost by E (Figure 12.1). This emphasizes the importance of the evaporation of sweat in a hot environment and highlights the difference between the dry or sensible (measurable) routes of heat exchange and evaporative or insensible heat exchange (E).

If the body does not remain in heat balance, then, by definition, S will change and will be reflected in a change in mean body temperature (T_b) according to the equation

$$S = c_p m (d\overline{T}_b / dt)$$

where c_p is the specific heat of the body (in J/g/°C) and is about 3.5 kJ/kg/°C (0.83 kcal/kg/°C), m is the mass of the body (in kg), T_b is the mean body temperature (in °C; see below) and t is time (in s).

The terms in the heat-balance equation are considered in the following section.

[1]Body surface area can be estimated from the DuBois equation: $A_D = 0.202 \times W^{0.425} \times H^{0.725}$, where A_D is the surface area (in m^2), W is the mass of the body (in kg) and H is the height of the body (in m). A value of 1.8 m^2 for a 'standard man' of 70 kg mass and 1.73 m height is sometimes used.

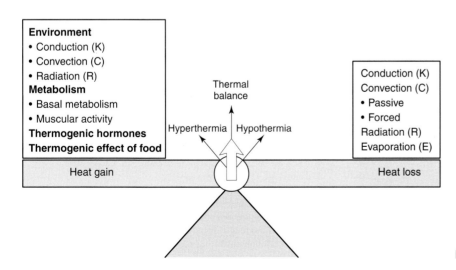

Figure 12.1 *Heat balance.*

METABOLISM

The catabolic chemical reactions of the body liberate energy, the sum total of which constitutes total metabolic energy utilization or rate (M). Some of this may be used when performing positive mechanical work ($+W$), but due to the chemical inefficiency of the body, much remains within the tissues as heat. Only 20–25 per cent of the chemical energy used during muscular contraction is converted into mechanical work; the remainder is liberated as heat. Normally, 67–85 per cent of an individual's total daily energy expenditure is due to the activities of the body that maintain vital functions. At complete rest, this basal metabolic rate (BMR) amounts to about 1 kcal/min (1440 kcal/day). The biggest cause of variation in energy expenditure comes with muscle activity, such as exercise and shivering.

Metabolic heat production can be measured by direct calorimetry. However, this requires time, engineering expertise and large and cumbersome equipment, such as a human calorimeter (a carefully controlled respiration chamber). An alternative and accurate approach is indirect calorimetry, which is based on the fact that all energy-releasing reactions in the body ultimately depend on oxygen, and a calorific value for oxygen can be determined if the steady-state non-protein respiratory quotient (RQ) is known:

$$RQ = V_{CO_2}/V_{O_2}$$

where V_{CO_2} is the carbon dioxide production (in litres/min) and V_{O_2} is the oxygen consumption (in litres/min).

Due to differences in the chemical structure of carbohydrates, fats and proteins, the amount of carbon dioxide produced per unit of oxygen consumed varies with nutrient mixture metabolized. Thus, measuring RQ is a way of estimating the mixture of substrates metabolized, on the basis of pulmonary gas exchange. From this, the thermal (energy) equivalents for oxygen consumption at different non-protein RQ can be obtained by reference to standard tables; some examples are given in Table 12.2. Alternatively, the following equation provides an estimation in kilojoules (divide by 4.1855 to convert to kilocalories):

$$21.168(0.23RQ + 0.77)$$

Table 12.2 *Thermal (caloric) equivalents for oxygen for non-protein steady-state respiratory quotient (RQ)*

Non–protein RQ	kcal/L O_2	% kcal from carbohydrate	% kcal from fat
0.707	4.686	0	100
0.82	4.825	40.3	59.7
1	5.047	100	0

Using the non-protein RQ assumes that no protein is being metabolized. Determining the contribution from protein metabolism requires urinary nitrogen analysis. However, in most cases, not doing this results in only a minimal error ($\approx$0.5 per cent) because the contribution of protein to energy metabolism is normally small, but it can increase in survival (starvation) situations (see Chapter 13).

Once the thermal equivalent has been established, energy expenditure can be determined from the following equation:

Energy expenditure (in kcal/min) $= V_{O_2} \times$ caloric equivalent per litre of O_2 at the given steady-state RQ

However, for activities ranging from complete rest to mild aerobic exercise, if it is assumed that about 40 per cent carbohydrate and 60 per cent fat are being metabolized, and an RQ of 0.82 is used to determine energy expenditure, then the maximum error possible in the estimation from steady-state oxygen consumption is only 4 per cent.

Various indirect calorimetry methods exist to measure oxygen consumption, all of which have a variety of logistical and theoretical pros and cons. Closed-circuit spirometry requires the subject to rebreathe from a spirometer filled with 100 per cent oxygen. Soda lime (potassium hydroxide) removes exhaled carbon dioxide, while oxygen removal from the system is recorded. This approach requires cumbersome equipment and is not suitable for exercising subjects.

Open-circuit spirometry is a simpler way of measuring oxygen consumption by measuring the oxygen removed from inspired air. This technique can be very accurate – within 0.2 per cent of that obtained by direct calorimetry. The subject inhales ambient air, and the concentration of their exhaled air is analysed for carbon dioxide and oxygen. Changes in these concentrations reflect metabolism and, with the additional measure of ventilation, can be used to calculate oxygen consumption and estimate energy expenditure as follows:

$$\dot{V}O_2 = (F_{I_{O_2}} \times V_I) - (F_{E_{O_2}} \times V_E)$$

where $\dot{V}O_2$ is the oxygen consumption (in l/min, STPD[2]), F_{IO_2} is the fractional concentration of oxygen in the inspired air, V_I is the inspired volume (in l/min, STPD)[3],

[2]STPD is the volume at standard temperature (0 °C), pressure (760 mmHg), dry (no water vapour).

[3]Fractional concentration of carbon dioxide in the expired air is required to determine V_I from V_E when the RQ is not 1 (1 − %O_2 expired − %CO_2 expired = %N_2 expired, then *Haldane transformation*). When RQ is less than 1, slightly more O_2 is being consumed than the amount of carbon dioxide being produced (RQ = V_{CO_2}/V_{O_2}) and therefore V_E is smaller than V_I.

F_{EO_2} is the fractional concentration of oxygen in the exhaled air, and V_E is the expired volume (in l/min, STPD).

The classic method for measuring oxygen consumption involves collecting expired air via a mouthpiece in a Douglas bag for subsequent analysis of gas concentrations and volume. Various automated portable devices also exist that measure and report oxygen consumption. These are particularly useful during activity and in the field.

Another technique worthy of note is an isotope-based method that employs double-labelled water (i.e. water containing a known concentration of the stable isotopes of hydrogen – ^2H, or deuterium – and oxygen – ^{18}O, or oxygen-18). This technique is useful in that subjects can be free-living and are not required to wear a mouthpiece for respiratory data collection. However, the technique measures CO_2 production, and this must be related to O_2 consumption via an estimation of RQ. This technique does not provide highly accurate estimations of the energy expenditure of an individual; it is within three to five per cent of directly measured energy expenditure in a controlled setting. This discrepancy probably increases in the field.

RADIATION

Thermal radiation is part of the electromagnetic spectrum that ranges from gamma rays and X-rays (short wavelength: 0.1–100 Å), through visible light (wavelength 0.4–0.8 μm), to radio waves (long wavelength: 1 mm–100 km). The ultraviolet (UV) portion of the spectrum is divided into UV-A (wavelength 320–400 nm), UV-B (wavelength 290–320 nm) and UV-C (wavelength 200–290 nm). Although comparatively little UV-B radiation reaches the Earth, it is very efficient at causing sunburn and has been shown to cause cancer in laboratory animals and humans. Over the shortwave radiation spectrum, white skin absorbs about 60 per cent of the incident radiation, while dark skin absorbs about 80 per cent. However, dark-skinned individuals are less susceptible to sunburn: dark skin allows less penetration than white skin of solar radiation, as some radiation is absorbed in the pigmented melanin layer.

All objects possessing heat emit thermal radiation from their surfaces in the form of a wave of energy containing particles (photons) within the red–infrared range (between visible light and shorter radio waves) of the electromagnetic spectrum (wavelength 0.8–80 μm). The peak wavelength of the emitted radiation is inversely proportional to the absolute temperature of the emitting surface; this is the basis for estimating the temperature of a hot object by its colour. The energy from these particles is absorbed by, and transferred to, the atoms of objects they come into contact with. No medium is required for the transfer of heat by radiation (it occurs across a vacuum), it is independent of air movement, and the temperature of any air through which heat radiates has little effect on the heat transferred.

Radiation can be a major route of heat loss in certain specific scenarios: it is the process that enables heat to be gained from the sun on a cold day (direct, scattered or reflected solar radiation) and lost to a cloudless sky at night in the desert. Solar radiation refers to radiation in the 400–750-nm wavelengths emitted and received directly from the sun; it can provide in excess of 1000 W/m^2. Indirect solar radiation is an additional component due to reflections from the ground and clouds and from sunlight scattered throughout a clear sky: it can increase net solar radiation by 20–30 per cent compared with direct solar radiation.

Radiant heat is also responsible for high cockpit temperatures: the relatively short wavelength of solar radiation passes through cockpit transparencies and heats up internal surfaces. These, in turn, emit radiant heat, but at a longer wavelength, which is unable to pass through the canopy. As a consequence of this 'greenhouse effect', the cockpit temperature can increase significantly.

The quantity of heat transferred from one object to another by radiation depends on the following:

- Effective radiating surface area: when standing with the arms and legs extended away from the body, the radiating surface area is maximal, at about 75 per cent of the total body surface area. This reduces to about 50 per cent when the body is curled up in the fetal position.
- Difference between the mean surface temperatures of both objects.
- Emissivity (ε) of the surface: this is the ratio of heat emitted by the surface to that emitted by a perfect emitter (blackbody) at the same temperature. The Stefan–Boltzmann law defines the emission of a perfect blackbody.

Heat exchange between two surfaces by radiation is proportional to the difference in the fourth powers of their absolute temperatures. For practical purposes in human heat exchange, this is simplified to:

$$R = h_r(\overline{T}_{sk} - \overline{T}_R)A_r/A$$

where R is the radiant heat exchange (in W/m^2), h_r is a radiant heat transfer coefficient (5.4 W/m^2/°C is often used), $\overline{T}_{sk}$ is the mean skin temperature (in °C; see below), $\overline{T}_R$ is the mean radiant temperature of the surroundings (in °C), and A_r/A is the ratio of the surface area of the body available for radiant heat transfer to the whole body surface (DuBois formula). Fanger (1970) gives this ratio as 0.73 for a standing man and 0.7 for a sitting man.

CONVECTION

Convection is the exchange of heat by molecular mass transfer within a fluid medium (normally air or water), during which molecules retain their heat energy but move within the confines of the medium, carrying heat with them. It is often the most significant route of heat loss from the body in cold environments.

The rate of heat exchange between a body and its environment through convection depends on the following:

- Temperature gradient between the two: this determines the amount of heat absorbed or donated by a given mass of air that comes into contact with the skin.
- Density, pattern and relative movement of the fluid in which the body is placed.
- Surface area exposed.

These factors are represented in Newton's law of cooling, from which heat loss by convection from the skin may be quantified as follows:

$$C = h_c(\overline{T}_{sk} - T_a)$$

where C is the convective heat loss (in W/m^2), h_c is the convective heat transfer coefficient, T_{sk} is the mean skin temperature (in °C) and T_a is the ambient temperature (in °C).

h_c is a complex function of fluid density, viscosity, specific heat capacity, flow and body shape and posture. Therefore, it is not a constant but is calculated from a series of dimensionless variables (Nusselt, Grashof, Prandt and Reynolds numbers). h_c has been calculated by numerous authors for a range of environments; it varies between about 1–4 $W/m^2/°C$ in still air to 60–100 $W/m^2/°C$ in still water, and rising to about 400 $W/m^2/°C$ in water with a velocity of 0.5 m/s.

It follows that two basic types of convection are recognized: free (natural) and forced. Free convection is important only in environments with very low fluid flow rates. In a naked person standing in cool air, body heat is transferred to the molecules in contact with the skin, giving rise to a warmer layer next to the skin: the boundary layer. The Brownian motion of these molecules increases, forcing them further apart and making them less dense and more buoyant; due to Archimedes' principle, thermal currents begin to rise. The resulting bulk movement represents a stream of molecules possessing thermal energy and rising away from the heat source.

For a naked individual in a room at 25 °C and with a mean skin temperature of 33 °C, the boundary layer is about 180 mm thick at the face and, 20 mm away from the skin, it has a velocity of 0.5 m/s, resulting in about 10 l/s of air passing over the head. This plume of free convectional currents facilitates heat exchange, as cooler air moves into the vacated space. In spite of this, overall, the boundary layer of rising and relatively warm air reduces the skin to environment temperature gradient and thereby provides some insulation to the body in still air conditions in an upright posture.

The boundary layer is destroyed when the fluid in which the body is placed moves, or the body moves in the fluid (relative movement). As a result, convectional heat exchange is increased through forced convection. Such heat loss is a function of the velocity of the fluid up to maximum levels. The forced convective heat transfer coefficient may be approximated as follows:

$$h_c = 8.3V^{0.5}$$

where h_c is the forced convective heat transfer coefficient (in $W/m^2/°C$) and V is the wind speed (in m/s).

In humans, free and forced convection assume approximately equal importance between 0.1 and 0.2 m/s wind speed. Forced convection in air is maximized with air movements above 4.2 m/s; the equivalent velocity for water is 0.5 m/s.

CONDUCTION

This term is used to describe heat exchange between two solid surfaces in direct contact or in solid–fluid interfaces. With this form of energy exchange, there is no physical movement of material within the respective objects; rather, energy is exchanged directly via collisions caused by the vibrational motions of free electrons (solids) and molecules (liquids and gases).

The rate of conductance depends on the following:

- temperature gradient between the skin and the surface with which it is in contact
- surface area in contact
- thermal conductivity (ease with which heat moves through a substance) and specific heat capacity of each object
- distance through which the heat is conducted.

This can be expressed mathematically as follows:

$$K = (k/l)(\overline{T}_{sk} - T_a)$$

where K is the conductive heat transfer (in W/m^2), k is the conductance of the material (in $W/m^2/°C$), l is the distance through which the heat is conducted (in m), T_{sk} is the mean skin temperature (in °C) and T_a is the ambient temperature (in °C).

Usually, the amount of heat exchanged with the environment in this way is small. For an upright naked person in air, the only surface area available for conductive heat exchange is that of the soles of the feet and the ground on which the person is standing. This represents a small percentage of the surface area of the body and a small percentage of the total heat exchange with the environment.

However, there are circumstances in which conduction can become a more major route of heat exchange. If the individual lies down, the surface area of the body in contact with the ground increases; depending on the temperature, this can significantly increase conductive heat exchange. Conduction is an important route for heat exchange within the body and when considering contact freezing and burning injuries.

The inverse of conductance (resistance to heat exchange by conductance) is thermal insulation (thermal resistance). This is a term that is in common usage, describing an important characteristic of items ranging from sleeping bags to immersion suits (see the next chapter). The most common units associated with insulation are the Clo and tog: 1 Clo = 1.55 tog = 0.155 °C m²/W.

EVAPORATION

Evaporation is the process by which energy transforms a mass of liquid to a gas. This mass transfer results in fluid being lost down the water-vapour pressure gradient. The phase change from liquid to water vapour requires 2.4 kJ/g (0.576 kcal/g) of energy – the latent heat of vaporization – and is not associated with an increase in the temperature of the liquid. Evaporative heat exchange occurs only within a gaseous medium and when liquid evaporates from the surface of an object.

With regard to sweating, no sweat can evaporate when relative humidity (rh) is 100 per cent (air saturated with water vapour); this is the only impact that rh has on evaporation. When rh is below 100 per cent, the rate of evaporation is determined by the ratio of water vapour pressure at the skin (P_s) to that of the environment (P_a); both pressures are determined by, and proportional to, temperature. When $P_s > P_a$, evaporation will occur; when $P_a > P_s$, no evaporation will occur.

Thus, the rate of evaporation depends on the following:

- skin surface area that is wet
- air movement around the body (wind or body movement)
- difference between the vapour pressure at the skin surface and that in the air.

The rate of heat loss by evaporation (E) can be predicted from the following:

$$E = h_e(P_s - P_a)$$

where E is the rate of heat loss by evaporation (in W/m²), h_e is the coefficient of evaporative heat exchange (in W/m²/kPa), P_s is the water vapour pressure at the skin (in kPa) and P_a is the water vapour pressure of the environment (in kPa).

The rate of evaporation is influenced by air movement: in still air, the water vapour pressure next to the skin rises as sweat is produced and lowers the gradient between P_s and P_a. Air movement prevents this boundary effect, and thus the coefficient of evaporative heat exchange can be estimated from the following:

$$h_e = 124V^{0.5}$$

where V is the wind speed (in m/s).

Although the processes of convection and evaporation have things in common (a coefficient and a gradient), the gradient for heat loss by evaporation ($P_s - P_a$) is a vapour pressure gradient that determines the mass transfer of vapour. In contrast, the gradient in the equations for dry heat exchange is a thermal gradient that determines the mass transfer of heat. Although vapour pressure is influenced by temperature, there are no temperature terms in the evaporative heat loss equation. The fact that P_s can still be greater than P_a when ambient temperature is higher than mean skin temperature (approximately 33 °C) is the physical basis for evaporation being the only route for heat loss in a hot environment.

Although sweat evaporation more usually is associated with heat balance in hot environments, the phase change from liquid to vapour and back has implications for heat balance in cold temperatures. Even in a cold environment, the body is constantly losing water by evaporation from the lungs and skin to the surrounding environment. For example, on a cold day, the moisture vapour in expired air is readily visible as a fog, as is the condensation formed on the inner surface of waterproof clothing, which reduces insulation. This insensible water loss, which is outside the body's control, amounts to about 1 l/day, which, if evaporated, will dissipate approximately 24 kcal/h (28 W) (Figure 12.2).

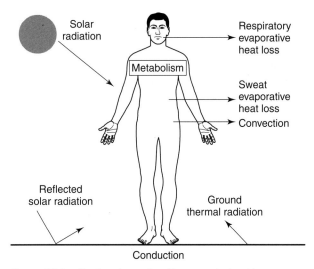

Figure 12.2 *Heat exchange in a thermoneutral outdoor environment (25 °C, relative humidity 50 per cent).*

THE THERMAL ENVIRONMENT AND ITS ASSESSMENT

Air temperature

Air temperature can be measured using a thermometer, which works by relating a change in its intrinsic properties to the mean kinetic energy of the substance being measured. In 1595, Galileo invented a simple but unreliable gas thermometer known as the thermoscope. Fifty years later, glass bulb thermometers containing alcohol appeared. In 1714, Fahrenheit developed the mercury-in-glass thermometer. Today, common types of thermometers include mercury- (or alcohol, for low temperatures)-in-glass, thermistors and thermocouples. The latter two are electronic and, when associated with appropriate circuitry, generally are faster and more accurate than direct-read thermometers. They are also compatible with data-logging devices, enabling automated data collection from otherwise inaccessible places such as cockpits.

Liquid-in-glass thermometers rely on the linear expansion of a liquid with temperature. Thermistors are semiconductors, the impedances of which decrease as temperature increases; they require voltage across the device. Thermocouples do not require an imposed voltage; they include junctions of two different metals (usually copper and constantan). If two such junctions are connected in a circuit, they will produce a potential difference that is related to their temperature (the Seebeck thermoelectric effect) and that causes a current to flow, which can be measured and converted to a temperature.

All devices and associated equipment require calibration, as no devices, particularly thermistors, are completely linear across a wide temperature range. When measuring air temperature, especially when thermal radiation is significant, the device should be shielded from direct sunlight, have low emissivity, be dry and have good air circulation.

As with all measuring instruments, what is measured is critical. For the measurement of air temperature, this translates into where the measurement is taken. With regard to thermal balance, the air temperature of most interest is that close to the surface of the skin, whether that is the macroclimate temperature of the environment or the microclimate temperature under clothing. There can be a large vertical gradient in air temperature in extreme environments, indoors or outdoors, e.g. standing on snow, standing on rock heated by the sun, in a cockpit, during fire-fighting. Variations in air temperature of over 20 °C have been measured between the ground and at a height of 2 m in the desert. Variations of over 200 °C may also be seen over similar vertical distances indoors during fire-fighting. Such thermal gradients necessitate the measurement of air temperature at several different heights. In more uniform environments, air temperature at head height is often used as the single measure of air temperature. All measurements should be made in close proximity to the subject under investigation to reduce the effect of lateral variations in temperature, i.e. both the site of measurement and the number of measurements taken should provide as close an approximation of the conditions being experienced by the subject as possible.

Radiant temperature

Radiation, particularly direct solar radiation, can represent a significant thermal load on an individual outdoors, or indoors behind a window or in a cockpit. The radiation from a source such as electronic equipment can also add significantly to the thermal stress of an environment. The measurement of radiant temperature therefore is an important aspect of the assessment of the thermal environment.

For most physiological studies, measurement of the mean environmental radiant temperature (T_R) is sufficient. This is defined as the temperature of a uniform enclosure within which a small black sphere (or human body) at its test point would have the same radiant heat exchange as it does with the real environment. It is usually measured using a globe thermometer, consisting of a metal sphere painted matt black and with an air-temperature-measuring device at its centre. The globe is traditionally 150 mm in diameter, a reflection of the fact that the first devices were made from 6-inch ball-cocks used in plumbing. Smaller globes can be used in confined spaces with appropriate corrections for surface area.

The standard black copper globe requires about 20 minutes to reach equilibrium. This is reduced slightly with air movement and the use of thermistors, which respond faster than mercury-in-glass thermometers. After stabilization, the mean radiant temperature is given by the equation:

$$\overline{T}_R = T_g + 2.44 V^{0.5}(T_g - T_a)$$

where $\overline{T}_R$ is the mean radiant temperature (in °C), T_g is globe temperature (in °C), V is the wind speed (in m/s) and T_a is the environmental temperature (in °C).

The equation identifies a weakness in this approach, in that the measurement is dependent on the accurate measurement of wind speed: an error in this measurement will result in an error in the measurement of T_R. The black globe provides a good approximation in most situations, but it may not be representative for non-uniform (directional) radiation. For example, radiation longitudinal to the body (e.g. heated ceilings) may be assessed better using a cylindrical-shaped measuring device. For outdoor conditions with solar radiation, a black globe will overestimate the effects of radiation on an individual and a correction should be made, or the globe should be given the colour of the clothing being worn. Indoors, the mean radiant temperature can be calculated from the temperature of the surrounding surfaces, angle factors, and the shape, size and relative position of the surface in relation to a person.

Altitude

Air temperature falls by approximately 1 °C with every 150-m increase in altitude. However, higher altitudes receive more solar radiation, because the radiation must travel through a smaller mass of air before reaching the surface of the Earth. The reduction in air density with altitude reduces the rate of convective heat transfer (the opposite of what happens in hyperbaric environments). h_c is a power function of barometric pressure according to the equation:

$$h_c' = h_c (P_b/760)^{0.55}$$

where h_c' is the convective heat transfer coefficient at elevation (in $W/m^2/°C$), h_c is the convective heat transfer coefficient at sea level (in $W/m^2/°C$) and P_b is the barometric pressure (in Torrs).

An increase in evaporative heat transfer at altitude is related to the change in thermal diffusivity (D). The mass transfer coefficient (h_m) is adjusted for pressure according to the equation:

$$h_m' = h_m(760/P_b)^{0.45}$$

where h_m' is the mass transfer coefficient at elevation (in $W/m^2/Torr$), h_m is the mass transfer coefficient at sea level (in $W/m^2/Torr$) and P_b is the barometric pressure (in Torrs).

The differing directions of change of these coefficients with decreasing barometric pressure explains why the relationship (Lewis) between convective and evaporative heat exchange is uncoupled as pressure is significantly reduced.

Air movement

Air movement has an important influence on convective and evaporative heat exchange, and its accurate assessment can be important in the determination of heat balance. It can be laminar or turbulent. Laminar flow is linear (unidirectional) in parallel currents. Turbulent flow has eddies or other confusing currents. The pattern of airflow has an influence on the type of device used to measure it. Near-laminar unidirectional flow may be measured using a vane or cup anemometer. These devices include either a vane wheel or hollow cups that are turned by the wind (Figure 12.3). The speed of rotation is measured and displayed as wind velocity on a calibrated scale or as a digital readout. A disadvantage of this type of device is inertia, caused by

friction in the mechanism and the mass of the vane or cups; this limits their use in winds below 0.2 m/s and, as a consequence, in certain studies. Humans can perceive air velocities below 0.1 m/s.

The pitot-static tube is an accurate way of measuring unidirectional air velocity, particularly when airspeed is quite high. The device consists of two tubes, one inside the other, which are bent at right-angles. The outer tube has a series of circumferential holes (static pressure holes) back from the nose piece. The open end of the tube must face directly into the airflow. The outlets of both the central and the outer tubes are taken independently to either side of a manometer. The difference between the pressure of the nose piece (velocity pressure) and the static pressure can be related to air velocity by the Bernoulli equation. This method is similar to that used to measure air speed in aircraft. It is inexpensive and adequate for gross estimations of wind speed.

If airflow is turbulent, then it is more usual to measure wind speed by determining its cooling effect. The Kata thermometer can be used to measure air movement in ventilated areas, particularly when the air is slow-moving. It has also been used as a 'comfort-meter' to assess the cooling power of the environment. It consists of an alcohol-in-glass thermometer with a large bulb. It is heated in hot water until the spirit fills the column and reservoir at the top of the stem. It is then dried and suspended in air. The time taken for the thermometer to cool from 38 to 35 °C is used to determine the rate of cooling of the thermometer. This rate is affected by radiation and convection from the heated globe. The thermometer may also be used as a wet-bulb device by placing a wet silk sleeve over the bulb. The cooling rate is then also influenced by evaporation.

Although simple observation is not precise, if undertaken carefully, it can be as accurate as a single measurement taken with a handheld device in a poorly selected location. The simplest and one of the earliest scales for approximating wind speed was that developed by Beaufort in 1806. Originally designed to assess the effect of wind pressure on sails in order to determine the amount of canvas a ship should carry, the Beaufort scale (Table 12.3) is now used to estimate wind speed on the basis of the observable effects of the wind on the outdoor environment.

COMBINATIONS OF MEASURES AND INDICES

In order to assess some aspects of the environment (e.g. humidity), two or more measures are taken simultaneously, as the relationship between them correlates with the variable being assessed. In other cases (e.g. heat stress indices), a variety of measurements are taken in order to compute a single value that gives an index of the stress represented by the environment.

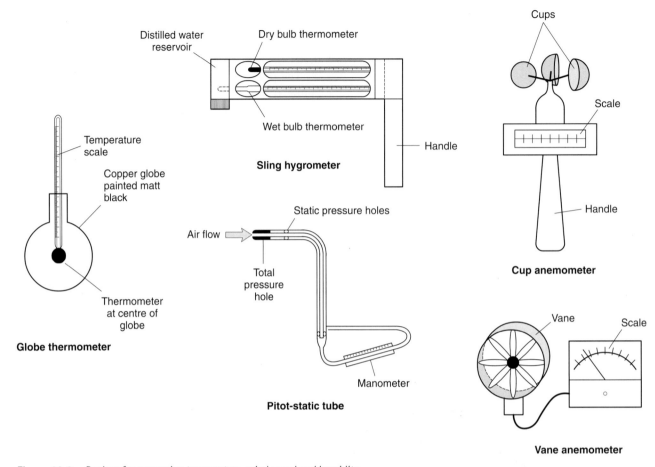

Figure 12.3 *Devices for measuring temperature, wind speed and humidity.*

Humidity

Humidity is the amount of water vapour present in a gaseous atmosphere. It can be expressed in several ways, including as:

- water vapour pressure in the environment (P_a)
- dew-point temperature, i.e. the temperature of air at which dew will begin to form if the air is cooled slowly
- relative humidity, i.e. the ratio (usually expressed as a percentage) of P_a to the saturated water pressure at that dry-bulb temperature (P_{sa}).

Humidity is an important determinant of the capacity for heat loss (see Evaporation) and comfort in both natural and artificial environments such as aircraft cabins.

The instrument used to measure humidity is the hygrometer. This comes in several types (hair, corona-discharge, whirling/sling). Of these, the most common is the sling hygrometer, which consists of two mercury-in-glass thermometers that are rotated vigorously in air by holding a handle attached to one end of their casing and whirling them to expose the thermometers to rapid air movement. The bulb of one of the thermometers is covered by a silk or muslin sleeve kept wet with clean or distilled water. The extraction of latent heat by evaporation from the wet bulb gives it a lower temperature than the dry bulb. The difference in temperature between the wet and dry bulb thermometers, for a given air temperature, correlates inversely with the humidity of the environment (the bigger the difference, the lower the humidity). Humidity is obtained from the ventilated wet and dry bulb temperatures by use of a psychrometric chart such as that shown in Figure 12.4. When temperatures are above freezing, partial pressure of water vapour (P_a) and relative humidity (rh) can be calculated from the dry-bulb (T_{db}) and ventilated (aspirated) wet-bulb (T_{wb}) temperatures using the following equations:

$$P_a = P_{swb} - 0.667(T_{db} - T_{wb})$$

$$rh = P_a/P_{sa} \times 100$$

where P_{swb} is the saturated water vapour pressure (in millibars, mb) at ventilated wet-bulb temperature and P_{sa} is the saturated water vapour pressure (in millibars) at air temperature.

Other devices are ventilated automatically by fans or pumps. It is important that the wet bulb is aspirated at

Table 12.3 *Beaufort scale of wind force*

Force	Description	Sea state	Speed knots	km/h	mph
0	Calm	Sea like a mirror	< 1	< 1	< 1
1	Very light	Ripples with appearance of scales; no foam crests	1–3	1–5	1–3
2	Light breeze	Wavelets small but pronounced; crests with glassy appearance but do not break	4–6	6–11	4–7
3	Gentle breeze	Large wavelets; crests begin to break; glassy-looking foam; occasional white horses	7–10	12–19	8–12
4	Moderate breeze	Small waves becoming longer; frequent white horses	11–16	20–29	13–18
5	Fresh breeze	Moderate waves of pronounced long-form; many white horses; some spray	17–21	30–39	19–24
6	Strong breeze	Some large waves; extensive white foam crests; some spray	22–27	40–50	25–31
7	Near-gale	Sea heaped up; white foam from breaking waves blowing in streaks with the wind	28–33	51–61	32–38
8	Gale	Moderately high and long waves; crests break into spindrift, blowing foam in well-marked streaks	34–40	62–74	39–46
9	Strong gale	High waves; dense foam streaks in wind; wave crests topple, tumble and roll over; spray reduces visibility	41–47	75–87	47–54
10	Storm	Very high waves with long overhanging crests; dense blowing foam; sea surface appears white; heavy tumbling of sea, shock-like; poor visibility	48–55	88–101	55–63
11	Violent storm	Exceptionally high waves, sometimes concealing small and medium-sized ships; sea completely covered with long white patches of foam; edges of wave crests blown into froth; poor visibility	56–63	102–118	64–73
12	Hurricane	Air filled with foam and spray; sea white with driving spray; visibility very seriously affected	> 64	> 119	> 74

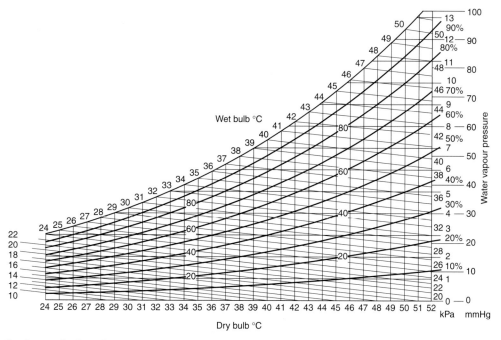

Figure 12.4   *Psychrometric chart. The chart is entered with ventilated wet-bulb and dry-bulb temperatures. The point of intersection can be read on the right-hand scale as absolute humidity, or as relative humidity (rh) by interpolation between the lines of equal rh given in ten-per-cent steps.*

about 5 m/s; unaspirated or 'natural' wet-bulb temperature is not used in the measurement of humidity. All devices become less accurate at low humidity (< 20 per cent). Electronic humidity sensors can be used to log humidity data automatically, although, many of these sensors are limited by their slow response time and lack of precision.

Operative temperature

Operative temperature (T_o) was introduced as a means of expressing all the parameters of dry heat exchange as a single variable for human subjects. It is the integrated value of air temperature and mean radiant temperature, weighted according to values of the convective and radiative heat transfer coefficients. It is defined as the uniform temperature of an imaginary isothermal 'black' enclosure in which an individual at thermal equilibrium would exchange the same amount of heat by radiation, convection and conduction from the skin surface as they would in the real non-uniform environment.

$$T_o = \frac{(\text{hc}T_a + \text{hr}\bar{T}_R)}{(\text{hc} + \text{hr})}$$

where hc is the convective heat transfer coefficient (in W/m²/°C), hr is the radiant heat transfer coefficient (in W/m²/°C), T_a is the ambient air temperature (in °C) and T_r is the mean radiant temperature (in °C).

Indices and models of heat and cold stress

A large number of indices and thermal models attempt to predict the thermal stress and consequent physiological strain associated with an environment. These tools continue to be developed and refined, some of the most recent being molecular markers of heat stress (Kumar *et al.* 2003). A summary of some of these indices is presented in Table 12.4. For more details, refer to Clarke and Edholm (1985), Parsons (1993) and Golden and Tipton (2002).

Heat stress indices have been derived from the physics of heat exchange (e.g. heat stress index, index of thermal stress), empirical observations from physiological experiments (e.g. wet-bulb globe temperature, predicted four-hour sweat rate), and subjective impressions (temperature sensations, comfort) in different environments (e.g. effective temperature, corrected effective temperature). The rational indices are derived from a selection of the following: air temperature, radiant temperature, relative humidity, air velocity, clothing insulation, metabolic rate and external work.

Thermal models usually are derived from a combination of the physics of heat exchange and empirical observations from a wide range of studies on a variety of species, or from stimulus–response data obtained from studies with humans. While the ability to model and predict the thermal responses of individuals is attractive and can assist understanding, the thermoregulatory system is a complex system to represent either physically (manikins) or mathematically (computer models). For this reason, it is easier to model heat exchange with an environment than the thermoregulatory response to this heat exchange and its consequence for body temperature.

THE RESPONSE: THE PHYSIOLOGICAL RESPONSE TO THERMAL STRESS

Having discussed the physics of heat exchange with the environment, we now turn to the physiology of temperature regulation. The two, along with behavioural response, are linked inextricably in a dynamic equilibrium, such that they all contribute to the magnitude of each term in the heat balance equation. For example, the amount of heat lost from the body by the evaporation of sweat depends on the physiological responses that control peripheral blood flow and sweat production and on the physical characteristics of the environment, such as temperature, relative humidity and air velocity. Behavioural responses such as removing clothing, moving to shade and fanning will also influence the level of heat loss.

The human thermoregulatory system combines peripheral and central sensors, afferent and efferent pathways, and central integrating and controlling centres in an attempt to achieve thermal homeostasis, or a deep body temperature that remains stable at about 37 °C. The major components and functions of the thermoregulatory system are described below and in Figure 12.5.

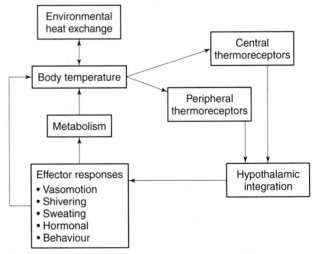

Figure 12.5 *Schematic of the temperature regulation system.*

Table 12.4 *Indices of heat, cold and comfort*

Name	Formula	Comment
Heat stress		
Heat stress index (HSI)	$HSI = E_{req}/E_{max} \times 100$ Maximum sweat rate taken to be 1 L/h for 8 h $AET = 2440/(E_{req}) - E_{max}$	Based on comparison of evaporation required to maintain heat balance (E_{req}) with the maximum evaporation that could be achieved in the environment (E_{max}). At HSI = 100, required sweating is the maximum that can be achieved and therefore represents the upper limit of body temperature control. HSI > 100 results in body heat storage and an allowable exposure time (AET, minutes) is then calculated. HSI < 0 results in mild cold strain. HSI is identical to the required skin wettedness value (W_{req})
Index of thermal stress (ITS)	$ITS = (H - (C + R) - R_s)/0.37\,\eta_{sc}$ H is metabolic heat production, R_s is solar load, $S_w = E_{req}/\eta_{sc}, \eta_{sc}$ is efficiency of sweating, and 0.37 converts W/m^2 to g/h	Improved version of HSI. Recognizes that not all the sweat produced evaporates
Required sweat rate (SW_{req})	$SW_{req} = E_{req}/r$ E_{req} is required evaporation, r is sweating efficiency	Improvement on the HSI and ITS. Calculates sweating required for heat balance from an improved heat balance equation, against what is possible in humans. Accepted as ISO 7933 (International Organization for Standardization 2004b)
Predicted 4-h sweat rate (P4SR)	$P4SR = B4SR + 0.37 I_{clo} + (0.012 + 0.001 I_{clo})(M - 63)$ B4SR is basic 4-h sweat rate, obtained from nomogram, I_{clo} is clothing insulation, M is metabolic rate	Scale based on sweating response of individuals. Allows prediction of 4-h sweat rate from measurement of dry- and wet-bulb temperatures plus air movement. Adjustments (oversimplified) are made for clothing and metabolic activity. Useful in hot and humid conditions. Scale determined using young, fit, acclimatized subjects – therefore can overestimate sweating. Also, outside the zone in which thermal balance can be achieved (prescriptive zone), sweat rate is not a good indicator of thermal strain. P4SR of 4.5 = limit of no incapacitation of fit acclimatized young men
Wet-bulb globe thermometer index (WBGT)	With solar radiation, $WBGT = 0.7 T_{wb(n)} + 0.2 T_g + 0.1 T_{db}$ Under indoor conditions, with no solar radiation, $WBGT = 0.7 T_{wb(n)} + 0.3 T_g$ $T_{wb(n)}$ is naturally ventilated wet-bulb temperature, T_g is globe temperature (150 mm diameter), T_{db} is dry-bulb temperature (shielded)	Most widely used index. Originally designed to determine whether environmental conditions were too severe for military exercises. Becomes ineffective if $T_{db} > 40\,°C$. Various instruments exist, with an array of sensors that will automatically provide WBGT. WBGT can vary greatly over short distances and in unpredictable ways. See also Chapter 13
Fighter index of thermal stress (FITS)	$FITS = 0.83 T_{wb} + 0.35 T_{db} + 5.08$ T_{wb} and T_{db} are ventilated wet- and dry-bulb temperatures, respectively, on the ground	Based on WBGT, to provide an index that predicts thermal stress within a fast-jet cockpit during low-level (< 3000 feet) flight. Assumes that 1.5–2 Clo of insulation is being worn (i.e. not applicable if CBRN, immersion or cold weather clothing are being worn). 'Caution' and 'danger' zones are identified and appropriate protective measures are recommended, including recovery intervals, shading cockpits, fluid intake and flight cancellation (Nunneley and Stribley 1979)

Table 12.4 *continued*

Name	Formula	Comment
Environmental stress index (ESI)	$ESI = 0.62T_a - 0.007rh + 0.002SR + 0.0043(T_a \times rh) - 0.078(0.1 + SR)(-1)$, T_a is ambient temperature (in °C), rh is relative humidity (in %), SR is solar radiation (in W/m^2)	High correlation between ESI and WBGT ($r = 0.899$). ESI (refined), which is constructed from fast response and commonly used weather sensors (T_a, rh, SR), has potential to serve as an alternative to WBGT for heat category assessment
Physiological strain index (PSI)	$PSI = 5(Tret - Tre_0)(39.5 - Tre_0) - 1 + 5(HR_t - HR_0)(180 - HR_0) - 1$ Tre_t and HR_t are simultaneous measurements taken any time during exposure; Tre0 and HR0 are initial measurements	Rates physiological strain on universal scale of 0–10
Heat shock protein 70 (Hsp70) as a biomarker of heat stress in humans	Six volunteers exposed to T_{db} 55 °C dry-bulb temperature in a simulated cockpit, rh 30%, air velocity 20 feet/min	Hsp70 significantly induced in leucocytes on exposure to heat stress and correlates with other indicators of strain (Kumar *et al*. 2003)
Thermal comfort		
Effective temperature (ET) index		ET of an environment is the temperature of still unsaturated air that gives rise to an equivalent sensation
Corrected effective temperature		ET modified (black-globe temperature replaces dry-bulb temperature) to include factor for radiation in nomograms. Rarely used as index of comfort, but still used as heat stress index. Effective in moderate warm environments (28–40 °C). Cannot be used in temperatures < 20 °C
Bedford scale	Much too warm Too warm Comfortably warm Comfortable Comfortably cool Too cool Much too cool	Comfort scale derived from preferred temperatures of people working under a variety of conditions in different parts of the world
American Society of Heating, Refrigeration and Air-conditioning Engineers (ASHRAE) scale	Hot (+ 3) Warm (+ 2) Slightly warm (+ 1) Neutral (0) Slightly cool (− 1) Cool (− 2) Cold (− 3)	Sensation scale used with and without numbers shown in parentheses

Cold air stress

Index	Formula / references	Description
Wind chill index (WCI)	$WCI = (10\sqrt{v} + 10.45 - v)(33 - T_a)$ v is wind speed (in m/s), T_a is air temperature (in °C)	Originally determined from observation made in the Antarctic of times taken for water to freeze in various climatic conditions. Emphasizes effect of air movement on cooling. Simple to use and therefore most popular of the cold-air indices. See also Chapter 13
Equivalent still air temperature (ESAT)	$I_a = I_{sa} - W$ I_a is insulation of the boundary air layer of a nude person, I_{sa} is standard value (1 Clo) for insulation of still air, W is decrement in I_{sa} due to air velocity	Presents the still air temperature that gives the equivalent thermal demand as that represented by air temperature plus wind. Also developed equivalent shade temperature (EST) and still shade temperature (SST), which take into account effects of radiation
Required clothing insulation index (IREQ)	$IREQ = (T_{sk} - T_{cl})/(M - W - E_{res} - C_{res} - E)$	$IREQ_{min}$ defines minimum thermal insulation required to maintain mean body temperature at subnormal but acceptable temperatures. $IREQ_{neutral}$ is thermal insulation required to provide thermal neutrality. If insulation is less than $IREQ_{min}$, then a maximum acceptable exposure time is provided. Assumes insulation is distributed evenly over the body. Does not take into account problem of insulating the extremities. ISO TR 11079 provides a method for calculating IREQ and guidance on its practical application (International Organization for Standardization 1993)
Cold strain index (CSI)	$CSI = 6.67[T(core_t) - T(core_0)][35 - T(core_0)](-1) + 3.33[T(sk_t) - T(sk_0)][20 - T(sk_0)](-1)$ $T(core_0)$ and $T(sk_0)$ are initial measurements; $T(core_t)$ and $T(sk_t)$ are simultaneous measurements taken at any time t. T_{core} = core (deep body) temperature	Rates cold strain on a universal scale of 0–10

Cold water stress

Index	Formula / references	Description
Prediction of survival time: analysis of accidental immersions	Molnar survival curve (Molnar 1946) Barnett survival curve (Barnett 1962) UK National Immersion Incident Survey (1979)	Data obtained from shipwrecks and boating accidents (Golden and Tipton 2002)
Prediction of survival time: laboratory-based models	Keating (Keating 1969) Golden (Golden 1976)	Based on experimental data and case studies (Golden and Tipton 2002)
Prediction of survival time: mathematical models	Hayward (Hayward et al. 1975) Wissler model (Nunnely and Wissler 1980) RAF Institute of Aviation Medicine Model (adaptation of the Wissler model) (Hayes and Cohen 1987) Tikuisis (Tikuisis 1994)	Simple equations to complex mathematical models of human thermoregulation, underpinned by laboratory experimentation (Golden and Tipton 2002)

CBRN, chemical, biological, radioactive and nuclear.

Cutaneous thermosensors

The surface of the body is well supplied with sensors that are extremely sensitive to temperature and increase their firing rate when cooled (cold sensors) or warmed (warm sensors). The static frequency response of both receptors as a function of temperature describes a bell-shaped curve. Cold sensors are active between about 10 and 40 °C, with a static maxima at about 25 °C. Warm sensors are active from around 30 to 50 °C and have a static maxima at about 44 °C. The static firing frequencies of the two populations of thermal receptors are roughly equivalent at 37 °C, i.e. normal deep body temperature. Cold receptors are inhibited by warming, and warm sensors are inhibited by cooling. Both types of sensor show a strong dynamic response to changing temperature (Figure 12.6).

The anatomy of the cutaneous thermosensors is better understood than the mechanism by which they transduce thermal energy into neural-coded information, although cold sensitivity has been associated with thermal effects on the electrogenic Na+/K+ pump. Both cold and warm sensors exist as free nerve endings (C-fibres); there are also thinly myelinated (Aδ-fibres) cold sensors. There are three to four times more cold than warm sensors in the skin, and cold receptors are located more superficially (immediately beneath the epidermis) than warm receptors (dermis). Psychophysiological studies suggest that the cutaneous thermosensors are not distributed evenly. For example, five times more cold points per square centimetre have been reported on the fingers than on the broad surfaces of the body, and four times more on the lips than on the fingers. This variation is also reflected in the autonomic response, e.g. cooling the forehead is three times more effective in decreasing sweating than cooling a corresponding surface area of the lower leg.

Thermal information is carried to the brain along the same general pathways as pain. Afferents enter the spinal cord via the spinal ganglion and the dorsal root. In the cor-responding segment, the afferents are connected to second-order neurons in laminae I, II and III of the dorsal horn. Spinal thermosensitive afferents are conveyed mainly in the long ascending contralateral anterolateral (spinothalamic) tract. There may also be projections via the ipsilateral dorsolateral (spinocervical) tract.

The spinal and trigeminal thermoreceptive pathways terminate in third-order neurons in the ventrobasal complex of the thalamus, the reticular areas of the brainstem (via the spinoreticular bundle) and possibly in the intralaminar nuclei of the thalamus along with pain signals. A few signals are relayed to the somatosensory cortex from the ventrobasal complex.

Central reception and processing

On the basis of information obtained from a range of animal species, several sites have been identified within the body that are capable of eliciting generalized thermoregulatory responses. For example, local cooling or warming of the spinal cord can produce a wide range of thermoregulatory responses. However, the primary centre of thermoregulatory integration and control is the preoptic nucleus–anterior hypothalamus (POAH). Sites of maximum thermoregulatory response to warming and cooling are highly localized in the posterior part of the area preoptica. Warming of the anterior hypothalamus in thermoneutral environments activates heat loss efferents. In a cold environment, local heating of the anterior hypothalamus can reduce cold-induced vasoconstriction and shivering and activate panting. Hypothalamic cooling in a hot environment can inhibit panting and vasodilation and activate shivering. The posterior hypothalamus has little thermosensitivity, but it has been implicated in the integration of thermoregulatory responses and in behavioural thermoregulatory responses.

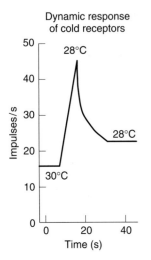

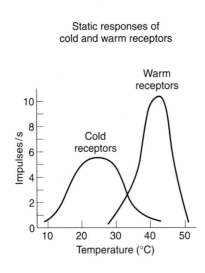

Figure 12.6 *Static and dynamic responses of thermoreceptors.*

Possible connections between spinal and cutaneous afferents and the POAH are via midbrain raphe nuclei, via ascending fibres from the reticular formation, and an extralemniscal connection from the mesencephalic reticular formation via the reticulothalamic fibres to the non-specific medial thalamic nuclei and from there to the hypothalamus.

In a variety of species, inputs from cold-sensitive peripheral neurons connect to cells that excite noradrenergic neurons in the subcoeruleus region projecting to cold-sensitive neurons in the POAH. Peripheral warm-sensitive neurons connect to serotonergic cells in the nucleus raphe magnus, which project to warm sensitive cells in the POAH.

Warm sensitivity is probably an inherent property of some POAH neurons. In contrast, cold sensitivity in this area appears to require synaptic input and, 'cold reception' therefore may be a function of the response of interneurons. About half of the POAH thermosensitive neurons also respond to non-thermal stimuli such as osmotic pressure and glucose concentration. This is important and may represent the neurophysiological basis for interactions between different control systems and help to explain conditions such as the impairment of thermoregulation caused by hypoglycaemia in the cold.

Thermoregulation thus is achieved via a complex network of pathways between neurons that are sensitive to local temperature (thermosensitive) or respond to changes in temperature (thermoresponsive) occurring elsewhere. In order to understand how such a system controls body temperature, it must, inevitably, be simplified. For teaching and conceptual purposes, a useful but limited early model for understanding thermoregulatory control was a simple homeostatic feedback loop with a thermostat, or set point, analogous in many ways to a home central heating system. A proportional controller initiated the effector mechanisms of the thermoregulatory system in proportion to the extent to which the controlled variable (body temperature) deviated (error signal) from a set point (reference temperature). Later models allowed for an adjustable set point to cater for the variations seen in the controlled body temperature, with factors such as circadian rhythm, menstruation and fever. More than one set point was introduced to allow for the fact that the thermoregulatory system is clearly a multiple loop system, with inputs and effector responses that can be changed independently of each other as a result of procedures such as acclimatization to heat or cold.

Perhaps the major problem with models requiring a set point is the fact that a structure that could establish a reference signal indicative of normal body temperature has eluded discovery. An alternative approach to conceptualizing thermoregulation, and one that complies more closely with known physiological mechanisms, replaces a set point with Sherrington's (1906) theory of reciprocal inhibition. In this case, cold afferent pathways stimulate heat production/conservation, while those associated with heat stimulate heat loss. Additionally, each pathway inhibits the other (cross-inhibition), preventing simultaneous stimulation of both sets of effector responses (Figure 12.7). Such a model can stabilize at a temperature that equates to the body temperature observed in thermoneutral environments.

Model with reference temperatures

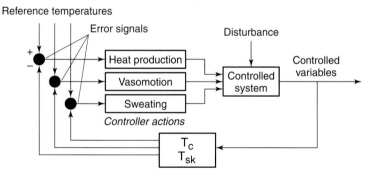

Model in which cross-inhibition replaces reference temperatures

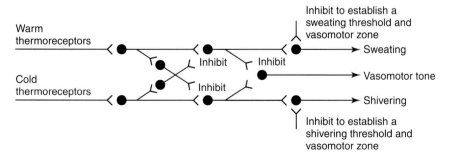

Figure 12.7 *Two possible models for the central control and integration of thermoregulation (adapted from Mekjavic et al. 2003).*

Inhibitory input to both pathways creates a region between shivering and sweating in which thermoregulation is achieved by alterations in peripheral blood flow (vasomotor zone, thermoneutral zone).

The inputs from the various peripheral and central thermosensors are combined in the POAH, and appropriate effector responses are initiated. In humans, it is usual to measure skin and deep body temperature as representations of peripheral and central inputs. Even with the addition of muscle temperature, this remains an oversimplification but the best that can usually be achieved. From the concept of a multiple-input system, it follows that several combinations of these inputs can result in a similar magnitude of effector response. Thus, in humans, evaporative heat loss of about 100 W/m^2 results from various combinations of mean skin temperature and deep body temperatures (Figure 12.8).

With larger animals such as humans, the thermal drive from the deep body sites is greater than that from the skin, i.e. skin temperature has to change by a greater amount than deep body temperature to have the same impact on the thermoregulatory effector response. For small animals, the thermal drives from the skin and body core are approximately equal. This is important, as these animals have smaller body mass and therefore less thermal inertia, and changes in skin temperature can result quickly in changes in deep body temperature if appropriate thermoregulatory responses are not initiated rapidly.

For a given effector response, the combination of two thermal drives (e.g. skin and anterior hypothalamus) has

been found to be either additive or multiplicative. For example, the change in metabolism with cooling in humans can be estimated from the equation:

$$\text{Change in metabolism} = 70W(36 - T_{ty})(34.1 - \overline{T}_{sk})$$

where T_{ty} is the tympanic temperature and $\overline{T}_{sk}$ is the mean skin temperature (both in °C) (Stolwijk and Hardy 1996).

Although the deep body sensors are often reported to respond to absolute temperatures rather than the rate of change of temperature, experiments with rapid intragastric cooling and the release of occlusion in the cold suggest that a rate component of central temperature contributes to regulatory responses.

EFFECTOR RESPONSES

Behaviour

The primary autonomic thermoregulatory responses of the body are vasomotion, sweating and shivering. More powerful and therefore more important than these are the behavioural responses, which are driven by the conscious perception of temperature and comfort, resulting from the thermoregulatory pathways to the somatosensory cortex. It is the behavioural responses, underpinned by intellect, that have enabled humans to move away from their equatorial origins and to inhabit the rest of the planet. A given skin temperature can be perceived as either pleasant or unpleasant, depending on whether it is assisting deep body temperature return towards normal values. The effector responses themselves contribute towards the perception of thermal comfort; for example, during intermittent shivering, individuals feel more uncomfortable when they are shivering than when they are not.

Vasomotion

Microcirculatory structures influencing cutaneous blood flow include capillaries, metarterioles, arteriovenous anastomoses and venous plexus. Flow through these vessels is controlled by smooth muscle, with local factors (e.g. oxygen and carbon dioxide tensions, hydrogen ion concentrations) primarily influencing pre-capillary sphincters, and neuronal and humoral (adrenaline, histamine, angiotensin, vasopressin) inputs influencing receptors on the other vessels.

The neural control of blood flow is achieved by active vasoconstriction and vasodilation. Active vasoconstriction is achieved through a noradrenergic nervous pathway acting primarily through α_1 and α_2 adrenoceptors. When an individual is exposed to heat, the initial increase in skin

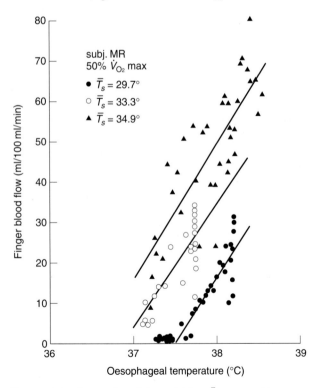

Figure 12.8   *Interaction of thermal drives. $\overline{T}_s$ = mean skin temperature (Wenger et al. 1975).*

blood flow is thought to be due to the withdrawal of vaso-constrictor tone. The subsequent increase in skin blood flow, which accounts for 85 per cent of the total increase observed in blood flow, is thought to be due to active vasodilation. The precise pathways and mechanisms for active vasodilation remain to be elucidated. They do not appear, however, as once thought, to be closely dependent on inflammatory agents released from sweat glands or on sweat-gland function. Cholinergic stimulation appears to participate in the initiation of active vasodilation in the early phase of heat stress, but other mechanisms are required to explain the full response. Prime candidates at the time of writing include nitric oxide and locally pro-duced peptides (Kellogg et al. 2002).

Homeothermic animals without fur, such as humans, depend heavily for their heat regulation on control of their skin circulation. The afferent inputs that determine skin blood flow are local temperature, mean skin temperature and deep body temperature. These inputs are integrated in the hypothalamus, and the capability of local, mean skin or deep body temperature to determine skin blood flow depends on the level of the other inputs. For example, in thermoneutral air with normal deep body temperature, skin blood flow is determined primarily by mean skin tem-perature and local temperature. However, when deep body temperature is raised or lowered by 1–2 °C, local tempera-ture no longer significantly influences local blood flow, although if only small changes in deep body temperature have occurred, mean skin temperature can still exert an influence.

The total skin blood flow in humans exposed to cold may be reduced to 20 ml/min; this maximizes the insulat-ing capability of the skin and subcutaneous fat. The reduc-tion in skin blood flow is not due solely to an increase in vascular tone: viscosity is more than doubled with a fall in blood temperature from 37 to 10 °C. During maximal vasodilation, skin blood flow may be as much as 3 l/min; at rest, in a thermoneutral environment, it is about 0.16 l/min, but it continually oscillates between vasocon-striction and vasodilation, with an overall periodicity of about 60 seconds.

At least three functionally different regions have been identified with regard to vasomotion:

- Extremities (hand, foot, ears, lips, nose): these tissues have a small mass in relation to their surface area, and therefore they facilitate heat transfer to and from the environment. These regions are rich in arteriovenous anastomoses with their associated bountiful neurovascular supply. The anastomoses control huge variations in blood flow through the limbs for thermoregulatory purposes, and their patency varies between complete closure and maximum vasodilation, with only small changes in sympathetic discharge.
- Trunk and proximal limbs.

- Head and brow: these lack significant vasoconstrictor input and consequently can be responsible for high heat loss in cold temperatures.

Vasomotor tone modulates heat loss. Intense vasocon-striction on exposure to cold maximizes tissue insulation and leaves skin, unperfused muscle and subcutaneous adi-pose tissue as the major sources of insulation. Human adi-pose tissue has similar thermal characteristics to cork; its in vitro thermal resistance is 0.0048 °Cm^2/W per 1 mm of tis-sue thickness. The insulation provided by adipose tissue (1.5 Clo/cm fat) is due to the fact that it is perfused poorly and contains relatively small amounts of water. It has a thermal conductivity that is about 35 per cent that of blood and less than 50 per cent that of skeletal muscle. However, because the body contains more muscle than fat, up to 70 per cent of total tissue insulation can be provided by unperfused muscle. This source of insulation is lost when exercise, including shivering, increases muscle blood flow. This occurs at relatively low levels of exercise (three times the resting metabolic rate). Thus, body adipose tissue can be regarded as fixed insulation, which changes little in the medium term, whereas muscle represents variable insula-tion, which is destroyed by exercise hyperaemia.

The loss of the insulation provided by muscle is not usu-ally of any consequence in a cold air environment, as the increase in heat production due to metabolism can more than balance heat losses to air. In contrast, exercise in water that is cooler than about 25 °C results in a faster fall in deep body temperature than that seen at rest. This is due not only to the loss of the insulation provided by muscle but also to the additional convective cooling caused by water agitation due to movement. The magnitude of this factor depends on whether the water is still or flowing. Some evi-dence suggests that in cold water, arm exercise is more detrimental than whole-body exercise, and that leg exercise may actually be beneficial (Golden and Tipton 1987). The arms are certainly more prone to heat loss than the legs: they have twice the surface area/mass ratio of the legs, a smaller conductive pathway from the centre to surface of the limb, and greater relative blood flow for a given work demand; also, when the arms are not used, they can oppose and therefore insulate the torso, the major area for heat loss in cold water.

When the skin circulation is cold-vasoconstricted, skin temperature falls towards environmental temperature. The extremities are the most susceptible to cooling due to their high surface area, small mass (little stored heat) and low level of inherent heat production. Therefore, they are highly dependent on blood flow to maintain their temper-ature and, when vasoconstriction occurs, are the areas most likely to suffer cold injury (see Chapter 13).

Vasodilation bypasses the insulating tissues of the body and transports body heat by mass flow directly to the skin. As a consequence, skin temperature rises; when environmental temperature is lower than body temperature, this increases the gradient down which heat can be lost. For each litre of blood at 37 °C that flows through the skin and returns to the deeper tissues at 36 °C, the body loses roughly 4.2 kJ of heat. As maximum skin blood flow can be as much as 3–4 l/min, the same 1 °C fall in the temperature of the blood will offload up to 16.7 kJ/min (280 W). High skin blood flow places a strain on the cardiovascular system and is associated with pooling of blood in compliant skin and subcutaneous vascular beds. This results in reduced cardiac filling and stroke volume and thus a higher heart rate to maintain cardiac output. Increased sympathetic nervous activity increases myocardial contractility. The redirection of blood from the viscera to skin and muscle during exercise in the heat can, if excessive, contribute to the development of heat injury.

Shivering

The central nervous pathway that initiates shivering leaves the posterior hypothalamus and runs caudally through the midbrain tegmentum and pons, close to the rubrospinal tracts. Shivering is controlled by the motor system – tractus cerebrospinalis and recticulospinalis and peripheral alpha and gamma motoneurons. It is the involuntary simultaneous asynchronous and rhythmic contractions of skeletal muscle motor units. These contract at a rate of about 9–20 per second (mean peak frequency 9 Hz) and out of phase with other units, such that little external work is done and most of the energy consumed is converted to heat.

Shivering is preceded by an increase in muscle tone and begins in the masseter or pectoral muscles. It moves from the proximal parts of the extremities to the central part of body (activity decreased in distal parts).

Heavy shivering may be interspersed with periods of light shivering or rest in the early phase of cooling, but later it becomes continuous before progressing into an almost tonic state. At its maximum, heat production from shivering can reach five or six times resting levels. Maximum shivering is related to maximum aerobic capacity ($\dot{V}_{O_2 max}$), with individuals able to shiver at a maximum of about 46 per cent of their $\dot{V}_{O_2 max}$. However, this level of shivering heat production cannot be maintained for very long, as it is fatiguing and extremely uncomfortable.

Shivering is attenuated (i) if blood glucose levels fall, (ii) with reduced oxygen levels in the inspired air, or (iii) if carbon dioxide levels increase. Shivering uses the same skeletal muscles as voluntary exercise, and the two can coexist up to moderate levels of voluntary activity. With mild cooling, shivering is inhibited progressively, as exercise intensity increases. With severe cooling, the increase in muscle tone associated with shivering can inhibit coordinated movement and impair activities such as swimming and walking.

Sweating

Humans have a total of about 2.5 million sweat glands – more per unit area than any other mammal. These are distributed in densities ranging from 100 to 600 per square centimetre, with more on the forehead, neck, trunk, hands and forearms, and fewer on the thighs. The gland itself consists of coiled glandular portion in the dermis; from this, a duct extends through the epidermis to a pore on the skin surface.

Thermoregulatory (eccrine gland) sweating in humans is controlled by cholinergic sympathetic pathways activating muscarinic receptors. The sweat glands are activated within seconds of the commencement of exercise or exposure to heat and reach maximum output after about 30 minutes. When sweat is secreted in the sweat glands, it has the same tonicity as extracellular fluid. However, as it ascends through the duct towards the surface of the skin, active ion-exchange pumps reabsorb much of the sodium and chlorine, making sweat more hypotonic. Therefore, sweat can be the most dilute of all body secretions (0.3–0.6 per cent NaCl, 10–70 mmol/l), depending, in part, on the rate of sweating and thus the transit time of the sweat through the duct and time available for ion reabsorption.

Maximum sweat rates are around 2 l/h; maximum sustainable rates are about 1 l/h. The disadvantage of sweating is loss of salt and water. The accumulation of sweat on the skin, for example in high-humidity environments, can cause osmotic swelling of the cells around the pores and block the duct, a process called hidromeiosis. People acclimatized to heat produce a greater volume of sweat, but its salt content is less than in those who are unacclimatized, helping them to conserve salt.

Like the other thermoregulatory responses, sweating is evoked by a combination of both skin and deep body thermoreceptors, and thus skin cooling can inhibit sweating. With increasing thermal stimulation, sweat appears on the extremities and proceeds centrally. Thus sweat output is increased by the progressive recruitment of more glands. In addition, there is a capability to increase the amount of sweat produced from each sweat gland.

FACTORS INFLUENCING THERMOREGULATION

Heat exchange with the environment via conduction, convection, radiation and evaporation will be determined by environmental factors such as humidity and air movement and whether an individual is immersed in air or water. Clothing ('external' insulation), depending on its characteristics (see Chapter 13), will also influence heat exchange with the environment. With regard to the body, factors such as fat content, muscle mass and its perfusion ('intrinsic' insulation), fitness and the performance of exercise alter heat balance. There are also a variety of factors, often referred to as 'non-thermal factors', that influence heat balance via an effect on the thermoregulatory system. These include the following:

- Ageing: delayed initiation of the shivering response, less sensitive response.
- Gender: females have a smaller thermogenic response, higher surface area/mass ratio, more body fat.
- Anaesthesia: decreased shivering.
- Dehydration: decreased sweating.
- Hyperbaria: inert gas narcosis decreases shivering and thermal perception.
- Hypobaria/hypoxia: impaired shivering response.
- Hypercapnia: impaired shivering response.
- Hypoglycaemia: delayed initiation of the shivering response, less sensitive response, decreased thermal perception.
- Trauma: varies with type of trauma.
- Motion illness: diminished vasoconstrictor response in the cold, faster deep body cooling.
- Acclimation:

  - Cold: decreased shivering response over body temperatures experienced during acclimation (beyond these temperatures, response returns to normal), no change in sensitivity of shivering response, increased thermal comfort.
  - Heat: earlier and increased production of more dilute sweat, more effective distribution of sweat, increased plasma volume, decreased cardiovascular strain, increased work capacity, increased thermal comfort.

- Medical/genetic conditions: varies with condition, e.g. metabolic and neuromuscular disorders (muscular dystrophy, diabetes mellitus, myasthenia gravis) impair heat production.
- Drug intoxication: varies with drug:

  - Alcohol (75 ml in 200 ml water): diminishes thermal perception and vasoconstrictor response in cold air. In water, alcohol does not appear to alter the average fall in rectal temperature over a 30-minute immersion in 15 °C water when compared with controls. Thus, the greater cold stimulus represented by water appears to override the vasodilatory action of alcohol.
  - Marijuana: despite increasing metabolic rate to a higher level than in control subjects, marijuana (0.739 g) smoked immediately before immersion does not alter the average rectal temperature response over a 60-minute immersion in water at 28 °C.
  - Ecstasy: the available literature suggests that the prolonged use of ecstasy (methylenedioxymethamphetamine, MDMA) damages 5-hydroxytryptamine (5-HT) nerve terminals in the central nervous system and delays both the onset and the magnitude of the thermoregulatory effector mechanisms. As a consequence, the thermoneutral zone is widened, and hypo- and hyperthermia occur more easily.

MEASURING THE BODY'S TEMPERATURE AND THERMOREGULATORY RESPONSE

Body temperature

Although the thermoregulatory system has multiple inputs, central nervous thermoreception and integration and a range of effector responses, thermoregulatory studies in humans are limited to the assessment of body temperatures and effector response. Usually, skin and deep body temperatures are measured; muscle temperature is measured in a smaller number of studies. The effector responses measured most often are shivering, sweating and cutaneous blood flow.

Skin temperature can be measured using a variety of techniques, including thermistors, thermocouples and infrared thermography. Individual skin temperatures are normally combined to produce a mean skin temperature for the purpose of calculating the gradient for heat exchange between the surface of the skin and environment. For this, a weighting is given to each skin temperature site that equates to the fraction of the total surface area of the body represented by that site. The greater the number of skin sites sampled, the smaller the fraction of the total body surface area represented by each site, and the higher the accuracy of the estimation of mean skin temperature (International Organization for Standardization 2004a).

Skin and mean skin temperature are easy to measure and calculate but often misused. Frequently, mean skin calculations, developed and area-weighted in one environment, are employed in other, inappropriate and unvalidated, conditions. Therefore, careful consideration should be given to the number of skin sites sampled and the locations measured; these will vary depending on the nature of the environment, the clothing worn and the response being investigated. For example, on immersion in water, skin temperature is 'clamped' close to water temperature and varies little between immersed sites. As a consequence, fewer sites need to be measured in order to obtain an estimation of mean skin temperature. In air or when clothing is being worn, more skin temperature sites must be measured in order to obtain an accurate estimation of mean skin temperature. Olesen (1984) compared ten equations for estimating mean skin temperature with the temperature obtained from 14 unweighted skin sites chosen to represent an equal area of the body surface. It was concluded that the number of sites necessary to obtain an accurate estimation of mean skin temperature correlates with the non-uniformity of skin temperature. Thus, in warm conditions, two to four sites may be sufficient; in thermoneutral conditions, four to eight sites are necessary; and in cold conditions, eight to twelve sites are recommended.

Usually, the weightings used in the calculation of mean skin temperature reflect surface area. However, if skin temperature is being correlated with the shivering or sweating response rather than heat exchange, then other sites and weightings, e.g. related to cutaneous thermoreceptor distribution, may be more appropriate.

As skin temperature can be the same for a variety of combinations of exercise, clothing and environmental temperature, this variable does not always reflect heat exchange with the environment. Heat transfer from the skin or clothing to the environment can be measured using heat-flux transducers. These include two thermistors that measure the surface temperature of a disc made from material of known conductivity. They have a fixed and known surface area. The temperature difference across the disc is used to determine the direction of heat flow and its magnitude in Watts per square metre.

Muscle temperature, typically measured at a depth of 2–3 cm, can be obtained from needle thermistors or thermocouples or fine-wire thermistors inside a guide cannula. Usually, only a limited number of sites are measured, and it is difficult to determine how representative are the data being collected.

Deep body temperature can be measured at several different sites using a variety of techniques, including thermometers (mercury-in-glass, alcohol-in-glass, infrared), thermistors, thermocouples and gastrointestinal radio-pills. Each site and technique has benefits and disadvantages. Some of these are reviewed in Table 12.5.

As with skin temperature, the site used to measure deep body temperature should be given careful consideration and will depend on the nature of the study being undertaken. Particular thought should be given to the rate of change of deep body temperature likely to be induced and the speed of response of the sites being considered. It is also clear that no single deep body temperature exists.

For thermoregulatory studies, mean skin and deep body temperature are often combined to produce mean body temperature. The rationale for this is that as thermoregulatory responses can be initiated by alterations in both skin and deep body temperature, a combination of both of these

Table 12.5 *Sites for measurement of deep-body temperature*

Site	Comment
Oral	Most commonly used site clinically. Affected by breathing, speaking, eating and dinking. May take up to 5 minutes to obtain a representative reading. Too inaccurate for use in thermoregulatory studies
Rectum	Robust site. Rectal probe should be inserted at least 10 cm. Slow-responding: appropriate for cooling/steady-state studies, but less useful under dynamic conditions, such as rapid heating. Can be up to 0.5 °C higher than other deep-body sites. Aesthetically displeasing but generally tolerated well
External auditory meatus/ tympanic membrane	Thermistor or thermocouple must be close to the tympanic membrane, and the ear canal must be insulated (1–2 cm thick) from the environment to minimize the thermal gradient along it. Influenced by facial skin temperature and external carotid artery temperature. Can be painful and aggravating, but when accurate gives a good estimation of hypothalamic temperature: internal carotid artery supplies tympanic membrane (in part) and hypothalamus. Infrared devices have become used more widely but are too inaccurate (in part, due to user error) for thermoregulatory studies
Oesophagus	Probe passes in through nose, usually to level of the heart (probe length 25% of height). Accurate but uncomfortable to introduce and remove. Provides good index of blood temperature with short time lag (< 1 min). Can be influenced by food, drink and swallowed saliva
Urine	Same temperature as bladder if measured when being voided (e.g. thermistor in urine flow). Can be used only when subject can urinate. Easy to use inaccurately
Gastrointestinal tract	Measured using radio-pill, the transmitted frequency of which is correlated with pill temperature according to a calibration curve established before use. Good for field studies. Tolerated well by subjects now that pills are disposable. Some find the pills difficult to swallow, and battery decay can alter calibration. Temperature may increase as the pill enters the rectum. Should not be used until it has left the stomach. Transit through the gastrointestinal tract usually takes 24–36 h
Transcutaneous temperature	Insulated disc is placed on body (usually chest). Contains two thermistors and a heating circuit that is warmed until no thermal gradient exists across a pad. At this point, deep-body temperature has been exteriorized and can be measured. Acceptable to subjects, responds to changing temperature, and results are independent of environmental temperature. Gives slightly lower temperatures than those recorded in rectum. Requires power supply

temperatures will give a closer approximation of the actual temperature of the 'controlled' variable within the system. The most accurate mathematical representation of this variable would require terms for tissue temperature at several sites as well as allow for threshold, rate and non-linear effects. In practice, it is more straightforward, but still useful, to combine the most easily measured temperatures (skin, deep body) in the following linear equation:

$$\overline{T}_b = \alpha T_{db} + (1 - \alpha)\overline{T}_{sk}$$

where $\overline{T}_b$ is the mean body temperature, T_c is the deep body temperature and $\overline{T}_{sk}$ is the mean skin temperature (all in °C). α is a factor that determines the weighting between the deep body tissues and the skin, i.e. how much of the body is regarded as deep or superficial tissue. The weightings are only approximations and differ between subjects and conditions according to body build, distribution of fat, and state of vasomotion (peripheral blood flow). For example, in the heat, when blood flow is high and deep body temperature is exteriorized, α often is given a value as high as 0.92; with cold-induced vasoconstriction, however, a value of 0.64 can be used for α.

As described at the beginning of this chapter, mean body temperature, and thus deep body and skin temperature, are also used in the calculation of the heat content of the body in order to determine heat storage.

Measuring effector responses

Peripheral blood flow can be measured and estimated by a large number of methods, the most commonly used of which are laser Doppler, infrared photoplethysmography, strain gauge and venous-occlusion plethysmography. In constant environments, heat flux and skin temperature can be used. Forearm–fingertip skin temperature difference seems to be a useful, easy and robust way of determining the onset of vasoconstriction and vasodilation (House and Tipton 2002). All of these techniques have advantages and disadvantages, and the method chosen will depend on the specific circumstances. In all cases, it is worth remembering that the techniques sample only a small portion of total skin blood flow and that significant regional variations exist in this response. Laser Doppler flowmetry is used widely in clinical practice and scientific investigations; it has been shown to produce values in proportion to those obtained by other methods such as [133]xenon washout, plethysmography and video microscopy.

Shivering is normally assessed by measuring oxygen consumption (see Metabolism), the assumption being that shivering causes any increase seen in this variable in a resting individual in the cold (Figure 12.9). Electromyography is also used to identify shivering; a popular muscle for this purpose is the sternomastoid.

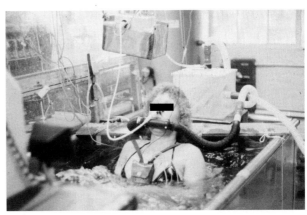

Figure 12.9   *Measuring shivering by open-circuit spirometry.*

In naked individuals, sweat production and evaporation normally are assessed by the change in naked body weight before and after exposure, making appropriate allowances for any fluid or food consumed and any urine or faeces produced. Any unevaporated sweat can be wiped from the skin with tissues and measured as an increase in the weight of the tissues. In clothed subjects, naked weight before and after exposure indicates sweat production, and the difference between clothed weight and naked weight before and after gives a value for sweat evaporation, the assumption being that the sweat that was not evaporated remains in the clothing. This is a whole-body but gross measure; it takes no account of respiratory water loss or substrate utilization during prolonged experiments.

Onset of sweating and changes in sweat rate can be recorded using a sweat capsule. This device includes a capsule of known surface area through which air is passed at a low flow rate (e.g. 1 litre/min). The humidity and temperature of the air are measured on entry and exit from the capsule. Sweat onset is seen as an increase in humidity, and sweat rate can be calculated from temperature, humidity, flow rate and capsule surface area. In theory, sweat capsules can be positioned anywhere on the body; the forehead is used frequently, and the forearm provides the best indication of whole-body sweat rate.

Having reviewed the thermal environment and thermoregulation, in the following chapter the impact of thermal stress on the body is examined in terms of threats and solutions.

REFERENCES

Barnett PW. Field tests of two anti-exposure assemblies. Arctic Aerospace Laboratories report no. AAL-TDR-61-56, 1962.

Clarke RP, Edholm OG. *Man and His Thermal Environment*. London: Edward Arnold, 1985.

Fanger PO. *Thermal Comfort.* Copenhagen: Danish Technical Press, 1970.

Golden FS. Hypothermia: a problem for North Sea industries. *Journal of the Society of Occupational medicine* 1976; **26**: 85–88.

Golden FS, Tipton MJ. Human thermal responses during leg-only exercise in cold water. *Journal of Physiology* 1987; **391**: 399–405.

Golden FS, Tipton MJ. *Essentials of Sea Survival.* Champaign, IL: Human Kinetics, 2002.

Hayes PA, Cohen JB. Further developments of a mathematical model of immersion clothing insulation. Institute of Aviation Medicine report no. 653. Royal Air Force, MoD, UK, 1987.

Hayward JS, Eckerson JD, Collis ML. Thermal balance and survival time prediction of man in cold water. *Canadian Journal of Physiology and Pharmacology* 1975; **53**: 21–32.

House JR, Tipton MJ. Using skin temperature gradients or skin heat flux measurements to determine thresholds of vasoconstriction and vasodilatation. *European Journal of Applied Physiology* 2002; **88**: 141–5.

International Organization for Standardization. Evaluation of cold environments: determination of required clothing insulation (IREQ). ISO TR11079. Geneva: International Organization for Standardization, 1993.

International Organization for Standardization. Ergonomics: evaluation of thermal strain by physiological measurements. ISO 9886. Geneva: International Organization for Standardization, 2004a.

International Organization for Standardization. Ergonomics of the thermal environment: analytical determination and interpretation of heat stress using calculation of the predicted heat strain. ISO 7933. Geneva: International Organization for Standardization, 2004b.

Keatinge WR. *Survival in Cold Water.* Oxford: Blackwell Scientific, 1969.

Kellogg DL, Jr, Liu Y, McAllister K, Friel C, Pergola PE. Bradykinin does not mediate cutaneous active vasodilatation during heat stress in humans. *Journal of Applied Physiology* 2002; **93**: 1215–21.

Kumar Y, Chawla A, Tatu U. Heat shock protein 70 as a biomarker of heat stress in a simulated hot cockpit. *Aviation, Space, and Environmental Medicine* 2003; **74**: 711–16.

Mekjavic IB, Tipton MJ, Eiken O. Thermal considerations in diving. In: Brubak AO, Neuman TS (eds). *Barnett & Elliot's Physiology and Medicine of Diving*, 5th edn. Saunders, Elsevier Science, 2003.

Nunneley SA, Stribley RF. Fighter index of thermal stress (FITS): guidance for hot weather aircraft operations. *Aviation, Space, and Environmental Medicine* 1979; **50**: 639–42.

Nunnely SA, Wissler EH. Prediction of immersion hypothermia in men wearing anti-exposure suits and/or using life rafts. Advisory Group for Aerospace Research and Development, AGARD-CP-286, A1-1–A1-8, 1980.

Oakley EHN, Pethybridge R. The prediction of survival during cold immersion: results from the UK National Immersion Incident survey. INM report no. 97011, Institute of Naval Medicine, MoD UK, Gosport, 1997.

Olesen BW. How many sites are necessary to estimate a mean skin temperature? In: Hales JRS (ed.). *Thermal Physiology.* New York: Raven Press, 1984; pp. 33–8.

Parsons KC. *Human Thermal Environments.* London: Taylor & Francis, 1993.

Sherrington C. *The Integrative Action of the Nervous System.* New Haven, CT: Yale University Press, 1906.

Stolwijk JAJ, Hardy JD. Temperature regulation in man. Plüger's Archiv: *European Journal of Physiology* 1966; **291**: 129–62.

Tikuisis P. Prediction of survival time for cold exposure. In: Frim J, Ducharme MB, Tikuisis P (eds). *Proceedings of the 6th International Conference on Environmental Ergonomics.* Canada: Montebello, 1994; pp. 160–61.

Wenger CB, Roberts MF, Nadel ER, Stolwijk JAJ. Thermoregulatory control of finger blood flow. *Journal of Applied Physiology* 1975; **38**: 1078–82.

FURTHER READING

Moran DS, Pandolf KB. Wet bulb globe temperature (WBGT): to what extent is GT essential? *Aviation, Space, and Environmental Medicine* 1999; **70**: 480–84, 720.

Moran DS, Shitzer A, Pandolf KB. A physiological strain index to evaluate heat stress. *American Journal of Physiology* 1998; **275**: R129–34.

Moran DS, Castellani JW, O'Brien C, Young AJ, Pandolf KB. Evaluating physiological strain during cold exposure using a new cold strain index. *American Journal of Physiology* 1999; **277**: R556–64.

Moran DS, Pandolf KB, Laor A, *et al.* Evaluation and refinement of the environmental stress index for different climatic conditions. *Journal of Basic and Clinical Physiology and Pharmacology* 2003; **14**: 1–15.

Siple PA, Passel CF. Measurement of dry atmospheric cooling in subfreezing temperatures. *Proceedings of the American Philosophical Society* 1945; **89**: 177–99.

13

Thermal stress and survival

MIKE TIPTON

INTRODUCTION

Having described the physics and physiology associated with the achievement of thermal balance in Chapter 12, we will now examine what happens when such balance is not achieved and what can be done to prevent and treat the most common thermal injuries. An understanding of these areas should enable individuals to appreciate the limitations of the human thermoregulatory system and to recognize the early signs of the various thermally related illnesses. Such knowledge enhances the capability to take preventive action and to administer appropriate treatment. In the context of a flying mission, any member of the flight team – i.e. not just the aircrew – may experience thermal problems. Indeed, often it is the ground crew who are placed at greatest risk; for example, it is this group that are most likely to have to undertake tasks requiring physical work in hot conditions.

THREATS

Whenever possible in air, the human thermoregulatory system moderates heat exchange with the environment so as to maintain deep body temperature within about 1 °C of 37 °C and mean skin temperature at about 33 °C. In thermoneutral conditions, these body temperatures can be achieved by alterations in skin blood flow. Thus, this zone is often referred to as the 'thermoneutral zone' or 'vasomotor zone'. In warmer or colder conditions, the autonomic thermoregulatory responses, primarily sweating and shivering, are evoked to help maintain a stable deep body temperature; hence, this zone is referred to as the 'thermoregulatory zone'. Thermoregulation in this zone is possible as long as sweating and shivering can proceed at the required rate; anything that impairs these processes (e.g. dehydration, starvation/hypoglycaemia) may prevent the body remaining in the thermoregulatory zone (Figure 13.1). When the thermal stress of an environment overwhelms the thermoregulatory capability of the body, deep body temperature will rise or fall uncontrollably and result in hyperthermia or hypothermia. Humans can survive a fall in core temperature of around 10 °C (but note that this figure can vary dramatically) and an increase of about 6 °C. Before these lethal body temperatures are reached, thermal

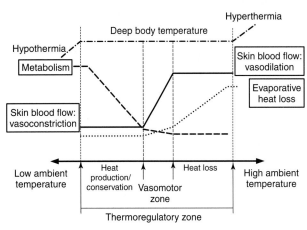

Figure 13.1 *Thermoregulatory zones.*

strain can have a significant impact on physical and mental performance.

Even in temperate environments, heat illness and dehydration can represent significant problems when exposure is associated with exercise and the requirement to use protective clothing and equipment. These problems are compounded in hot environments. In cold environments, the combination of low ambient temperatures and peripheral vasoconstriction can lower tissue temperatures to the levels at which freezing and non-freezing cold injuries become possible. Although not immediately life-threatening, these injuries are serious and have lifelong sequelae. In the sections that follow, hyperthermia, hypothermia and cold injuries are examined in more detail.

HYPERTHERMIA

Many occupational groups, such as fire-fighters, divers and military personnel, can be presented with a combination of physical and environmental demands that push them to their physiological limits. During sustained vigorous exercise, heat production by the body can increase 20–25 times above the resting levels, reaching in excess of 80 kJ/min. This heat must be removed from the body to prevent an undesirable rise in body temperature. For example, most individuals will be unable to tolerate a deep body temperature of 42 °C with a skin temperature of 38 °C without suffering heat illness. These body temperatures represent an increase in the amount of heat stored in the body of a 70-kg human of about 1045 kJ. If the body were prevented from losing any of the heat it produced, then a fatal level of heat storage would be reached in about four hours when at rest, and after just 25 minutes with moderate exercise.

Clothing, especially specialist protective clothing, can significantly impede heat loss. Such clothing includes that used by fire-fighters and by civilian and military groups, such as immersion coveralls. Indeed, the most commonly reported cause of heat strain in Royal Navy (RN) aircrew is the impermeable immersion suit. Modern extended coverage anti-G clothing, chest counter-pressure garments and chemical, biological, radioactive and nuclear (CBRN) protective clothing all impede heat loss from the body. The combination of insulative garments and high metabolic heat production can result in heat illness in temperate conditions. The effects can range from impairment of performance to death. In 2000, 112 fire-fighters lost their lives in the USA, with the single largest cause of death (46 cases) being cardiac problems related to hyperthermia caused by the inability to lose metabolic heat.

Heat strain is recognized as a limitation in military air operations. In a review and questionnaire survey of 121 RN helicopter aircrew (House 1999), 53 per cent reported that heat strain reduced operational capabilities and 37 per cent

reported that it reduced flight safety. The heat load on a pilot within a cockpit comes from metabolism, the outside environment and the cockpit environment. Ambient thermal conditions have been related to cockpit temperatures and pilot mean body temperature in helicopters and Harrier and Buccaneer fast jets. Aircrew metabolic heat production varies from sedentary levels (60–80 W/m²) during straight and level flight to moderate levels (180–240 W/m²) during demanding flight, such as that requiring anti-G manoeuvres. A military pilot may start a flight with a raised body temperature due to the exertion associated with donning flying and protective clothing. Pre-flight checks in hot environments can add to the thermal load. Initial cockpit temperatures can be high if the aircraft has been parked in direct sunlight. Cabin dry-bulb temperatures as high as 50 °C have been measured in Mk8 Lynx helicopters in such conditions, with dashboard temperatures exceeding 61 °C when external temperature was 25 °C. Taxiing and standby also can result in high cockpit temperatures in hot (33 °C) environments (cockpit wet-bulb globe temperature (WBGT) of approximately 30 °C; from globe 45 °C, dry bulb 36 °C, wet bulb 25 °C), as air-conditioning systems are usually at their least effective at this time. In fast jets, cockpit temperatures tend to fall during flight, as air temperature falls with altitude, air-conditioning becomes more effective and stored heat is removed from the materials of the cockpit. In two-seater jets (F4 Phantom), the front cockpit cools more than the rear, which remains hot during flight. A thermal challenge can also arise in aircraft operating at low level with inadequate air-conditioning (Nunneley et al. 1981).

The sources of heat arising from aircraft include the avionic systems within the cockpit and aerodynamic friction (Table 13.1). This friction can raise the fuselage temperature to several hundred degrees during low-altitude high-speed flying due to the combined factors of higher air temperature and density.

The heat load on a pilot is but one of several stressors that can be experienced in the cockpit; others include noise, vibration, G, motion illness and confinement. These stressors can interact, e.g. both motion illness and hyperthermia-induced dehydration can reduce G-tolerance by 0.5 to 1 G.

Table 13.1 *Sources of heat in the cockpit of a Tornado aircraft flying at mach 0.9 at sea level and ambient air at 40° C*

Heat source	Heat production (kW)
Pilot's metabolism	0.06
Aerodynamic heat load	9
Avionics	1.2
Solar radiation	2.5
Total	12.76

Heat: effects on performance

It is unusual for the tasks associated with flying to increase metabolism to much higher than moderate levels. However, even this intensity of activity in the heat places an additional strain on the cardiovascular system. Heat dissipation occurs more by repartitioning cardiac output than by increasing it: 15–25 per cent of cardiac output is directed to the skin to assist in heat loss; constriction of splanchnic and renal vascular beds aids the majority of this increase in cutaneous blood flow. Compromised muscle blood flow and decreased hepatic blood flow result in an earlier onset of anaerobic metabolism and blood lactate accumulation. Muscle glycogen utilization is increased and fatigue occurs earlier during prolonged moderate exercise in the heat. There is also a diminished central drive to exercise in hyperthermic individuals. Heating does not decrease maximum strength, but it does reduce muscle endurance and time to fatigue. Aerobically fit individuals are able to perform for longer in hot environments and tolerate higher levels of hyperthermia than less fit individuals. However, abnormally high core temperatures impair performance in all individuals in the heat.

With regard to psychological function, mild heat strain can result in deterioration in attention and vigilance, memory registration and recall, reasoning and decision-making. Mental performance is degraded on the most boring, monotonous and repetitive tasks and tasks requiring concentration, attention to detail and short-term memory. Vigilance performance will degrade slightly after 30 minutes and markedly after two to three hours. These decrements are due, in part, to thermal discomfort. A dose–response relationship has been reported (Froom *et al.* 1991, 1993) between ambient heat stress and pilot error in Israeli military helicopter pilots operating in the field; error rates were lower when the ambient dry-bulb temperature was 25–29 °C and increased to high-risk levels when it exceeded 35 °C. This was the first study outside a laboratory to identify this relationship.

The above physiological and psychological changes mean that even mild to moderate levels of heat strain can cause aircrew to be more likely to tire and make errors.

During exposure to heat, body fluid loss, due primarily to sweating, increases by an amount that depends on several factors, including environmental temperature, level and duration of any activity undertaken, state of fitness and level of acclimatization. Maximum sweat losses of about 2 l/h are possible. Without adequate fluid replacement, dehydration occurs; this can also affect performance. It is important to recognize the signs of dehydration, which include fatigue, headache, irritability and insomnia. In comparison with the responses seen when hydrated, dehydration between 1.9 and 4.3 per cent of body mass can reduce physical endurance by 22–48 per cent. Dehydration equivalent to five per cent of body mass increases rectal temperature due to decreased sweating and cutaneous blood flow and is associated with weariness and nausea. Thirst is not a reliable indicator of hydration status, and the satiation of thirst is not a reliable indicator of rehydration. Although sodium is also lost in sweat, the high salt intake of the average Western diet usually prevents the muscle cramps, vomiting and nausea associated with sodium depletion.

It is not possible to adapt to reduced fluid intake, and the risk of heat illness is increased if exercise is undertaken in the heat in a dehydrated state (Figure 13.2).

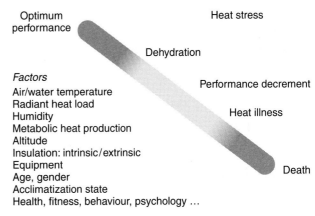

Factors
Air/water temperature
Radiant heat load
Humidity
Metabolic heat production
Altitude
Insulation: intrinsic/extrinsic
Equipment
Age, gender
Acclimatization state
Health, fitness, behaviour, psychology …

Figure 13.2 *Effects of heat on the body. See also colour plate 13.2.*

Heat illness

If the heat load on the body is greater than that which can be ameliorated by the thermoregulatory system (i.e. above the thermoregulatory zone), then deep body temperature will rise uncontrollably and dangerous levels of hyperthermia are possible. The problems caused by heat result from decreased circulating blood volume and consequent alterations in regional blood flow, increased blood viscosity, and a direct effect of temperature on the respiratory centres and proteins. Heat illness can occur in cool or temperate conditions if humidity is high (sweat evaporation impaired) or, as mentioned above, if the individual is unable to offload the heat produced from high work rates due to clothing. The conditions recognized as heat illness include heat cramps, heat exhaustion and heat stroke (Table 13.2).

The prognosis for a person suffering heat illness appears to be related to the length of time that the deep body temperature remains above about 40 °C. Initial treatment should focus on resuscitation, reducing deep body temperature, fluid replacement, treatment of any seizures and evacuation.

Table 13.2 *Heat illness*

Condition	Description
Heat cramps	Usually occur in the specific muscles exercised due to an imbalance in the body's fluid volume and electrolyte concentration, and low energy stores. Core temperature remains in normal range. Aetiology unknown. Can be prevented by appropriate rehydration strategy. Treated by stretching and massage
Heat syncope	Faint caused by a combination of lowered circulating blood volume as a consequence of dehydration and increased thermal demand for peripheral blood flow. Can be exacerbated by venous pooling in the lower limbs due to remaining stationary in an upright posture. Heart rate increases, but blood flow to the brain can fall, producing syncope. Casualty should be kept horizontal, removed to a cool environment and rehydrated
Heat exhaustion	Most common form of heat illness, defined as the inability to continue exercising in the heat. Usually seen in unacclimatized individuals. Caused by ineffective circulatory adjustments and reduced blood volume. Characterized by breathlessness, hyperventilation, weak and rapid pulse, low blood pressure, dizziness, headache, flushed skin, nausea, paradoxical chills, irritability, lethargy and general weakness. Deep body temperature is raised, but not excessively, sweating persists and there is no organ damage. Heat-exhausted individuals should stop exercising, lie down, control breathing if hyperventilating and rehydrate; failure to do so can result in progression to severe heat illness. Heat exhaustion is a predominant problem when body water loss exceeds 7% of body mass
Heat stroke	Medical emergency resulting from failure of thermoregulatory system due to high deep body temperature (> 40.5 °C). Characterized by confusion, absence of sweating, hot and dry skin and circulatory instability. If not treated by immediate cooling, results in death from circulatory collapse and multi-organ damage. Aggressive steps should be taken to cool the casualty, as mortality is related to degree and duration of hyperthermia. Consider using 'artificial sweat' (spraying with tepid water/alcohol) and fanning; fluid replacement (do not overinfuse/overload, as can result in pulmonary oedema). Consider colder water immersion/ice packs if no peripheral circulation

A large list of factors influence thermoregulation in the heat and an individual's susceptibility to heat illness, including:

- air temperature, humidity, movement, radiant heat load
- body size (mass, skin-fold thickness): heat stroke occurs 3.5 times more frequently in excessively overweight young adults than in individuals of average body mass; children are also at greater risk, due to their relative large surface area/mass ratio
- state of training/sudden increase in training (military recruits with low aerobic fitness (> 12 min for 1.5-mile run) and high body mass index (> 26 kg/m²) have a nine-fold greater risk of heat illness)
- degree of acclimatization
- hydration status
- heat production (metabolic intensity/duration)
- clothing worn (vapour permeability, fit, colour)
- state of health, e.g. fever, viral illness, cold, 'flu, diabetes mellitus, cardiovascular disease, gastroenteritis/diarrhoea)
- genetic disorders, e.g. mutations for cystic fibrosis, malignant hyperthermia
- skin disorders, including sunburn over five per cent of body surface area
- use of medication, e.g. diuretics, antihistamines, ergogenic stimulants
- sweat gland dysfunction, e.g. prickly heat
- salt depletion
- age
- sleep deprivation
- glycogen or glucose depletion
- acute/chronic alcohol/drug abuse
- psychology: perception of thermal environment/ motivation to continue exercising in the heat.

Because some of these factors can operate acutely (e.g. infection), an individual may suffer heat illness in circumstances in which previously they have been unaffected.

Severe heat illness is unlikely to occur in the cockpit, but it may occur in ground crew in hot environments. The more subtle effects of heat strain on performance, as noted above, are much more common. Indeed, heat stress is accepted widely as 'part of the job' of a military aviator. However, it is critical that the resulting level of heat strain remains below a level at which flight safety is compromised. In connection with this, there are no specific rules about the thermal conditions in cockpits, and the recommendation remains that thermal stress should be kept as low as possible.

Heat strain: protection and prevention

In this section, the strategies and technologies that can be used in order to reduce heat stress, increase heat tolerance and thereby help maintain performance in the heat are considered.

Pre-flight

The risk associated with a warm environment can be assessed using one of the heat stress indices introduced in Chapter 12. These include the fighter index of thermal stress (FITS), which is an attempt to provide an operational index that would predict, based on the environmental conditions on the ground, the thermal stress in a fast-jet cockpit during low-level flight. It is derived from the most widely used heat stress index, the WBGT index:

$$WBGT = 0.1T_{db} + 0.7T_{wb} + 0.2T_{g}$$

where T_{db} is the dry-bulb temperature, T_{wb} is the wet-bulb temperature and T_{g} is the globe temperature. The weightings emphasize the importance of humidity for heat stress.

WBGT meters are relatively inexpensive. They consist of a thermometer/thermistor (dry bulb), a thermometer/ thermistor covered with a dampened wick (wet bulb), and a thermometer/thermistor enclosed on a black metal sphere that absorbs radiant energy from the surroundings (globe temperature). To reduce the chance of heat injury in lightly clothed individuals, the limits given in Table 13.3 are recommended.

Acclimatization to heat increases the permissible WBGT threshold values for continuous activities, as demonstrated in Table 13.4, which was designed for UK military personnel wearing a single-layer uniform and working for one hour with a minimum of 30 minutes' rest. If CBRN, body armour or similar protective clothing is worn, WBGT values for unacclimatized personnel at low or medium work intensity should be reduced by 5 °C.

Although used widely, the WBGT index can be cumbersome and is more suited for a fixed site than a mobile site. The modified discomfort index (MDI), compiled from ambient temperature and wet-bulb temperature, correlates highly with WBGT ($r > 0.95$) and is easier to use and calculate. If the only information available is air temperature and relative humidity (rh), then the heat stress index gives an indication of the heat stress of the environment (Table 13.5).

The period before takeoff or between sorties can be the most thermally stressful for aircrew and ground crew. With regard to aircrew, it is desirable to reduce the thermal

Table 13.3   Recommended action for different wet-bulb globe temperatures (WBGTs)

WBGT (°C)	Recommendation
26.5–28.8	Use discretion, especially if untrained or unacclimatized
29.5–30.5	Avoid strenuous activity in the sun

Table 13.4   Wet-bulb globe temperature (WBGT) limits for acclimatized and unacclimatized individuals

Acclimatized (°C)	Unacclimatized (°C)	Level of maximum permitted work
No limit	32	Low, e.g. lying down, driving
30	26	Medium, e.g. marching at 2.25 mph with 30-kg load
27	24	High, e.g. marching at 3.5 mph with 20-kg load
25	20	Very high, e.g. marching at 5 mph with no load, or at 3.5 mph with 30-kg load
20	20 (maximum 30 min)	Extreme, e.g. running in sports kit

Table 13.5   Heat stress index (shaded numbers represent 'heat sensation'). See also colour plate table 13.5.

Relative humidity (%)	Air temperature (°C)										
	46.1	48.9									
	21.1	23.9	26.7	29.4	32.2	35	37.8	40.6	43.3	46.1	48.9
0	17.7	20.6	22.8	25.6	28.3	30.6	32.8	35	37.2	39.4	41.7
10	18.3	21.1	23.9	26.7	29.4	32.2	35	37.8	40.6	43.9	46.7
20	18.9	22.2	25	27.8	30.6	33.9	37.2	40.6	44.4	48.9	54.4
30	19.4	22.8	25.6	28.9	32.2	35.6	40	45	50.6	57.2	64.4
40	20	23.3	26.1	30	33.9	38.3	43.3	50.6	58.3	66.1	
50	20.6	23.9	27.2	31.1	35.6	41.7	48.9	57.2	65.6		
60	21.1	24.4	27.8	32.2	37.8	45.6	55.6	65			
70	21.1	25	29.4	33.9	41.1	51.1	62.2				
80	21.7	25.6	30	36.1	45	57.8					
90	21.7	26.1	31.1	38.9	50						
100	22.2	26.7	32.8	42.2							

32.2–40.6 °C: possibility of heat cramps during exercise.
40.6–54.4 °C: heat cramps or heat exhaustion likely; heat stroke possible.
54.4 °C+: heat stroke a definite risk.

load incurred at this time by as much as possible, as this load may not be dissipated during flying. Provision of air-conditioned buildings for briefings and for changing into flying clothing and of air-conditioned transport to the aircraft is clearly beneficial. Sufficient recovery time between sorties allows return to normothermia.

A particularly stressful time can be entry into the cockpit of an aircraft that has been parked in CBRN defence posture ('closed down') in sunlight. In such a situation, a Lynx helicopter pilot has reported being unhappy to fly after 80 minutes, by this time his rectal temperature had risen to 38.25 °C (House and Davies 2002). As mentioned above, in such situations, even with reflective coating, cockpit temperatures can rise above 50 °C. One solution to this is to cover the aircraft or ensure that it is parked in the shade wherever possible. Small further reductions can be obtained in cabin temperature by wetting the cabin cover to facilitate evaporative cooling (House and Davies 2002). Another possible partial solution involves spraying a fine mist of water over the aircraft cabin; this absorbs some of the solar infrared radiation and increases evaporative cooling. Alternatively, mobile air-conditioning units can be used to precondition the cockpit.

FITS (measured in degrees Celsius) can be calculated using the formula

$$\text{FITS} = 0.83 T_{wb} + 0.35 T_{db} + 5.08$$

where T_{wb} and T_{db} are, respectively, aspirated wet-bulb and dry-bulb ambient temperatures on the ground. The equation assumes that normal (not CBRN) aircrew clothing is worn. If the value exceeds 38 °C, thermoregulatory mechanisms will be inadequate to cope with the heat stress in the cockpit.

Acclimatization and fitness

The biological adaptations to repeated heat stress include heat acclimatization and acquired thermal tolerance. Repeated exposures to hot environments that produce increases in deep body and skin temperature, and profuse sweating, result in acclimatization to heat; this improves exercise capacity and comfort. It is important to exercise during these exposures, gradually increasing activity each day until at the required intensity, because resting in the heat provides only partial acclimatization. The acclimatization acquired is specific to the climate and activity level: people acclimatized to a hot dry environment will require additional time to acclimatize if they move to a hot humid environment.

The process requires exposure to representative environmental temperatures for at least two hours per day and takes a total of 10–14 days. No more than three days should elapse between successive exposures. The adjustments to the raised body temperatures associated with exercise mean that fitter individuals can acclimatize more quickly (seven to ten days). However, even fit individuals need to exercise in a hot environment in order to achieve full acclimatization.

The exposures can be in the field (acclimatization) or in a suitable climatic chamber (acclimation). Using sweat-suits (impermeable/semipermeable clothing) or saunas is partially effective. The beneficial changes associated with heat acclimatization include the following:

- aldosterone secretion increases and increases sodium reabsorption in sweat ducts and renal tubules. This results in lowered salt content in sweat (e.g. sweat sodium reduced from 50 to 25 mmol/l) and increased osmotic retention of water, producing increased plasma volume
- less cardiovascular strain, perfusion pressure better maintained
- more effective distribution of cardiac output
- improved cutaneous blood flow
- earlier onset and greater rate of sweating
- possibly more effective distribution of sweat over skin surface
- lower skin and deep body temperatures for given level of exercise
- improved physical work capacity
- increased comfort
- decreased reliance on carbohydrate metabolism.

Because an acclimatized individual can produce more sweat, there is a greater fluid requirement in order to maintain hydration. Following return to a temperate climate, the major benefits of heat acclimatization are retained for a week; 75 per cent are then lost within three weeks.

Acquired thermal tolerance occurs at the cellular level and refers to adaptations that protect the tissues from heat injury. It is associated with increased synthesis of heat-shock proteins, which provide protection and accelerated repair of cells from heat exposure. Acquired thermal tolerance can be induced by heat exposure or physical exercise, the largest benefits being seen when both occur. The time course for induction and decay of the heat-shock-protein responses are similar to those for heat acclimatization. Pre-induction of heat-shock proteins as a way of protecting personnel from stressful conditions is worthy of further investigation. Other cellular systems (e.g. antioxidant enzymes, stress kinase pathways) and genes have been suggested to be involved in acquired thermal tolerance, but precise contributions are yet to be elucidated.

Fluid and salt replacement

Much has been written about fluid replacement, most of it of direct relevance to prolonged athletic performance when the opportunities to drink fluids are limited. When fluid is freely available, the actual composition of a rehydration beverage is less critical. Nevertheless, it is worth understanding the basic principles of fluid replacement.

Because sweat is hypotonic in comparison with body fluids, water rather than mineral replacement is the primary concern in the heat. Water absorption occurs mainly in the upper part of the small intestine and depends on osmotic gradients. Adding small amounts of glucose and sodium to a rehydration drink has little negative effect on gastric emptying. The presence of glucose may accelerate fluid uptake due to the active co-transport of glucose and sodium across the intestinal mucosa. Adding sodium will help to maintain plasma sodium concentrations, reduce urine output and sustain the sodium-dependent osmotic drive to drink. Drinks with low sugar content (two to four per cent, 20–40 g/l) will not supply much energy, but if they are hypotonic and have a high sodium content (40–60 mmol/l, 1–1.5 g/l), then they will give the fastest water replacement. Gastric emptying slows when ingested fluids have high osmolality (plasma osmolality 280 mosm/l) or caloric content. A drink containing glucose polymers rather than simple sugars minimizes this negative effect.

Gastric volume influences gastric emptying, with emptying rate increasing with volume in the stomach. Consuming 400–600 ml immediately before exposure optimizes the transfer of fluids into the intestine. Drinking 150–250 ml at 15-minute intervals during exposure maintains gastric volume and fluid uptake at maximal levels of about 1 l/h. A drink that tastes good is more likely to be drunk. Highly carbonated beverages retard gastric emptying.

Although it is important to avoid dehydration, excessive volumes of fluid should not be ingested, as this can lead to overhydration and hyponatraemia (low blood sodium), which, if severe enough, can produce symptoms of central nervous dysfunction, lung congestion and muscle weakness. Hyponatraemia and dehydration-mediated heat exhaustion share many symptoms, and laboratory tests are required to distinguish between the two. Patients with dehydration-mediated heat exhaustion respond fairly quickly to fluid replacement, whereas hyponatraemia will be aggravated by the administration of hypotonic fluids. The International Marathon Medical Directors Association (IMMDA) has stated that blanket hydration recommendations for athletes are incorrect and unsafe and that athletes should drink as needed but not exceed 400–800 ml/h: lesser amounts for slower, smaller athletes in mild environments and greater amounts for faster athletes in warmer environments. Other than in exceptional circumstances, daily fluid intake should not exceed 12 litres. Hydration status can be monitored by measuring urine specific gravity or by noting the colour and volume of urine produced; frequent and large volumes of light-coloured urine indicate that fluid intake is sufficient.

If personnel are heat-acclimatized and eating, then the salt obtained from and added to food usually is adequate to meet the body's needs, except in extreme conditions. Sodium intake is likely to range between 170 mmol/day (average UK diet) and 380 mmol/day (UK military ration pack). Thus, a sodium deficit will occur if daily sweat losses exceed 3.5–7.5 litres for unacclimatized individuals and exceed 7–15 litres for acclimatized individuals. Salt tablets are not recommended without medical supervision, as their use has been associated with gastrointestinal discomfort and incapacitating nausea.

Clothing and personal cooling systems

From a thermal perspective, clothing can be a major advantage or disadvantage, depending on whether it is providing protection against a thermal load (e.g. fire-fighting clothing) or preventing the loss of metabolic heat from the body (e.g. exercising in CBRN protective clothing). Ideally, the extrinsic insulation provided by clothing will help to achieve the same objective as that of the intrinsic insulation of the body, which is to maintain body temperature within the vasomotor zone.

Clothing impedes all routes of heat loss to the environment. Evaporative heat loss can occur from the surface of clothing but is less effective than at the skin surface. It also requires the clothing to be saturated with sweat; this delays the onset of evaporative cooling and makes most garments uncomfortable to wear.

To minimize the thermal burden, clothing in hot environments should be:

- lightweight/open-weave, in order to minimize insulation and increase the exchange of air between the microclimate (beneath the clothing) and environment with body movement ('bellows effect')
- light-coloured, in order to reflect more radiant heat in the visible and ultraviolet bands (colour is largely irrelevant for infrared wavelengths)
- loose, in order to facilitate the bellows effect
- vapour-permeable, in order to facilitate evaporative heat loss by preventing the clothing microclimate becoming saturated
- made from materials that readily absorb water (e.g. linen, cotton) in order to facilitate evaporative heat loss.

In space, clothing designed to reflect radiant heat is essential, as this is the only pathway for heat exchange.

In some scenarios, there is a limit to what can be achieved through basic clothing design; in response, personal cooling systems (PCSs) have been developed. These are important in countering the thermal burden in the cockpit and the resistance to heat loss from the body caused by specialist garments, such as immersion coveralls and anti-G ensembles. PCSs are cooling garments designed to be worn next to the skin; they can be divided broadly into air-cooled and liquid-cooled garments.

Air-cooled PCSs enable both convective and evaporative heat loss from the body. The convective component is related inversely to the temperature of the air flowing through the suit, and high heat losses by this route require low air temperatures, although humidity levels are irrelevant. In severe conditions, suit air inlet temperatures down to 5 °C may be required at flow rates of 1 kg/min. For convective heat loss, a high mass flow of air is required; this is usually directed preferentially over the limbs (88 per cent) rather than the torso (12 per cent), in order to help maintain the normal thermal gradient (5–6 °C) between the trunk and the extremities and thereby maintain thermal comfort.

In contrast, the use of evaporative cooling is less thermally comfortable, as it requires sweating; it also increases the likelihood of dehydration. The temperature of the air supply is less critical; there is still a net loss of heat by evaporation up at air temperatures of 45 °C. However, the efficacy of this approach is related inversely to the humidity of the air supply. A high-volume flow of air is required (about 0.5 kg/min); this is normally distributed evenly over the surface of the body in recognition of the more or less even distribution of sweating over the body surface. Suit air supply systems include (i) aircraft supply systems, which use engine air and therefore require the engine to be active, or a ground-supplied source; (ii) reverse-flow ventilation, which uses an electric fan to suck air through a ventilated suit; and (iii) portable air conditioners.

On the basis of such comparisons, it has been concluded that convective cooling is preferable to an evaporative approach. Both types of suit require filtration if operated in a chemically contaminated environment; this can represent a major drawback and engineering challenge for this type of PCS.

The first liquid-conditioned suits were developed in the UK in the 1960s. They can be used for heating or cooling. They comprise a stretch fabric undergarment with fabric tunnels containing 50–120 m of tubing. The greater the length of tubing, the better the heat extraction but the greater the resistance to flow and therefore the greater the pumping power required. To maintain normal thermal gradients, cool water can enter the suit at the wrists and ankles and then flows to the trunk, where it is collected and returned to the supply system in a closed-circuit system, thereby avoiding contamination problems. In purely physical terms, the heat removed from the body is a function of the gradient between the water temperature and skin temperature and the flow rate. However, the optimum setup is that which produces the lowest skin temperatures commensurate with the avoidance of peripheral vasoconstriction; it is better to have body heat delivered to the skin surface by mass flow than to have to drag it out from the deep tissues by conduction. Due to the way in which the thermoregulatory system functions (see Chapter 12), lower inlet temperatures will be possible when the body temperature is raised, but there is no well-established and generally applicable relationship between these two variables. In general, an inlet temperature below 15 °C is not recommended. Due to the heat-transfer characteristics of the tubes within the suit, there is a limit to the relationship between flow rate and heat extraction, such that the maximum useful flow rate in a suit containing 50 m of tubing is about 600 ml/min. Suit-cooled liquid supply systems include aircraft systems (vapour cycle refrigeration plus circulation pump) and portable systems (ice bottle plus battery-powered pump).

A suit that covers only the torso and arms is usually adequate for aviation purposes and can extract about 150 W. A suit that covers the whole body can extract around 400 W. Head cooling has been given a good deal of attention. Its attraction is the relatively weak vasoconstrictor input to the scalp and the consequent possibility of extracting large quantities of heat from this region. Liquid-conditioned hoods have been shown to improve thermal comfort during heat stress, but there are integration problems with flying helmets and they have low cooling rates.

Body–cooling after and between sorties

Returning body temperature to normal levels between repeated bouts of heat exposure helps to maintain performance, decreases physiological strain and extends work time. One of the quickest and simplest ways of doing this is by immersing the hands in cold water: the large surface area and high cutaneous blood flow of the hands make them ideal for heat exchange. The rates of heat exchange achieved by this method compare favourably with those achieved by the use of ice-vests and forced convective cooling (House 1996). Unfortunately, extremity cooling is much less effective when cooling is applied to the wrists or forearms, probably due to the dearth of arteriovenous anastomoses in these regions (see Chapter 12). Thus, the need to leave the hands free for flying tends to preclude the possibility of using extremity cooling during flight as a method of reducing thermal strain. However, the possibility of using cooled gloves or controls deserves further consideration.

Appropriate work–rest schedules, the provision of shaded cooled areas, and the availability of hand cooling and fluid for rehydration are the best ways of ensuring that busy ground crew operating in hot environments remain healthy and effective.

Environmental control systems

It would be exceptional for any of the severe heat illnesses described above to be produced in the cockpit environment, although they may be experienced by ground crew. However, the more subtle manifestations of heat stress are much more common in the cockpit. To protect occupants against thermal and pressure effects, most aircraft are equipped with an environmental control system (ECS), which conditions the air within the cockpit. These systems serve a number of functions, such as cabin pressurization, temperature control to provide cooling (or heating in cold conditions) for both avionics systems and cabin occupants, demisting, pressure for canopy seals, and provision of air supplies to anti-G and on-board oxygen generating systems. The details of ECS design vary considerably between aircraft, but Figure 13.3 shows a typical layout.

The requirement for the air to be pressurized is achieved by bleeding it from the compression stage of the engines. However, the pressure is greatly in excess of that required for cabin pressurization, and the temperature of the air may be in excess of 500 °C. The ECS, therefore, operates to lower both the pressure and the temperature of this compressed air to the required values. The air is passed through a pressure-reducing valve and cooled by bringing it into proximity with ambient ram air in the primary heat exchanger. It then passes to a bootstrap cold-air unit (CAU), which consists of a compressor, secondary heat exchanger (or intercooler) and downstream turbine (Figure 13.4). The air in the CAU is compressed, which raises its temperature; this increases the temperature gradient between it and the ambient air as it passes through the intercooler, thus increasing heat loss from the conditioned air to the environment. As the air passes into the turbine, the air expands, which further lowers its temperature; it also loses energy by driving the turbine blades that work the compressor; both of these physical processes remove heat from the air, and the air leaves the CAU at a temperature of around −20 °C. Fine control of the desired temperature is achieved by mixing this cold air with warm air that bypasses the CAU. Water vapour condenses out

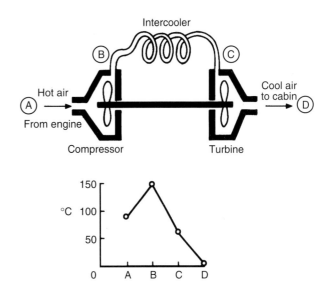

Figure 13.4 *Diagram of a cold-air unit. The graph shows typical temperatures at four points throughout the unit.*

and is removed by centrifugation before the air is distributed via ductwork to the avionics and the cabin.

Control systems have a number of inherent design limitations. They add weight to the aircraft and their requirement for bleed air from the engines reduces engine performance. Some aircraft require the ECS to be turned off for a high all-up-weight takeoff. Control systems are a potent source of cabin noise, which can be a problem particularly in commercial passenger aircraft. To counteract the high heat loads that are present, conditioning of the entire cockpit interior to the desired temperature may require extremely low air temperatures, which paradoxically can lead to problems of localized cold discomfort. This can be largely avoided by careful design of the outlet nozzles, such that the cooled air is directed on to the cockpit occupants, optimizing its effectiveness. As water extraction

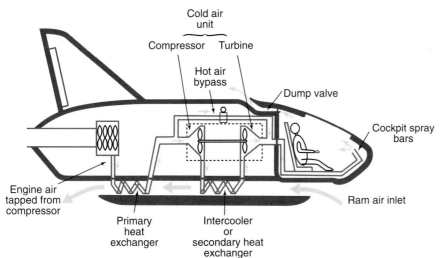

Figure 13.3 *Schematic diagram showing the arrangement of the main components of a typical environmental control system. See also colour plate 13.3.*

is rarely totally efficient, cooling the air to sub-zero temperatures will cause the remaining water to freeze, with the undesirable result that ice may be blown into the cockpit.

Determining the air temperature that is required in the cockpit is difficult as it depends on many variables. It is important that the ECS has a means of allowing the manual selection of the temperature of the conditioned air. The effectiveness of the ECS varies dramatically between aircraft types. Generally, in commercial aircraft, the ECS provides a comfortable 'shirtsleeves' environment throughout the aircraft. The temperature within military transport aircraft is less uniform, and the ECS in a number of these aircraft is unable to maintain comfortable temperatures on the flight deck and in the rear of the aircraft at the same time. The problem is even worse in most helicopters, particularly if required to fly with open doors or hatches, when the heating or cooling system may be unable to counteract the effects of the environment. The effectiveness of the fast-jet ECS is highly dependent on the phase of flight and on the clothing worn by the aircrew. If the ECS is unable to provide adequate cooling to prevent a degree of heat strain that has the potential to interfere with aircrew performance, then there is a strong argument for the provision of a personal cooling system, as described previously.

HYPOTHERMIA AND COLD INJURY

In recent years in the military, there has tended to be a preoccupation with heat and hot environments. However, there are many regions of the world and survival scenarios in which both aircrew and ground crew may be exposed to the threats associated with cold environments. As with heat, in normal circumstances it is likely that ground crew will be at greater risk than aircrew.

In most situations in air, when appropriate clothing is worn, the heat produced by the body via activity or shivering is sufficient to offset that lost to a cold environment. In air, therefore, problems with cooling tend to arise only when heat production is reduced due to injury or exhaustion or when heat loss is accelerated due to inappropriate thermal protection.

Although air can reach lower temperatures than water, water represents the greater threat because of its higher thermal conductivity and specific heat (see Chapter 12). Skin temperature cools rapidly on immersion in cold water, and the deep body temperature of an individual immersed in cold water will cool about four times faster than when in air at the same temperature. In contrast to the situation in air, exercise in cold water tends to accelerate rather than prevent cooling because the heat produced by the exercise does not balance that lost as a result of moving in the water (increased convection) and increasing blood flow to the peripheral musculature (loss of inherent

variable insulation). The major threat associated with immersion in cold water is drowning; in air it is hypothermia and cold injury. Other problems associated with cold include the significant extent to which shivering and bulky protective garments can interfere with various activities, particularly those involving fine motor skills.

Cold: effects on performance

In air or water, the first tissue to be affected on exposure to cold is the skin. Skin cooling is accentuated by the peripheral vasoconstriction initiated by the body in order to reduce heat loss. It is the extremities (hands and feet) that are most affected owing to their high surface area/mass ratio and the fact that their major source of heat – blood flow – is restricted by vasoconstriction. This, in part, explains why it is the extremities that normally become cold-injured.

Rapid skin cooling on immersion in cold water evokes a set of cardiorespiratory responses that include uncontrollable hyperventilation, hypertension and increased cardiac workload, which can be precursors to cardiovascular accidents and drowning. This 'cold shock' response is not seen on exposure to cold air, due to the slower rates of skin cooling evoked in air. For a more comprehensive review of the specific responses associated with immersion in cold water, and the protection and treatment of immersion casualties, see Golden and Tipton (2002).

After the skin, the next tissues to cool are the superficial nerves and muscles; this can result in physical incapacitation (Figure 13.5). The time taken for this to occur depends on the exact nature of the environment (air/water, temperature, wind speed). The conduction of action potentials is slowed (15 m/s per 10 °C fall in local temperature) and their amplitude reduced. Below a muscle temperature of 27 °C, the contractile force and rate of force application is reduced and fatigue occurs earlier: maximum power output falls by three per cent per 1 °C fall in muscle temperature. As a consequence, speed of move-

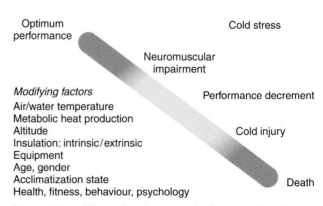

Figure 13.5 *Effects of cold on the body. See also colour plate 13.5.*

ment, dexterity, strength and mechanical efficiency are reduced with cooling.

Shivering is initiated by a combination of peripheral and central drives, with the central drive being the most potent. Thus, as deep body temperature falls, shivering is intensified. The contractile force generated by these contractions may be 15–20 per cent of that elicited during maximal voluntary muscle activation; this is reflected in an increased metabolic rate, which during intense shivering can be elevated by approximately five to six times the resting metabolic rate.

Acute cold stress stimulates sympatho-adrenal secretion; this has potent effects on energy utilization. Catecholamines stimulate lipolysis, hepatic glycogenolysis and gluconeogenesis. Thus, cold exposure increases lipid and carbohydrate metabolism. The contribution of carbohydrate oxidation to total energy consumption during strong shivering is increased and equals that of lipid metabolism. In such situations, it is hypoglycaemia acting on central nervous thermoreceptors, rather than depletion of muscle glycogen, that can inhibit shivering. This helps to explain the frequent coexistence of hypoglycaemia and hypothermia (for a review, see Stocks *et al.* 2004).

Hypothermia is defined as a deep body temperature below 35 °C. The condition affects cellular metabolism, blood flow and neural activation due to the temperature dependence of membrane ionic pumps. The signs and symptoms of hypothermia vary between individuals, and within individuals between scenarios, but the general responses are shown in Figure 13.6.

With a deep body temperature below about 28 °C, the following responses can be observed:

- decreased spontaneous depolarization of pacemaker cells of the heart
- fluid shift out of the vascular space
- depressed renal function: decreased glomerular filtration, augmented osmotic diuresis – hypovolaemia, increased blood viscosity

- impaired hepatic metabolism
- slowed activity of membrane channels (opening/closing)
- decreased sodium channel conduction
- impaired potassium ion regulation
- impaired function of brainstem
- reduced enzyme reaction times
- decreased gastrointestinal smooth-muscle motility
- cold-induced collapse of the microvasculature
- cessation of insulin's gluco-transport role.

At a deep body temperature of around 28 °C, the specialist conductive pathways of the heart lose their refractory advantage over cardiac muscle and spontaneous ventricular fibrillation can occur, a common cause of death in hypothermia.

The rate at which an individual cools in cold air or water is influenced significantly by the many thermal and non-thermal factors discussed in Chapter 12. It is these sources of variability that make the prediction of survival time, and the mathematical modelling of the thermal response to a cold environment, so difficult; this area remains more of an art than a science.

Dehydration is common in cold environments because thirst is blunted, water is not always easily available (as it may be frozen) and respiratory water loss can be high in cold dry environments. Furthermore, cold exposure can result in a cold-induced diuresis due to raised central venous pressure, suppression of antidiuretic hormone (ADH, vasopressin), secretion of atrial natriuretic hormone and, with more profound cooling, reduced renal tubular reabsorption of water and decreased sensitivity of the tubules to ADH.

The combination of exhaustion, hypoglycaemia, dehydration and hypothermia can represent a significant threat during exposure to the cold.

Cold injury

Cold injuries can be classified as freezing cold injury (FCI; frostnip, frostbite) and non-freezing cold injury (NFCI) (Figure 13.7). The first symptom of freezing cold injury is numbness; this is an important sign that should be watched for. As the superficial tissues freeze, they become white, hard and waxy in appearance. Superficial and reversible freezing is called frostnip; this can be identified early using a 'buddy system' (i.e. watching out for others) and treated by placing the affected part against a warm area of skin. Human tissue freezes at around −0.55 °C. Depending on the rate of freezing, intracellular crystals may form (rapid cooling), causing direct mechanical disruption of the tissues. The more common slow cooling and freezing results in predominantly extracellular water crystallization, which increases plasma and interstitial fluid osmotic pressure. The

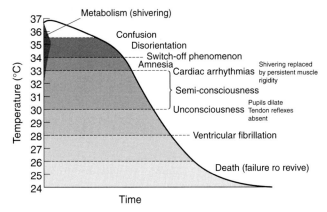

Figure 13.6 *Signs and symptoms of hypothermia. Adapted from Golden (1973).*

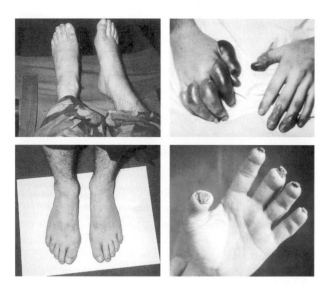

Figure 13.7 *Non-freezing (left) and freezing cold (right) injuries. See also colour plate 13.7.*

resulting osmotic outflow of intracellular fluid raises intracellular osmotic pressure and can cause damage to capillary walls. This, along with the local reduction in plasma volume, causes oedema and reduced local blood flow and encourages capillary sludging. These changes can produce thrombosis and a gangrenous extremity. The risk of frostbite is low above air temperatures of −7 °C, irrespective of wind speed, but increases below this temperature, becoming pronounced when ambient temperature is below −25 °C, even at low wind speeds.

NFCI describes a range of conditions that result from protracted exposure to low ambient thermal conditions but in which freezing of tissues does not occur. Immobility, posture, dehydration, low fitness, inadequate nutrition, constricting footwear, fatigue, stress, anxiety and concurrent illness or injury can all increase the likelihood of NFCI. NFCI can occur in temperatures as high as 12 °C and after exposures from 6–24 hours and beyond.

Moderate to severe cases present in four stages:

1. Cold exposure (one day to one week): loss of sensation, extremities initially bright red but then becoming paler.
2. Following cold exposure (hours to days): small increase in peripheral blood flow; extremities become mottled blue. Cold and numb injured area with loss of sensory and motor function, oedema and weak peripheral pulse.
3. Hyperaemia (days to weeks, usually six to ten weeks): injured part hot and flushed, full peripheral pulse but sluggish microcirculation, intense pain, oedema or blistering.
4. Post-hyperaemia (weeks to lifelong): 'cold sensitivity' (protracted cold vasoconstriction following a cold stimulus) and hyperhidrosis (local increased sweating), both of which accentuate local cooling and thus increase future risk of cold injury; persistent pain.

The precise pathophysiology of NFCI is poorly understood. The injury appears to be to the neuroendothelio-muscular components of the walls of local blood vessels. Opinions vary as to whether the primary damage is vascular or neural in origin, or whether the aetiology is primarily thermal, ischaemic, post-ischaemic reperfusion or hypoxic in origin.

Prevention and protection

ASSESSING THE RISK OF A COLD ENVIRONMENT

The cooling power of the environment is the result of air temperature, air movement or movement through air (e.g. as when skiing). These factors are combined into the wind chill index, which illustrates the cooling effect of temperature and wind on bare skin and predicts the associated danger of cold injury (Table 13.6). This index is used

Table 13.6 *Wind chill chart: effect of increasing wind speed on degree of cooling at different ambient temperatures. The equivalent temperature is the environmental temperature that would have the same effect on bare skin in the absence of any wind (equivalent cooling power)*

Ambient temperature (°C)	4	−1	−7	−12	−18	−23	−29	−34	−40	−46
Wind speed (mph)	Wind chill (equivalent) temperature (°C)									
5	2	−4	−12	−15	−21	−26	−32	−37	−43	−48
10	−1	−9	−15	−23	−29	−37	−34	−51	−57	−62
15	−4	−12	−21	−29	−34	−43	−51	−57	−65	−73
20	−7	−15	−23	−32	−37	−46	−54	−62	−71	−79
25	−9	−18	−26	−34	−43	−51	−59	−68	−76	−84
30	−12	−18	−29	−34	−46	−54	−62	−71	−79	−87
35	−12	−21	−29	−37	−46	−54	−62	−73	−82	−90
40	−12	−21	−29	−37	−48	−57	−65	−73	−82	−90
	Less danger			Increasing danger: flesh may freeze within 1 min			Great danger. Flesh may freeze within 30 s			

widely but is misunderstood. The chart does not display actual temperatures; rather, it displays the cooling power of the environment expressed as an equivalent temperature. This is the temperature that the environment would have to be at in order to have the same effect on bare skin in the absence of any wind. It is a physical impossibility for air movement to reduce temperature below ambient levels, but wind increases cooling so that skin temperature falls more quickly and closer to ambient levels.

The wind chill index is of little use in predicting time to hypothermia or clothing requirements in the cold. It is of more use in assessing the risk of exposed poorly perfused skin, but even in this case the fact that the index was developed from the cooling time of canisters of water means that it is likely to overestimate the effect of cold air on skin temperature; however, at least it errs on the side of caution.

PROTECTIVE CLOTHING

Protective clothing should alter the physical routes of heat exchange with the environment in order to create the optimum conditions next to the skin (microclimate) for the activity being undertaken. Cold environments can be wet or dry, still or windy; for each combination, there is an appropriate clothing assembly.

The primary defence against cold is insulation. As a general rule, and because still air is an effective insulator, clothing insulation depends more on clothing thickness and the consequent volume of trapped still air ('dead air') than on the nature of the fibres from which the clothing is made. Thus, clothing does not have to be heavy to insulate, but it must contain trapped dead air to be effective. Clothing insulation is often measured in Clo.[1] In a still-air environment, clothing insulation is equivalent to about 1.6 Clo per 1 cm of clothing thickness, when the air in the clothing is confined to narrow spaces and therefore 'dead'. To be most effective, air should be trapped in clothing within small pockets (< 0.5 cm in diameter); this minimizes the build-up of convective currents within each pocket.

The total insulation of a clothing assembly (I_t) is the result of the intrinsic insulation of the clothing (I_{cl}) and that of the air trapped in the microclimate (I_a), such that

$$I_t = I_{cl} + I_a/f_{cl}$$

where f_{cl} is a clothing area factor represented by the ratio of the clothed to nude surface areas of the body. This term is necessary to account for the increased surface area for

heat exchange created by wearing clothing (particularly important with hand protection; see below). Certainly, as garments increase in insulation, they become thicker and bulkier. The practical upper limit for insulation due to bulk is a thickness of about 3 cm (4.8 Clo). Greater insulation (up to 8 Clo) can be provided by sleeping bags. Clothing insulation can be bypassed if cool environmental air is pumped as a result of movement in and out of the clothing (i.e. the bellows effect) through the wrist, ankle and neck openings. Most garments provide adjustable apertures in these parts to prevent or facilitate this effect and consequent heat exchange by forced convection.

The insulation provided by clothing falls as a result of any factor that reduces the amount of stationary air trapped within the clothing assembly. Thus, although from the point of view of insulation the material from which clothing is made is relatively unimportant, its response to compression can make a significant difference. If the material is compressed easily and stays deformed, then much of the insulation will be lost with compression, as the insulating air is squeezed out of the garment. A strong wind can act as the compressive force and also can increase convective heat loss. Therefore, in cold windy conditions, an outer windproof layer of clothing should be worn. Water may also enter the clothing from the environment and displace air, thereby reducing insulation. In wet conditions, an outer waterproof fabric will be required to help preserve the insulative integrity of the undergarments; this is often combined with windproofing. The value of such protection can be seen in the fact that clothing insulation is reduced by 30 per cent in a 9-mph wind, by 50 per cent by wetting, and by 85 per cent by a combination of wind, wetting and exercise (the bellows effect).

The water vapour produced by sweat represents a source of water in clothing assemblies. The higher the vapour permeability of a clothing assembly, the greater the volume of water vapour that can pass though it and leave the microclimate. Thus, the vapour permeability of a clothing assembly can significantly influence undergarment wetting and, therefore, insulation and comfort.

HEAD PROTECTION

As a result of the absence of cold constrictor fibres in the blood vessels of the scalp, head protection is important in the cold. Heat loss from the head can account for over half of the resting metabolic heat production. For the same reason, the head can be used to vary overall clothing insulation for thermoregulatory purposes, when the removal of other items of clothing may not be convenient.

HAND AND FOOT PROTECTION

The hands and feet do not produce much heat and have high surface area/mass ratios. The temperature of these areas is dependent primarily on the heat delivered by blood

---

[1] 1 Clo is equivalent to the amount of insulation required to keep a seated subject comfortable in air at a temperature of 21 °C and a relative humidity of less 50 per cent, with 0.1 m/s air movement (about the insulation provided by a 1940s business suit).
1 Clo = 0.18 °C m^{2}h/kcal = 0.155°Cm^2/W. The textile industry uses the tog as the unit of insulation; 1 tog = 0.645 Clo.

flow. When this is reduced by vasoconstriction in the cold, the hands and feet cool quickly. The resulting low local tissue temperatures make the extremities particularly prone to cold injury. Thus, the best way to protect the hands and feet is, in addition to insulating them, to keep the body warm and thereby maintain their blood supply. Gloves and footwear will insulate but will not maintain local blood flow if deep body temperature is falling. In this situation, insulating the extremities will merely slow the rate at which they cool. The hands are particularly difficult to protect. As the thickness of gloves increases, so does the surface area for heat loss (hence the term f_{cl} in the equation for clothing insulation). It is for this reason that fingerless mitts are preferred to gloves when air temperature falls below about −10 °C. Heated gloves are becoming more widely available. While these may raise skin temperature locally and thereby improve thermal comfort, a danger lies in the fact that they are heating relatively bloodless tissue, which can be harmful.

PROTECTION AGAINST COLD-WATER IMMERSION

Suits designed for protection against immersion are defined as wet or dry. Dry suits can be insulated (include inherent insulation) or uninsulated. For comfort in warm air, aviators use uninsulated suits (immersion coveralls), which, as their name implies, have little inherent insulation. They are usually constructed from a tri-laminate waterproof material composed of a synthetic membrane bonded to two layers of nylon facing fabric. Often, a breathable waterproof membrane is bonded to the nylon facing fabrics. These suits usually incorporate waterproof zips and wrist and neck/face seals.

Uninsulated dry suits are designed to keep the insulation of the clothing worn beneath them dry. In so doing, such a suit can increase insulation from 0.06 immersed Clo for everyday clothing to 0.33 immersed Clo when everyday clothing is worn with a dry suit. That everyday clothing is normally worn beneath a dry suit means that insulation is affected adversely by water leakage into the suit: as little as 500 ml of water can produce a 30 per cent reduction in the insulation provided by such clothing. To reduce the impact of leakage, a thermal liner can be worn with the suit. These liners tend to cover the torso and upper parts of the limbs and are constructed from a water-resistant (hydrophobic) insulating material.

Although important, avoiding or minimizing undergarment wetting is not the sole determinant of retained insulation. With submersion, the pressure of the water surrounding the body (hydrostatic pressure) will compress the clothing, displace air and, consequently, reduce insulation. This, along with the differing physical properties of air and water, explains why clothing assemblies have lower clo values in water (immersed Clo) than in air.

Finally, no matter what clothing is being worn, and what weather conditions prevail, because the cooling power of water is much greater than that of air, an immersion victim is always better off out of the water than in it, even when it feels colder in air.

In summary, clothing for cold conditions should:

- prevent flushing of cold air/water beneath the garment, i.e. have airtight/watertight seals
- provide insulation by trapping a large volume of dry air in small sections close to the skin
- enable adjustments in insulation to cater for times of increased/decreased metabolic heat production
- be windproof
- wick moisture away from the body for comfort
- be vapour-permeable to prevent accumulation and condensation of moisture under the clothing, which, because of its high thermal capacity, will reduce clothing insulation. It should also dry quickly.

It is generally considered that when exercising in cold temperatures, several layers of lighter clothing are better than one large bulky garment. The former approach enables air to be trapped between and within clothing layers, thus increasing insulation. It also allows clothing insulation to be adjusted more easily and variably.

ACCLIMATIZATION TO COLD

There is still a good deal of debate about whether humans can acclimatize to cold. Various forms of adaptation have been described in the literature, none of which appears to be particularly beneficial. The most frequently reported adaptation to cold is characterized by a reduced shivering response (habituation), a faster fall in deep body temperature (hypothermic adaptation) and increased thermal comfort.

The hazardous initial responses to immersion in cold water can be reduced by as much as 50 per cent by as few as five two-minute immersions in cold water. A large part of this habituation appears to last for months.

Treatment

OUT-OF-HOSPITAL TREATMENT OF HYPOTHERMIA

A profoundly cold casualty will have a very low pulse rate and slow and shallow respiration. Both of these are difficult to detect in adverse conditions, and it is easy to assume death erroneously. Any intervention that irritates the heart or increases the demand for cardiac output should be avoided unless essential. The following is offered as a guideline:

1 Lay the casualty flat, give essential first-aid, and if possible enquire about coexisting illness.
2 Prevent further heat loss with blankets/sleeping bag, cover head and leave airway clear.

3   Insulate from the ground and place in the recovery position.
4   If possible, provide shelter from the wind and rain, but avoid unnecessary movement of very cold individuals.
5   If the casualty is unconscious or semiconscious, allow slow spontaneous rewarming to occur. Rewarming too quickly can result in collapse of arterial pressure as the peripheral vasculature opens up prematurely (rewarming collapse).
6   Maintain close observation of pulse and respiration.
7   Obtain help as soon as possible and transport the casualty to hospital.
8   If breathing is absent, becomes obstructed or stops, standard expired air ventilation should be instituted.
9   Chest compression should only be started if:

   – there is no carotid pulse detectable after palpating for at least one minute (the pulse is slow and weak in hypothermia), and
   – cardiac arrest is observed, or there is a reasonable possibility that a cardiac arrest occurred within the previous two hours, and
   – there is a reasonable expectation that effective cardiopulmonary resuscitation (CPR) can be provided continuously until the casualty reaches more advanced life support. This is likely to mean being within two hours of a suitable hospital.

10 The rates of expired air ventilation and chest compression should be the same as for normothermic casualties. Hypothermia may cause stiffness of the chest wall.

Although reflective blankets can, theoretically, reduce radiant heat loss in warm environments (e.g. hospital wards), they are of little use in cold environments. This is because when skin temperature approaches ambient temperature, heat loss via radiation is minimal. Also, water vapour in the microenvironment from insensible perspiration will condense quickly on the cool inner surface of the reflective blanket and reduce its reflectivity to almost zero. In a survival situation, it is better simply to enclose the casualty in some appropriate vapourproof- and windproof barrier (e.g. a heavy-duty polythene bag) and help to prevent continued heat loss through the primary routes of convection and evaporation.

Cold injury

It is important to establish whether the dominant injury is freezing (FCI) or non-freezing (NFCI) in nature. This determines the preferred method of rewarming. In all cases, shelter should be sought. As casualties with cold injury are likely to be hypothermic, they should be kept warm.

All patients with freezing injury should be rewarmed thoroughly by immersion of all of the chilled part in stirred water at 38–42 °C. A topical antibacterial should be added to the water. Rewarming should be delayed if there is a chance that refreezing may occur. Thawing an FCI can be intensely painful. Conventional and narcotic analgesics should be provided as necessary. Continuing treatment for FCI is a twice-daily, 30-minute immersion of the affected part in a 38–42 °C whirlpool bath containing an appropriate antibacterial.

In contrast to patients with FCI, patients with NFCI should have the affected extremities rewarmed slowly, by exposure to warm air alone, and must not be immersed in warm water. The early period after rewarming can be very painful in NFCI, even in patients without any obvious tissue damage. Amitriptyline (10–50 mg given as a single dose at night) is the drug of choice for the treatment of pain following NFCI and should be given as soon as pain is felt. Amitriptyline may cause drowsiness and hypertension.

With either form of injury, once rewarmed the affected extremities should be treated by exposure to air and early mobilization. The patient should be not be allowed to smoke.

SURVIVAL

The information provided in this and the previous chapter should enable a survival strategy to be developed for use in hot dry, hot humid, cold dry, and cold wet climates. Tools have been identified that enable the thermal threat posed by an environment to be assessed. In heat, the importance of proper hydration and rehydration has been emphasized. The routes of heat loss in the cold have been identified and their relevance for deep body and peripheral temperatures discussed. The principles that should govern the selection of protective clothing for use in heat and cold have been outlined. The early signs and symptoms of thermal injuries have been described and guidelines for initial treatment suggested.

The survival hierarchy in terms of the body's requirements is:

1   Adequate air: failure to maintain this results in a survival time measured in minutes.
2   Cardiovascular stability: failure to maintain results in a survival time measured in minutes.
3   Stable body temperature: failure to maintain results in a survival time measured in hours.
4   Fluid balance (fluid): failure to maintain results in a survival time measured in days.
5   Energy balance (food): failure to maintain results in a survival time measured in weeks.

In terms of thermally related threats, it can be concluded from the above that sudden immersion/submersion in cold water represents the greatest threat to the aviator, as the initial responses to immersion (cold shock) reduce breath-hold time and increase the likelihood of aspirating water and drowning. The cardiovascular strain associated with such immersions also represents a significant threat. Thus, the aviator at risk of ditching in cold water should be provided with an immersion suit and lifejacket. The shortfall between maximum breath-hold time on immersion in cold water when wearing an immersion suit (average 25 s) and that required to escape from a ditched inverted aircraft (about 60 s) provides the rationale for the provision of some form of emergency breathing aid. Whether a rebreather or source of compressed air is used will depend on specific requirements (Tipton *et al.* 1997). It is essential that, as with all forms of survival equipment, the combination that is provided for the aviator to protect him or her from the various thermal threats constitutes an 'integrated survival system' in which the components complement and assist each other rather than negate performance.

In both hot and cold environments, the survival benefits of shelter cannot be overstated. This may be in the form of a natural feature such as a cave or may be crafted from snow or branches. Alternatively, it may be provided for non-emergency situations, such as a place for ground crew to rest and cool or rewarm between sorties. A shelter, for example a life-raft, may be provided for emergency situations. Whatever the nature of the shelter, it significantly increases the chances of survival by reducing wetting (which increases conductive and evaporative heat loss) and wind (convective heat loss) and providing shade (reducing radiant heat gain).

Once protection has been achieved, location becomes a priority. The job of the search-and-rescue team can be assisted by the filing and adherence to a flight plan. Clearly, Mayday calls and personal locator beacons and global positioning systems are an advantage in this regard.

The availability of food and water are not immediate issues, but they must be addressed once the more immediate threats have been countered, with water taking the higher priority. In a survival situation at complete rest in a thermoneutral environment, the body requires about 1 litre of water and 1400 kcal a day. In a survival situation in optimum conditions, water intake can be reduced to 110–220 ml per day and calorific intake to 600–1400 kcal per day for a short period. In hot and cold environments, these values must increase to cater for fluid lost in sweating or via the respiratory tract in cold dry air and increased metabolism to support shivering. Water can be obtained from many sources, but not seawater, as this accentuates dehydration. Desalination kits and reverse-osmosis pumps are available to increase the volume of water available. When water is in short supply, none should be drunk for the first 24 hours; this causes the body to adjust to mild dehydration by reducing urine production.

Historically, fat has been a favourite constituent of survival rations. However, in order to maintain blood glucose levels, a high-carbohydrate diet is preferable. Short-chain glucose polymers are absorbed as quickly as pure glucose but are more palatable. Protein is not recommended if water is likely to be in short supply, as there is obligatory water loss (2–3 ml per 1 g of protein to combine with urea) during the breakdown of protein. Also, the digestion, absorption and assimilation of a high-protein meal elevates metabolic rate by a greater amount than a carbohydrate or fat meal, which is disadvantageous in a hot environment. During starvation, the body begins to metabolize its own protein. One of the major functions of a survival ration is to prevent this from happening and thereby preserve function and body fluid. The survival ration should comprise a variety of food composed predominantly of carbohydrate. This might include chocolate, biscuits, oatmeal blocks or high-energy bars, and boiled sweets.

It is concluded that in order to maximize the chances of survival all the threats associated with a particular environment must be identified and suitable policies, equipment and training put in place to, first, avoid the threats and, second, to deal with them when they arise. Thus, the onus is not simply on the individual who finds him- or herself in a survival situation; it is also incumbent on equipment manufacturers to test their equipment properly and appropriately. Too often, so-called 'survival' equipment designed and tested in air-conditioned offices fails to perform in an emergency.

For many individuals, the equipment and know-how that they take with them into a survival situation is the result of a management decision. This may involve the type of life-raft or location device they are given or the training they receive. Therefore, there is also a requirement for the managerial chain to put in place policies that will ensure that due consideration is given to the impact of an environment on performance and safety. This will include the dissemination of information and training on subjects such as altitude, heat and cold. Appropriate facilities, tools and equipment should be provided and used. Agreed protocols for the treatment of thermal injuries should be established for use both in the field and in hospitals. Policies for the medical evacuation of casualties should be established, rehearsed and updated regularly. In short, the number of individuals who find themselves in a survival situation, and what they are able to do for themselves in such a situation, is as reliant on good management as it is on good survival skills. The incentive for all concerned is not only health and safety; it has been shown time and time again, over the centuries, that ignorance of the possible adverse impact of the environment can have catastrophic implications for individuals and operations.

DEDICATION

This and the previous chapter are dedicated to the memory of Dr Mike Harrison.

REFERENCES

Froom P, Caine Y, Shochat I, Ribak J. Heat stress and helicopter pilot errors. *Journal of Occupational Medicine* 1993; **35**: 720–24.

Golden FS. Recognition and treatment of immersion hypothermia. *Proceedings of the Royal Society of Medicine* 1973; **66**: 1058–61.

Golden FS, Tipton MJ. *Essentials of Sea Survival.* Champaign, IL: Human Kinetics, 2002.

House JR. Reducing heat strain with ice-vests or hand immersion. In: Shapiro Y, Moran DS, Epstein Y (eds). *Proceedings of the 7th International Conference on Environmental Ergonomics.* London: Freund Publishing House, 1996; pp. 347–350.

House JR. Heat strain in Royal Navy helicopter aircrew. *Journal of the Royal Naval Medical Service* 1999; **85**: 84–109.

House JR, Davis M. Reducing aircrew heat stress by wetting or covering parked (or 'at alert') helicopters. In: Tochihara Y, Ohnaka T (eds). *Proceedings of the 10th International Conference on Environmental Ergonomics.* Tokyo: Elsevier, 2002; pp. 143–4.

Nunneley SA, Stribley RF, Allan JR. Heat stress in front and rear cockpits of F-4 aircraft. *Aviation, Space, and Environmental Medicine* 1981; **52**: 287–90.

Stocks JM, Taylor NAS, Tipton MJ, Greenleaf JE. Human thermoregulation during exposure to cold: acute and chronic responses. *Aviation Space and Environmental Medicine* 2004; **75**: 444–57.

Tipton MJ, Franks CM, Sage BA, Redman PJ. An examination of two emergency breathing aids for use during helicopter underwater escape. *Aviation, Space, and Environmental Medicine* 1997; **68**: 906–13.

FURTHER READING

Defence Medical Services Department. Climatic injuries in the armed forces: prevention and treatment. JSP 539. Camberley: Army Medical Directorate (Defence Medical Services Department), 2003.

Faerevik H, Reinertsen RE. Effects of wearing aircrew protective clothing on physiological and cognitive responses under various ambient conditions. *Ergonomics* 2003; **46**: 780–99.

Francis TJR, Golden FS. Non-freezing cold injury: the pathogenesis. *Journal of the Royal Naval Medical Service* 1985; **71**: 3–8.

Francis TJR, Oakley EHN. Cold injury. In: Tooke JE, Lowe GDO (eds). *A Textbook of Vascular Medicine.* London: Arnold, 1996; pp. 353–70.

Froom P, Shochat I, Strichman L, Cohen A, Epstein Y. Heat stress on helicopter pilots during ground standby. *Aviation, Space, and Environmental Medicine* 1991; **62**: 978–81.

Gibson TM, Cochrane LA, Harrison MH, Rigden PW. Cockpit thermal stress and aircrew thermal strain during routine Jaguar operations. *Aviation, Space, and Environmental Medicine* 1979; **50**: 808–12.

Golden FS, Handley AJ, Keatinge WR, Lloyd EL, Tipton MJ. Report of the working party on out of hospital management of hypothermia. Medical Commission on Accident Prevention. London: Royal College of Surgeons, 1992.

Harrison MH, Higenbottam C, Rigby RA. Relationships between ambient, cockpit, and pilot temperatures during routine air operations. *Aviation, Space, and Environmental Medicine* 1978; **49**: 5–13.

Oakley EHN. A review of the treatment of cold injury. Institute of Naval Medicine report no. 2000.026. Gosport: Institute of Naval Medicine, 2000.

14

Vibration

J.R. ROLLIN STOTT

INTRODUCTION

Vibration is defined as motion that repeatedly alternates in direction. The motion of tides and ocean waves, the shaking of the Earth's crust during earthquakes, the movement of pistons within the cylinders of engines, the disturbances generated in aircraft flying through turbulent air, and the disturbances in vehicles travelling over uneven terrain are all forms of vibration. They are also examples of vibration that can be transmitted to humans and may result in a range of physiological and psychological effects. Vibration generally is transmitted to the body through direct contact with a vibrating structure. In these conditions, significant levels of vibrational energy can be transferred to the body, with potentially harmful consequences. Vibration may also reach the body by transmission through air. Airborne vibration, if in the appropriate frequency range, is perceived as sound, but at low sonic and subsonic frequencies it may exert other physiological effects.

Much of human exposure to whole-body vibration occurs through transport in vehicles of various sorts. Although engineering solutions have been found to reduce the physiological hazards of vibration in many types of vehicle, undesirably high levels of vibration can be encountered in helicopters, fixed-wing aircraft during low-level flight, and high-speed sea-going craft and land vehicles traversing rough terrain. Vibration is of operational significance in aviation because it may, among other things, impair visual acuity, interfere with neuromuscular control, including speech, and lead to fatigue. The human body is mechanically complex, and the pattern of vibration to which it is subjected in, for example, low-level turbulence in an aircraft or travelling over a rough track in a road vehicle is also complex. Some understanding of the effects of vibration can be gained by considering the body as an assemblage of simpler mechanical subunits and by analysing a complex vibration waveform in terms of its constituent sinusoidal components.

PRINCIPLES OF VIBRATION

Natural vibration

The simplest example of a vibrating system is provided by a mass hanging from a fixed point by a spring. When displaced from its rest position, the mass oscillates about this position for some time before it comes to rest. This vibration involves a repeated interchange of energy between the mass and the spring. The mass has gravitational energy when it is at the highest point of its travel and kinetic energy when it is in motion. The spring stores energy when it is extended. If no energy was lost from the system, then oscillations would continue indefinitely. In practice, the mass encounters some resistance to motion from the surrounding air, and further energy is lost within the spring in the form of heat. If the displacement of the mass from its rest position is plotted against time, the resulting graph will be sinusoidal in shape. Sinusoidal motion can be quantified by two pieces of information: (i) the frequency, defined as the number of cycles of oscillation that occur in one second (1 cycle/s = 1 Hz), and (ii) the amplitude, generally defined as the maximum displacement, measured in metres, from the rest position.

The frequency at which an ideal mass spring system will oscillate when it is disturbed is termed the natural frequency, f_n (Hz). The natural frequency depends on two quantities: the size of the mass, m (kg) and the stiffness of the spring, k (N/m). A greater mass will oscillate more slowly, i.e. at a lower natural frequency, whereas a stiffer spring stiffness will lead to oscillations at a higher natural frequency. The formula that links these quantities is as follows:

$$2\pi f_n = \sqrt{(k/m)}$$

The loss of mechanical energy in a vibrating system as heat, with consequent decay in the amplitude of oscillation, is known as damping. As a discrete entity, a damper is exemplified by the shock absorber of a car. This typically consists of a piston in an oil-filled cylinder. A force on the piston causes it to move at a rate determined by the ease with which oil is able to flow from one side of the piston to the other, either through orifices in the piston or through an external channel connecting one end of the cylinder with the other.

A system that incorporates only a small degree of damping continues to oscillate for a long time after an initial disturbance. As the amount of damping is increased, so the oscillations that follow an initial disturbance decay more rapidly. With further increases in damping, the mass returns to its rest position without any overshoot. The minimum degree of damping required to produce this result is termed critical damping, C_c (kg/s). Its magnitude can be calculated from the size of the mass, m (kg), and the spring stiffness, k (N/m), as follows:

$$C_c = 2\sqrt{(km)}$$

The amount of damping in a system is commonly expressed as a proportion of critical damping, termed the damping factor. Thus, a system that has a damping factor of 1 is critically damped. If the damping factor is less than 1, the system is underdamped; if the damping factor is greater than 1, the system is overdamped.

Forced vibration

The previous section dealt with the behaviour of a mass/spring/damper system left to vibrate following an initial mechanical disturbance, i.e. so-called natural vibration. It is necessary to consider how such a system behaves when it is subjected to an external source of sustained vibration at various frequencies. Figure 14.1 shows a mass supported on a vibrating surface through a spring and a damper. The amplitude of motion of the mass is expressed as a proportion of the motion of the base in the graph. The response of the mass is determined by the frequency of the imposed vibration. At low frequencies, the mass and the base share the same amplitude of vibration (amplitude ratio 1). As the frequency of vibration is increased, the mass begins to vibrate to a greater extent than the base. Its vibration relative to the base reaches a maximum at the resonant frequency (fo). With further increases in the frequency of vibration, the relative amplitude of vibration falls until a frequency is reached above which the vibration of the mass becomes progressively less than that of the base.

The amount of damping in the system determines the extent to which vibration is amplified at the resonant frequency. Figure 14.2 shows a family of graphs of the frequency response of a mass/spring system plotted for different values of damping. With less damping in the system, the amplification of vibration at resonance increases. (In theory, it is infinite if there is no damping at all.) Even with critical damping, there is some amplification of vibration at the resonant frequency. The resonant peak occurs at a somewhat lower frequency in a more damped system compared with a system with little or no damping. However, irrespective of the degree of damping, the response of the mass becomes identical in amplitude with that of the base at a frequency that is $\sqrt{2}$ times the undamped natural frequency. As the frequency of applied vibration is increased above this point, the vibration of the mass becomes increasingly small compared with that of the

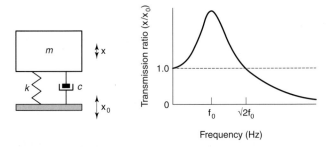

Figure 14.1 *A mass/spring/damper system mounted on a vibrating surface, where m is the mass (kg), k is the spring stiffness (N/m) and c is the coefficient of damping (kg/s). The graph shows the ratio of the sinusoidal motion of the mass (x) to that of the base (x₀) as the frequency of vibration of the base is increased. f₀ represents the resonant frequency of the system.*

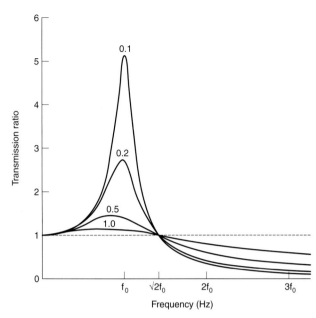

Figure 14.2 *Graphs showing the response to forced vibration of a mass/spring system with different degrees of damping. The figure adjacent to each graph is the damping factor. f_0 is the undamped resonant frequency.*

base. In this frequency range, the effect of the spring is to isolate the mass from the vibration of the base.

In a system with a low degree of damping, the motion of the mass at or near the resonant frequency may be many times that of the external vibration and may result in structural damage. However, such a system gives a high degree of vibration isolation of the mass at frequencies well above the resonant frequency. In the design of a vibration isolation system such as the suspension of a motor car, some compromise level of damping (achieved through the vehicle's shock absorbers) has to be found that is low enough to obtain adequate vibration isolation of the vehicle at frequencies generated by the normal roughness of the road surface but not so low that the vehicle bounces out of control if it hits a pothole that excites the resonant vibration frequency of the suspension. The damping factor that best achieves this compromise is generally about 0.7, which limits the amplification at resonance to a factor of about 1.3.

The concept of resonance is particularly important in understanding some of the harmful effects of vibration both in engineering structures and in the human body. The presence of inadequately damped resonances within a complex structure means that comparatively small vibrational accelerations can, at certain frequencies, build up much higher accelerations and, hence, forces on component parts of the structure, with potentially damaging consequences. A large part of vibration engineering involves the avoidance or the suppression of resonant vibration.

When a structure contains multiple masses resiliently coupled together, the behaviour of the system under vibration is correspondingly complex. Figure 14.3 shows two masses linked in series by springs and dampers to a vibrating base. The graph shows the motion of the lower mass as a proportion of the vibration of the base at different frequencies of applied vibration. Two resonant peaks are now evident at frequencies that differ from the resonant frequencies of each individual mass/spring system. Between these two resonances is a frequency region in which the vibration of the lower mass relative to the base is much reduced, although there is increased vibration of the upper mass relative to the lower mass. This principle of reducing the vibration of a mass by coupling to it a second vibration system is used in the design of the dynamic vibration absorber, a device fitted to some helicopters.

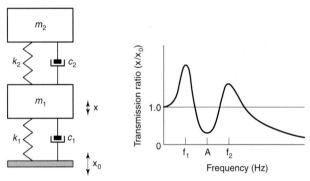

Figure 14.3 *Response to forced vibration of two linked mass/spring/damper systems, where m is the mass (kg), k is the spring stiffness (N/m) and c is the coefficient of damping (kg/s). The graph shows the ratio of vibration amplitude of the lower mass (x) with respect to the base (x_0). Two resonances are present, f_1 and f_2, with attenuation of vibration at an intermediate frequency (A). At this frequency, the upper mass is resonant relative to the lower mass.*

MECHANICAL PROPERTIES OF BIOLOGICAL TISSUES

Although it is of value to identify mass, elasticity and damping in a vibrating system, these constituents are better regarded as properties possessed by the components of the system rather than as discrete entities. For example, elasticity is the principal property of a steel spring, but the spring also has mass. Similarly, many springy materials, such as rubber and connective tissue, possess significant degrees of damping generated by friction at a molecular level within the material. In the human body, it is possible, with varying degrees of precision, to identify mass/spring systems, i.e. structures that are loosely coupled to the rest of the body by connective tissue, which, by virtue of its springiness, may cause the structure to resonate when vibrated at a particular frequency. Important in this regard are the head, the torso, the shoulder girdle, the liver and mediastinum, and the limbs.

The springiness of connective tissue is not modelled so easily as that of an ideal spring. The force required to stretch an ideal spring is proportional to its increase in length. The spring is said to possess uniform stiffness. The collagen of tendon and ligament is non-uniform in stiffness. It becomes stiffer the more it is stretched (Figure 14.4). The implication for a vibrating system that has collagen as the spring component is that the resonant frequency depends on the underlying tension within connective tissue. This connective tissue tension is determined mainly by muscle activity and by the static loading that results from the gravitational environment.

Damping occurs by several mechanisms within the body. In addition to the internal friction within tissue as it is stretched, there is an important damping effect from active skeletal muscle. When active muscle is made to lengthen by the application of an external force, the muscle generates an opposing force, which, for a given degree of neural activation, is proportional to its rate of lengthening. This is the property of an ideal damper. It is, therefore, not surprising that the state of muscle tension and the consequent body posture are major variable factors governing the mechanical response of the body to vibration. Increased tension in muscles has the effect of stiffening the vibrating system to which the muscles are attached. This tends to raise the resonant frequency and at the same time, by generating increased damping, tends to reduce the degree of resonant amplification.

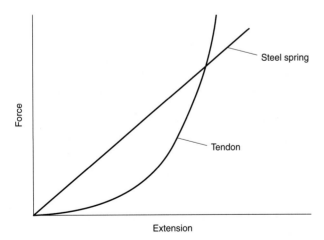

Figure 14.4 *Relationship between force and extension for a steel spring compared with that for tendon. Stiffness is given by the slope of the graph. Tendon becomes increasingly stiff as it is stretched.*

VIBRATION SOURCES

Vehicles are a major source of human exposure to whole-body vibration. In most vehicles, there are two principal sources of vibration to be considered. The first originates within the vehicle, in particular the engine; the second is derived from the environment, i.e. the terrain over which the land vehicle is travelling, the turbulent air through which the aircraft is flying, or the sea state in which the ship is sailing.

All machinery is liable to generate vibration. In the internal combustion engine, the impulse as each cylinder fires and the reciprocating motion of the pistons provide a source of vibrational energy that is propagated to the vehicle through the mountings of the engine and gearbox. Gas turbines and electric motors in good condition are inherently less likely to generate vibration, but any mass imbalance of a rotating component or looseness in its bearings may result in significant vibration. The detailed analysis of vibration records from accelerometers mounted on the fuselage of a helicopter and the casing of engines and gearboxes is an important technique for detecting wear in these components during their working life.

The vibration generated from an engine is at a frequency that can be predicted from the rotational speed of the machinery. A piston engine rotating at 60 revolutions per second (3600 rpm) is likely to propagate vibration at this frequency (60 Hz). The rotor of a helicopter typically revolves at four revolutions per second and, therefore, potentially generates vibration within the helicopter at 4 Hz. However, generally the intensity of vibration in helicopters at this frequency is low. This is achieved by accurate matching of the mass of each blade on the rotor and by aerodynamically trimming the blades so that they rotate in the same plane. This fundamental rotor frequency is often referred to as the 1R frequency. Generally, the vibration produced at the blade-pass frequency is of greater amplitude. This frequency is the 1R frequency multiplied by the number of rotor blades and in many helicopters is in the region of 15–25 Hz. In addition, components of vibration are generated at higher harmonics (i.e. integer multiples) of the blade-pass frequency and also at a frequency related to the tail rotor speed. Figure 14.5 shows the spectrum of vertical vibration recorded from a Chinook helicopter. The repetitive pattern of vibration gives rise to discrete peaks in the spectrum. That at 1R (3.8 Hz) is small: the principal components are at the blade-pass frequency, 6R (22.75 Hz) and the first harmonic of the blade-pass frequency, 12R (45.5 Hz). Other peaks in the spectrum at frequencies unrelated to the main rotor frequency may originate from gearboxes and transmission systems within the aircraft.

Helicopter vibration occurs with broadly similar intensity in all three axes of motion, vertical, lateral and fore–aft. Although there may be large differences in the amplitudes

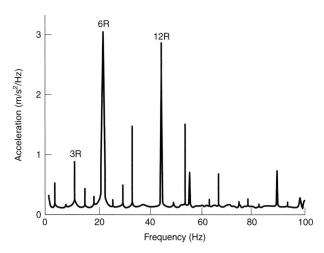

Figure 14.5 *Vertical vibration amplitude spectrum of the Chinook helicopter. Peaks labelled 3R, 6R, 12R are harmonics of the fundamental rotor frequency at 4 Hz. In this case, the highest peak occurs at the blade-pass frequency (6R), but there is much variation in the relative amplitude of the different harmonics recorded under different flight conditions.*

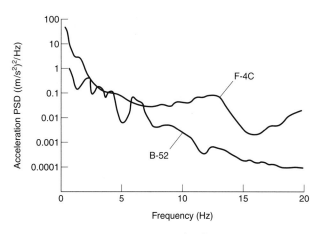

Figure 14.6 *Power spectral density (PSD) of G_z vibration from two fixed-wing aircraft, the F-4C fighter and the B-52 bomber, during high-speed low-level flight. Note the logarithmic scale on the vertical axis, which emphasizes the lower vibration amplitudes at the expense of the higher amplitudes. The levels of vibration are greater at the low frequencies (< 1 Hz) and decline sharply at increasing frequencies. Redrawn from Speakman et al. (1971).*

of specific harmonics in different modes of flight, the overall amplitude of vibration tends to increase with airspeed and with the loading of the aircraft. Vibration usually is worse during transition to the hover. The measured levels of vibration may differ quite widely between helicopters of identical type operating under similar conditions, although the source of these differences is often elusive.

In fixed-wing aircraft, any vibration arising from the power source tends to be at a higher frequency than in helicopters. In a propeller-driven aircraft, the blade-pass frequency is in the region of 100 Hz, although lower frequencies of vibration may be generated by the beating effect of two propellers running at different speeds. A single-stage turbine of a fixed-wing jet aircraft typically rotates at about 8000 rpm (130 Hz); the high-pressure stage of a dual-stage turbine rotates at about 13 000 rpm (230 Hz). The main source of vibration encountered in fixed-wing aircraft arises from the atmospheric turbulence through which the aircraft is flying. In consequence, the most severe vibration tends to occur during storm-cloud penetration or during high-speed low-level flight. It reflects the random disturbances of turbulent air modified by the aerodynamic characteristics of the aircraft and by the control actions of the pilot (Figure 14.6). Most of the vibrational energy of fixed-wing aircraft is found at low frequencies in the vertical axis. In atmospheric turbulence, the vertical vibration of the aircraft at 1 Hz may exceed by a factor of 100 that at 10 Hz. The sharp peaks that are characteristic of the spectrum of helicopter vibration are not seen in fixed-wing aircraft, although the vibration spectrum may reflect the flexural resonances of the wings and

fuselage by showing broad maxima at these frequencies. These features are less evident in the spectrum of high-performance fighter aircraft, whose wings and fuselage are constructed more rigidly. However, during buffet, which occurs, for example, in maximum-rate turns that require the greatest degree of aerodynamic lift from the wings, vibration is imposed on the airframe over a narrow frequency range that varies according to aircraft type between about 8 and 20 Hz.

The response of the aircraft as a whole to atmospheric turbulence is determined by the aerodynamic loading on the wings. An aircraft with a large wing area relative to its weight undergoes greater amplitude low-frequency excursions from level flight as a result of turbulence. Such motion is predominantly in the frequency range of 0.1–1 Hz. The firing of machine guns from military aircraft transmits to the airframe a series of mechanical shocks. These may be attenuated to some degree by gun mountings that allow the gun to recoil. Such shocks vibrate the airframe not only at the frequency of firing of the gun but also over a broader range of frequencies. The firing of a missile produces a single shock disturbance that evokes a transient vibrational response from undamped resonances within the aircraft.

MEASUREMENT AND ANALYSIS OF VIBRATION

Complex oscillatory motion can be described in terms of the changes in position with respect to a fixed point, the changes in velocity relative to a constant or zero velocity, or changes in acceleration in relation to an inertial frame of reference. Displacement, velocity and acceleration are related mathematically. In principle, one may be derived if the others are known (Figure 14.7). Vibration intensity is most frequently quoted in terms of the amplitude of the acceleration in units of m/s^2, but it may also be expressed in units of G, i.e. multiples of the acceleration due to gravity (1 G = 9.8 m/s^2). Vibration at a single frequency can be quantified in terms of its half-peak amplitude, but for a complex vibration containing multiple frequency components the root mean square (RMS) amplitude is used. This can be considered as a type of average amplitude for a complex waveform. The RMS level of a single frequency sine wave is 0.707 ($1/\sqrt{2}$) of its half-peak amplitude.

An additional descriptor of a vibration waveform is provided by the crest factor. If vibration is generated from an impulsive source such as a mechanical hammer or from weapons firing in a military aircraft, then the recorded vibration will show short-duration high peaks of acceleration,

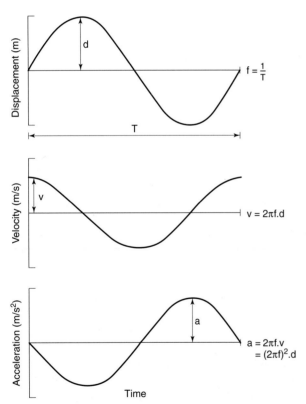

Figure 14.7 *Relationship between displacement, velocity and acceleration for sinusoidal vibration. With respect to displacement, the phase of velocity is advanced by one quarter-cycle and acceleration by one half-cycle. The duration of one cycle of motion T (s) is known as the period. The reciprocal of the period, 1/T, gives the frequency f (Hz). The velocity amplitude v is obtained from the displacement amplitude d by multiplying by 2πf. The amplitude of the acceleration a is found from the velocity amplitude by a further multiplication by 2πf.*

termed mechanical shocks, whose presence makes the perceived severity of vibration much greater than its RMS level would indicate. The crest factor is defined as the ratio of the peak acceleration amplitude of a vibration record to its RMS amplitude. For vibration in which the crest factor exceeds a value of 6, the RMS level of vibration is a poor indicator of its subjective severity, and a form of averaging is used that gives extra weight to the peak levels. The most widely used device in the measurement of vibration is the accelerometer. Accelerometers vary from rugged units designed to measure the high accelerations that occur during an impact to fragile devices that will measure well below the threshold of human perception. For the measurement of angular motion, accelerometers are manufactured that are insensitive to linear acceleration and respond only to angular acceleration. Also available are devices that measure angular velocity, from which angular acceleration can be derived.

When accelerometers are used on the human body, the need for high sensitivity and small size are often conflicting requirements. There are very few places on the body surface where good fixation of an accelerometer can be achieved and where the mass of the accelerometer and the springiness of the underlying soft tissue cannot form a resonant system and, thereby, generate misleading information. The teeth provide a useful fixation point, and small accelerometers can be mounted on a dental bite to measure accelerations of the head. Elsewhere on the body, unless fixation is achieved by screwing into bone, accelerometers have to be strapped to the overlying skin. It is often desirable to measure the level of vibration at the point of entry to the body, and this may be achieved in a seated subject by enclosing small accelerometers in a thin seat pad on which the subject sits. Accelerometers have a directional sensitivity. For a full description of the vibration of a structure, three linear accelerometers are needed, with their sensitive axes at right-angles to each other. Additionally, if angular motion is to be measured, a further three transducers are required.

The direction of vibration accelerations acting on the body is specified on the same three-axis system with reference to the trunk as used in relation to long-duration accelerations. G_x acceleration acts in the anteroposterior direction, G_y in the lateral direction and G_z in the craniocaudal direction. Angular accelerations about these axes are generally referred to in terms of roll, pitch and yaw.

Vibration waveforms can be divided into two main types: those that have repetitive or periodic features, typically generated by machinery, and those that are irregular or aperiodic, such as the vibration of an aircraft in atmospheric turbulence. Any complex vibration waveform can be considered as the summation of a series of increasing frequency sinusoidal components, or harmonics, of appropriate amplitude and phase relationship. The technique of breaking down a vibration signal into its constituent frequencies (Fourier analysis) is important, since the effects of vibration on the body are critically dependent on the frequency. A plot of the amplitude of each component versus frequency is known as the vibration spectrum. Periodic vibration generates a spectrum that has narrow discrete peaks with little or no activity in the intervening spectral components. Aperiodic, or random, vibration yields a continuous spectrum that may show broad peaks in specific regions of the spectrum.

BIOMECHANICAL EFFECTS OF VIBRATION

Mechanical impedance of the body

In order to transmit vibration to an object, a source of vibration has to exert an alternating force at its point of contact. The amount of force that is required to produce a given vibration response is known as the mechanical impedance. More specifically, mechanical impedance is defined as the ratio of the peak oscillatory force exerted on an object by a vibration source to the resulting peak velocity of vibration measured at the point of contact. The concept of mechanical impedance is directly analogous to that of electrical impedance, which relates an alternating electromotive force (voltage) to the resulting flow of alternating current in a circuit component. When the human body is in direct contact with a source of vibration, mechanical energy is transferred, some of which is degraded into heat within those tissues that have damping properties. Mechanical impedance also gives an indication of the capacity of the body to absorb vibrational energy. The mechanical impedance of the human body is dependent on the frequency of vibration. If the body was a simple mass, then its mechanical impedance would increase linearly with frequency. For a seated human subject, this is true only for frequencies of vibration up to about 2 Hz (Figure 14.8). Thereafter, there is a disproportionate increase in mechanical impedance, which reaches a maximum at 4–5 Hz. When vibrated at this frequency, a 70-kg man has an apparent mass of 130 kg. This effect is the result of a major resonance within the body. Above a vibration frequency of 7 Hz, the impedance of the body falls below that of a simple mass, indicative of the vibration isolation effects of compliant body tissues. Of principal importance is the flexibility of the lumbar spine and, at higher frequencies, the compressibility of intervertebral discs and the soft tissues of the buttocks, which allow the upper trunk to be relatively isolated from the source of vibration. Mechanical impedance diminishes with increasing frequency, but this trend is interrupted by a second peak at about 12–15 Hz, indicative of a second resonance. The shape of the impedance curve is modified by posture, the type of seating and restraint system, and G loading. At 3 G, the peak in mechanical impedance is shifted upwards to about 8 Hz (Vogt *et al.* 1968).

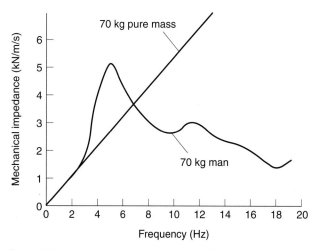

Figure 14.8 *Mechanical impedance of a 70-kg seated subject at vibration frequencies up to 20 Hz. The two peaks in the curve occur at the frequencies of the first and second body resonances. Also shown is the impedance of a pure mass of 70 kg.*

Body resonances

Measurement of mechanical impedance gives little indication of the body structures that are involved in the principal resonances. It is likely that several resonances contribute to the impedance peak at 4–5 Hz. During vertical vibration of a seated subject, the flexibility of the lumbar spine and its associated musculature provides a compliant link between the mass of the torso and the pelvis and, thus, allows resonance of the upper trunk. There is also amplification of motion in the shoulder girdle at these frequencies. Less evident, but of greater relevance to human tolerance to vibration, is the resonance of the liver, diaphragm and mediastinum within the body cavity. Animal experiments suggest that this mass moves as one unit against the restraints of compliant connective tissue and of the fluid- and gas-filled abdominal contents. The associated movement of the diaphragm promotes oscillatory airflow in the respiratory tract as well as abdominal wall movement (Coermann *et al.* 1960) and intra-abdominal pressure changes. All these measures show a peak at 3–4 Hz in humans.

The additional energy required to vibrate the body at the frequency of maximum mechanical impedance is absorbed in the supporting connective tissue associated with these resonant structures, both by frictional heating and, under more severe vibration, by mechanical disruption of tissues. Animals exposed to lethal levels of vibration (10–15 G) at frequencies in the region of their internal body resonance have developed pulmonary congestion with haemorrhage and collapse, diffuse intestinal bleeding and, occasionally, superficial brain haemorrhage. Electrocardiogram (ECG) changes indicative of myocardial damage often preceded death (Nickerson and Paradijeff 1964).

The origin of the second major resonance of the body at 12–15 Hz is less clear. It has been postulated that this resonance is the result of axial compression of the torso controlled by the elastic properties of the spinal column and its supporting musculature, although direct experimental evidence for this is lacking. Both the first and second resonances (4–5 Hz and 12–15 Hz) are evident as peaks in the transmission of vibration from the seat to the head and the shoulders (Figure 14.9). At 4–5 Hz, resonant vibration of the shoulders predominates, whereas at 12–15 Hz, resonant vibration of the head is the principal effect (Rowlands 1977). The transmission of vertical vibration to the head in seated subjects is affected by body posture, whether slouched or erect, and by the configuration of the seat and the degree of mechanical coupling between the backrest and the trunk. The presence of a backrest allows vibration to bypass the vibration-attenuating effect of the trunk and the levels of head vibration at around 6 Hz for G_x, G_z and pitch head movements are increased (Paddan and Griffin 1988a). Vibration of the head in these axes is increased by the presence of a backrest over a broader frequency range, 4–16 Hz, in response to vibration in the fore–aft direction (Paddan and Griffin 1988b).

The mechanical response of the head under vertical vibration involves not only linear but also angular motion, particularly in pitch. This occurs because the centre of gravity of the head lies anterior to the atlanto-occipital joint and the consequent tendency to forward flexion of the head, readily observed in somnolent rail passengers, has in the waking state to be opposed by continuous activity in the neck extensor muscles. The relationship between head-pitch acceleration and linear vertical seat acceleration

tends to reach a peak at 5–6 Hz. A further effect often seen in response to vibration at these frequencies is that the motion of the head contains components at twice the frequency of the input vibration. The effect of wearing an aircrew helmet is to increase the mass of the head and, in consequence, the stiffness of the neck muscles that hold the head upright. Measurement of the motion of a well-fitted aircrew helmet shows that it remains coupled well to the head at frequencies of vertical vibration up to about 4 Hz, but at 7 Hz the pitch motion of the helmet can be more than twice that of the head.

At different frequencies of vibration, other resonances become apparent within the body. Although the maximum oscillatory airflow is produced by frequencies of vertical vibration around 3–4 Hz, speech is not impaired at these frequencies unless vibration levels are severe. From about 6 Hz to 20 Hz, the oscillatory airflow persists, probably as a result of chest-wall resonance, and produces loudness modulation of speech. This may give rise to loss of intelligibility at some frequencies (Nixon and Sommer 1963) and may pose problems for automatic speech-recognition systems. A two- to three-fold increase in error rate has been measured in the operation of such a device on speech from subjects undergoing vertical vibration at 20 Hz, a typical vibration frequency for helicopters (Leeks 1986).

Subjects vibrated at frequencies between about 2 Hz and 6 Hz experience difficulty in controlling the position of the outstretched hand, which may pose problems in the operation of switches and controls in an environment vibrating at these frequencies. Tracking-tasks in which the arm is supported and the hand operates a joystick control show most disruption by vibration in the frequency range 4–8 Hz. As frequencies of vibration are increased, progressively smaller structural units in the body may resonate – at lower frequencies (4–8 Hz) the muscles of the thigh, at higher frequencies muscle groups of smaller mass, and at 15–20 Hz the facial tissues, often accompanied by mild irritation in the skin of the face.

The possibility of mechanical resonance of the eye has been investigated. Early experiments showed visual acuity for stationary targets to be impaired under whole-body vibration in the frequency ranges 20–40 Hz and 60–90 Hz (Coermann 1940). An indirect method of tracking the retinal image during vibration applied direct to the head has also shown resonant peaks at 30–40 Hz ($\times 1.3$) and at 70 Hz ($\times 3$) (Stott 1984). In practice, whole-body vibration applied through a seat at these frequencies is much attenuated within the trunk, and relatively little reaches the head. It seems likely that any resonance of the eye involves intraocular structures rather than movement of the eye globe as a whole. The effect of vibration on vision is considered in more detail below.

The response of the body to vibration transmitted through the feet of a standing subject is little different from that of a seated subject, the straight legs acting as rigid

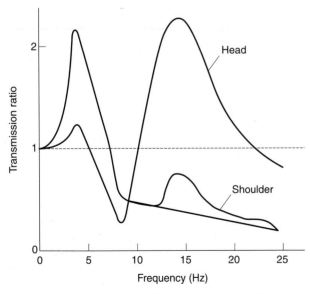

Figure 14.9 *Transmission of vibration to the head and shoulders of a seated subject. Redrawn from Rowlands (1977).*

columns. Flexion of the legs brings into play the compliance and damping properties of striated muscle and produces increasingly effective vibration isolation of the trunk to frequencies above about 5 Hz, a fact appreciated, if not understood, by charioteers and downhill skiers. When vertical vibration is applied to supine subjects, the attenuating effect of the trunk on vibration reaching the head is absent. In supine subjects vibrated in the anteroposterior direction (G_x), some amplification of vibration was found at the head at frequencies above 10 Hz and a resonant peak ($\times$ 2) at 60 Hz. There was also amplification of vibration at around 8 Hz on the abdomen, sternum and knee, with attenuation above about 16 Hz (reviewed in Dupuis and Zerlett 1986).

EFFECTS OF VIBRATION ON VISION

There are two principal requirements to enable the eye to view objects with a maximum degree of visual acuity. First, the image formed on the retina must be focused correctly; second, the eyes should be directed such that the image remains essentially stationary on the fovea. This second requirement of a stable retinal image may have to be achieved either when the object of regard is in motion or when the head itself is moving. Two important reflexes, the vestibulo-ocular reflex and the pursuit reflex, promote stability of the retinal image. The vestibulo-ocular reflex uses sensory information derived primarily from the semicircular canals to generate angular eye movements that compensate for head movements. The pursuit reflex is mediated visually and uses the error of visual fixation to generate eye movements, which maintain the retinal image on the foveal region. The shortest neural pathway between the vestibular system and the eye muscles comprises only three neurons and, consequently, enables the eye to respond rapidly to changing head movement. By contrast, the pursuit reflex comprises more complex visual processing and is relatively slow in response.

Thus, if a stationary subject views an oscillating complex display, the visual acuity for details of the display will be reduced if this motion exceeds an angular velocity of 40 degrees per second or if its frequency of oscillation exceeds about 1 Hz. The subject's performance at this task is limited by the pursuit reflex (Figure 14.10). By contrast, if a subject with normal vestibular function undergoes angular oscillation while viewing a stationary display, good visual acuity is maintained up to frequencies of 8 Hz or more. That this ability depends on an intact vestibulo-ocular reflex is indicated by the fact that a subject who lacks vestibular function loses visual acuity when either the subject or the display is oscillated at frequencies above 1 Hz (Benson and Barnes 1978). It is likely that the vestibulo-ocular reflex is able to generate eye movements that are

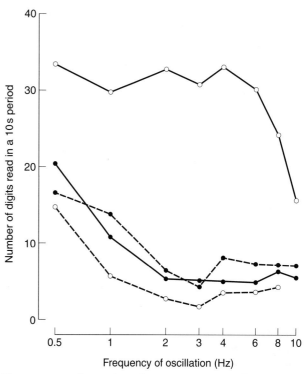

Figure 14.10 *Comparison of reading performance (mean of eight subjects) when subjects undergoing sinusoidal oscillation in yaw were required to read a stationary numerical display (●–●) and when stationary subjects were required to read an oscillating display (○–○). The dotted lines indicate the performance of a subject who lacked labyrinthine function. Redrawn from Benson and Barnes (1978).*

compensatory for angular head movement at frequencies up to 20–25 Hz.

Whole-body vertical vibration generates angular movement of the head principally in pitch. The highest angular accelerations are generated by vertical vibration between about 3 Hz and 10 Hz. Such angular head movement is within the frequency range in which the vestibulo-ocular reflex will promote compensatory eye movements, although with high intensities of vibration at these frequencies subjects may be aware of some visual instability of earth-fixed objects.

The pilot of an aircraft undergoing vibration needs to maintain visual acuity under two principal conditions – when the world outside the aircraft is observed and when reading instruments or displays that are, like the pilot, undergoing vibration. The outside world is at optical infinity and is space-stable, although the pilot may need to track objects moving within it, such as other aircraft. Under these conditions, the eye is stabilized to angular head movement by the vestibulo-ocular reflex, and purely linear movements of the head will produce no retinal image motion. Objects that the pilot wishes to track within this field of view are unlikely to move so fast that they exceed the angular velocity limitations of the pursuit reflex. When viewing objects within the aircraft, however, the pilot may experience problems. The aircraft vibration will, at certain frequencies, be amplified at the pilot's head; at frequencies above 1–2 Hz, head motion is likely to be out of phase with the motion of the instrument panel, owing to transmission delays through the body. This relative linear motion between the eye and the instrument panel will result in retinal image motion and degraded visual acuity, since, unlike the outside scene, the instrument panel is not at optical infinity. Also, in these circumstances, any eye movements generated by the vestibulo-ocular reflex in response to angular head motion may not improve retinal image stability. The mechanism by which unwanted vestibular-induced eye movements are suppressed has the same frequency and velocity limitations as the pursuit reflex. (It is likely that vestibulo-ocular suppression and ocular pursuit involve the same neural pathways.) Thus, vestibular-induced eye movements resulting from head vibration at frequencies above 2 Hz cannot be suppressed and may, therefore, contribute to a decrement in visual acuity when both subject and visual target are undergoing vibration.

A further circumstance in which the vestibulo-ocular reflex produces inappropriate eye movements occurs in the use of helmet-mounted display systems, which generate images that are coupled to, and, therefore, move with, the head. The legibility of a helmet-mounted display is particularly impaired by vibration at frequencies between 4 Hz and 6 Hz (Figure 14.11) but can be improved if the projected visual image of the display is stabilized by moving it in anti-phase to the sensed pitch and yaw rotations of the helmet (Wells and Griffin 1984). The legibility of flight instruments in helicopters is a subject that has received insufficient attention. Pilots are often aware that at certain phases of flight, e.g. transition to hover, the levels of vibration render instruments difficult to read. In addition to the relative motion between observer and visual target, many other factors are involved in the legibility of symbolic information, including size, line width, colour, brightness and contrast.

CARDIOVASCULAR EFFECTS OF VIBRATION

Exposure to moderate levels of whole-body vibration produces no consistent changes in simple measures of cardiovascular function. There may be an increase in pulse rate at the start of vibration exposure, but this is not sustained. A rise in blood pressure after periods of vibration lasting one to two hours has been reported. In response to whole-body vibration, there is an increase in muscle activity, both in order to maintain posture and, possibly, to reduce the resonant amplification of body structures. This is reflected in an increase in metabolic rate under vibration and a redistribution of blood flow, with peripheral vasoconstriction (Hood *et al.* 1966). More severe levels of vibration have provoked transient cardiac rhythm changes in humans and fatal dysrhythmias in laboratory animals exposed to high intensity vibration.

RESPIRATORY EFFECTS OF VIBRATION

The increase in metabolic rate during vibration is comparable with that seen in gentle exercise, and respiration is increased in order to achieve the necessary increase in elimination of carbon dioxide. However, true hyperventilation may occur, leading to reduced CO_2 tensions within the body (Ernsting 1961). The mechanism for this hyperventilation is not understood fully. High levels of vibration may give rise to alarm with consequent hyperventilation. Alternatively, vibration may stimulate stretch receptors in the lung to promote increased pulmonary ventilation. Vibration over a wide range of frequencies promotes an oscillating airflow superimposed on the normal respiratory air movements. The maximum oscillating volume is found with G_z vibration at 3–4 Hz, corresponding to the frequency of internal body resonance. Although this oscillating volume is less than the anatomical dead space, it has a disproportionate effect on gas exchange on account of the convective mixing of gases promoted by vibration of the air within the bronchial tree. This effect may be maximal at higher frequencies of oscillatory airflow (George and Geddes 1985).

Individual differences in the degree of hypocapnia induced by vibration may be related to the individual's responsiveness to CO_2. In subjects with a low CO_2 responsiveness, minute ventilation is regulated less tightly by arterial CO_2 levels. It has been suggested that the increased ventilation provoked by vibration is not compensated in

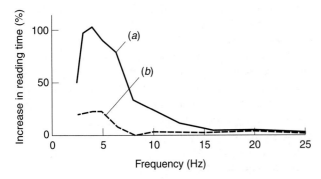

Figure 14.11 *Effect of vibration on reading performance from a helmet-mounted display, (a) when the display image is fixed in position relative to the helmet and (b) when the image is stabilized in space. Redrawn from Wells and Griffin (1984).*

these individuals by a reduction in CO_2-mediated ventilatory drive (Lamb and Tenney 1966). Generally, vibration levels in helicopter operations are insufficient to produce overt symptoms of hyperventilation, but end-tidal P_{CO_2} levels of 30 mmHg have been measured in the laboratory during repeated two-hour exposures to the simulated noise and vibration environment of the Chinook helicopter (Figure 14.12).

NEUROMUSCULAR EFFECTS OF VIBRATION

Vibration in the frequency range 20–100 Hz applied directly to a skeletal muscle or its associated tendon provokes a reflex contraction, the tonic vibration reflex, accompanied by an erroneous perception of increased muscle stretch. Local vibration can be regarded as a rapid sequence of mechanical stimuli provoking a succession of stretch reflexes. The effect is mediated through the stimulation of muscle spindles and Golgi tendon organs, whose receptors are responsible for the sense of proprioception. Thus, vibration applied to the Achilles tendon or the soleus muscle in a standing subject is perceived as a lengthening of this muscle, which is interpreted as ankle dorsiflexion and a forward tilt of the whole body. The subject, in an attempt to remain upright, generates an inappropriate backward movement of the body, to the point where he or she may fall. Similarly, local vibration applied to the neck extensor muscles provokes an illusion of forward flexion of the head, and vibration to the rectus abdominis provokes an illusion of extension of the upper trunk. When vibration is stopped, there is a transient illusion of motion in the opposite direction. Furthermore, if during vibration of muscle groups the subject views a stationary light in the dark, there is a visual illusion of movement of the light in the direction of the illusory body motion, and it may be possible to record an associated nystagmus (Lackner and Levine 1979). In contrast to vibration applied to individual muscles, whole-body vibration provokes a reflex inhibition of tendon reflexes. The effect seems to be mediated peripherally, since inhibition of leg reflexes can be produced as readily when vibration is applied through the feet of seated subjects (Roll et al. 1980).

VIBRATION AND MOTION SICKNESS

Whole-body vibration at frequencies around 0.2 Hz can induce the symptoms of motion sickness in susceptible subjects. This effect occurs to a diminishing extent at frequencies up to about 0.7 Hz. In seated subjects, susceptibility is greater for a stimulus in the G_x (fore–aft) direction than for the same stimulus applied in the G_z (craniocaudal) direction. The effect of a supine posture is to reduce susceptibility to low frequency oscillation, but in this posture the effect on susceptibility of stimulus direction relative to the axis of the body is still present (Golding et al. 1995). The frequency range over which motion sickness is provoked lies well below any internal body resonance, so that there is no direct mechanical cause for the stomach-awareness that characterizes the onset of motion sickness. This stimulus to motion sickness is discussed more fully in Chapter 29.

INFRASONIC VIBRATION

Aircraft engines and rocket motors generate airborne vibration over a very broad range of acoustic frequencies. Airborne vibration is perceived mainly as sound when it lies within the frequency range of the ear. Acoustic frequencies below 25 Hz, nominally the low-frequency threshold of hearing, can still be heard if they are of sufficient intensity, but the sensitivity of the ear falls off rapidly in this frequency range. Below a frequency of about 18 Hz, sounds are heard not as a continuous tone but as a series of pulses. At even lower frequencies (5–10 Hz), pressure pulsations are still sensed by the ear, although possibly through nerve endings in the tympanic membrane, which convey a sense of fullness in the ear and of pain if acoustic vibration is of sufficient intensity (> 155 dB at 5 Hz). There is evidence that the feeling of fullness or pressure in the ear is the result of indrawing of the tympanic membrane. It can be relieved, but only temporarily, by venting the middle ear using the Valsalva manoeuvre. The Eustachian tube appears to be acting as a one-way valve, so that large excursions of the tympanic membrane force air out of the mid-

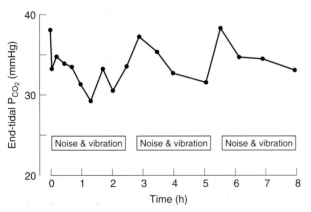

Figure 14.12 Vibration-induced hyperventilation. End-tidal PCO_2 levels measured in one subject during exposure to laboratory-reproduced noise and vibration from the Chinook helicopter over an eight-hour period. End-tidal CO_2 levels return to near-normal following each 20-minute rest period.

dle ear more readily than it can be drawn back in. After exposure to intense infrasound, vascular injection of the eardrum may be observed and audiometry may show a small degree of temporary threshold shift (von Gierke and Nixon 1977).

Other symptoms reported by subjects exposed to high-intensity infrasound include nausea and impairment of balance, symptoms that suggest an involvement of vestibular receptors. Vertical nystagmus has been recorded, its onset related to the frequency, intensity and duration of infrasonic vibration. No objective evidence of equilibratory disturbance has been obtained. Infrasonic vibration over the frequency range 2–15 Hz can be felt as pressure pulsations on the chest and abdomen, often associated with a sense of tightness in the chest. Because of the disparity in density (more strictly, acoustic impedance) between air and body tissues, much of the pressure wave is reflected and very little movement is imparted to the chest wall. However, the fluctuating air pressure generates an alternating mass flow of air in and out of the chest. If the gas flow is measured at different frequencies and constant sound pressure level, a peak in flow is seen at around 50 Hz, which is indicative of an acoustic resonance of the chest cavity at this frequency. Dogs exposed to acoustic vibration of 0.5 Hz at 172 dB can cease spontaneous respiration without ill effect. Such observations have led to the use of oscillatory gas flows at frequencies between 0.5 Hz and 6 Hz as a technique for assisting alveolar ventilation in patients with respiratory disease. Tiredness and an inability to concentrate are also symptoms that may be reported during exposure to infrasound. These effects are indicative of the psychological stressor effects of infrasound.

HUMAN TOLERANCE TO VIBRATION

In the investigation of vibration tolerance, animal studies have yielded information on the anatomical sites that are vulnerable to vibration, and at what frequencies. Because of differences in body mass and posture, extrapolation of the results of animal studies to humans leads to uncertainties. The nearest approach to carrying out a similar experiment in humans required 15 well-motivated volunteers to submit to steadily increasing amplitudes of vibration until they thought they would sustain bodily harm by any further increase (Magid *et al.* 1960). The results of this experiment (Figure 14.13) indicate that the human body is least tolerant of vertical vibration between the frequencies of 4 Hz and 8 Hz. The main symptoms for which vibration was discontinued were precordial and central abdominal pain. The acceleration levels of vibration that were tolerated at 1 Hz were roughly twice those at 4–8 Hz. At 1–3 Hz, the main symptom was difficulty in breathing. After one minute of exposure to vibration at 8 Hz, one subject

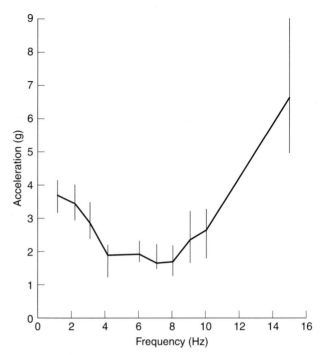

Figure 14.13 *Limits of voluntary human tolerance to G_z sinusoidal vibration at frequencies between 1 Hz and 15 Hz. The graph shows the mean of the results from ten subjects. Vertical bars indicate the range at each test frequency. Redrawn from Magid et al. (1960).*

fainted and was found to have developed a nodal tachycardia. The general shape of the vibration tolerance curve derived from this experiment has also emerged from psychophysical studies to find the levels of vibration at different frequencies and in different directions that produce equivalent levels of discomfort (Miwa 1967).

VIBRATION STANDARDS AND ASSESSMENT OF VIBRATION SEVERITY

The process of standardization seeks to define a terminology and to specify techniques for the measurement of vibration and procedures for the analysis of recorded vibration data. More contentiously, it may attempt to define limits for what is safe or acceptable to humans in a range of different circumstances. Standards have to be based on current knowledge and, therefore, may evolve as new information becomes available. However, a standard may be more dogmatic than is warranted by the tenuous data on which it is based. An important reason for the recording of vibration levels in a particular environment is to determine the likely effect on individuals who have to operate in that environment. By comparison with the assessment of a noise environment, the assessment of vibration poses additional complexities. First, the effect of vibration depends on its direction relative to the orientation of the body. Second, different vibration effects may be relevant to specific circumstances. For example, a vehicle designer may be concerned with the level of passenger discomfort, while a designer of high-rise buildings may be concerned with the likelihood that its upper-floor occupants perceive any sway of the building in high winds. In more hazardous environments, the concern may be the effect on physical health of exposure to whole-body vibration or to hand–arm vibration from handheld tools. Other effects may be the impairment of manual control, the loss of visual acuity or the development of motion sickness. For all of these effects, there is a dependence on the frequency of vibration; some frequencies are more relevant than others. The approach taken in British Standards BS6841:1987 (British Standards Institution 1987a) and BS6842:1987 (British Standards Institution 1987b), and adopted by the corresponding International Standards ISO 2631-1:1997 (International Organization for Standardization 1997a) and ISO/CD 5349-1:1997 (International Organization for Standardization 1997b), is the use of frequency-weighting functions. These can be thought of as soft-edged windows that are applied mathematically to the spectrum of recorded vibration in order to allow through vibration frequencies to the extent that they contribute to the effect under consideration. There are six weighting functions defined for whole-body vibration and one for hand-transmitted vibration.

In the assessment of vibration, the ultimate aim is to arrive at a single number that represents the vibration severity, much like the Richter scale for earthquakes or the dB(A) scale for noise. The first step in this direction is to measure the vibration at the appropriate location, usually at the interface between the body and the source of vibration, and to record from transducers in the appropriate orientation, which may require up to six transducers to measure linear and, where necessary, angular motion in the three body-related axes. The duration of recording also has to be assessed in relation to the variability of vibration over time. The second step involves the Fourier analysis of the recorded time histories of vibration acceleration to convert them to the equivalent frequency spectra and then to apply a weighting function appropriate to the direction of vibration, body posture and the vibration effect of concern (hand control, vision, motion sickness, perception, discomfort, health). The final step is to summate the components of the weighted spectrum in order to give a single figure, the vibration dose value (VDV). The formula for this is

$$\text{VDV} = \left[\int_0^T a_w^4(t)\,dt\right]^{1/4}$$

This formula has two useful properties. It introduces a dependence of vibration dose on the duration of vibration exposure that is consistent with experimental data on the relationship between severity and exposure duration. Also, if the vibration source contains high-intensity spikes of acceleration (mechanical shocks), then the summation of the fourth power of the weighted acceleration a_w^4 gives an appropriately greater emphasis to these in the derived value of VDV.

In 2002, the European Commission issued the Physical Agents (Vibration) Directive, which came into force in the UK in July 2005. This document sets out the requirements for the protection of workers from the adverse health consequences of vibration. The directive requires employers to assess the levels of vibration to which their employees are exposed. Employers have a duty, if certain levels are exceeded, to take steps to mitigate the effects of vibration either by reducing the levels of vibration at source or by limiting the time for which employees are exposed.

The directive is concerned with both whole-body and hand-transmitted vibration and lays down two levels of vibration, the exposure action value and the exposure limit value, measured in terms of the eight-hour equivalent weighted root mean square (RMS) level. It could be argued that for certain types of vibration, the VDV would give a more reliable measure, but use of the weighted RMS level has the merit that it is directly analogous to the method for determination of noise exposure. For whole-body vibration, the exposure action value is set at 0.5 m/s^2 RMS A(8) and the exposure limit value at 1.15 m/s^2 RMS A(8). For hand-transmitted vibration, the corresponding values are 2.5 m/s^2 RMS A(8) and 5 m/s^2 RMS A(8), respectively.

These limits are likely to pose problems in relation to military activities, particularly for personnel in long-range insertion craft and the crews of tanks. Some helicopter operations may also exceed the limit. Calculations based on vibration data recorded in the Chinook helicopter in cruise show a weighted RMS level of 1.9 m/s^2. If continued for eight hours, this level of vibration would be well in excess of the exposure limit value. In fact, this limit would be reached after about three hours of flight.

PROTECTION AGAINST VIBRATION

The effects of vibration on the body can be reduced by attention to the source of vibration, by modification of the transmission pathway, and by alteration of the dynamic properties of the body. If the source of vibration is turbulent air, this can be avoided by the appropriate routing of commercial aircraft away from storm-cloud activity or by choosing a different cruising altitude. Reduction of vibration emanating from aircraft engines is a task for the design and maintenance engineers of the aircraft.

Several methods have been used in helicopters to reduce the vibration reaching the aircrew and passengers.

Dynamic vibration absorbers are fitted to the cockpit floor in the Chinook helicopter. This device consists of a minimally damped mass/spring system that is fixed to the airframe and has a natural frequency that corresponds to the predominant vibration frequency of the helicopter. Vibration of the aircraft induces relatively large-amplitude resonant oscillation in the mass of the dynamic vibration absorber, which, in consequence, exerts an alternating force tending to oppose, and thus reduce, the input vibration. Such a device works only over a narrow frequency range and will amplify vibration at frequencies immediately above and below (see Figure 14.3, p. 233).

Another engineering approach to the reduction of vibration is by means of vibration isolation of the aircrew seat. This has been achieved in the Lynx helicopter by connecting the seat-pan and backrest to the body of the seat through steel springs. Provided the resonant frequency of the system formed by the body mass and the sprung seat is low relative to the predominant vibration frequency of the aircraft, increasing attenuation of vibration can be expected at frequencies greater than 1.4 times the resonant frequency. However, the apparent mass of the human body when vibrated at 20 Hz is much less than its static mass, and for this reason such a seat does not give the degree of vibration isolation that simple theory would predict. The heavier the occupant of the seat, the lower is the resonant frequency of the seat. Therefore, the vibration isolation at higher frequencies is more effective for heavier subjects. In practice, the seat and its occupant have a resonance at 3–4 Hz, close to the principal body resonance. Although in flight there is little vibration input at these frequencies, in a crash a sprung seat will amplify the impact forces at these frequencies and, consequently, may worsen the chances of survival. The same principle of vibration isolation is used in the civilian passenger-carrying version of the Chinook helicopter, in which the whole floor of the passenger compartment is mounted on a spring suspension.

A further technique for the reduction of vibration is the use of active vibration absorption. This has been implemented on the Merlin (EH101) helicopter. The technique involves the use of active struts between the rotor head and the top of the fuselage. Each strut incorporates a force-sensing element and an actuator that can apply rapidly changing longitudinal forces to lengthen and shorten the strut. By this means, vibrational forces generated at the rotor head can be sensed and actively cancelled out. This technique is particularly relevant for the attenuation of vibration at the blade-pass frequency, which is not amenable to reduction by mechanical balancing of the rotor blades.

Mention has already been made of the effects of posture and muscle tension on body resonances. Under severe vibration, muscle tensing is an involuntary response tending to increase damping within the body and to stiffen the spring component of vibrating structures and so alter their resonant frequency. Subjects tend to adopt a posture that minimizes vibration reaching the head.

The evacuation of casualties by helicopter has the advantage of speed of access to appropriate medical facilities, which is unlikely to be outweighed by the stress of helicopter vibration. Nonetheless, pre-flight assessment should, ideally, take account of the effects of vibration and, for example, ensure adequate analgesia in patients with fractures. A casualty lying on the floor of the aircraft is exposed to more vibration, particularly to the head, than is a sitting subject. An air mattress is effective in attenuating vibration at frequencies above about 5 Hz. A degree of vibration isolation is also provided by the compliance of the hanging stretcher mountings installed in some helicopters.

OCCUPATIONAL HAZARDS OF VIBRATION

Apart from the hazards of acute exposure to high levels of vibration, long-term exposure to vibration has been suspected as a causative factor in a number of conditions. The causal link between local vibration to the hand and arm from hand-held vibrating tools and the development of Raynaud's disease ('vibration white finger') was first reported in 1911. The condition is not likely to be seen in aviators, but it may occur in people working in manufacturing industries related to aviation, in particular workers who use handheld grinding and chipping tools for metal-finishing. Vibration white finger is a prescribed disease. This means that its occurrence in certain groups of workers can lead to the payment of financial compensation (Taylor 1985). Vibration to the hand in the frequency range 20–200 Hz is probably most liable to lead to the condition. Symptoms appear after months or years of vibration exposure and consist initially of episodes of tingling or numbness in the fingers. Later, attacks of finger blanching, usually provoked by cold, occur with increasing frequency. Touch and temperature sensations are impaired, and the loss of finger dexterity interferes with work and leisure activities. With further vibration exposure, blanching attacks are replaced by a more continuous dusky cyanosis. Atrophic changes in the finger pulps may be followed by necrosis of the skin over the fingertips. Progression of the condition may be halted by the affected individual ceasing to carry out work involving exposure to vibration, but the condition can be reversed only if it is caught in its early stages.

Whole-body vibration has been implicated as a factor in the development of disorders of the lumbar spine, particularly in drivers of tractors, earth-moving vehicles and trucks. Lumbar backache is also a common complaint among helicopter pilots. Direct measurement of the movements of the lumbar spine in seated subjects during vertical vibration using markers fixed into the spinous processes indicates that at about 4 Hz, there is a peak in amplification not only of vertical motion but also of fore–aft and rotational motion of lumbar vertebrae. The major body resonance occurs at this frequency, and therefore mechanical stress on the lumbar spine is likely to be at a maximum in this frequency range. The epidemiological surveys conducted on drivers of tractor and earth-moving vehicles (reviewed in Dupuis and Zerlett 1986) indicate that degenerative disorders of the lumbar spine occur at an earlier age in these groups of workers and that vibration is implicated as an aetiological factor. It is not certain whether the same is true for helicopter pilots. The predominant vibration frequency of helicopters tends to be above the major body resonance, and the unvarying slightly bent sitting posture that the disposition of cyclic and collective imposes on the pilot may be of greater importance in provoking back pain during flight. Evidence for a greater incidence of radiological abnormalities of the lumbar spine in helicopter pilots is inconclusive. The subject is reviewed by Bowden (1987).

Epidemiological studies have also shown a higher than normal incidence of stomach-related disorders in drivers of tractors and earth-moving vehicles. The relationship of these disorders to vibration exposure is far from certain, although it is of interest that the incidence of stomach ailments in operators of tracked vehicles is half that of drivers of wheeled earth-moving vehicles. Although the lifestyles of the two groups of workers could be expected to be similar, the vibration exposure in wheeled vehicles is likely to be much greater.

REFERENCES

Benson AJ, Barnes GR. Vision during angular oscillation: the dynamic interaction of visual and vestibular mechanisms. *Aviation, Space, and Environmental Medicine* 1978; **49**: 340–45.

Bowden T. Back pain in helicopter aircrew: a literature review. *Aviation, Space, and Environmental Medicine* 1987; **58**: 461–7.

British Standards Institution. Guide to measurement and evaluation of human exposure to whole-body mechanical vibration and repeated shock. BS 6841:1987. London: British Standards Institution, 1987a.

British Standards Institution. Measurement and evaluation of human exposure to vibration transmitted to the hand. BS 6842:1987. London: British Standards Institution, 1987b.

Coermann R. Investigation into the effect of vibration on the human body. Library translation no. 217. London: Ministry of Defence, 1940.

Coermann RR, Ziegenruecker GH, Wittwer AL, Von Glerke HE. The passive dynamic properties of the human thorax–abdomen system and of the whole-body system. *Aerospace Medicine* 1960; **31**: 443–55.

Dupuis H, Zerlett G. *The Effects of Whole-Body Vibration.* Berlin: Springer, 1986.

Ernsting J. Respiratory effects of whole-body vibration. RAF Institute of Aviation Medicine report no. 179. London: Ministry of Defence, 1961.

European Commission. Directive 2002/44/EC of the European Parliament and of the Council of 25 June 2002 on the minimum health and safety requirements regarding the exposure of workers to the risks arising from physical agents (vibration). *Official Journal of the European Communities* 2002; **L177**: 13–19.

George RJD, Geddes DM. High frequency ventilation. *British Journal of Hospital Medicine* 1985; **33**: 344–9.

Golding JF, Markey HM, Stott JRR. The effects of motion direction, body axis, and posture on motion sickness induced by low frequency linear oscillation. *Aviation, Space, and Environmental Medicine* 1995; **66**: 1046–51.

Hood WB, Murray RH, Urschel CW, Bowers JA, Clark JG. Cardiopulmonary effects of whole-body vibration in man. *Journal of Applied Physiology* 1966; **21**: 1725–31.

International Organization for Standardization. Mechanical vibration and shock: evaluation of human exposure to whole-body vibration. Part 1: general requirements. ISO 2631-1:1997. Geneva: International Organization for Standardization, 1997a.

International Organization for Standardization. Mechanical vibration: measurement and assessment of human exposure to hand-transmitted vibration. Part 1: general guidelines. ISO 5349-1:1997. Geneva: International Organization for Standardization, 1997b.

Lackner JR, Levine MS. Changes in apparent body orientation and sensory localization induced by vibration of postural muscles: vibratory myesthetic illusions. *Aviation, Space, and Environmental Medicine* 1979; **50**: 346–54.

Lamb TW, Tenney SM. Nature of vibration hyperventilation. *Journal of Applied Physiology* 1966; **21**: 404–10.

Leeks C. Operation of a speech recogniser under whole body vibration. Royal Aircraft Establishment technical memorandum FS(F) 634. London: Ministry of Defence, 1986.

Magid EB, Coermann RR, Ziegenruecker GM. Human tolerance to whole-body sinusoidal vibration. *Aerospace Medicine* 1960; **31**: 915–24.

Miwa T. Evaluation methods for vibration effect: part 1. Measurements of threshold and equal sensation contours of whole-body for vertical and horizontal vibrations. *Industrial Health* 1967; **5**: 183–205.

Nickerson JL, Paradijeff A. Body tissue changes in dogs resulting from sinusoidal oscillation stress. Technical documentary report AMRL-TDR-64-58. Wright-Patterson Air Force Base, OH: USAF Aerospace Medical Research Laboratories, 1964.

Nixon CW, Sommer HC. Influence of selected vibrations upon speech. III. Range of 6 cps to 20 cps for semi-supine talkers. *Aerospace Medicine* 1963; **34**: 1012–17.

Paddan GS, Griffin MJ. The transmission of translational seat vibration to the head. I. Vertical seat vibration. *Journal of Biomechanics* 1988a; **21**: 191–7.

Paddan GS, Griffin MJ. The transmission of translational seat vibration to the head. II. Horizontal seat vibration. *Journal of Biomechanics* 1988b; **21**: 199–206.

Roll JP, Martin B, Gauthier GM, Mussa Ivaldi F. Effects of whole-body vibration on spinal reflexes in man. *Aviation, Space, and Environmental Medicine* 1980; **51**: 1227–33.

Rowlands GF. The transmission of vertical vibration to the heads and shoulders of seated men. Royal Aircraft Establishment technical report no. 77088. London: Ministry of Defence, 1977.

Speakman JD, Bonfili HF, Hille HR, Cole TN. Crew exposure to vibration in the F4C aircraft during low altitude high speed flight. AMRL-TR-70-99. Wright Patterson Air Force Base, OH: Aerospace Medical Research Laboratory, 1971.

Stott JRR. The vertical vestibulo-ocular reflex and ocular resonance. *Vision Research* 1984; **24**: 949–60.

Taylor W. Vibration white finger: a newly prescribed disease (editorial). *British Medical Journal* 1985; **291**: 921–2.

Vogt HL, Coermann RR, Fust MD. Mechanical impedance of the sitting human under sustained acceleration. *Aerospace Medicine* 1968; **39**: 675–9.

Von Gierke HE, Nixon CW. Effects of intense infrasound on man. In: Tempest W (ed.). *Infrasound and Low Frequency Vibration*. London: Academic Press,1977; pp. 115–50.

Wells MJ, Griffin MJ. Benefits of helmet-mounted display image stabilization under whole-body vibration. *Aviation, Space, and Environmental Medicine* 1984; **55**: 13–18.

FURTHER READING

Boff KR, Lincoln JE. Engineering data compendium: human perception and performance. Wright-Patterson Air Force Base, OH: Armstrong Aerospace Medical Research Laboratory, 1986.

Griffin MJ. *Handbook of Human Vibration*. London: Academic Press, 1990.

Guignard JC, King PF. Aeromedical aspects of vibration and noise. AGARDograph AG-151. Neuilly-sur-Seine: AGARD/NATO, 1972.

Harris CM, Crede CE. *Shock and Vibration Handbook*, 2nd edn. New York: McGraw-Hill, 1976.

Mansfield NJ. *Human Response to Vibration*. Boca Raton, FL: CRC Press, 2005.

Speakman JD, Rose JF. Crew compartment vibration environment in the B52 aircraft during low altitude high speed flight. AMRL-TR-71-12. Wright-Patterson Air Force Base, OH: Aerospace Medical Research Laboratory, 1971.

15

Anthropometry and aircrew equipment integration

ALISTAIR J.F. MACMILLAN

INTRODUCTION

The primary task of military aircrew is to ensure that the complete operational envelope of the aircraft and its weapons system are exploited fully. Other than individual flying skills and experience, a pilot's ability to fly an aircraft to its peak performance as safely as possible depends on optimum integration of the components comprising the pilot's personal aircrew equipment assembly (AEA) and its compatibility with the cockpit in which the pilot operates. These crucial demands require the skilled interpretation and application of appropriate anthropometric data obtained from surveys of the aircrew population. The information that this provides allows aircrew equipment manufacturers to produce the smallest, and therefore the cheapest, range of clothing sizes and helmets that will fit the aircrew population. In addition, the information can be used to aid the design of aircraft cockpits that will accommodate as large a range as possible of human body shapes and sizes, concomitant with the safe operation of the aircraft. The final, and in military aviation probably the most important, stage in the union of the aircrew members with their aircraft is an assessment of a representative size range of aircrew, fully clothed with correctly fitting assemblies in the cockpit of the required aircraft.

Aircrew clothing and equipment comprise those items worn, carried or used by aircrew personnel in the normal performance of their duties in flight and for emergency escape, location and survival. Some items of equipment are on the aircraft inventory, e.g. restraint systems and survival aids, such as the dinghy, survival rations, etc.; these are not considered further in this chapter. The items worn or car-

ried comprise the AEA and are intended to meet the demands of physiological wellbeing in flight, to ensure operational effectiveness, to provide protection of the person against the hazards of escape and survival, and to be there always, ready for use should the need arise.

Accordingly, current AEAs are multi-layered sets of garments, each having its own particular function and capable of being worn in various combinations appropriate to the mission and prevailing conditions. The range of equipment and clothing typically available in high-performance aircraft is illustrated in Figure 15.1.

AEAs may be subdivided conveniently into four categories:

- Life support: oxygen equipment, anti-G protection, chemical/biological/radiological/nuclear (CBRN) warfare protection, personal conditioning.
- Operational: communication facilities, vision enhancement, displays and pockets, etc. in the flying coverall or other outer garment.
- Escape and survival: restraint and parachute harness, head protection, flotation, immersion protection.
- Personal.

The equipment and clothing that lie in the first three of these categories are described in detail in other chapters. The final category, which consists of underwear, shirt, socks and flying boots, should need no further depiction. It is essential that all the items that comprise the assembly should fit snugly upon each other in order to ensure comfort and do nothing to hamper integration between aircrew, equipment and workspace. This integration can be assessed systematically and objectively by appropriate

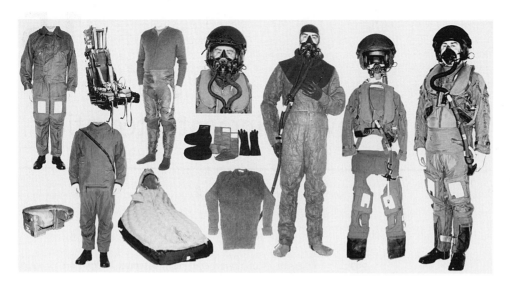

Figure 15.1 *Example of aircrew clothing and equipment available for one aircraft type.*

appraisal in a laboratory, other appropriate facilities, and the aircraft cockpit. Although determination of comfort is subjective, it may be considered to have been achieved when the individual is in physical, physiological and psychological harmony with his or her environment.

The development of aircrew equipment is achieved in stages. The three generally recognized phases include (i) definition of the requirement, (ii) assessment of form fit and function in the laboratory or specialist test facilities, and (iii) determination of operational acceptability to the user by means of appropriate flight appraisal in the required aircraft. The achievement of close fit, inter-compatibility and optimum operational function depends on precise definition of the requirement, together with a common philosophy for sizing and fitting of the layers that is based on the application of anthropometry for the derivation and development of the basic size rolls. Continuous assessment of the acceptability of each item must be conducted at each phase in the development of the assembly, irrespective of whether it is a replacement for, or an additional component in, an existing AEA schedule or an entirely novel ensemble for a new aircraft.

The information required, along with an outline of the processes that are necessary to ensure optimum integration of AEAs, is described in this chapter. Details of procedures and techniques of assessment are specified elsewhere (ASCC 1996a,b; Ministry of Defence 1999). In the context of aircrew clothing, it is important that the commonly used terminology is understood fully. It is customary in the UK to use the following terms:

- *Sizing:* the process of development aimed at determining the appropriate dimensions for the clothing, the number of sizes required in the size roll

to accommodate the predetermined population, and the nomenclature with which each size can be identified.
- *Fitting:* the process of bringing together the garment with the wearer to facilitate an evaluation of its size and suitability for the purpose intended.
- *Functional fit:* used to ensure that the wearer and clothing, when combined, can each fulfil their intended function.

DEFINITION OF REQUIREMENT

The requirements of the user must be stated in some detail so that the developer knows exactly the hazards to which the user are to be exposed and those to which the user might be exposed in a survival situation. Description, therefore, of the working environment must include information on altitude, acceleration, toxic threats, mission duration, thermal profile and cockpit workspace. Post-escape factors such as flotation requirements, thermal protection and other aspects of the theatre of operations that might influence provision of survival aids must also be considered. Generally, the definition of requirement results in the provision of a family of garments and equipment, which the user may wear in a number of permutations. In the UK, the combinations recommended in order to permit worldwide operations are grouped into AEA schedules for each aircraft type. These schedules comprise combinations of garments and equipment suitable for operations over land and sea, both in winter and in summer. Typical AEA schedules for such conditions are shown in Table 15.1. If CBRN protection is required, appropriate

Table 15.1 *Typical range of leading garments available for aircrew flying high altitude fast jet aircraft in world-wide operations. Additional items will be required if CBRN protection is necessary*

Item	Summer	Winter Land	Winter Sea
Underwear	✔	✔	✔
Personal conditioning garment	✔		
Thermal protection garment(s)		✔	✔
Immersion protection coverall			✔
Cold weather flying suit		✔	
Anti-G trousers	✔	✔	✔
Chest counterpressure garment	✔	✔	✔
Lightweight flying coverall	✔		
Life preserver	✔	✔	✔

additional protective layers must be added to each schedule of clothing.

Additional elements that contribute to overall user/operational acceptability include specification of the aircrew population and definition of the size roll of garments. Both of these rely heavily on the extent and accuracy of available anthropometric details.

ANTHROPOMETRY

Anthropometry is the measurement of the human body and its segments. However, as the application of anthropometry is not a precise science, it is necessary to conduct a comprehensive survey of the overall aircrew population from time to time and to regularly update the anthropometric data held for each individual aircrew, in order that individual size can be checked against aircraft cockpit size limits when personnel are reassigned from one aircraft to another. Anthropometric surveys are costly, labour-intensive exercises that tend to be undertaken at infrequent intervals, mainly owing to the impact of rigid selection limitations. At the time of writing, the last Royal Air Force (RAF) survey to cover the (at the time, exclusively male) aircrew population was carried out in 1970–71. More recently, the anthropometry of female RAF personnel has been surveyed, although very few of these women were aircrew.

Techniques for measurement of the human body

With any anthropometric survey, it is essential to develop a detailed methodology with care and to conduct extensive training in order to ensure accuracy and reproducibility of measurements between and within different measurers to minimize variance. Most measurements must be taken with the subject unclothed in order to locate points on the skin corresponding to landmarks on the underlying skeleton. The posture of the subject is extremely important, and the measurer must ensure that the subject does not slump during measurement or inflate the chest unduly when the chest circumference is being measured.

Traditional measuring techniques

Previously, the standard method for recording body size parameters was by simple measurement using a tape measure, a measuring rig or anthropometer, the reduced scale or spreading calliper, or the sliding calliper to identify the distance between two anatomical points or around a body segment. A typical rig is described in an RAF survey (RAF IAM 1973). With varying degrees of success, several alternatives have been attempted, but reproducibility and calibration can be a problem.

PHOTOGRAMMETRY

Photogrammetry, in which the body is photographed and the dimensions are measured from the photograph, is well established and can be used in several areas. It has a number of advantages, including the fact that it reduces the time required of both the subject and the measurer, it produces a permanent record of the raw data from which additional measurements can be taken in the future without recourse to seeing the subject again, and movement is frozen so that all measurements relate to one posture. This latter feature makes the technique particularly useful for measurement of the head, as small movements can make appreciable changes in certain measurements where the anatomical landmarks are indistinct, such as the top and back of the head. In order to ensure accuracy, it is important to use extremely long focal length lenses, either directly or via a multiple mirror optical pathway (to shorten rig/room size). In this way, parallax errors, in which parts of the anatomy nearer the camera appear slightly larger than those further away, can be minimized. Clearly, numerous measurements do not fall within the capabilities of photogrammetry, particularly those that involve circumferences and measurements along curves at a certain axis. A preliminary assessment against conventional measuring equipment will identify measurements suitable for this technique by verification of conformity. However, both of these techniques are not very satisfactory in providing information on the shape or changes of the surface curvature between anatomical landmarks, and especially where these landmarks are few and far between, such as the top and back of the head. Three-dimensional (3-D) surface scanning overcomes this inadequacy by providing accurate contour data in addition to the majority of the traditional landmark data.

THREE-DIMENSIONAL SCANNING TECHNIQUES

There are two main methods of providing 3D anthropometric information by surface scanning. The first involves the projection of white light through an interference (diffraction) grating on to the surface being scanned, which results in the production of Moiré fringe interference patterns on the surface of the human body. These patterns, which are spaced regularly on a flat surface, are distorted by the contours of the body in a manner that is related directly to the shape of the contour. The patterns are photographed for later analysis. The subject can be stationary or can be rotated. The information from twin Moiré measuring units is fed through a pre-processor to a powerful dedicated graphics computer loaded with image-processing software that produces an accurate 3-D image of the surface being scanned. Scans take approximately two seconds.

A more versatile and accurate technique involves the use of a laser. During a laser scan, a helium/neon laser beam is projected via an optical system that converts the beam into a line of laser light on to the surface of the subject being scanned. The precise position in 3-D space where this line is projected on the surface of the subject is recorded by a camera, which by means of a sophisticated optical system views the laser light from two different angles, allowing triangulation. In the majority of systems, the scanner rotates around the subject, who remains stationary. The information acquired by the scan, which can take 15 seconds or more, is fed via a pre-processor to a very powerful graphics computer using highly sophisticated, complex software. This is used to produce very accurate 3-D images of the surfaces scanned, with resolutions better than 1 mm. Furthermore, these images can be rotated around all three axes and manipulated in a number of ways in order to extract the required anthropometric information. Because of the mass of information produced, where every point of the surface scanned (at very high resolution) is recorded in 3-D, only recently have advances in computer hardware and software permitted its successful analysis and manipulation.

The advantages of scanning techniques are numerous, including the fact that they are less labour-intensive, the data produced are of a much higher quality and have less measurer error, they provide higher resolution with more 3-D points, and they are able to give accurate information on curves. Furthermore, the extraction of more information from existing data is easy, as are further processing and combination and comparison with other data. In addition, it is possible to transfer this information directly to computer-aided design/modelling (CAD/CAM) systems. There are some disadvantages: scanning technology is still in a relatively early stage of development, scans are not entirely 3-D (e.g. when the laser beam strikes the surface exactly at a tangent, the information becomes sparse or non-existent), and laser light can cause blinking, which produces movement artefacts. Furthermore, it is difficult for subjects to remain perfectly still for the duration of the scan, and any movement reduces resolution, although the image-processing software compensates for this to a large extent. In addition, anatomical landmarks that rely on palpation rather than observation cannot be identified by the scan directly but can be marked before the scan.

The availability of increasingly powerful computers has allowed the development of 3-D modelling techniques to simulate both the human form and the cockpit workspaces into which it must fit. Separately, sophisticated 3-D models of the body and of the aircraft cockpit can be built up. However, problems arise when attempts are made to combine the two in order to derive meaningful information about, for example, the ability of a given size of body to reach or operate specific controls or to visualize specific areas of cockpit displays and controls or the outside world. In particular, interference algorithms have to be extremely complicated to be fully representative and provide usable results.

As a general principle, any geometric or mathematical modelling techniques must be suitably validated by extensive real-life experimentation before any reliance can be placed on the data obtained. Once validation has been achieved, modelling affords the distinct advantage of rapidly reviewing alternative combinations without having to undertake further live subject evaluation.

Common misconceptions in anthropometry

It is important to appreciate that there is no general descriptor of overall body size, other than large/small, thin/fat, short/tall, etc. Percentile values, which are often misunderstood and misapplied, pertain to a single body size parameter. It may well be that a cockpit design goal (in anthropometric terms) may specify several size parameters, e.g. sitting height, functional reach, leg length. However, since there is a relatively poor correlation between separate body size parameters within and between individuals across the aircrew population, the specification of a combination of parameters can have a profound effect. Assuming for a moment that all individual body size parameters are correlated perfectly, then any person who is a ninetieth percentile in stature would have a 90th percentile sitting height, a 90th percentile leg length, and so on. In such a situation, a cockpit design specification to include the third to the 99th percentiles across all selected size parameters would exclude only four per cent of the aircrew population. At the other extreme, if all body size parameters were totally uncorrelated and the same design specification limits were applied across n body size parameters, then the percentage of the aircrew population excluded on size alone would be $(4 \times n)$ per cent. Reality lies between these two extremes. There is, therefore, no such being as a 90th percentile person. Any one individual could exhibit a 95th percentile stature, an 80th percentile leg length, a 75th percentile functional reach and a 50th percentile chest circumference. As a practical example, the design specification for the Typhoon aircraft required the cockpit to accommodate (nominally) the 5th to 95th percentiles across eight body size parameters. At the extremes of the argument outlined above, this would exclude either ten per cent (parameters correlated, $r = 1$) or 80 per cent (parameters uncorrelated, $r = 0$) of the aircrew population. When the design parameters were compared sequentially with the RAF anthropometric database to identify those individuals who fulfilled all eight criteria, it was found that (in theory) 23.5 per cent of RAF aircrew would be excluded on size. In order to ensure that the specification requirements were met, the design engineers have made the cockpit marginally larger, so that, in practice, only some 12–15 per cent of aircrew members should be too small or too large to operate the aircraft. A dedicated aircrew cockpit size limitation assessment will identify the precise proportion.

Common misconceptions in anthropometric surveys

Another common pitfall is comparison between anthropometric surveys. Unless individual body size parameters common to different surveys have been measured using exactly the same methodology, it is unsafe to assume direct comparison. Provided each measurement was carried out in similar fashion, then statistically it is possible to state that there is no significant difference between the values for each survey, but only in terms of that specific size parameter. Only when a sufficient number of specific comparisons have been made in this way can one begin to consider the two populations described in each survey as similar. In this manner, work by Turner in the 1970s established that the descriptors of aircrew size for the UK and US Air Force (USAF), and for UK and German aircrew populations, were essentially similar. Over the years, the methodology for anthropometric measurement has become increasingly consistent between nations as a result of compliance with the recommendations of international working parties such as the Air and Space Interoperability Council (ASIC), formerly the Air Standardization Coordinating Committee (ASCC).

The practice of taking specific percentile values for selected size parameters from surveys conducted by several different nations, selecting the smallest (e.g. the 5th percentile) and greatest (e.g. the 95th percentile) value for each parameter, and then stating that these two composite values (possibly from different national databases) repre-

sented the 5th and 95th percentile values, respectively, for all the aircrew included in the contributing surveys as a composite whole is statistically indefensible. In such a situation, one must revert to specifying the numerical value in absolute terms for each of the selected parameters. Given these absolute values, each nation involved can then assess the impact of the derived limits on its own survey of the aircrew size range.

Application of anthropometric survey data

COCKPIT WORKSPACE DESIGN

In view of the often conflicting requirements between optimizing the performance of an aircraft and the ability to accommodate the overwhelming majority of the aircrew population, it is essential that aircraft manufacturers are provided with accurate information about the anthropometry of the aircrew population that will be required to fly the aircraft. The cross-sectional area of the cockpit significantly influences the aerodynamic drag of an aircraft, so most aircraft designers attempt to minimize the size of the cockpit while ensuring that they meet the specified requirement to accommodate the full aircrew size range. The design of an aircraft cockpit is complicated by the limited range of seat/other adjustment that is possible in military (especially combat) aircraft; by the wide range of clothing that may be worn, depending on the operational scenario; by the restrictive multipoint harnesses that are used; and by the extensive range of controls, pedals, switches, handles, levers, displays and other avionics that need to be reached. Furthermore, the cockpit of a fast jet military combat aircraft will be very different to that of a helicopter.

AIRCREW SELECTION

It is not practical from a size point of view to recruit aircrew from all of the available population. Most of the anthropometric measurements of a given population will have a normal distribution, with the majority of individuals having measurements near the median of the distribution and with progressively fewer people towards the extremes. Attempting to accommodate the whole population would require an unacceptably large range of adjustment of the seat or pedals, as indicated in Table 15.2.

Table 15.2 shows the range of aircrew sitting heights, taken from an anthropometric survey of 2000 aircrew (RAF IAM 1973), expressed as both measurements and percentiles. It can be seen that to cater for all aircrew personnel, the range of up and down adjustment of the seat (before making allowances for the seat-back angle, etc.) would have to be 202 mm. By excluding two per cent of the aircrew, the range of adjustment could be reduced by almost one-third to 142 mm. Even if the range of adjust-

Table 15.2 *Sitting height of UK aircrew expressed both as measurements and percentiles*

Percentile (%)	Measurement (mm)
Minimum	824
1	865
5	883
10	895
90	974
95	986
99	1007
Maximum	1026
Overall range	202
1st–99th percentile	142
5th–95th percentile	103

Source: Anthropometric Survey of 2000 RAF Aircrew (RAF IAM Report 531).

ment were to be halved to approximately 100 mm only ten per cent of aircrew would be excluded.

Since aircraft are built to accommodate a specified range of sizes, it follows that aircrew must be selected to conform to these parameters to ensure, as far as is possible, that any individual selected for aircrew training will, ultimately, be able to safely operate and 'fit' any aircraft type to which he or she may be assigned. Thus, a recruit's measurements must fall between well-defined minimum and maximum values in certain critical dimensions. Sitting height, arm length (or functional reach), leg length (buttock–heel) and thigh length (buttock–knee) are the dimensions normally considered. More recently, weight restrictions have been introduced, due in part to the greater weight of the ever-increasing AEA worn under certain circumstances. To ensure that fully equipped aircrew members are within the all-up weight limitation imposed by the ejection seat, allowable nude body weight must be decreased as the weight of the AEA increases. An excessively high ejecting mass (aircrew + AEA + ejection seat) may slow the ejection to the point where the seat may not clear the tailfin under certain circumstances. Conversely, the introduction of female aircrew and people from ethnic groups of small size and light build has raised concerns about the injury potential of an excessively light ejecting mass and, therefore, correspondingly rapid ejection.

These limitations can present problems during recruiting, because allowances must be made for growth changes in younger aircrew in order to prevent problems occurring at a later stage. Theoretically, if aircrew selection limits are applied rigorously, then the extremes of the aircrew population size range should not exceed the upper and lower selection limits. However, for a variety of reasons, this is not so; in virtually all cases, the lower and upper percentile values of (selection criteria) body size parameters measured during the RAF IAM (1973) anthropometric survey

exceed the associated selection limits. That said, existing selection limits have stood the test of time, with relatively few aircrew being unable to operate any aircraft based on size factors alone.

Although the overall size range of the general population from which aircrew candidates are selected may change with time (e.g. growth trends) and may be skewed by ethnic and gender size and shape differences, it does not follow that the size range of the aircrew population will reflect these changes, such as an overall aircrew size increase as the general population becomes 'bigger'. It is probably safe to state that the basic descriptors of aircrew size will not change, due to the application of selection limitations, provided these are applied rigorously. However, ethnic and gender considerations may influence changes to the aircrew population within the selection parameters, particularly in areas concerned with the sizing and fitting of flying clothing.

SIZING AND FITTING OF AIRCREW CLOTHING

Having recruited an aircrew population, which should conform to the imposed anthropometric selection limitations, a range of aircrew clothing must be provided. It is unacceptably expensive to manufacture tailor-made clothing for each individual, not only in respect of the individual tailoring that this would entail but also with respect to the logistic problems of having replacement garments readily available in cases of loss or damage. Hence, a range of sizes of clothing needs to be manufactured to fit, ideally, the whole aircrew population. Furthermore, in order to keep costs low and to reduce logistic and supply problems, the number of sizes should be kept to a minimum. The normal approach in devising a sizing scheme is to take two control measurements, typically stature and chest circumference for a one-piece garment, and to plot a scattergram. Sizing grids can then be superimposed to include the majority of individuals. The current UK system is a 9-size roll, details of which are shown in Figure 15.2.

The measurements given in Figure 15.2 are the nude data. The clothing manufacturer makes the necessary adjustments when drafting the patterns. The system is designed in such a way that, depending on the item of clothing and where it is worn in relation to other items of clothing, different adjustments are made to the nude body data when drafting the patterns. This ensures that most aircrew will take a given size for all or most of their different layers of clothing. For example, a pilot requiring a size 5 flying coverall will probably take a size 5 external immersion coverall, the latter of which will be slightly larger but designed to fit comfortably over the former.

The fit of garments that are less dependent on stature than on other body dimensions may result in the use of an

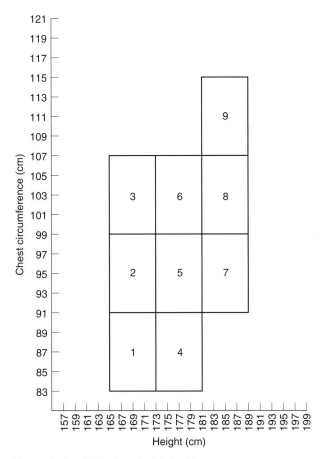

Figure 15.2 *UK 9-size role sizing grid.*

alternative control measurement. For example, because the successful operation of the active arm restraint system in the Tornado aircraft necessitates correct fitting of the life-preserver sleeves, arm length replaces stature as the control measurement when sizing aircrew for this garment.

The use of more than two control measurements can result in a very large and logistically unacceptable size roll. However, the availability of accurate anthropometric data for the aircrew population, and a sensibly designed sizing system, has ensured that the number of individuals that cannot be fitted with clothing from the standard size roll is low. These aircrew are referred for special-measure clothing that is tailor-made to their body dimensions.

ASSESSMENTS OF AIRCREW EQUIPMENT ASSEMBLY INTEGRATION (FORM FIT AND FUNCTION)

Ideal integration of AEA is achieved when the equipment is comfortable to wear, there is no compromise of the functions of any items worn, there is no impairment of the wearer's ability to see and/or operate controls, switches,

etc. in the cockpit, and there is no degradation in the operational capability of the aircraft or its escape system. The adequacy of the integration should be assessed by a series of tests, which can be subdivided as follows: effect on aircrew procedures, effect on escape and survival, dynamic tests and environmental tests. The schedule of tests adopted in the UK and the precise pass/fail criteria demanded in a schedule of tests adopted by the UK, and used by other nations, are detailed in documents from ASIC, formerly ASCC (ASCC 1996a; 1966b); similar procedures have been recommended for use by other nations in ASCC (1996b).

Laboratory test and evaluation

The second of the three phases in AEA development requires a comprehensive assessment in an appropriate integration laboratory. If possible, representative cockpit mock-ups should be used with final confirmation of AEA acceptability conducted during the final flight assessment phase of AEA development. The primary objectives of an integration laboratory are as follows:

- to integrate various developmental items with all existing or other new items of AEA
- to validate fit and function of the AEA at an early stage to preclude the need for expensive equipment or even aircraft modification during or after equipment production
- to focus efforts on increasing the probability of mission success, increasing combat effectiveness/survivability, ensuring cost-effectiveness and reducing logistic requirements.

The schedule of integration tests is normally apportioned between the laboratory, the aircraft and other environmental facilities. The tests require the participation of subjects at the extremes of the acceptable anthropometric range for the aircraft and are subdivided as follows:

- effect on aircrew procedures
- effect on escape and survival
- dynamic tests
- environmental tests.

Effect on aircrew procedures

DRESSING AND UNDRESSING

The purpose of this test is to assess any interaction between the items of AEA that could cause wear and tear or snagging to any part of the assembly. Dressing should be carried out in a simulated crew facility (particularly important in the assessment of CBRN protective equipment) and should follow the current service procedures, including assistance if available. The test must be deemed a failure if consistently one or more items of the AEA interacts adversely with the remaining items of the assembly to impair function or cause wear in an unreasonably short time.

WALK-OUT AND COCKPIT ENTRY

This test is intended to confirm that the AEA does not interfere with normal access to the aircraft or impair any external or on-board pre-flight checks. If any interaction between AEA and the aircraft structure inhibit the completion of checks or entry into the aircraft, then the test is deemed a failure.

STRAPPING-IN PROCEDURES

Any adverse interaction between the AEA and the seat-restraint system or aircraft controls or impairment of accessibility to the person/seat connection that prevents the agreed strapping-in procedures from being carried out is considered a failure.

WORKSTATION MANOEUVRES

This test demonstrates that none of the items of AEA interferes with the ability of the aircrew to carry out normal and emergency procedures during takeoff, landing and flight. Qualified aircrew participate or advise in these assessments in order to ensure that the full range of movements and activities required in a typical sortie is covered.

Effect on escape and survival

A series of tests is required to demonstrate that the AEA under development does not inhibit the aircrew from escaping from the aircraft either on the ground or in the air.

EMERGENCY EGRESS ON THE GROUND

This test must be simulated with the subjects having donned any appropriate survival aids and commence from the strapped-in position. If any component consistently and across the subject size range causes a hindrance to exit from the aircraft, then the test should be considered a failure.

ESCAPE FROM EJECTION-SEAT AIRCRAFT

A comprehensive battery of tests is required to confirm that aircrew members can operate the escape facilities available in the ejection seat and utilize the post-escape survival equipment and amenities. These tests include assessment of the ability of the aircrew to operate the seat emergency controls, e.g. operating handle with a aircraft out of control and inverted; confirmation that an aircrew member of maximum critical dimensions and dressed in the bulkiest AEA will have sufficient clearance within the cockpit for a clean ejected exit; simulated automatic and manual separation from the seat following ejection; and assessment of the security of the items of AEA and any interactions between the AEA and the parachute harness that could potentially be hazardous during and after parachute deployment. The first requires a drop test, with the subject representatively settled into his or her harness and then allowed to drop in the harness, thus simulating the opening loads of the particular parachute being used. This drop can be followed by the second assessment, suspension in the harness, which is used to check that the AEA does not interfere with the actions that may be required under the canopy. The ability of a subject, dressed in the AEA under test, to release and divest the harness while being dragged by the parachute on the land is also required. The effect of the AEA on escape and survival at sea completes the assessments in this phase of the schedule of tests. These tests are conducted at sea or in a suitable wave tank and comprise harness release and flotation; parachute dragging at sea; and life-raft operation and boarding followed by the final action in the crew member's survival sequence, i.e. winching into a helicopter.

Dynamic tests

EJECTION TEST

The most comprehensive way of assessing the behaviour of a fast-jet AEA under airborne escape conditions is for it to be incorporated as part of an ejection seat test programme. Generally, when new aircraft are introduced, the AEA can be included in the test schedule, which has the additional advantage that the number of tests and dummy sizes is defined by that programme.

The AEA must complete the defined ejection test without damage to those items that are required to function either during or following ejection. Other non-essential items of the AEA should not become detached under the influence of the ejection forces.

ALTERNATIVES TO THE EJECTION TEST

The cost and complexity of ejection tests may not be justified when a new item of AEA is introduced retrospectively. In these circumstances alternative dynamic tests can be considered acceptable. The effect of entry into the airstream during ejection can be studied by the use of an air-blast test facility. Such equipment should be capable of simulating the airspeed and decay profiles experienced by a seat and crew member emerging from the aircraft during an ejection. However, this alternative cannot re-create all the dynamic forces of an ejection, and the results must be interpreted with caution. Testing of those items of the AEA that are required to function just before or at the initiation of ejection, e.g. separation of night-vision-enhancement devices, arm restraint, etc., can be tested on an ejection-seat test ramp. The ramp must be capable of projecting a seat and the occupant at similar accelerations to those of a genuine ejection. Additional dynamic tests to simulate person/seat separation and the activation of facilities that are required to function, e.g. locator beacon activation, etc., may be checked on a rig that is capable of extracting a manikin from the seat by the parachute-deployment system at a velocity similar to that which occurs during an ejection. In the absence of such a device, simple roll-out tests using human subjects may suffice. Pass/fail criteria for these alternatives are similar to those mandated for the ejection test. Thus, all the components of the AEA that are required to function during and after the ejection sequence is complete must operate successfully after each test.

Environmental tests

Tests to demonstrate the effects of the operational environment on the various items that comprise an AEA must also be carried out. These assessments normally require the participation of human subjects and can readily be included with appraisal of other items that constitute the life-support system, e.g. oxygen delivery equipment, acceleration protection facilities, etc.

Flight acceleration profiles similar to those experienced operationally can be produced on a human subject-carrying centrifuge. However, most human subject-rated machines cannot reproduce realistic acceleration onset rates, and it is essential that these tests are complemented by appropriate flight trials. Exposure to the vibration spectrum simulating aircraft flight should be conducted with a subject dressed in the AEA under test and strapped into an appropriate seat. A frequency sweep is also conducted in order to identify any critical frequencies that cause interactions between the components of the AEA. The full altitude profile of the aircraft can be simulated in a decompression chamber and must include rapid decompression (simulating sudden loss of cabin pressure) related to the operational use of the aircraft.

The acceptability of the AEA must be assessed in a range of operationally representative thermal conditions. These tests would normally be conducted in appropriate environmental chambers in which air temperature, humidity, radiant heat load and air movements corresponding to the operational environmental conditions can be produced.

Wear and comfort of the AEA are best assessed by experienced subjects. In the short term, the test is intended to ascertain whether interaction between various components of the AEA, both before and during flight, is sufficient to cause unacceptable discomfort. The test requires full inflation of any pressure garment components and would normally simulate standby and maximum sortie duration. Longer-term assessments of comfort following

repeated donning and doffing of the AEA together with evaluation of wear and tear can be achieved only by flight trials, ideally before authorizing full production; however, if the AEA is required urgently, then careful and detailed monitoring following introduction into service is essential.

FLIGHT TRIALS

In-flight assessment is the final and most crucial phase in the evaluation of AEA. It constitutes the critical verification of satisfactory integration of all items under test in realistic operational environments using experienced aircrew members. The primary objectives of in-flight evaluation are as follows:

- to confirm the characteristics demonstrated during the earlier phases of assessment (laboratory, etc.)
- to verify the essential performance and safety features examined on the ground
- to validate the intrinsic compatibility of each item comprising the assembly and their integration with the aircraft systems and facilities
- to confirm that the AEA enhances and does not diminish aircrew performance and operational effectiveness
- to obtain information from both aircrew and equipment maintenance personnel on the effectiveness, safety, comfort, ease of operation and maintainability of the AEA under test.

The methods adopted for flight evaluation depend on the equipment under test. Thus, assessments can be purely subjective and data recording can be achieved from simple questionnaires. On the other hand, if detailed information regarding the physiological protection afforded by the equipment or other performance measures is required, then appropriate instrumentation and recording facilities will be necessary. When the latter is desired, the data are obtained most conveniently by dedicated flights using an aircraft suitably instrumented for capture of the desired data.

Dedicated flights have the additional advantage of affording repeatability of flight manoeuvres within structured sorties as well as encompassing the unpredictable actions that might arise during combat exercises. Recommendations on some aspects of in-flight test and evaluation are described by Sears et al. (1983).

REFERENCES

ASCC. Methodology for assessing fit of aircrew clothing. ADV PUB 61/105/14. Air Standardization Coordinating Committee, Washington, 1996a.

ASCC. Methodology for integration testing of aircrew clothing and equipment. ADV PUB 61/105/12. Air Standardization Coordinating Committee, Washington, 1996b.

Bolton CB, Kenward M, Simpson RE *et al*. An Anthropometric Survey of 2000 Royal Air Force Aircrew 1970/71. RAF IAM Report 531, Farnborough 1973. FPRC Report 1327. HMSO London 1973.

Ministry of Defence. Specification for integration testing of aircrew equipment assemblies. Specification MAP 34/007. Ministry of Defence, London, 1999.

Sears WJ, Searist GE, Moore AA. *Aircrew Personal Protective Equipment: Test and Evaluation Guide*. Brooks AFB, TX: Aerospace Associates and Technology Incorporated, 1983.

Turner GM. Anthropometric Survey of 2000 Royal Air Force Aircrew, 1970/71 – Comparison of British and American Measuring Techniques. RAF IAM Report 556, Farnborough 1974.

FURTHER READING

Aplin JE. The application of anthropometric survey data to aircrew clothing sizing. Royal Aircraft Establishment technical report 84050, Royal Aircraft Establishment, Farnborough. 1984.

Aplin JE, Nammari H. DRA/AS/MMI report CR95076/1. Anthropometric survey of UK military females, Defence Research Agency, Farnborough, 1995.

Boff KR, Lincoln JE. *Engineering Data Compendium*. New York: John Wiley & Sons, 1987.

DEF STAN 00–970. Design and airworthiness requirements for military aircraft. Ministry of Defence, London, 2003.

Hobbs PC. RAE Technical Report 73137. An Anthropometric Survey of 500 Royal Air Force Heads. Royal Aircraft Establishment, Farnborough, 1972.

Ministry of Defence. Specification no. DTD 1321. Acceptance tests for aircrew helmets. Ministry of Defence, London, 1983.

Turner GM. RAF IAM AEG. Report no. 525. Aircrew size limitations RAF policy and procedures. RAF Institute of Aviation medicine, Farnborough, 1986.

16

Physiology of sleep and wakefulness, sleep disorders, and the effects on aircrew

J. LYNN CALDWELL

INTRODUCTION

Several reports have indicated that pilots and crews frequently experience shortened sleep, reduced sleep efficiency and/or changes in sleep architecture that prevent full recovery from preceding periods of wakefulness (Bisson *et al.* 1993; Boll *et al.* 1992; Dement *et al.* 1986; Neville *et al.* 1994; Nicholson *et al.* 1986; Rosekind *et al.* 1994; Sasaki *et al.* 1986). Needless to say, these sleep troubles often lead to serious problems with on-the-job sleepiness (Akerstedt and Folkard 1995). Anything that disrupts the quality and quantity of restful sleep creates a potential safety hazard on the flight deck. Fatigued pilots suffer from increased lethargy and distractibility, decreased willingness to work cooperatively with other crew members, degraded ability to integrate incoming information, and impaired capacity to make the higher-level cognitive decisions that are often crucial for flight safety (Petrie and Dawson 1997; Ritter 1993).

Once a certain level of sleepiness occurs, pilots begin to experience involuntary micro-sleeps (short involuntary sleep episodes) even during critical periods such as the time span from top-of-descent to landing (Rosekind *et al.* 1994).

Since optimum sleep is necessary to maintain alertness in the flight environment, every effort should be made to ensure that sleep is of the best quality and of sufficient duration. This chapter will address the physiology of sleep and the variables that disturb sleep quality, including medically recognized sleep disorders.

HISTORY OF SLEEP RESEARCH

When German psychiatrist Hans Berger recorded electrical activity in the human brain in 1928, the door opened to the measurement of sleep brain patterns and the science of sleep began. Even after the discovery of rapid-eye-movement (REM) sleep by Eugene Aserinsky and Nathanial Kleitman in the early 1950s, the other non-rapid-eye-movement (NREM) sleep stages were not described fully. Most of the research focused on REM sleep and its cyclical pattern. The idea that REM sleep and non-REM sleep were qualitatively different first developed after many years of research, but the duality of sleep was not established until 1960. Sleep research blossomed in the 1960s and was the precursor of sleep medicine and clinical polysomnography. In 1957 William Dement and Nathanial Kleitman categorized sleep stages solely on the basis of the electroencephalogram (EEG) and electro-oculogram (EOG), but in 1968 criteria were modified to include muscle activity based on research by Michel Jouvet, which showed the importance of muscle atonia in classifying REM sleep. This now-standard sleep-staging system (Rechtschaffen and Kales 1968) officially defined the sleep stages. The formalization of the practice of sleep medicine evolved in the 1970s with the 1979 publication of the Association of Sleep Disorders Centers' (ASDC) *Diagnostic Classification of Sleep and Arousal Disorders* (DCSAD). It is from these decades of research that the knowledge of sleep and sleep disorders has grown.

RECORDING AND CLASSIFYING SLEEP STAGES

To monitor sleep stages it is necessary to first attach a series of electrodes to the scalp according to the international 10–20 system (Jasper 1958). Most researchers and sleep clinicians use one or two central recording sites – C3 and/or C4 – and one or two occipital recording sites – O1 and/or O2. These sites are referenced to the contralateral mastoid or ear lobe to record the EEG. Additionally, the EOG is recorded from two eye-monitoring sites – one at the outer canthus and slightly above the horizontal plane of one eye and one at the outer canthus and slightly below the horizontal plane of the other eye. Both of the EOG electrodes are referenced to either the right or the left mastoid or ear lobe (both eyes are referenced to the same point). Electromyography (EMG) is recorded in a bipolar fashion from two electrodes placed beneath the submentalis muscle underneath the chin. A third electrode can be placed on the chin as a backup in the event that one of the other EMG signals is lost during recording. Of course, more electrodes or transducers are necessary to record respiration, limb muscle activity, etc. for clinical diagnosis of some sleep disorders, but these are not necessary for staging normal human sleep. Figure 16.1 shows the placement sites for the EEG, EOG, and EMG sensors discussed above.

By recording and classifying sleep into specific stages in a standardized way, information collected from many different laboratories can be compared and quantified, and sleep recordings from the same individual, collected at different points in time, can be compared. Through the use of such recordings, it is possible to determine exactly when an individual falls asleep and wakes up, to calculate total sleep time, and to determine changes in sleep quality by examining the different sleep stages as well as the frequency of

disruptions throughout the sleep period. This information can in turn be used to identify impediments to optimal sleep and to evaluate the effectiveness of sleep-promoting strategies that may be useful in operational contexts.

Stages of sleep

NREM AND REM SLEEP

Sleep is separated into two distinct states: NREM and REM. NREM sleep is divided further into four stages that progress from the lightest (stage 1) to the deepest (stage 4). Each of these stages is discussed below.

Awake

When a person is awake and active, the EEG activity is fast and desynchronized. These activated EEG waveforms, characterized by oscillations of 12 or more cycles per second, are called beta activity. When a person closes his or her eyes and relaxes, the EEG activity changes to a pattern of activity ranging between 8 and 12 cycles per second called alpha-activity. Alpha activity is more uniform and synchronous than beta activity. Usually, when a person relaxes with the eyes closed, the eyes become relatively still and overall muscle tension is reduced. However, a relaxed person is not necessarily asleep, and the patterns observed in the EEG, EOG and EMG reflect this. Figure 16.2 shows the EEG, EOG and EMG patterns that normally occur when a person is relaxed but awake with the eyes closed. This recording is more than 50 per cent alpha activity; EMG is high and EOG is relatively inactive.

Stage 1 sleep

When sleep onset begins to occur, the brain activity slows even more than it did under conditions of relaxation. This slower EEG pattern, called theta activity, is characterized by waveforms that oscillate at about four to eight cycles per second. When the EEG recording contains a combination of alpha and theta activity, with the majority of the activity in the theta range, the epoch is labelled stage 1 sleep. The EOG pattern shows slow movements as the eyes roll from side to side in a pendulum fashion. However, muscle activity remains similar in magnitude to that under conditions of relaxation (indicating the continued presence of muscle tone), even as the EEG and EOG features suggest sleep onset. Figure 16.3 shows the EEG, EOG and EMG patterns typical for stage 1 sleep.

Stage 1 sleep is the transition between wakefulness and sleep. During this stage, the sleeper may still be aware of activity in the surrounding environment. Conversations might still be heard, even though the eyes are closed and the brain is transitioning into sleep. A person who is awakened from this very light stage of sleep might not even remember being asleep, which is part of the reason why sleepiness can be hazardous in the operational environ-

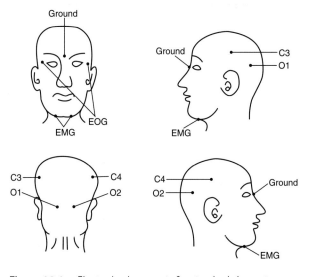

Figure 16.1 *Electrode placements for standard sleep-stage recordings.*

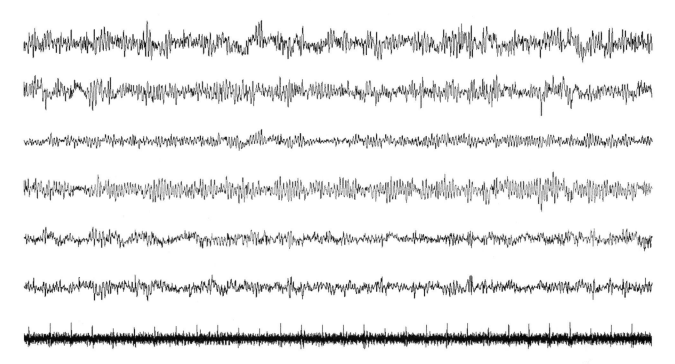

Figure 16.2 *Electroencephalogram (EEG), electro-oculogram (EOG) and electromyogram (EMG) activity during wakefulness. The figure represents a 30-second epoch of data, which equates to one page of a written polysomnograph record. A 20-second epoch is also used in some sleep laboratories. When scoring an entire episode of sleep, each epoch of the record is staged to evaluate sleep quantity and quality. Diagram is C3/A2, C4/A1, O1/A2, O2/A1, EOG-L, EOG-R, and EMG. The figure represents a 30-second epoch of data.*

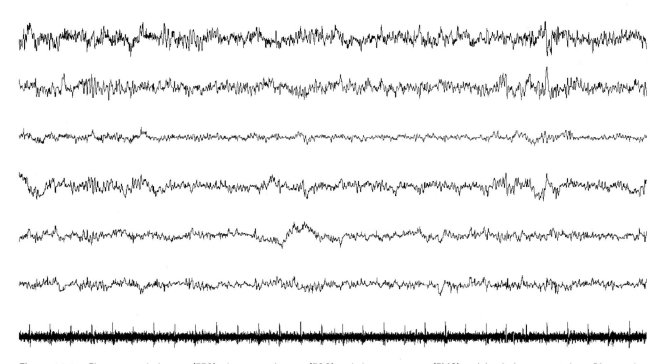

Figure 16.3 *Electroencephalogram (EEG), electro-oculogram (EOG) and electromyogram (EMG) activity during stage 1 sleep. Diagram is C3/A2, C4/A1, O1/A2, O2/A1, EOG-L, EOG-R, and EMG. The figure represents a 30-second epoch of data.*

ment. People who 'nod off' during a meeting, while watching TV or even while driving or flying are usually in stage 1 sleep. When evidence of stage 1 sleep is observed in a person who is supposed to be awake, it is often referred to as a micro-sleep or a micro-lapse (Dinges *et al.* 1987; Harrison and Horne 1996; Porcu *et al.* 1998). While relaxing at home, these short lapses are of little or no concern, but on-the-job micro-sleeps can be very dangerous. Obviously, falling asleep while flying an aircraft, even for a few seconds, can cause a pilot to miss navigational checkpoints, warning indications or hazards to safe flight. Disturbingly, micro-sleeps often occur involuntarily, even in people who are trying to stay awake; upon awakening from a micro-sleep, there often is no recognition that a sleep episode has occurred.

Stage 2 sleep

During a normal night-time sleep period, stage 1 sleep lasts about five minutes before sleep progresses to the deeper stage 2. From an electrophysiological standpoint, this stage of sleep is characterized by unique EEG waveforms called k-complexes and sleep spindles. Most researchers and clinicians believe that the occurrence of stage 2 (rather than stage 1) sleep is actually the true onset of sleep (Carskadon and Dement 2000). During stage 2 sleep, generally the eyes are still, but they may show some movement. The muscles are somewhat relaxed but still taut. The major change between stage 1 and stage 2 sleep is found in the EEG tracing. An example of stage 2 sleep is shown in Figure 16.4; notice the sleep spindle and k-complex in the middle of the recording.

Stages 3 and 4 sleep

In normal night-time sleep, stage 2 lasts about 10–20 minutes as sleep becomes deeper and the brain activity slows even more. As time progresses, these deeper stages of sleep are signalled by the appearance of slow high-amplitude delta-waves, which have a frequency of between 0.5 and two cycles per second and an amplitude of at least 75 µV. Together, stages 3 and 4 constitute slow-wave sleep (SWS), also called delta-sleep, because the brain's patterns consist mostly of delta activity, as can be seen in Figure 16.5. Stage 3 sleep is separated from stage 4 sleep by the amount of delta activity in the sleep epoch. When more than 50 per cent of the epoch is composed of delta-activity, the epoch is considered to be stage 4 sleep. When the epoch consists of only 30–49 per cent delta activity, it is considered to be stage 3 sleep. From a behavioural standpoint, it is much more difficult to awaken someone from SWS than from either stage 1 or stage 2 sleep. Furthermore, once someone is awakened from SWS, they tend to be very groggy, and it may take several minutes for them to overcome this sleep inertia.[1] Note that in Figure 16.5, the eyes are still relatively inactive and the muscles are still taut but a little more relaxed than they were in the lighter sleep stages.

[1]Sleep inertia is always a consideration when using strategic naps to sustain performance in operational contexts. Although the degree of sleep inertia appears to depend partially on the previous amount of sleep deprivation and the time of day at which sleep occurs, the primary factor is the depth of sleep obtained immediately before waking up. This is why some experts recommend only short naps, since this often minimizes the transition to SWS. However, a better approach is to let the crew sleep for as long as possible and to provide a 30-minute 'wakeup buffer'.

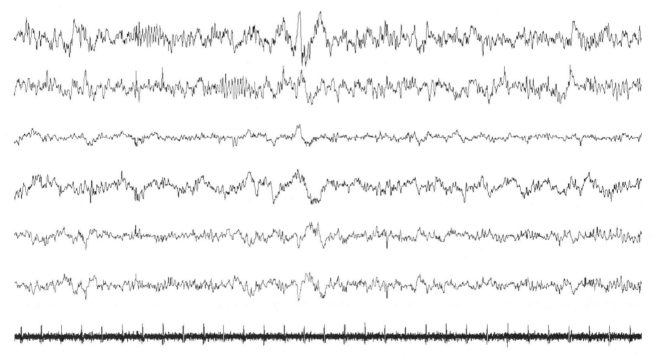

Figure 16.4 *Electroencephalogram (EEG), electro-oculogram (EOG) and electromyogram (EMG) activity during stage 2 sleep. Diagram is C3/A2, C4/A1, O1/A2, O2/A1, EOG-L, EOG-R, and EMG. The figure represents a 30-second epoch of data.*

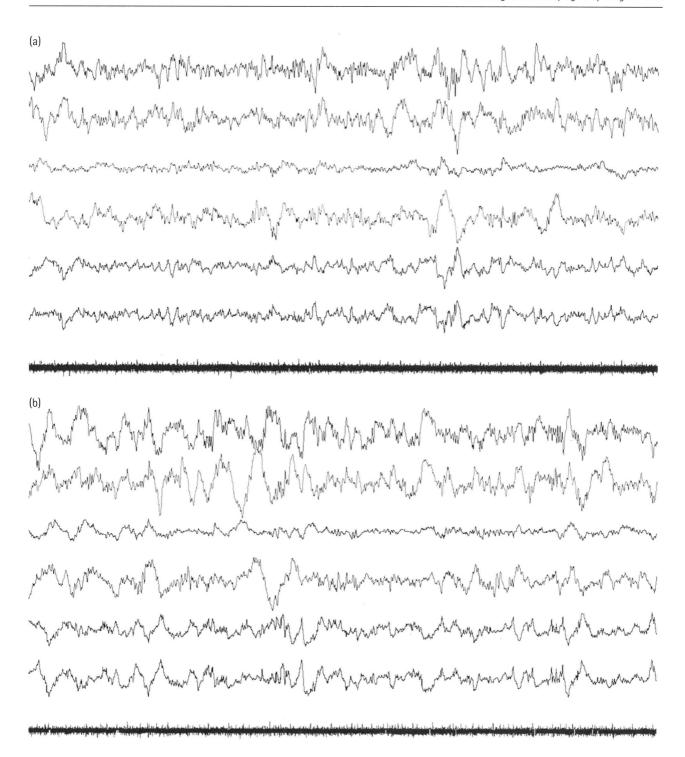

Figure 16.5 *Electroencephalogram (EEG), electro-oculogram (EOG) and electromyogram (EMG) activity during stage 3 (a) and stage 4 (b) sleep. Diagram is C3/A2, C4/A1, O1/A2, O2/A1, EOG-L, EOG-R, and EMG. The figure represents a 30-second epoch of data.*

REM sleep

After spending about 30 minutes in SWS, brain activity begins to become more active as a transition is made back into stage 2 sleep for several minutes. The next progression of sleep is into REM sleep. During REM sleep, the eyes move rapidly from side to side, usually in bursts, as shown in the EOG tracing in Figure 16.6. In addition to the quick eye movements, the EEG is characterized by higher-frequency low-voltage desynchronous activity. A novice looking at a polysomnographic representation of REM sleep could mistake it as being indicative of wakefulness, which is why some authors refer to REM sleep as 'paradoxical sleep'. Another factor that classifies this period of sleep as REM is the relative lack of muscle tone.

There are four to six episodes of REM sleep during each eight-hour sleep period. The first REM period is very short, but the length of each REM period increases as the sleep episode progresses. REM sleep is when most dreaming occurs, as evidenced by the fact that dreams are reported about 80 per cent of the time when subjects are awakened from REM sleep but only eight per cent of the time after subjects are awakened from non-REM stages of sleep (Pivik 2000). Since REM periods tend to occupy more of the sleep architecture just before awakening, many people awake from the night out of REM sleep and, as a result, can remember the dream that was occurring just before waking.

Distribution of stages throughout a period of sleep

The progression of sleep through the stages identified above occurs predictably during the night. Sleep begins in stage 1 and then progresses to stages 2, 3 and 4, before returning back to stage 2 and then to REM. This pattern of activity recurs in approximately 90-minute cycles. SWS dominates the first half of the night, while REM sleep dominates the second half. Throughout the night, brief transitions to stage 1 sleep and/or brief awakenings are often observed. The progression of sleep stages over an eight-hour sleep period is shown in Figure 16.7.

WHAT AFFECTS SLEEP ARCHITECTURE?

The average amount of sleep needed by most adults is eight hours (Drake *et al.* 2001). However, a small percentage of people need less sleep than this and are able to function normally with only five or six hours of sleep a night. There also are some people who require more than the average person, requiring as much as nine or ten hours of sleep to feel fully rested and alert during the day. While the need to sleep for more than eight hours a day may be inconvenient, it is not a pathology and should not be considered as such.

Regardless of the length of the individual's sleep requirements, sleep structure can be affected by a number of factors, including age, time awake, time of day, environmental characteristics, medications and sleep disorders. These factors can influence the overall structure of sleep, and many exert a noticeable subjective affect on the quality of sleep.

Age

Age affects the sleep cycle (Bliwise 1993; Van Cauter *et al.* 2000). Infants sleep much longer than adults; children and adolescents require less sleep than infants but more sleep than adults. Most of an infant's sleep time is spent in REM sleep. The amount of SWS increases with age until adulthood. Around the third decade of life, the amount of SWS begins to decline until around age 60–70, when almost all

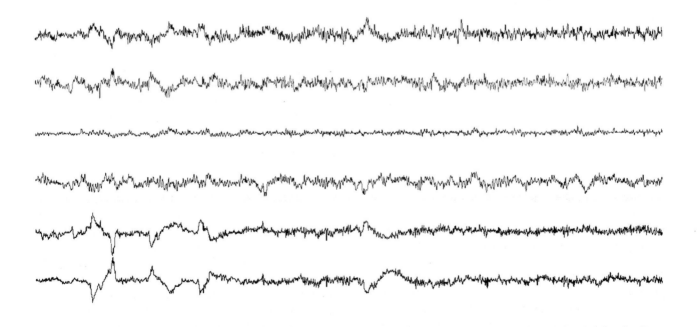

Figure 16.6 *Electroencephalogram (EEG), electro-oculogram (EOG) and electromyogram (EMG) activity during rapid-eye-movement (REM) sleep. Diagram is C3/A2, C4/A1, O1/A2, O2/A1, EOG-L, EOG-R, and EMG. The figure represents a 30-second epoch of data.*

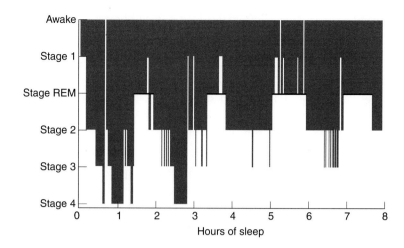

Figure 16.7 *Hypnogram of an eight-hour sleep period in a normal young adult.*

SWS is gone. Frequent night-time awakenings are more common in older people. Since the sleep of older individuals is no longer deep, noises occurring during the night and other disruptive factors such as light and caffeine are more likely to disturb sleep than when the person was younger.

Sleep deprivation

When job requirements entail sleep loss because of extended duty periods, the sleep that occurs in the first rest opportunity often contains significantly more slow-wave activity throughout the night, while REM sleep is pushed either much later in the sleep episode or sometimes even into the next night of sleep (Borbely 1982; Carskadon and Dement 2000). The brain shows a preference for recovering SWS first and REM sleep afterwards, which has led some scientists to believe that SWS probably conveys a greater survival advantage than REM sleep (Sejnowski and Destexhe 2000). However, the exact roles of the different stages of sleep have not been determined precisely (Nicolau *et al.* 2000).

The extent of changes in sleep characteristics will depend in part on how long the person has been awake before recovery sleep occurs. Typically, a subject enters SWS much faster than normal after periods of prolonged wakefulness. This type of change in sleep architecture is important to note in situations in which a sleep episode occurs immediately before the onset of work, such as when strategic napping is used as a countermeasure against workplace fatigue. As noted earlier, sleep inertia will be greater when a subject is awakened from SWS than from a lighter stage of sleep (Balkin and Badia 1988; Borbely 1982; Naitoh *et al.* 1992). If a previously sleep-deprived pilot is taking a nap before resuming duties at the controls, then it is important to remember that the nap probably contains a higher than normal amount of SWS, and extra time

should be allotted in order for sleep inertia to dissipate before resuming command of the aircraft.

Timing and duration of sleep

The time at which a subject sleeps can affect the structure of the sleep cycle. With night-time sleep, the preponderance of REM sleep generally occurs later in the sleep period and most of the SWS occurs at the beginning of the night. When sleep onset is delayed until the early morning, when the temperature rhythm is at its nadir, most of the REM activity usually occurs in the first part of the sleep period, while SWS shifts to the second half of the sleep cycle (Czeisler *et al.* 1980a,b). Shift workers who change from night sleep to day sleep may show this reversed sleep pattern on the first few days before their circadian cycle adjusts to the new schedule. Such a change can noticeably affect the restorative quality of sleep during the transitional period, particularly if the sleep period is truncated.

In situations in which the majority of sleep occurs in the form of napping, there are characteristic effects on sleep architecture that should be borne in mind. Naps that are placed early in a period of sustained operations (prophylactic naps) will differ markedly from those occurring after lengthy periods of sleep deprivation (recovery naps). Earlier-placed naps tend to contain more of the lighter stages of sleep, whereas later-placed naps will likely contain significantly more SWS, largely because of differences in the levels of the homeostatic sleep drive. Both types of nap are helpful for improving subsequent performance, but recovery naps should be longer than prophylactic naps in order to derive the same performance benefit (Gillberg 1984; Haslam 1985; Nicholson *et al.* 1985). The quality of a nap also will be affected by the time of day at which the napping occurs. Sleep tendency is highest when core body temperature is in its trough (early morning hours) and lowest when core body temperature is at its peak (early evening hours). Thus, there may be significant problems initiating and/or maintaining a nap during times when core temperature is high, a period that has been termed the 'forbidden zone' for sleep (Lavie 1986). Naps are easier to maintain if taken at times when body temperature is low, and they will likely bestow a greater benefit on later performance. However, sleep inertia is highest following these naps, because the sleep is deeper. Naps taken at any time of day (during circadian peaks or troughs) will improve performance measured later in the day in comparison with having no sleep at all, but naps taken in the temperature trough will produce the most benefit (Carskadon and Dement 1982; Dinges et al. 1985; Dinges 1986; Lavie 1986) and will likely contain more restorative sleep than naps taken at other times.

Environment

Environmental factors are a common cause of sleep difficulties. An unfamiliar environment, noise, light, heat and cold will interfere with sleep, as will a bed that is either too hard or too soft, a pillow that does not support the head and neck properly, or a sleep partner, bunk mate or room mate who is restless, snores or otherwise disturbs the tranquillity of the sleep setting. Deployed military pilots are especially susceptible to the adverse effects of a poor sleep environment. Sharing a tent with several other people, and trying to sleep in a cot, in the desert, in the middle of the day, while listening to the sounds of aircraft departing and landing, trucks driving through the area, and people talking as they walk from one place to another, can thwart even the best efforts to sleep before the next duty cycle.

In some situations, aircrew are given space and opportunity to nap on board the aircraft during certain portions of the flight. While this strategy to combat fatigue is very helpful, one must remember that the sleep that occurs in the aircraft is not the same quality as the sleep that occurs at home in a comfortable bed. With regard to the on-board bunk sleep of long-haul pilots, Rosekind et al. (2000) reported that 71 per cent of pilots who identified themselves as 'good home sleepers' reported difficulty with sleeping in the aircraft bunk 'often' or 'the majority of the time'. Five areas were identified that interfered with sleep: environmental disturbance (e.g. background noise, turbulence), luminosity (e.g. lighting), personal disturbances (e.g. bathroom trips, random thoughts), environmental discomfort (e.g. low humidity, cold) and interpersonal disturbances (e.g. bunk partner). Pilots attempting to sleep on board an aircraft in a regular reclining passenger seat cannot obtain the same level of sleep quality that is possible when lying flat. Nicholson and Stone (1987) found that subjects experienced reductions in total sleep time, decreased sleep efficiency and increased awakenings when they attempted to sleep in a more upright sitting position

(17.5 degrees from the vertical angle) compared with either lying flat or reclining at 49.5 or 37 degrees. Similar results were reported by Aeschbach et al. (1994), who discovered that subjects who slept in reclining chairs rather than lying flat in bed experienced reduced sleep efficiency, less REM sleep and increased stage 1 sleep. The section below on insomnia discusses the impact of environmental effects on sleep along with some potential solutions.

Medications and herbal remedies

Medications or herbal substances can change the sleep cycle. Although pilots generally do not use many prescription drugs, it is worthwhile for the flight surgeon/physician/aeromedical examiner (AME) to note which medications affect sleep. Some medications inhibit the amount of SWS or REM sleep, some interfere with the ability to go to sleep or to stay asleep, and others lead to excessive sleepiness. It is necessary not only to consider the effects of prescription medications but also to warn aircrew of the effects of over-the-counter (OTC) medications, since many of these can affect sleep and alertness. Several OTC pain/headache remedies contain caffeine, some as much as 65 mg per tablet; a subject taking a recommended dose of two tablets will thus consume sufficient caffeine to interfere with sleep onset and sleep maintenance (Boutrel and Koob 2004). Many OTC cold medications contain pseudoephedrine, another central nervous system stimulant that can lead to sleep difficulties.

Due to the popularity of herbal supplements, it is worth knowing which of these alter sleep and alertness. The major alerting herbal agents that may affect sleep adversely include ephedra, ma huang, Indian sida, bitter orange, yohimbe and ginseng. In addition to these herbs, many tea and green tea beverages contain caffeine, which may disrupt sleep in some individuals. Herbs that have been shown to possess sleep-inducing properties include valerian, kava and lavender. For a comprehensive review of the efficacy and safety of these and a variety of other herbal stimulants and sedatives, see Gyllenhaal et al. (2000).

INSOMNIA

Clearly, there are a number of factors that can impact the content or characteristics of sleep episodes. However, pilots (and others) also may suffer from some type of insomnia, which will severely limit sleep duration. There is no specific objective definition of insomnia such as defines other sleep disorders (Sateia 2002). However, generally insomnia is defined as the inability to initiate sleep and/or to maintain sleep throughout the night. The diagnosis of insomnia is made by acquiring a medical history and discussing life events and sleep patterns. It is important that the flight surgeon/physician/sleep specialist rules out respiratory disorders, including sleep apnoea and neurological disorders, some of which are discussed later in this chapter. Some of the reasons for insomnia may be identified quickly and thereby rectified once the specific circumstances under which the sleep problems occur are discovered. However, if physiological causes are ruled out, then the underlying cause of the insomnia sometimes is not easy to identify and treat. As detailed below, there are many common possibilities that must be considered. Especially within the aviation arena, stress, environmental factors and circadian factors should be explored when insomnia occurs in an otherwise normal healthy individual. Aircrew members, who are, by definition, in positions of responsibility and who find themselves often taken away from home and/or away from standard work schedules, can easily relate to difficulties in all three of these areas. Once the source of the problem is clear, a specific treatment option can be identified and implemented.

Transient insomnia

Insomnia occurs in most people at some time or another. If the problem occurs regularly, i.e. for more than three weeks, then it falls into the category of chronic insomnia; if the problem is short-term, then it is classified as transient insomnia. Both types of insomnia often are symptomatic of another problem, such as stress, anxiety, apprehension, pain or new surroundings (Hauri 1993). In addition, short-term insomnia can be caused by environmental factors and circadian disruptions (Gander et al. 1998; Gander and Graeber 1987). People with insomnia usually seek treatment either because of their frustration over the inability to take advantage of sleep opportunities or because their sleep problems are impairing alertness during waking hours. In the aviation context, numerous factors can cause frequent short-term bouts of insomnia, especially since frequent shift changes, long duty hours and rapid time-zone transitions are commonplace (Rosekind et al. 1994, 2000; Gander et al. 1998; Nicholson 1987). Flight surgeons and other physicians should work with pilots and crew members to help resolve mild to moderate cases of insomnia or other sleep difficulties before these disturbances threaten operational readiness.

INSOMNIA DUE TO STRESS

Everyone lives with stress to some extent on a daily basis, but pilots seem to be facing an escalation in job-related stress due to, for example, work pressures and downsizing. Although the sources of stress can be either negative (tight deadlines, long work hours, expanded responsibilities) or positive (increased pay or rank, desirable transitions into larger or faster aircraft), stressful events can temporarily disrupt sleep, until either the source of the stress is removed or the individual has learned to deal adaptively with the stressful situation. If sleep suddenly becomes difficult for no apparent reason, then a psychological stressor may be the underlying source.

Treating insomnia due to stress

To prevent this temporary problem becoming chronic, the individual should try to alleviate the source of the stress, or their negative reaction to the stress, as early as possible. The crew member should be advised to take stock of the current situation and implement one of many strategies designed to cope with psychological stress. A plethora of advice is available on how to overcome worry and transient anxiety, and some techniques are immediately effective for minimizing the impact of stress on sleep. For instance, progressive relaxation exercises (systematically tensing and relaxing the body's muscle groups) have been proven to be very effective for dealing with temporary anxiety or psychological pressure, because these quick and easy self-help strategies bring the body's natural relaxation response under more voluntary control (Lushington and Lack 2002; Smith and Neubauer 2003). In addition, the act of focusing on producing a relaxation response may be all that is necessary to divert attention away from an anxiety-provoking situation towards a sleep-conducive state long enough to fall asleep. This may sound overly simplistic, but it is true that people can consciously identify and cope with a previously unrecognized problem once they focus energy in this direction. In the meantime, and at a minimum, it would be worthwhile to engage in some type of aerobic exercise three to four hours before bedtime, because this has been shown to improve the onset and quality of sleep later on (Youngstedt 2003). If psychological stress is producing transient sleeping problems, then self-help techniques, relaxation exercises, aerobic exercise or some other stress-management strategy may offer a solution.

INSOMNIA DUE TO ENVIRONMENTAL CHANGE

Environmental factors are a common cause of transient insomnia. As discussed earlier, a pilot may have particular difficulty in sleeping in constantly changing environments. This is in part why Comperatore et al. (1996) have recommended a systematic approach to planning crew rest that includes daylight management, environmental management and living-quarters planning, as well as coordination of scheduled events such as meetings, meals and flight schedules, in such a way as to minimize the impact on available sleep opportunities.

Treating insomnia due to environmental factors

Treatment of insomnia due to environmental factors usually involves alleviation of the noise, light, etc. that is interfering with sleep. If the environmental problems are temporary, such as is often the case in aviation with a short layover, then a hypnotic may be prescribed to induce sleep despite conflicting factors. However, when this strategy is used for pilots, it should be kept in mind that there are post-drug grounding times designed to avoid subsequent impairments in on-the-job alertness. For example, current US Air Force (USAF) policy specifies a post-drug grounding time of 12 hours for temazepam, six hours for zolpidem and four hours for zaleplon (Department of the Air Force 2001). For civilian pilots, the US Federal Aviation Administration does not permit the use of temazepam or zaleplon; however, it does specify that zolpidem may be used (maximum twice a week) as long as the pilot waits 24 hours before resuming flight duties (Silberman 2003). As noted in Chapter 52, sleep-promoting medications can be a very beneficial short-term method for enhancing sleep quality and, as a result, enhancing subsequent alertness and performance.

As well as the use of a pharmacological approach, sleep difficulties associated with new environments also can be overcome with behavioural types of intervention. Sometimes, adjustment to a new environment can be facilitated simply by making the new setting more familiar. Bringing along a comfortable pillow, a family picture or minor convenience items that might not be available in a typical hotel room or temporary military quarters can make the situation more comfortable and, therefore, more sleep-conducive. Improving the environment itself (lighting, temperature, etc.) is also an option. Although this is difficult in military field settings and in-flight environments, the use of sleep masks can block light, foam ear plugs can attenuate noise, and cooperative agreements with tent/bunk/room mates can minimize the disruptive effects of conversation and other disturbing activities in the sleeping quarters. In hotel rooms, and often in on-board in-flight bunks, environmental control is somewhat easier than it is in the field.

INSOMNIA DUE TO CIRCADIAN DISRUPTIONS

Another source of short-term insomnia is related to the sleep schedule. Shift workers often have a very difficult time maintaining sleep due to the timing of their sleep opportunities. Work/rest cycles that vary frequently often are associated with sleep difficulties because the body cannot establish a consistent routine (Akerstedt 1988, 2003; Costa 1997). In addition, travelling across multiple time zones can produce sleep difficulties similar to those experienced by shift workers (Stone and Turner 1997; Waterhouse et al. 1997; Waterhouse 1999). Long-haul pilots are constantly confronted with disagreements between their circadian rhythms and the environmental cues present at their destination. Military pilots likewise must face these problems when they are deployed across multiple time zones, especially when travelling in an east-

erly direction. A pilot working a normal daytime schedule in London may be in the habit of waking up early in the morning and going to sleep at 22:00 or 23:00 each night; such a schedule means that the time span from approximately 17:00 to 21:00 will be associated with a high degree of alertness. This is fine in the UK. However, when pilots travel from London to Tokyo, they cross eight time zones in less than a day, and when they attempt to stick to the 23:00 local bedtime in Tokyo, they are actually trying to initiate sleep at 15:00 according to the body's internal clock. In addition to the problem of getting to sleep, there is also the problem of waking up at a time that is eight hours before the usual body-clock wakeup time. In this example, the Tokyo wakeup time of 07:00 is only 01:00 according to the body's clock.

Treating insomnia due to circadian disruptions

Insomnia due to circadian disruption is difficult to manage, particularly in aviation settings. The body cannot adjust quickly to changes in schedules, and sleep is generally one of the casualties of a new schedule. In some situations, hypnotics may be prescribed in the short term. However, implementation of behavioural countermeasures also represents a successful alternative. The application of countermeasures depends in part on the length of time that the person will be in the new time zone or on the new work schedule. Generally, it will be necessary to combine several strategies to promote optimal adjustment. For instance, a traveller might be advised to use a hypnotic during the early part of a departure flight to promote sleep (only useful for non-pilots), caffeine during the later part of the flight and/or after arrival at the destination to sustain wakefulness (pilots and non-pilots), varying degrees of sunlight exposure to help shift the body's rhythms (pilots and non-pilots), and rapid adjustment to new meal/activity times to facilitate more effective time-zone adaptations (pilots and non-pilots). For the first few days in the new time zone, it may be necessary to continue the use of either a short-acting or a long-acting sleep medication (depending on the direction of the travel and the number of time zones crossed) to promote night-time sleep. Many of these strategies are covered in Chapter 52.

FLIGHT STATUS AND INSOMNIA

There are no specific criteria under which insomnia will impact the ability to secure and maintain flight status. Many cases are relatively mild and therefore have an inconsequential effect on routine alertness levels. Also, even when transient insomnia is more severe, the short duration of the sleep difficulty is unlikely to result in any chronic impairment. However, it should be remembered that any degree of sleep loss translates into some decrement in alertness later on. Because of this, countermeasures for sleep difficulties, shift lag and jet lag should be implemented.

Chronic insomnia

Chronic insomnia is a sleep disturbance that lasts for more than three weeks. It is much more difficult to treat than transient insomnia, due to the various reasons for its occurrence. Sometimes, the sufferer has developed habits that are not conducive to sleep or is taking a medication that interferes with sleep. If the problem is as simple as this, then the insomnia can be treated fairly successfully. However, if the insomnia results from a less identifiable cause, then a more complex solution may be needed. Regardless of the source, chronic insomnia is a serious condition due to its adverse effects on health and safety.

TREATMENT OF CHRONIC INSOMNIA

Pilots who experience chronic insomnia may be treated successfully with behavioural interventions (Manber and Kuo 2002). Relaxation techniques may be helpful in some situations; stimulus control therapy is helpful in those people in whom poor habits interfere with sleep. In some cases, sleep-restriction therapy is successful in breaking the insomnia cycle. Sleep restriction works by increasing the homeostatic sleep pressure by limiting time spent in bed until the effects of sleep deprivation accumulate to the point that sleep efficiency improves. Cognitive-behavioural therapy is used widely to treat insomnia successfully, combining behavioural treatments with cognitive therapy to educate the patient and resolve dysfunctional thought processes that lead to insomnia. Generally, cognitive and behavioural therapies require several treatment sessions to overcome the problem behaviours or thoughts. In addition, chronic insomnia due to environmental factors often can be rectified by modifying the characteristics of the sleep setting. Chronic insomnia due to circadian factors can be corrected without medication, although it is difficult to eliminate the adverse effects of constant schedule changes in transcontinental pilots or frequently deployed military aviators. Chronic sleep disturbances often can be corrected without affecting fitness for full flying duty. Once the physician or sleep specialist has ruled out the possibility of a sleep disorder, then persistence and time on the part of the physician and the patient are required to work through the behavioural interventions that will break bad sleep hygiene habits and alleviate the insomnia.

FLIGHT STATUS AND INSOMNIA

As with transient insomnia, there are no specific criteria under which chronic insomnia will impact the ability to secure and maintain flight status. Although chronic sleep loss will seriously impair on-the-job alertness/performance, it is true that many individuals seem to continue functioning at some marginal level despite the problem. Nevertheless, it is desirable to treat such sleep difficulties, because the daytime sleepiness associated with night-time sleep restriction represents a serious threat to flight safety. The strategies outlined above should be effective in most cases.

SLEEP DISORDERS

It is important to recognize that some alertness difficulties are a function of medically recognized sleep disorders rather than more controllable factors such as the environmental conditions and medications mentioned above. Sleep disorders can impair alertness because of their interference with the sleep cycle, either by causing frequent awakenings or by disrupting the phases of sleep (Aldrich 2000; Bonnet and Arand 2003). The *International Classification of Sleep Disorders* (ICSD), first published in 1990 by the joint efforts of the European Sleep Research Society, the Japanese Society of Sleep Research and the Latin American Sleep Society, was developed for diagnostic and epidemiological purposes (Thorpy 2000). There are 84 sleep disorders described in the text; these disorders are classified into four major categories:

- *Dysomnias:* disorders of initiating or maintaining sleep and disorders of excessive daytime sleepiness.
- *Parasomnias:* disorders that are characterized by problems that occur during sleep, but do not lead to insomnia or excessive sleepiness.
- Other sleep-disrupting disorders associated with medical or psychiatric problems.
- *Proposed sleep disorders:* sleep-related disorders that are understood too poorly to be classified.

Of these sleep disorders, only dysomnias will be discussed here.

As with any disorder, the first step in treating it is to diagnose it correctly. Proper diagnosis of a sleep disorder occurs after the sleep specialist/physician interviews the patient for medical and family history review, conducts a thorough physical examination, and usually studies an overnight sleep record from the sleep laboratory. The overnight stay in a sleep laboratory involves a polysomnography, in which the EEG, ECG, EMG, respiration, limb and muscle movements, and oxygen saturation are monitored while the patient sleeps. Following documentation of the magnitude of the problem, treatment options can be investigated. In many cases, an interview with the patient's partner may be highly informative, since he or she may be aware of the behaviours that occur while the patient is sleeping.

Once the sleep specialist determines that a sleep disorder is present, and once the exact nature of the disorder is known, proper treatment can begin. Although the prevalence of sleep disorders is likely to be small in young, healthy and physically fit aviators, they can be a problem for a small percentage of the pilot population. When working with pilots, it is important to note that some of these disorders can be treated successfully in a way that does not affect flying status. A few of the most common sleep disorders along with their treatments are discussed here.

Sleep apnoea

The diagnosis of obstructive sleep apnoea syndrome (OSAS) is defined by repetitive apnoeas (cessation of breathing) during sleep, each of which last at least ten seconds (Butkov 2002). The sleep of a normal person contains as many as five short sleep apnoeas per hour (the apnoea index), generally without any residual effects on health or daytime alertness. However, if the apnoea index increases to as many as 20 or more per hour, if an individual apnoea event lasts for many seconds, or if the oxygen desaturation falls significantly, then both health and daytime alertness will subsequently suffer. Apnoea events cause sleep disruptions because the oxygen-deprived sleeper usually reacts to the lack of oxygen with a jerk, which precipitates an awakening or a shift into a lighter sleep stage. As these events occur throughout the night, sleep becomes fragmented and non-restorative. The severity of the symptoms is linked to the severity of the apnoea. A person with severe sleep apnoea can stop breathing more than 100 times an hour, with episodes lasting 60 seconds or more. A person with minor sleep apnoea may stop breathing ten times an hour, with each episode lasting only a few seconds.

People with sleep apnoea often do not awaken fully every time they experience an apnoea event, so they may not complain of a 'sleep problem'. However, they sometimes will complain of restless sleep, and usually they complain of excessive daytime sleepiness, headaches in the morning, depressed mood or personality change, possibly impotence, inability to control the bladder and/or a decline in mental performance. Their partners may complain of loud snoring, which often ends in a snort and awakening (or partial awakening) from sleep. Many people with apnoea are overweight, and the incidence of apnoea increases with age. Sleep apnoea is more common in men than women. A random sample of 602 people in Wisconsin, USA, studied by overnight polysomnography indicated a prevalence of sleep-disordered breathing in two per cent of women and four per cent of men (Young *et al.* 1993). A telephone study conducted in the UK (with no examinations or sleep recordings) indicated a similar prevalence of up to 4.6 per cent in males and 2.2 per cent in females (Ohayon *et al.* 1997). Untreated apnoea that worsens progressively over time can lead to serious health problems, such as high blood pressure, stroke and increased risk of accidents due to increased sleepiness. Treatment of apnoea can significantly mitigate these associated problems.

Identification/diagnosis of sleep apnoea usually begins with complaints from the person's partner about loud snoring, which prompts the sufferer to seek treatment. Following the person's visit to a sleep laboratory, the physician or sleep specialist determines from the polysomnographic record the magnitude of the problem and investigates various treatment options.

TREATMENT OF SLEEP APNOEA

Sleep apnoea can be treated in a number of ways, depending on the severity of the problem, the physical construction of the nose and throat, and the weight of the patient. The most successful treatment is through continuous positive airway pressure (CPAP). This consists of a small mask that fits over the patient's nose and mouth and is linked to a small air pump. The pump sends air through the mask and acts as a splint to the airways, holding the airway open during inspiration. Prevention of airway collapse alleviates snoring as well as the apnoeas, which leads to less disrupted sleep during the night. As sleep becomes less fragmented, daytime sleepiness diminishes, the heart and brain have a continuous flow of oxygen, and the patient's mood and personality return to normal. Compliance is usually the biggest problem with CPAP success. A proper-fitting mask and appropriate air pressure are essential to the comfort of the device, both of which will encourage compliance.

Another mechanical treatment option for sleep apnoea is a dental appliance that can be fitted by a qualified dentist. The appliance modifies the position of the mandible, allowing better airflow in some cases.

Other treatments for sleep apnoea include surgery on the upper airway, which can be as minor as removal of the tonsils and adenoids, straightening of the nasal areas or uvulopalatopharyngoplasty (UPPP) or as major as reconstruction of the jaw and tongue. Usually, any surgical treatments involve a series of operations, each of which is followed by a re-evaluation designed to determine the extent of the improvement after each treatment. The success of any of the procedures varies depending on the type, size and location of the obstruction.

Another treatment for some apnoea patients is weight loss. Overweight people have additional fatty tissue surrounding the airways, which can obstruct proper breathing. In some situations, weight loss can resolve the problem entirely. Often, when overweight sufferers of sleep apnoea are placed on CPAP, they reap a secondary gain in terms of weight loss once their improved energy leads to increased physical activity. Many people can lose enough weight so that CPAP is no longer needed or the pressure required to keep the airways open can be decreased, making the CPAP more comfortable.

There are three different types of sleep apnoea. The most common is the obstructive sleep apnoea described above. This derives its name from the fact that the breathing difficulties result from a physical airway obstruction. The person exerts the effort to breathe, but inadequate air gets through. Another type of sleep apnoea is central sleep apnoea. This occurs when the signals from the respiratory control centres of the brain fail to evoke stimulation of the peripheral respiratory system, and the patient does not breathe for several seconds. In contrast to obstructive sleep apnoea, patients with central apnoea fail to exert any effort to breathe. The problems associated with this type apnoea are the same as for obstructive apnoea – including poor sleep and excessive daytime sleepiness. The treatment is usually either CPAP or medication. Sometimes, central sleep apnoea is associated with other medical disorders, such as congestive heart failure, cerebrovascular disease and some endocrine disorders; when these disorders are treated, the central apnoea often improves. The third type of sleep apnoea is mixed, i.e. a combination of obstructive and central apnoea. Treatment for this type of apnoea usually focuses on the obstructive part of the apnoea, which, when treated, also may lessen the central apnoeas. In some cases, a patient suspected of sleep apnoea but who does not show apnoeas on the polysomnogram is diagnosed with upper-airway resistance syndrome. The symptom of daytime sleepiness is due to the increased breathing effort during the night, which creates brief arousals from sleep. When this diagnosis is made, CPAP is a good treatment choice.

FLIGHT STATUS AND SLEEP APNOEA

In military aviation, a pilot diagnosed with sleep apnoea often cannot continue their flying career if the apnoea is treated with CPAP. However, successful treatment via surgery or weight loss typically can be waived. If CPAP is required, the pilot may not be deployable if their health and alertness depend on the use of an electrically powered CPAP machine, because electricity may be unavailable in a field environment. Successful treatment with surgery or weight loss resolves the issue without complications.

In the civilian aviation community, a pilot may still fly if diagnosed with sleep apnoea as long as treatment is successful and compliance with treatment can be demonstrated. Usually, after diagnosis is made and treatment has begun, the pilot is brought into a sleep laboratory for the maintenance of wakefulness test (MWT), which provides an objective measure of how well a person can stay awake. If the pilot is able to pass this test, then they are considered fit for flight duty. However, the regulatory agency, the physician and/or the airline will probably require a record of compliance with CPAP treatment and/or proof that the apnoea has been treated successfully through surgery. Most CPAP machines now have the ability to track the hours of use, so compliance is easy to verify. A second overnight sleep test following surgery often proves that the surgery was successful.

Periodic limb movements in sleep

Periodic limb movements in sleep (PLMS) is another sleep disorder that disrupts and fragments sleep. The disorder can disturb sleep to the point that its restorative value is degraded significantly, leading to problems with daytime sleepiness (Tabbal 2002).

PLMS involves periodic contraction of the tibialis anterior, with muscle dorsiflexion of the ankle and toes, which results in a leg jerk or twitch, usually lasting between 0.5 and 5 seconds and with a frequency of one every 20–40 seconds. Usually these movements are associated with short EEG arousals. The severity can range from a mild toe movement to a full kick of the leg. The most common type of PLMS involves the legs, but there are cases in which the arms are affected. Often the person is not aware of the limb movements during sleep, so frequently the problem is reported by a partner. The rhythmic jerks of PLMS should not be confused with hypnic jerks (also called hypnic myoclonus and sleep starts), which are brief contractions of the muscles of the arms and legs that occur at sleep onset and are a normal feature of falling asleep.

In order to diagnose PLMS, the patient should stay overnight in a sleep laboratory while EEG, EMG, ECG and respiration are monitored. Bilateral EMG electrodes attached to the anterior tibialis muscles are used to identify and count the muscle movements associated with PLMS. A PLMS index (average number of limb movements per hour of sleep) of greater than 5 is considered pathological; however, the number of leg movements varies from night to night.

RESTLESS LEGS SYNDROME

A similar disorder that may occur with PLMS is restless legs syndrome (RLS), characterized by limb discomfort that occurs while the person is awake and is of sufficient intensity to prevent or delay the onset of sleep. The symptoms of RLS vary from mild tingling in the legs to severe discomfort and pain that becomes pronounced when sitting or lying down. To eliminate or reduce the unpleasant sensations, the sufferer usually needs to move the legs, which adversely affects sleep. Some patients fall asleep rapidly but wake up frequently with paraesthesiae that are relieved only by walking. Many people with RLS also have PLMS. The treatments for both disorders are the same.

TREATMENT OF PERIODIC LIMB MOVEMENTS IN SLEEP AND RESTLESS LEGS SYNDROME

Sometimes sleep is not disrupted by these movements, and in such cases no treatment is necessary. However, if there are disruptions in sleep architecture, the physician or sleep specialist may prescribe appropriate medication in an effort to reduce or eliminate the limb movements. In a small percentage of people, large doses of vitamin E are effective at alleviating the symptoms. Prescription medications used include a levodopa/carbidopa combination and other medications that are prescribed for other types of movement disorder, such as Parkinson's disease. (Even though the treatments are the same for these two problems, there is no indication that people with PLMS are susceptible to Parkinson's disease.) Some physicians prescribe a benzodiazepine to treat PLMS; this may not stop the limb movements, but it can increase the depth of sleep enough to protect it from movement-related disturbances.

FLIGHT STATUS AND PERIODIC LIMB MOVEMENTS IN SLEEP OR RESTLESS LEGS SYNDROME

Unless pilots with these disorders are fortunate enough to respond to vitamin E therapy, some type of prescription medication may be necessary. Since these medications are likely not waiverable, there may be problems maintaining flight status. The administration of benzodiazepines or levodopa/carbidopa usually requires a grounding period after dosing due to the sedative characteristics of the drugs. Some other antiparkinson medications do not have the sedative qualities of the more common medications, but they may have some other side effects that are not compatible with flying and thus are not allowable under civil aviation or military regulations.

Narcolepsy

Narcolepsy is a sleep disorder characterized primarily by excessive daytime sleepiness. The prevalence of narcolepsy in the general population varies among the different countries, with a very low estimate in the Israeli population of about 0.002 per cent to a relatively high estimate in the Japanese population of about 0.18 per cent. The incidence in the US population is estimated at about 0.05 per cent. Overall, more males are affected than females (Brooks and Mignot 2002). This is a fairly serious disorder that is often resistant to complete alleviation. Patients with narcolepsy usually begin to experience symptoms during adolescence or young adulthood, but symptoms can start as late as the fifth decade. The classic tetrad for narcolepsy is excessive daytime sleepiness, muscle weakness (cataplexy), which is usually brought on by emotions, sleep paralysis (unable to move for several seconds when falling asleep or upon awakening), and hypnogogic hallucinations. In addition, automatic behaviours and disturbed night-time sleep have also been noted in patients with narcolepsy. Some or all of these symptoms may be present, from mild to severe levels.

The diagnosis of narcolepsy requires an overnight stay at a sleep laboratory, during which EEG, EMG, EOG, ECG and respiration are monitored. Since sufferers often seek treatment because their excessive daytime sleepiness is impairing their ability to function in day-to-day activities, other possible sources for their impaired alertness are ruled out first. Once an overnight stay indicates that other disorders such as sleep apnoea and PLMS are not present, the patient is required to stay an additional day for a multiple sleep latency test (MSLT). The MSLT requires the patient to lie down for 20 minutes every two hours and attempt to fall asleep while the standard physiological parameters are measured. The time it takes to fall asleep on each occasion is recorded, and the type of sleep is assessed. Typically, four or five nap periods are used in the evaluation. If sleep occurs within 20 minutes across most of the naps, and if REM sleep occurs during at least two of these 20-minute naps, then a diagnosis of narcolepsy is made and treatment options are discussed.

TREATMENT OF NARCOLEPSY

Depending on the severity of the disorder, naps can sometimes be used to alleviate the excessive daytime sleepiness, but usually stimulant medication is required. If cataplexy occurs, medication is prescribed for this as well. Usually all symptoms can be alleviated or reduced with proper medication.

FLIGHT STATUS AND NARCOLEPSY

A diagnosis of narcolepsy will end the flying career of a pilot, whether civilian or military. Even with medication, neither the civil aviation authorities nor the military will allow a person with narcolepsy to pilot an aircraft, because the possibility of falling asleep or experiencing cataplexy during flight is too dangerous. The prevalence of narcolepsy within the pilot population is no doubt virtually insignificant. However, it can occur, and the diagnosis and treatment of this disorder in anyone who is responsible for operating complex machinery (especially in the transportation industry and the military) is important to the safety of both the patient and others who are dependent on their actions.

SUMMARY AND CONCLUSIONS

Although sleep is a poorly understood process, it nonetheless has clear implications for the performance, alertness and wellbeing of pilots, aircrew and others associated with military and commercial aviation. Unfortunately, many factors can disturb the sleep process, ranging from job-related scheduling problems and environmental issues, to an individual's poor sleep habits, to the presence of a severe sleep disorder. If a pilot or crew member indicates that he or she is experiencing sleeping difficulties, then various reasons for the problem must be considered by the flight surgeon or physician. Recognizing the complexities of the normal sleep process provides a basis for understanding disruptive influence of a variety of factors on the recuperative nature of sleep. Inappropriate sleep environments, poor sleep habits, changes in schedules and sleep disorders all interfere with the ability to obtain a restful period of sleep. Offering behavioural and/or pharmacological treatment for the individual experiencing sleep difficulties will improve mood, performance, safety and overall health, as well as the welfare of the entire unit. Improved sleep quality and duration will maximize the safe and successful completion of the mission.

REFERENCES

Aeschbach D, Cajochen C, Tobler I, Dijk D, Borbély AA. Sleep in a sitting position: effect of triazolam on sleep stages and EEG power spectra. *Psychopharmacology* 1994; **114**: 209–14.

Akerstedt T. Sleepiness as a consequence of shift work. *Sleep* 1988; **11**: 17–34.

Akerstedt T. Shift work and disturbed sleep/wakefulness. *Occupational Medicine* 2003; **53**: 89–94.

Akerstedt T, Folkard S. Validation of the S and C components of the three-process model of alertness regulation. *Sleep* 1995; **18**: 1–6.

Aldrich MS. Cardinal manifestations of sleep disorders. In: Kryger MH, Roth T, Dement WC (eds). *Principles and Practice of Sleep Medicine*, 3rd edn. Philadelphia, PA: W.B. Saunders, 2000; pp. 526–33.

Balkin T, Badia P. Relationship between sleep inertia and sleepiness: cumulative effects of four nights of sleep disruption/restriction on performance following abrupt nocturnal awakenings. *Biological Psychology* 1988; **27**: 245–58.

Bisson RU, Lyons TJ, Hatsel C. Aircrew fatigue during Desert Shield C-5 transport operations. *Aviation, Space, and Environmental Medicine* 1993; **64**: 848–53.

Bliwise DL. Sleep in normal aging and dementia. *Sleep* 1993; **16**: 40–81.

Boll PA, Storm WF, French J, *et al.* C-141 aircrew sleep and fatigue during the Persian Gulf conflict. In: NATO/AGARD (ed.). *Nutrition, Metabolic Disorders and Lifestyle of Aircrew*. Neuilly-sur-Seine: NATO/AGARD, 1992; pp. 29.1–11.

Bonnet MH, Arand DL. Clinical effects of sleep fragmentation versus sleep deprivation. *Sleep Medicine Reviews* 2003; **7**: 297–310.

Borbely AA. A two process model of sleep regulation. *Human Neurobiology* 1982; **1**: 195–204.

Boutrel B, Koob GF. What keeps us awake: the neuropharmacology of stimulants and wakefulness-promoting medications. *Sleep* 2004; **27**: 1181–94.

Brooks SN, Mignot E. Narcolepsy and idiopathic hypersomnia. In: Lee-Chiong TL, Satela MJ, Carskadon MA (eds). *Sleep Medicine*. Philadelphia, PA: Hanley & Belfus, 2002; pp. 193–202.

Butkov N. Polysomnography. In: Carskadon MA (ed.). *Sleep Medicine*. Philadelphia, PA: Hanley & Belfus, 2002; pp. 605–37.

Carskadon MA, Dement WC. Nocturnal determinants of daytime sleepiness. *Sleep* 1982; **14**: 307–15.

Carskadon MA, Dement WC. Normal human sleep: an overview. In: Kryger MH, Roth T, Dement WC (eds). *Principles and Practice of Sleep Medicine*. 3rd edn. Philadelphia, PA: W.B. Saunders, 2000; pp. 15–25.

Comperatore CA, Caldwell JA, Caldwell JL. *Leader's Guide to Crew Endurance*. Fort Rucker, AL: US Army Aeromedical Research Laboratory and US Army Safety Center, 1996.

Costa G. The problem: shiftwork. *Chronobiology International* 1997; **14**: 89–98.

Czeisler CA, Weitzman ED, Moore-Ede MC, Zimmerman JC, Knauer RS. Human sleep: its duration and organization depend on its circadian phase. *Science* 1980a; **210**: 1264–7.

Czeisler CA, Zimmerman JC, Ronda JM, Moore-Ede MC, Weitzman ED. Timing of REM sleep is coupled to the circadian rhythm of body temperature in man. *Sleep* 1980b; **2**: 329–46.

Dement WC, Seidel WF, Cohen SA, Bliwise NG, Carskadon MA. Sleep and wakefulness in aircrew before and after transoceanic flights. *Aviation, Space, and Environmental Medicine* 1986; **57** (suppl.): B14–28.

Department of the Air Force. Memorandum: revised duty limitation times for the ground testing and operational use of temazepam, zolpidem and zaleplon in aviators and special duty personnel. Bolling AFB, DC: Air Force Medical Operations Agency, 2001.

Dinges DF. Differential effects of prior wakefulness and circadian phase on nap sleep. *Electroencephalography and Clinical Neurophysiology* 1986; **64**: 224–7.

Dinges DF, Orne MT, Orne EC. Assessing performance upon abrupt awakening from naps during quasi-continuous operations. *Behavior Research Methods, Instruments, and Computers* 1985; **17**: 37–45.

Dinges DF, Orne MT, Whitehouse WG, Orne EC. Temporal placement of a nap for alertness: contributions of circadian phase and prior wakefulness. *Sleep* 1987; **10**: 313–29.

Drake CL, Roehrs TA, Burduvali E, *et al.* Effects of rapid versus slow accumulation of eight hours of sleep loss. *Psychophysiology* 2001; **38**: 979–87.

Gander PH, Graeber RC. Sleep in pilots flying short-haul commercial schedules. *Ergonomics* 1987; **30**: 1365–77.

Gander PH, Rosekind MR, Gregory KB. Flight crew fatigue. VI: a synthesis. *Aviation, Space, and Environmental Medicine* 1998; **69**: B49–60.

Gillberg M. The effects of two alternative timings of a one-hour nap on early morning performance. *Biological Psychology* 1984; **19**: 45–54.

Gyllenhaal C, Merritt SL, Peterson SD, Block KI, Gochenour T. Efficacy and safety of herbal stimulants and sedatives in sleep disorders. *Sleep Medicine Reviews* 2000; **4**: 229–51.

Harrison Y, Horne JA. Occurrence of 'microsleeps' during daytime sleep onset in normal subjects. *Electroencephalography and Clinical Neurophysiology* 1996; **98**: 411–16.

Haslam DR. Sleep deprivation and naps. *Behavior Research Methods, Instruments, and Computers* 1985; **17**: 46–54.

Hauri PJ. Consulting about insomnia: a method and some preliminary data. *Sleep* 1993; **16**: 344–50.

Jasper HH. The ten–twenty electrode system of the International Federation. *Electroencephalography and Clinical Neurophysiology* 1958; **10**: 371–5.

Lavie P. Ultrashort sleep-waking schedule. III: 'gates' and 'forbidden zones' for sleep. *Electroencephalography and Clinical Neurophysiology* 1986; **63**: 414–25.

Lushington K, Lack L. Non-pharmacological treatments of insomnia. *Israel Journal of Psychiatry and Related Sciences* 2002; **39**: 36–49.

Manber R, Kuo TF. Cognitive-behavioral therapies for insomnia. In: Lee-Chiong TL, Satela MJ, Carskadon MA (eds). *Sleep Medicine*. Philadelphia, PA: Hanley & Belfus, 2002; pp. 177–85.

Naitoh P, Kelly T, Babkoff H. Sleep inertia: is there a worst time to wake up? Naval technical report no. 91-45. San Diego, CA: Naval Health Research Center, 1992.

Neville KJ, Bisson RU, French J, Boll PA, Storm WF. Subjective fatigue of C-141 aircrews during Operation Desert Storm. *Human Factors* 1994; **36**: 339–49.

Nicolau MC, Akaârir M, Gamundi A, González J, Rial RV. Why we sleep: the evolutionary pathway to the mammalian sleep. *Progress in Neurobiology* 2000; **62**: 379–406.

Nicholson AN. Sleep and wakefulness of the airline pilots. *Aviation, Space, and Environmental Medicine* 1987; **58**: 395–401.

Nicholson AN, Stone BM. Influence of back angle on the quality of sleep in seats. *Ergonomics* 1987; **30**: 1033–41.

Nicholson AN, Pascoe PA, Roehrs T, *et al.* Sustained performance with short evening and morning sleeps. *Aviation, Space, and Environmental Medicine* 1985; **56**: 105–14.

Nicholson AN, Pascoe PA, Spencer MB, Stone BM, Green RL. Nocturnal sleep and daytime alertness of aircrew on transmeridian flights. *Aviation, Space, and Environmental Medicine* 1986; **57**: B42–52.

Ohayon MM, Guilleminault C, Priest RG, Caulet M. Snoring and breathing pauses during sleep: telephone interview survey of a United Kingdom population sample. *British Medical Journal* 1997; **314**: 860–63.

Petrie KJ, Dawson AG. Symptoms of fatigue and coping strategies in international pilots. *International Journal of Aviation Psychology* 1997; **7**: 251–8.

Pivik RT. Psychophysiology of dreams. In: Kryger MH, Roth T, Dement WC, (eds). *Principles and Practice of Sleep Medicine*, 3rd edn. Philadelphia, PA: W.B. Saunders, 2000; pp. 491–501.

Porcu S, Casagrande M, Ferrara M, Bellatreccia A. Sleep and alertness during alternating monophasic and polyphasic rest-activity cycles. *International Journal of Neuroscience* 1998; **95**: 43–50.

Rechtschaffen A, Kales A. *A Manual of Standardized Terminology: Techniques and Scoring System for Sleep Stages of Human Subjects*. Los Angeles, CA: UCLA Brain Information Service/Brain Research Institute, 1968.

Ritter RD. 'And we were tired': fatigue and aircrew errors. *AES Systems Magazine* 1993; **March**: 21–6.

Rosekind MR, Gander PH, Miller DL, *et al.* Fatigue in operational settings: examples from the aviation environment. *Human Factors* 1994; **36**: 327–38.

Rosekind MR, Gregory KB, Co EL, Miller DL, Dinges DF. Crew factors in flight operations XII: a survey of sleep quantity and quality in on-board crew rest facilities. NASA/TM report no. 2000-209611. Moffett Field, CA: NASA Ames Research Center, 2000.

Sasaki M, Kurosaki Y, Mori A, Endo S. Patterns of sleep-wakefulness before and after transmeridian flight in commercial airline pilots. *Aviation, Space, and Environmental Medicine* 1986; **57** (suppl.): B29–42.

Sateia MJ. Epidemiology, consequences, and evaluation of insomnia. In: Carskadon MA (ed.). *Sleep Medicine*. Philadelphia, PA: Hanley & Belfus, 2002. pp. 151–60.

Sejnowski TJ, Destexhe A. Why do we sleep? *Brain Research* 2000; **886**: 208–23.

Silberman WS. Certification issues and answers. *Federal Air Surgeon's Medical Bulletin* 2003; **41**.

Smith MT, Neubauer DN. Cognitive behavior therapy for chronic insomnia. *Clinical Cornerstone* 2003; **5**: 28–40.

Stone BM, Turner C. Promoting sleep in shiftworkers and intercontinental travelers. *Chronobiology International* 1997; **14**: 133–43.

Tabbal SD. Restless legs syndrome and periodic limb movement disorder. In: Lee-Chiong TL, Satela MJ, Carskadon MA (eds). *Sleep Medicine*. Philadelphia, PA: Hanley & Belfus, 2002; pp. 225–36.

Thorpy MJ. Classification of sleep disorders. In: Kryger MH, Roth T, Dement WC (eds). *Principles and Practice of Sleep Medicine*, 3rd edn. Philadelphia, PA: W.B. Saunders, 2000; pp. 547–57.

Van Cauter E, Leproult R, Plat L. Age-related changes in slow wave sleep and REM sleep and relationship with growth hormone and cortisol levels in healthy men. *Journal of the American Medical Association* 2000; **284**: 861–8.

Waterhouse J. Jet-lag and shift work. 1: circadian rhythms. *Journal of the Royal Society of Medicine* 1999; **92**: 398–401.

Waterhouse J, Reilly T, Atkinson G. Jet-lag. *Lancet* 1997; **350**: 1611–16.

Young T, Palta M, Dempsey J, *et al.* The occurrence of sleep-disordered breathing among middle-aged adults. *New England Journal of Medicine* 1993; **328**: 1230–35.

Youngstedt SC. Ceiling and floor effects in sleep research. *Sleep Medicine Reviews* 2003; **7**: 351–65.

17

Optics and vision

PAUL WRIGHT AND ROBERT A.H. SCOTT

SCIENCE OF LIGHT

The energy from a light source can be considered as a stream of discrete particles – photons – or as a continuous stream of energy along a ray or wave. Both theories are equally valid, and together they form the 'duality of light' hypothesis. The concept of the photon is useful when considering light in terms of quantum physics, as used in the investigation of the origin of light and how light interacts with matter. Generally, the concept of the propagation of waves of light gives useful insight into classical optical phenomena and underpins the majority of visual optics.

Characteristics of light

A wave of light can be described by various characteristics, including wavelength, frequency, phase, polarization and coherence. The wavelength and frequency of a wave are related to the speed of light in a vacuum as

$$c = f\lambda$$

where c is the speed of light, f is the frequency of the wave and λ is the wavelength.

Visible light is a small part of the electromagnetic spectrum found between 380 and 780 nm (Table 17.1). Wavelengths outside of this band are not seen, but their energy can have significant effects on visual function.

Table 17.1 *Electromagnetic spectrum*

Light	Wavelength (nm)
UV(A)	315–380
UV(B)	295–315
UV(C)	200–295
Visible	380–780
Near-IR	780–1400
Far-IR	1400+

IR, infrared; UV, ultraviolet.

The energy contained within a given wavelength is defined by

$$E = \rho f = \rho/\lambda$$

where E is energy, ρ is Planck's constant and f is the frequency of the wave.

Therefore, the higher-energy wavelengths are located in the ultraviolet (UV) to blue end of the spectrum.

PHASE

Light waves travel in a straight optical path, but particles in the wave oscillate in a sinusoidal pattern perpendicular to this line. At a given point along the optical path, light waves are said to be in phase if the position of oscillation is the same, i.e. if the particle is found at the peak, in a trough or at a point in between. Two waves are said to be in antiphase when the positions of the particles are diametrically opposite each another, e.g. one wave is at a peak and the other is in a trough. The points between in-phase and anti-phase are normally described by the angle of phase. The angle of phase when the waves are in phase is zero (or 360 degrees) and when the waves are in anti-phase 180 degrees.

POLARIZATION

A wave follows a sinusoidal motion in one plane. That plane can be in any one of 360 degrees, and so a wave can also be described by its angle of polarization. Conventional light sources emit unpolarized light, and so the waves of light are emitted through all 360 degrees. It is possible to control polarization by using a filter that allows passage of only a single plane. If two polarizing filters are placed perpendicular to each other, they halt transmission of light completely. Polarized light occurs when light in a given wave has only one orientation. Polarized light arises from filtering unpolarized light or can be created from coherent light sources such as lasers.

COHERENCE

When two waves of light of the same frequency arrive at a given point along their optical paths, there is a constant phase relationship between the waves, and the energy intensity of the combined wave is equal to the sum of the individual amplitudes. A source of light does not emit a continuous wave train but emits a succession of wave trains of finite and varying lengths and with no fixed phase relationship between the successive wave trains, i.e. the source emits light with random variations in phase. The combination of light of the same wavelength from two independent sources will vary in intensity due to the endless phase-changing effect. These variations are both too small and too fast for the eye to perceive. Light with a constant phase relationship between two or more wave trains of light is said to be coherent; if this condition is not met, then the light is described as being incoherent. Coherent light can occur only with monochromatic (single-wavelength) light. With current technology, the laser is the nearest we have come to achieving a fully coherent light source. Conventional light sources, such as the tungsten light bulb, emit many different wavelengths, including infrared (IR) (heat), and therefore are described as incoherent light sources.

Attributes of a medium

The speed of light in a medium is different from that in a vacuum. If the velocities are v and c, then the ratio c/v is called the refractive index, usually denoted by n. When light enters a medium of greater refractive index, light is 'bent' towards the perpendicular of the surface. Refraction of light is greater with larger differences in refractive index at the boundary between two media. For example, most refraction in the eye occurs at the air–cornea surface, because the relative refractive index between these two media is greater than that at the lens, which, surrounded by the humours, has a smaller relative refractive index. Most media used in optics are chosen for their refractive-index-dependent properties. Frequently, there can be problems with birefringence, wherein the refractive index of the media varies in two directions of orientation. Combinations of different media can be used to reduce this property.

Refraction is used to bend light to a focus and is the basis for lens design. The ability of a lens to bend light is known as the refractive power and is described as the inverse of the focal length of the lens, i.e. the larger the power of refraction, the shorter the focal length. The unit of refractive power is the dioptre (D), e.g. a 1-D lens has a focal length of 1 m and a 2-D lens has a focal length of 0.5 m.

EFFECTS OF A MEDIUM ON LIGHT

When light is incident upon a material medium, the medium exerts a number of effects on light. These are related to the refractive index properties of the material. In particular, light is reflected at the medium boundary, changing its optical path combined with potential changes in polarization and phase. Most material boundaries have reflective properties, with light being reflected in a given direction or diffusely in all directions as a function of the surface. If one considers light in terms of energy, then the total incident light energy on contact with the material medium boundary is split into two components. Some light energy is reflected at the surface, while the rest is refracted through the material medium. The energy being refracted continues to lose energy in the material due to the material both absorbing and scattering energy away from the optical path.

Light scatter is the dispersion of light through a medium as a result of light interaction with particles that make up the material. For example, light entering the eye usually passes through the pupil; however, additional light can transilluminate the iris and sclera. The photo-pigments melanin and haemoglobin absorb some of this light, but the majority of light can pass through into the humours. In addition, some light is also scattered by the humours, resulting in 'stray light' reaching the retina. Stray light reaching the fovea decreases the contrast of foveal images, resulting in disabling glare. Rayleigh scattering of light is due to interaction with small particles (cf. wavelength of light) that make up the medium. Light affected by Rayleigh scattering is scattered in all directions; it tends to affect shorter wavelengths. This is observed when solar light travels through the Earth's atmosphere and accounts for the blue appearance of the sky, except in the direction of the sun, and the red sky around the sun at the rising of the sun or at sunset. Mie scatter of light is due to interaction with large particles within the medium and results in a forward scatter, i.e. it can produce a blurring effect in an optical device. Mie scatter is not wavelength-dependent, as Rayleigh scattering is, and typically is found in foggy conditions, where image focus and contrast are reduced.

MEASUREMENT OF LIGHT

When dealing with any form of radiant energy, it is usual to define its measurement in terms of radiometry. When dealing with visible light, the principles of radiometry are used, but the energies measured are weighted according to the visual response that the energy can produce in the eye. The measurement of visible light energy is called photometry. For illustration, we can consider a basic optical system such as a slide projector illuminating a display screen that is observed by a viewer. The luminous flux describes the rate of flow of photon energy from the source, again weighted according to its efficiency in producing a visual response. The unit of luminous flux is the lumen. The luminous intensity of the source is defined as the amount of luminous flux emitted per unit solid angle (a three-dimensional angle, giving rise to a conical shaped beam). The unit of luminous intensity is the candela, approximately equivalent to the intensity emitted by a domestic candle. These two terms describe the source. Moving through our optical system, the next term we come across is that of illuminance. This is the amount of luminous flux received over a unit area on any point on the surface of the screen. In other words, it describes the concentration of light energy on a given area of the screen: the greater the illuminance level, the brighter the image will appear on the screen. The unit of illuminance is the lux. In the same manner as for all radiant energy, the energy level in the beam drops with distance from the source, in accordance with the inverse square law. In addition, the energy level drops with deviation from the centre of the beam, in line with the cosine law of illumination. The illuminant energy is incident upon the screen; some energy will be absorbed into the screen, but the remainder will be reflected back towards the viewer. The term 'reflectance' (or albedo) describes the amount of light energy reflected as a fraction or percentage of the illuminating energy. The greater the level of reflectance, the brighter the image will appear to the viewer. Finally, the light energy received by the viewer is called the luminance and is the concentration of light energy over a unit surface area in a stated direction. Not all surfaces reflect equally in all directions or all in one direction, which can give rise to variations in luminance. The unit is candelas per square metre. For a stated direction, it can also be considered as the product of the illuminance and the screen reflectance in a given system. Again, luminance is considered as a concentration of light energy. To perceive an object to be bright, the viewer needs to receive a high luminance level from the object together with a retina sensitive to that light level. For example, if two individuals, one having been in a dark room for an hour and the other having been outside in the sunshine for the same time, view a dimly lit cathode-ray tube (CRT) display, then the dark-adapted individual would perceive the display to be brighter than would the light-adapted individual. Therefore, brightness of an object is a factor of both the luminance and the light sensitivity of the retina.

SCIENCE OF COLOUR

Different wavelengths of light produce different sensations of colour (hue). A stimulus that does not contain a marked excess of any one group of wavelengths produces the sensation of white light. If one wavelength is slightly dominant, then the sensation is of a pale or desaturated colour. An alternative term is 'chroma', which defines the amount of white light in the mixture. As the proportion of dominant wavelength is increased, the colour is said to become more saturated. Monochromatic light is said to have complete saturation.

An additive mixture of red, green and blue light can produce a wide range of coloured lights. From these colours, it is possible to match an additive mixture against many colours that are not highly saturated. This is true only for coloured light sources and not for paint or dye pigments. A mixture of red and green light can create additive mixtures of fairly saturated orange, yellow and yellow-green light, depending on the relative amounts of each additive. Additive mixtures cannot match very saturated colours, especially in the blue-green region. When an additive mixture of two colours produces white light, then these colours are said to be complementary. If red, green and blue light are mixed to give white light, and then the blue is removed, the resultant colour is yellow. When yellow light is mixed with blue light, the resultant light colour is white, and so blue and yellow are complementary.

Opponent system of colour vision

The human retina contains photoreceptors. These consist of light-sensitive pigments (photo-pigments), which absorb photons of light, and neural elements, which help to channel nerve impulses to the brain. There are two main classes of photoreceptors: rods and cones. Rods function in scotopic (low light) conditions and cones operate in photopic (normal daylight) conditions, with an overlap between the groups in mesopic (intermediate) conditions. Rods are not colour-sensitive or sensitive to fine detail, but cones are sensitive to colour and fine detail.

There are three types of cone photo-pigment, each type having a maximum absorbance in a different part of the visible spectrum, although there is a considerable spectral overlap. The different cone types traditionally have been referred to as 'red', 'green' and 'blue', but the maximum absorbance values, or peak wavelength sensitivities, of the photo-pigments lie in the yellow-green (approximately 570 nm), green (approximately 542 nm) and blue (approximately 442 nm) parts of the spectrum. It is, therefore, more appropriate to label them long-wave (L-cones), medium-wave (M-cones) and short-wave (S-cones) sensitive photo-pigments.

The molecules of the photo-pigments in the retina are excited when light is absorbed, causing a signal to be generated and transmitted along nerve fibres to the brain. The process of this signal transmission is not understood completely. It is, however, known that there are not four different types of signal, one for each type of receptor (rods and three types of cones), but that different combinations of these signals are transmitted along nerve fibres. It is most likely that photoreceptor signals are combined to form three channels – the achromatic channel and two colour difference channels. The achromatic signal is composed of inputs from the rods and all three cone types. The two colour difference signals are composed of the three possible basic difference signals:

$$L - M = C1$$
$$M - S = C2$$
$$S - L = C3$$

When these are added up, they equal zero, and so they do not need to be transmitted separately. It has been suggested that the signals transmitted resemble $C1 = L - M$ and $C2 - C3 = M - S - (S - L) = L + M - 2S$. These two colour difference signals are referred to broadly as the opponent system of 'red minus green' and 'yellow minus blue', where $L + M$ is labelled as yellow. From this system, the ratio of the signal C1 to that of $C2 - C3$ can be used to indicate hue and the strength of these two signals to indicate colourfulness. For achromatic 'colours' (white, grey, black) the signals from each cone type are equal, and so the colour difference signals C1, C2 and C3 would be zero (as would be the colourfulness).

Trichromatic theory

The trichromatic theory is based on two well-established experimental outcomes: (i) that the proper mixture of three-coloured stimuli can match any given colour and (ii) that colour matching is predictable provided the relative amount of coloured stimuli is known. The unit trichromatic equation defines this principle as follows:

$$(C) \equiv r(R) + g(G) + b(B)$$

where C is the desired colour, and r, g and b are the relative amounts of red, green and blue light, respectively.

The units are chosen so that equal amounts of red, blue and green stimuli are required to produce white light. Many different chromaticity charts are available, allowing any colour to be defined by its degree of saturation and red, blue and green content. Examples of these include the International Commission on Illumination (CIE) (x,y) chromaticity diagram, the Munsell system and the CIE L*a*b* system.

If a light source emits a spectrum containing equal amounts of energy for each constituent wavelength and it illuminates an object that reflects all wavelengths, then the object will appear white. If the object absorbs some wavelengths and reflects others, then it will appear coloured. The colour that an object appears to have is determined by the wavelengths it reflects to the eye.

The additive mixture laws relate to the mixing of coloured light. However, the laws for colour mixing of paint pigments are different. A paint pigment of a specified colour absorbs some wavelengths and reflects the rest. By varying pigments in a mixture, one can vary the intensity of the wavelengths it absorbs but not necessarily those that it reflects, as these remain at maximum intensity. One obtains control of the red, blue and green light entering the eye by varying the proportions of those pigments that absorb the spectral region corresponding to these three colours, i.e. by subtracting the complementary colour from the white mixture. The primary pigment colours may be referred to as minus red, minus green and minus blue. With the naked eye, these pigments appear to be blue-green, magenta and yellow, respectively.

In summary, with additive mixing of light, one starts with no light and adds the chosen amounts of red, blue and green light in order to produce the desired colour. However, with subtractive mixing of pigments, one starts with light of all wavelengths (white) and subtracts chosen amounts of red, blue and green in order to produce the desired colour. The subtraction is the loss of a colour absorbed into the pigment.

THE FOCUSING SYSTEM

Basic anatomy

Each eye is roughly spherical, measuring approximately 25 mm in diameter and lying within the bony orbit of the skull. The bony orbit protects the eye in all directions apart from the front, where protection is limited to the eyelids. The eye is hollow and maintains its own shape by means of controlling its internal pressure. The outer wall consists of three layers, modified at the front to admit light. The outermost layer, the sclera, is a tough fibrous outer coating modified at the front to become the cornea. The middle layer is mainly vascular, as it consists of the posterior choroid layer and the anterior ciliary body and iris. The inner layer is the retina and is associated closely with the coverage of the choroid. The globe is divided into two main compartments separated by the lens–iris diaphragm: the smaller anterior chamber filled with a clear liquid called the aqueous humour and a large posterior compartment filled with a jelly-like substance called the vitreous humour. Figure 17.1 shows the anatomy of the eye.

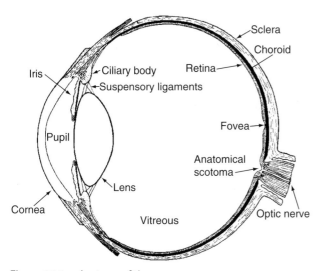

Figure 17.1 *Anatomy of the eye.*

EYE MOVEMENT

The globe rotates in the orbit about its own centre in response to the pull of three pairs of extraocular muscles. The two eyeballs are yoked together, and their axes remain parallel in all conjugate movements. Their axes are, by necessity, not parallel in the disjunctive movements of convergence and divergence.

Refractive surfaces

Most refraction occurs at the air–cornea junction (38–48 D) due to the large difference in refractive index between the air and the corneal media. In addition, as the amount of refraction occurring at a curved surface increases with an increase in the degree of curvature, so the cornea is capable of even larger refractive power than if it was a flat surface. The cornea can be considered as having three layers – endothelium, internal stroma and epithelium. The endothelium faces the aqueous humour, while the epithelium faces the tear film. The corneal stroma has a high colloidal pressure, and the resultant water ingress increases the overall refractive index. This influx of water is countered by a water pump, which maintains a state of

equilibrium. The cornea is 1 mm thick at its edge (limbus), thinning to approximately 0.7 mm in the centre. The cornea is avascular and achieves oxygenation by a number of means. The outer epithelium is oxygenated by gas diffusion from the atmosphere, while the inner endothelium is oxygenated by the aqueous humour. This accounts for sea-level oxygen tensions of 150 mmHg at the epithelium, 100 mmHg in the mid-layer and 55 mmHg at the endothelium. Use of contact lenses that result in a reduction in corneal oxygen tension might, therefore, have profound effects on vision at altitude.

The physiology of the lens is very similar to that of the cornea. However, the lens does not have the same degree of refractive power, due to the smaller differences in refractive index either side of it. The lens is capable of changing its refractive power by changing the degree of curvature of the anterior surface and so controls the amount of refraction (19–34 D). The eye uses this lens system to focus an image on a light-sensitive screen, the retina (Figure 17.2).

Accommodation is the process that enables the eye to change focal length from the furthest point of vision to the nearest point. To focus on objects at the far point of vision (infinity) the ciliary muscles relax, which in turn pull taut the zonular fibres connected to the lens. This places the lens under tension and reduces the lenticular degree of curvature. To achieve vision at the near point, the opposite occurs, i.e. the ciliary muscles contract and the zonular fibres relax, resulting in a less tense lens and enabling the lens to take up a more natural rounded shape. The range of accommodation is about 15 D at best, but this tends to degenerate with age, up to a maximum rate of 1-D loss per year in middle age. For most people over the age of 60 years, the eye is effectively a fixed-focus device. It takes

Helmholtz equation $h' = -x'\theta' = -x'(n/n')\theta$

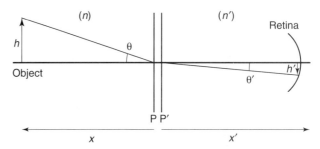

Figure 17.2 *Helmholtz optical diagram. An object of height h is at a distance x from the eye and subtends an angle θ at the eye. Points P and P′ are the principal points of the eye optical system. The image in the retina has height h′ at a distance x′ from the eye optics and subtends a visual angle of θ′. The apparent size of an object is determined by the relative size of its retinal image. Mathematically, it can be shown that the apparent size of an object is directly proportional to the angle that the object subtends at the eye.*

time to change the shape of the lens; in aviation in particular, this transit time to the next focal point results in unfocused vision over this period. To accommodate the lens fully, i.e. to move the focus of vision from the far point to the near point, takes 0.8 seconds; to change focus from the near point to the far point takes 0.5 seconds. The combination of time taken to achieve focus with typical aircraft speeds means that significant distances are travelled in the air without the pilot having any focused sight.

Role of the pupil

The pupil plays an important role in image formation. First, the pupil restricts the total amount of light reaching the retina, protecting it from dazzle and bright daylight conditions. The time taken to constrict the pupil is much quicker than the time taken to dilate it. Second, the pupil acts as an aperture stop, restricting the number of rays reaching the retina. This is beneficial as it improves the sharpness of the image by reducing the degree of image aberration and increases the depth of focus. Depth of focus is the maximum range of movement away from the focal plane with which deterioration of image quality is not serious. It is often confused with the depth of field, which is the permissible movement of an object in the object plane resulting in the image being moved to an out-of-focus location on the retina. At night, when the pupil widens, there is a reduction in the depth of field of the eye, which can exaggerate the visual decrement caused by refractive error. Third, the pupil is associated with the Stiles–Crawford effect – light entering the eye near the centre of the pupil is more effective in producing a visual response than that entering near the periphery. In daylight conditions this effect occurs across the full visible spectrum, but at night it appears to be limited to wavelengths above 580 nm (green to red).

INHERENT ERRORS IN EYE FOCUSING

Chromatic aberration

With transparent materials, the refractive index of the material usually decreases with increasing wavelengths of light. Therefore, a shorter focal length occurs for shorter wavelengths. For example, after refraction in a lens, incident white light spreads out into its constituent wavelengths – the prismatic effect. There is no focal point for the white light source, and therefore each wavelength will form a separate image. This defect is called longitudinal chromatic aberration (Figure 17.3). As well as different focal lengths, different levels of magnification will also occur, so each coloured image will be a different size. This

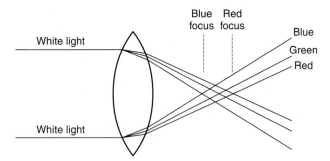

Figure 17.3 *Chromatic aberration. A lens can be considered as two prisms placed base to base. White light is split into its component wavelengths, resulting in a range of focal lengths from the blue end to the red end of the visible spectrum.*

is known as chromatic difference of magnification. Both focal length and magnification effects of chromatic aberration severely degrade the image quality.

Chromatic aberration is thought to play a large part in rapid focusing. When one accommodates in white light, if the image is too close red fringes predominate; if the image is too far away, then there is a predominance of blue fringes. Therefore, using such a system of aberrations it is possible to determine whether accommodation needs to be increased or relaxed.

Spherical aberration

With optical systems, including the eye, an aperture stop (iris) produces an edge effect at the pupil, resulting in a change in focal length. Rays of light in the centre of the pupil will be focused on the retina, whereas rays affected by the edge effect will come to a focus before reaching the retina (Figure 17.4). An optical system with spherical aber-

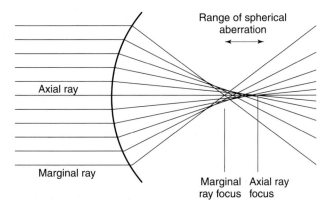

Figure 17.4 *Spherical aberration. When the pupil widens, spherical aberration increases, resulting in defocusing of the image. The location of the aberrant images is found anterior to the retina, in the same region as the uncorrected myope.*

ration has no point where all the rays intersect to produce a classical focal point. The dispersion of focal lengths due to spherical aberration is directionally proportional to the square of the aperture height, i.e. spherical aberration worsens as the pupil gets larger. This in part reduces image quality in the eye in night conditions.

DEFECTS AND CORRECTION OF FOCUS

There are four types of focusing defect: myopia, hypermetropia, presbyopia and astigmatism.

Myopia

In myopia, parallel rays of light are brought to a focus in front of the retina in the un-accommodated eye. This is usually due to an enlarged eyeball, from either congenital or pathological aetiology. As a result, the range of accommodation is very much reduced, with the far point becoming nearer the observer. Very frequently, myopes may find that they need corrective flight spectacles at night although their vision is adequate by day. This is due to the effect of a wide pupil at night and the concomitant loss of depth of field. For some individuals, the near and far points can be collocated. Correction of myopia is with a negative lens.

Hypermetropia

In hypermetropia, parallel rays of light entering the eye are brought to a focus behind the retina in the un-accommodated eye. Generally this is due to a hereditary cause, with the lens being closer than usual to the cornea. The range of accommodation is reduced, with the near point moving further away from the observer. Correction of this condition is with a positive lens (magnifying glass).

Presbyopia

Presbyopia is a physiological condition related to age. The lens is said to have elastomeric properties, i.e. it has both elastic and plastic properties, but with increasing age elastic tissue is lost gradually, resulting in loss of accommodation power. This causes a progressive inability to focus on near objects, similar to hypermetropia. In addition, another ageing effect is a yellow discolouration of the lens, which can result in intraocular haze when viewing light sources with a high yellow content.

Astigmatism

The refractive power of a surface is related directly to the degree of curvature of the surface. Frequently, the cornea has different degrees of curvature occurring in different planes. Therefore, dissimilar refractive power exists and the resultant image can be focused in one plane but will be out of focus in the other. This is known as astigmatism. If the maximum and minimum powers are in orthogonal planes, then the astigmatism is said to be regular. This type of refractive error is corrected with a cylindrical lens. A cylindrical lens focuses not to a point but to a line. Therefore, in order to correct astigmatism, both the power of correction and the angle to which the line is placed need to be determined.

Positioning of spectacles

The positioning of spectacles is not arbitrary. A lens placed anywhere in front of the eye will have a magnifying effect, except if the lens is placed at the front focal point of the eye, at which point the magnification factor will be unity. This means that widely different lens powers can be placed in front of each eye without affecting the image size. Contact lenses work by different means. They are worn on the surface of the cornea and are used to correct myopia by flattening out the curvature of the cornea, hence reducing refractive power.

THE DETECTION SYSTEM

Retina

The retina is divided into two layers, the retinal pigment membrane and the neural retina. The retinal pigment epithelium is the outermost layer of the retina. It lays on the choroid and contains melanin for absorption of stray light. The neural retina has five main types of photoreception and retinal image processing. Rods and cones are the light detectors, while horizontal cells, bipolar cells, amacrine cells and retinal ganglionic cells have image-processing functions. The photo-detector cells are found adjacent to the retinal pigment layer, while the image-processing cells form the innermost layer. This means that retinal imagery is degraded as it passes through the neural layer before reaching the rods and cones.

The rods are monochromatic receptors. They have no central visual function, as they are found mainly in the periphery of the retina. Rods are used in low light levels and can be sensitive to individual photons. They may, in part, be responsible for detecting object movement, but they are incapable of good image resolution. The cones provide the means of colour perception but require daylight levels of light to function, the ability improving with increasing ambient light levels. Cones are distributed universally in the retina and are responsible for the high image resolution associated with central visual function. The area of greatest cone concentration in the retina is in the macula lutea; at its centre, the fovea centralis, only cones are present. When fixating on an object, the image is centred on the fovea. There are approximately seven million cones in the retina; there are 20 times as many rods.

The retina is a concave light-sensitive screen that contains blind spots – scotomata – areas devoid of light detection. Two non-pathological scotomata are found in the retina. The anatomical scotoma (blind spot) occurs at the head of the optic nerve and subtends a small proportion of the visual field – it subtends a visual angle of five degrees and is found lateral to the point of fixation by 15 degrees. The physiological (functional) scotoma is located at the fovea and occurs when there is not enough light for this pure cone region to function.

Light and dark adaptation

The visual system is a sensitive detector for the discrimination of small differences in luminance across the retinal image (Figure 17.5). It is capable of operating over large changes in ambient illumination with a dynamic range of about 12 orders of magnitude. It has been said that this range equates to the ability to sense light from quantum levels up to tissue-damaging levels. The visual system compensates automatically and involuntarily for changes in ambient illumination level, and even a 100-fold change in luminance in daylight would go largely unnoticed by the observer. The purpose of adaptation is to keep the retinal response to visual objects constant when ambient illumination levels are changing. This does, however, break down at high light intensities.

The visual threshold is approximately 10^{-6} cd/m^2, corresponding to faint starlight conditions; the maximum limit is as high as 10^6 cd/m^2, equivalent to bright sunlight over fresh snow. Photopic, or cone, vision occurs above 1 cd/m^2; scotopic, or rod, vision occurs below 10^{-3} cd/m^2. Mesopic vision is the intermediate stage between photopic and scotopic vision, when both rods and cones function. Night driving and night flying are considered to be mesopic tasks.

When the eye adapts from photopic to scotopic conditions, dark adaptation is slow. Dark adaptation occurs in two stages, the initial stage commensurate with lowering of stimulus threshold in the cone cells and the second stage affecting the rods (Figure 17.6). The time to dark adapt is variable, as it depends on both the start and end-point luminances. The term 'dark adaptation' should be considered as a laboratory condition, because its measurement is performed in initial light levels that are bright enough to bleach a significant amount of photo-pigments while the end-point illumination level is the equivalent of the photographer's dark room. For these conditions, cone adaptation takes approximately seven minutes and full rod adaptation takes 30–40 minutes. In nature, these levels of illuminance do not usually occur, and so the time to adapt is much shorter.

Colour vision

Human colour perception is a complex topic. It can be discussed both in terms of colour stimulus based on the science of colour and in terms of colour perception based on psychophysical science. Colour sense is mediated by the cones in photopic light conditions and spatially by the rel-

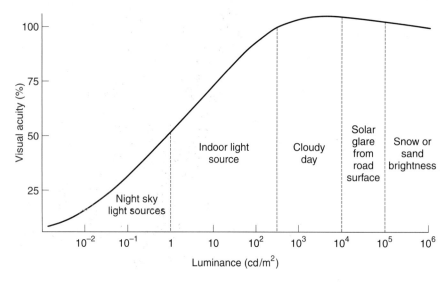

Figure 17.5 *Effect of ambient illuminance on visual acuity.*

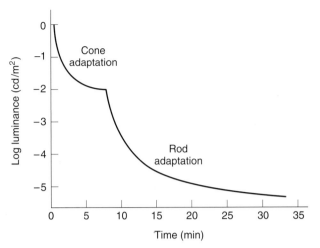

Figure 17.6 *Dark-adaptation curve.*

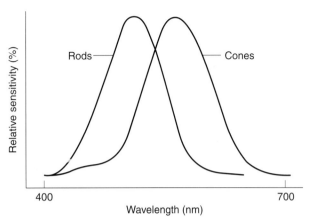

Figure 17.7 *Spectral sensitivity of the eye. Different wavelengths produce different intensities of colour. The sensitivity for the cones (a composite curve for the three classes of cone) is called the V_λ curve, with its maximum sensitivity occurring at 555 nm (yellow-green). The rods are also wavelength-sensitive but do not contribute to colour perception. The sensitivity curve for the rods is called as the V_λ' curve; its maximum sensitivity is 510 nm (blue-green). The difference in wavelength sensitivity between the rods and cones is the basis for the Purkinje phenomenon.*

ative positioning of cones in the retina. The three-receptor theory is the essential basis of the Young–Helmholtz trichromatic theory of colour vision. There are three classes of cone – red, green and blue – each with different sensitivity to a given wavelength. The cones are found in the ratio of ten red cells to ten green cells to one blue cell. The perception of colour is, in part, the relative activation of the three cone types. Cone output travels in three channels, one channel for summated brightness information and two colour channels – red-green (R-G) and blue-yellow (B-Y). The two chromatic channels have complex interactions. Some colours, e.g. brown, do not exist in the visible spectrum, and the perception of brown is the effect of colour image processing in the brain. In order to perceive all colour potential, one needs to have normally functioning R-G and B-Y channel systems. The perception of colour is complex, as it depends on a number of factors, including the hue, colour brightness, contrast and degree of saturation, which in turn are influenced by other factors.

PURKINJE SHIFT PHENOMENON

A problem with mesopic vision is that the transition from one light detector to another results in an overall change in sensitivity to visible light. When blue and red objects with the same light energy in daylight are viewed at dusk or dawn, the colour brightness of the objects appears to change. Viewing a blue object in daylight correlates to the cone sensitivity for that wavelength sensitivity for that wavelength on the V_λ curve, and as light levels continue to fall rod function begins to increase (Figure 17.7). Consequently, blue objects stimulate rods to a greater degree than cones, and so blue objects appear to glow. The reverse is true with the appearance of red objects in diminishing light levels. A red object in lighter conditions stimulates the cones more than the rods in darker conditions, and so red objects will appear darker. At dawn and dusk, this phenomenon can be

troublesome for aviators, as changing colour brightness can lead to misperceptions when judging depth.

AMBIENT RED LIGHTING

In theory, red-light illumination reduces the problem of rod desensitization before night operations and so negates the need for dark adaptation. The advantage of preserving rod vision is, in fact, illusory, as the night-flying task is in mesopic conditions. In aviation, the disadvantages of red cockpit lighting negate its use in the aviation setting. The eye loses its ability to rapidly change focus by means of chromatic aberration adjustment when the spectrum is limited from the full visible spectrum to only the red end of the spectrum. In addition, poor colour discrimination makes it difficult to interpret conventional maps. Other disadvantages include decreased accommodation cues and distortion of relative brightness of objects, which can result in errors of depth judgement and lead to visual illusions.

Defects in colour vision

In general, a colour-defective subject is one whose powers of colour discrimination between lights of different wavelengths are more limited than normal. The complete failure of colour discrimination is known as monochromatism; dichromatism is the loss of one class of cone cell. Colour-anomalous people have all three classes of cone but one class is relatively insensitive and requires more stimulation to achieve equivalent perception in the colour-normal individual. The most common defect in colour vision is red-green deficiency. People who cannot perceive either red or green merge both colours into yellows, and any differences that are perceived are due to brightness, which is not a reliable indicator for colour discrimination. Impaired or atypical colour perception can be categorized into three groups, as follows.

MONOCHROMATISM

Monochromatism is complete loss of colour sensation. There are two varieties of monochromatism – rod monochromatism and cone monochromatism. Rod monochromats have no functioning cones; the prevalence of this condition is one in 30 000. Cone monochromats possess both rods and cones, but central image processing is lost; this very rare condition has a prevalence of one in 100 000 000.

DICHROMATISM

Dichromatism is loss of function of a single colour cone. Protanopes do not have red cones; clinically, they are found to have a red-green colour defect and a perceived loss in image brightness. The prevalence is one in 100. Deuteranopes have a conjoined red-green cone with a red-green colour defect but do not suffer a loss of image brightness. The prevalence is one in 100. Tritanopes do not possess blue cones; the condition has a prevalence of one in 65 000. Only three per cent of cones in the fovea are blue, and so it can be considered that fovea-only vision is very close to being tritanopic.

TRICHROMATISM

In trichromatism, all three cone types are present in the retina, but one type of cone cell requires a greater stimulus than normal to function. Protanomalous individuals have relatively insensitive red cones and require greater red stimulus than normal; the prevalence is one in 100. Deuteranomalous trichromats have insensitive green cones and require greater green stimulus. This is the most prevalent colour deficiency in the population, occurring in one in 20 individuals. Tritanomalous trichromats have insensitive blue cones and require greater blue stimulus; it is thought to have a prevalence of about one in 4000.

As well as congenital causes of colour defects, colour sense can be lost as a result of ocular disease, drug reactions and light hazards. In addition, coloured filters placed in front of the eye can induce loss of colour sense, which is a particular concern for designers of aircraft coloured multi-function displays.

IMAGE PROCESSING

The retina contains other cell types in addition to the photo-detector cells. In human embryology, the retina develops from tissue that also forms elements of the brain, so the retina itself can be thought of as brain tissue. Retinal output can be considered as image-processed visual information, which in turn is passed via the optic nerve to the brain for higher-level processing, modelling and interpretation.

Recognition of targets is influenced by the inductive state of the retina. One part of the retina modifies the function of another part, and this is known as spatial induction. When a signal from a cone cell passes through a bipolar cell to a ganglion, an excitatory nerve from the ganglion is also activated. This increases the likelihood of an action potential in a nearby ganglion occurring. Therefore, if light falls on a specific area of the retina, specific ganglia will be stimulated. This has given rise to the mapping of the retina in terms of the receptive field of a ganglion. This lateral activation of ganglia is known as lateral summation. In the fovea, there are very small receptive fields, indicating a one-to-one cone/ganglion association. In the distal reaches of the retina, the receptive fields are much larger, signifying a larger cone/ganglion ratio. This may also account for reduced visual acuity in the retinal periphery, as a specific ganglion is managing a much larger spatial area of the retina.

When a signal from a cone passes through a bipolar cell to a ganglion, an inhibitory nerve from the ganglion can also be activated. This decreases the likelihood of an action potential occurring in a nearby ganglion. This lateral inhibition has been associated with enhanced border-contrast image processing. This would make the identification of a dark aircraft against a uniformly bright sky easier to recognize (Figure 17.9).

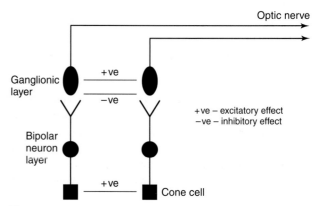

Figure 17.8 *Retinal micro-circuitry.*

DIFFERENTIATION OF MOTION

The eye makes never-ending unconscious movements, even if it is staring fixatedly on an object. This creates the problem of how to keep this moving image placed on the fovea. Objects that are constantly moving further complicate the situation. It has been postulated that the amacrine cells are involved in the process of motion detection and differentiation. Major advances in the understanding of amacrine cell function have occurred in the past few years. Most research in this area has been animal-based, but there is strong scientific opinion that it is also valid for humans. The amacrine cell is a polyaxonal cell with many axons spread across the whole retina. It receives visual information from the rods and cones and compares signals across the whole retina. If a fixated object and its background move together, then the apparent movement of both the object and its background must be due to eye movement. This could, potentially, confuse the individual with artefact object motion information, and so a terminating signal from the amacrine cell aborts the firing of the retinal ganglion cells, thus preventing retinal output of this signal. If an object moves independently of its background, then the amacrine cells perceive differentiated image movement, thereby allowing an output signal to be generated from the retina.

PERFORMANCE OF THE EYE

Contrast sensitivity

The Snellen visual acuity specifies the smallest spatial detail that can be resolved for high-contrast stimuli. It does not provide information about the ability to detect and discriminate between objects of different sizes and contrast. Sinusoidal grid patterns of different contrast against an even background are used to measure the contrast sensitivity. The human visual system varies in the amount of contrast needed to detect a grating pattern for different spatial frequencies or sizes of light and dark bars. Intermediate spatial frequencies are visible at lower contrast levels than low spatial frequencies or high spatial frequencies, and this gives an inverted U-shaped appearance to the contrast sensitivity curve. Contrast sensitivity is affected particularly by media opacities such as cataracts, corneal disease including refractive surgery, and macular disease. Certain charts may also be used to assess contrast sensitivity. These include the Vistec contrast sensitivity chart, the Bailey–Lovie visual acuity chart, and the Pelli–Robson contrast sensitivity letter chart.

Contrast-sensitivity measurement of retinal image degradation is not easy to carry out, and its effect on visual performance is difficult to quantify. A new test based on

contrast acuity assessment (CAA) has been developed to identify subjects who fall out of the normal range of visual function. This test is based on a study of modern aircraft cockpit design and has allowed a normal range of contrast acuity for aviators to perform their roles safely (Figure 17.9).

Weber's law (Figure 17.10) describes the liminal contrast as being a constant in photopic light levels. In other words, the brighter the background, the brighter the light stimulus (ΔB_ε) increment has to be for the disc to be seen. This law is true for all photopic conditions, apart from very high light levels, when the law breaks down due to excessive photoreceptor pigment bleaching. The implication of Weber's law in retinal light adaptation is to maintain the retinal response to visual objects when ambient illumination levels are changing. De Vries' law (Figure 17.10) describes liminal contrast in scotopic conditions and shows that ε varies with

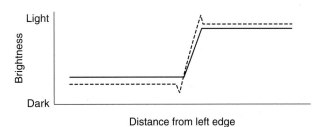

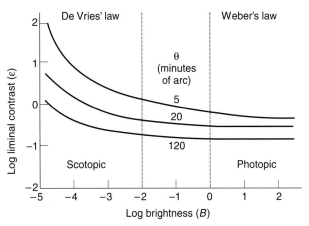

Figure 17.9 *Edge enhancement. Consider an image consisting of a bright area with a sharp border to a darker area. When the image is formed on the retina, the ganglia near the boundary and 'in the dark' will have their ganglia inhibited from the ganglia in the bright region. This has the net effect of increasing the perceived contrast of the border above that of the actual pattern.*

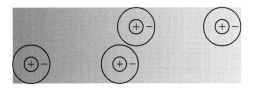

Figure 17.10 *Weber's and De Vries' laws.*

the background brightness B in an inverse square-root relationship. This means that in darker conditions, greater differences in brightness between disc and background are needed to maintain a 50 per cent detection rate.

Other experiments have looked at the relationships between disc size and liminal contrast. In general, the larger the disc, the less contrast is required to maintain the 50 per cent detection rate (Figure 17.11). The disc experiments have important implications in aviation, as contrast is an important flight safety factor, e.g. mid-air collision avoidance (much worse at night), identifying the edge of the runway in a desert strip, and design of aircraft instrumentation.

The second type of experimentation relates to the use of spatial gratings. In this case, a computer monitor is used to show a sinusoidal light- and dark-striped (grating) display. In a similar manner to the testing of hearing, the fundamental frequency of a given wave can be used to test the eye. Using different frequencies, the contrast sensitivity of the eye can be determined; this is probably the most sensitive measure of acuity. Under photopic conditions, the liminal contrast is directly proportional to the frequency of the spatial grating. In other words, the larger the spatial frequency (and, consequently, the smaller the wavelength), the greater contrast is needed to maintain a 50 per cent detection rate.

VISUAL ACUITY

Vision is a sensory outcome of integration between the refracting system, the retina and the visual pathways, including the central nervous system. The resolving power of the eye is the smallest angle of separation between two distinct points that allows the formation of two discernable images, empirically 1 min of arc. The theoretical two-point discrimination of the eye is directionally proportional to the wavelength of light and inversely proportional to the pupil radius (Rayleigh's equation). As a result, the best theoretical resolution of the eye is 0.5 min of arc (1/120 of 1 °). This is commensurate with a linear image separation of 4 μm on the retina. Since photoreceptors are approximately 1.5 μm in diameter, it supports the idea that two stimulated cones are separated by an unstimulated receptor. With line-detection acuity, the eye can resolve down to 0.5 s of arc (1/7200 of 1 °), as long as the line is longer than 1 ° of arc and there is 100 per cent contrast. This equates to the detection of a pencil-thick wire a mile away against a uniformly bright sky. Vernier acuity measures the degree of misalignment between two lines; the eye is capable of achieving a detection of misalignment at 4 s of arc (1/900 of 1 °).

The Snellen test type is the most common chart used to measure visual acuity. It bears letters constructed so that each letter subtends a total visual angle of 5 min of arc when viewed from the specified distance. Each component of the letter is separated by 1 min of arc. The chart bears letters of diminishing size, the largest having a viewing distance of 60 m and the smaller letters having viewing distances of, respectively, 36 m, 24 m, 18 m, 12 m, 9 m, 6 m and 5 m. The patient is positioned 6 m from a backlit chart. A normal eye reads the 6-m letters from a distance of 6 m and is said to have 6/6 vision. A weaker eye may be able to resolve only the larger letters, e.g. an eye that resolves the 36 m letters is said to have 6/36 vision. A normal eye would resolve the 36 m letters at 36 m. If the patient reads the chart from a different distance, the numerator of the Snellen angle is amended accordingly, e.g. 2/60 if the 60 m letter is read at 2 m.

A number of factors affect visual acuity, including ambient luminance level, spectral composition of illumination, pupil size, retinal location of the stimulus, refractive errors and pathological changes. Visual acuity improves with increasing luminance up to 10^3 cd/m², where acuity remains optimal, until 10^5 cd/m², at which point glare will start to reduce it. The relationship between Snellen acuity and contrast sensitivity is not tenuous and relates to the association between a pure frequency and a complex mix of frequencies, in the same manner as pure tone frequency relates to a complex sound. A complex sound, such as from a musical instrument, is made up of a fundamental frequency note together with a series of harmonics that are related mathematically to the fundamental. The same principle is true with vision, as a visual image can be considered as consisting of fundamental frequencies and their harmonics. Contrast-sensitivity measurement using sinusoidal gratings determines the ability to sense fundamental

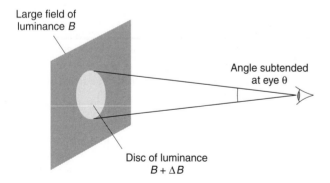

Figure 17.11   *Disc experiments. A target disc is placed against a uniform background. The size of the disc is controlled and usually defined in terms of the angle subtended at the eye. The brightness of the background, B, can be varied as can the brightness of the target disc, B + ΔB. The contrast is defined as C = ΔB/B. Liminal contrast, ε, is defined as the contrast corresponding to a 50 per cent detection rate, i.e. ε = ΔB$_ε$/B, where ΔB$_ε$ is the increment of brightness above the background brightness level seen 50 per cent of the time.*

frequencies, while Snellen acuity is founded on a square-wave pattern, i.e. the border between a black letter and the white background is a sharp distinct border in the same manner as a light/dark square wave. The Snellen chart is, in essence, the visual equivalent of the measurement of hearing with a musical instrument, i.e. the sum of the fundamental frequency and its harmonics. Despite this, Snellen acuity remains an excellent visual measure, as it is easy to perform, the results are easy to replicate, and the results relate well to overall visual function.

Visual acuity reduces with increasing eccentricity due to a number of reasons (Figure 17.12):

- The number of cones reduces with distance from the fovea.
- The number of photoreceptors per bipolar cell and retinal ganglion increases with distance from the fovea.
- Effects of spherical aberration.
- Stiles–Crawford effect.

Depth perception

Depth or distance judgement consists of two stages: the receipt of perceptual cues to depth followed by the interpretation of the cues to form a judgement of distance. The loss of any cue leads to riskier decision making, as the decision will be made with less information. There are two types of cue, monocular (psychological) and binocular (physiological). Monocular cues consist of the following:

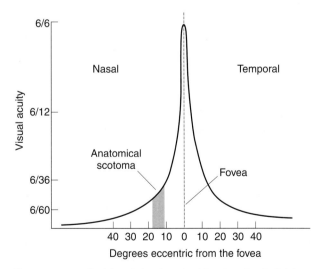

Figure 17.12 *Peripheral visual acuity. Visual acuity diminishes rapidly away from the foveal image, so the observer has to continually scan the surroundings in order to keep the image of a moving object on the fovea. The acuity found 5° eccentric from the fovea is approximately one-quarter that found at the fovea and one-twentieth that found at 20° eccentricity.*

- *Relative size:* the apparent size of an object appears to get smaller with greater distance from the observer, as the visual angle gets smaller.
- *Perspective:* the convergence of parallel lines to a point on the horizon. Classically used by artists to create the impression of depth in two-dimensional images.
- *Overlapping of objects:* suggests that the distant object is being partly hidden by a nearer object.
- *Position in visual field:* as an object moves into the distance, it appears to be closing in on the horizon.
- *Aerial perspective:* a depth cue arising from Rayleigh scattering of light in the atmosphere. As a result, similarly coloured objects in the foreground appear to be intensely coloured whereas those in the distance take on a desaturated appearance.
- *Parallax:* on viewing two objects, head movement in one direction results in the nearer object appearing to move in the opposite direction while the distant object moves with the head.
- *Motion parallax:* when an observer moves, objects near the viewer appear to move faster than more distant objects. In aviation, this explains the height cue – the blur zone – with lower altitude, there appears to be greater blurring of the approaching terrain.

The binocular cues comprise of lens accommodation, eyeball convergence and stereopsis. The eyeballs should be in the anatomical position when viewing distant objects. As an object comes closer to the observer, the eyes rotate medially, converging on to the object. The angle between the two optical axes is known as the convergence angle. As a general rule, the larger the convergence angle, the nearer the object is to the observer. Both lens accommodation and eyeball convergence are under muscular control, so afferent signals are relayed to the brain, detailing the degree of muscular tone. This information gives indirect indication of depth. The brain considers optical infinity to be anything more than 6 m away from the observer, and so accommodation and eyeball convergence are limited to within a 6-m range. In aviation, these cues are useful only inside the cockpit and in the immediate surrounds of the aircraft.

As an individual's eyes gaze on the world, they do so from slightly different positions and so have slightly different views of the world. Binocular vision relates to vision from two eyes with overlapping fields of view. Stereopsis is the exploitation of binocular vision for the purposes of three-dimensional perception (Figure 17.13). The angle subtended at an object between the two optic axes is known as the binocular parallax. The closer the observer to the object, the larger the angle of binocular parallax. When comparing the relative distances between two objects, the brain effectively is judging the difference in angle at each object. We do not understand how this is achieved. Fixating on an object places the image on both foveae, and

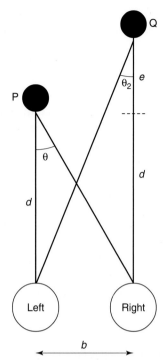

Figure 17.13 *Stereopsis. Consider a pair of eyes looking at point P. The distance between the pupils is* b *and the object P is at a distance* d *from the observer. The angular disparity between the left and right eye at P is* $\tan\theta = b/d$. *The object at point Q is at a distance* (d + e) *from the observer, and so the angular disparity* θ_2 *between each eye at point Q is* $\tan\theta_2 = b/(d + e)$. *The angle of disparity* θ_{dis} *is the difference between these two angles, i.e.* $\theta_{dis} = \theta - \theta_2$. *So,* $\theta_{dis} = (b/d) - (b/[d + e])$. *If the angle of disparity* θ_{dis} *is zero, then* e *must also be zero, and so points P and Q are equidistant from the observer. If the angle of disparity* θ_{dis} *is constant, then the larger* d *becomes, the larger* e *has to become in order to maintain the disparity. When* $d = b/\theta_{dis}$ *then* e *must equal infinity, i.e. stereopsis ceases to exist. In this case,* d *is the stereoptic range.*

objects close to the fixated object will have their images on non-corresponding parts of each retina. The brain perceives the extent (disparity) to which different images fall on non-corresponding parts of the retinas and can estimate the relative object distance. We do not know how the brain fuses these two images in order to perceive a three-dimensional image. The role of retinal image disparity in stereopsis is central to our current understanding of this process.

Taking the theoretical limit for two-point discrimination of the eye as being 0.5 min of arc and using this as the minimum angular separation the eye can resolve together with an inter-pupillary distance of 75 mm, then from Rayleigh's equation, the range of stereoscopic vision is 450 m.

About 12 per cent of the population does not have stereopsis. In part, this is related to the childhood incidence of strabismus (four per cent) and amblyopia (two to three per

cent). Stereopsis can also be compromised or lost with age. At 65 years of age, approximately a third of individuals have no stereopsis, a third have reduced stereopsis and a third retain stereoptic ability.

There are other factors that affect stereopsis and as a result reduce the range of stereopsis, including the following:

- *Poor illumination:* visual acuity reduces in darker conditions.
- *Refractive errors*, e.g. myopia.
- *Different magnification of an image presented to each eye*, e.g. with a poor optical device: magnifications less than 0.5 per cent present no problems, up to two per cent can result in eye strain, between two and five per cent can seriously degrade stereopsis, and above five per cent can result in a temporary amblyopia.
- *Different colouration an image presented to each eye:* if a red filter is placed in front of one eye and a blue one in front of the other, then the brain has difficulty in fusing both images. In addition, chromatic aberration effects give rise to different states of lens accommodation in each eye, compounding the visual confusion.
- *Different brightness of an image presented to each eye:* if the brightness of an image in each eye differs by more than ten per cent, then significant degradation in stereopsis occurs. In extremis, this can result in motion illusions, i.e. the Pulfrich effect (Figure 17.14).

AVIATION HAZARDS TO VISION

Light hazards

Glare is defined simply as an intrusive light source, irrespective of whether it is viewed directly or indirectly. Glare can reduce visual acuity and contrast sensitivity and can be considerably uncomfortable. It is classified into two types, discomfort glare and disability glare. Discomfort glare does not impair visual performance but can cause blinking, squinting and aversion and can impair individual performance, as it is distracting and fatiguing. There are three types of disability glare, each type having a significant impact on visual performance. Veiling disability glare occurs when a diffuse light source superimposes its image over the retinal image, resulting in a reduction in image contrast. A classic example of this is the reflected image of a map placed on the instrument panel in the cockpit, reducing the contrast of outside world images. Dazzle disability glare occurs when a bright glare source is imaged on an extra-foveal location, e.g. flying when the sun is low on the horizon. This glare scatters in the ocular media and strays into the retinal image at the fovea, again reducing

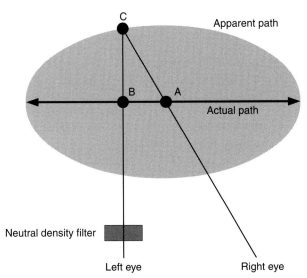

Figure 17.14 *Pulfrich effect. Consider a pendulum swinging in a straight horizontal line and viewed by an observer with a neutral density filter over the left eye. The signal from the left eye is delayed, because it has a dimmer image and so takes longer to process. When the pendulum is at A, moving from left to right, the right eye will see it in real time, at A. The left eye however, perceives the pendulum at B, as the time taken to process has image has been longer than for the right eye, even though the pendulum has moved to A. The disparity in retinal position creates the illusion that the pendulum is at C and moving in an elliptical path.*

image contrast at the point of fixation. Finally, scotomatic disability glare occurs when a brilliant light source reduces the retina's sensitivity to light, as seen with flash photography. In this case, retinal sensitivity falls rapidly during the period of light exposure and then regains its sensitivity more slowly after the exposure. Photo-stress is another term for scotomatic disability glare and its resultant retinal pigment bleaching and regeneration. The time to recover from photo-stress worsens with age.

OTHER RISKS FROM SOLAR LIGHT

Apart from light intensity, the main risk from solar light is wavelength-dependent. The energy contained within different wavelengths of light increases with shorter wavelengths; therefore, the blue end of the spectrum has the potential to be more damaging than the red end. There is more blue and UV content in the atmosphere with increasing altitude, and so aviators encounter specific risks to their vision. Wavelengths in the blue end of the visible spectrum – 400–500 nm – risk accelerated retinal ageing and have been linked with macular degeneration. Outside of the visible spectrum, long-term exposure to UV(A) – 315–380 nm – can cause cataract formation, while shorter-

wavelength UV(B) – 295–315 nm – can lead to episodes of acute keratoconjunctivitis.

PROTECTION FROM SOLAR LIGHT DAMAGE

It is recommended that either sunglasses or a helmet-mounted tinted visor be used to protect the eyes from high intensity solar light. In general, the filter (tint) needs to reduce the overall energy being transmitted through the tint to 10–15 per cent of the incident level. The overall aim is to reduce light levels at the eye to a value at which the eye can obtain maximum visual information. This system is limited, as the incident light level will always vary, so the aviator may find that the level of tint is not dark enough in very bright conditions and yet is too dark in dimmer conditions. Technologies that can dynamically change the level of tint as a function of the ambient light levels are also limited. The time taken to darken the level of tint in bright conditions is rapid, but lightening of tint when conditions darken, e.g. on entering cloud, takes much longer, thus reducing the visual performance of the aviator until the lag period has passed.

Wavelength-specific protection is also required, especially as the amount of blue light and UV radiation in solar light increases with increasing altitude. Ideally, the tint needs to reduce the transmittance of UV(A) and UV(B) to below one per cent and the blue end of the spectrum to below five per cent. Technically, this is difficult to achieve without affecting the rest of the visible spectrum, but it remains an objective in future filter development. A consequence of filtering the visible spectrum from a tint would be to affect the aviator's ability to discriminate colour and so make coloured displays potentially more difficult to read. The physical and optical properties of aircrew optical devices such as sunglasses or visors should be within International Organization of Standardization (ISO) standards; it may be advisable to consider the application of both quarter-wavelength anti-reflection coatings and anti-abrasion coatings.

Lasers

The term LASER is an acronym for Light Amplification by the Stimulated Emission of Radiation. When energy is applied to an atom, the electrons of the atom are raised to a higher energy level. Higher-energy levels are inherently unstable; consequently, the electrons fall back to a lower energy level, with the release of surplus energy as light. The emitted wavelength is dependent on the energy loss between high- and low-energy states, which in turn is dependent on the type of atom. If the atoms are contained in a tube lined with mirrors, then the emitted light can be reflected back and forth through the atoms, exciting even more light emission. The laser light is allowed out of the tube through a small aperture in one of the mirrors. There are three characteristics of laser light:

- *Monochromatic:* laser light is a single wavelength, unlike conventional light sources, which are heated and thus emit visible and IR wavelengths.
- *Collimation of beam:* the light travels in the same direction as a beam that can be focused to a tiny spot, with all the energy of the source transmitted to that area.
- *Coherence:* laser light consists of light waves emitted in phase with each other. When two waves of light are in phase, the sum of the wave amplitudes (energy) are at a maximum; if the two waves are in anti-phase with each other, then the sum of the wave amplitudes is zero and the beam has no energy. Conventional light sources emit only very small amounts of coherent light and so are less powerful.

A laser is normally described by the type of laser media (type of atom), its energy output and the type of output. The type of output can be continuous-beam (beam lasts for more than one second), pulsed-beam (small packets of beam energy released every second) or Q-switched (very short, very high-energy pulse of laser light).

Lasers are being used increasingly frequently in the aviation environment, especially in non-destructive testing of aircraft components. There is also the risk to military aviators, as lasers have the potential to be used as weapons. For damage to occur in the eye, energy must be transferred from the laser beam to the energy-absorbing tissue. The degree of tissue damage depends on the energy output from the laser and the wavelength of the laser radiation. Different tissues within the eye absorb different wavelength bandwidths; if enough energy is applied, tissue damage will result (Figure 17.15). The magnitude of damage from a laser ranges from transient photo-stress (low-energy continuous lasers), to burning (continuous or low-energy pulsed lasers), to photo-acoustic damage (high-energy pulsed or Q-switched lasers). The cornea is vulnerable to wavelengths in the far-UV(B) and UV(C)

(200–315 nm) and far-IR(B) and IR(C) (1400 nm–1 mm) spectrum and can result in either acute keratitis or corneal opacity. The lens can develop cataracts chiefly from wavelengths in the near UV(A) region (315–380 nm). The retina is at risk from visible light (380–780 nm) and near-IR radiation (780–1400 nm). An additional risk with retina-damaging lasers is that the optical components of the eye can concentrate the beam into a very small area of the retina, exacerbating the damage.

Loss of vision for even a short period of time during flight can be extremely hazardous. To protect people in the vicinity of lasers, the nominal ocular hazard distance (NOHD) has been determined for each type of laser. The NOHD is the distance along the axis of the laser beam beyond which eye exposure is acceptable, i.e. may result only in temporary photo-stress effects. Generally, protection is best afforded by distance, as energy falls in line with the inverse square law. The calculation is based on the knowledge of the limit of safe exposure, the maximum permissible exposure (MPE), together with factors such as the maximum beam output energy and the degree of beam divergence in the atmosphere. NOHD does not take into account atmospheric conditions that allow hotspots, i.e. areas of atmosphere having lens-like effects.

Additional protection is possible with the use of appropriate filters placed in front of the eyes, such as laser-protective glasses or goggles. The filter needs to attenuate the laser energy reaching the eye to a safe level, with an appropriate wavelength-matched filter corresponding to the laser. The filter substrate also has to have the mechanical characteristics to withstand the laser energy and not to be damaged itself.

Eye hazards in flight

EMPTY FIELD MYOPIA

The empty field myopia phenomenon occurs when an aviator has nothing to focus on outside of the aircraft. Flying in a fixed-wing aircraft in featureless conditions such has high altitude, over flat desert or at night can give rise to this phenomenon. It tends not to occur in rotary-wing aircraft because of the continual visual interest created by each pass of a rotor blade. The eye attempts to locate an object in the distance to focus upon but is unable to locate a target. In this situation, the ciliary muscles are unable to stay in the relaxed state and will assume some degree of contraction. As a result, the far point of the eye becomes nearer to the aviator, producing a physiological myopia, with a focal length down to 1.5 m from the aviator's eyes. This phenomenon can occur within seconds, especially if the aviator is fatigued or if the only outside object of interest is dirt on the windscreen or canopy. The pilot needs to be able to focus to infinity to scan the skies for other aircraft and other

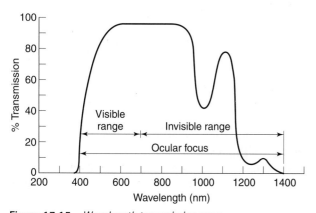

Figure 17.15 *Wavelength transmission curve.*

flight hazards. To correct empty field myopia, the aviator needs to be aware of the risk in featureless scenes and to be able to return his or her focus to the horizon. To restore focus to infinity, the pilot needs to either focus on the aircraft wingtips, if they are in view and more than 6 m away from him or her, or focus on the head-up display (HUD).

HIGH-SPEED FLIGHT

Large distances may be travelled during the time taken to perceive and react to objects appearing in the visual field, and this effectively increases the reaction time. Supersonic flight creates the greatest potential visual problems. For example, while travelling in an aircraft at 700 knots, if the pilot observes a flight hazard, in order to react appropriately, i.e. identify the problem, make a decision about the correct course of action, and then physically undertake that action, takes time and five to six seconds may have elapsed. Over this time period, a distance of more than one nautical mile has been travelled, which may not be distant enough to avoid the hazard. In addition, the need for the pilot to scan the skies for hazards is interrupted at irregular intervals as he or she checks the aircraft instruments. It takes time to change the focal length of the eyes and also to read and register the information from the flight instruments. At the previous example speed of 700 knots, this whole process, taking say three seconds, results in a flight distance of 0.5 nautical miles being travelled with the pilot not focusing on anything outside the aircraft.

DYNAMIC VISUAL ACUITY

When a target moves across the visual field, the eye must track it in order to maintain foveal fixation. The ocular pursuit mechanism is capable of maintaining steady fixation where the angular velocity does not exceed a value greater than 30 °/s. At an angular velocity of 40 °/s, visual acuity may drop to half its static value, the decrement increasing further with increasing angular velocity. This phenomenon gives rise to the 'blur zone' around the aviator, in which objects become less distinct due to their relative speed of movement.

CANOPIES AND WINDSCREENS

Most flying today is performed within a fully enclosed cockpit. As a result, windscreens and canopies need to be designed to protect the aviators from meteorological conditions whilst having the optical properties to minimize the effects of magnification, distortion, prismatic effects and multiple reflections. Many modern aircraft transparencies incorporate various coatings in order to reduce these problems. Any transparency placed in front of a pilot's eye has the potential to create visual difficulty for the pilot. These problems include multiple reflections between the canopy or windscreen and other reflective surfaces within the cockpit, e.g. HUD, mirrors, helmet visor and spectacles. In addition, any light traversing a medium will result in light scatter, especially if the surface is dirty or oil-stained. This can give rise to image distortion and glare. Precipitation, especially rain, can be troublesome, as a rain-swept windscreen can act like a lens. The image distortion through a rain-swept windscreen occurs more readily at higher air speed. The lens effect results in objects appearing closer than they are, giving the pilot the tendency to undershoot on a visual landing approach.

Visual illusions

The most important visual illusions, such as the Coriolis effect and oculogravic and oculogyric illusions, are discussed in Chapter 28. Autokinesis is an illusion that would appear to be attributed solely to the eyes. When a single light source is watched against a dark background, such as the night sky, after a short period the light source will start to wander spontaneously, even if it is a stationary source. The movement observed can be linear, circular or elliptical, but how it moves appears to be constant for a given individual. The cause of this is phenomenon is unknown, but there is conjecture that involuntary eye movements produce an apparent motion of the image on the retina.

Flicker effects, such as those produced by helicopter rotor blades and strobe lighting systems, can lead to systemic problems in susceptible aviators. For most people, flickering acts as a distraction, but occasionally it can cause headaches, dizziness or nausea. Most significantly, and least commonly, flicker can induce epileptiform episodes. Flicker photo-stimulation can induce seizures, especially if the flicker occurs at a frequency between 5 and 20 Hz. The maximal frequency for photo-induced epilepsy is 12 Hz. The strobe lighting used in aircraft anti-collision light strobes at the much slower rate of around 1 Hz is safe. The incidence of photo-induced epilepsy is relatively small, as it affects only approximately five per cent of epileptic people. Normal medical screening procedures for epilepsy before flying training normally preclude such individuals from controlling an aircraft in the first place.

Mechanical hazards

BIRD-STRIKE

Bird-strikes are a demanding hazard in low-altitude aviation. Approximately 95 per cent of bird-strikes occur below 750 feet above mean sea level and usually result in the bird being ingested into an engine intake or colliding with the airframe. Sixteen per cent of bird-strikes result in a collision with the canopy or windscreen. The canopy or windscreen transparency needs to be made of a substrate capable of withstanding these considerable forces. However, to prevent bird penetration absolutely would be very costly in terms of weight, manufacture and optical degradation. The amount of energy lost as a result of a bird penetrating a windscreen is significant, and windscreen design does impart a considerable amount of protection for the aviator. That said, not all of the energy is lost, and so another protection layer is required for the pilot, particularly those involved in low-altitude high-speed flight, such as military aircrew. The most common solution is the use of a helmet-mounted visor to protect the eyes from blunt trauma. Visors are generally made from 3 mm polycarbonate material. Polycarbonates have a very high tensile strength and can withstand very high forces. Visors generally cover most of the area of the face not protected by an oxygen mask. The combination of visor and mask gives almost full-face protection from blunt injury. The helmet must be fitted properly to the individual, and the gap between the inferior edge of the visor and the upper edge of the oxygen mask must be minimized in order to reduce the risk of penetration through to the aviator.

Aerodynamic blast protection

With high-performance fast-jet aircraft, the risk of high-speed ejection is always present. On ejection, the head may be subject to very high aerodynamic forces, risking both acceleration injury and blunt trauma to the eyes. The helmet-mounted visor, as currently used by the Royal Air Force (RAF), is designed to withstand blast winds up to 650 knots indicated air speed (IAS). Again, it is vitally important that the helmet, visor and oxygen mask are appropriately fitted, so as to remain in place with ejection.

Canopy fragmentation devices

With the initial stages of ejection from a fast-jet aircraft, the canopy needs to be removed and in some cases fragmented. Miniature detonating cord (MDC) is an explosive material, lined on its internal surface by a layer of lead that is designed to fragment the canopy. On detonation, the lead directs the explosion through the substrate of the canopy, shattering it and ensuring that downward explosive forces towards the aviator are limited. A consequence of this design is that the explosion creates enough heat to melt the lead, which can then fall on to the aviator. This results in lead splatter to unprotected skin and eyes, risking penetrating eye injury in particular. Linear cutting cord has a very similar mechanism to MDC but is designed to cut the canopy (usually in half), which then falls away. This system has the same risk of lead splatter to the eyes. Canopy jettison rocket motors use rockets to remove the intact canopy

away from the fuselage. This system risks rocket propellant splatter, which may include a burns risk. A polycarbonate helmet-mounted visor together with oxygen mask provides adequate protection, and it is recommended that the visor is down and the eyes closed for ejection.

NIGHT–VISION GOGGLES

Given the poor-resolution qualities of the naked eye at night, systems were designed to improve visual quality, primarily to gain military advantage. Night-vision goggles (NVGs) are helmet-mounted electro-optical image intensifiers used primarily in military aviation. They operate by amplifying light and near-IR radiation by means of an image-intensifier tube and present the image on a phosphor display (Figure 17.16). The perceived ambient brightness through the goggles is dependent on the level of near-IR illumination in the night sky. IR content varies according to the presence and height of the moon and starlight and is reduced by the presence of clouds and adverse weather conditions. There are also incandescent light sources on the ground from cultural lighting (e.g. roads, railways, housing), contributing to the overall illumination level in addition to ground-reflected night-sky illuminance. Different terrains will reflect different amounts of illuminant energy back into the sky, e.g. flying over soil will appear darker than flying over sand or snow.

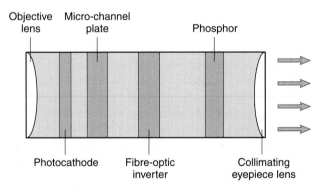

Figure 17.16 *Schematic diagram of night-vision goggles tube. Night radiation is focused on a gallium-arsenide photocathode with an objective lens. The radiant energy is capable of ejecting an electron from the inner surface of the photocathode. The photocathode is most sensitive to wavelengths in the near-infrared (IR) region and the red end of the visible spectrum. The electrons are then accelerated in an electric field towards the multiplying element, the micro-channel plate (MCP). There are millions of micron-sized channels at a small angle of inclination to the electron beam. As an electron enters a channel, it hits a channel wall and dislodges another electron. This multiplying effect occurs along the full length of the channel and is capable of generating 100 000 electrons from the incident electron.*

The NVG phosphor output is a narrow band in the green part of the spectrum (530–545 nm), and the illumination level is commensurate with mesopic vision. Most goggles are focused to absolute infinity, but some can be nearer focused. As a result, the aviator needs to view under the goggles to view cockpit instrumentation. There must be adequate lighting in the cockpit for the aviator to see instrumentation, but this light must be compatible with the use of NVGs. No amplification is desired from cockpit lighting sources, since this would give rise to an intra-cockpit glare source, thus negating any advantage gained by using NVGs. NVG-compatible lighting systems (Figure 17.17) use a narrow band of green wavelengths, either by filtered white light bulbs or electroluminescent panels. The NVG photocathode is largely insensitive to green wavelengths, and the cones have maximum sensitivity, thereby maximizing both direct and NVG viewing.

With NVG, visual acuity is 6/9 at best, and the field of view is limited to a circular 40 degrees, compromising normal daytime visual assumptions. There are continuing developments in NVG technology, improving both visual acuity and field of view. However, a significant risk to the aviator is the loss of visual cues to depth perception, with a resultant overestimation of clearance distances. Stereopsis appears to be degraded significantly, while some of the monocular cues are lost. After prolonged use, some aviators have 'magenta'-coloured after-effects on returning to white-light conditions. This is believed to be a result of desensitization of the green-sensitive cones, resulting in the perception of the complementary colour on viewing white objects. This effect is transient and normal colour vision returns.

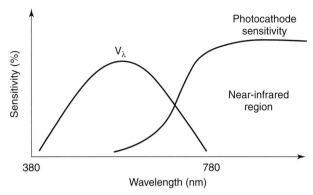

Figure 17.17 *Night-vision goggles-compatible lighting. V_λ represents the cone sensitivity curve.*

mounted sensors can be shown. Presently, monocular systems predominate, which can create additional problems with depth information, visual field loss and binocular rivalry. Binocular rivalry occurs when there is competition between the two disparate images to each eye, and the aviator may have to learn how to focusing of attention in order to switch from one view to the other. Binocular systems are under development, but there are technological difficulties in fusing the two images. As a result, bi-ocular systems that present the same image to each eye could be used. These systems do not address the issue of loss of depth information, as a stereoptic image is not produced.

HELMET-MOUNTED DISPLAYS

Aircraft instrumentation is displayed primarily either on the instrument panel or on an HUD, but the latest technologies have allowed for instrumentation to be displayed on a helmet display visor. Both colour and monochromatic displays helmet-mounted displays (HMD) are currently in use, coupled with head-tracking systems to provide a head-stabilized display. As well as aircraft status displays, both near- and far- (thermal) IR imagery from aircraft-

FURTHER READING

Abrams D. *Duke-Elder's Practice of Refraction*, 10th edn. London: Churchill Livingstone, 1993.

Davson H. *Physiology of the Eye*, 5th edn. London: Macmillan, 1990.

Falk DS, Brill DR, Stork DG. *Seeing the Light: Optics in Nature, Photography, Colour, Vision and Holography.* New York: John Wiley & Sons, 1986.

Gregory RL. *Eye and Brain: The Physiology of Seeing*, 5th edn. Oxford: Oxford University Press, 1998.

Olveczky BP, Baccus SA, Meister M. Segregation of object and background motion in the retina. *Nature* 2003; **423**: 401–8.

Wilson J, Hawkes JFB. *Optoelectronics: An Introduction*, 2nd edn. London: Prentice Hall, 1988.

18

Spatial orientation in flight

ALAN J. BENSON

INTRODUCTION

The ability of humans to sense or, more correctly, to perceive orientation in three-dimensional space depends on a learned ability to interpret the continuous input of signals from many sensory receptors (Figure 18.1). Some of these receptors are grouped together to form a specialized sense organ, such as the eye or the vestibular apparatus of the inner ear. Others are distributed more generally in the body and are found in the skin, capsules of joints and supporting tissues. The 'seat of the pants' (i.e. the gluteal area) is not endowed with any special sensory receptors; among

aviators, however, this phrase has come to mean not only cutaneous sensations but all non-visual sensory mechanisms that contribute to the perception of spatial orientation in flight.

In our natural environment, i.e. when standing, sitting or moving about on the ground, adequate and accurate perception of the spatial orientation of our own body (ego-orientation) relative to the immediate surroundings is achieved readily by the use of visual cues. These cues, along with those from non-visual receptors, also allow the sensing of bodily position, attitude and motion relative to a stable frame of reference, namely the surface of the Earth

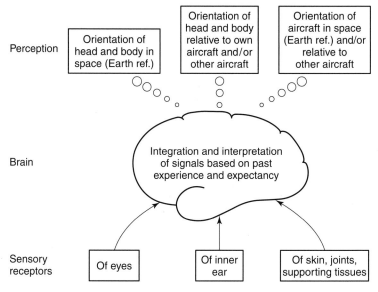

Figure 18.1 *Diagram showing the sense organs used by humans to determine spatial orientation and components of perception of spatial orientation in the flight environment.*

and the gravitational vertical. In flight, the perceptual task is somewhat more complicated, for the aviator's immediate surrounding is the aircraft, which has a changing orientation relative to the Earth's surface and to the vertical (Figure 18.2). The cues that allow the aviator to perceive orientation of self with respect to the aircraft are very strong; part of the aircraft is nearly always visible and the aviator is in physical contact with aircraft structures. This close perceptual bond means that the pilot's appreciation of the orientation of his or her own body in space is rarely separated from the perception of the orientation of the aircraft: the pilot and the aircraft are as one. The motion and attitude of the aircraft, as indicated by cockpit instruments, are perceived by the pilot as motion and attitude of both the aircraft and self. Similarly, signals from the inner ear that signal attitude and motion of the head are perceived as attitude and motion of both self and the aircraft.

Accurate perception of aircraft orientation, which is essential if adequate control of the aircraft is to be achieved, is dependent primarily on the correct interpretation of visual cues, whether obtained from outside the aircraft or from cockpit instruments. These visual cues can be supported by information from non-visual sense organs, although in normal flight operations these play a subservient, but not insignificant, role in the correct perception of aircraft orientation and contribute to the pilot's dynamic control, particularly in high-performance aircraft.

VISION

As noted above, the visual system is of prime importance in spatial orientation. Although the eye is a single sense organ, it is now recognized that functionally there are two visual systems – or, more precisely, two modes of processing spatially distributed visual information: the focal mode and the ambient mode. In everyday life, it is the ambient visual system that is used to determine our orientation to our surroundings, usually without conscious awareness of the visual cues employed. Ambient vision is mediated by relatively large stimulus patterns in the peripheral visual field and is relatively uninfluenced by the brightness or optical quality of the image. Indeed, the ambient visual system is part of what may be termed an ambient orientation system, for there is convergence at centres within the brain of signals from the peripheral retina with those from vestibular and somatosensory receptors signalling body orientation and movement. In contrast, the focal visual system is concerned with object recognition and identification. It requires the resolution of relatively fine detail of the visual image and, hence, is best represented in the central visual fields (fovea and parafoveal areas of the retina). The information processed by this visual system is usually well represented in consciousness and can be critically dependent on image quality.

The distinction between focal and ambient vision is important when considering the role of vision in determining spatial orientation in flight. When there is good aerial visibility and a clearly defined horizon (visual meteorological conditions, VMC), the pilot employs his or her ambient visual system for spatial orientation. The task requires little conscious processing, as it is but an extension of the way in which spatial orientation is achieved in normal everyday life, a process that is well entrenched from experience since early childhood. However, when reliable ambient cues are degraded or absent, as when flying in cloud or at night (instrument meteorological conditions, IMC), the aviator must determine the orientation of the aircraft from flight instruments. These symbolic displays require focal vision, for they have to be scanned, read and interpreted. The task has to be learned and involves considerably greater cortical processing than when external ambient visual cues are employed. Pilots acquire considerable skill in the use of flight instruments; with experience,

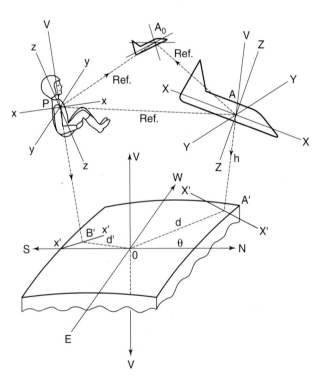

Figure 18.2 *Spatial references used during orientation in flight. The pilot has been separated from the aircraft to emphasize the fact that perception of the attitude of the aircraft relative to the gravitational vertical is determined by the pilot's perception of his or her own attitude relative to the vertical and the orientation of the body with respect to the aircraft. Correct orientation also depends on the correct perception of the height of the aircraft above the surface of the Earth, of the heading of the aircraft and of the projected position of the aircraft on the surface of the Earth, with respect to known coordinates.*

the task is achieved without undue obtrusion in consciousness. Nevertheless, by necessity, it involves the focal system, which is not the 'natural' orientational mechanism; as such, this is more susceptible to impairment. Spatial disorientation is thus more likely to occur during flight in IMC than when external visual cues are unambiguous (as in good VMC) and are processed by the ambient visual system.

Ambient visual cues, although allowing the aviator to sense the attitude and change of attitude of the aircraft in pitch and roll, in general provide inadequate cues for the perception of distance, such as altitude and height above the ground. Nor do they give good cues about derivatives of distance, such as air speed and rate of climb/descent. It is necessary for information about these variables to be provided by flight instruments, which have to be scanned and, hence, processed by the focal visual system. Traditionally, information about attitude, air speed, altitude, etc. is presented on separate instrument dials, but more spatially integrated displays that can be scanned more quickly are now more prevalent. These may be located below the cockpit coaming – a 'head-down display' – or on a fixed transparency through which the pilot can view the scene ahead – a 'head-up display'. Head-mounted displays allow the pilot to see essential flight information in the extreme head positions required in air combat.

The focal visual system is also involved in the judgement of distance, a task that is of critical importance during low-altitude ('nap of the Earth') flight and during approach and landing. One cue for distance perception is the retinal image size of an observed object, although for this to be of value the observer must have prior knowledge of the size of the surface feature (e.g. building, tree, aircraft, runway) for the percept to be correct. Errors occur when the observed object is larger or smaller than expected. Other monocular cues employed in distance perception are geometric and aerial perspective, overlapping contours and displacement parallax. Binocular cues of stereopsis mediate the perception of relative distance, i.e. one object is in front or behind another, at distances of up to about 60 m but are only of value for the perception of the absolute distance of objects that are about 10 m or less away from the observer.

THE VESTIBULAR SYSTEM

The vestibular apparatus is about the size of a pea, and yet within this small volume are sensory receptors that are stimulated by angular accelerations as low as $0.5\,°/s^2$ ($0.9\ mrad/s^2$) and linear accelerations of less than $0.01\ g$ ($0.1\ m/s^2$). In form and function, the vestibular apparatus may be divided into two parts – although not without reason is it called the labyrinth. The semicircular canals contain the receptors responding specifically to angular accelerations; the sac-like utricle and saccule house the otolith organs – the specialized receptors of linear acceleration. Figure 18.3 shows the arrangement of the membranous structure that forms the vestibular apparatus. There are three ducts – the semicircular canals – which open into the sac of the utricle. Below and in connection with the utricle lies the saccule. The membranous labyrinth is filled with a watery fluid, the endolymph, and is attached securely within the labyrinthine cavity of the petrous temporal bone. The space between the membranous labyrinth and bone is occupied by perilymph, a fluid of low viscosity that is like endolymph but with a different ionic constitution. Because the membranous labyrinth is coupled firmly to the skull, it experiences the same angular and linear accelerations as those at the head and, by virtue of the inertial properties of the sensory apparatus, it can signal angular and linear movements of the head.

The semicircular canals

The three membranous ducts are roughly semicircular and lie in bony canals having an internal diameter approximately four times that of the duct itself. Perilymph fills the space between duct and canal. Each semicircular duct has a swelling, the ampulla, where the sensory cells are congregated in a ridge, the crista. These cells have many hair-like projections arising from them and are covered by a gelatinous structure, the cupula. As shown in Figure 18.4, the cupula fills a cross-section of the ampulla and can be considered as a watertight swing-door that is deflected by movement of the endolymph within the membranous duct by the resulting difference in pressure across it. The activ-

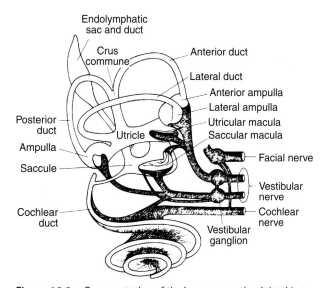

Figure 18.3 *Representation of the inner ear on the right side to show the relative positions of the semicircular canals and the utricular and saccular macula.*

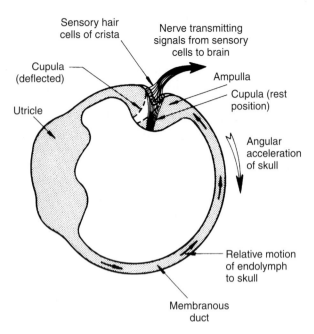

Figure 18.4 *Diagram showing how the cupula is deflected by an angular acceleration in the plane of the semicircular duct. The ring of endolymph, because of its inertia, resists angular acceleration, and a force is exerted that deflects the flexible cupula.*

ity of the sensory cells is determined by the bending of the hair-like processes, which in turn is dependent on the position and movement of the deformable cupula.

The sensory cells in the ampulla of each semicircular canal are maximally stimulated by an angular acceleration in the plane of the canal. As the three semicircular canals on each side of the body are arranged approximately at right-angles to each other (Figure 18.5), then an angular

acceleration in any plane will always stimulate the sensory cells of at least two 'canals'. The canals work as functional pairs in a push–pull type of configuration. The two horizontal canals (l in Figure 18.5) work as a pair and sense angular motion in yaw. The vertical canal pairs lie at 45 degrees to the conventional roll and pitch axes, so that the anterior (av) canal of one side works in conjunction with the posterior (pv) canal of the opposite side. Although this arrangement does not correspond with the orthogonal pitch and roll axes in which the aviator conventionally senses and appreciates angular motion, the brain is well able to sort out the signals from these three pairs of canals in order to allow accurate perception of the plane, direction and magnitude of an angular movement, provided the movement is within the dynamic range of the sensory system (i.e. the end organ and central neural processing).

The way in which the sensory receptors of the semicircular canal provide information about angular motion of the head may best be understood by considering what happens when the head is turned suddenly (Figure 18.4). During such a movement the semicircular canals and the whole of the membranous labyrinth will move with the head, but in those semicircular ducts that lie in the plane of the angular movement the rings of endolymph will tend to remain in their original position because of their inertia. Thus, during angular acceleration, a force will develop between the cupula and its associated ring of endolymph. The cupula will be deflected and the activity of the sensory cells altered. During normal head movement, in which angular acceleration is followed shortly by deceleration, the dynamics of the hydromechanical system are such that the cupula deflection and the associated signal from the sensory cells closely match the angular velocity of the head. Although the effective stimulus is the angular acceleration

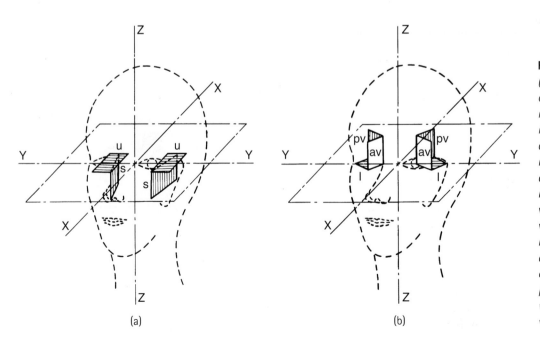

(a) (b)

Figure 18.5

(a) Approximate planes of the otolithic maculae, where u and s identify the utricular and saccular maculae, respectively. (b) l, av and pv identify the horizontal, anterior vertical and posterior vertical canals, respectively. X, Y and Z are the principal axes of the head; the XY plane is horizontal when Z is Earth-vertical.

of the head and not its velocity, the semicircular canal acts as a rapidly responding rate-of-turn transducer. Indeed, it works well for the type of head movements made in normal life on the ground. It has a good frequency response (up to at least 10 Hz), and so it is able to respond accurately to the rapidly changing angular motions of the head that occur during normal locomotor activities, such as walking, running and jumping, as well as to quick voluntary movements of the head.

The semicircular canals provide accurate information about angular movements of the head in the natural environment. Errors of transduction occur, however, when the speed of rotation is held steady for several seconds or when the rate of turn increases or decreases at a steady rate (i.e. a constant angular acceleration). In order to illustrate how the semicircular canals provide erroneous information, consider their response to a prolonged rolling or spinning manoeuvre in flight (Figure 18.6). Before the pilot begins a roll, the cupulae of the semicircular canals are in their neutral positions, provided that the aircraft has been in a straight and level flight for half a minute or more. As soon as the roll begins, the cupulae of the semicircular canals in the plane of the roll motion will be deflected by the angular acceleration in the roll axis and will generate a signal that reflects accurately the increasing angular velocity in roll. As soon as the rate of roll becomes constant, the cupulae of the stimulated canals begin to return to their neutral position, because there is no longer any angular acceleration and, hence, no deflecting force. The rate of return of the cupulae and the decay of the evoked sensation of turning are determined primarily by the hydrodynamic properties of the canal–cupula–endolymph system. Typically, in a roll at,

say, 100 °/s (2 rad/s), the sensation of roll dies away in some 10–15 seconds. Thereafter, roll at a constant rate can continue indefinitely without any sensation of angular motion in roll being engendered by the semicircular canals, provided the position of the head with respect to the axis of rotation is not altered. If, after rotating at a constant rate for 20–30 seconds, the pilot recovers from the roll, there is an angular acceleration in the opposite direction to that which occurred on entering the roll. The cupulae of the 'roll-axis' canals will be deflected and will signal turning in the opposite direction, with an intensity equal to the change in roll velocity of the aircraft. But once the aircraft is in straight and level flight, the angular acceleration is zero and there is no inertial force to deflect the cupulae, so they return slowly to their normal positions. The lack of information about rolling at a constant rate, as well as the erroneous signal of rolling in the opposite direction on recovery from a constant rate of roll, is brought about entirely by the hydromechanical properties of the semicircular canals. These are normal physiological responses.

CROSS-COUPLED (CORIOLIS) STIMULATION OF THE SEMICIRCULAR CANALS

Illusory and apparently bizarre sensations also can be produced when angular movements of the head are made in an aircraft that is turning. These cross-coupled responses, due to the stimulation of the semicircular canals by the interaction of angular motion in two planes, can be analysed in terms of the Coriolis forces induced by the complex motion. However, it is conceptually much simpler to consider each canal as an angular velocity sensor

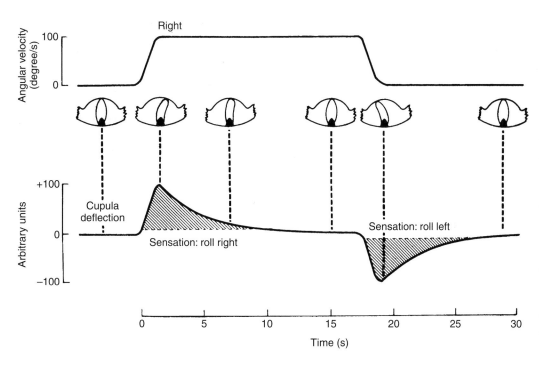

Figure 18.6
Response of the semicircular canal and sensation of turning during prolonged rotation. The upper graph shows the angular velocity during a sustained rolling manoeuvre. The lower graph shows the deflection of the cupula of a vertical semicircular canal stimulated by the angular motion.

and to analyse how the angular velocity in the plane of each canal changes with the head movement.

As an initial simplification, let us examine the response of a single, yaw-axis, semicircular canal to angular movement of the head in roll, in an individual who is rotating in yaw at a steady speed (ω_z) (Figure 18.7). Further, assume that rotation at this speed has continued for a minute or more, so that the cupula, deflected by the initial angular acceleration in yaw, has returned to its neutral position. If the head is now moved, in a second or so, from the initial vertical position through 90 degrees to the left-ear-down position, the yaw axis canal is taken out of the plane of rotation and the angular velocity in the plane of canal changes from ω_z to zero; the cupula is deflected in just the same manner as if the yaw axis rotation was stopped without any movement of the head in roll. The sensation is, therefore, one of rotation in the yaw axis of the head in the opposite direction to that of the sustained rotation. As with the normal post-rotary sensation, this dies away slowly as the cupula returns to its neutral position. Once steady-state conditions are established, if the head is returned to the vertical position the yaw canal is brought back into the plane of rotation and it 'sees' a change in velocity from zero to ω_z, which of course stimulates the receptors and gives rise to a correct sensation of rotation in yaw to the right. This subsequently dies away as rotation is at constant speed, and there is no force to deflect the cupula. In this example, a head movement through a right-angle in roll to the left was used, but the same effect is produced for such an idealized yaw axis canal by a 90-degree head movement

to the right or by movements of comparable magnitude in pitch to the nose-down or nose-up position.

If movements of a smaller magnitude are made, then the change in velocity 'seen' by the canal is also smaller. The angular velocity in the plane of the canal is $\omega_z \sin\theta$, where θ is the angle between the plane of the canal and the axis of rotation. Thus, if the head is moved through 45 degrees from the vertical (where $\theta = 90°$), then the effective stimulus (ω_e) is:

$$\omega_e = \omega_z \sin 90 - \omega_z \sin 45 = \omega_z (1 - \sin 45) = 0.3\,\omega_z$$

If the head is moved from a left-ear-down position ($\theta = 0°$) through 45 degrees towards the vertical:

$$\omega_e = \omega_z \sin 0 - \omega_z \sin 45 = -\omega_z \sin 45 = 0.7\omega_z$$

Now consider not one canal but three canals. Although in life the vertical canals do not lie in the pitch and roll axes of the skull, the brain is able to resolve the rotation transduced by these receptors into these orthogonal axes, so it is justifiable to represent all six canals as three orthogonal canals in the pitch, roll and yaw axes of the head. Figure 18.8 represents the angular velocity in the plane of each canal when the head is moved in roll from the vertical to the left-ear-down position while rotating at a steady speed in yaw. During the head movement, the roll axis canal 'sees' the rise and fall of angular velocity in roll (ω_z); this movement is executed within a few seconds, so the stimulus is transduced correctly by the receptors. The yaw axis

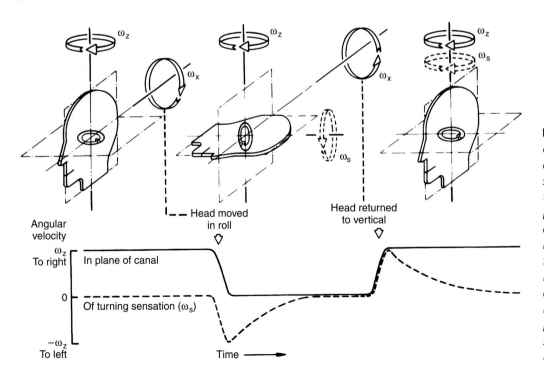

Angular velocity
ω_z To right
In plane of canal
0
Of turning sensation (ω_s)
$-\omega_z$ To left
Time

Head moved in roll
Head returned to vertical

Figure 18.7 *Cross-coupled stimulation of an idealized semicircular canal in the transverse (xy) plane of the head. An angular head movement in roll (ω_x) from the vertical to the left-ear-down position during sustained rotation in yaw (ω_z) produces an illusory sensation in the orthogonal axis.*

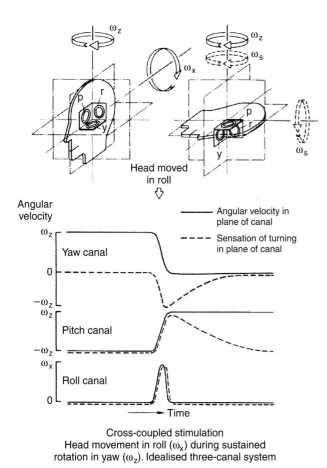

Cross-coupled stimulation
Head movement in roll (ω_x) during sustained
rotation in yaw (ω_z). Idealised three-canal system

Figure 18.8 *Examples of cross-coupled stimulation produced by head movements in roll (a, b) and in pitch (c) during sustained rotation in yaw (ω_z). Simplification is afforded by the representation of the semicircular canals by three orthogonal canals that lie in the pitch, roll and yaw axes of the head. Note how in each example the illusory sensation is orthogonal to the axes of the two imposed angular movements.*

canal is taken out of the plane of rotation and 'sees' a velocity change of ω_z, while the pitch axis canal is brought into the plane of rotation and its receptors are stimulated by the velocity change, also of magnitude ω_z. The sensation evoked by the 'stopping' stimulus to the yaw canal and the 'starting' stimulus to the pitch canal are, with respect to the skull, rotation in yaw to the left and forward rotation in pitch. The presence of gravity, however, allows the individual to perceive these sensations of angular motion in an Earth reference system rather than a head reference system, so the signal from the pitch canal is reported as an increase in the rate of rotation about the vertical (z) axis, while the yaw canal signal is sensed as a pitching motion about a y body axis.

After the head movement, the sensations of yaw and pitch die away as the deflected cupulae return to their neutral positions, although characteristically the distracting and illusory sensation of pitching forward dies away more

quickly than that evoked by a simple stopping stimulus to the canals without movement of the head. The principal reason for this accelerated decay is the absence of correlated information from the canals, which signal rotation in pitch, and from the otoliths, which signal no movement of the head with respect to gravity. This conflict between canal and otolithic cues, whilst bringing about a more rapid attenuation of the illusory sensation, is disturbing and is a cause not only of disorientation but also, if repeated, of motion sickness.

A head movement in roll from 45 degrees right to 45 degrees left while rotating at a steady speed (ω_z) about the z body axis may be shown to be a potent stimulus to the pitch axis canal. When the head is in the tilted position, both the yaw and pitch canals 'see' an angular velocity of $0.7\,\omega_z$, but as the head is moved in roll (ω_x) the yaw canal is brought fully into the plane of rotation and then out of it again to an effective velocity of $0.7\,\omega_z$ when the head is tilted 45 degrees to the left. There is no overall change in angular velocity, so there is no sustained cupular deflection. However, the pitch axis canal receives a stimulus of $2 \times 0.7\,\omega_z$ as it is taken from $0.7\,\omega_z$ in the pitch-back direction to $0.7\,\omega_z$ in the pitch-forward direction. There is, thus, a strong stimulus in the pitch-forward direction of greater magnitude than could be achieved by simply stopping rotation from a speed of ω_z in the pitch axis.

As a further example, consider the nature of the stimulus to the semicircular canals when the head is moved in pitch during rotation about the z-axis. This movement takes the yaw axis canal out of the plane of rotation and brings the roll axis canal into the plane of rotation. The dominant illusory sensation is thus one of rotation (roll) relative to gravity, due to the effective deceleration of the yaw axis canal.

The foregoing analysis shows that the principal effect of a head movement in one axis during rotation about another orthogonal axis is to produce an illusory sensation of rotation in the third orthogonal axis. It should be emphasized that the effects of dynamic cross-coupling are not due to the presence of endolymph flow in two canals 'inducing' flow in the third, as is suggested in some texts, but to a change in the orientation of the canals with respect to the axis of the sustained rotation. It is important, also, to recognize that the false sensations associated with cross-coupling arise because the imposed rotation is sustained, and that the cupulae of the canals in the plane of the steady turn have had time to return to their neutral positions. When a head movement out of the plane of rotation is made during deceleration from a sustained turn, the erroneous sensations are even more potent and disturbing than when the same head movement is made during the sustained rotation. In contrast, head movements made during the initial few seconds of the start of rotation in another axis do not give rise to inappropriate sensations because the time course of the rotational stimuli fall within the normal dynamic range of the semicircular canals. Each canal correctly transduces the angular velocity to which it is exposed, so both the imposed rotation and the angular motion of the head are sensed correctly.

THE OTOLITH ORGANS

Two endolymph-filled sacs, the utricle and saccule (see Figure 18.3, p. 295), lie below the semicircular ducts and contain plate-like congregations of sensory cells, the maculae (Figure 18.9). These cells, like those found in the ampulla, have many hair-like projections, which, when deflected, alter the activity of the sensory cells. In both the utricular and saccular maculae, the cells are grouped together in an irregular saucer-shaped area and are covered with a gelatinous layer, the outer surface of which is invested with small calcium carbonate crystals. In life, this has the appearance of a white stony plaque and is called the otolithic membrane, hence the common name for these specialized sense organs – otoliths. Because the otolithic membrane has a density nearly three times as great as that of the endolymph that fills the utricle and saccule, the sensory hairs are bent as the attitude of the head alters relative to the force of gravity (Figure 18.10). Figure 18.10 also shows how an imposed linear acceleration of the head acting in a plane parallel to that of the otolith organ (i.e.

acting in shear) will, by virtue of the inertial mass of the otolith membrane, cause displacement of the membrane, deflection of the cilia of the sensory cells and an alteration of their neural activity. Movement of the otolith membrane, unlike movement of the cupula, is not damped heavily, and so the otolith organs are, in effect, transducers of linear accelerations of the head.

There are two otolith organs on each side of the head. Those of the utricle lie in an approximately horizontal plane when the head is upright, and those of the saccule lie in a vertical plane (see Figure 18.5, p. 296). The sensory cells in each macula have an organized pattern of directional sensitivity, which allows the neural resolution and perception of the direction and intensity of the linear acceleration of the head, provided the time course and intensity of the stimulus are within the dynamic range of the otolith sensory system. Figure 18.10 shows that the effective stimulus to the otolith organ, namely the acceleration acting on the plane of the macula, is similar when the orientation of the head to gravity is changed by ± 27 degrees in the pitch (sagittal) plane and when the head is subjected to a linear acceleration in the x (anteroposterior) axis of $\pm 0.5\,G_x$ that is associated with a deviation of the resultant of 27 degrees from the gravitational vertical. Normally, we can readily differentiate head tilt from a G_x acceleration, because the former is accompanied by signals from the semicircular canals that are stimulated by the

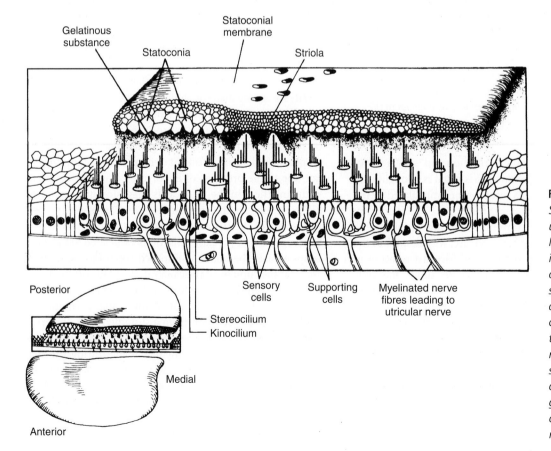

Figure 18.9
Structure of the utricular macula. The lower part of the figure is a general view of the organ. The upper part shows the sensory cells and the irregular crystalline structure of the otolithic membrane. The saccular macula differs only in shape and the grouping of the crystals of the otolithic membrane.

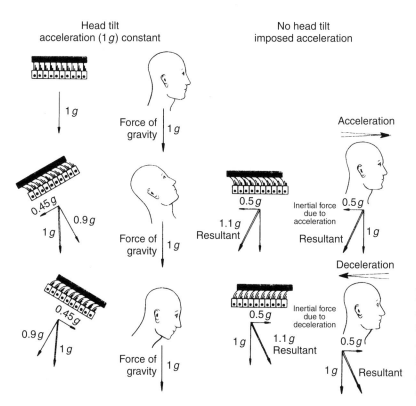

Figure 18.10 *Representation of the utricular macula, showing how the sensory cells are stimulated by displacement of the otolithic membrane (solid black) when the head is tilted in a fore–aft plane (left side of figure) and under the influence of linear accelerations (G_z) in the fore–aft direction (right side of figure).*

angular movement of the head. It is not surprising, however, that in the less familiar force environment associated with a G_x acceleration, particularly one that is sustained, the otolithic signal is interpreted as a change in the pitch attitude of the head and not just a change in linear velocity (i.e. a linear acceleration) (see also Chapter 28).

HAPTIC, KINAESTHETIC AND PROPRIOCEPTIVE SENSORY SYSTEMS

A variety of sensory endings in the skin, muscle, tendons, capsules of joints and deeper supporting tissues are stimulated by forces acting upon them and, hence, the linear accelerations to which the body is exposed. They provide static and dynamic information about the orientation of the body to the gravitational vertical as well as about the magnitude and direction of imposed linear accelerations, as when 'pulling G'. These various mechanoreceptors complement otolithic signals, although they lack the sensitivity and specificity of the vestibular receptors. Furthermore, most exhibit rapid adaptation and so are more responsive to a change in acceleration (jerk) than to one that is sustained. Like the otoliths, they are not stimulated by angular motion unless it is of a magnitude to induce a supra-threshold change in the force environment of the tissues in which the receptors are located.

The past decade has seen a heightened interest in the use of cutaneous receptors to provide the aviator with information about aircraft orientation or other important flight variables. In contemporary systems, a number of small electromechanical or pneumatic vibrators – 'tactors' – are assembled in a matrix that surrounds the torso and is held in contact with the skin by a form of jacket or vest. Information about aircraft orientation is given by the spatial configuration of tactors activated within the matrix, while rate of change of orientation can be coded by the frequency of tactor vibration or the sequential activation of tactors to give a sensation of movement. Simulator experiments have shown that when a pilot was loaded by a secondary audio task, the presence of a tactile torso display improved performance without increasing ratings of mental effort. These findings give substance to the claim that a tactile display can provide intuitive cues for spatial orientation that do not make demands on high-level processing within the central nervous system.

AUDITORY SYSTEM

Audio cues are, in general, of minor importance in spatial orientation in flight. Nevertheless, there are times when audio communications can give the pilot critical information about orientation and flight trajectory, as during approach and landing. Audio warnings, presented as either voice messages or audio tones, can inform about certain components of spatial orientation, such as airspeed and proximity to the ground, as well as many other variables contributing to situational awareness.

Audio displays have been developed to provide the pilot with information about spatial orientation. Binaurally presented signals are used to generate a three-dimensional (3-D) acoustic space in which aircraft orientation is indicated by the localization of a sound source within the envelope. It has been shown that such a 3-D audio cue can be used to maintain orientation, but the audio display, unlike a haptic display, has to compete, and at times conflict, with other information sources using the sensory modality.

THRESHOLDS OF PERCEPTION OF BODILY MOTION

Linear thresholds

Experiments carried out on subjects secured in seats that could be moved in either pitch or roll from an Earth-vertical position have shown that 75 per cent of judgements of verticality fell within ± 2.2 degrees of the vertical. This corresponds to the detection of a component of gravity acting in the transverse (xy) plane of the head that has a magnitude of 0.35 m/s². Determinations of thresholds for the detection of whole-body oscillatory motion have shown that these vary with the frequency of the stimulus. As shown in Figure 18.11, the threshold falls from about 1 m/s² at 0.01 Hz to about 0.02 m/s² at 10 Hz. The low sensitivity (i.e. high threshold) at low frequency underlies the observation that when tilted very slowly from the vertical, large deviations from an Earth-vertical attitude can develop before the tilt is detected. In one experiment involving lateral tilt (roll) from the vertical at 3 °/min, subjects on average did not detect deviation from the vertical until they had been rotated through 16 degrees.

The sensory processes mediating perception of the subjective vertical also exhibit appreciable adaptation. For example, when a person is tilted in roll from the vertical to, say, a left-ear-down position and kept in that position for 30 seconds, on being returned towards the upright the individual feels to be vertical some 10–15 degrees before reaching Earth vertical and once actually vertical feels as if tilted a few degrees towards a right-ear-down position.

Angular thresholds

Thresholds for the perception of whole-body angular motion are determined by the sensitivity and dynamics of the semicircular canals and their afferent projections, for when the axis of rotation is close to the body signals from

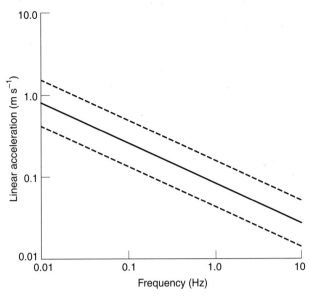

Figure 18.11   *Graph showing how the threshold for detection of whole-body linear motion varies with the frequency of the linear acceleration of the stimulus. The increase in sensitivity with frequency indicates that the sensory system transducing the stimulus is influenced by both the acceleration and the rate of change of acceleration (jerk). The interrupted lines represent ± 1 standard deviation (SD).*

the otoliths and other mechanoreceptors (gravireceptors) make little or no contribution to detection of the angular stimulus. As stated above, the physiological function of the canals is to transduce the angular velocity of the head during normal locomotor activities on the ground. Thus, for angular movements in yaw (i.e. about a z body axis) having a duration of some five seconds or less, the angular velocity must exceed a median value of 1.5 °/s for the motion to be detected. The median threshold for the detection of rotation about the x and y body axes is slightly higher at 2 °/s. When rotation is sustained, its detection is dependent upon the angular acceleration, which, typically for motion in yaw, must exceed a median value of 0.3 °/s². The way in which threshold varies with the frequency and plane of the angular stimulus is shown in Figure 18.12. Threshold changes little in the frequency domain 0.1–5 Hz but increases rapidly with decreasing frequency in the decade below 0.1 Hz. At these frequencies, the slope of the graph approaches −1 log unit/decade, a figure that implies that threshold is governed by the angular acceleration of the motion rather than its velocity, as at the higher frequencies. When the axis of rotation is Earth vertical, thresholds for the detection of motion in pitch and roll are similar to that shown for yaw. However, when the movement involves a changing orientation to gravity, as when the axis of rotation is horizontal, threshold decreases at frequencies below about 0.2 Hz. This is due to the detection by otolithic and other gravireceptors of the increasing

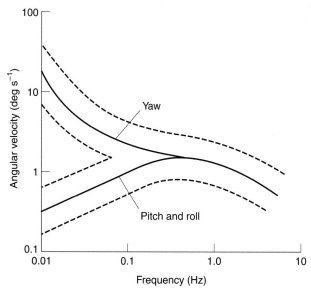

Figure 18.12 *Graph showing how the threshold for detection of whole-body angular motion varies with the frequency of the angular velocity of the stimulus. At frequencies below 0.2 Hz, thresholds for motion in pitch and roll, involving tilt from the vertical, depart from those in yaw because the displacement is detected by the otoliths and other gravireceptors. At frequencies below about 0.1 Hz, the gradient steepens and at 0.01 Hz is close to −1 logunit/decade, which indicates that threshold is determined by the angular acceleration rather than the velocity of the stimulus. The interrupted lines represent ± 1 standard deviation (SD).*

which the task of the subjects was solely to attend to and report the detection of specific whole-body motion stimuli. In flight, the aviator is rarely able to devote undivided attention to bodily sensations. Indeed, at times, workload may be so high that there is no spare capacity for processing sensory information to engender a conscious perception and awareness of changes in aircraft attitude or motion, even though the magnitude of the motion may be an order of magnitude or more greater than the sensory threshold. On the other hand, knowledge about sensory thresholds and adaptation provide a basis for understanding why so many aviators experience an erroneous perception of attitude – 'the leans' – when flying in IMC (see p. 447 in Chapter 28).

VISUAL–VESTIBULAR INTERACTIONS

So far, the discussion of vestibular mechanisms has been concerned with the sensations produced by signals from the semicircular canals and otolith organs. However, the prime function of the vestibular apparatus is the maintenance of equilibrium, an activity that is normally achieved without willed or volitional control through postural reflexes. The way in which the vestibular system controls the muscles of the body to maintain equilibrium is complex and need not concern us here, except to note the powerful control exercised over the eye muscles. The function of this vestibular reflex is to stabilize the position of the eye, relative to an object fixed in space, when the head moves. Thus, when the head is turned suddenly, the eye is reflexly moved in the opposite direction to that of the head in order to stabilize the image of the outside world on the retina (Figure 18.13). If the eyes were to move with the

amplitude of tilt from the gravitational vertical at these low frequencies.

It should be emphasized that the sensory thresholds quoted above are based on laboratory experiments in

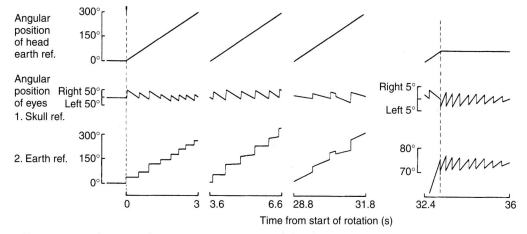

Figure 18.13 *Eye movements (nystagmus) during prolonged rotation. At the beginning of rotation, the eye movements compensate accurately for the angular motion of the head. After a few seconds, the signal from the semicircular canals no longer matches the stimulus, and eye stabilization is impaired. After 30 seconds, semicircular canal information is all but absent, the eye is not stabilized and there may be impairment of vision for objects outside the aircraft. When rotation stops, nystagmus in the opposite direction develops, which, although of low velocity (note change in scale), can degrade the pilot's vision both inside and outside the aircraft.*

head, then the retinal image would also move and vision would be seriously degraded by smearing of the image over the retinal mosaic. During natural head movements the semicircular canals correctly transduce the instantaneous angular velocity of the head, and therefore the reflex eye movements also have an angular velocity that is approximately equal to, but in the opposite direction to, that of the head. This is true irrespective of whether the motion is in pitch, yaw or roll. Vestibular stabilization is remarkably accurate, particularly for the rapid small angular movements of the head that occur during natural movements. Indeed, without a vestibulo-ocular reflex, an individual is not able to see clearly and resolve fine visual detail when walking, running or exposed to vibration.

During prolonged angular movement of the head, the compensatory eye movements take on a characteristic form (Figure 18.13). When the head begins to turn, say to the right, the eyes initially move in the opposite direction (relative to the skull) in order to compensate for the head movement. Once they have deviated about ten degrees from their initial position, they quickly flick in the direction of the turn and then begin another slow compensatory movement. In this way, the characteristic vestibular nystagmus is generated. The speed of the slow component of the eye movement – the one that is physiologically significant in the stabilization of the eye with respect to an object fixed in space – is related closely to cupula deflection. Accordingly, during a prolonged spin or rolling manoeuvre, the compensatory eye movement is correct only during the initial change in angular velocity. Once a steady angular velocity is achieved, the signal from the stimulated canals decays and with it the velocity of the nystagmus. On recovery from the manoeuvre, the semicircular canals signal rotation in the opposite direction. The information is inappropriate, as is the associated nystagmus, which serves only to degrade the vision for objects both inside and outside the aircraft.

Other than when in darkness, these eye movements are usually suppressed quickly and acuity restored, although erroneous perception of the location of a visual target can persist. A visual target (either inside or outside the aircraft) that is fixed with respect to the observer appears to be displaced in the direction and plane of the sensed turn. The magnitude of the illusion mirrors the vestibular signal, and so displacement decreases as the sensation of turning decays. This so-called oculogyral illusion also occurs at the beginning of an angular movement when the canals accurately signal the change in angular velocity. It can be elicited by very weak stimuli. Indeed, the presence of an observer-fixed visual input – whether an isolated target light or sight of an illuminated cockpit – lowers threshold for the detection of whole-body angular motion by about 50 per cent. In the oculogyral illusion, the direction of the apparent displacement always corresponds to the plane of the rotation signalled by the semicircular canals, and thus

rotation in yaw induces apparent lateral displacement, rotation in pitch vertical displacement, and rotation in roll displacement in the vertical (roll) plane. The latter may often be observed as a passenger in a civil transport when the pilot initiates a coordinated turn. As the aircraft banks, the view ahead of a cabin bulkhead or divider appears to rotate through a few degrees in the same direction as the roll motion.

Emphasis has been placed on the nystagmus engendered by the semicircular canals, but changing linear accelerations also generate eye movements, which, although compensatory in nature, are matched less accurately to the stimulus than the nystagmus produced by angular motion. When the linear acceleration stimulus is constant, as when the head is tilted on one side, a sustained deviation of the eye from its rest position may be observed. These sustained eye movements (called ocular counter-rolling) occur in the expected compensatory direction but in amplitude are only five to ten per cent of the angular deviation of the head. The inadequacy of this 'static' vestibulo-ocular reflex stresses the essential dynamic nature of the control of eye movements by the vestibular apparatus.

The apparent movement and displacement of observer-fixed visual targets also occur in response to changes in the magnitude or direction of the linear acceleration vector. These so-called oculogravic illusions have similar characteristics to oculogyral illusions insofar as the apparent displacement is in the same direction as the perceived motion. For example, during sustained linear acceleration in the line of flight, the change in direction of the resultant acceleration can engender a sensation that the aircraft is pitched nose-up (i.e. a somatogravic illusion). This is accompanied by the apparent upward movement and displacement of the visual environment, both within and outside the aircraft. Transient changes in the magnitude but not direction of the acceleration vector, as when a lift (elevator) accelerates or decelerates, can also induce an apparent movement of the visual scene within the lift in the same direction as the sensed bodily motion. This 'elevator illusion' is but a specific manifestation of the oculogravic illusion.

SPATIAL ORIENTATION: A COMPONENT IN CLOSED-LOOP CONTROL

Figure 18.14 illustrates the important elements in the sensory systems and central (brain) mechanisms involved in the perception of spatial orientation and its pivotal role in closed-loop control of the aircraft by a human operator, the pilot. Feedback about aircraft attitude and motion is provided by several sensory systems whose afferent signals are processed within the brain to yield a percept of spatial orientation. If this differs from that required, it allows the

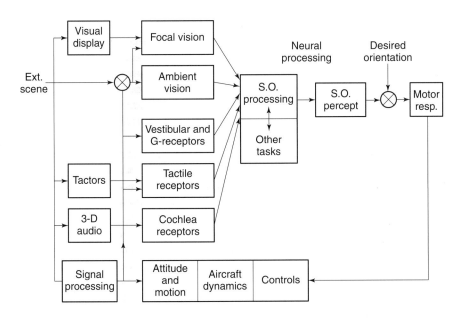

Figure 18.14 *'Black-box' model of components in the pilot's closed-loop control of aircraft spatial orientation (SO).*

pilot to initiate or modify his or her input to the aircraft controls in a manner that would reduce the disparity between perceived and desired orientation. The attitude and motion of the aircraft in response to a control input are dependent upon its aerodynamic characteristics, but if the changes are above threshold intensity they will stimulate the sensory receptors either directly or indirectly via visual, tactile or audio displays. A veridical percept of aircraft orientation should ensure correct control, but if the pilot has an erroneous percept or fails to be aware of its spatial orientation, (i.e. the pilot is suffering from spatial disorientation), then feedback is degraded and control of the aircraft may be inappropriate or even lost.

The sensory systems that provide information about spatial orientation are described in some detail earlier in this chapter, but in the context of closed-loop control distinction should be made between those systems, namely vestibular, ambient visual and haptic, that are stimulated directly by changes in aircraft attitude and motion, and those, such as focal visual, auditory and vibrotactile, in which information about orientational variables is derived from displays only after electronic or electromechanical transduction of signals from aircraft sensors. Although delay in transduction may be short, the orientational variable displayed, whether visual, tactile or auditory, is usually aircraft attitude in pitch and roll. This the aviator has, in effect, to differentiate in order to perceive rate of change of attitude, i.e. angular velocity, and so optimize manual control of a system in which stick position governs angular velocity in pitch and roll. In contrast, signals from vestibular and other mechanoreceptors provide information about angular velocity and linear acceleration to which the operator can respond with less delay than to visual cues. Consequently, these non-visual orientational

cues can contribute to the precision and stability of control, particularly in high-performance responsive aircraft. Simulator studies have shown the presence of whole-body motion cues improved the pilot's ability to cope with perturbations when flying such a 'high-gain' aeroplane. However, simulator motion did not significantly enhance control when a less responsive aircraft, such as a civil transport, was simulated.

In Figure 18.14, the complex neural processes involved in the elaboration of a percept of spatial orientation are but a part of the total processing capacity of the central nervous system. The proportion of the total resources devoted to spatial orientation is probably not fixed but varies with the neural load imposed by other tasks, i.e. workload. This variability is indicated in the figure by the arrows on the line that separates the component of processing resource devoted to spatial orientation from the total available. Part of the allocation of resources may be achieved by some form of attentional filter. There is experimental and anamnestic evidence for the restriction of the field (coning) of attention in high-workload, often emergency, situations, in which the aviator fails to be aware of certain sensory inputs. The susceptibility of a sensory modality to attentional filtering appears to depend on the complexity of the neural system involved. Thus, most examples of coning of attention relate to focal vision and hearing, whereas the perception of vibrotactile cues seems to be relatively resistant to degradation by high workload.

In the pilot/aircraft closed-loop control task, the motor output of the pilot is determined by the difference between the desired and the perceived orientation of the aircraft. Perception implies a conscious awareness of sensory events, but in routine flight, just as when driving a car, adequate control is maintained without awareness of the sensory cues that are being employed. With experience, the task is learned and is executed by subcortical pathways within the central nervous system; it has, in effect, been automated. The sensory cues employed are accessible to introspection and conscious awareness, but in the normal course of events in flight that is routine they do not obtrude upon consciousness. This is not without hazard, for when orientational cues are atypical, erroneous or deficient, the pilot may be unaware that control is compromised. In such circumstances, the pilot is, in effect, spatially unoriented, a condition that is embraced within the definition of spatial disorientation (see p. 433 in Chapter 28).

FURTHER READING

Guedry FE. Psychophysics of vestibular sensations. In: Kornhuber HH (ed.). *Handbook of Sensory Physiology*, vol. 6. Berlin: Springer-Verlag, 1974; pp. 3–154.

Howard IP. *Human Visual Orientation*. Chichester: John Wiley, 1982.

Previc FH, Ercoline WR, *Spatial Orientation in Aviation*. Reston, VA: American Institute of Astronautics and Aeronautics, 2004.

NATO Symposium. Spatial disorientation in military vehicles, causes, consequences and cures. Report no. HFM-085, TP/42. Neuilly-sur-Seine: NATO Research and Technology Agency, 2003.

Wilson VJ, Melville Jones G. *Mammalian Vestibular Physiology*. New York: Plenum Press, 1979.

PART II

Operational aviation medicine

PART

Operational aviation medicine

19

Selection and training

JOHN W. CHAPPELOW AND CHRIS ELSHAW

SELECTION

It is self-evident that organizations have a responsibility to ensure that the best employees are selected. Individuals bring a variety of characteristics, such as abilities, attitudes and motivations, to the workplace; therefore, ensuring that the most suitable people fill jobs is good not only for the organization, in terms of lower costs, but also for the individuals. Time devoted to training for a job for which an individual might prove to be unsuitable may be costly in terms of wasted time and loss of self-esteem. Although costs to the individual might be difficult to calculate, some attempts have been made to estimate costs to the organization. For example, for the US Air Force (USAF), the cost of each person who fails undergraduate pilot training is estimated to be $50 000–80 000. With a failure rate of around 20–30 per cent, which is typical for military pilot training, and 1100 new pilots per year (in 2004–05), the annual cost is $30–48 million. In the UK, there is a need for 250 military pilots (in 2000), and on average it costs £3.8 million to train each one. It is evident that small improvements in selection could result in significant savings, and so it is not surprising that many military training organizations wish to maintain and improve their selection systems. Equally, there are potential cost savings to be made with commercial aircrew if careful selection reduces the rate of failure in training.

PRINCIPLES OF SELECTION

Although completely new selection systems are developed, it is more often the case that an existing system is modified to meet some change or problem in the organization. Whatever the reason, for any selection system to work, a number of questions need to be answered, including: What should be measured? How should it be measured? And is the system effective? This can be represented by the model shown in Figure 19.1.

What should be measured?

Before a selection system can be designed and implemented, the first question that needs to be answered is: What selection criteria is the system designed to assess? This is best answered by means of job analysis. The pur-

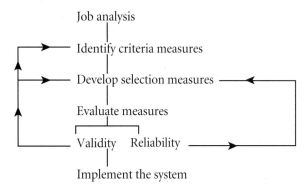

Figure 19.1 *Model for developing a selection system.*

pose of the analysis is to specify the relationship between the selection criteria (the predictors) and the training and performance criteria (the variables to be predicted). The results from such an analysis should be used to identify both requirements (outputs – what the holder does) and personnel requirements (inputs – the skills, knowledge and abilities that the holder needs).

Measuring requirements

Two approaches used widely to identify requirements are hierarchical task analysis and functional analysis. In task analysis, the job is broken down into discrete phases of activity. Within these phases, the individual tasks can be identified and broken into subtasks. For example, in the case of flight crew, the task can broken down into pre-take-off, takeoff, climb, cruise, approach and landing. Within these phases, the individual tasks are broken down into the actions performed, such as the use and interpretation of instruments. A hierarchy of tasks is produced, starting at a top-level task and descending to detailed subtasks.

In functional analysis, the work is broken down from the organizational perspective, taking more account of roles. Jobs within the organization are identified and defined in terms of the competencies required to carry them out. Some competencies will be common across the organization, while others will be specific.

Task analysis, therefore, is more suitable in the design of equipment and training, while functional analysis is used more in defining managerial roles.

Personnel requirements

A number of different methods have been developed for determining the aptitudes that a person needs. The essential differences lie in the degree of structure that each involves, but each has its own advantages and all have been used widely. The first method is the *critical incidents technique* (CRT). This is, essentially, a qualitative technique, but it can be used to produce rating scales for designing performance, training and selection measures. CRT is used to provide examples that can be used to define good and bad performance. This is done by asking subject-matter experts (SMEs), e.g. pilots and instructors, for examples of poor and good performance. For example, in the case of a pilot, the SME might be asked to think of how a pilot might exercise judgement while flying an approach. The SME provides examples of behaviour that he or she has witnessed that are representative of good and poor judgement and that were critical to a successful or unsuccessful outcome. The incidents obtained are classified for each task. The data can be checked by other experts, and any anomalies can be resolved. The resulting information can be used to identify those behaviours that differentiate performance and to create rating scales of performance. A drawback of this technique is that large numbers of critical incidents are required.

A similar technique that can be used to provide a shortcut is the *repertory grid technique*. Although designed originally as a tool in counselling, this technique is used widely as a means of eliciting job knowledge. The first step in the analysis is to determine a set of statements that characterize the domain (known as elements). SMEs are asked to give examples of tasks or activities that can be differentiated in terms of, for example, complexity and frequency and to identify individuals who are good, average or poor performers. Each of the elements is summarized and written on cards or some other convenient means of presentation. The cards are presented in threes to the SMEs, who are asked to decide in which way two of the elements are similar to each other but different from the third. The factors (known as constructs) that differentiate the elements are recorded. The process of comparison continues until all combinations of three cards have been processed. Many constructs can be elicited from a small number of interviews. The constructs are then summarized and classified into dimensions. The repertory grid has been used to identify the qualities required for success in the training of Royal Air Force (RAF) aircrew. Interviews produced 17 dimensions, and these were rated in terms of importance by a larger group of trainers. Statistical analysis showed that the ability dimensions (planning and organization, problem solving) were more important than trait dimensions (courage, extroversion). The results have been used to review the extent to which the assessment procedures used in training have covered all those qualities identified as important.

The final set of techniques uses methods that are structured and involve standard sets of descriptors. The approach is known as the task taxonomy technique. Information from psychometrics, experimental psychology and human factors research has been used to develop scales to rate the abilities needed to perform jobs. Abilities are classified into domains such as cognitive (information processing, problem solving), perceptual and spatial (attention, spatial orientation), physical (flexibility, strength, stamina) and psychomotor (coordination, reaction time). The advantage of this method is that the results can map directly on to existing tests and offer the possibility of off-the-shelf tests. Such tests have been identified, although some important measures are not available commercially. An example of the application of this technique is in the selection of fast-jet navigators. The approach has also been used in a North Atlantic Treaty Organisation (NATO)-wide study of the aptitude requirements for military fast-jet pilots.

Crew resource management (CRM) training is now an important feature of both initial and refresher aircrew training (see Chapter 20). Consideration at the selection stage can give guidance on understanding and attitude or relevance to CRM.

Measuring abilities

In the early days of aviation, it was generally believed that the best predictor of success in flying training was the ability to ride a horse. However, it soon became apparent that this was not an effective selection procedure, as many individuals failed to acquire the complex skills of a pilot, with expensive and time-consuming consequences. In the UK, selection procedures based on medical examination of the physiological systems most affected by altitude and on simple tests of coordination were introduced. The system adopted in the USA examined emotional stability, perception of tilt and mental alertness. Although the psychology of selection developed further after the First World War, there was little change in selection procedures until the early 1940s. The increased demand for pilots during the Second World War, together with the serious consequences of poor selection, stimulated the development of more rigorous criteria. However, although there have been rapid developments in aircraft technology in recent years, the basic techniques developed in the 1940s are still used, although new tests are evaluated and introduced into modern selection schemes. In this context, it is useful to recall the writings of Goodman et al. (1983):

The successful tactical air mission of yesteryear depended predominantly upon a pilot's psychomotor abilities in guiding his aircraft and its projectiles, success for the modern-day counterpart relies also upon his ability to process vast arrays of complex information, make rapid, highly consequential decisions, *and* execute a large number of co-ordinated responses.

Having completed the job analysis and derived a specification, it should be possible to answer the question: What needs to measured? Most published studies in this domain have been related to the question of military *ab initio* pilot selection. Little published work has been sponsored or conducted by civil aviation. Hunter and Burke (1990) reported 254 studies dealing with pilot selection, but only seven referred to non-military studies. Consequently, much of what follows refers to military pilot selection. Essentially, a well-designed selection system needs to fulfil a number of different criteria. First, it needs to be fair; this may include the need to meet legal requirements with the ability to demonstrate that the measures are ethnically and gender-neutral. Second, it must be valid and effective; however, the practical consideration remains to balance the cost of the selection process against the cost of the benefits. For example, if applicants are in plentiful supply, then the cost penalties associated with training failure are low and it might not be cost-effective to employ an elaborate and costly selection system.

Cognitive ability

Selection measures are derived from general models of human ability. One model that has had a large influence on the development of selection systems is that of Vernon (1961). It is based on experimental evidence that suggests that scores on specific ability tests tend to cluster together to form ability factors. For example, verbal, numerical and general reasoning cluster together, as do spatial, mechanical and motor abilities. These in turn aggregate to form the higher factors of verbal, numerical and educational (v-ed) and practical, spatial, mechanical (k-m). At the highest level, there is a general factor (g) underlying human ability, which has led to the development of general ability tests. However, it is recommended that selection procedures based on general abilities should sample multiple abilities in order to ensure accuracy and fairness of assessment.

Typical of the classical abilities test is the Air Force Officer Qualifying Test (AFOQT) of the USAF, which includes measures of verbal, quantitative and spatial abilities, and perceptual speed and aviation knowledge. Some of the measures are found in selection tests of many occupational groups, although others are specific to aviation. A number of composite scores are derived. The pilot composite is made up of verbal analogies, mechanical comprehension, scale reading, instrument comprehension, table reading and aviation information. Studies have shown that the g component is by far the best predictor of the ten training criteria, while the specific ability components made little contribution beyond that measured by g. Similar tests can be found in the selection systems of most military air forces and occasionally can be found in the selection of commercial pilots.

Computer-based assessment

Developments in cognitive psychology have identified the significance of information-processing, coordination and attention to pilot performance. The ready availability of personal computers has led to the development of computer-based assessment systems. An advantage of such testing is that it can provide dynamic measures of information-processing using both single- and multiple-task performance. A computer-based selection centre for pilot selection is established at the Officer and Aircrew Selection Centre of the RAF. Although the original tests were adaptations of existing paper-and-pencil and electromechanical tests, new cognitive measures have been added. Within the battery are a control-velocity test (anticipatory tracking), a test of the sensorimotor apparatus (compensatory tracking), instrument comprehension, vigilance (visual attention) and digit recall (short-term memory). Recent studies of the battery involving fixed-wing and helicopter training have reported validity correlations of 0.3–0.5 measured against success in flying training.

An early computer-based assessment battery was the MICROPAT system. This was developed for military aircrew in the UK and has been extended to the civil sector. Measures include tracking tasks, attention and discrimination, and simulation of an aircraft-landing task. A third battery, TASKOMAT, includes measures of reaction time, memory search, visual and auditory selective attention (ASA) and dual-task performance (DT). Both the ASA and DT have been shown to predict performance in military and civil flight training. The basic attributes test (BAT), a computer-based system developed by the USAF, comprises 13 tests covering coordination, visualization, memory, time-sharing, speed of information-processing, memory, attitudes towards risk and an aircrew personality profile. Correlations of 0.29 have been reported between the composite score and performance in flying training. These are four of the available computer-based systems. A more comprehensive overview of computer testing within NATO is given by Burke and Van Raay (1993).

Work–sample and simulation–based assessment

The use of cognitive abilities to measure pilot aptitude is based on the assumption that the skills and abilities underlie pilot performance. A more direct approach is to measure performance on measures of the actual task. Work-sample testing has a good record in a number of occupations and has been shown to be ethnically and gender-fair. Applicants are given basic instruction, and the time taken to reach some criterion of performance is measured. Alternatively, a fixed amount of training is given, and performance at the end of this period is measured. The most obvious approach for aircrew training is the use of light aircraft. The applicant is given instruction in basic light-aircraft manoeuvres and is tested on his or her ability to reproduce them. Scoring is, generally, in terms of errors in reproducing the set manoeuvres, although measures of character and attitude are also gathered, often informally. Despite the susceptibility of such assessments to poor reliability, these measures can produce high predictive validities.

While the predictive validities of such methods can be good, high costs are a drawback. This has led to studies to capitalize on the techniques of flight screening, but at a reduced cost through the use of simulation. Early studies to investigate the use of simulation were carried out by the USAF using a link general aviation trainer (GAT-1). This was used to administer a six-hour syllabus of flight instruction before entry into flight training. Subjects learned to perform straight and level flight and turns and descents by reference to flight instruments. Validities reported for flight screening and the GAT-1 selection were remarkably similar when performance in initial jet training was used as the criteria. This led to the automated pilot aptitude measurement system (APAMS), in which all instruction and performance measurements were completely automated. Although the system showed great promise as a selection method, it was not thought to be sufficiently economical for operational use.

These studies had an impact on the Canadian forces, which developed the APAMS system into the Canadian automated pilot selection system (CAPSS). CAPSS uses a light-aircraft simulator and involves the learning and demonstration of eight flight manoeuvres. For each manoeuvre, ten flight measures are recorded. A great deal of data are generated and processed in order to produce the final score. Validation against success in initial flying training showed a gain of ten per cent in the classification of training success over existing measures. The system became operational in 1997, and it is claimed that the use of CAPSS will save around $4 million for every 100 pilots who graduate. The cost of development was $4–7 million. A similar approach has been taken by the Royal Netherlands Air Force, with their simulator-based assessment.

Other assessment methods

Finally, there is the question of measuring the non-cognitive aspects of pilot performance. These can be described broadly as measures of personality. It is interesting to note that the most common way in which people are described in everyday life has proved to be elusive to measurement. People are often described in terms of their personality, but they are seldom described as having good hand–eye coordination. Many terms are difficult to define and, when subjected to investigation, have proven to be unreliable. Personality is assessed in many selection systems, but the procedure is seldom formalized. Implicit measures are often made during interviews but are seldom subjected to rigorous investigation. Standardized personality questionnaires are available, such as Cattell's 16PF (16 personality factors), but the results from such studies have been mixed. There is a great deal of debate about the reliability of personality questionnaires. However, there are other approaches to personality assessment based on the exercise of clinical judgement and a variety of personality theories, such as that proposed by Freud.

The value of such techniques is beyond the scope of this chapter; in any case, the cost of such in-depth procedures generally rules them out for selection purposes. Nevertheless, some significant findings have been reported. For example, there are differences between samples of successful and unsuccessful helicopter pilots on three of the 16 scales of the Cattell system. Some results from pilot-related studies have shown that stable introverts have a higher success rate in advanced military flying training, although other results suggest that pilots score higher on emotional stability and extroversion. It has also been reported that pilots tend to score more highly on achievement orientation, group orientation, precision, dominance, adventurousness and the need for esteem. The question arises as to whether these reported differences are a function of selection, attraction of particular individuals towards being a pilot or the ability of individuals to give the correct impression. It is noteworthy that in the USA, there is a renewed interest in personality testing of military aircrew, although generally the results have not been promising.

Clinically based methods of personality assessment have gained prominence. In the defence mechanism test (DMT), pictures similar to those used in the thematic apperception test are presented at decreasing exposure times, and responses are scored for accuracy. Deviations are said to indicate the presence of defence mechanisms. The theory is that the presence of defence mechanisms is perceived as threatening and prevents the timely processing of information and, thus, will interfere with the performance of piloting an aircraft or other hazardous activities. However, trials in the UK on the usefulness of this approach have been disappointing. There have been difficulties in scoring, and the reliability of the scores from procedures is poor. A meta-analysis of 15 available studies obtained a mean correlation of 0.22. Different results were obtained when the studies were divided into those from Scandinavian countries and those from non-Scandinavian countries. The mean correlation for Scandinavian countries was 0.3, while that for non-Scandinavian countries was only 0.05. These differences have been attributed to difficulties in translation of the original procedures, and it has been suggested that the role of the psychologist as administrator and interpreter of the results may have had an influence. Scandinavian psychologists have a tradition of using tests as a tool for individual assessment, whereas tradition in the USA and the UK is one of strict empiricism.

Most of the major studies investigating personality have used *ab initio* pilot training measures as their criteria. However, beyond individual performance, personality may contribute significantly towards crew performance, and the measures have a significant impact on training in crew coordination. Work on personality has been summarized by Hunter and Burke (1994). They concluded that meta-analysis confirmed what simple inspection revealed, i.e. that the mean simple weighted correlation between personality measures and flying performance (usually pass/fail measures) for 46 personality measures was 0.1. However, the results show much poorer levels of predictive validity than the use of biographical inventories, which continue to be used in Europe and the USA. Clearly, a limitation of this work is that the results are based almost entirely on *ab initio* pilot training. Personality measures may well have an influence on post-training performance and in an operational setting, as indicated by studies on CRM.

EVALUATING SELECTION

Selection tests must satisfy the criteria of reliability and validity.

Reliability

The reliability of a test reflects the consistency of its scores. A test would be reliable if it yielded the same score on two separate occasions. In practice, however, such consistency is unlikely, because error is introduced by extraneous factors, such as changes in emotional state and differences in environmental conditions. To minimize error, tests are administered under standardized conditions. Test reliability can be estimated by several methods, all based on the statistical technique of correlation. This procedure expresses the level of agreement between two sets of scores as a correlation coefficient. All coefficient values fall between -1 and $+1$. A correlation of $+1$ indicates perfect agreement, 0 indicates independence, and -1 indicates an inverse relationship.

Reliability can be assessed in the following ways:

- *Test–retest reliability:* the same test is given to the same people on two occasions, either with no inter-test interval (immediate test–retest) or after a specific time interval (delayed test–retest). Not surprisingly, the immediate retest method generally produces the higher estimate of reliability because virtually everything is held constant over the two test sessions. In fact, the level of reliability may be artificially high because testees are likely to remember and repeat their responses on the second occasion.
- *Split-half reliability:* the internal consistency of a single test is assessed by examining the degree to which the different test items measure the attribute in question. Items are allocated to one of two groups (e.g. odd- versus even-numbered questions); scores on the two halves are then correlated.
- *Equivalent-forms reliability:* sometimes, it is desirable to develop more than one test. The correlation of results on these different versions is equivalent-forms reliability.

Validity

Validity reflects the degree to which a test is able to measure what it intends to measure. Although a test cannot be valid unless it is reliable, it can be reliable without being valid. Different forms of validity are recognized:

- *Face validity:* a test has face validity if it appears to measure the attribute in question. A test that has face validity is not necessarily a good selection tool. Thus, a test of the theoretical aspects of flight might appear to be relevant to pilot selection, although it would not necessarily provide any information about an individual's aptitude. Face validity is usually adduced from the reaction of those sitting the test. If a test has little face validity, then candidates may fail to take it seriously. This in turn can affect reliability.
- *Content validity:* when a test is designed to examine the ability to perform a complex task, all aspects of that task must be included for it to have validity. Validity is established through job analysis (a procedure that identifies constituent parts) rather than by a statistical procedure.
- *Predictive validity:* this is concerned with the ability of a test to predict the outcome on some independent criterion. In aircrew selection, the criterion usually is the successful completion of training. Predictive validity can be assessed by all candidates proceeding into the training programme, regardless of performance on the test. Success during training can be correlated with selection test scores.
- *Concurrent validity:* if a test can distinguish between different levels of performance attained by current incumbents (rather than applicants), then it is said to have concurrent validity.

PRACTICAL ASPECTS OF SELECTION

Typically, selection is based on a battery of tests that measure a number of attributes, including intelligence, ability and aptitude. Figure 19.2 represents a situation in which both selection and training criteria have been established. The ellipse represents a positive correlation between selection and success in training. If there was a perfect relationship between the two sets of results, then the ellipse would be replaced by a straight line and all those who were selected would have satisfied the training criterion. This demonstrates two problems. First, some of those who do well on overall selection do not satisfy a subsequent training criterion. These false positives are in sector C. Second, some of those rejected would have succeeded if they had been selected. These false negatives appear in sector A. The selection ratio is calculated by dividing the number selected (B + C) by the number of candidates (A + B + C + D). This ratio is approximately 33 per cent. However, the success ratio (calculated by comparing the number who succeed (B) with those who are selected

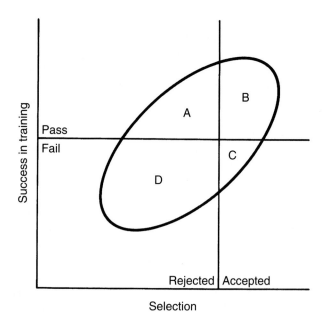

Figure 19.2 *Relationship between selection and success in training.*

(B + C)) is only two to three. In other words, a third of the selected applicants fail to perform satisfactorily during training. When training costs are high, as in aviation, such a substantial proportion of 'failures' is unacceptable.

When a large number of applicants is available (Figure 19.3), the selection criterion can be set higher, thus reducing the number of training failures. However, when too few high-scoring candidates are available, a decision has to be taken either to accept fewer people into training or to

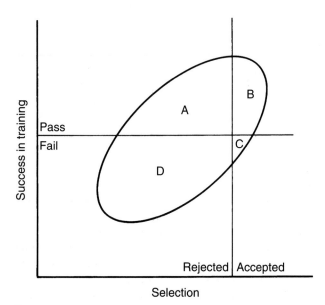

Figure 19.3 *As a result of raising the selection criterion, fewer candidates enter training. A higher success ratio is achieved, but the proportion of false negatives (area A) is increased.*

lower the entry standard. If the standard is lowered (Figure 19.4), fewer of the able candidates (sector A) will be ignored, but the number of training failures will increase to approximately 60 per cent of those selected. The optimum selection ratio depends on cost of training and the number of suitable applicants. If the validity of the selection criterion is increased, then the proportion of individuals falling into sectors A and C is reduced. In other words, fewer acceptable candidates are lost, and fewer unsuitable candidates are passed into training. Selection tests must be validated continuously for this reason. Content validity, once established, can be maintained by frequent job analysis, but the investigation of predictive validity poses a more difficult problem because of the cost and potential danger in allowing unselected candidates to go forward into pilot training. The predictive validity of a test, therefore, is generally evaluated by comparing its success ratio with that of existing tests. This ignores the problem of denying able candidates the opportunity for training but represents the best practical solution to a difficult problem.

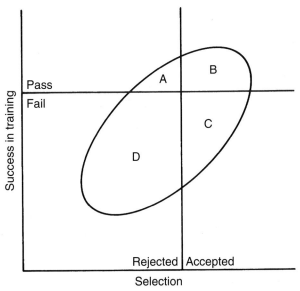

Figure 19.4   *When the entry standard is lowered, the proportion of false negatives is reduced, but the success ratio is also affected negatively.*

TRAINING

Contemplation of the complexities of training necessarily requires some understanding of the learning process. What is learning? The answer to this question is not as straightforward as it appears at first. Clearly, objective evidence of learning can be obtained only if there is an observable change in behaviour. But it is obvious that other processes (maturation, fatigue, disease) also change behaviour. Changes due to learning tend to be relatively permanent

and to result from experience or practice. In general, they are not likely to occur unless the student is motivated to learn. Several paradigms of learning have been explored experimentally. These may reflect different types of learning or different aspects of the same underlying processes.

Paradigms of learning

CLASSIC CONDITIONING

Pavlov established many of the basic principles of conditioning. He observed that some stimuli (e.g. sight and smell of food) elicited simple responses (e.g. salivation). By repeatedly presenting the unconditioned stimulus (food) in conjunction with another stimulus (e.g. sound of a bell, usually presented just before the food), Pavlov found that it was possible to elicit the response by presenting the bell alone. The strength of the conditioned response (the amount of saliva produced at the sound of the bell) increased as training progressed. Pavlov also demonstrated several other phenomena common to many learning situations:

- *Extinction:* if, after training, the conditioned stimulus (the bell) is presented repeatedly without the unconditioned stimulus (i.e. without reinforcement), then the strength of the conditioned response will decline and eventually disappear.
- *Spontaneous recovery:* if, after a period of extinction, the subject is returned to the experimental situation, then the conditioned response is often found to have recovered some of its former strength. This suggests that the extinction procedure does not simply weaken the original conditioning but that either the extinction procedure interferes with the response (the subject learns not to respond) or the conditioned response is suppressed by a temporary inhibition.
- *Stimulus generalization:* this is an important characteristic of all learning. Once a response has been conditioned to a stimulus, other similar stimuli also acquire the power to elicit the response in proportion to their similarity to the original conditioned stimulus.
- *Higher-order conditioning:* once a conditioned response has been established, it may be used as the basis of further conditioning, so that the conditioned response can be associated with other stimuli. In this type of experiment, the first conditioned stimulus provides secondary reinforcement and no primary reinforcement is given.

Although these studies illuminated some characteristics of learning, the classic conditioning paradigm has not proved to be an adequate model for the rich variety of learned behaviours observed in humans. An attempt to cope with this is embodied in the instrumental conditioning paradigm.

INSTRUMENTAL CONDITIONING

The responses learned in instrumental conditioning have one or both of two objectives. They may result in a positive reinforcement (food, water, sexual activity) or the avoidance of a negative reinforcer (pain, fear). In both instances, the reinforcer may be secondary, i.e. a stimulus that has been associated with a primary positive or negative reinforcer. A typical instrumental response is that of pressing a lever to obtain food. An animal that is motivated (has been deprived of food) may, in the course of general exploratory activity, press the lever that causes a food pellet to be delivered. After a few such accidental responses, the rate of responding increases. The animal has learned a response that is instrumental to the attainment of a goal, although the goal need not necessarily be linked to a physiological drive. Thus, instrumental responses can be learned to satisfy curiosity. In this manner, apparently incidental (or latent) learning can occur, which becomes apparent only when a reward is provided to motivate performance. Long and complex sequences of responses can be established by careful training, as can discriminations between classes of stimuli or even concepts. Extinction, stimulus generalization and secondary reinforcement can be demonstrated in a manner similar to that for classic conditioning. Partial reinforcement has been found to be an important manipulation of the experimental conditions. By requiring several responses for each reinforcement, high rates of responding and a resistance to extinction can be established, particularly if a variable ratio of responses to reinforcements is used.

INSIGHT

Although the paradigm of instrumental conditioning is relevant to many aspects of learning and training, there are some varieties of learning that require more complex formulations. Humans seem to be able to learn in a way that involves sudden solutions to a problem rather than blind trial and error and reinforcement of simple responses. Such solutions may be obtained by covert (conceptual) trial and error based on previously learned habits. The notions of motivation and reinforcement are by no means irrelevant. It is worth noting, however, that humans will undertake such hypothesis testing out of sheer curiosity and that the only reinforcement they receive may be the knowledge of their success. The informative aspects of reinforcement may have an important function – perhaps the critical one – in apparently simpler forms of learning. It is certainly true that feedback of information on accuracy or speed of performance is essential to the development of skills of all types.

VERBAL LEARNING

The earliest systematic studies of learning used verbal materials such as poems, lists of words and nonsense syllables (meaningless, but pronounceable, combinations of letters). Although verbal material presents special problems in experimentation (covert rehearsal and interaction with experiences outside the experiment), it represents an important area of learning with wide relevance. The more significant findings from this type of study include the following:

- Forgetting is most marked immediately after training.
- Forgetting is caused at least partly by interference from other learning activities.
- The beginning and the end of a list or lesson are learned more easily than the middle.

Human learning

Examples of human learning may be found that can be described adequately by the simplest instrumental or classic conditioning paradigm. Although much human behaviour seems far removed from simple responses and basic drives, differences appear to be of complexity rather than of kind. This applies even to complicated training objectives, such as learning to fly. A systematic analysis of the task can often simplify the trainee's – and the trainer's – job by identifying component skills that can be learned separately and by setting objective standards of performance to aim for. Crucial factors are motivation and the reinforcement of correct responses (with emphasis on the informing role rather than the rewarding role of reinforcement).

MASSED VERSUS DISTRIBUTED PRACTICE

Is it better to learn by practising for relatively long periods or to have frequent short rests? This question was once of considerable theoretical interest in connection with the role (and varieties) of inhibition in learning. Many experiments gave results like those shown in Figure 19.5. Two groups were trained on a tracking task with 18 trials of 30 seconds each day. One group had 90-second rests between practice trials (spaced or distributed practice), while the other group had only two-second breaks (massed practice). Several effects are apparent in the results:

- Improvement shown by the massed-practice group on any one day was less than for the spaced-practice group.
- The massed-practice group showed an overnight improvement on the first trial of each day. This effect (reminiscence) suggested that they had learned more than was evident in their previous day's performance.
- The spaced-practice group needed some time to 'warm up' on each new day before attaining the level of performance of the previous day.
- On the final day, both groups were given spaced practice, and the difference between them reduced markedly.

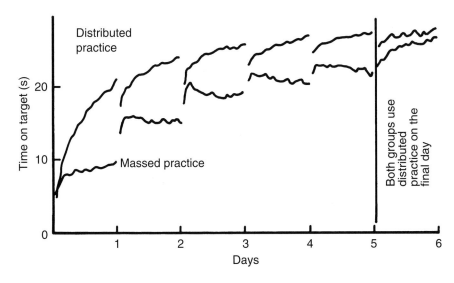

Figure 19.5 *Effects of massed and distributed practice. Adapted from Digman (1959).*

Some experiments seem to show a residual benefit of spaced practice. This may be due to a number of factors that are difficult to control. For example, the spaced-practice group may get more practice by rehearsing mentally during the rest periods. The massed-practice group may get less practice, owing to lapses of concentration resulting from fatigue. Overall, it appears that the detrimental effects of massed practice are confined to immediate levels of performance, with little long-term effect on learning. However, from a practical point of view, if spacing practice has no drawbacks (such as disruption of the training programme), then there may be some advantages. The student's motivation may be enhanced if his or her performance shows obvious improvement. In complex tasks, adequate performance on elements of the task allows the student to tackle more advanced procedures (positioning the aircraft in the circuit requires a certain minimum of skill in attitude flying). Finally, it is obvious that the effects of massed and spaced practice should be familiar to trainers so that they can make sensible assessments of a student's progress in comparison with others or with the required standard.

WHOLE VERSUS PART PRACTICE

Some activities are naturally divisible into component parts. Map-reading and basic attitude flying are both required for cross-country navigation, but each can be divided into simpler subtasks. To what extent is it advisable to decompose tasks into simple constituents for the purposes of training? There is no clear-cut answer to this question. Practising part tasks seems to be advantageous when the whole is too complex or too large for a novice to tackle conveniently (e.g. learning a long part in a play). It may also have the advantage of maintaining the trainee's interest, as progress is more obvious when subtasks are being mastered. In general, however, whole-task practice is

advantageous, especially when the whole forms a meaningful unit and when the trainee is capable of rapid progress. For practical purposes, it must be stressed that a systematic task analysis may reveal ways in which the trainee's job could be simplified by separating components of the task but that care must be taken not to destroy important interrelationships that have to be learned in due course.

PHASES OF LEARNING

If a measure of performance in a complex skill is plotted against time in practice, then some features commonly emerge. In the early stages there may be little improvement, but later performance may improve rapidly. In the final stages, the rate of improvement slows down. For many skills, the trainee faces an initial conceptual task. The trainee must learn to organize the requirements of the skill and the information into easily understood units. Little change in performance may be evident until this task is completed. In the next phase, psychomotor coordination improves and the trainee becomes skilled in subtasks. In the final phase, the various components of the skill are integrated into a smooth operation, and improvements in timing, speed and ease of performance are evident. Some skills, especially those with a strong hierarchical structure, tend to show rather discontinuous improvements in performance, and for considerable periods the trainee may show little or no progress. Good examples are learning to play a musical instrument and learning to receive Morse code. In the latter case, having achieved a certain standard (speed) receiving letter by letter, the trainee will show no improvement for a while. Eventually, a further improvement occurs when the trainee learns to interpret whole words. A further increase in speed may be apparent eventually when whole phrases are received as a unit. Obviously, there is a risk of discouragement and loss of motivation for the trainee who has reached such a plateau in performance. However, many skills are not especially susceptible to this phenomenon, and erratic performance may be more of a problem.

KNOWLEDGE OF RESULTS

One of the most important features of any training situation is feedback provided to the student. The role of feedback can be viewed in two ways. It furnishes the information that the trainee needs in order to adjust his or her actions to match those required, and it reinforces correct responses. The former is essential to the development of a skill, but the style in which feedback is presented can also have important effects on the trainee's motivation. Feedback of one sort or another is intrinsic to many tasks. Most vehicle-control tasks rely on visual feedback such as the distance of the car from the kerb and the rate of closure on the vehicle in front. Skilled movements in tasks requiring manual dexterity involve not only visual feedback but also internal proprioceptive feedback. The trainee may be assisted in learning to use the feedback intrinsic to the task by additional, artificial feedback. Such knowledge of results can be manipulated in several ways that have an influence on learning and performance. One possible drawback is that it may distract attention away from intrinsic cues.

Artificial feedback in an air-to-air gunnery trainer has been provided in the form of a buzzer sounding when the target is correctly ranged and sighted. Although a group trained using this method appeared better than one trained without it, removing the buzzer caused a large drop in their performance. The trainees had used the artificial cue to guide their actions rather than to evaluate their results. In this particular experiment, the artificial feedback was concurrent with the task. Delaying the feedback until the completion of an action (terminal feedback) may lead to better results in training relatively on uncomplicated tasks. Simply delaying the feedback even further (within reasonable limits) has little effect on learning. This is in contrast to the dramatic effects on performance induced by even small delays in intrinsic feedback. There are advantages in elaborating feedback beyond the simple report of success or failure. Graphical presentations of, say, control movements could allow the trainee to compare his or her technique with that of an expert and to modify it accordingly. Similarly, the verbal feedback traditionally used by instructors can, in the hands of a competent instructor, be both informative and highly motivating. In addition, by presenting feedback not only on current responses but also on accumulated progress, the trainee's performance can be set in context by comparison with long- or short-term goals or with others' rates of progress. This feedback can influence the trainee's motivation and efforts to improve, particularly when combined with detailed analysis of his or her strengths and weaknesses.

Transfer of training

The fundamental purpose of training is to effect a change in behaviour or capabilities in situations remote from that in which the training occurs. The assumption that skills once acquired will transfer to the real world, which may be very different from the classroom, is implicit in all training. Over what range of differences does such an assumption hold true? Early interest in this question centred on the notion of ability training. For example, is it possible to improve one's memory simply through practice in memorizing? In general, little transfer seems to occur between unrelated tasks (learning poems and learning lists of nonsense syllables) unless the trainee is also given instruction on, in this case, general techniques of memorization. In some circumstances, the trainee may 'learn to learn' without special prompting (particularly if exposed to a variety of tasks); in this case, a degree of non-specific transfer of training may be evident, i.e. the trainee can learn other tasks in the same broad category more quickly. The saving in training time required to reach a criterion performance on one task produced by practice on another is the standard measure of training transfer. Variables with an important influence on transfer of training include the following:

- *Stimulus similarity:* the phenomenon of stimulus generalization was mentioned in connection with simple conditioning. Many skills require the same response to a general class of stimuli. The definition of that class may require the trainee to learn to discriminate between what initially appear to be very similar stimuli (e.g. detecting spin on a cricket ball). In general, the greater the similarity between the stimulus elements of two tasks, the greater will be the transfer of training between them.

- *Response similarity:* when the responses required by two tasks are identical or very similar, the transfer of training between the tasks can be very high. If the responses are not similar, then little or no transfer would be expected, although there may be some due to the learning of stimulus discriminations. A third possibility arises when the tasks require basically similar responses with small but functionally significant differences. In this case, previous training with one task may hinder progress on the second task, i.e. negative transfer. The use of a tiller in steering a boat seems unnatural to many car drivers and they may make many mistakes before adjusting to the apparent reversal of control sense. Typically, it is intrusion of the previously learned, and now inappropriate, control movements that cause problems early in training. Mastering the new skill may have a retroactive effect on previously learned skills. Although the control movements required by the two tasks may quickly become differentiated in the trainee's mind so that he or she can perform adequately on both tasks, there remains the possibility of intrusions of inappropriate behaviour in times of stress or inattention. This can be particularly hazardous in aviation, where aircraft of the same class (fast jets, four-engined transports) have broadly similar cockpit and yet aircraft of the same type within a fleet or squadron may incorporate different modifications. Both states of affairs invite, and have caused, operation of controls in error.

- *Task difficulty:* transfer of training between two tasks may be unequal because the tasks themselves demand different levels of skill. Two opposing principles seem to apply. First, the more difficult task may give better transfer to the easier task because it allows the trainee a greater breadth of experience and may even, in some sense, include the easier task. Second, the easier task may permit more accurate learning and so show better transfer to the more difficult task.

Psychomotor skills

An important variety of learning is that used in the acquisition of psychomotor skills. Of particular significance in aviation is skill in tracking, such as is necessary for control of an aircraft's flight path. Two major types of tracking task are:

- *pursuit tracking*, in which the operator has to match the position of a controlled element (a pointer on a display or the position of his own vehicle) with that of a target, e.g. formation flying
- *compensatory tracking*, in which the operator's display shows only an error signal, which he or she should attempt to reduce to zero; flying an instrument landing system approach using a zero reader type display uses this type of tracking.

Experimental studies of tracking usually include manipulation of the forcing function, i.e. the path that the target or error signal follows. The operator's control may work in several different ways. Its position may be related directly to the position of the controlled element, or it may control its velocity. In some (generally more difficult) tasks, control position affects acceleration of the controlled element. The relationship between the direction of movement of the control and that of the displayed response can have a strong influence both on the level of performance attainable withthe task and on a typical operator's rate of learning. Incompatible control–display relationships (those that oppose previous learning) generally produce an initially poorer performance but allow greater gains to be made in training. However, studies indicate the persistence of a residual deficit due to incompatibility. Some

psychomotor skills, particularly those including manual dexterity, have been studied over long periods of time. The indications are that performance goes on improving indefinitely with practice unless physically limited by the equipment.

PRACTICAL ASPECTS OF TRAINING

The variety of training undertaken in pursuit of aviation is immense. In addition to the basic psychomotor skills used in control of an aircraft, aircrew are trained in procedural, problem-solving, social and managerial skills. Training continues throughout the person's career. Aircrew will occasionally receive conversion training for a new aircraft type and at regular intervals will undergo continuation training and assessments. Any generalization intended to cover this spectrum of activities must, necessarily, be broad. What follows obeys this dictum.

General principles

A primary requirement of successful training is adequate motivation on the part of the trainee. Maintaining such motivation should be an important concern of the trainer. Knowledge of results provides a significant source of motivation for most trainees. When the results are poor, there may be an immediate depression of performance, but this need not do lasting damage if the trainee's overall motivation is satisfactory and the feedback is both informative and relevant to the trainee's needs. In addition, feedback can be arranged in ways that make learning easier by drawing the trainee's attention to subtle distinctions or cues and by allowing comparison with ideal responses. The analysis of the trainee's performance is as important as the practice itself.

Most tasks in aviation are relatively complex. It should, generally, be possible to make the task of the novice easier by identifying subtasks that can be practised separately. Certainly, the task should be analysed and the goals of training specified in objective terms. This not only standardizes the basis on which the trainee is assessed but also permits another important form of feedback – assessment of the training system. Without such assessment and systematic evaluation of changes in the training programme, there is no rational basis for improvement of the training system. A formal analysis of the training task should also permit the balance between theory and practice to be optimized and appropriate training techniques to be selected (lecture, tutorial, group discussion, simulation) in order to maximize transfer to the real world.

Simulation

The widespread use of flight simulators brings into focus many training issues, particularly the maximization of transfer. Flight simulators could be regarded primarily as teaching machines, but the impetus for their use generally owes far more to economic and safety considerations than to a detailed analysis of training objectives. Nevertheless, simulators offer some important advantages over real aircraft:

- The task can be simplified and the level of difficulty matched easily to the trainee's capabilities. For example, instrument landing procedures can be introduced without cross-winds, turbulence and other traffic, which complicate the task and distract the trainee's attention from the essentials of the task.
- Discrete components of the job can be taught in part-task trainers without unnecessary distractions.
- Practice may be intensified on important aspects of the task by using the reset or reposition facilities available on modern simulators to eliminate, for example, flying the whole circuit in order to practice the approach and landing, or the preparatory manoeuvring necessary for air-combat training.
- Feedback can be optimized. Some simulators allow the instructor not only to arrest the flight for an immediate diagnosis of problems but also to replay short periods, so that the trainee can have a second opportunity to see what went wrong. In addition, graphical and numerical analyses of performance are provided readily.

It should be apparent that many of these training advantages are in direct opposition to the commonsense requirement for maximum fidelity in a flight simulator. A degree of fidelity is required for transfer of training to the real aircraft, but there are two major ways in which total fidelity is a needless (and, in some cases, impossible) target. First, there are many things to learn about the operation of a complex system. Some of them do not require that the system be fully functional or be accompanied by all the incidental stimuli available in flight. For example, the positions of displays and controls and the order in which they are used during a drill can be learned from a static cardboard mock-up. Second, even when an attempt is made to simulate important cues, only the psychologically important aspects need to be reproduced. Modern motion platforms now extend to the full six degrees of freedom (roll, pitch and yaw angular movements; surge, heave and sway translations). Common devices for making the limited travel available on such a platform seem like the unlimited freedom available in the air include washout, wash-back and subthreshold movements. Figure 19.6 compares the roll angles produced in an aircraft and in a simulator during a coordinated turn. The aircraft's initial acceleration in roll is matched fairly faithfully by the simulator, but eventually the simulator washes out the roll velocity in order to avoid reaching the end of its available travel. The cockpit is then washed back to a neutral position at an undetectable rate; as a result, the apparent normal acceleration vector rests where the pilot would expect it to be during the turn. Some of the sensations produced by longitudinal acceleration (surge) can be suggested by pitching the simulator up at an undetectable rate. With the pilot's impression of attitude stabilized by the simulator visual system or instruments, the resulting rotation of the gravity vector is interpreted as a longitudinal acceleration.

Although motion platforms are a common feature of modern simulators, their training advantages seem to be limited, since most flying tasks are controlled visually. In the aircraft, kinaesthetic motion cues provide concurrent feedback on the response of the aircraft to control movements. Providing such cues in a simulator seems to allow experienced pilots to employ control movements more like those they would use in the aircraft and to fly more accurately than they would in a fixed-base simulator. However, there appears to be little direct advantage in terms of training. Roughly equal transfer has been shown in three groups of *ab initio* students trained in a simulator with normal motion, no motion or motion randomly reversed in bank. Nevertheless, motion simulation probably serves some useful training functions. It can provide alerting stimuli such as yaw, signalling failure of an outboard engine. It can support a level of performance that may be necessary in order to practise advanced tasks or, at least, to reduce the pilot's workload in producing that performance. There is some evidence that intensive high-rate manoeuvring in a fixed-base simulator, particularly one with a wide-angle visual system, can provoke prolonged and unfortunate effects in pilots who adapt to this dynamically unrealistic regime. However, this is not a universal feature of using

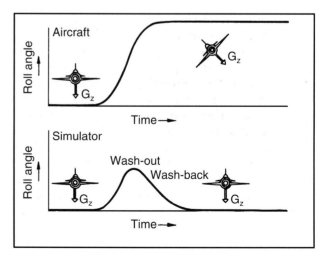

Figure 19.6 *Simulation of roll motion.*

such simulators, and the necessary conditions have yet to be explored fully.

Studies into the features required in visual simulations generally have lagged behind technical developments. Modern computer-generated visual systems have now attained high levels of performance in terms of dynamic response, angle of view and fidelity of screen content. Their limitations include low levels of brightness, less than realistic texturing and absence of stereoscopic information (which may be significant in some specialized tasks such as air-to-air refuelling). The complexity of the tasks undertaken using visual references and the ability of experienced pilots to adapt to manipulations of the cues provided make research using realistic tasks difficult. There is some evidence that pilots learn to use idiosyncratic repertoires of cues selected from the totality of redundant cues normally available in the visual world. This finding would go some way to explaining why some experiments show little performance decrement when cues are selectively manipulated and, incidentally, why some but not other pilots have accidents when faced with extra-wide or sloping runways or a dearth of cues (e.g. approaching over the sea at night).

REFERENCES

Burke EF, Van Raay P. *Computer-based Assessment in NATO: Final Report of Research Study Group 15.* Brussels: NATO, 1993.

Digman JM. Growth of a motor skill as a flinction of distribution of practice. *Journal of Experimental Psychology* 1959; **57**: 310–16.

Goodman L, McBride DK, Owens JM, Wherry RJ. The identification of processes underlying the skilled aviator. In: Jensen RS (ed.). *Proceedings of the Second Symposium on Aviation Psychology.* Columbus, OH: Ohio State University, 1983; pp. 541–6.

Hunter DR, Burke EF. An annotated bibliography of the aircrew selection literature. Research Report 1575. Alexandria, VA: US Army Research Institute, 1990.

Vemon PE. *The Structure of Human Abilities.* London: Methuen, 1961.

FURTHER READING

Anastasi A, Urbina S. *Psychological Testing*, 7th edn. London: Prentice-Hall, 1996.

Bailey M, Woodhead R. Current status and future developments of RAF aircrew selection. In: *Selection and Training Advances in Aviation.* AGARD conference proceedings 588. Prague: AGARD, 1996.

Fiffs PM, Posner MI. *Human Performance.* London: Prentice-Hall, 1973.

Hunter DR, Burke EF. Computer-based selection testing in the Royal Air Force. *Behaviour Research Methods, Instruments and Computers* 1987; **19**: 243–5.

Hunter DR, Burke EF. *Handbook of Pilot Selection.* Aldershot: Avebury Aviation, 1995.

Hunter DR, Thompson NA. Pilot selection development. AFHRL-TR-78-33. Brooks City-Base, San Antonio, TX: United States Air Force Human Resources Laboratory, 1978.

National Audit Office. *Training New Pilots.* London: The Stationery Office, 2000.

Stammers RB, Patrick J. *The Psychology of Training.* London: Methuen, 1975.

20

Crew resource management

ERIC W. FARMER

INTRODUCTION

Crew resource management (CRM) training was developed in response to growing evidence that interpersonal factors contributed to a substantial proportion of aviation accidents (Cooper *et al.* 1980) (Figure 20.1). This type of training, originally called cockpit resource management, is now used widely and indeed is mandated by many aviation regulatory authorities. It can be distinguished from the training of technical skills that is the subject of traditional aircrew instruction, but increasingly it is becoming integrated within technical training.

Early work that contributed to the development of CRM included National Aeronautics and Space Administration (NASA) studies of crew errors (e.g. Ruffle-Smith 1979), the line-oriented flight training (LOFT) developed by Northwest Airlines to improve crew coordination in simulators, and KLM's courses on leadership skills following the 1977 Tenerife accident (Beaty 1995). United Airlines

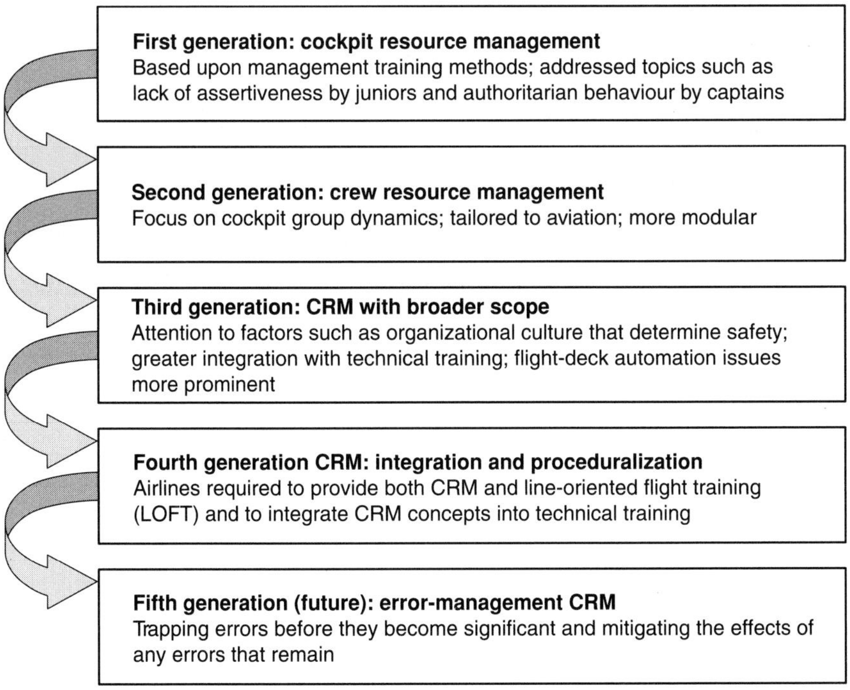

First generation: cockpit resource management
Based upon management training methods; addressed topics such as lack of assertiveness by juniors and authoritarian behaviour by captains

Second generation: crew resource management
Focus on cockpit group dynamics; tailored to aviation; more modular

Third generation: CRM with broader scope
Attention to factors such as organizational culture that determine safety; greater integration with technical training; flight-deck automation issues more prominent

Fourth generation CRM: integration and proceduralization
Airlines required to provide both CRM and line-oriented flight training (LOFT) and to integrate CRM concepts into technical training

Fifth generation (future): error-management CRM
Trapping errors before they become significant and mitigating the effects of any errors that remain

Figure 20.1 *Evolution of crew resource management (CRM) training. Based on data from Helmreich et al. (1999) and Helmreich and Merritt (2000).*

was responsible for the first comprehensive US CRM programme in 1981 (see Helmreich *et al.* 1999).

CREW RESOURCE MANAGEMENT TRAINING: IMPORTANCE AND OBJECTIVES

In a study of human error and CRM failures in US Navy aviation mishaps, Wiegmann and Shappell (1999) reviewed tactical jet (TACAIR) and rotary-wing class A flight mishaps in the period 1990–96. For each set of data, over 75 per cent of mishaps were partly or fully attributable to human error; 70 per cent of these mishaps were associated with aircrew human factors, of which 56 per cent involved at least one CRM failure.

Monitoring or challenging errors feature prominently in aircraft accidents involving human error (National Transportation Safety Board 1994). Hence, one of the aims of CRM training is to ensure that crew members provide mutual support (e.g. Fischer and Orasanu 1999). More specifically, the objectives of CRM training, as described by the Royal Aeronautical Society (1996), are:

- to enhance crew and management awareness of human factors that could cause or exacerbate air incidents
- to enhance knowledge of human factors and develop CRM skills and attitudes
- to apply CRM knowledge, skills and attitudes to aircraft operations and to integrate them within organizational culture
- to use CRM skills to integrate commercially efficient aircraft operations with safety
- to improve the working environment for crews and all those associated with aircraft operations.

CONTENT OF TYPICAL CREW RESOURCE MANAGEMENT COURSE

CRM is taught using a variety of methods, including lectures, practical exercises, role play, case studies and accident re-enactments on videotape (O'Connor and Flin 2003). Although CRM training is mandatory in the aviation industry, the specific content is not standardized. However, the syllabuses of most courses address aspects of communication and teamwork, situation awareness, decision-making, leadership and stress (e.g. Hatlestad 2005; Flin and Martin 2001; O'Connor and Flin 2003). For example, the syllabus defined by the UK Civil Aviation Authority (2003) comprises the following:

- human error and related topics
- company safety culture and standard operating procedures

- stress, stress management, fatigue and vigilance
- information-processing, including situation awareness and workload management
- decision-making
- communication and coordination
- leadership and teamwork
- automation issues (if appropriate)
- specific aircraft type-related issues
- case studies.

Since CRM is concerned essentially with the interactions between members of small groups, it will be convenient to begin by considering lessons learned from social psychology.

PSYCHOLOGY OF SMALL GROUPS

Experiments in social psychology have demonstrated powerful social influences within small groups. This research is clearly relevant to aviation, in which teams are prevalent, e.g. flight crew, cabin crew, team of planning and tactical air traffic controllers and maintenance teams.

Conformity

The term 'conformity' refers to behaviour that is consistent with social norms. Pressures to conform are exerted by social groups at all levels, from small groups to societies. Classic studies by Asch (1951, 1956) demonstrated that pressure to conform strongly influenced behaviour. The participant was one of a group asked individually to perform a task of indicating which of three lines matched a reference line, unaware that the other 'participants' were in fact confederates of the experimenter (Figure 20.2). On some occasions, the confederates gave responses that were incorrect. Individuals differed in the extent to which they yielded to this social pressure, but overall about one-third of the responses conformed to the group's clearly erroneous judgement. When the responses of the confederate group were not unanimous (e.g. one confederate always

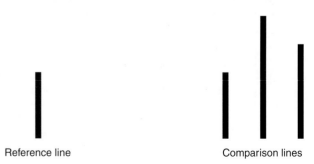

Figure 20.2 *Line judgement task used by Asch.*

giving the correct answer), conformity was reduced greatly. Further examination showed that some participants conformed, despite knowing their responses to be incorrect, whereas others appeared to have undergone a distortion of their perception.

Group size was found to determine the likelihood of conformity. A single confederate was unable to influence the participant's behaviour, but conformity increased with confederate groups of up to three or four individuals, no further increase being observed with larger groups. Research has shown that individuals are slower to express opinions when they are in a minority (Bassili 2003), and that this effect increases as a function of the difference between the sizes of the majority and the minority.

Bond and Smith (1996) performed a meta-analysis of studies using line judgement tasks similar to that of Asch. The results indicated that conformity in US studies had declined since the 1950s, and cross-cultural comparisons revealed that conformity was related to a country's 'individualism–collectivism', i.e. the extent to which its population tends to favour individual or group solutions to problems.

Asch's experiments illustrate the potency of 'normative influence' upon behaviour. However, we are also subjected to 'informational influence', in which the views of others provide information that is used to inform our own decisions. An example of this type of influence was demonstrated by Sherif (1936) in experiments on the autokinetic effect, an illusion whereby a stationary spot of light in an otherwise dark room appears to move randomly. Participants were asked to estimate the amount of movement individually and then in groups of three. Sherif found that the groups established norms on which their judgements converged; participants conformed to these norms even when they were again tested individually. Small groups, such as flight-deck crews, when faced with unfamiliar and ambiguous circumstances may too readily converge on a false interpretation of the evidence.

Compliance

The term 'compliance' refers to behaviour that is consistent with another individual's request. Research has demonstrated the conditions under which compliance is likely to occur. Cialdini *et al.* (1975), for example, provided an example of the 'door-in-the-face' technique, in which an initial unreasonable request is followed by a more modest request. Only 17 per cent of students who were asked to chaperone inmates from a juvenile detention centre on a daytrip to a zoo agreed to do so. However, students who were first asked – and refused – to make a much greater commitment (spending two hours per week for two years acting as counsellors for the inmates) were almost three times more likely to comply with the later request to act as chaperone for a day. The opposite approach ('foot-in-the-door') is also effective in some circumstances. A small request is made first in an attempt to induce the individual to comply with later, more substantial requests (e.g. Freedman and Fraser 1966; Pliner *et al.* 1974). This technique does not depend on personal contact; for example, compliance can be increased using emailed requests (Guéguen 2002).

Obedience

The work of Milgram (1974) demonstrated the ease with which individuals can be induced to obey authority. Milgram's experiments ostensibly were concerned with the effects of punishment on learning. The participant was designated a 'teacher' and was asked to administer increasingly intense electric shocks when a 'learner' committed errors in a word-pair learning task. The learner was, in fact, a confederate of the experimenter, and no shocks were actually delivered. Teachers were given a sample 45-V shock to ensure that they believed the punishment to be genuine. The learner exhibited increasing signs of distress as the voltage increased, leading ultimately to an agonized scream followed by silence. Despite predictions from experts such as psychiatrists that only one participant in 1000 would be prepared to administer the highest voltage, Milgram found that about 60 per cent of Yale undergraduates were prepared to do so. The finding was replicated for a wide range of other groups; in a study conducted in Munich, for example, the incidence of obedience was 85 per cent. In a variation of the experiment, 30 per cent of participants delivered 450 V even when they had to forcibly push down the learner's hand on the electrode. Other findings included the following:

- Most participants were prepared to acquiesce in delivery of the highest voltage when someone else was responsible for pulling the lever.
- Participants delivered much lower voltages when they were free to choose the intensity.
- Obedience was much lower when the experimenter was not physically present but gave orders by telephone, when two experimenters gave incompatible orders, and when actors playing the roles of other teachers disobeyed the experimenter.

Milgram's findings are clearly relevant to the flight deck. In this formal and highly structured environment, there is often a marked 'cockpit authority gradient' (CAG) (Edwards 1975). A junior first officer may find it very difficult to disobey an experienced and dominant captain, even if the order compromises safety (many of Milgram's participants were apparently prepared to countenance administering fatal electric shocks on the basis of poor performance on a trivial task).

Anderson *et al.* (2001) noted the importance of the command structure on the flight deck. The captain, whether acting in the role of pilot flying or pilot not flying, has responsibility for major decisions. However, other crew members play a significant role in monitoring the progress of the flight and must be prepared to challenge questionable decisions. They may fail to do so if the CAG is too steep. Conversely, a CAG that is too flat may imply weak leadership, with all its inherent risks. A major contribution of CRM training is to provide guidance on optimizing the CAG.

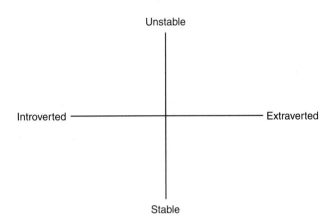

Figure 20.4 *The two major dimensions of personality.*

Personality and leadership

STRUCTURE OF PERSONALITY

The term 'personality' refers to enduring predispositions to behave in particular ways. These predispositions, or traits, can be distinguished from more transient moods, or states. One approach to discovering the underlying dimensions of personality is to compute the correlations between individuals' responses to questions about behaviour. Figure 20.3 shows hypothetical correlations between two variables, which can be expressed quantitatively as a correlation coefficient from −1 (perfect negative correlation), through zero (no correlation), to +1 (perfect positive correlation). The approach favoured by Eysenck (1970) and other personality theorists was to use the statistical technique of factor analysis to reduce a complex set of intercorrelations to a small number of factors accounting for much of the underlying variance in the scores.

Two major factors of personality have emerged: introversion–extraversion (E) and neuroticism (N), also known as trait anxiety. The typical extravert is sociable and impulsive, whereas the introvert is more socially withdrawn and cautious. People low in neuroticism are emotionally stable, whereas those high in neuroticism tend to worry and to be easily upset. Eysenck argued that these were orthogonal factors, i.e. that they were uncorrelated with each other and, hence, the position on one dimension did not predict position on the other (Figure 20.4). Another prominent personality researcher, Raymond Cattell, argued for the existence of 16 personality factors. The discrepancy between these positions is accounted for by the fact that Cattell was prepared to accept factors that were intercorrelated. When his set of factors is subjected to further factor

analysis, second-order factors emerge that clearly include those identified by Eysenck as E and N.

Eysenck posited the existence of a third factor, which he called psychoticism or tough-mindedness. However, there is growing consensus (e.g. Wiggins 1996) that the 'big five' personality dimensions are E and N, together with conscientiousness (C), openness to experience (O) and agreeableness (A). Since E and N account for the greatest variance in behaviour, the Eysenck personality inventory (EPI), which produces a score on these factors, is still used widely. For those who wish to obtain a measure on all of the big five dimensions, tests such as OCEAN (openness to experience, conscientiousness, extraversion, agreeableness and neuroticism; Collis 1997) are available.

PERSONALITY AND ACCIDENTS

There is some evidence relating personality to accidents. For example, in classic studies of South African bus drivers, unstable extraverts appeared to be most liable to accidents (Shaw and Sichel 1971). More recently, Robertson and Clarke (2002) reported a meta-analysis of personality and accidents in high-risk occupations using the 'big five' framework. Accidents were found to be associated with openness, low agreeableness and low conscientiousness. However, Cellar *et al.* (2000) found only limited evidence that agreeableness was associated negatively with vehicular accidents, and Salgado (2002) was unable to demonstrate a reliable association between any of the big five factors and

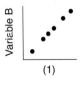 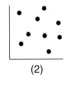 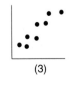 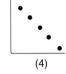

Figure 20.3 *Correlations between variables A and B. (1) perfect positive correlation; (2) no correlation; (3) strong positive correlation; (4) perfect negative correlation.*

accident rates. Levine *et al.* (1976), in a study of accident involvement in US Navy fast-jet pilots and support personnel on board an aircraft carrier, found that those with a history of accident involvement were more adventurous and risk-taking. Sanders *et al.* (1976), in an attempt to cross-validate earlier findings that three factors from the Cattell 16PF (personality factors) personality test were predictive of pilot-error accident involvement, reported that 'individual differences in personality characteristics of the aviators prevent consistent identification of traits associated with pilot-error groups'. Although there does appear to be some association between personality and accidents, it is unlikely that a single 'accident-prone' personality exists (Sümer 2003; Farmer 1984). A more useful approach may be to consider the possible effects of extreme positions on particular personality dimensions and to determine whether certain types of error can be associated with them. For example, the extreme extravert may be error-prone owing to a tendency towards risk-taking, whereas the extreme introvert may be overcautious and hesitant.

Personality is relevant to CRM not only because it influences individual performance but also because it helps to determine the quality of social interaction. An important manifestation of the latter is leadership style.

LEADERSHIP STYLES

In group interactions, a fundamental distinction can be drawn between task-oriented behaviour that is concerned with goal achievement and socioemotionally oriented behaviour that seeks group maintenance (Bales 1950; Cartwright and Zander 1968). This distinction often features in CRM courses, since it has a great effect on group performance and decision-making.

The major aspects of task-oriented leadership (Casimir 2001) are pressure (exhorting subordinates to work hard, imposing deadlines) and instruction (issuing orders, specifying procedures). Socioemotional leadership, on the other hand, refers to encouraging, friendly and fair treatment of subordinates. Clearly, both types of leadership have a place on the flight deck, and the appropriateness of each will depend on the circumstances. In an emergency, for example, an autocratic, task-oriented approach is likely to be more effective.

It has been argued that leaders should emphasize both task-oriented and socioemotional behaviour. However, this assumption has been labelled the 'hi-hi leader behaviour myth' (Larson *et al.* 1976). Casimir's study suggested that combinations of leadership style are important. Employees' perceptions of leadership statements indicated that task-oriented leadership should not be provided in the absence of socioemotional leadership, and that socioemotional leadership is most effective immediately before task-oriented leadership.

Group decision making and performance

APPROACHES TO DECISION MAKING

The traditional approach – classical decision making (CDM) – assumes that individuals weigh up all possible courses of action and select the one that is most appropriate. Thus, the individual is assumed to perform a series of activities, typically identifying the problem, developing alternatives, assessing the advantages and disadvantages of each, choosing a solution, and testing its effectiveness.

Real-life decision making in dynamic time-critical environments where information may be ambiguous or lacking does not conform to the rational, exhaustive processes assumed by CDM. Such naturalistic decision making (NDM) is particularly applicable to experts who draw upon a considerable amount of past experience. In Klein's (1989, 1998) recognition-primed decision model, for example, the expert matches the current situation to similar past experiences, selecting an adequate course of action rather than exhaustively comparing all possible solutions and selecting the one that is optimal. This process is called 'satisficing'. There is growing interest in NDM within aviation, since aircrew activities, particularly in emergencies, are performed under adverse conditions appropriate to the naturalistic approach. However, although the principles of NDM have received support in the literature, they are not yet sufficiently mature to form the basis of aircrew training.

In response to evidence that many aircraft accidents can be attributed at least in part to poor decision making, aeronautical decision-making (ADM) was developed by Jensen and his colleagues (e.g. Jensen and Benel 1977). The distinction between ADM, sometimes called judgement training, and CRM training has largely disappeared (Diehl 1991), since they have many common components. The rationale for ADM training is that sound judgement can be taught, contradicting the notion that judgement is acquired only by experience in performing the task (Federal Aviation Administration 1991). The ADM process is intended to build upon conventional decision making, primarily by recognizing that decision making depends not only on the 'headwork' (rational analysis) emphasized in CDM but also on attitudes.

In the context of aviation, five hazardous attitudes have been identified (Berlin *et al.* 1982) (Table 20.1). ADM courses try to help aircrew to develop 'attitude management', the ability to recognize these hazardous attitudes in themselves and to counteract them. The aircrew are taught to label thoughts as hazardous and to recall an appropriate antidote thought that has been memorized. They participate in antidote-recall exercises and reinforcement exercises based on scenarios likely to lead to hazardous thoughts in an attempt to make this behaviour automatic.

Table 20.1 *Hazardous attitudes and their antidotes (Federal Aviation Administration 1991; Jensen and Biegelski 1989)*

Attitude	Description	Antidote
Anti-authority	Resentful of being told what to do	'Follow the rules'
Impulsivity	Feeling the need to do something quickly	'Think first'
Macho	Taking risks to impress others	'Taking chances is foolish'
Invulnerability	Feeling that accidents happen only to others	'It could happen to me'
Resignation	'What's the use?'	'I'm not helpless; I can make a difference'

The elements of good decision making (Federal Aviation Administration 1991) are:

- identifying hazardous attitudes
- learning methods of modifying behaviour
- learning to recognize and cope with stress
- developing skills in risk assessment
- using all the resources available to the crew
- evaluating the effectiveness of one's ADM skills.

THE DECIDE MODEL

ADM is often delivered using the DECIDE model (Jensen 1988; Jensen and Biegelski 1989). This acronym represents a sequence of actions intended to help pilots make effective decisions (Table 20.2). There was some empirical support in Jensen's study for this approach. Five aircrew participants received training in the DECIDE method; five others did not receive this training. All participants flew a flight simulator, during which unexpected events occurred, such as a failure of the attitude indicator. Although this was only an exploratory study, it provided evidence that trained participants had a greater explicit regard for safety. A larger-scale study (Connolly 1990) provided further evidence that simulator-based ADM training was effective.

GROUPTHINK

The term 'groupthink' was coined by Janis (1972) to describe a tendency for members of a group to seek to reach consensus, often resulting in poor decisions. When groupthink emerges, individuals tend to suppress their doubts about a possible course of action, creating a misleading sense of unanimity. Dissent is considered an act of disloyalty, alternative decisions are rejected out of hand, and any negative consequences of the favoured course of action are rationalized. Sometimes, a 'mindguard' is appointed to prevent dissent and to shield the group from material that might lead it to question its chosen decision.

This phenomenon must be avoided on the flight deck. Fortunately, a variety of strategies to avoid groupthink can be incorporated within CRM training. The group leader, such as the airline captain, can encourage free discussion and the generation of ideas. The consequences of each decision can be discussed, and contingency plans can be put in place to deal with unexpected outcomes.

POLARIZATION AND THE RISKY SHIFT

A related phenomenon is the polarization that is often observed in collective decision making: the group's decisions are more extreme than those of its individual members. Originally, it was thought that groups tended to undergo a 'risky shift'. Stoner (1961) asked business graduates to complete a choice dilemma questionnaire (CDQ) and then to discuss the problems in small groups. In most cases (92 per cent), the group decisions were riskier than the average decisions reached by the individual group members.

The notion of the risky shift was undermined by the finding that two of the CDQ items tended to produce group decisions that were more cautious than those of individuals (Stoner 1968). Further research suggested that decisions related to factors such as personal safety tended to produce a shift towards caution. The notion of the risky shift was, hence, replaced by the more neutral term 'group polarization' (e.g. Moscovici and Zavalloni 1969; Myers and Lamm 1976), which suggested that groups adopt a more extreme position in the direction of their initial bias. These findings support Sherif's notion that small groups converge towards consensus but do not support his argument that the consensus view is roughly the mean of the individual judgements.

Communication

Research on communication has uncovered the characteristics of effective flight crews. It has been reported, for example, that crews that engage in more frequent operational communications and exchange of information com-

Table 20.2 *The DECIDE approach to decision making*

D	Detect	Detect that a change has occurred
E	Estimate	Estimate the need to react to the change
C	Choose	Choose a desired outcome
I	Identify	Identify appropriate actions
D	Do	Take the necessary action
E	Evaluate	Determine the effects of the action

mit fewer errors and distribute workload more evenly during critical phases of flight (Foushee and Manos 1981).

Communication can be made more effective in a number of ways (Huey and Wickens 1993), such as standardizing and restricting vocabulary, using short messages, and presenting redundant information (e.g. both visual and auditory). The number of pilots' requests for full or partial repeats of air traffic controllers' taxi instructions increases with complexity, as do errors in read-back, and longer message lengths can overload the pilot's working memory (Morrow and Rodvold 1993; Morrow et al. 1993). Errors in communication were starkly revealed in a study by Rantanen and Kokayeff (2002), in which experienced pilots listened to taped air traffic control clearances and copied them down on to paper. The authors reported 'astonishingly poor performance' on this task. Errors of commission were much more frequent than errors of omission and were influenced strongly by habit and past experience. The errors typically made by pilots during communication with air traffic controllers are the use of non-standard phraseology, truncation of read-back, failure to issue read-back, and failure to request clarification when appropriate (Spence 1992; Prinzo and Britton 1993).

CREW RESOURCE MANAGEMENT COMMUNICATION SKILLS

Jensen and Biegelski (1989) summarized the communication skills that should be nurtured by CRM training:

- *Enquiry:* crew members may be reluctant to seek clarification, lest it call into question their professional skills or hearing.
- *Advocacy:* aircrew members, even if they occupy a relatively junior position, must be prepared to state their beliefs.
- *Listening:* Jensen and Biegelski emphasized that listening is a skill that must be learned.
- *Conflict resolution:* when crew members express their opinions and beliefs, conflicts are likely to emerge. They must be taught how to resolve conflicts effectively, using them to arrive at better solutions.
- *Critique:* this is an important form of feedback that can be used to improve a variety of flight deck skills.

FACTORS INFLUENCING EFFECTIVENESS OF CREW MEMBERS

Situation awareness

Perhaps the most widely accepted definition of situation awareness (SA) is that of Endsley (1988), illustrated in Figure 20.5: the perception of the elements in the environment within a volume of space and time (level 1), the comprehension of their meaning (level 2) and the projection of their status in the near future (level 3). A large number of aircraft accidents have been attributed to lack of SA (Durso and Gronlund 1999), including 74 per cent of accidents involving controlled flight into terrain in the period 1978–92.

It has proved difficult in practice to measure SA. Two of the most widely used measures are the situation awareness global assessment technique (SAGAT) and the situational awareness rating technique (SART). SAGAT (Endsley 1988) attempts to measure SA objectively, freezing and blanking the operator's displays and presenting queries to test knowledge of the current state of the system (e.g. location of other aircraft). SAGAT has been found to have good reliability, and there is evidence for its validity, such as significant correlation with aircrew performance in a combat simulation (Endsley 2000). However, SAGAT perhaps relies too heavily on memory as an index of SA and does not appear to provide a means of assessing the implicit (and non-verbalizable) knowledge that is a characteristic of the highly skilled operator. SART (e.g. Selcon and Taylor 1990) adopts a different approach, eliciting subjective ratings on a number of scales related to demand for mental resources, supply of resources, and understanding of the situation. Like SAGAT, SART has been found to be related to aircrew performance (Selcon and Taylor 1990) but is subject to the disadvantages associated with subjective techniques, including the effects of possible errors in the individual's mental model.

In aviation, there is particular interest in team SA (Rousseau et al. 2004). SA at the level of the team is assumed to be a function of both individual SA and team cognition. Therefore, it cannot be estimated only by meas-

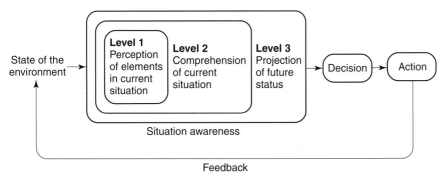

Figure 20.5 *Simplified version of Endsley's (1999) model of situation awareness.*

uring the SA of the individual crew members. Additional factors such as communication and coordination must be considered. Since the emphasis is on shared knowledge, team SA is extremely relevant to CRM. Although SA is a product of many factors (Banbury *et al.* 2004), it can to some extent be trained and therefore is suitable as a component of a CRM course (Prince 1998). Prince provided a detailed framework for SA training, which included:

- discussion of the high frequency of SA-related incidents
- the CRM-related activities that support SA (leadership, communications, preparation and planning, adaptability)
- inferring SA from observable behaviours
- the role of team SA in accident prevention
- the conditions under which SA is likely to be compromised (high workload, fatigue, equipment malfunction).

Stress

The term 'stress' refers to unfavourable conditions to which an individual must adapt. A distinction can be drawn between the following types of stress:

- *Life stress:* life events such as bereavement or divorce.
- *Environmental stress:* both the external environment in which a task is performed (e.g. excessive heat, vibration, altitude) and the internal environment (e.g. fatigue).
- *Cognitive stress:* stress imposed by the task itself (see Workload below).

Life stress typically is measured by questionnaires that attempt to quantify the individual's exposure to particular life events in the recent past (e.g. Holmes and Rahe 1967). Of interest in the present context is the work of Alkov and colleagues (Alkov and Borowsky 1980; Alkov *et al.* 1985), suggesting that life stress may be a factor in some aircraft accidents. A study of US Coast Guard helicopter pilots reported by Fiedler *et al.* (2000) supported the notion that domestic stress can contribute to the stress experienced in the working environment. Crew members should be made aware that colleagues who have recently experienced significant life events may be more liable to error.

Many studies have demonstrated that environmental stressors affect performance. One possible underlying mechanism is alteration of the individual's level of arousal, a continuum that extends from deep sleep to frantic excitement. The Yerkes–Dodson law (Yerkes and Dodson 1908) attempts to relate arousal to performance. It is assumed that there is an optimal arousal level for the performance of any task and that performance declines if arousal increases or decreases from this level, producing an

inverted-U relationship. A further assumption is that this optimal level varies inversely with task difficulty, such that easy tasks require a relatively high level of arousal for best performance (Figure 20.6).

Although the Yerkes–Dodson law is oversimplistic, it can explain some findings reported in the literature, such as Farmer and Green's (1985) observation that the performance of sleep-deprived aircrew, who were naturally in a state of low arousal, declined more sharply on simple repetitive tasks than on a more challenging reasoning task. It also predicts correctly that the combined effect on performance of sleep loss and noise, which have opposing effects on the level of arousal, is lower than that of either in isolation (Corcoran 1962). However, it cannot account easily for the finding that states of low and high arousal are associated with different patterns of performance; for example, attention becomes more focused than normal in an arousing noisy environment but becomes less focused when the individual is sleep-deprived (Hockey 1970a,b). Indeed, each stressor appears to have its own unique 'footprint' of effects on cognition, a finding that is impossible to reconcile with a simple inverted-U model of arousal and performance (Hockey 1986).

It is important that aircrew be familiarized during CRM training with the changes in performance that are likely to occur when they or their colleagues are subjected to sources of stress. Flight safety can be maintained by effective teamwork in which errors committed by individual crew members are identified and rectified.

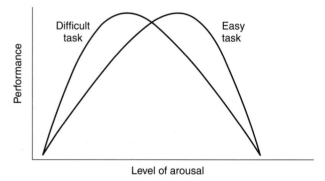

Figure 20.6 *Yerkes–Dodson law.*

Workload

DEFINITION OF WORKLOAD

Workload is a concept that is notoriously difficult to define (e.g. Gartner and Murphy 1979). Sometimes, workload is defined operationally in terms of factors such as the requirements of the task. However, a complete definition must also consider the effort required to perform the task and the level of performance achieved. Clearly, for example, the workload imposed by a given task will be influenced by the expertise of the operator and the level of performance that the operator strives to achieve. However, performance measures alone cannot serve as an adequate metric of workload, since the individual may compensate for increased demand by increasing the level of effort in order to maintain performance. In practice, therefore, a battery of measures typically is used in order to characterize the workload imposed by a particular task or system.

MEASUREMENT OF WORKLOAD

The most common types of workload measure are summarized in Table 20.3. They include performance on the primary task (the task whose workload is of interest) or on a secondary task introduced to determine less directly the demands imposed by the primary task. Subjective measures also have been developed, many specifically for application to aviation. Finally, physiological measures such as pupil size have been used with some success to estimate the effort required to perform flight tasks. For an overview of workload measures and their applications, see O'Donnell and Eggemeier (1986).

EFFECTS OF HIGH WORKLOAD

The flying task is characterized by the need to share attention between several subtasks. In general terms, four types

of task must be performed: aviation, navigation, communication and systems management (e.g. Wickens 2002). By observing airline flights and examining incident reports, Loukopoulos et al. (2003) noted not only that pilots must often perform several tasks concurrently but also that they are frequently interrupted. Flight training does little to prepare pilots to cope with these demands.

Even the highly skilled pilot may perform suboptimally under conditions of high workload, such as dealing with an emergency. With mastery of a task comes the development of 'motor programmes', automated behavioural routines that require little conscious attention (compare with the experienced car driver, who often is unaware of routine actions such as changing gear). Many everyday errors are the result of well-practised but inappropriate behaviour, or 'actions not as planned' (Reason 1990). High workload, which reduces the opportunity to monitor behaviour that has been delegated to the control of motor programmes, makes such errors more likely.

A further possible consequence of overload is an increase in attentional selectivity, i.e. a focusing of attention on particular elements of the task. Such an effect has been demonstrated in noisy environments, which, like overload, tend to increase the individual's level of arousal (Hockey 1970b). Faced with increased task demands, the operator may choose to act quickly at the expense of accuracy or may even shed some subtasks completely, with

Table 20.3 *Major types of workload measure*

Type of method	Rationale	Examples	Advantages	Disadvantages
Primary-task performance	Performance on the task in question indicates the demands that it imposes	Reaction time, accuracy	Provides direct measure of performance, which is often of primary concern	Performance may be insensitive to workload change if operators compensate by varying the effort expended
Secondary-task performance	Performance on a secondary task indicates the operator's 'spare capacity', declining as a function of the demands of the primary task	Time estimation, memory search, manual control task	Useful measure of spare capacity (e.g. ability to respond to emergencies)	Some secondary tasks may be insensitive to the demands of the primary task
Subjective measures	Operators can assess the demands of a task by introspection	Various questionnaires are available, such as the DRA Workload Scales and the NASA task load index	High 'face validity' and hence acceptance by operators; most operators find it fairly easy to assign ratings	Difficult to compare workload on qualitatively different types of task; methods differ in terms of scales used to assess aspects of workload
Physiological measures	Physiological changes are associated with variation in workload	Heart-rate variability (power at 0.1 Hz), pupil size, blink rate	Often, can be recorded continuously, with little intrusion on work activities	Often, a large volume of data is generated, requiring sophisticated analysis

DRA, Defence Research Agency; NASA, National Aeronautics and Space Administration.

obvious implications for safety. As Wickens (2002) has noted, high workload is also likely to impair the pilot's awareness of both the environment and the state of the aircraft; hence, workload and situation awareness are intimately related.

Several approaches have been adopted in the aviation industry to manage workload more effectively. An obvious example is automation. However, Bainbridge (1983) has drawn attention to 'ironies of automation', such as the fact that monitoring an automated system may itself impose significant mental demands. Moreover, new technology has led to a reduction in crew complement. Although the demands upon aircrew have evolved over time, the problem of workload remains.

Training is a powerful method of managing workload. Flying training attempts to automate skilled behaviour as far as possible, producing 'over-learning' by continued practice after proficiency has been achieved. The individual may, therefore, have more spare capacity to deal with other tasks (Farmer et al. 2000). Personnel selection also offers a means of ensuring that aircrew will be able to cope with high task demands. Those who succeed in flying training are more emotionally stable than those who do not (Bartram and Dale 1982), possibly because anxiety impairs the ability to perform concurrent tasks (Eysenck 1982).

In the context of CRM, an important issue in workload management is effective sharing of activities among the crew members. As Huey and Wickens (1993) note, maintenance of team performance under high workload requires effective CRM, including sharing of information and coordination of monitoring and task responsibilities.

EVALUATING CREW RESOURCE MANAGEMENT TRAINING

Measurement issues

Helmreich et al. (1999) summarized the problems of validating CRM training. Validation criteria such as the accident rate per one million flights are precluded because of the low incidence of accidents and the variability of training programmes. Hence, more indirect measures must be used. Incident reports represent a more plentiful source of data but are compromised by the voluntary nature of such reporting. Helmreich et al. suggested that observation of behaviour on the flight deck and acceptance or rejection of CRM concepts are the most appropriate basis for validation. It can be assumed that those people expressing negative attitudes are unlikely to alter their behaviour following CRM training; however, acceptance of CRM concepts does not imply behavioural change.

The validity of typical evaluation methods such as written examinations and simulator evaluations was also questioned by Wise (1996). He advocated the evaluation of real changes in behaviour, rather than role-playing or written responses, particularly since many aircrew have become 'test-wise', giving the officially endorsed answer rather than describing actual behaviour. A solution proposed by Wise was analysis of cockpit voice-recorder data by a human factors practitioner, a pilot and a psycholinguist, in order to search for utterances that were appropriate or inappropriate in terms of CRM principles.

An important development is the use of behavioural marker systems such as NOTECHS to measure the non-technical skills that are central to CRM training (Klampfer et al. 2001). Behavioural markers represent a set of required skills, with examples of the observable behaviour characteristic of each. They are derived from a number of sources, including incident reports, task analysis and interviews (Flin and Martin 2001), and may allow more objective analysis of CRM training.

Effectiveness of crew resource management

Despite finding that CRM training usually had positive outcomes such as promoting appropriate behavioural changes, Salas et al. (2001) concluded from examination of 58 published accounts of CRM training that it was impossible to determine whether CRM achieved its ultimate goal of improving flight safety. It has been claimed that CRM and ADM training reduce the incidence of accidents involving human error by 81 per cent (Diehl 1991). An advisory circular on ADM (Federal Aviation Administration 1991) drew attention to research showing that ADM training reduced in flight judgement errors by 10–50 per cent and that an operator flying about 400 000 hours annually had effected a 54 per cent reduction in accident rate after using ADM materials for recurrency training.

Less positive outcomes have emerged from a number of studies. In Wiegmann and Shappell's (1999) review, the incidence of CRM-related mishaps was found to be comparable to that observed before the introduction of aircrew coordination training. Initial benefits of CRM had, thus, not been enduring. Johnson (2000) drew attention to accident reports in which prior participation in CRM training had no observable effect on crew performance. He attributed failures of CRM to factors such as crew fatigue and the cockpit authority gradient and argued that greater attention should be given to the underlying causes of high workload, distraction and poor decision-making, rather than attempting to counteract their effects by means of CRM training. There is also evidence that CRM has failed to ensure adherence to automation-related procedures (Helmreich et al. 1996); that acceptance of CRM deteriorates over time, even when recurrent training is provided (Helmreich and Taggart 1995); that a small proportion of pilots consistently reject CRM concepts (Helmreich and

Wilhelm 1991; Helmreich and Merritt 2000); and that courses originating in the USA are unsuitable for cultures that discourage the questioning of the judgement of superiors (Helmreich and Merritt 1998).

It is clear that CRM training has not met its objectives fully. Nevertheless, it has become a well-established method of encouraging the effective teamwork that is central to flight safety, and the efforts of dedicated researchers and industry practitioners will ensure its continued evolution.

REFERENCES

Alkov RA, Borowsky MS. A questionnaire study of psychological background factors in U.S. Naval accidents. *Aviation, Space, and Environmental Medicine* 1980; **51**: 860–63.

Alkov RA, Gaynor JA, Borowsky MS. Pilot error as a symptom of inadequate stress coping. *Aviation, Space, and Environmental Medicine* 1985; **56**: 244–7.

Anderson M, Embrey D, Hodgkinson C, *et al*. The human factor implications for flight safety of recent developments in the airline industry: a research study for the JAA: final report. London: Icon International Services Limited, 2001.

Asch SE. Effects of group pressure upon the modification and distortion of judgements. In: Guetzkow H (ed.). *Groups, Leadership, and Men*. Pittsburgh, PA: Carnegie Press, 1951; pp. 177–90.

Asch SE. Studies of independence and conformity: a minority of one against a unanimous majority. *Psychological Monographs* 1956; **70**(9).

Bainbridge L. Ironies of automation. *Automatica* 1983; **19**: 775–9.

Bales R. *Interaction Process Analysis: A Method for the Study of Small Groups*. Cambridge, MA: Addison-Wesley, 1950.

Banbury SP, Croft DG, Macken WJ, Jones DM. A cognitive streaming account of situation awareness. In: Banbury S, Tremblay S (eds). *A Cognitive Approach to Situation Awareness: Theory and Application*. Aldershot: Ashgate, 2004; pp. 117–34.

Bartram L, Dale M. Personality and pilot performance. *Psychological Reports* 1982; **31**: 65–9.

Bassili JN. The minority slowness effect: subtle inhibitions in the expression of views not shared by others. *Journal of Personality and Social Psychology* 2003; **84**: 261–76.

Beaty D. *The Naked Pilot: The Human Factor in Aircraft Accidents*. Shrewsbury: Airlife Publishing, 1995.

Berlin JI, Gruber EV, Holmes CW, *et al*. Pilot judgement training and evaluation, vol. 1. Report no. DOT/FAA/CT-82/56-1. Atlantic City Airport, NJ: Federal Aviation Administration Technical Center, 1982.

Bond R, Smith PB. Culture and conformity: a meta-analysis of studies using Asch's (1952b, 1956) line judgment task. *Psychological Bulletin* 1996; **119**: 111–37.

Cartwright D, Zander A. Leadership and performance of group functions: introduction. In: Cartwright D, Zander A. (eds). *Group Dynamics: Research and Theory*, 3rd edn. New York: Harper and Row, 1968; pp. 301–17.

Casimir G. Combinative aspects of leadership style: the ordering and temporal spacing of leadership behaviors. *Leadership Quarterly* 2001; **12**: 245–78.

Cellar DF, Nelson ZC, Yorke CM. The five-factor model and driving behavior: personality and involvement in vehicular accidents. *Psychological Reports* 2000; **86**: 454–6.

Cialdini RB, Vincent JE, Lewis SK, *et al*. Reciprocal concessions procedure for inducing compliance: the door-in-the-face technique. *Journal of Personality and Social Psychology* 1975; **31**: 206–15.

Civil Aviation Authority. Crew resource management (CRM) training guidance for flight crew, CRM instructors (CRMIs) and CRM instructor-examiners (CRMIEs). CAP 737, issue 1. London: Civil Aviation Authority, 2003.

Collis JM. The OCEAN personality inventory: administrator's guide and test manual. Report no. DERA/CHS/HS3/CR97072/1.0. Farnborough: Defence Evaluation and Research Agency, 1997.

Connolly TJ. Pilot decision-making: training. AFHRL technical paper 88-67. Daytona Beach, FL: Air Force Human Resources Laboratory, 1990.

Cooper, GE, White MD, Lauber JK. Resource management on the flightdeck: proceedings of a NASA/industry workshop. NASA report no. CP-2120. Moffett Field, CA: NASA/Ames Research Center, 1980.

Corcoran DWJ. Noise and loss of sleep. *Quarterly Journal of Experimental Psychology* 1962; **14**: 178–82.

Diehl AE. Does cockpit management training reduce aircrew error? Paper presented at the 22nd International Seminar International Society of Air Safety Investigators, Canberra, Australia, 4–7 November, 1991.

Durso FT, Gronlund SD. Situation awareness. In: Durso FT, Nickerson R, Schvaneveldt R, *et al*. (eds). *The Handbook of Applied Cognition*. Chichester: John Wiley & Sons, 1999; pp. 283–314.

Edwards E. Stress and the airline pilot. Paper presented at the BALPA Technical Symposium: Aviation Medicine and the Airline Pilot. Loughborough: Department of Human Sciences, University of Technology, Loughborough, October 1975.

Endsley MR. Design and evaluation for situation awareness enhancement. In: *Proceedings of the Human Factors Society 32nd Annual Meeting*. Santa Monica, CA: Human Factors Society, 1988; pp. 97–101.

Endsley MR. Situation awareness in aviation systems. In: Garland DJ, Wise JA, Hopkin VD (eds). *Handbook of Aviation Human Factors*. Mahwah, NJ: Lawrence Erlbaum Associates, 1999; pp. 257–76.

Endsley MR. Direct measurement of situation awareness: validity and use of SAGAT. In: Endsley MR, Garland DJ (eds). *Situation Awareness Analysis and Measurement*. Mahwah, NJ: Lawrence Erlbaum Associates, 2000; pp. 147.

Eysenck HJ. *The Structure of Human Personality*, 3rd edn. London: Methuen, 1970.

Eysenck MW. *Attention and Arousal: Cognition and Performance*. Berlin: Springer-Verlag, 1982.

Farmer EW. Personality factors in aviation. *International Journal of Aviation Safety* 1984; **2**: 175–9.

Farmer EW, Green RG. The sleep-deprived pilot: performance and EEG responses. In: Sorsa M (ed.). *Report of the Sixteenth Conference of the Western European Association for Aviation Psychology*. Helsinki: Finnair, 1985; pp. 155–62.

Farmer EW, van Rooij J, Riemersma J, Jorna P, Moraal J. *Handbook of Simulator-Based Training*. Aldershot: Ashgate, 2000.

Federal Aviation Administration. Aeronautical decision making (ADM). Advisory circular no. 60-22. Springfield, VA: National Technical Information Service, 1991.

Fiedler ER, Della Rocco P, Schroeder DJ, Nguyen KT. The relationship between aviators' home-based stress to work stress and self-perceived performance. Report no. DOT/FAA/AM-00/32. Washington, DC: Federal Aviation Administration, Office of Aviation Medicine, 2000.

Fischer U, Orasanu J. Say it again, Sam! Effective communication strategies to mitigate pilot error. Presented at the 10th International Symposium on Aviation Psychology, Columbus, OH, USA, 3–6 May 1999.

Flin R, Martin L. Behavioural markers for CRM: a review of current practice. *International Journal of Aviation Psychology* 2001; **11**: 95–118.

Foushee HC, Manos KL. Information transfer within the cockpit: problems in intracockpit communications. In: Billings CE, Cheaney ES (eds). Information transfer problem in the aviation system. NASA technical paper no. 1875. Moffett Field, CA: NASA/Ames Research Center, 1981; pp. 63–71.

Freedman J, Fraser S. Compliance without pressure: the foot-in-the-door technique. *Journal of Personality and Social Psychology* 1966; **4**: 195–202.

Gartner WB, Murphy MR. Concepts of workload. In: Hartman BO, McKenzie RE (eds). Survey of methods to assess workload. AGARDograph no. 246. Neuilly-sur-Seine: AGARD, 1979; pp. 1–2.

Guéguen N. Foot-in-the-door technique and computer-mediated communication. *Computers in Human Behavior* 2002; **18**: 11–15.

Hatlestad D. Flying lessons: adapting the CRM as a model for airway resource management. *RT: The Journal for Respiratory Care Practitioners* 2005; March. www.rtmagazine.com/Articles.ASP?articleid=R0503F04

Helmreich RL, Merritt AC. *Culture at work: National, Organizational, and Professional Influences.* Aldershot: Ashgate, 1998.

Helmreich RL, Merritt AC. Safety and error management: the role of crew resource management. In: Hayward BJ, Lowe AR (eds). *Aviation Resource Management.* Aldershot: Ashgate, 2000; pp. 107–19.

Helmreich RL, Taggart W. CRM: where are we today? Presented at the CRM Industry Update Workshop, Seattle, WA, USA, 12–13 September 1995.

Helmreich RL, Wilhelm JA. Outcomes of crew resource management training. *International Journal of Aviation Psychology* 1991; **1**: 287–300.

Helmreich RL, Hines WE, Wilhelm JA. Common issues in human factors and automation use: data from line audits at three airlines. Report 96-1. Austin, TX: NASA/University of Texas/FAA, 1996.

Helmreich RL, Merritt AC, Wilhelm JA. The evolution of crew resource management training in commercial aviation. *International Journal of Aviation Psychology* 1999; **9**: 19–32.

Hockey GRJ. Changes in attention allocation in a multi-component task under loss of sleep. *British Journal of Psychology* 1970a; **61**: 473–80.

Hockey GRJ. Effects of loud noise on attentional selectivity. *Quarterly Journal of Experimental Psychology* 1970b; **22**: 28–36.

Hockey GRJ. Changes in operator efficiency as a function of environmental stress, fatigue, and circadian rhythms. In: Boff KR, Kaufman L, Thomas JP (eds). *Handbook of Perception and Human Performance*, vol. 2. New York: Wiley–Interscience, 1986; pp. 1–49.

Holmes TH, Rahe RH. The social readjustment rating scale. *Journal of Psychosomatic Research* 1967; **11**: 213–18.

Huey BM, Wickens CD. *Workload Transition: Implications For Individual And Team Performance.* Washington, DC: National Academy Press, 1993.

Janis I. *Victims of Groupthink.* Boston, MA: Houghton Mifflin, 1972.

Jensen RS. Creating a '1000 hour' pilot in 300 hours through judgement training. Presented at the Workshop on Aviation Psychology, Institute of Aviation, University of Newcastle, Newcastle, Australia, 1988.

Jensen RS, Benel RA. Judgment evaluation and instruction in civil pilot training. DOT/FAA report RD-78-24. Washington, DC: Department of Transportation, 1977.

Jensen RS, Biegelski CS. Cockpit resource management. In: Jensen RS (ed.). *Aviation Psychology.* Aldershot: Gower, 1989; pp. 176–209.

Johnson CW. Reasons for the failure of CRM training in aviation. In: Abbott K, Speyer J-J, Boy G (eds). *HCI Aero 2000: International Conference on Human–Computer Interfaces in Aeronautics.* Toulouse: Cepadues-Editions, 2000; pp. 137–42.

Klampfer B, Flin R, Helmreich RL, et al. *Enhancing Performance in High Risk Environments: Recommendations for the Use of Behavioural Markers.* Ladenburg: Daimler-Benz Shiftung, 2001. www.abdn.ac.uk/iprc

Klein G. Recognition-primed decisions. *Advances in Man–Machine Systems Research* 1989; **5**: 47–92.

Klein G. *Sources of Power: How People Make Decisions.* Cambridge, MA: MIT Press, 1998.

Larson LL, Hunt JG, Osborn RN. The great hi-hi leader behavior myth: a lesson from Occam's razor. *Academy of Management Journal* 1976; **19**: 628–41.

Levine JB, Lee JO, Ryman DH, Rahe RH. Attitudes and accidents aboard an aircraft carrier. *Aviation, Space, and Environmental Medicine* 1976; **48**: 82–5.

Loukopoulos LD, Dismukes RK, Barshi I. Concurrent task demands in the cockpit: challenges and vulnerabilities in routine flight operations. In: Jensen R (ed.). *Proceedings of the 12th International Symposium on Aviation Psychology.* Dayton, OH: Wright State University, 2003; pp. 737–42.

Milgram S. *Obedience to Authority.* New York: Harper & Row, 1974.

Morrow D, Rodvold M. The influence of ATC message length and timing on pilot communication. NASA contract report 177621. Moffett Field, CA: NASA Ames Research Center, 1993.

Morrow D, Lee A, Rodvold M. Analyzing problems in routine controller–pilot communication. *International Journal of Aviation Psychology* 1993; **3**: 285–302.

Moscovici S, Zavalloni M. The group as a polarizer of attitudes. *Journal of Personality and Social Psychology* 1969; **12**: 125–35.

Myers DG, Lamm H. The group polarization phenomenon. *Psychological Bulletin* 1976; **83**: 602–27.

National Transportation Safety Board. Safety study: a review of flightcrew-involved, major accidents of U.S. air carriers, 1978 through 1990. Report no. NTSB/SS-94/01. Washington, DC: National Technical Information Service, 1994.

O'Connor P, Flin R. Crew resource management training for offshore oil production teams. *Safety Science* 2003; **41**: 591–609.

O'Donnell RD, Eggemeier FT. Workload assessment methodology. In: Boff K, Kaufman L, Thomas JP (eds). *Handbook of Perception and*

Human Performance, vol. II. New York: John Wiley & Sons, 1986; pp. 42/1–49.

Pliner P, Hart H, Kohl J, Saari D. Compliance without pressure: some further data on the foot-in-the-door technique. *Journal of Experimental Social Psychology* 1974; **10**: 17–22.

Prince C. *Guidelines for Situation Awareness Training*. Orlando, FA: NAWCTSD/FAA/UCF Partnership for Aviation Team Training, 1998.

Prinzo OV, Britton TW. ATC/pilot voice communications: a survey of the literature. Report no: DOT/FAA/AM-93/20. Washington, DC: Federal Aviation Administration Office of Aviation Medicine, 1993.

Rantanen EM, Kokayeff NK. Pilot error in copying air traffic control clearances. In: *Proceedings of the 46th Annual Meeting of the Human Factors and Ergonomics Society*. Santa Monica, CA: Human Factors and Ergonomics Society, 2002; pp. 145–9.

Reason J. *Human Error*. Cambridge: Cambridge University Press, 1990.

Robertson I, Clarke S. Personality and accidents in high-risk occupations: a meta-analysis. Presented at the International Congress of Applied Psychology Conference, Singapore, 7–12 July 2002.

Rousseau R, Tremblay S, Breton R. Defining and modelling situation awareness: a critical review. In: Banbury S, Tremblay S (eds). *A Cognitive Approach to Situation Awareness: Theory and Application*. Aldershot: Ashgate, 2004; pp. 3–21.

Royal Aeronautical Society. Quality CRM: an HFG working paper. London: Royal Aeronautical Society, 1996.

Ruffle-Smith HP. A simulator study of the interaction of pilot workload with errors, vigilance, and decisions. NASA technical memorandum no. 78482. Moffett Field, CA: NASA/Ames Research Center, 1979.

Salas E, Burke CS, Bowers CA, Wilson KA. Team training in the skies: does crew resource management (CRM) training work? *Human Factors* 2001; **43**: 641–74.

Salgado JF. The Big Five personality dimensions and counterproductive behaviours. *International Journal of Selection and Assessment* 2002; **10**: 117–25.

Sanders MG, Hofmann MA, Neese TA. Cross-validation study of the personality aspects of involvement in pilot-error accidents. *Aviation, Space, and Environmental Medicine* 1976; **47**: 177–9.

Selcon SJ, Taylor RM. Evaluation of the situational awareness rating technique (SART) as a tool for aircrew systems design. In: Situational awareness in aerospace operations. Report no. AGARD-CP-478. Neuilly-sur-Seine: NATO/AGARD, 1990; pp. 5/1–8.

Shaw L, Sichel HS. *Accident Proneness*. Oxford: Pergamon Press, 1971.

Sherif M. *The Psychology of Social Norms*. New York: Harper & Brothers, 1936.

Spence C. Communications recurrent ASRS problem, seminar attendees told. *Air Safety Week* 1992; **27 April**: 1–2.

Stoner JAF. A comparison of individual and group decision involving risk. Master's thesis. Cambridge, MA: Massachusetts Institute of Technology, 1961.

Stoner JAF. Risky and cautious shifts in group decision: the influence of widely held values. *Journal of Experimental Social Psychology* 1968; **4**: 442–59.

Sümer N. Personality and behavioral predictors of traffic accidents: testing a contextual mediated model. *Accident Analysis and Prevention* 2003; **35**: 949–64.

Wickens CD. Situation awareness and workload in aviation. *Current Directions in Psychological Science* 2002; **11**: 128–33.

Wiegmann DA, Shappell SA. Human error and crew resource management failures in naval aviation mishaps: a review of U.S. Naval Safety Center data, 1990–96. *Aviation, Space, and Environmental Medicine* 1999; **70**: 1147–51.

Wiggins JS. *The Five-Factor Model of Personality: Theoretical Perspectives*. New York: The Guilford Press, 1996.

Wise JA. CRM and 'The Emperor's New Clothes'. Presented at the Third Global Flight Safety and Human Factors Symposium. Auckland, New Zealand, 9–12 April, 1996.

Yerkes RM, Dodson JD. The relation of strength of stimulus to rapidity of habit-formation. *Journal of Comparative Neurology and Psychology* 1908; **18**: 459–82.

21

Air traffic control: aeromedical aspects and human factors

SHEILA STORK AND SUSAN M. BAKER

INTRODUCTION

Air traffic control (ATC) dates back to the Second World War, when the requirements for air operations at night and in poor visibility led to the compilation of rudimentary procedures based on principles similar to those still followed for aircraft beyond radar coverage (Hopkin 1995). At that time, standard practices in all aspects of civil aviation management, including ATC, were being formulated, and this led to the formation of the International Civil Aviation Organization (ICAO) as the body concerned with common ATC procedures and practices. Aeronautical, technical and navigational advances had made long flights feasible, aircraft construction had become a major industry, airfields that could handle many large aircraft had been built, and experienced pilots were keen to continue flying. A judicious balance between national sovereignty and the regulation of air traffic was reached, taking into account differences in geography, traffic demand and political and financial priorities.

ICAO (2001a) defines an ATC service as a:
'service provided for the purpose of:

(a) Preventing collisions:
 1. between aircraft, and
 2. on the manoeuvring area between aircraft and obstructions; and

(b) Expediting and maintaining an orderly flow of air traffic.'

In the modern commercial world, cost-effectiveness also has to be taken into account. However, the foremost consideration remains the safety of the system as a whole. Aircraft must remain separated from each other at all times and must not collide with the ground or with other obstacles. Pilots must be guided to their destinations and warned of hazards such as severe weather. Much of the task of the air-traffic controller involves effective communication with other elements in the system. The controller has to take account of the actions and wishes of the pilots, the performance of the aircraft, and the constraints imposed by the nature of the airspace. Problems arise from the deterioration of skills that have already been acquired or inadequate training. ATC has been described as 'three-dimensional chess', to which the fourth dimension of time could well be added. This is meant to convey the complexity of the situation and the fact that controllers have to take account of not only the movement of aircraft in vertical and horizontal planes but also their relative positions and the time at which they are expected to cross particular locations. While this description has a certain appeal, it probably does little to clarify the real nature of the task, and it tends to be a term used more by those who talk about ATC than those who carry it out.

ATC has developed into two major disciplines: area control and airfield control. Area control provides air traffic services to en-route or transiting aircraft, while airfield control provides approach and aerodrome control services to aircraft operating in the vicinity of an aerodrome (Figure 21.1). Controllers are licensed according to the disciplines in which they operate. Controllers working at the area control centres hold ratings equivalent to a combined ICAO area control and an ICAO area radar control licence. Extensive radar coverage, such as that which exists over the UK, means that aircraft are controlled using radar skills; for areas outside radar cover, other techniques are used, which are referred to as procedural control.

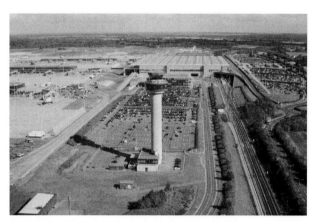

Figure 21.1 *Air traffic control tower environment.*

THE ENVIRONMENT

Controllers have to take into account a plethora of information originating from a variety of sources and involving different sensory modalities. Considerable information is presented visually on radar displays (Figure 21.2), flight-progress strips, maps and charts and closed-circuit television screens and through the window of the visual control room (VCR). Auditory information arrives via the radiotelephony (RTF) link with the aircraft or the telephone, as well as from conversation and information exchange with colleagues in the immediate vicinity. All controllers in the en-route environment, and many controllers in control towers, wear headsets, although in some towers information may be broadcast over a loudspeaker system. The sequence in which this information arrives is not predictable and can be conflicting, with more than one aircraft calling at once or the telephone ringing when the controller is engaged in conversation.

Changes to an aircraft's position or estimated time of arrival on the sector have to be recorded on a flight-progress strip. This may be done by the controller, supervisor or coordinator. The information has to be drawn to

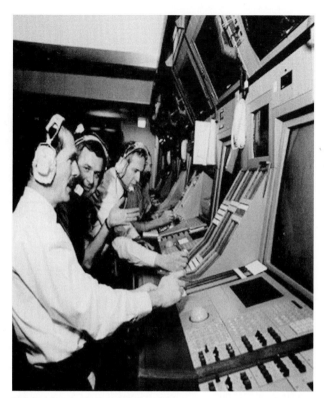

Figure 21.2 *Typical radar environment.*

the attention of the controller concerned; the scope for error is self-evident. The paper flight-progress strip (PFPS) is a commonly used method of recording ATC operational data at airfield and area air traffic services units (ATSUs) throughout the world. Paper strips have been used in various forms since the beginning of ATC, and there is no other system that can so flexibly and tangibly record the movement of aircraft in three dimensions. The typical flight-progress strip display, which contains the aircraft's call sign, height, time, route details and control instructions (Figure 21.3), must be kept up to date, since it represents the traffic situation for the controller. Electronic coordination could be viewed as a more efficient method of data transfer, and transition from the traditional paper strip to an electronic version is currently under way in the UK. Although there are undoubted advantages inherent in electronic strip displays, the ability to annotate, manipulate and position the paper strips by hand serves as a powerful aide memoir to controllers. It can represent the physical position of an aircraft in the air traffic environment and is an active reminder to a controller of decisions already taken and of those that need to be made. These physical and flexible aspects of the PFPS make it a unique and well-liked method of operational data-recording, and many advantages may be lost with the advent of paperless formats.

The environment is seldom quiet. Large centres can have up to 100 controllers working at any one time, with addi-

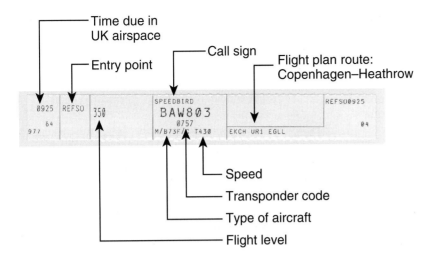

Figure 21.3 *Flight-progress strip.*

tional supervisory staff, assistants and support personnel. The controller who is distracted easily does not survive long. Conversely, the controller cannot afford to become too focused on any one aspect of the task. Incoming information has to be attended to and/or logged and communication maintained with the aircraft and other controllers. In the radar environment, the controller has to monitor the radar display, checking aircraft routes and levels to ensure that the process is going according to plan. The radar display usually presents the traffic picture in plan, with north at the top, and traffic headings are given in terms of the 360-degrees clock. Aspiring controllers who cannot tell left from right or who fail to appreciate that a southbound aircraft turning left is actually going right on the radar display do not progress very far through the system.

SELECTION AND TRAINING

The lifecycle of the controller begins with a selection process. The age at which a student can begin training is within a specific band. Applicants usually require educational qualifications to the level of university entrance. They must have aptitude in visuospatial skills and decision-making as well as certain personality traits that have an influence on health and wellbeing. Psychometric testing is used to highlight individuals who can work in a team and are logical, anxiety-resistant and emotionally stable. Pathological personality traits and significant psychiatric history are unacceptable. Criminal offenders and the possibility of drug or alcohol misuse must be assessed carefully.

Training may be considered in three phases. Initial training is usually carried out at a dedicated college, where students are given basic instruction in the theory and application of procedures. This leads to a student licence, which enables the trainee to progress to the next phase. Pre-on-the-job training (pre-OJT) and on-the-job training

(OJT) are carried out at a unit. Pre-OJT is designed to bridge the knowledge and skills gap between what has been already taught and what will be required before commencing OJT and thus plays a fundamental part in the development of control skills. Experienced controllers monitor trainees. In the early stages, the trainee will do little more than issue instructions to aircraft under the guidance of a mentor. As training progresses, the trainee will act more and more on their own initiative until they are able to perform the whole task, but still under supervision. When the trainee is considered competent, they are given a certificate of competence to work solo. With increasing experience, the controller will train on other sectors or functions in the en-route environment.

Illness requiring the student to have more than one week's absence from training usually necessitates a full recourse as it has been found that students are unable to catch up satisfactorily on the missed coursework. Good health and fitness throughout training therefore are of paramount importance; in addition, the trainees should be counselled regularly with regard to healthy eating. Trainees should be encouraged to live 'sensibly' with regard to their lifestyle and the pursuit of risky physical activities. Trainee controllers often find the regime of study, continuing assessment and validation stressful, and there may be a need for further guidance and counselling.

OJT is not without its problems for the instructor or mentor. During the early stages of training, alertness is maintained by an awareness of the lack of skill of the trainee and the high probability of error. However, as training progresses and fewer mistakes are made, attention may wane and errors pass unnoticed. Mentors frequently assert that one of the more difficult aspects of training is maintaining close supervision as the trainee approaches the validation standard; a concomitant issue is that of preserving their own operational expertise. Many mentors feel that facets of their own skills, notably those involving rapid reactions and prompt decision making, suffer from the lack of hands-on work. It is, therefore, important to restrict the amount of supervision any one individual carries out; nevertheless, problems do occur occasionally.

After validation, the continued competence of the controller is ensured by means of competency checks. Typically, these are conducted by a suitably qualified member of the same unit who has undergone training in competency checking. It might be argued that the dual roles of colleague and competency checker are too close for comfort, but the checker is in the position of seeing the controller's work on a regular basis and should, therefore, be in a good position to notice and monitor any changes in performance. A one-off check by an outsider, although ostensibly more impartial, is less likely to reveal a gradual deterioration in performance, since, at best, a one-off check can be only a snapshot and probably would not provide a fair assessment of the controller's abilities or any degradation over time.

DECISION-MAKING AND FLEXIBILITY

The controller must have the ability to make effective positive decisions within a relatively short timescale: one of the facets of ATC that distinguishes it from many other safety-related professions is the speed at which many decisions have to be made. In many industries, operators have time to deliberate on potential courses of action and perhaps even to discuss them with other, more experienced colleagues. For the controller, the luxury of lengthy deliberation is not available. This is not to suggest that controlling is a question of snap decisions, but the time available to get it right is limited – sometimes to seconds – as, for example, in the case of a potential collision between two aircraft. While the time available for making decisions may be limited, there is also often little time for dwelling on the effects of decisions once they have been made. Although controllers have to ensure that their decisions have been accurate and effective, there is little or no time available to scrutinize those decisions after the event, since the traffic situation will have moved on and new demands will be presenting.

The second important feature that has implications for decision making and problem solving is the dynamic nature of the environment. The scenario that faces the controller is changing constantly, often predictably but occasionally in ways that are totally unanticipated. Not only is the situation dynamic, but also its contributory elements are interactive. The movement of any one aircraft is likely to have implications for others in the vicinity, not only in the short term but also possibly at some time in the future. Controllers often speak of 'having the picture' – essentially, situational awareness – or of 'losing the picture' – when their grasp of the situation is flawed. However good the 'picture' may be at any given time, it is changing constantly, and the controller has to be aware of, and respond

to, those changes. The dynamism of the situation is not, however, altogether outside the controller's influence. He or she will contribute to the changing pattern by means of the instructions given to the aircraft. This should bring an element of order and predictability to the situation, since the controller will be working to a formulated plan.

The controller has to be capable of positive, relatively rapid decision making and must be sufficiently flexible to adapt to the changing scene. One of the skills of effective controlling is the ability to adapt to a changing situation while, at the same time, maintaining the overall picture and the way in which the parts of that picture interact. The controller will be subject to a number of pressures, including responding to requests from pilots for level changes, taking account of the weather and the routes of other aircraft, and assimilating information from a variety of sources, all of which can have implications for the decision-making process.

The normal age for retirement of air traffic controllers is 60 years, although some controllers experience difficulty in coping with the job from the late forties onwards. Whether a controller approaching 60 years of age is equipped to cope with the demands of modern ATC is open to question, although it has to be said that age, per se, has been a contributory factor in relatively few incidents within the UK. Nevertheless, older controllers do experience problems that differ from those of their younger colleagues. Rapid decision making places demands on controllers and may pose particular problems for older controllers, whose speed of reaction may not be optimum. Greater experience and knowledge may compensate, to an extent, for this reduction in response time, but the situation can be difficult for older controllers, a fact of which they are only too aware. Another difficulty is maintaining skills and competence. This is especially the case with respect to those positions in which the controller may work relatively infrequently. Some older controllers may be able to find other non-operational positions in which their knowledge and long experience can be put to good use, but the number of such positions is dwindling. In addition, the task itself is changing, becoming more automated and making use of new high-technology equipment. Such innovation can cause problems of adaptation, particularly for older personnel, who may be less familiar and comfortable with computerization.

COMMUNICATION

Communication in ATC can be verbal, written or, increasingly, electronic, such as by data link. Communication takes place between controllers at the same unit, with controllers at other units, and with aircraft both on the ground and in the air. There are various safeguards to ensure that communication proceeds as planned. Since a large element of ATC involves communication, it is not surprising that breakdown of communication figures so prominently in the occurrence of incidents and near-incidents. Communication breakdown can occur at any phase of the operation. It can turn an otherwise normal operational sequence into an incident, or an incident into an accident.

The first aspect of verbal communication to be considered is that between controllers and the pilots of the aircraft under their control. The international language of aviation is English, or, more accurately, 'aviation English', which has its own structure and syntax. To reduce the possibility of misunderstanding, standard phraseology should be adopted during radiotelephony interchange. This involves the use of not only standard terms and phrases but also the internationally recognized phonetic alphabet. Despite these safeguards, mistakes do happen, especially when the situation is non-standard for some reason, such as during an emergency. Verbal communication is fraught with problems. Apart from the more obvious, such as language and technical difficulties leading to poor transmission and/or reception of messages, slips of the tongue and misunderstandings also occur.

A pilot in receipt of an instruction is required to read back that instruction so that the controller can verify that the message has been received and understood properly. This process can be considered as a communication loop, albeit, unfortunately, one that both controller and pilot can break. Most if not all possible verbal communication problems are evident in the read-back situation. These include hearing what one wants or expects to hear, forgetting to give or request a read-back, distraction from any one of a number of sources, language problems, slips of the tongue, low vigilance when errors are not noticed, and reluctance to give a read-back, preferring instead to use the term 'Roger' or simply to repeat the call sign of the aircraft. Technological advances such as data-link systems that ensure that the message is transferred accurately to the flight deck or even directly into the aircraft's flight-management system may help to alleviate some of these difficulties, although such innovations are likely to bring their own peculiar problems. One of the more perplexing communication problems is that of the pilot who gives a complete and accurate read-back of the executive instruction but subsequently, for whatever reason, goes on to do something different.

If communication is vitally important during normal operation, it is even more crucial during emergencies, when a situation can be rendered critical by communication breakdown. While an emergency persists, pilots and controllers will be working under a high level of stress, a factor that is not likely to be conducive to good performance. For this reason, a number of safeguards are built into the system, such as the use of emergency checklists and procedures designed to support the individuals concerned

in what is an unanticipated and, for most, a rare event. Training in what to expect and how to cope is essential. It is argued sometimes that adequate training in emergency handling cannot be provided, since no two emergencies will be alike and thus it is impossible to build a training programme to cover all contingencies. This line of argument misses the point: while it may be possible to train for specific and anticipated failures, such as radio or radar failure and engine fires, the aim of emergency training is not to rehearse a shortlist of known events but rather to inculcate a method and attitude for dealing with the unexpected in a prompt and effective manner. Air traffic controllers in the UK have to undergo annual refresher training in the handling of such unexpected events. This training in unusual circumstances and emergencies (TRUCE) is designed to provide controllers with experience of rare and possibly stressful events in order to learn how to cope better should the need arise.

TEAMWORK AND HANDOVER

Although each controller is responsible individually for his or her decisions and for the precise manner in which the task is carried out, controllers nevertheless work as a part of a team. The team may be self-evident, such as other controllers in the same operations room or the same control tower, but sometimes the rest of the team is not so obvious, as it involves controllers at other units and the pilots receiving the control service. To consider all of these individuals as part of the same team may appear to be stretching a point, but if they fail to work together, serious consequences can result. Until recently, little or no recognition has been given to the need to train controllers to function as a team. This situation is changing, however, and initiatives are under way to develop and provide training courses in team resource management (TRM). Although advantage can be taken of the work already accumulated in connection with crew resource management (CRM) on the flight deck, it is not advisable simply to graft CRM on to the control community. Having said this, the fundamentals of a TRM course will resemble CRM in many ways, and they contain a number of the same basic elements such as situational awareness, decision-making, communication, leadership, stress management and training in teamwork itself.

It is often difficult to pinpoint a time during a shift when controller-related incidents are most likely to occur. Experience has shown that the handover from one controller to another can be a vulnerable time. Although there will be a procedure that most controllers follow in handing over, there is often no formal method and no written procedure for transferring responsibility. Typically, in the radar environment, the outgoing controller will pass information to the person taking over by correlating the traffic visible on the radar display with that indicated on the flight-progress strips. During this time, any particular problems should be pointed out, together with an idea of the pending traffic. It is the responsibility of the incoming controller to be satisfied that the complete picture has been assimilated before assuming control of the position.

It is evident that the dynamic nature of ATC renders this handover and takeover process vulnerable to confusion and error. Information is being transferred and assimilated on a dynamic and varying situation. In addition, the picture that is being handed over is created, to a certain extent, according to the preferences and methods of working of the outgoing controller. Variations in controlling style may mean that a controller accepts traffic that is not configured as he or she would wish and that may entail a certain amount of rearranging after the handover has taken place. The potential for error can be exacerbated by time pressure. The situation may be so busy that it is not possible for the optimum amount of time to be devoted specifically to the handover, and so errors of omission and misunderstanding could occur. UK incident data indicate that the most vulnerable time is not, as quoted frequently in the literature, the period immediately following the handover, as controllers are very much on their guard during this phase; rather, it is some 15–30 minutes after assuming control, possibly because the controller has started to relax a little, with a concomitant reduction in vigilance.

WORKLOAD AND FATIGUE

The workload of the controller is made up of several elements. The most evident, and probably the easiest to estimate, is the number of aircraft on a frequency over a given time period. It is not unusual for controllers to have 15–18 aircraft on the frequency at the same time, and they may have as many as 60–70 through a sector in the space of an hour. Nevertheless, perceived workload is not governed by the number of aircraft alone. The configuration of aircraft, traffic complexity and the specific constraints of a particular piece of airspace all contribute to perceived workload, and the situation is likely to be complicated further by the weather, organizational problems and availability of staff.

Although it is true that mistakes do occur at times when workload is high, this is by no means always the case; errors are also made during quiet periods. It is rather too simplistic to attribute this to boredom. Often, it is the transition in workload from high to low and vice versa that causes problems. The transition from high to low workload allows the opportunity to relax a little after what may have been a demanding time. It is precisely during this period that mistakes may occur. The reduction in work-

load sometimes appears to bring with it a reduction in vigilance and alertness. Conversely, the controller coping with a rapid transition from low to high workload may fail to anticipate or plan ahead to accommodate the change. Workload changes due to traffic volume are often relatively predictable, but a sudden increase in workload due to an incident or emergency is, by its very nature, impossible to foresee.

There are means by which high workload levels can be handled. Sectors can be split so that more than one controller works a particular piece of airspace or the flow of traffic through the airspace may be restricted. Some years ago traffic flows were characterized by marked seasonal peaks and troughs, but in more recent years these fluctuations have not been nearly so pronounced. This means that workload is likely to be high over a more prolonged period, with less opportunity to recover, since the troughs are infrequent.

The aviation industry operates around the clock, thus necessitating shift systems. Many controllers enjoy the freedom and flexibility of the lifestyle facilitated by rotating shifts, though some people are not suited and some older controllers experience fatigue and sleep problems. Sleep deprivation impairs performance, and the detrimental effects are greater when the required response is unfamiliar, e.g. an unpractised emergency. Furthermore, although motivation can improve performance, sleep deprivation reduces motivation and so is doubly detrimental. Personality has a link with performance: people who have been shown to be 'morning types' have their peak of performance earlier than those who are 'evening types'. However, introversion or extroversion seems to have little effect.

Apart from sleep difficulty associated with night work, a controller's social life is also disrupted by a work/rest pattern that differs from that of the majority of the population and, importantly, that of their family. Shift workers often rate the detrimental effects of their unusual work times on their family and social life as of greater importance than the adverse effects on their sleeping patterns. When designing work schedules, social needs must be considered if the controller is to remain content. It is difficult to design a suitable schedule for all involved in work outside the 'normal' working day, since tolerance to disrupted sleep varies considerably among individuals. Some people perform better in the evening than in the morning; others are simply better able to tolerate night work; and some manage well until middle-age and then find coping increasingly difficult. Older people may be able to tolerate early-morning starts better than younger colleagues but may find night work more difficult. Constant night work would allow some entrainment of the circadian rhythms to a new schedule, but this is not usually acceptable for social reasons, even if it were operationally convenient. Where shifts are worked, the cycle should move to become progressively later during the day, and no more than two consecutive night shifts should be worked. In the UK, the shift patterns of controllers are regulated by law under the Scheme for the Regulation of Air Traffic Controllers Officers Hours (SRATCOH), which covers such aspects as length of shifts, rest periods and number of consecutive night shifts.

What is perceived as fatigue has been used to describe a state following physical or mental effort, lack of sleep, boredom, stress or anxiety, or any combination of these. Individuals differ in their tolerance, so what is exhausting for one is only tiring for another. Tiredness may be detrimental, since a controller may fall asleep under situations of low arousal and he may fail to appreciate a situation that might later result in an emergency. Low levels of performance attributed to fatigue cause errors that may remain uncorrected and include reduced flexibility of approach, increased likelihood of errors in flight-management decisions, mood changes (increased hostility/irritability) detrimental to teamwork, tunnelling of attention (fascination) and decreased powers of concentration.

STRESS

In the late 1980s the Royal Air Force Institute of Aviation Medicine carried out a survey of controllers and their sources of stress (Farmer *et al.* 1990). The survey did not support the popular notion that ATC is an inherently stressful occupation but indicated that issues such as dissatisfaction with equipment, staff shortages and lack of participation by the workforce in decision-making were stressful. Sources of stress in the workplace included involvement in airproxes or incidents, difficulties among older controllers in learning to use new technology and procedures, relocations and personality differences. Stress-related illness was often associated with domestic crises, shock of accidents and injury, and health concerns regarding relatives.

More recently, controllers have been subject to much technological and organizational change. Increase in air traffic movements, coupled with staff constraints, has caused increased pressure, and managers and controllers are encouraged to look for signs of stress, both in themselves and in colleagues. Some examples include heavier than usual smoking and drinking, sudden overeating or loss of appetite, sleeplessness (particularly early wakening), unusual tiredness and lack of energy, short temper, difficulty in making decisions that previously posed no problem, and difficulty in concentrating. If a controller is considered to be fit and safe to remain at work, then they may do so, even while attending counselling groups or individual sessions with a clinical psychologist.

It is, of course, appropriate to consider the operational consequences of stress and the effects that stress, from whatever source, may have on the performance of the controller. Effective decision-making depends to a very large extent on the breadth and quality of the information used by the individual in arriving at a decision, and this is where the first problems arise. Under stress, the range of information intake can become limited. There is a tendency to focus on what may appear to be the most salient aspects of a task or situation at the expense of other inputs. On occasion, the input that appears to be most salient is often only the input that is most attention-getting or easily available. If the quality of the information used in making the decision is deficient, then the decision itself is almost certain to be flawed. Decisions made under stress are often premature. The very act of making a decision or arriving at a plan of action is, in itself, stress-reducing, allowing the individual to turn his or her attention to other tasks. A plan made in a hurry and based on inadequate information is a poor plan.

In the dynamic situation of ATC, it is essential that plans, once formulated, are monitored to ensure that the planned course of action is still relevant to the changing situation. In a stressful situation, the monitoring of plans is often faulty, since the stressed worker finds it difficult to stand back and take a broad view of the situation. Consequently, the plan is adhered to and, even though the changing situation has rendered it inappropriate, the individual stays with the plan and is unwilling, or unable, to amend it. Sometimes, the situation progresses to a point at which even the individual realizes that the plan is no longer suitable or has broken down. The possibility is that the person will not try another plan but will dispense with planning altogether and take each situation as it comes on an ad hoc basis. Controllers whose plans have failed sometimes revert to a form of 'reactive controlling', in which each aircraft is dealt with as a separate entity, and an overview of the interactions among them – essentially, the overall picture – or situational awareness is lost.

One of the ways in which workload can be managed is by prioritization of tasks. If workload is very high, then this may involve shedding those tasks deemed to be of lesser importance. Unfortunately, under stress, the decisions regarding those tasks that should be shed may not be correct. Consequently, important tasks are left undone while less important tasks are given undue priority. There is also a tendency to solve the easy problems first, i.e. to devote effort to simpler tasks that are well within the scope of the individual rather than focusing attention on more serious, but more difficult, jobs. When a problem presents itself, the individual has to choose an appropriate means of dealing with it. However, under stress, there can be a tendency to revert to a tried and tested course of action. The difficulty arises when the problem to be solved resembles, but is not precisely the same as, one encountered before. The individual fails to recognize this and tries to impose an inappropriate solution on the problem.

INCIDENTS AND INVESTIGATIONS

It should, by now, be evident that the controller needs to be confident and self-reliant, capable of positive but flexible decision-making, and able to assimilate and utilize a range of information from a variety of sources, while maintaining careful monitoring of the traffic situation and without becoming distracted or overly focused on any one element of the task. In other words, the controller has to build and maintain a good grasp of the air traffic picture. In the light of these demands, together with what we have said already about the environment and the nature of the task, incidents can be expected to occur. The situation is always dynamic, often very busy and, at least up to the present time, reliant to a great extent on the human element. Incidents can occur and, when they do, need to be investigated and appropriate remedial action taken if a repetition is to be avoided.

The watch manager is responsible for the input of their team's contribution to the safety of the system. Therefore, in the event of an incident, it is his or her responsibility to remove the controller from operational duty and offer initial support and counselling. An on-watch investigation then takes place, which involves collection of RTF tapes, flow-management data and reports from the controllers involved, supervisors and the controller's local competency examiner. It is evident that in addition to the incident, the investigation procedure itself could be extremely stressful. Therefore, at any stage in the process, the controller may be referred directly for immediate counselling or for medical advice.

The decision to investigate incidents, as well as the more attention-getting accidents, is not one that can be taken lightly, since it is a specialized resource-intensive activity. The first and most obvious reason for investigating incidents and accidents is that it allows investigators to build up a wider picture of what problems exist and also to gain an understanding of any trends. The more information available, the firmer the basis on which conclusions and decisions can be made. From the human factor perspective, the behaviour manifested by individuals or groups involved in incidents may not differ greatly from that observed in accident scenarios. Admittedly, the gravity of an accident will add another dimension to the situation, but generally the cognitive failures, problems in decision-making, communication breakdown, distraction and all the other factors that contribute to the sum total of behaviour in an accident are present in incidents.

It is important not to underestimate the effect of incidents on controllers, who may well try to cover up their feelings. A macho ethos is still sometimes evident, and many controllers, especially older men, feel that it is a weakness to admit to stress-related symptoms. With better training of managers and employees, promotion of attitude change and facility for consultation, it is hoped that controllers will feel less isolated and will utilize the support system. It is by now generally accepted that accidents and incidents are often the result of an accumulation of events rather than the outcome of one single causal factor. In addition, the contributory and causal factors are often found in the system, even though they are manifested in the performance of an individual. Therefore, to focus on errors committed by individuals rather than looking at the system as a whole is to miss an opportunity to make system-related improvements, which are likely to be far more effective in the longer term than simply identifying an individual and leaving untouched the underlying problems.

MEDICAL STANDARDS AND LIMITATIONS

Throughout the operation of every form of public transport, there is an expectation that the highest standards of safety will be maintained, and so it is important to ascertain whether the employee has the mental and physical attributes to carry out the job (Figure 21.4). The air traffic controller must be physically fit, free of serious degenerative illness, and conform to the medical standards set by the regulatory authority. The preferred body mass index (BMI) is between 20 and 25. Candidates with a BMI greater than 30 should be investigated; if found to be free of physical pathology, they should be encouraged to lose weight. The necessary attributes for both tower and radar work include good visual acuity with full peripheral and colour vision, normal hearing and clear diction without speech impediment. Good verbal and visuospatial skills are also important. An intact memory is necessary, as flight-progress strips may not have current data; this is especially relevant in tower work at some airfields, where landing aircraft may be at different stages in the circuit while others are pushing back from the stands. Additionally, the individual must not be vulnerable to sudden or subtle incapacitation. ICAO (2001b) promotes global medical standards for controllers; the class 3 medical standards refer to controllers. Within the spirit of ICAO and the European Joint Aviation Authorities Requirements (JAR-FCL3) for commercial pilots, there has been a move to harmonize the European medical requirements for controllers in the formulation of a European class 3 medical certificate. These new requirements apply to states that have signed up to membership of the European Civil Aviation Conference (ECAC).

At various stages in the career of a controller, it may be necessary to exercise some flexibility in the application of medical standards. Applicants for ab initio medical certification must conform to the standards, however certain limitations may be acceptable at this stage, the most common being for visual acuity i.e. the individual may be

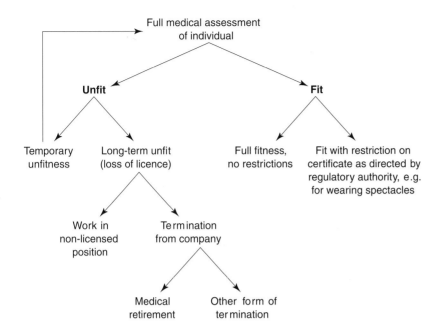

Figure 21.4 *Decision-making process regarding medical certification of air traffic control officers.*

required to wear spectacles correcting for distance. Contact lenses are also permitted, provided that spare correcting spectacles are available. Very rarely, and only after careful assessment, it may be necessary to impose medical assessment more frequently than usually specified. Examples include applicants with non-progressive disabilities, who are able to carry out the job safely and efficiently. Occasionally, an individual may be deemed fit to work at ground level but not, for professional flying, at altitude, e.g. a person with a history of asthma. In certain circumstances, whereby an individual does not comply fully with the ATCO medical standards, it is possible to grant a waiver, although it is necessary to ensure that the individual can carry out their work without compromising the safety of the operation. In this context, once all the information is to hand, it may be useful to arrange an assessment of the individual, at work, involving all tasks that may have to be carried out during training, qualification and job placement. Examples of individuals who might be involved in this process are people with paraplegia or amputations. Each case will then be assessed on the findings, on an individual basis, for certification purposes.

For many years, medical standards have struck a balance between ensuring that controllers do not operate when unfit and avoiding the unnecessary bureaucracy associated with short-lived and minor illnesses. However, it must be emphasized that developments in medical practice have resulted in more rapid investigations with markedly reduced periods of hospitalization and time off work for investigation and treatment of fairly serious pathologies. In such circumstances, a controller may not be aware of the flight-safety implications of their illness and thus they must obtain qualified medical advice. Particular examples are day surgery, medical investigations showing abnormal results, regular use of medication, brief loss of conscious-

ness, ultrasound treatment of kidney stones, coronary angiography, apparent transient ischaemic attacks, and abnormal heart rhythms, including atrial fibrillation and flutter. Some conditions render the controller permanently unfit; these include certain cardiovascular, neurological and psychiatric conditions, certain malignancies and severe pathologies. Each case must be assessed in the light of all the information available. A controller may have limitations placed upon them or, in the extreme case, may be rendered 'long-term unfit', with loss of licence.

Since the mid-1980s, there has been an increase in the recruitment of female controllers. In the UK, the current proportion of male to female controllers is four to one. A large number of these controllers are of childbearing age and they may continue to work up to the time stipulated by the regulaory authority. Regular antenatal care is essential, and the controller is required to report symptoms of faintness, dizziness, vertigo, nausea and vomiting. Anaemia (haemoglobin $\leq 10\,\text{g/dl}$), glycosuria, proteinuria, urinary tract infection, vaginal bleeding, abdominal pain and high blood pressure must be monitored closely.

POSTURE AND MOBILITY

Currently, good mobility is required for tower work, as most towers have narrow winding stairs leading to the visual control room and, once there, the tasks involve twisting and turning movements. Although mobility is not such an issue in the radar room, and new centres are being designed to accommodate wheelchairs, it still remains true that strong, supple vertebral spines are necessary to tolerate various ergonomic problems. The tower controller may be required to work alone, especially at night, and therefore bowel or bladder irregularities could be a major problem. In the radar room, good visual accommodation is needed to assimilate information from screens and keyboards at varied distances. Extreme hypermetropia or presbyopia can be a problem, and multifocal spectacles may be necessary for older controllers. The ambient lighting in the radar room is often lower than that in the tower, and 'eyestrain' may be experienced. In a confined atmosphere where close supervision may be required, body odour and dermatological problems may be offensive.

Improved working practices and ergonomic design of equipment have been incorporated into work areas helping to alleviate the adoption of awkward postures. However, it is still possible that upper-back and neck pain may occur if controllers are not instructed fully in the correct use of the work area or if they do not comply with such practice. Fully adjustable chairs with good lumbar support are required. It is important for individuals to be aware of correct posture, the need to adjust the chair at the start of each work cycle, the benefit of physical exercise to maintain strength and suppleness of the spine, and the necessity to report problems early before pathology has developed. Advice at an early stage may be appropriate regarding the workstation, work practice, specific treatment regimens such as physiotherapy, and the possible modification of home lifestyle, especially with regard to gardening, housework, home repairs and the concentrated use of personal computers. Nevertheless, even with preventive measures, conditions such as cervical spondylosis, osteoarthritis of the spine and ankylosing spondylitis may lead to 'long-term' unfitness.

VISUAL FATIGUE

Although the use of display-screen equipment neither makes existing visual defects worse nor is associated with damage to the eyes, some workers experience visual fatigue, red or sore eyes and headaches. Radar controllers appear to have particular problems especially at the onset of presbyopia. The variety of visual distances involved in carrying out their work and the need for rapid accommodation often necessitate the use of multifocal lenses; these must be adjusted for the individual's task, as excess tilting of the head may lead to neck and upper-back discomfort. Aerodrome controllers working in the visual control room of a tower may experience problems with glare, especially if it is sunny, and it may be difficult to reduce this problem without compromising visibility. Much can be achieved by shielding and replacing or repositioning sources of light and equipment. As a last resort, antiglare screen filters may be used. Controllers are permitted to wear contact lenses but, as individuals tend to stare and blink less when concentrating, the surface of the eye is prone to drying.

Encouraging controllers who wear contact lenses to increase their individual blink rate and maintaining good ventilation and humidity in the room tend to diminish this problem. Controllers should be encouraged, both when taking rostered breaks and when working, to rest their eyes at infinity by gazing into the distance whenever possible.

MEDICATION AND ALCOHOL

With the increasing availability of over-the-counter drugs, more controllers are taking self-prescribed medications, to the possible detriment of their work and health. The ideal situation is that anyone requiring medication should not be on duty, but this is not practicable. The illness may be relatively mild and may not seriously affect the performance of a controller's duties, and the medication in any case may not conflict with the standard of fitness required. Nevertheless, since many common drugs and remedies have important adverse effects, all ATC personnel must be aware of the potential pitfalls of self-medication. Controllers must assure themselves that they are fit for work and that the medication is free of adverse effects. Many medications may impair performance. It is essential to seek expert advice before the use of hypnotics, and controllers should not take tranquillizers or antidepressants while undertaking operational work. Antibiotics may have short-term or delayed effects; in addition, their use indicates an infection, which will usually render the controller unfit for work. Antihistamines, which may be sedative, are used widely in 'cold cures' and in the treatment of hayfever, asthma and allergic skin conditions, and expert advice should be sought regarding their safe use. Stimulants cannot be permitted. Antihypertensive and antimalarial agents must be approved. Oral contraceptives and hormone replacement therapy in standard doses are acceptable. Analgesics such as paracetamol, aspirin and ibuprofen are acceptable, provided there are no side effects. Slimming pills should not be taken.

Controllers are covered by legislation with respect to alcohol and drugs. For reasons of safety alone, it is necessary to be concerned about problems with drinking. Governments in many countries, including the USA and many European countries, have introduced specific upper limits for blood alcohol levels. Individuals found to be above the prescribed limit may be criminally prosecuted. Obvious drinking usually attracts management attention or causes concern in fellow controllers, but it is not always easy to identify a chronic drinker who is able to cope with routine work but is unable to react in an emergency. An alcohol problem often involves unacceptable behaviour, impaired performance, lateness, inexplicable accidents or errors and high absenteeism. Once diagnosed, such a controller is withdrawn from work. However, after successful treatment, often as an inpatient, they may be reinstated with close supervision. In the case of dependency, controllers must be totally abstinent from alcohol for the rest of their career. This abstinence must be substantiated by line management, their partner or family and friends, and the family doctor should see the controller at regular intervals. The controller must attend regular mandatory psychiatric consultations with long-term supervision.

THE FUTURE

In the world of ATC, technological advances are being applied to established units as well as new projects. Such innovations place demands on controllers for regular retraining and updating of skills and procedures. One of the most important changes that has occurred is direct interaction with a computer via a keyboard or touch-screen, and further innovations, such as wider use of data link, are likely to lead to a greater distancing of controllers from the system. Older controllers may well feel threatened by the increasing influence of computers, leading to dependence on, and possible lack of confidence in, the system. It is important that managers and medical personnel are fully aware of future challenges to controllers, so that remedial measures can be taken at the appropriate time to ensure efficient, effective and safe controllers in an efficient, effective and safe service.

REFERENCES

Farmer EW, Belyavin AJ, Berry A, Tattersall A, Hockey GRJ. Stress in ATC. 1: survey of NATS controllers. Report no. 689. Farnborough: RAF Institute of Aviation Medicine, 1990.

Hopkin VD. *Human Factors in Air Traffic Control.* London: Taylor & Francis, 1995.

ICAO. Air traffic services. Annex 11 to the Convention on International Civil Aviation, 13th edn. Montreal: International Civil Aviation Organization, 2001a.

ICAO. Personal licensing. Annex 1 to the Convention on International Civil Aviation, 9th edn. Montreal: International Civil Aviation Organization, 2001b.

22

Error and accidents

JOHN W. CHAPPELOW

INTRODUCTION

The technology used in aviation has changed markedly over the past 50 years, particularly in terms of its reliability. As a result, although aircraft fly faster, lower, higher, over greater distances, and with larger loads, they are also safer. The intrinsic reliability of humans has not improved noticeably over the same period, so, as engines, airframes and systems have contributed progressively less to the accident rate, the proportion of accidents attributable to human error has necessarily increased. Estimates vary according to the way accidents are classified by different agencies. About 40 per cent of military accidents in the UK are attributed to aircrew human factors, and many of the 17 per cent classified as 'not positively determined' are likely to have a strong human factor component. Elsewhere, as much as 80 per cent has been claimed for 'aircrew error'. Human error clearly is a major factor in accidents. Although it is probably the most important single causal group, it comprises a wide variety of factors of different types, and in a typical accident investigation three or four are likely to be described as at least possible contributory factors. These factors can be classified according to the general scheme shown in Figure 22.1. A more detailed list of factors is given in Table 22.1.

An investigation naturally begins by identifying the errors contributing immediately to the accident. Three types are distinguishable:

- *Errors of perception: important piece of information is misinterpreted or not detected.* Visual illusions and disorientation are examples of misinterpretation; failure to see a conflicting aircraft in time to avoid collision is an example of a detection failure.

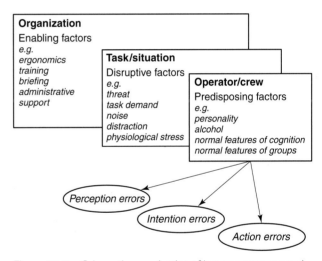

Figure 22.1 *Schematic organization of human error types and contributory factors.*

- *Errors of intention: the crew formulates a plan that entails risks.* Deliberate violation of rules is an obvious example, but more often the crew's intentions are based on a misunderstanding of the situation or of the regulations or instructions governing their activity.
- *Action errors: appropriate plan is executed inappropriately.* Simple slips and lapses, such as forgetting an item in a well-practised drill or inadvertently operating the wrong control, are common examples. In stressful or demanding circumstances, performance may be disrupted. Slow, disorganized or precipitate responses are likely.

Irrespective of type, these errors typically represent items of behaviour lasting from less than a second to a few

Table 22.1 *Error types and contributory factors*

Error type	Predisposing factor	Disruptive factor	Enabling factor
Perception errors	*Trait*	*Stressors*	*Equipment design*
Visual illusion	Personality	Noise	Ergonomics: displays
Disorientation	Lack of talent	Physiological stresses	Ergonomics: controls
Misinterpreted display	Inexperience	Operational pressure	Ergonomics: layout
Communication failure	Excess zeal	Time pressure	Personal equipment
Threat not detected	Lack of airmanship	Task demand: high	Logic in automatic systems
	Sensory limitations	Task demand: low	Aircraft handling characteristics
	Normal features of group behaviour	Distraction	
	Normal features of cognitive function	Threat	
Intention errors	*State*		*Process failings*
Deliberate violation	Alcohol/drugs		Training
Inappropriate model	Fatigue		Briefing
	Hypoglycaemia		Administrative support
	Life stress		Selection criteria
Action errors	Low morale		
Slip/lapse	Underarousal		
Slow response	Overarousal		
Precipitate response	Social factors: crew coordination		
Disorganized response	Locally condoned practice		
Mishandling	Social context		
	Social factors: mutual complacency		

seconds and contribute immediately and obviously to the causation of the accident. To understand why such errors occur, and to formulate remedies, it is necessary to examine the precursors of the errors, which are not immediate causal factors and may be less obviously implicated. These lie in three domains:

- *The crew itself: predisposing factors.* Two classes of predisposing factor can be identified, both of which distinguish individuals more at risk than others within the population of potential candidates for the accident. These are traits and states. Traits are relatively unchanging characteristics of individuals or groups. They include normal characteristics of human cognition that entail a risk of error. These are necessarily difficult to combat. The personality of individual crew members appears, in some cases, to be associated with particular types of risk. Although selection methods would seem to offer a remedy in this case, training and management are more likely to provide an effective approach. Similarly, any group, team or crew is likely to behave in predictable ways that normally facilitate personal interactions at the cost of introducing risk in some circumstances. In principle, these risks can be reduced by training. In addition to these relatively permanent characteristics of individuals and crews, other factors of a more transient nature (states lasting minutes or hours to weeks) also have a potential impact on crew

performance. For the purposes of this classification, states are considered to be normally more or less within the control of the individuals involved. They include the effects of fatigue, drugs and alcohol, and the response to chronic stress (life stress), immediate threat (overarousal), and boredom (underarousal).

- *The task or situation: disruptive factors.* These factors generally are effective for periods of minutes to hours. They are usually beyond the control of the crew. In principle, any crew may be affected by such factors, but the effect may be enhanced by interaction with predisposing factors. For example, a particular type of personality may be especially affected by high task demand or the threat of an emergency. Disruptive factors include excessive or insufficient task demand, the threat caused by malfunctions or operational circumstances, time pressure, and physiological stresses such as heat and acceleration.
- *The organization: enabling factors.* All aviation operations take place within a complex organizational context. Inevitably, that context embodies factors that make errors more likely. Again, the risk is, in principle, increased for all potential candidates. Some of these factors are identifiable in the design of equipment, such as confusing display formats or awkward arrangements of controls. More subtle factors are probably more ubiquitous in the form of, for example, misinterpretable rules, poorly designed procedures and badly written manuals. In principle,

such problems are easier to rectify than any others, but their identification may be difficult, and overcoming organizational inertia may be more difficult still.

Although many accidents involve several errors, sometimes made by more than one individual, characteristic patterns of factors associated with particular error types are discernible. Because investigations traditionally have concentrated on the crew's behaviour, and because it takes a long time to collect sufficient data to identify common patterns, the process of describing those patterns is only just beginning in earnest. Nevertheless, some important patterns and the underlying psychology can be described.

PREDISPOSING FACTORS

Three important classes of trait factors are the normal features of cognitive function, the normal characteristics of group processes, and personality. Important state factors are overarousal, usually due to the threat of an emergency, and life stress.

Cognition

An important feature of human behaviour is that some activities seem to require little or no mental effort and so can be performed in parallel with other activities, while others seem to absorb all our mental capacity. This is not only a matter of conflicting motor actions: it is a central mental resource that is implicated. Most adults can ride a bicycle and talk or do mental arithmetic at the same time but would have difficulty multiplying two two-digit numbers during a hard-fought game of squash or badminton. The unpredictability of the overtly physical game precludes unrelated mental effort. It is also significant that activities can be moved from the mentally demanding group to the low-mental-effort group simply by practice, i.e. there is no hard and fast categorization. Indeed, encountering a puncture or unexpected obstacle at high speed can suddenly but temporarily reverse the process and change riding a bicycle into the sort of task that excludes all other thought.

Introspection offers an indication of the nature of this limited mental resource. When we perform a difficult or novel task, it demands our attention. The task becomes the principal thing of which we are conscious. And attention seems to be flexible, both in terms of the sensory modalities to which it refers and temporally. The contents of consciousness need not be the results of current stimulation; they can be formed from memories of past events or imaginative constructions. Attention has the character of memory for the present. It enables information of present interest, from a variety of sources, to be held in the con-

sciousness while it is evaluated or used in decision-making or computation. There is good experimental evidence for this separate short-term form of memory. Indeed, three qualitatively different types of memory store have been identified: short-term or working memory, long-term memory, and sensory stores. These differ in terms of capacity, the duration of storage, and the mechanisms involved in forgetting.

WORKING MEMORY

Working memory appears to have three components. The best understood, known as the articulatory loop, handles phonological (i.e. speech-based) information. Its capacity is limited to only a few items – about enough for a telephone number – and decay takes only a few seconds. The memory can, however, be maintained more or less indefinitely by rehearsal using articulatory processes connected with speech. There appears to be an independent but structurally similar component used for storing spatial information. Like the articulatory loop, this involves a passive information store and an active rehearsal mechanism, in this case possibly based on the system that controls eye movements.

The least well-understood component of working memory is known as the central executive. This is believed to be capable of handling any type of information and to be responsible for the integration of information from disparate sources as well as scheduling the allocation of mental resources. Its capacity is believed to be limited but has so far defied measurement. The central executive's rather grand title reflects the importance attached to its functions. It has also been aptly described by Baddeley (1986) as an 'area of residual ignorance'. It is, perhaps, inevitable that all the (so far) experimentally inaccessible functions of working memory should seem to reside in one enigmatic block. If any progress can be made in this area, then a more complex and more satisfying picture should emerge. For the moment, some important features of working memory are clear: although both spatial and phonological information can be stored, the overall capacity is limited, and maintaining the memory for more than a few seconds demands effort and consumes precious resources. Information in working memory is also vulnerable to interference from new inputs. These limitations demand effort-saving strategies in gathering information from the world and controlling our actions.

LONG-TERM MEMORY

In contrast to working memory, long-term memory appears to have an enormous capacity and to store information indefinitely. However, we are aware of this information only when it is transferred to working memory. Long-term memory seems to involve several subsystems, but the distinctions involved are not always clear-cut. For example, it is clear that some of the information in long-term memory can be described as semantic: it involves knowledge about the world: Julius Caesar was a Roman, the tyre pressures on my car are 32 psi (front) and 30 psi (rear), and so on. Other information is best described as episodic: it relates to the individual's own personal experience. It is not clear, however, that different processes are involved in forming these two types of memory, and sometimes the distinction between them is difficult to make. For example, recalling the tyre pressures also brings to mind incidents involving flat tyres, while any episodic recall also entails semantic knowledge.

It is interesting to note that the interviewing of accident survivors often reveals an apparent change in the way the story is told after several repetitions from a detailed, possibly confused pattern that seems to invoke actual impressions of the event, to a more coherent, sparser account that is often less informative and sometimes at variance with other evidence. This may reflect a change in the way the information is stored, semantic coding being more economical. The change that takes place in fishermen's tales with retelling probably involves a similar shift in balance between the more veridical episodic encoding and the more 'meaningful' semantic encoding.

Another useful distinction is between declarative knowledge (which embraces both semantic and episodic memory) and procedural knowledge. Procedural knowledge is of particular interest in the context of error because it involves the mechanisms that control or guide performance of a task without reference to underlying factual knowledge. Knowing how to ride a bicycle is a good example of procedural knowledge. Once attained, the knowledge persists indefinitely and is available instantly should the opportunity to exercise it arise. It is also peculiarly difficult to communicate the fundamentals of the skill verbally. This latter point is not true of all procedural knowledge, however, and the distinction from declarative knowledge is not entirely clear-cut.

In the context of error analysis, some authors have found it useful to classify tasks according to the type of knowledge involved in their execution (Reason and Mycielska 1982). The most automatic activities are described as skill-based; they demand little conscious attention and verbalization of the processes involved may be difficult. Rule-based behaviour involves more easily described procedures, e.g. '"i" before "e" except after "c"'; 'to change a wheel, first loosen the wheel nuts, then jack up the car, remove the nuts and the wheel, and then reverse the process with the new wheel.' It demands a little more conscious monitoring if actions are to be performed in the correct order and without omissions. The most demanding activities are described as knowledge-based. Here, the activity is largely non-automatic, the mental load is considerable, and artificial memory aids may be required, e.g. checklists, computational notes, diagrams and maps.

Again, it is often difficult, if not impossible, to make precise distinctions in practical cases.

Most complex tasks involve more or less unconscious procedural elements and overall strategies based on explicitly definable knowledge. With increasing experience, the trainee's behaviour on some aspects of his or her tasks might be said to progress from one level to the next as less and less conscious attention is required. This is surely not a general description of skill or expertise acquisition, however. It is, for example, possible to describe the sequence of actions involved in changing gear in a car. Some people are even capable of explaining in detail the mechanical consequences of these control movements. For most people, however, gear-changing is simply a knack, and attempting to convey it in words to a learner driver can be almost pointless. With a little practice, however, the knack is acquired, regardless of whether the learner understands the mechanical details. Nevertheless, the distinction between skill-, rule- and knowledge-based behaviours does have the merit of reflecting an important aspect of a task in terms of the degree of conscious attention that it demands of the operator.

The cognitive failures known as slips and lapses involve a mismatch between intentions and actions. The correct drill is selected, but items are omitted, confused with others from a similar drill, or operated in reverse (e.g. raising rather than lowering a lever). Such cognitive failures often are associated with distractions or preoccupation in otherwise normal and undemanding circumstances. Where knowledge-based errors are identified in an investigation, very often they are associated with failures in training or briefing or the administrative support (which includes the framing of orders, manuals and instructions).

SENSORY STORES

Very little of the information available at any moment in the sensory domain is allowed into the focus of attention. But that focus can shift very quickly, from reading this text to sounds coming from another room, say, or the sensations produced as your hands support the book. When the impetus for a shift of attention is produced by an unexpected external event, such as your own name cropping up in the conversation in the next room, some antecedents of that stimulus (e.g. the beginning of the sentence) may also be noticed. Experimental evidence suggests that this remarkable and useful feat is achieved not through prescience but by routine, very short-term storage of sensory information. Sensory stores seem to have unlimited capacity but retain information for, at most, a second or so. This allows not only selection of the information to be processed but also some interpretation on the basis of past experience and current context.

Perception is, therefore, in part driven by expectation. This is a labour-saving ruse that takes advantage of redundancy and predictability in the real world in constructing a representation of it. The advantages are considerable: it reduces the resources required to interpret the world and allows some flexibility in selection and interpretation based on succeeding as well as preceding information. The disadvantage is, of course, a risk of misperception or misinterpretation by placing too great a reliance on previous experience and present expectations. In a novel situation, where visual cues are distorted or reduced by comparison with previous experience, a visual illusion may result. Reality may also be distorted when expectations are based on a well-practised routine in which an error has occurred due to cognitive failure. For example, the pilot is distracted or preoccupied during the pre-landing checks. The checks, which the pilot has done so often that he or she hardly need think about them, are completed, but with an omission. The pilot 'knows' that they have lowered the undercarriage, and so a routine glance at the undercarriage indicator gives the expected result rather than the true state of affairs and the landing continues without wheels. Even after landing, the pilot may not correctly diagnose the cause of the strange noises and bumps as the aircraft slides down the runway, so strong is the expectation.

OVERVIEW

The system described above is flexible and efficient. In familiar situations, the effort required is minimized: well-practised routines and rules of thumb operate almost automatically, and the signals required to direct actions or initiate new responses are selected without much deliberation. In taxing or problematic situations, a more effort-intensive approach can be adopted. The environment is scanned for the signs that identify the problem or situation, and previously effective solutions are recalled from past experience and implemented. When the situation is novel, a deliberate, more or less systematic exercise in information-gathering and conceptual reasoning may be required. The expert approaches the task with all three strategies at his or her disposal. Long-term goals may be set consciously, and these define the skills required and the experience that the expert will have to draw on in executing shorter-term plans.

The weaknesses of the system are characteristic of the resources deployed in each type of approach. The capacity of working memory is an all too evident limit on efficiency in conceptual reasoning. When diagnosis and response are required in a fairly short time, and aide-memoires are not available, then it is common that some relevant information is overlooked or given insufficient weight, particularly if it does not fit the first tenable hypothesis that comes to mind. Solutions may be proposed that are focused on the observable symptoms but without thought for possible side effects of the solutions (a trivial example is replacing a blown fuse with one of higher rating). When there is just too much to think about, there is a strong temptation to test hypotheses in a concrete manner without considering the possible consequences of the intervention. When disruptive factors such as threat and high task demand cause overarousal, then disorganized, slow or precipitate responses are likely.

In more routine circumstances, minor slips and lapses are more likely. Monitoring may fail to detect the signs, and the situation is seen as normal and as expected. About two-thirds of slips and lapses happen in routine undemanding circumstances (underarousal). Often all that is required is a minor distraction. The consequences seem out of proportion to the precipitating event. It is an important finding for flight safety that normal behaviour in normal circumstances carries a significant risk of serious error.

Group processes

Even in single-seat operations, the pilot is a member of a team. This team may include other members of a formation or air traffic controllers and will certainly include supervisors, authorizers and others involved in briefing and preparing the sortie. Simple communication failures are not unknown, but it is more common for decision-making to be less effective than might be expected. In principle, the more people that are involved in a decision process, the more likely it is that unnecessary hazards will be detected. In practice, this benefit is not realized fully. This is a general feature of group decisions, but some specific factors can be identified. First, when a group of people of similar outlook are required to work together, not only do their attitudes tend to conform to a group norm but also that norm is often more extreme than any individual member's attitude. This is known as 'risky shift' and can result in the hazards attaching to small modifications of an accepted operational plan going unnoticed. This effect may, arguably, be more likely in a disciplined organization where ranks and roles are well defined and mutual trust is a necessity. It is likely to operate when small novel changes are made to well-established patterns of operation. Large changes inevitably attract scrutiny, but the risks associated with small changes may receive less attention from a group working together than from an individual alone.

Excessive mutual trust can arise between individuals when, for example, two flying instructors are flying together. If one makes a mistake, then the other may be slower to point it out or take control than would be the case with a student, because the instructor does not wish to cause offence, trusts the other pilot's skill to handle the situation, and may want any problems to be unequivocal so as to avoid dispute in the debrief. The handling pilot, meanwhile, may be experiencing difficulty in controlling the aircraft as a result of his or her error but is less concerned than they might be otherwise because the instructor has not passed any comment. This situation is best described as mutual complacency.

Organizational factors can put specific small groups at risk. The key appears to be a degree of isolation. This can be achieved by sending a small detachment to a remote location, by generating an inappropriate sense of elite status, or by a failure to ensure normal functional control of a specialist unit by higher echelons, or any of these in combination. The result is a gradual re-interpretation of rules and procedures to suit the perceived special needs of the isolated group. This results in locally condoned procedures being adopted, which are justified by the specialist nature of the unit and its particular expertise. If effective, these practices may even be unofficially sanctioned by higher authorities or at least may benefit from passive acquiescence.

Crew resource management training is implemented in both military and civil operations. It deals directly with issues of crew cooperation and decision-making and, ideally, should also address the more difficult problem of organizational factors.

Life stress

A popular lay explanation for pilot error involves domestic and other pressures. The association between stressful life events (both positive and negative) and heart disease and other illnesses is well known. A similar statistical association between the incidence of life events and involvement in flying accidents has been reported at least once, but this is clearly a difficult area for research and further analysis can suggest other interpretations (Alkov and Borowsky 1980; Alkov *et al.* 1982). Close examination of Royal Air Force (RAF) accidents in which life stress was arguably present has revealed very few cases in which a link between life events and the causes of the accident can be claimed confidently. These were rather special cases and did not involve a general depletion of the pilots' ability to cope with the stresses of work. In addition, any sample of pilots is bound to reveal some burden of life stress. What is unknown is whether the sample based on accident involvement carries a greater burden than aircrew in general.

It is also possible that military aviation allows greater compartmentalization than some other professions. The crews are isolated from other distractions and pressures while performing the task, and, in many cases, the critical parts of the task (i.e. while airborne) last for relatively short periods. Many individuals can cope under these circumstances, unless the stress is causing noticeable sleep disruption. It is also likely that individual differences play a large part in determining the impact of life events. In addition, individual differences in cognitive functioning may play a part in determining liability to accidents. Broadbent *et al.* (1986) suggested that the ability to cope with chronic mild stress and liability to cognitive failure may be related to sta-

ble biases in cognitive style, people with a more obsessional style being less vulnerable to stress and less prone to cognitive failure. These authors also suggested that under stress, cognitive styles may become more extreme. Thus, cognitive style may identify those who are vulnerable to life stress and even, possibly, mediate a relationship between life stress and accident involvement.

Personality

The scientific description of personality can be approached in a variety of ways. Two dimensions that have proved useful in many fields of investigation are extraversion and neuroticism (Eysenck and Eysenck 1964). Questionnaire tests of extraversion and neuroticism distinguish different types of deviant personality and psychiatric disorder and also show reliable differences between professional groups. In addition, scores on such tests account for some of the variation in the way people approach tasks, cope with a range of stressors, and behave generally. Extraverts are assumed to require more stimulation than introverts to excite the central nervous system. As a result, extraverts are active, sociable and impulsive while introverts are passive, reserved and thoughtful. A high neuroticism score indicates a labile autonomic nervous system; it would be associated with an emotional or moody disposition. A low score would indicate stability. Introverts tend to work in a methodical manner and, hence, to be slower than extraverts, who may make more mistakes in the interests of speed. Stimulants and threatening circumstances, by raising arousal level, would tend to be detrimental for introverts (by overarousal) but may improve the performance of extraverts, since the latter tend to be chronically underaroused. Introverts perform better, however, when sustained vigilance is required.

A high neuroticism score has implications for performance in threatening circumstances. Anxiety may divert mental resources into unproductive worry and degrade performance. Psychosomatic illness can result from prolonged exposure to such stress. A high score may also accentuate the differences between introverts and extraverts in terms of liability to accidents. Several studies in aviation and road safety have implicated neuroticism or some form of maladjustment. High extraversion scores have also been found to be associated with accident involvement. Contradictory results and failures to find any association are by no means unknown, however, and it is not possible to claim that a clear picture has emerged. Bearing in mind that not all accidents are likely to involve an important contribution from personality variables, it is obvious that large numbers would be needed to establish any correlations. It is also likely that some attention should be given to classifying types of accident, thus further increasing the numbers required.

About one-fifth of aircrew-error accidents in the RAF have a possible association with personality. It has been possible to classify about two-thirds of these on the basis of descriptors used in personal records. Two groups have emerged. One is described as underconfident, nervous and prone to overreaction; the other is described as overconfident, reckless and heedless of rules. It is tempting to apply the labels 'unstable introvert' and 'unstable extravert', respectively, but more evidence is required. It is clear, however, that the former group tends to be associated with accidents involving mishandled emergencies (i.e. threat, high task demand, and disorganized, slow or precipitate responses) while the latter group tends to be associated with accidents involving unauthorized or risky manoeuvres (deliberate violation) or failure to appreciate risk (slow response or undetected threat).

It is clear that future research should not be expected to produce simple correlations between personality measures and accident involvement. It would be wise to expect a bipolar relationship with extraversion mediated by neuroticism and to classify accidents according to the types of error involved. Personality tests can provide some guidance in selecting aircrew and are used by many airlines. They are, however, relatively imprecise instruments, and their utility in selection depends on the ratio of suitable candidates to vacant posts. In most aviation contexts, differences in personality remain a management issue.

DISRUPTIVE FACTORS

Military aircrew have to contend with a variety of environmental stresses but, in general, these contribute little to accident causation, since heat, vibration, noise, acceleration, etc. are catered for with special equipment. The acute reactive stress and high task demand associated with life-threatening emergencies contributes to about one-quarter of aircrew error accidents in the RAF.

Stress and task demand on performance

The effects of stressors on performance are complex and varied. To some extent, the concept of arousal simplifies (perhaps oversimplifies) discussion of these effects. It implies a continuum of activation from extreme drowsiness to extreme excitement. Psychological indicants of arousal level include alertness, sensitivity to stimulation and performance on tests. Physiological indicants, such as heart rate, skin resistance, etc., sometimes but not always, show useful correlations with psychological variables. Figure 22.2 embodies two ideas that have proved a useful, if incomplete, description of the relationship between arousal level and performance for many years (Yerkes and

Dodson 1908). The first idea is that there is an optimum arousal level for any task. This implies an inverted 'U' relationship with performance. This is a difficult hypothesis to test experimentally. The second idea is that easy tasks are more tolerant than difficult tasks of high arousal levels. Difficulty level in this context depends on the training and experience of the operator. Further individual differences (see Personality, above) also complicate the picture. Variations in arousal level seem to affect performance largely by changing attentional capacity and processing speed. To some extent, these changes are moderated by learned strategies in the control of attention.

At low levels of arousal, such as might occur after a long period of work at night, particularly if the work is unstimulating or monotonous, responses take longer and lapses of attention and omissions are more likely to occur. Given noise, stimulants (such as caffeine or interesting conversation) or sufficient motivation, apparently normal levels of efficiency can be achieved, although the less important tasks may be neglected. Fatigue and sleep deprivation are, to a large extent, controlled well in military aviation operations and make only a minor contribution to aircrew error accidents. In civil aviation, some of which routinely involves long periods on duty, time-zone shifts and disruption of circadian rhythms, there may be more scope for fatigue and sleep deprivation to affect performance. In both the military and civilian sectors, however, duty cycles and rest periods are governed by firm regulation and are monitored closely.

At high levels of arousal, such as might be provoked by an emergency, information may be processed more quickly, but at the expense of a reduction in the capacity of working memory. Control of attention becomes more of a problem. The reduction in capacity of working memory can be compensated for by increased attentional selectivity, focusing intently on the important information, but impairment of perceptual discrimination may allow superficially relevant stimuli to become distracting, thus disrupting performance. The main causes of acute reactive stress are mechanical problems, e.g. engine fires, bird strikes, etc. Prior mishandling by the pilot and disorienta-

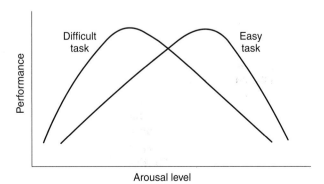

Figure 22.2 *Yerkes–Dodson law.*

tion make a small contribution. The main results (about 30 per cent) are best described as a disorganization of response: the wrong drills are selected or the pilot's analysis of the emergency is haphazard and ineffective. Slow responses and precipitate action are about equally likely (about ten per cent of the total each). Narrowing of attention and slips and lapses together account for another 30 per cent of cases.

ENABLING FACTORS

About 40 per cent of RAF accidents conventionally described as due to 'aircrew error' involve one or more enabling factors, such as poor equipment design, inadequate training or briefing, or poor administrative support. The potential for such system-induced errors increases with the sophistication and power of the systems employed. Aviators increasingly rely on indirect apprehension of important data and indirect control of the aircraft systems. There are obvious benefits in the use of technology to supplement human capabilities, but the designer of equipment faces real challenges in devising suitable interfaces. Conflicting requirements have to be met. Both the novice and the expert require easily interpretable displays and accessible simple controls. The expert, however, may require more detailed information or a more flexible operating style than the novice. Ease of operation in controls is obviously desirable but may facilitate mis-selections. In addition, the training and administrative background set the context in which the operator works, and both can easily provide opportunities for misinformation and confusion.

The following example illustrates both the interaction of different enabling factors and how what appear to be simple engineering design decisions can have serious human factors implications. A fly-by-wire airliner was designed with the following features: Control of both slats and flaps was embodied in one lever with five possible positions (0–3 plus 'FULL'); to compensate for changes in handling characteristics with different configuration settings, the gain of the control stick varied according to the configuration selected (not that achieved); and a computer monitor replaced the flight reference cards and automatically displayed instructions relevant to any malfunctions detected by the system. On the approach, the aircraft encountered a severe gust and the flaps system locked with the flaps at 'FULL'. The crew overshot and attempted a second approach. This time, following guidance displayed on the flight deck monitor, they selected configuration 3. As they lowered the undercarriage, the aircraft rolled uncontrollably; they overshot again. The third approach was downwind. Late in the approach, the aircraft rolled and pitched uncontrollably and the ground-proximity warning was

activated. They overshot again. By this time, they were short of fuel and performed a short circuit to position for another downwind landing. Control difficulties were experienced from 1200 feet down to touchdown. Although the landing was successful, the aircraft departed the runway and minor damage was sustained before it was brought to rest.

The crew's control problems were caused by the mismatch between the stick sensitivity resulting from their selecting configuration 3 and that required for the full-flap configuration they actually had. Although this potential problem was known, the computerized flight-deck monitor had not been updated to provide more appropriate guidance. Such guidance was available in paper form (not on board the aircraft) and was not known to the crew. The crew's attempts to interpret their problems were not helped by an overly complex configuration display, which confused them and added to their workload. Basic design decisions, poor ergonomics and inadequate administrative support and training all combined to put the crew in a demanding and alarming situation, which could easily have had a more costly outcome.

The variety of enabling factors is enormous. One unifying aspect is the fact that such problems are identifiable before they cause an accident and, in contrast with most of the psychological factors discussed above, in principle are amenable to relatively simple remedies. The inquiries into many major disasters (e.g. Chernobyl, *Challenger*, the *Herald of Free Enterprise*) have provided examples. The failure of senior management to remedy this type of problem may be due to lack of imagination, error of judgement or an unfortunate ordering of priorities. The failure of professionals operating the system to demand action may be due to a perceived lack of influence or, perversely, to an aspect of the 'professional' attitude. Professionals expect to be able to cope. Performing under less than optimum conditions does afford some satisfaction. Complaining about inadequate equipment or questioning common practice may seem 'unprofessional', particularly if it involves an admission that something is not understood. In both military and civilian aviation, steps have been taken to circumvent this problem in the form of confidential or open incident reporting schemes.

CONCLUSIONS

Individual accidents often involve a complex interaction of factors, some of which have been described here. Usually, however, it is possible to identify the critical errors and to trace the precursors of those errors in individual predispositions, situation-specific factors and organizational failings. These links are important because they identify the targets for remedial action and demonstrate the benefits to be gained. Table 22.1 (p. 350) is a more or less comprehensive list of factors that have proved useful in understanding RAF and other accidents over the past 25 years.

REFERENCES

Alkov RA, Borowsky MS. A questionnaire study of psychological background factors in US Navy aircraft accidents. *Aviation, Space, and Environmental Medicine* 1980; **51**: 860–63.

Alkov RA, Borowsky MS, Gaynor JA. Stress coping and the US Navy aircrew factor mishap. *Aviation, Space, and Environmental Medicine* 1982; **53**: 1112–15.

Baddeley A. *Working Memory.* Oxford: Clarendon Press, 1986.

Broadbent DE, Broadbent MHP, Jones JL. Performance correlates of self-reported cognitive failure and obsessionality. *British Journal of Clinical Psychology* 1986; **25**: 285–99.

Eysenck HJ, Eysenck SBG. *Manual of the Eysenck Personality Inventory.* Sevenoaks: Hodder & Stoughton, 1964.

Reason J, Mycielska JD. *Absent Minded?* Englewood Cliffs, NJ: Prentice Hall, 1982.

Yerkes RM, Dodson JD. The relation of strength of stimulus to rapidity of habit formation. *Journal of Comparative Neurological Psychology* 1908; **18**: 459–82.

23

The flight deck and cockpit

MICHAEL BAGSHAW

INTRODUCTION

The navigation and operation of an aircraft are executed by the crew members from the flight deck or cockpit. The systems to operate engines and aerodynamic control surfaces govern the progress of the aircraft on the ground and in flight, while the instrumentation provides information on direction, speed, altitude and orientation, as well as information for the management of the flight, such as navigation, fuel and warning systems.

This chapter deals with the operation of the aircraft, particularly the interface between the flight crew members and the aircraft instrumentation and operating systems. The psychological aspects of personality, behaviour and interaction between crew members (e.g. crew resource management) and life-support equipment and personal protection are considered in Chapters 20 and 15, respectively.

DEFINITIONS

When the crew are normally unable to leave their seats during the course of a flight, the aircrew compartment is usually referred to as the 'cockpit'. This encompasses primarily, but not exclusively, military fast jet aircraft, helicopters and trainers, where the crew may require personal life-support equipment and/or may be restrained in an armoured or ejection seat.

The term 'aircraft flight deck' describes the compartment housing the crew when they may leave their seats during flight and do not require personal life-support equipment during normal operations. This applies generally, but not only, to civilian aircraft and military transports. In smaller aircraft and helicopters, the cabin can house the flight crew and the passengers in the same compartment, and the pilot's operating space may then be referred to as the cockpit.

The terms 'aircrew' and 'flight crew' are interchangeable, but military crew members are usually known as 'aircrew' whereas the term 'flight crew' generally refers to civilian crew members. In the USA the term 'flight crew' can also include flight attendants working in the passenger cabin, but in Europe it is usually exclusive to flight-deck technical crew (pilots and flight engineers).

ROLE OF FLIGHT CREW

Although there are similarities in the roles of military, commercial airline and general aviation flight-crew members, the tasks can be very different. It is axiomatic that selection and training of these different groups should differ, although the basic fundamentals are similar. Within these groups there are subdivisions of operation. For example, military aviation includes:

- basic and advanced flying training
- interdiction and ground attack

- airborne interception
- close air support
- tactical and strategic airlift and transport
- maritime fleet defence and attack
- air-to-air refuelling
- casualty evacuation
- airborne early warning and electronic countermeasures
- photo-reconnaissance
- air–sea rescue
- antisubmarine warfare.

The design of aircraft is optimized for the role, although whenever possible a multi-role function is incorporated in the design and development, e.g. air-to-air refuelling tankers can act as transport aircraft, battlefield support helicopters may be used for casualty evacuation, and light aircraft can be used for police or military surveillance or for training. However, the basic concepts of aircraft control and flight instrumentation are similar, regardless of the role of the aircraft, and they evolve throughout their service, leading to modifications and changes to cockpit instrumentation and equipment.

Just as the aircraft is optimized for a particular role or roles, so the crew members are selected and trained for particular specialist areas, after generic basic flying training. The prime operational grouping is between rotary and fixed wing, with further selection within those groups, e.g. support/transport/maritime/fast jet. Crew members initially are selected according to aptitude and service requirements for employment as pilots, navigators, weapons-system operators, radar operators, fighter controllers, flight engineers or loadmasters. Although the captain of the aircraft is usually (but by no means exclusively, particularly in maritime and early-warning operations) a pilot, there is no hierarchy of skill or knowledge. Some aircraft, chiefly fast jets, are operated by a single pilot, whereas others, such as long-range transport, refuelling and airborne early warning, require a larger crew complement. It is usual for military crews to be 'constituted', which means that they train and operate together and gain an understanding of individual personalities and foibles, so enhancing operational effectiveness.

In military single-seat and two-seat roles, crews operate within a squadron environment and fly together in tactical formations. Although not flying in the same cockpit or flight deck, the development of mutual understanding and trust between individual pilots enhances operational effectiveness in the same way as for constituted crews.

In two-seat combat aircraft, the crew of pilot and navigator/weapons-system operator is usually constituted.

Military aviation takes place in a dynamic strategic and tactical environment, with a need for ongoing situational analysis and appropriate reaction. The environment may be hostile as a result of climate and/or enemy activity, and the aircraft is very much a vehicle to achieve a particular military objective. The operation of the aircraft, its equipment and (if appropriate) its weapon system should make minimal demands on the crew, so they can concentrate on the tactical scenario to complete the task safely and effectively. Cockpit and flight-deck design should follow this maxim, but this ideal is not always achieved.

In airline operation, the driving force is commercial pressure. The aim is to carry as many passengers and as much freight as possible, safely and at the cheapest fare compatible with providing adequate revenue and meeting passenger service expectations. The revenue must cover the costs of the operation, including direct operating costs such as fuel, airports, navigation, maintenance and staff, as well as providing a margin for future investment and an adequate return on investment for the shareholders.

In the mid-twentieth century, the flight crew of a long-range commercial airliner or transport aircraft included two pilots, a flight navigator, a flight engineer and a radio operator. By the beginning of the twenty-first century, the crew generally consisted only of two pilots, the roles of navigator, radio operator and, more recently, the flight engineer having been supplanted by technology.

The task of the crew on a flight deck is to work together safely and effectively. This is influenced by the role or job of the individual crew members, the status and experience of the individuals, and their personalities.

The reason for having more than one pilot on the flight deck of an airliner or transport aircraft is to reduce workload by task sharing, to produce consensus decision making, and to ensure cross-checking of actions in order to minimize error and enhance safe operation.

The role of the pilot will depend on whether he or she is a nominated handling pilot for the particular sector of the flight. The captain retains command and ultimate responsibility for the conduct of the flight, but duties are shared. In general, the handling pilot ('pilot flying', PF) is concerned with the physical control of the aircraft, while the non-handling pilot ('pilot non-flying', PNF) is responsible for communication with air traffic control, actioning checklist items, inputting data to the flight management system, and monitoring the actions of the handling pilot. It is common practice for these roles to alternate between the pilots on consecutive flight sectors.

The monitoring role can be demanding, particularly if the non-handling pilot is junior or less experienced than the handling pilot. There has to be an understanding and acceptance by both pilots that it is entirely in order for the non-handling pilot to question the actions of the other and, if necessary, take over control. This aspect is explored in more detail in Chapter 20.

For long-range military logistics and transport operations and for ultra-long-haul commercial flights, it is common to carry additional flight crew members to allow periods of rest during the cruise. In the commercial operation, these are referred to as the 'heavy crew'.

It is the task of airline management to control the long-term risks of the company as a whole and the task of flight crew to control short-term risks encountered on individual flights to achieve a safe and efficient operation. The coordination of these tasks is achieved partly by the development and use of standard operating procedures (SOPs). These SOPs marry the needs of the particular operator with the checklists and standard drills issued by the aircraft manufacturer and also incorporate the requirements of the appropriate regulatory authority, such as the Civil Aviation Authority (CAA), Federal Aviation Administration (FAA) or European Aviation Safety Agency. In large airline companies, individual crew members rarely fly together on a regular basis and, indeed, may never have met before a particular flight, and so it is essential that they all follow and understand the SOP for any given operation or phase of flight. The crew interface with the cockpit and flight-deck instrumentation forms part of the critical pathway for consistent use of SOPs.

SOPs are equally essential in military operations to ensure safety and efficiency.

The term 'general aviation' encompasses flying activities other than military or commercial operations, including fixed- and rotary-wing (helicopter) aircraft. Gliding, micro-light and ultra-light flying activities usually are not classified as general aviation but are categories in their own right and are not considered in this chapter. General aviation includes a whole spectrum of fixed- and rotary-wing aircraft, from single-seat light aircraft with little or no instrumentation up to business jets with flight decks as sophisticated as any found in a commercial airliner. Similarly, the qualifications of general aviation pilots range from a basic national private pilot licence through to an airline transport pilot licence, with a wide range of experience. Civilian flying training, private recreational flying, sports flying, air ambulance and police support flying, and corporate aviation are all considered to be general aviation activity. Single-pilot operation is common in general aviation, particularly in light aircraft and light helicopters.

AIRCRAFT CONTROLS

The flight path of a fixed-wing aircraft is determined by the aerodynamic control surfaces. In basic form, the elevators control movement in pitch, the ailerons control roll (also controlled by spoilers in high-performance aircraft) and the rudder controls motion in yaw. Deflection of the elevators, ailerons and spoilers is controlled by movement of the control column or control wheel or side-stick, and the rudder is controlled by movement of the foot pedals.

In smaller aircraft, control surface deflection is effected via direct cable or rod links from the cockpit controls. However, in larger and high-performance aircraft, deflection is achieved by servo actuators, which respond to hydraulic or electrical signals derived from cockpit control deflection or autopilot guidance.

Engine thrust is managed by the power lever(s). In a jet engine, this is a function of the speed of rotation of the engine, which in turn is influenced by fuel flow. In a propeller-driven aircraft, power is delivered as a function of the speed of engine rotation and the pitch angle of the propeller blades, controlled by the throttle and the propeller pitch levers. In a piston-engined aircraft, the fuel/air mixture ratio is also controlled manually in order to take account of air density being a function of altitude.

Modern aircraft incorporate sophisticated engine management systems (such as full authority digital engine control, FADEC), in which automation can simplify engine control for the different phases of flight.

The flying controls of a helicopter are different. The flight path is determined by a combination of the power delivered by the rotor and the effective angle of attack presented to the relative airflow by the rotor disc. The tendency of a single-rotor helicopter to rotate opposite to the motion of the rotor disc is counteracted by sideways thrust produced by the tail rotor. In a twin-rotor helicopter, this is achieved by counter-rotation of the two rotor discs.

The collective lever changes the lift on the aircraft by altering the blade pitch and hence the angle of attack of the disc as a whole, i.e. collectively. An increase in the angle of attack results in increased drag and requires a linked increase in power to the rotor to maintain a constant rotor speed (rotor rpm). Conventionally, the collective lever is operated by the pilot's left hand and is the prime control for the vertical flight dimension.

Control of the horizontal flight direction is effected by the cyclic stick in the pilot's right hand, which varies the blade angle of attack as it rotates, i.e. cyclically, to create differential lift either laterally or fore/aft, thus rolling or pitching the aircraft.

The power delivered to the tail rotor, and thus motion in yaw, is controlled via the pedals.

Any change in deflection to one of the controls requires a compensatory adjustment to the input of the other two controls. Thus, flying a helicopter requires a high degree of cognition and physical coordination.

Unless specifically designed otherwise (e.g. agile high-performance fighter aircraft, light aerobatic competition aircraft), most fixed-wing aircraft are inherently stable in flight. The aircraft will usually continue on a given flight path until a control input modifies this. However, a helicopter is inherently unstable, requiring constant control input from the pilot, which may be assisted by automation in modern sophisticated helicopters.

FLIGHT-DECK DESIGN

The design of the flight deck or cockpit is necessarily a compromise between economics, the need to accommodate the range of flight crew shapes and sizes, and the positioning of instruments and controls for optimum functional reach without compromising lookout and the operation of the aircraft. The layout of the flight deck is designed to suit a population falling between the five per cent confidence limit for females and the 95 per cent limit for males, for key static, dynamic and contour measurements (see Chapter 15). For a military aircraft, the design will be influenced by the population demography of the sponsoring country. However, civilian aircraft are designed for worldwide sales, and some compromise is necessary to take account of the fact that different populations throughout the world are of different physical stature.

The key reference point on the flight deck for the safe and efficient operation of the aircraft is the eye datum point or the design eye position. When the pilot adjusts his or her seat to achieve this point, there should be optimum vision of controls and instrumentation and external reference without the need for excessive head movement. Sitting below the eye datum point decreases downward vision over the aircraft nose, and on the final stages of the landing approach sight of the runway undershoot may be lost. It is also essential that full deflection of all the flight controls, including rudder and toe-operated brake pedals, is possible when the pilot is strapped into the seat.

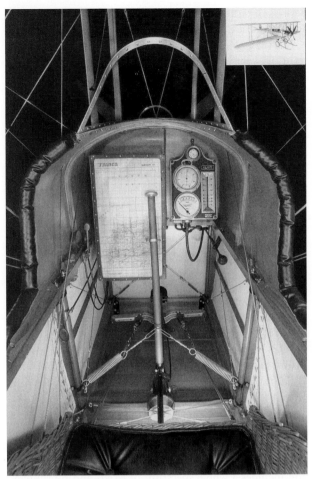

Figure 23.1   *BE2b cockpit.*

Instrumentation

To operate any type of aircraft safely and efficiently, the pilot needs to control its progress through the air from the point of departure to the destination. In the early days of flying, aircraft were flown in sight of the Earth's surface and duration of flight was relatively short within a limited aircraft performance envelope. Orientation was provided by visual cues from the ground, the horizon and the sky.

Figure 23.1 shows the cockpit of the Royal Aircraft Factory BE2b, which served as a light bomber and reconnaissance aircraft in the early months of the First World War (1914–18). The very basic cockpit arrangement includes a throttle and a map case at the left, a simple control column, and an instrument panel housing an air speed indicator, engine revolution counter and an altimeter. The pilot maintained orientation and navigated by reference to external visual cues.

Even at the end of the First World War, when the Vickers Vimy was introduced by the Royal Air Force (RAF) as the first purpose-built heavy bomber, the cockpit was cramped and had only basic instruments. Figure 23.2 con-

firms what a great feat of airmanship was achieved by Alcock and Brown in 1919, when they completed the first crossing of the Atlantic Ocean in this aircraft without the benefit of sophisticated instrumentation.

With the continuing development of both military and civil aviation, aircraft flew faster, further and higher and out of sight of the surface. The properties of the gyroscope were utilized to develop the artificial horizon, which assisted the pilot to determine orientation when flying 'blind' in cloud or at night. Application of the laws of gyrodynamics also enabled the development of the turn indicator and the gyrocompass.

Properties of the atmosphere and the physics of aerodynamics were utilized in the design of altimeters, airspeed indicators and vertical speed indicators, and compasses became more sensitive and sophisticated. Development of electronics and microprocessors has led to great advances in flight-deck instrumentation and technology.

A major problem in the provision of information to assist orientation is that the aircraft flies in a four-dimensional environment (the fourth dimension being time),

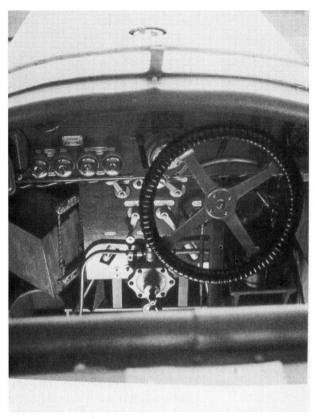

Figure 23.2 *Vickers Vimy cockpit.*

whereas it is possible to display information in only two dimensions.

Figure 23.3 shows an artificial horizon (also known as a gyro-horizon or attitude gyro; it is known as an attitude indicator when the instrument face is calibrated with

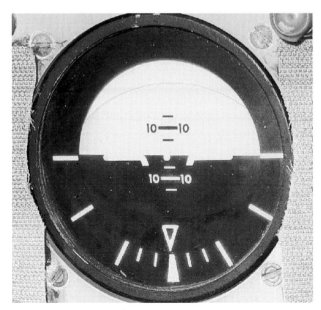

Figure 23.3 *Artificial horizon.*

degrees of pitch). The heart of the instrument is a horizontally mounted gyroscope, which maintains position while the aircraft (and the instrument case) moves around it. The artificial horizon line is attached to the gyroscope, and this will always represent the real horizon when the instrument is operating correctly. The fixed model in the centre represents the aircraft, and this moves with respect to the artificial horizon in the same way as the real aircraft moves in respect to the real horizon. (Russian aircraft instrument display works in the opposite sense, with the aircraft symbol moving around the fixed horizon line.) However, the instrument indicates the position of the aircraft only relative to the horizon, a concept known as the aircraft attitude. It does not indicate whether the aircraft is climbing, descending, turning or in level flight, although it does give an accurate representation of bank angle.

The only way to confirm what the aircraft is actually doing is to cross-refer to other instruments. This process is referred to as 'scanning' the instrument panel, and the pilot learns techniques of selective scanning according to the phase of flight.

Thus, with an indicated high-nose attitude, the aircraft might be in a climb, descending or maintaining level flight. Figure 23.4 shows the instrument panel of an aircraft descending with a high-nose attitude. The attitude indicator would suggest that the aircraft is in a climb – reference to the vertical speed indicator shows a descent, which is confirmed by the altimeter indicating a reduction in altitude ('unwinding').

To maintain straight and level flight at a constant airspeed, using the aircraft controls the pilot selects the appropriate attitude on the artificial horizon (or attitude indicator) and then scans the altimeter to ensure that the aircraft is not climbing or descending, the turn instrument to ensure that the aircraft is not turning, the compass to ensure that the desired heading is being maintained, and the airspeed indicator to ensure that the appropriate speed is being flown, returning to the artificial horizon after each scan. Any deviation from the desired parameter(s) requires a control input and a continuation of the instrument scanning process. Thus, a simple feedback loop is established, involving visual perception, cognitive processing and motor output.

In the early stages of flying training, the emphasis is on the development of motor skills and simple judgement-making. The development of more complex judgement occurs as experience is gained, because motor skills are developed by handling items that can be seen, felt and moved, whereas cognitive judgement and decision making are more abstract, using intelligence, awareness and experience.

Cognitive judgement is the end result of perceiving a situation via the sensory system or memory. The situation is then assessed using the hierarchical order of the brain and a plan of action is decided. In doing this, the pilot uses knowledge gained from previous experience to evaluate

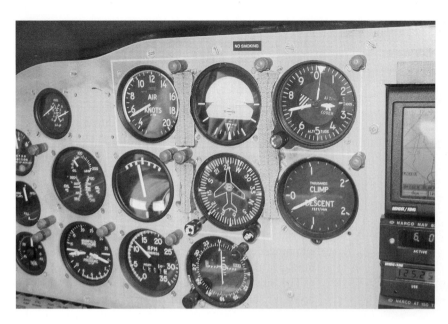

Figure 23.4 *Instruments showing aircraft in stalled descent.*

the plan based on information perceived. The development of motor memory proceeds from the basic cognitive phase to the associative phase, when events and procedures become linked with past experience involving some conscious thought process. Finally, the automatic phase is reached when no conscious thought is required. The acquisition of skill in this manner allows mental processing capacity to be freed for other tasks, such as maintenance of situational awareness, and the scanning process occurs at a lower conscious level.

During periods of high workload, or if the pilot is under stress, mental capacity may be reduced and the instrument scanning process can break down as a result of failure of the automatic phase, leading to loss of situational awareness (see below).

During the Second World War (1939–45), attempts were made to simplify the scanning process and improve the display of information within the cockpit. In the RAF, a standard instrument layout was adopted in which the main performance instruments were arranged in a 'T' shape, with the artificial horizon being placed in a central position. This standard 'T' was subsequently adopted throughout the Western world.

Figure 23.5 shows the development of the instrument panel up to 1963, with a notable similarity between the Hawker Hurricane panel of 1940 and the Hawker

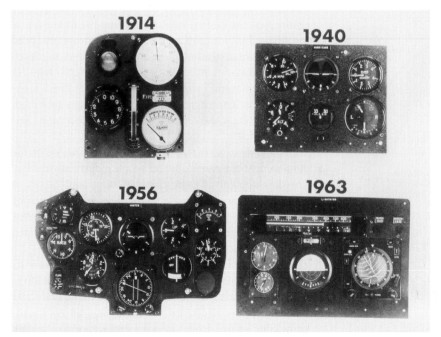

Figure 23.5 *Instrument panel development.*

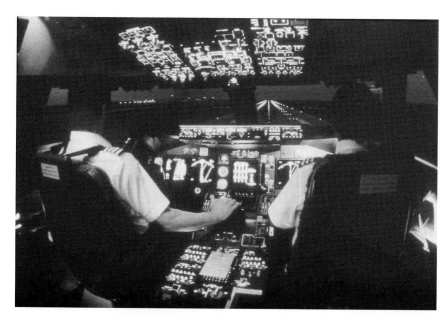

Figure 23.6   *Boeing 747-400 flight deck. See also colour plate 23.6.*

Hunter panel of 1956. Although the instrument designs and displays have changed slightly, the basic 'T' remains. With the introduction of higher-performance aircraft in the 1960s, attempts were made to improve instrument displays to reduce the amount of scanning required and to overcome the limitations of two-dimensional representation of the four-dimensional situation. The 1963 Lightning panel in Figure 23.5 shows the strip display of airspeed and a horizontal situation indicator; however, the attitude indicator is still the most prominent instrument.

Interpretation of strip displays compared with conventional dials takes a higher stage of mental processing, and it is more difficult to derive rates of change. They are still used sometimes for display of engine parameters and, in improved form, for the display of altitude and speed in modern electronic flight instrument displays. However, to overcome the difficulty in interpreting rate of change, modern strip speed displays incorporate an arrow to indicate the trend of speed change.

Strip displays of engine parameters in the Boeing 747-400 are shown in Figure 23.6 and can be compared with the conventional circular engine instruments of the C130 Hercules in Figure 23.7.

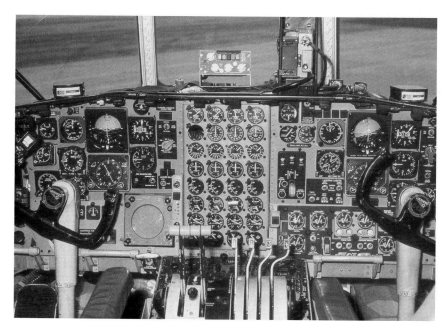

Figure 23.7   *C130 Hercules instrument panel.*

Altimetry

The altimeter is effectively an aneroid barometer calibrated to read in feet (or metres, in aircraft manufactured in Russia and Eastern Europe) rather than millibars (mb) or inches of mercury (inHg). It is calibrated for the International Civil Aviation Organization (ICAO) standard atmosphere (see Chapter 1), and an adjustment knob allows correction for local pressure, indicated on a subscale on the instrument display.

Altitude is defined as the elevation above mean sea level. Since atmospheric pressure varies at the surface of the Earth, a forecast is made of the pressure (mb or inHg) in a given geographical area for the next hour, and this is referred to as 'the QNH' (the Q code is a vestige of the early days in aviation, when information was transmitted in Morse code by telegraphy). Thus, altitude is measured with reference to the QNH datum and is a measure of the vertical distance (in feet or metres) of an aircraft above mean sea level. (In the USA, this is defined as 'true altitude', whereas 'absolute altitude' is the elevation above terrain.)

In aviation, height is a measure of the vertical distance of an aircraft above the airfield elevation. The atmospheric pressure is forecast at the airfield datum, and this is referred to as 'the QFE'. Thus, an aircraft altimeter set to this datum will indicate zero on the ground at the airfield, and not the altitude above mean sea level (unless the airfield happens to be at sea level).

Because of the continuously changing atmospheric pressure, and because at any one time the pressure varies at different points on the Earth's surface, the standard atmospheric pressure (1013.2 mb or 29.92 inHg) is used as the datum pressure for en-route flying above a certain altitude. This altitude is referred to as the transition altitude above which vertical elevation is referred to as a flight level (FL). The flight level is stated in three digits, representing hundreds of feet. Thus, FL290 means that the aircraft altimeter indicates 29 000 feet above the standard pressure datum of 1013.2 mb and ensures that appropriate vertical separation can be maintained between all aircraft flying in the vicinity, which will also be using the standard atmosphere datum. It does not necessarily mean that the aircraft is flying at an altitude of 29 000 feet above sea level (unless the surface atmospheric pressure at that point happens to be 1013 mb).

On descent to the aerodrome, the datum is changed from the standard setting to the appropriate QNH at the transition level. This ensures terrain clearance by the descending aircraft and allows an accurate approach profile to be flown to the runway.

The three-needle display altimeter (Figure 23.8) is easily misinterpreted, and the potential for fatal error is enhanced by the fact that the needle indicating tens of thousands of feet is smaller than that indicating thousands, which in turn is smaller than that indicating hundreds of

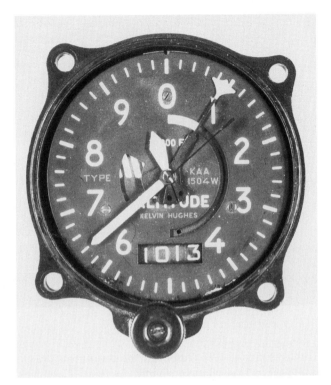

Figure 23.8 *Three-needle altimeter.*

feet. (The altitude indicated in Figure 23.8 is 9 640 feet, or just over FL96, as the datum is set as 1013 mb; a quick glance at the instrument might lead to an erroneous reading of 19 640 feet, with implications for safe terrain clearance.)

Modern altimeters have a digital display plus a single needle indicating hundreds of feet, giving the advantages of both display types (Figure 23.9).

Studies comparing the three-pointer altimeter display with a digital display show a difficulty factor of three to one and an error rate of 20 per cent over the digital (Campbell

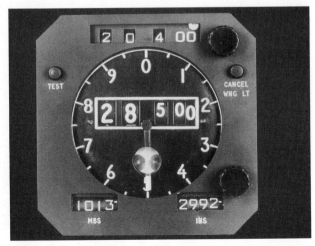

Figure 23.9 *Digital altimeter.*

and Bagshaw 2002). Although a small change in value is best displayed on a digital instrument, rate of change is best perceived on an analogue instrument (quantitative information is better suited to a digital display, while qualitative/comparative/rate information is more suited to an analogue display).

MULTIFUNCTION INSTRUMENT DISPLAYS

The development of modern cathode-ray tubes and liquid-crystal displays, requiring relatively little power and developing less heat than the earlier electronic instruments, enabled rapid advances to be made in multifunctional instrument displays. Figure 23.10 shows an example of an early cathode-ray tube, which brought together the functional performance instruments within a single display. Care is required to interpret the information from the clutter.

The flight deck shown in Figure 23.11 shows how progress has been made in improving the clarity of displayed information. However, the dominant feature of this flight deck is the number of keyboards and input devices. Pilots have to learn to adjust their workloads to a level that maintains a certain amount of intellectual activity and keeps them in the automation loop. Programming the system is time-consuming, and the pilot needs to know how to do the simple things in real time. All temporal sense can be lost when an individual becomes absorbed in programming a system.

Human error will always occur, and this applies as much in programming the system as in other activities involved in operating the aircraft, hence the importance of a mini-

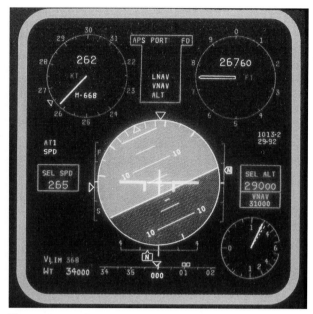

Figure 23.10   *Electronic instrument display. See also colour plate 23.10.*

mum two-crew operation, whereby one monitors the actions of the other.

It is not only modern airliners that have such sophisticated cockpits. Figure 23.12 shows the cockpit of the Augusta/Westland EH 101 Merlin helicopter. Essential flight information is presented on six multifunction display screens, with backup analogue instruments available in case of electronic display failure.

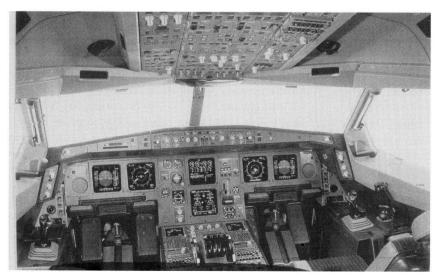

Figure 23.11   *Airbus flight deck. See also colour plate 23.11.*

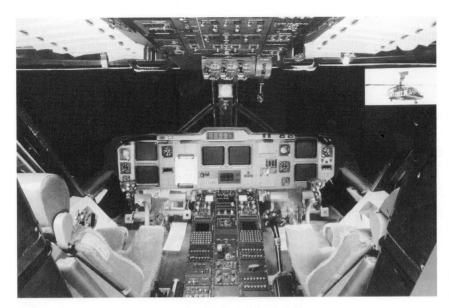

Figure 23.12   *EH 101 Merlin flight deck.
See also colour plate 23.12.*

HEAD-UP DISPLAYS

When involved in reading and interpreting the instrument displays, the pilot is looking inside the aircraft at the instrument panel with head down and eyes focused at the panel distance. It takes time for the gaze to be shifted to the external world seen through the windscreen, moving the head up and refocusing the eyes at infinity. This can be critical in an air combat situation or when delivering a weapon on to a target. It can also degrade flight safety when flying an instrument approach to a runway in poor visibility and a low cloud base, having to look up to visually acquire the runway at the instrument minimum descent height in the final stage of the approach.

Head-up displays (HUDs) originally were developed for military combat aircraft, but they are increasingly being used in corporate and commercial aircraft. Computer-generated information is projected on to a transparent screen in front of the windshield, which appears to the pilot to be superimposed at infinity on the external visual scene. The information duplicates that from the flight instruments as well as navigation and weapon systems (where applicable). Although reducing the need for head-down scanning, the symbology can be complex, and the operation of the HUD control system makes demands on cognitive processing, taking up mental processing capacity. Figure 23.13 shows the range of symbology used in a typical HUD.

Rather than projecting the image on to a fixed screen, the next stage in military combat aircraft and helicopters was for the information to be projected on to the helmet visor, giving a helmet-mounted display (HMD). This has the advantage of the information being visible wherever the pilot is looking, which can aid weapon aiming, but the design has to take account of weight, symbology and image contrast. Again, there is the consideration of complexity of interpretation and operation.

VISUAL ENHANCEMENT

When flying at night or in cloud, the pilot relies on information derived from the aircraft instrumentation, generally using external visual cues for takeoff and landing. Automatic 'blind' landings are now routine in airline and transport operations, although the problem in very low visibility remains of guidance on the ground once the landing is complete. The development of infrared and laser technology has allowed the pilot to 'see' in the dark or poor visibility and to visually acquire a target. Modern combat aircraft incorporate forward-looking infrared sensors, which superimpose the generated visual scene on the HUD. However, the pilot needs to cognitively process the image to translate the two-dimensional representation into four-dimensional situational awareness.

Visual enhancement can also be achieved by the use of night-vision scintillation tubes in the form of helmet-mounted goggles. Initially developed for use by military helicopter crews, night-vision goggles (NVGs) are now used routinely by the crew members of a range of military and civil aircraft. Their use requires special training in the interpretation of the perceived image, particularly with respect to judgement of depth and rate of relative closure between the aircraft and other objects. Because of the spectral sensitivity of the scintillation tubes, the cockpit lighting has to be adapted for use with NVGs.

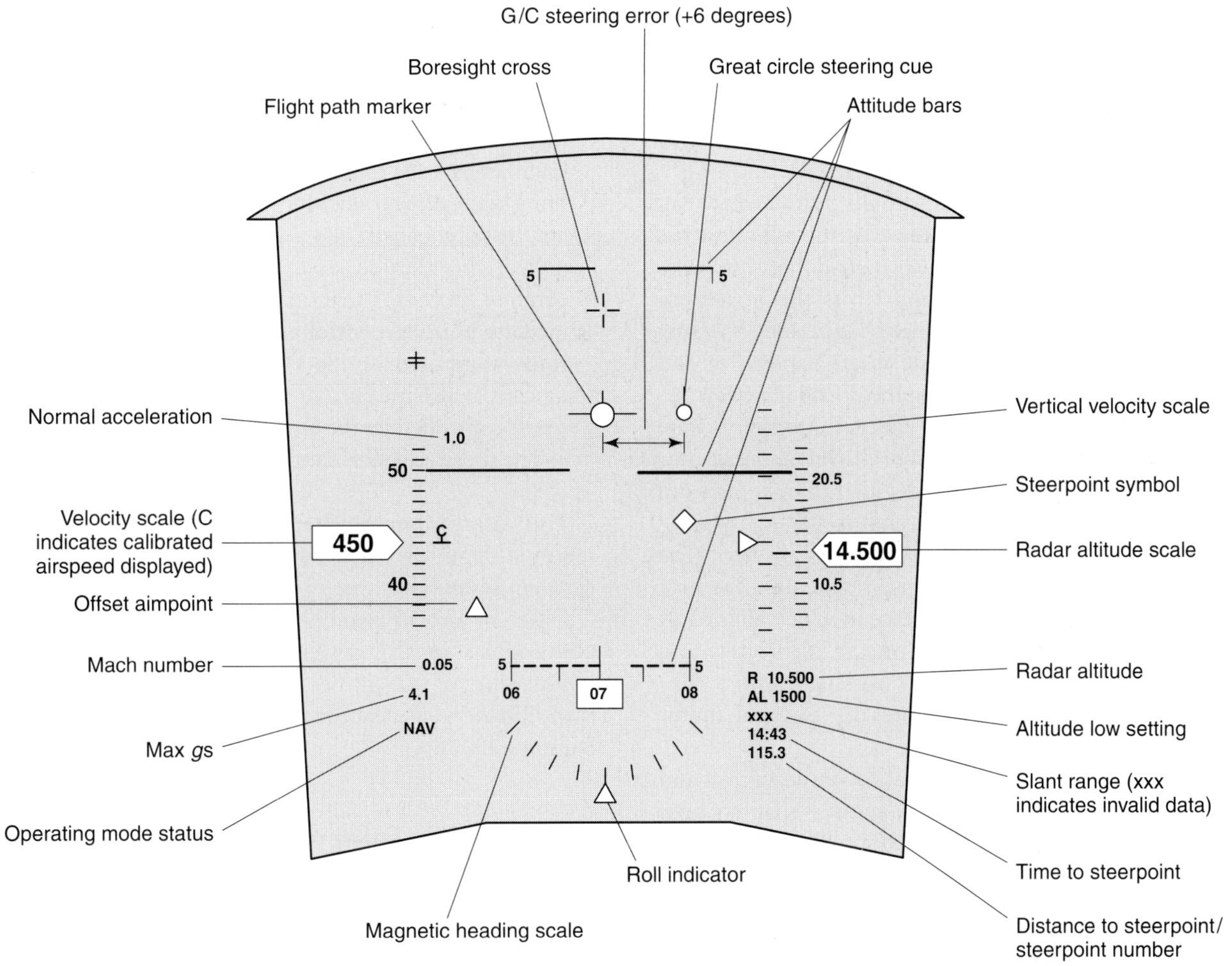

Figure 23.13 *Head-up display symbology.*

SITUATIONAL AWARENESS

Situational awareness is the state of knowing where the aircraft is, where it has been and where it is going in terms of the four dimensions of flight. Loss of situational awareness is a major causal factor in accidents associated with human error. It can be defined as the perception of the elements in an environment within a volume of time and space, the comprehension of their meaning, and the projection of their status in the near future. In practical terms, it is a state of mind encompassing a dynamic mental model of relevant aspects of the 'real' world. It is created and maintained by cognitive and physical activity, and it requires dynamic awareness of the operating environment, the aircraft modes and the state of the aircraft technical systems. The mental model is formed from perception, comprehension and projection to enable an active goal to be achieved.

When perception (and the mental model) matches reality, the crew member is situationally aware. This requires cognitive processing of the two-dimensional information on attitude, altitude, speed and time to give the four-dimensional picture, as well as continuing awareness of the progress of the navigational and operational plan.

AUTOMATION

The military tactical environment has become extremely complex, with large amounts of rapidly changing information needing to be processed and acted upon by the flight crew. The demands on crew members are such that the only way to operate efficiently is to use automation and computer technology. In civilian operations, a major driving force for technological development has been cost reduction: a microprocessor is cheaper than a human crew member; it is also more efficient at performing routine tasks, but only when under the control of a human being. Similarly, the evolution of electronic flight instrument displays has been driven as much by the fact that a liquid-crystal display is cheaper to build and maintain than a complex analogue mechanical instrument than by the multifunctional capacity of the electronic display itself.

Alone, these developments should not lead to an increase in workload or error. However, the pilot now has a range of functional tasks to perform, and there are fewer crew members to monitor and cross-check actions. Commercial and military pressures require long working hours, which can lead to fatigue (see Chapter 52) and reduced vigilance, thus increasing the possibility of error.

Automation itself is not a new concept. Autopilots were introduced before the Second World War and are now commonly found on most classes of aircraft, ranging from relatively unsophisticated light aircraft to the highly automated flight decks of modern commercial airliners. The technical complexities of modern aircraft, plus the ever increasing complexity of the airspace in which all aircraft operate, has increased demands on the flight crew and led to a steady increase in mental workload, with a concomitant reduction in the demands for physical motor skills.

As well as automating the navigation of the aircraft and its actual control via the autopilot, another goal has been to optimize flight performance and manage fuel consumption. Continuously monitored and computer-calculated throttle settings and flight paths can achieve significant fuel savings, which have commercial and military benefits.

All pilots undergo initial training on basic light aircraft or helicopters, utilizing simple control systems. When flying larger or more sophisticated aircraft, the perception remains that the physical deflection of an appropriate cockpit control is causing the appropriate response, even though the deflection has simply signalled the servomotor system to act. This applies regardless of whether the signal is generated by control input from the pilot or from programming the autopilot or flight system.

The operation of the human–machine interface has become more complex as the capabilities and capacity of the automated flight-management system have evolved. From the original suite of single-function switches and knobs, there is now a range of multifunction keyboards and controls. The following is an extract from the description of the autopilot controls in a modern passenger airliner (UK Air Accidents Investigation Branch 2004):

Fundamentally, the autopilot and auto throttle attempt to acquire or maintain target parameters determined either by manual inputs from the handling pilot or by computations from the flight management guidance system (FMGS). When the target parameter is set by the FMGS, the term 'managed' is used for the target parameter. When the target parameter is set by the flight crew, the term 'selected' is used.

The altitude and speed selection controls can be either pushed or pulled. When turned, the altitude selector knob adjusts the target altitude, and when pushed, the same knob allows the FMGS to 'manage' any intermediate altitude constraints entered into a route. When pulled, the altitude selector knob triggers an 'open' climb or descent. The term 'open' means that any intermediate altitude control constraints within the active route computed by the FGMS are ignored. When in descent, it also means that idle thrust is selected and airspeed controlled by the elevators.

The speed selection control has comparable functions.

This description illustrates the complexity and the required depth of understanding of modern flight-management systems.

Different aircraft manufacturers have evolved different philosophies in the development of automation. The philosophies of two of the major Western civilian aircraft manufacturers are summarized below (Campbell and Bagshaw 2002):

THE AIRBUS PHILOSOPHY IS:

- Automation must not reduce overall aircraft reliability but should enhance aircraft and system safety, efficiency and economy.
- Automation must not lead the aircraft out of the safe flight envelope, and it should be maintained within the normal flight envelope.
- Automation should allow the operator to use the safe flight envelope to its full extent, should this be necessary due to abnormal circumstances.
- Within the normal flight envelope, the automation must not work against operator inputs, except when absolutely necessary for safety.

THE BOEING PHILOSOPHY IS:

- The pilot is the final authority for the operation of the aircraft.
- Both crew members are ultimately responsible for the safe conduct of the flight.
- The order of priority of flight crew tasks is safety, passenger comfort, efficiency.
- Design for crew operations is based on pilots' past training and operational experience.
- Systems must be designed to be error-tolerant.
- Hierarchy of design alternatives is simplicity, redundancy, automation.
- Automation is a tool to aid, not replace, the pilot.

- Address fundamental human strengths, limitations and individual differences for both normal and abnormal operations.
- Use new technologies and functional capabilities only when they result in clear and distinct operational or efficiency advantages and there is no adverse effect on the human–machine interface.

It is recognized that there are advantages and disadvantages to aspects of both of these philosophies, but the products of both manufacturers are in safe and efficient worldwide service.

Advanced automation changes the nature of the human-factor considerations on the flight deck. The flight crew need to remain effectively 'in the loop' as part of the system, so the pilot–computer interface is crucial in keeping the pilots informed of the system operation and, conversely, keeping the computers informed of the condition and behaviour of the flight crew. Although on the one hand automation significantly reduces the pilot's workload, on the other hand new systems actually increase workload in the areas of programming, understanding and monitoring.

Advantages of humans over machines include:

- creativeness
- innovation
- aptitude to deal with novel situations.

Human qualities that cannot be replicated by automation include:

- the capability of quickly grasping logical connections in large complex quantities of data and filtering out the meaningless data;
- the ability to divide up memory into related data segments;
- the ability to identify errors when data are presented graphically;
- the possession of genuine flexibility in dealing with unforeseen events.

The irony of automation is that it does much better than the pilot those things that a pilot already knows how to do well; however, it does not know how to do those things that the pilot would like to do well (Bainbridge 1987).

Advantages of automation

The major advantage of automation is the reduction in pilot workload associated with the manual tasks of navigating and flying and the associated cognitive processing. There is high accuracy and reliability of the systems, and in general they are very cost-effective. The use of multifunctional displays allows increased sophistication of information presentation, enhancing accuracy, efficiency and the maintenance of situational awareness.

Disadvantages of automation

Although the workload associated with manually flying and navigating the aircraft is reduced, the programming and monitoring of the automated systems can significantly increase workloads during critical phases of flight. However, during long-range cruising, workload may fall to such low levels that boredom occurs and arousal levels can reduce significantly. This can influence performance, particularly of vigilance and monitoring tasks, and can reduce job satisfaction.

Difficulties in designing an effective pilot–equipment interface can relate to system opacity, autonomy and protection. System opacity increases with technology and gives poor mental representation of the underlying system function. It is based on the need-to-know principle, in that the display to the crew shows only a simple tree, which hides a forest of complexity. This is a great advantage for standard operations, but it can be a limitation when things go wrong and the crew are unclear as to what can be done to resolve the situation.

System autonomy means that the greater the technology, the more the system is able to adapt to a given situation without operator commands. This is particularly relevant in the function of the autopilot, which can initiate a chain of events without direction from the pilot. This again is not a problem during normal operation, but if the pilot workload is high, then he or she may be 'outside the loop'.

System protection is a built-in function to prevent errors from system malfunction. However, this can lead to the crew deviating from standard operating procedures because of fears that the system protection will lead the aircraft into dangerous modes of flight.

It has been suggested that these three problems can be resolved by increased training. However, adaptation is slow, particularly when a pilot is transferring to fly an automated aircraft from a conventional type, and the complexity of automated systems takes much experience for full understanding to develop.

Automation complacency

Automation has sometimes been seen as an end in itself, rather than as a tool to enhance the aircraft operation. Excessive reliance on automation can lead to automation complacency, where situational monitoring and cross-checking are reduced because of a belief in the infallibility of the automatic system. The very reliability with which automated systems normally perform can lead to overconfidence and complacency.

An error during data input may not be picked up and corrected at the time. Subsequent cross-checking of the flight progress may reveal a disparity, but automation complacency may reinforce the hypothesis or mindset that the system 'knows what it is doing'. Alternatively, the belief in the system reliability may lead to an absence of cross-checking and a breakdown in the crew's situational awareness.

Monitoring may become passive, whereby the inherent belief in the automated system's infallibility leads to the crew member simply watching what the system is doing, rather than analysing and constantly checking. However, the multifunctional capability of the automated cockpit can lead to a narrowing of concentration on to one particular aspect. This blinkered concentration leads to a breakdown in the monitoring of the whole system. Finally, the complexity of the automated system can lead to confusion and a loss of situational awareness. It is essential for the crew to maintain system mode awareness to remain in the automation loop.

Albert Einstein is credited with saying 'Computers are incredibly fast, accurate and stupid. Humans are incredibly slow, inaccurate and brilliant. Together, they are powerful beyond imagination.'

CONCLUSION

The cockpit or flight deck is a complex working environment. The practitioner of aviation medicine needs to understand the human factors as well as gain a basic knowledge of the technology involved. There is no substitute for gaining practical experience, and every opportunity should be taken to observe flight crew at work, either in the air or in a flight simulator.

REFERENCES

Bainbridge L. Ironies of automation. In: Rasmussen J (ed.). *New Technology and Human Error*. London: John Wiley & Sons, 1987; pp. 271–83.

Campbell RD, Bagshaw M. *Human Performance and Limitations in Aviation*, 3rd edn. Oxford: Blackwell Science, 2002.

UK Air Accidents Investigation Branch. *UK Air Accidents Investigation Branch Bulletin* 2004; **December**: EW/G2004/04/14.

24

Restraint systems and escape from aircraft

ALAN E. HEPPER

RESTRAINT SYSTEMS

Introduction

A restraint system may have more than one purpose. In normal and high dynamic flight, the restraint system keeps the individual within their workspace, so that control of the aircraft and equipment is maintained. However, during impact, the restraint system attempts to maintain the individual within a known volume, so that the crash dynamics may be attenuated and movement of the occupant restricted in order to avoid secondary impacts with equipment such as displays and controls.

In a crash, the occupants will obey Newton's first law of motion. They will stay at rest or move with uniform velocity in a straight line unless compelled to do otherwise by an external force. In this way, when a vehicle in motion decelerates, the occupants tend to continue in a straight line along the path of original motion. It is the function of the restraint system to resist this motion and thus decelerate the occupant. The system must apply this deceleration in the most appropriate direction, at sites over the human body that are most suitable to take the load.

A restraint system has different and often conflicting requirements. It must be comfortable to wear over the whole range of use, with easy adjustment, and it must protect the occupant from injury that may arise from multidirectional forces. Although each harness will be designed with particular impact dynamics in mind, it should protect the occupant under all foreseeable impact conditions; in aviation, this is likely to involve multiple directions. Care must be taken when a harness is integrated into a vehicle, in order to ensure that it provides the response require-ments for the expected dynamic and that the anchor points are capable of taking the maximum expected loading rather than just meeting an impact test standard. The system should provide maximum distribution of the forces over the body and should not lead to harness-related injury. It should not allow relative movement between the restraint system elements and the human body.

The system must be easy to put on, and release should be as simple as possible. A single-point mechanism is desirable, and it should be possible to operate under conditions of restricted vision, such as in a smoke-filled cockpit or cabin. The loads required to operate the mechanism should be in the range of 66–177 N (15–40 lbf) so that inadvertent operation is unlikely, single-handed operation should be possible, and two sequenced operations should be incorporated in order to avoid accidental opening. The system should allow enough movement for the occupant to operate the equipment and carry out all tasks and should be designed in such a way that it is just as efficient regardless of whether the occupant is sitting back, leaning forward or reaching for equipment. Active or inflatable restraint elements systems should operate without causing injury throughout the workspace.

The use of restraint systems relies upon a 'system approach', with the components regarded as elements. If certain elements require the use of other parts of the system, e.g. if an airbag also requires the use of a harness, then this should be clearly documented and demonstrated during training. In all systems, the seat should be regarded as an element of the restraint. It is the element of the vehicle that transmits the motion to the body and provides support to the buttocks and thighs during an impact with a vertical descent rate. It is essential that this is borne in mind when designing aircraft seating, as this will affect the transmission of impact energy to the body. For example, a soft cushion may appear to attenuate impact energy, but when the cushion is compressed to its maximum extent, it may impart a greater peak acceleration than would have been experienced if the person was sitting on a rigid seat. Elements of the support of the seat, such as braces, may localize the loading on the legs, back or buttocks, and these may create sufficient force to cause injury.

The ideal restraint system would lead to a uniform distribution of the forces experienced during an impact over the whole of the body and so eliminate the possibility of concentrated forces. Such a system would demand a fluid covering of the occupant to meet all possible impact situations. However, excellent restraint is provided by wide webbing straps or a harness or by using the clothing as part of the harness. The principle of ideal restraint is based purely on the ability to spread the loads evenly. Conversely, poor restraint occurs from concentrated loads, either from a poorly designed or poorly fitted restraint system or due to twisted straps.

The effectiveness of a restraint system must be considered in context with the other elements that affect the crashworthiness, such as the occupiable space, environment, energy absorption and post-crash survival aspects. These are summarized by the acronym CREEP: Container, Restraint, Environment, Energy absorption and Post-impact. Compromise of any of these aspects will affect the chance of survival. Loss of occupiable space (or reduction in the container volume, movement of the structure, or ingress of external objects into the compartment) may cause impact of the body against the interior surfaces. Harness failure or inadequate restraint will mean that the individual will continue in motion and impact the cockpit or cabin. Control of the environmental hazards, such as ensuring bulkhead-mounted equipment or stowed items, is necessary to prevent them becoming detached and causing injury. Energy absorption to alter the deceleration profile is necessary to reduce the severity of the impact and minimize the injury risks. Post-impact hazard reduction is also required with respect to fire, frost and drowning.

Lap–belts and diagonal straps

The simplest type of restraint system is the lap-belt (Figure 24.1). This is the conventional type of restraint system for most passenger aircraft. It requires two anchorage points, positioned on both sides of the body on either the seat itself or the floor. The belt is usually at a 45-degree angle with the seat base when observed from the side. This type of harness provides minimum restriction to the occupant, but the level of restraint is also poor. The torso is not restrained and will jack-knife under frontal or vertical impacts. Unless the head and chest trajectory is free of obstruction, or a brace position has been adopted, inca-

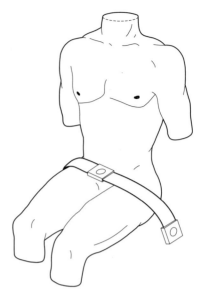

Figure 24.1 *Lap-belt.*

pacitating or fatal injuries may occur on impact. Furthermore, if the belt rises up over the iliac crests across the front of the abdomen, then abdominal and lumbar spine injuries may occur. Continued use in passenger aircraft owes much to simplicity and usefulness in providing restraint in turbulence. In any case, many aircraft seats are also incapable of taking a more sophisticated restraint system, as they are not stressed to take high-impact loading levels.

Another design involves a diagonal belt (Figure 24.2). This has the advantage of remaining a simple system, but as the pelvis is not restrained the occupant tends to rotate

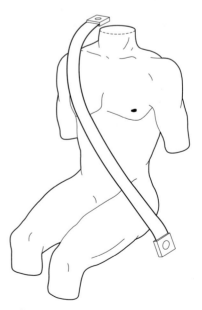

Figure 24.2 *Shoulder strap.*

out of the harness during impact. This can lead to a fatal whip action on the neck or internal chest injuries.

Multiple-point harnesses

The most widely used restraint is the three-point harness (Figure 24.3). This is used in cars. Although, if designed properly, it provides good restraint for frontal impacts, restraint during vertical impact is only moderate, and restraint in lateral impact is poor. It is important that this type of harness is fitted correctly and that the seat cushion is reasonably stiff, so that the lap-belt cannot slip over the iliac crests, with the possibility of abdominal injuries. Fitted correctly, this type of harness will give acceptable restraint up to accelerations up to 30 G_x.

The four-point harness involves lap restraint and a strap across each shoulder (Figure 24.4). It is an improvement on the three-point harness as it provides better restraint, due primarily to the larger spread of loading. The five-point harness provides the elements of the four-point harness along with a negative-g or tie-down strap, also called a lap-belt or harness-stabilizing strap (Figure 24.5). This strap, which is attached to the seat at the midline between the legs and joins the centre of the harness, prevents distortion of the harness. It is useful during manoeuvres that create vertical accelerations, which try to separate the occupant from the seat (negative G_z). This negative-g strap is also important during impact. It tends to maintain the position of the harness elements in a manner that reduces the amount of pelvis rotation (so-called 'submarining'), which in turn increases the loading in the abdomen and spine, increasing the risk and level of injury. Another use of the negative-g strap in the five-point harness is in ejec-

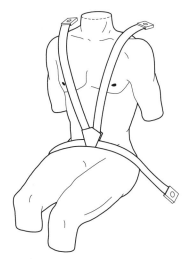

Figure 24.4 *Four-point harness.*

tion seats, where it is used to retain the personal survival pack in the seat-pan. The survival pack remains with the occupant on separation from the seat.

Multiple-point harnesses can be integrated into the seat, so that one harness per seat is required, or issued personally, in which case at least one harness per person is necessary (to account for clothing assembly and repair). The latter is usually an individually fitted four-point harness and referred to as a 'torso harness'. The choice of torso harness or seat-mounted harness has logistical implications and also gives rise to differences in performance under dynamic stresses in the aviation environment.

Rearward-facing and energy-absorbing seats

A restraint system should spread the impact loading over a wide area of the body. In this way, rearward-facing seats provide contact over most of the back. Rearward-facing

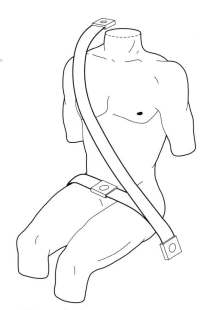

Figure 24.3 *Three-point harness.*

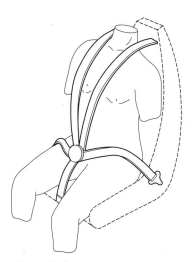

Figure 24.5 *Five-point harness.*

seats provide excellent protection from frontal impact. However, the seat structure must be sufficiently strong to withstand the forces of a body pressed against it, and a support is needed to prevent excess movement of the head. Rearward-facing seats have not been adopted, as they are disliked by some passengers, tend to cause discomfort on takeoff and landing, and have cost and weight implications. Such seats need to be constructed so that they can withstand the impact forces associated with aircraft crashes and should fail only once the whole-body tolerance has been exceeded.

Energy-attenuating seats may be used to reduce the magnitude of the deceleration imparted to the body by using elements in the seat that deform on impact. These act as a force-limiting mechanism and prolong the duration of the impact. Since the velocity change from the initial velocity to zero is constant for the aircraft and occupant, the increase in duration results in a reduction in the average deceleration, reducing the risk of injury (see Chapter 10).

AIRBAGS

Impact protection from airbags is becoming more common. Gas generation from small explosive devices has made this a viable technology, although some systems still use compressed air supplies. The release of gas into a woven nylon bag with an airtight coating (such as neoprene) is triggered from a deceleration sensor. The bag inflates, providing a soft structure that absorbs energy. Airbags are elements of a restraint system and do not replace the need for a harness. Covers that provide the stowage should be positioned so that they do not cause injury when the airbag is deployed.

ESCAPE FROM AIRCRAFT

The need to escape from an aircraft may arise on the ground or during flight. The means for escape must be available at all times and must take account of the forces that may be operating on the aircraft, e.g. aerodynamics, accelerations and rotations. For this reason, and because escape at speeds above 200 knots is problematic, most high-performance military and training aircraft have assisted escape systems, which use mechanical power for the escapee to leave the aircraft. Unassisted escape systems simply rely on physical strength. An assisted escape system must have sufficient thrust to eject the occupant clear of the aircraft structure at all speeds and provide sufficient ground clearance to enable full deployment and inflation of the main parachute before ground impact. The system should be fully automatic, relieving the occupant of any action after initiation of the ejection sequence. The system should restrain the occupant sufficiently and modulate any forces of the body, so that the risk of injury is minimized.

Ejection seats

The principal method of assisted escape is the open ejection seat, although some aircraft still have capsule escape systems. There is variability in the methods of operation between different seats, but the principles are similar. Ejection seats are tailored to the likely operational situation. Thus, aircraft that operate at relatively slow speeds, such as jet trainer aircraft, may have an ejection seat fitted without a rocket motor, as this would only subject the occupant to potentially hazardous and unnecessary accelerations. Correspondingly, supersonic aircraft may have blast protection in the form of deflector plates or screens in order to protect the occupant from dynamic air pressure.

In general, the seat is much more than an escape system. It is a seating platform for the aircrew and carries connections for part of the communications and life-support systems. It consists of a rigid framework supporting the seat-pan and is attached to the aircraft structure with one or more set of rails, which provide guidance for the initial part of the trajectory. The top of the seat is attached to a catapult- or gun-propulsion system, with the base of this catapult attached to the aircraft. In most modern systems, the catapult is a telescopic device that contains one or more explosive gas-generation cartridges, which provides and sustains the thrust as the seat leaves the aircraft. Nevertheless, some seats use a single rocket motor to cover the whole thrust from the aircraft. Some ejection seats have a rocket motor fitted to the base of the seat-pan to increase the final escape velocity. This motor may also be used to ensure divergence for the seats, so that front and rear seats travel in different directions and aid aircraft-fin clearance. However, increasingly, the divergent pathways for the seats are achieved using a symmetric rocket motor for the thrust and a small kicker rocket fitted to the seat-pan and facing laterally.

The seat also contains the drogue parachute, which is a small high-speed parachute deployed to decelerate and stabilize the seat, as well as the main parachute and harness to provide a steady final descent. The seat-pan is fitted with a personal survival pack, which contains the survival equipment and is retained with the occupant after the seat and escapee separate. The whole escape sequence is timed using explosive, mechanical or electromechanical devices. A typical ejection seat is shown in Figure 24.6.

OPERATION

An ejection seat sequence is shown in Figure 24.7. Essentially, ejection is initiated by the aircrew pulling the

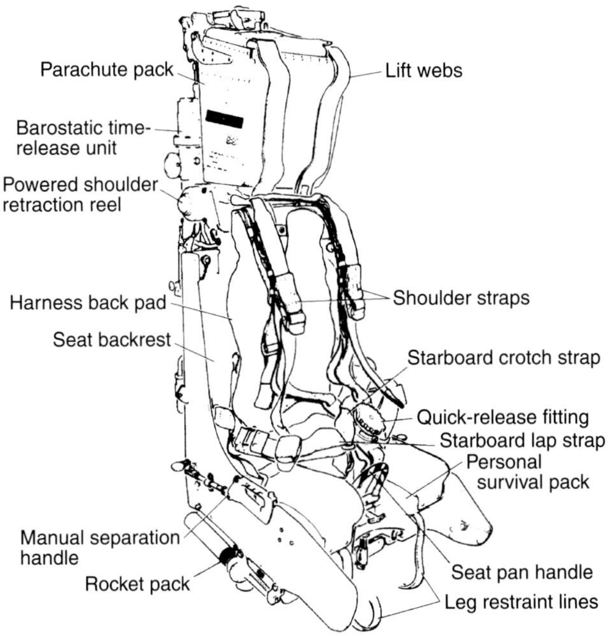
Parachute pack
Lift webs
Barostatic time-release unit
Powered shoulder retraction reel
Harness back pad
Shoulder straps
Seat backrest
Starboard crotch strap
Quick-release fitting
Starboard lap strap
Personal survival pack
Manual separation handle
Rocket pack
Seat pan handle
Leg restraint lines

Figure 24.6 *Anatomy of typical ejection seat.*

ejection handle situated between the legs. On early seats, the handle was positioned above the head, but it is now situated where it is easier to reach under $+G_z$ acceleration. On early tandem-seat aircraft, the pilot would inform the rear-seat occupant of an impending ejection so that, ideally, the rear seat may eject before the front seat. This would avoid collision between the two seats, but it introduced a potentially fatal delay. Modern aircraft therefore have an automatic 'command eject' system, whereby the operation of the front seat automatically ejects the rear seat, typically 0.3 s before the front seat moves. Operation of the rear seat may or may not operate the front seat with such a system, depending on the aircraft system or prior selection of the mode of operation.

Initiation of the seat activates a harness-retraction system and any necessary canopy-removal or destruction system, as well as, in the case of a multi-crew escape, command ejection systems to ensure the correct exit sequence. Activation of the seat catapult or gun starts the movement of the seat out of the aircraft and provides an escape velocity of 16–24 m/s. For slower catapults, this is often supplemented at the end of the stroke by a rocket. This maintains the seat–aircraft separation forces and produces a high relative velocity of up to 27 m/s. After catapult separation, a drogue parachute or stabilizing system is deployed to start to decelerate and steady the seat. This is essential, because the shape of an ejection seat and occupant is such that it is unstable in flight and can impart high rotational accelerations to the occupant.

The main parachute is deployed after a short period of deceleration of about 1.5 s. The occupant is released from the seat, and the shock force of the main parachute lines leads to separation from the seat. At high altitude, parachute deployment is delayed until descent has occurred to a specified altitude, which depends on the typical operating terrain but is intended to eliminate the possibility of hypoxia. Deployment of the parachute may also be limited to occur below a certain acceleration and/or velocity, so that the structural integrity of the parachute is not compromised and the occupant is not subjected to injury.

When the seat separates, the harness is usually attached to a personal survival pack by means of a lanyard. The pack contains survival aids, such as a life-raft, food supplies and emergency flares. The whole sequence from initiation to separation is in the order of 1.8 s with 2.65 s to parachute full inflation, provided parachute deployment is not

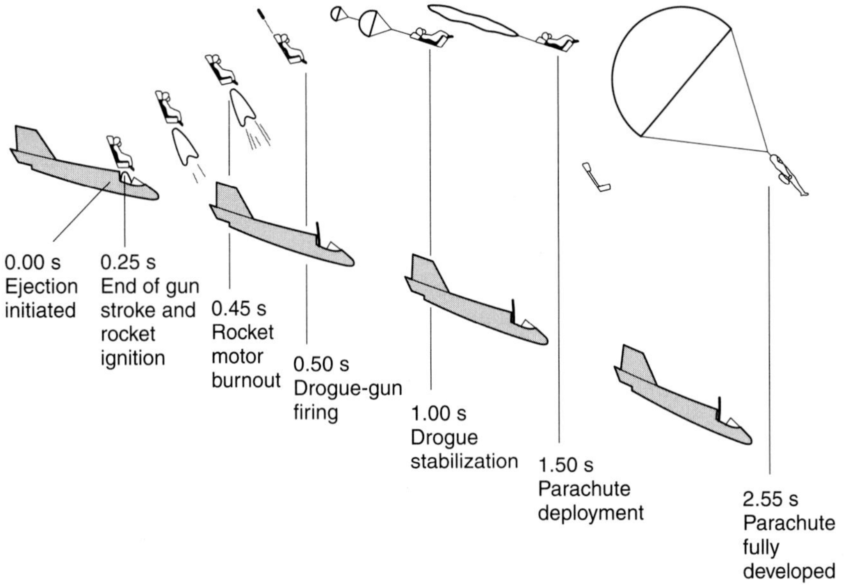
0.00 s Ejection initiated
0.25 s End of gun stroke and rocket ignition
0.45 s Rocket motor burnout
0.50 s Drogue-gun firing
1.00 s Drogue stabilization
1.50 s Parachute deployment
2.55 s Parachute fully developed

Figure 24.7 *Typical ejection seat sequence.*

delayed for the reasons outlined above. Some modern seats have more than one mode of operation, since at low speed deceleration to a safe velocity for release of the main parachute is not required. The seat velocity is monitored; at low speed, the main parachute is deployed and the occupant and seat separate at the time of drogue deployment. This has significant benefits in reducing the time to inflation of the main parachute and extending the safe working envelope.

Operation of the seat at high speed and under high rotational rates may impart instability, as the seat and occupant are a bluff body and in normal circumstances will fly in an unstable condition. The seat may tip forwards (speed less than 250 knots), tip backwards (speeds more than 450 knots) or rotate in yaw, depending on the ejection speed, seat design, mass, centre of gravity, inertial properties and occupant orientation – the seat may tumble and lead to rotational and flail injuries. There will also be the sensations of tumbling and disorientation. For these reasons, stabilizing techniques such as aerodynamic surfaces deployed on exit from the aircraft, and multi-strop bridles, which provide a stable attachment to the drogue, are being introduced. These should reduce the occurrence of rotational, flail and shear injuries. It must, however, be emphasized that the seat design and timings mean that seats have a limited operating range and will not save the occupants from all possible scenarios. In this context, aircrew must be aware of the limitations of the seat and must be aware of the safe operating envelope. A significant number of fatalities arise from the attempts of aircrews to eject too late.

Canopy

Cockpit canopy removal or destruction is a vital part of the escape process. The escape path may be cleared by physical removal, fracturing, fragmentation of the canopy itself, or using the seat and occupant to punch a path through the structure. The canopy is manufactured in a variety of methods. Traditional canopies have been made from stretched or cast acrylic but, in an attempt to increase strength and reduce weight, composite or sandwich materials are now being used in order to enhance protection against the effects of bird-strikes. These have benefits when it comes to structural strength and resilience, although they can be more difficult to break. The escape path clearance method can be chosen only when the canopy material composition, shape and strength are taken into account.

The most reliable method for escape path clearance from the point of ensuring minimum injury is canopy removal. The whole canopy is detached from the aircraft and separated using removal rockets or explosive charges. Forced removal is usually necessary to ensure that it occurs during a limited time interval, as aerodynamic forces alone may not lift the canopy. Indeed, under certain circumstances, such forces may keep the canopy in place. Typically, 0.3 s is allowed in the escape sequence for the removal of the canopy. Depending on the method used, the explosive reactions must occur within the airframe and the actuators placed to avoid burns to the aircrew from the explosive blast.

Another method of clearing the escape path is to fracture the canopy, so that the seat and occupant pass through it. This uses an explosive energy (either stored thermal or kinetic) system to fracture the canopy into small pieces. The process may not shatter the canopy or cut through it but may weaken the material so that lower forces are needed for the final breakthrough. The fracture pattern depends on the canopy shape, material properties and expected forces. For example, a material such as stretched acrylic, which is resilient to secondary crack propagation and breaks into large knife-edged pieces, will be broken in two or only weakened to allow the seat and occupant to push the resultant pieces out of the way. Other materials that fracture easily may be broken into small pieces to minimize injury. Depending on the form and power of the cutting device used to fragment the canopy, problems may occur from the miniature detonating cord (MDC) and linear cutting charge (LCC), as when the explosive sheathing is broken during combustion and sends molten sheath into the cockpit. This may cause burns and injuries to the eyes and compromise the effectiveness of the protective clothing of the occupant.

Ejection systems sometimes rely on the seat and occupant forcing their own path through the canopy. This is referred to as 'through-canopy ejection' and should not be used except where unavoidable, such as a backup system through the thinnest of canopies. There is a belief that canopy breakers fitted to the seat shatter the canopy, propagating cracks throughout the canopy. However, there is limited evidence that this happens, and experience in service has shown an unacceptable rate of head, neck, spinal, sternum and leg injuries. The chance of impairing the successful operation of the seat also exists, due to the impact damaging seat systems and from a reduced altitude of the seat trajectory due to the energy removed from the system.

Forces of assisted escape from aircraft

The ejection seat is the most commonly used form of aircraft in-flight abandonment, although it is available only to military fast-jet aviators.

The initiation mechanism and ejection from the cockpit applies acceleration in excess of 12 g for up to 500 ms, with an acceleration onset rate up to 300 g/s. The restraint system therefore is of vital importance, as it retains the position of the escapee. A properly fitted restraint system increases the coupling with the seat and should minimize the possibility of 'dynamic overshoot'. This can occur when a person sits on an elastic cushion; as the seat accelerates, the cushion depresses, until it is fully compressed. The seat can impart a sudden high-energy force, resulting in a very high-amplitude, short-duration impact, which may cause injury. Ideally, the seat and occupant should be attached rigidly to each other, so that the coupling moves as a single mass. This is impractical; therefore, invariably a well-damped thin foam pad is used between the occupant and the seat.

Although the main forces on the body are in the long axis of the spine, significant flexion forces are involved. These arise because the line of thrust of the seat does not coincide with the spinal axis, with the need to allow seat-height adjustment for the full anthropometric range and yet still maintain eye datum and reach of the controls. The included angle between the two axes may be as much as 18 degrees, which means with a 20 g vertical acceleration with the frontal component on the spine reaching 6 g. During ejection, this invariably results in spinal compression coupled with severe flexion. This commonly causes anterior lip wedge fractures to vertebrae in the lumbar and thoracic spine.

As the cockpit canopy is released from the aircraft, the occupant is subjected to windblast. Depending on the aircraft design, this may be quite small at the early stage of ejection. Within 0.2 s of the seat's first movement, the seat and occupant are subjected to the full blast of the air while still travelling at approximately the same speed as the aircraft. Windblast pressures vary with the density of the air and the square of the velocity; at 600 knots (308 m/s), there is a dynamic pressure of 58 kPa (8.4 psi) at sea level. The effect of the windblast is due to the sudden application of force to the chest and abdomen. The subject is 'winded' in mild cases, but in cases of high pressure an arterial pulse may be generated, which leads to subconjunctival haemorrhages. The threshold of injury for blast probably lies at about 31 kPa (4.5 psi; equivalent airspeed of 225 m/s or 440 knots) and for serious damage at about 55–62 kPa (8–9 psi; an equivalent airspeed of 300–320 m/s or 582–620 knots). Theoretically, very high blast pressures could lead to rupture of internal organs and death.

In ejections above 300 knots, the limbs and head may be subjected to severe windblast. Unrestrained legs may be forced over the side of the seat-pan, resulting in fracture or dislocation of the hip. The hands will tend to hold on to the firing handle, but at high speeds the force of the windblast may tear them free, with the arms flailing outwards, upwards and backwards. Positive restraint at the elbows or wrists is required at speeds above 500 knots. Furthermore, unless the head is located positively, it too may flail, but no satisfactory system of head restraint has yet been devised. It is fortunate that the majority of ejections are at moderate speed, and it is only with the highest speeds that head injury occurs, although usually compounded by the high

rotational rate of the seat that imparts shear. Addition of mass, such as night-vision, weapon-aiming and information equipment, to the headgear is an area of concern, and it is desirable that these systems are jettisoned before ejection. Failure to remove such equipment before ejection may impose injurious loads on the neck, depending on the level of restraint provided by the harness (and any energy attenuation that may be present).

During deceleration of the seat, the forces on the human body occur principally in the G_x direction, where the escapee is well-supported by the seat back. The decelerative forces are usually well within the whole-body tolerance limits and do not present a problem, apart from the possibility of flail.

Escape parachutes

Escape system parachutes are, on the whole, of fairly simple construction, being either round or conical. They are designed to withstand fairly high opening speeds, to open quickly, and to operate across a large range of aircrew masses. They are also fairly stable during descent and easy to control, since the escapees are not usually experienced parachutists. The steady-state vertical descent rate of escape parachutes is quite high, being of the order 8.5 m/s (28 feet/s) in still air conditions, and some landing injuries may be expected. When the parachute opens, the escapee is subjected to several loads, depending on the parachute method of the deployment. The first load is the snatch load of parachute rigging lines pulling tight, which is usually used to remove the escapee from the seat. The next loading happens while the parachute inflates and continues until it reaches full inflation. There is then an overinflation of the parachute, which produces another snatch load. The parachute thereafter starts to deflate and then re-inflate. The level of this oscillatory inflation depends on the design and the amount of in-built damping. Some designs of parachute also produce a level of oscillation during descent; others overcome this by adding drive. Both of these component velocities add to the descent rate of the parachute to give a higher actual velocity.

Escape under extreme conditions

The requirements of aircraft escape systems become more demanding as the aircraft operating envelope increases. High-altitude ejections mean more time on the parachute and lack of oxygen, while with vertical/short takeoff and landing (VSTOL) aircraft there is the potential requirement to operate at low level with a zero forward velocity, a high sink rate and potentially a high roll rate. Escape at high airspeed also involves blast. The new generation of unstable aircraft, which may fail in an even more dramatic manner compared with conventional aircraft, means that the operation of the escape system under high roll, pitch and yaw rates must also be considered, together with the effect on the initial seat dynamics.

Air density reduces as altitude increases, so that escape at high altitude produces lesser drag forces than at lower levels. The blast forces are correspondingly lower for a given aircraft. This benefit is offset by the reduced damping of seat motion with reduced air density. The seat will rotate at higher speeds, with 250 rpm having occurred, and the parachute opening shock is increased because the parachute opens quicker in the lower air density. The principal physiological problems of high-altitude ejection are hypoxia and cold. In view of this, emergency oxygen systems are invariably mounted on to the seat and protection from the cold is provided by clothing, although exposed skin, such as the face, may suffer frostbite. For these reasons, a drogue parachute or other stabilizing system is deployed, and withdrawal of the main parachute is delayed until a safe altitude is reached. This opening altitude depends on many factors, including parachute design, operating terrain and ejection seat; altitudes of 10 000 feet, 15 000 feet and 5000 m have been used.

High-speed ejections, especially those involving high blast pressures (high speed, low level), have special problems, which the seat design must be capable of withstanding. Many of the features of the seat cater for this type of ejection. These include sufficient thrust to exit the aircraft and miss the tail fin, with the gun/rocket system tailored to match this scenario. The blast and drag forces on the ejected package will be high, and the seat must decelerate as fast as tolerably possible to provide the maximum time on the main parachute. Time delays must be low, and a compromise must be reached to provide minimum delay without allowing the main parachute to deploy beyond its structural strength or beyond human tolerance. In some seats, this compromise is met with time delays; in others, it is augmented with an interdictor mechanism that delays the sequence.

Other cases are the zero–zero ejection (zero speed, zero altitude) and the low-speed, runway-level ejection. In early seat designs, the seat provided an initial thrust to force the occupant from the aircraft but failed to provide sufficient height for the main parachute to deploy and inflate. The addition of rocket motors has meant that enough altitude is provided to allow the main parachute to open, although, as this is at low speed, the parachute may not be deployed fully in a steady-state condition, and the landing velocity may be higher than normal. Similarly, with vertical takeoff and landing aircraft, which operate at low level with low or zero forward speed, the escape systems must be capable of operating under all failure conditions, including the possible 'fall off the hover' condition, in which the aircraft may roll violently due to a loss of power or high sink rate at low altitude.

Escape from helicopters

Although considerable effort has been spent on ejection seats for fixed-wing aircraft, there has been no parallel evolution of the escape systems for helicopters. The possibility of fitting ejection seats to rotary-wing aircraft has been considered, but the weight penalty and the problems associated with escape from helicopters have meant that autorotation is regarded as a preferred option, with the current exception of the Kamov Ka-50 'Hokum' Attack Helicopter. If escape is vertical, then the blades would need to have explosive elements fitted so that they are jettisoned and a clear escape path made. The operation of rotary-wing aircraft at low level realistically precludes the use of simple frontal or lateral ejection, since 95 per cent of helicopter accidents occur below 500 feet and 50 per cent below 50 feet altitude. However, the safety of helicopters has increased over the years, and in the case of power loss the possibility to autorotate usually exists. Loss of control does not have an escape possibility, and so improved crashworthiness is regarded as the most practical option. At high altitude, the bailout option exists if the rotational forces allow egress.

Unassisted escape

The precise procedure to be used in an emergency varies with the configuration of hatches, and type and role of aircraft, but certain general principles must be observed if the escape is to be successful. The first requirement is that the aircrew are fitted correctly with appropriate equipment and understand its operation and use. They must be familiar with the escape sequence and know the location and method of egress from emergency exits, escape hatches, tunnels or chutes. Unless these drills are practised, an escapee may not only prejudice their own chances of escape but also impede the progress of others. It is important for the escapee to enter the airstream without striking (or being struck by) the aircraft. This means that careful consideration must be given to the design and training in the use of the escape system. The exit routes must cater for the full physical strength ranges and anthropometric variation of aircrew with all of their escape and survival equipment. These issues must be taken into consideration when the aircraft is moving under any aerodynamic, inertial or vibration influences, as well as when it is stationary. Some degree of assistance may be incorporated into the system, e.g. explosive bolts and cutting charges to remove doors and escape hatches. The escape occurs in three phases: exit, parachute descent, and landing and recovery.

EXIT

Escapees usually must propel themselves through the escape exit with as much force as possible and then assume a compact shape without trailing arms or legs. Various techniques have been devised to suit the geometry of the different exit designs. For example, to leave a belly hatch, the escapee should squat at the rear edge of the hatch with their arms wrapped around their legs and their chin on their knees, and then roll forwards into the airstream in a 'cannonball' attitude. A modification is used in some aircraft that have belly escape tunnels. The person sits at the rear of the escape tunnel, holds on to a bar and pulls forward, allowing the legs and torso to fall down the tunnel. The escapee then releases the bar and falls out of the tunnel into the airstream with a cannonball attitude, until free from the aircraft slipstream. To escape from a side door, the escapee crouches, holding both sides of the door, and heaves themselves outwards and downwards, folding their arms across their chest. Where practical, the escape system should assist the escapee in directing the separation from the airframe. This may be with the use of aerodynamic windbreaks or even a scoop.

DESCENT

After successful separation from the aircraft, the escapee may either fall freely for a while or open the parachute immediately. This decision depends on many factors, including experience, equipment, escape speed and altitude. At altitudes below 500 feet, any delay is unacceptable and sufficient time should be allowed only to clear the aircraft structure (about 1 s). At altitudes below 200 feet, success will be problematic under the best of circumstances, as 3 s or less is available for the operation of the parachute. Escape at altitudes below 100 feet is invariably fatal, as the height lost during the parachute inflation is too great.

At altitudes between 2000 and 15 000 feet, the escapee should wait for some seconds before initiating the parachute, in order to ensure that they are clear of the aircraft and have lost some of the forward velocity. In this way, the parachute is not subjected to an airspeed that would create shocks beyond its structural strength. The time required between leaving the aircraft and operating the parachute depends on the initial aircraft velocity and the parachute capabilities. In unretarded descent, the escapee will fall approximately 1000 feet in the first 10 s of leaving the aircraft. The descent rate will then start to stabilize. At altitudes above 15 000 feet, factors such as high parachute opening shocks, hypoxia and low temperatures make it important to delay the deployment of the parachute. Free fall is advised from these altitudes, with some stabilization (with either clothing design or a small drogue), until the parachute can be deployed.

The safety and success of emergency escape systems on the whole can be increased by the use of automatic systems. The system is connected to the aircraft. When the person leaves the aircraft, the system is initiated with a static line.

The deployment mechanism is armed when the system is initiated. This deploys the parachute almost immediately at low altitude, but a barostat delays main parachute operation at high altitude in order to avoid the high forces, cold and hypoxia of high-altitude parachuting. The altitude for emergency escape parachute operation is usually set from 10 000 to 15 000 feet barometric altitude, which allows sufficient height to cater for most land heights.

The freefall descent of the human body subjects the body to the force of gravity, which causes the descent and the air drag, which opposes the direction of motion. Any initial velocity created by the aircraft motion will be lost due to the air drag, and so the descent will soon be vertical, with any lateral motion created purely by the aerodynamic position of the body. The magnitude of the air drag in steady-state descent will depend on the following relationship:

$$\text{Drag force} = \text{mass of body} \times g = 1/2 \, (\rho \times \text{velocity}^2 \times \text{drag area of body})$$

where ρ is the air density and g is acceleration due to gravity (9.81 m/s).

Since the density of the air reduces with altitude, the steady-state descent rate will increase with increasing velocity (Figure 24.8).

The position and shape of the human body contribute to the descent rate, a fact that is used by experienced parachutists to stabilize themselves during descent. Inexperienced parachutists may tumble during descent, leading to disorientation and possibly affecting drills and deployment with tangling of the canopy or lines. A tumbling individual may be subjected to a high opening shock as the parachute imparts rotational forces to the body with forcible alignment with the parachute. When the parachute is extracted and starts to inflate, it decelerates the escapee. The actual profile of the deceleration will depend

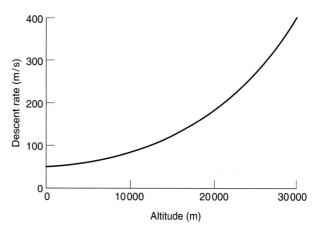

Figure 24.8 *Relationship between altitude and descent rate at terminal velocity for a freefalling person.*

on many factors, including the shape and size of the parachute, the deployment method, the parachute materials, the descent rate of the person, the mass of the person and the density of the air. The deceleration of a typical parachute is shown in Figure 24.9. This shows the different phases of the parachute inflation. Forces of the parachute inflation are highly variable and depend on the factors listed above, but they may reach a magnitude of 25 g peak acceleration. This is a short-duration shock and within the limits of human tolerance. Serious injury is improbable and is likely to be confined to some bruising under the straps of the harness.

The forces generated by a parachute increase with the square of the velocity. The opening shock generated by a parachute also increase as the air density reduces (i.e. as altitude increases). Care therefore should be taken, so that the structural strength of the parachute is not exceeded and that the survival equipment is sufficiently strong to withstand the parachute opening forces. Automatic operating systems for emergency escape parachutes take into account these compromises, so it is important that an escapee does not override these systems out of fear, unless they are certain that the system has failed. The actual final descent rate (referred to as the steady-state descent rate) depends on the parachute design (its drag coefficient and drag area), the air density and the weight of the person. Any wind or parachute drift will also produce a horizontal velocity. This will increase the impact velocity, which is a vector sum of the vertical and horizontal velocities.

LANDING AND RECOVERY

About 90 per cent of non-fatal injuries in unassisted escape occur during or immediately after landing. They are attributable largely to unfamiliarity with correct landing techniques, although the absence of still conditions and flat terrain increases the incidence. The principles of landing by parachute are simple to state but sometimes difficult to follow. The final stages of the descent should be as vertical as possible, and drift and oscillation should be cancelled. Some control can be achieved by pulling down on the appropriate parachute risers, distorting the canopy and imparting 'drive' in the required direction to counteract surface wind. Such manoeuvres slightly increase the rate of descent, but this introduces a much smaller hazard than that of an uncoordinated landing with a high lateral velocity. The hands and arms should be positioned over the head, which should be tucked well into the chest. The feet and legs should be together and the knees slightly bent to cushion the impact of landing. The line of vision should be in the direction of motion in order to avoid obstacles on the ground.

The landing shock should be spread over as long a time and as large an area as possible by allowing the body to collapse in the direction of motion as soon as the feet touch the ground and rolling from thigh to buttock to shoulder. During the roll, the legs must be kept in apposition. In the light of the limited opportunities for training and the wide range of conditions, including darkness, under which military aircrew must descend and land, the rate of injury is surprisingly low. Sprained and fractured ankles account for a high proportion of the ejection casualties; the overall current rate is about 40 per thousand descents. After landing, the parachute must be collapsed or released as soon as possible in order to avoid dragging and the risk of injury from rough terrain. If the descent is made into water, then there is the possibility of being dragged by surface winds or water currents with the head below water level. To avoid this hazard, some parachutes are fitted with water pockets, which collapse the canopy. Parachutists may be taught to undo the quick-release fastening of their parachute harness in the last seconds of the descent. They are then supported by the buttock loop of the harness and by grasping the parachute risers. By throwing up their arms and straightening their thighs, they can, as their feet touch the water, fall freely from the encumbrance of the parachute and, by inflating their life-preservers, float away safely.

PARACHUTES AND ASSOCIATED EQUIPMENT

The design of the parachute harness varies according to its use. Some harnesses are installed as part of the seat, some as part of the aircrew clothing, and some as a separate bailout system worn either throughout the flight or only during an emergency. The actual designs vary, but they all have similar elements. The harnesses are made from webbing straps, usually nylon approximately 50 mm wide,

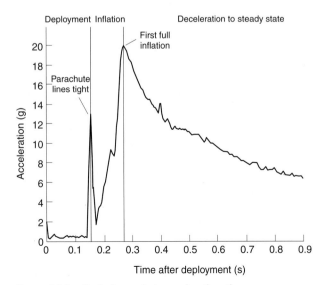

Figure 24.9 *Typical parachute acceleration–time curve.*

which spread the loads. The straps are routed to support the wearer comfortably beneath a deployed parachute with a sling passing under the buttocks and around the top of the thighs. Vertical loops pass up the back and over the shoulders to a central fitting. Some degree of lateral restraint is necessary. The harness is extended upwards from the shoulders to suspension strops that connect to the parachute. Four of these are usually fitted to each harness, two on each side of the body.

The parachute pack

The use of a pack to contain the parachute ensures that it is stowed in a manner that will allow reliable and predictable operation. It also protects the parachute from inadvertent operation and environmental conditions. The pack shape, construction and design vary according to use. A pack that is fitted permanently to the back of a seat or worn during flight will use the space available to store the parachute and deployment lines and attempt to provide some comfort for the seat occupant. The pack that comes into contact with the occupant will need to withstand everyday wear. A pack that is worn at the last moment will not need such design refinements.

Parachute packing is a skilled procedure that uses a variety of different methods depending on the intended use of the parachute. For example, a low-level, low-speed parachute will need to be packed in a manner that allows quick deployment and inflation. A high-level, high-speed parachute may employ packing methods that delay the inflation of the parachute in order to minimize the high shocks. On the whole, however, the parachute is retained in the pack in beckets or loops that allow sequential deployment of the lines and canopy. The lines and canopy may be stowed in separate compartments in order to ensure this deployment sequence, folded in S-folds and retained in place with break ties retaining the fabric. The whole pack is closed with a securing flap held in place with pins or loops. The parachute operation is initiated with a release line, which withdraws the initiation pins and allows the closure flap to open. The line is initiated either from a handle on the chest or by an automatic operating system. The flap will open due to aerodynamic forces, pack pressure or a mechanical assistance (spring), which will allow the parachute to deploy and inflate. Often, the withdrawal of the parachute is assisted with a small pilot or drogue parachute.

Parachute design

Parachutes typically are made up from a series of triangular panels (gores) that radiate from the vent situated at the apex. The gores terminate at the parachute periphery (peripheral hem), which is reinforced, since it takes most of the inflation load. The parachute rigging (or suspension) lines are fitted to the periphery at the junction between the gore seams and hem. These lines, in some designs, are extended up the gore seams and over the apex to provide continuous strengthening. The lines run from the hem to the harness suspension strops (risers). Parachutes tend to be manufactured from nylon, polyester or cotton, although some are made from fire-resistant materials. The canopy itself can be made from either plain woven nylon or rip-stop nylon, which has better resistance to damage. The design of a parachute depends on many factors, including the range of speeds at which it will be expected to work and the weight range of the personnel. Emergency escape parachutes tend to be smaller and produce a higher descent rate than military paratrooper canopies, because the rate of exposure is lower and the requirement for paratroopers is usually a 'fit-to-fight' rather than 'fit-to-survive' capability. The maximum mass of aircrew with survival aids is lower than paratroopers with full equipment.

The complexity of designs of emergency escape parachutes has increased with time. Modern parachutes are invariably aeroconical in design, whereas a system designed in the 1960s was more likely to use a simple flat circular design. Modern designs have increased performance, reduced shock and greater stability than their predecessors. Some parachutes are designed to take a degree of damage during inflation by using stretch materials and sacrificial gores for high-speed deployments without a dramatic increase in descent rate. The parachute is usually designed with a degree of drive, which is achieved by allowing slots in the rear of the parachute to spill air and push the canopy forward, increasing parachute stability.

Steering of emergency escape parachutes can be a problem, especially for inexperienced parachutists. This can lead to an increased risk of injury; therefore, wherever possible, training in the use of a parachute should be provided. The issue of gliding and high-performance parachutes to inexperienced personnel is not recommended, because the chance exists of a very high descent rate. Furthermore, gliding parachutes tend to have a restricted operating range compared with conventional round parachutes.

Some degree of steering is possible with conventional round parachutes by pulling down on riser pairs (usually the rear risers). This distorts the shape of the parachute, allowing a degree of drive or steering. With some designs, simple modification is possible to the shape of the parachute in order to allow direct distortion of the drive slots, producing a simple steering mechanism. This does not tend to increase the descent rate of the parachute and is simple to use, and these systems are recommended wherever possible.

FURTHER READING

Glaister DH. *Biodynamic Response to Windblast*. NATO AGARD Conference Proceedings CP170. Neuilly-sur-Seine: NATO AGARD, 1975.

Knacke TW. *Parachute Recovery Systems Design Manual*. Santa Barbara, CA: Para Publishing, 1992.

NATO Research and Technology Organization. *Injury Prevention in Aircraft Crashes: Investigative Techniques and Applications*. Lecture series 208. Neuilly-sur-Seine: NATO AGARD, 1998.

25

In-flight communication

GRAHAM M. ROOD AND SUSAN H. JAMES

INTRODUCTION

Historically, the primary form of communication in aviation has been speech. Since the sender and receiver usually are humans, speech has been a very effective medium. In aviation, English is used as the international communicating language, but there are a number of potential problems, e.g. regional accents and non-native English-speakers, which can affect the intelligibility of messages. This type of communication can be referred to as man-to-man communication.

With the increasing sophistication of radio and electronic systems, the ability of a machine to communicate with the pilot, either through relaying a verbal message or by using an auditory warning, became more commonplace, with many of these systems supplementing or complementing the visual warning systems. Often, the audio warning was used in a higher-urgency case (e.g. ground-proximity warning system, GPWS), when the likelihood of missing the visual-only signal was an unacceptable probability. This is a form of machine-to-man communication.

Currently, the final communication channel is from human to machine, where a person uses speech to talk to the machine, which 'understands' the contents of the message and activates the avionic systems to act appropriately. This requires sophisticated speech-recognition systems, which, in the harsh world of the aircraft cockpit, have only recently reached sufficient maturity to be incorporated in operational aircraft.

In day-to-day life, communication between people is predominantly speech-based, but the use of non-verbal methods such as gesticulation and facial expression normally provides added meaning and emphasis. In most aircraft, however, the only possible form of communication between crew may be speech: non-verbal methods of communication are not possible when military aircrew are physically separated and dressed in flight-clothing assemblies. This may represent a very significant loss.

COMMUNICATION IN AIRCRAFT

There are, effectively, two interface sites between the person and the aircraft communications system:

- human output device (mouth, throat)
- human input device (ear).

The goal at both of these locations is to transduce the signal as faithfully as possible and to maximize the exclusion of ambient noise. The acoustic merit of a mask or helmet will depend on how well it performs these two functions.

Output from the person

Speech may be transduced from a pressure wave (speech) signal into electrical signals by a microphone. In aviation, the most common types of microphone are those incorporated in the oronasal oxygen mask (used in most fast jets), noise-cancelling boom microphones (used in helicopters and transport types) and, in special circumstances, throat- or bone-conduction microphones.

MASK–MOUNTED MICROPHONES

The acoustic attenuation properties of oxygen masks are similar to those of flying helmets, i.e. poor at low frequencies but improving with rising frequency. Like most acoustic systems, the mask system may have resonances, which are a function of interactions between different parts of the mask structure and which will reduce attenuation, sometimes to the point of producing higher sound-pressure levels inside the mask compared with outside. However, the speech signal-to-noise ratio is generally more than adequate to provide good intelligibility at the mask-microphone output. Even in the noisiest aircraft, the quality of the signal from a microphone mounted in an oronasal mask is good. Nevertheless, there may be cases of poor design in the impedance matching of the microphone to the communication avionics and other distortions that may be introduced downstream of the mask, where aircrew can, often unjustly, put the blame for inadequate communications on this piece of equipment.

NOISE-CANCELLING BOOM MICROPHONES

This form of microphone transduces speech very well and generally performs its function perfectly satisfactorily. The noise-cancelling properties are a function of frequency and provide better cancelling properties at low frequencies than at high frequencies. The quality of design and the type of construction of these microphones affect their noise-rejection properties. This enables some microphones to have noise discrimination (or rejection) of up to 10 dB at 4 kHz, while others have none. At lower frequencies, noise rejection can be up to 30 dB, with a theoretical maximum of 45 dB at 100 Hz.

Owing to the low-frequency content of helicopter noise, noise-cancelling boom microphones are well suited to this type of vehicle and generally provide an acceptable solution for noise reduction. However, in order for the microphone to work efficiently, the microphone must be placed as close as possible to the lips. Even minor movement away from the lips, in the order of 2–3 mm, will significantly degrade the speech signal-to-noise ratios.

THROAT MICROPHONES

A throat microphone is inherently less sensitive to airborne noise and generally can provide a better signal-to-noise ratio than a noise-cancelling microphone. However, the overall frequency response is limited, and the microphone output has a preponderance of low-frequency components, which give good signal-to-noise ratios but do not contribute significantly to high intelligibility.

The transducer of the throat microphone is pressed against the pharynx and is sensitive to the powerful vibrations that occur here in voiced phonemes (see below). If one places the fingers on the larynx and says 'aaaah', these vibrations can be felt clearly; however, if one says 'sss' or any other unvoiced consonant, nothing will be felt. In a similar way, the throat microphone does not respond to unvoiced phonemes. Because of this, a throat microphone leaves a lot of speech to be 'filled in' or inferred by the listener. The throat microphone does, however, have excellent rejection of normal airborne sound, so what is lost in quality of speech transduction may be gained in terms of noise rejection. This form of transducer was once commonly worn in helicopters, where the rejection of noise is invaluable in some situations (e.g. the winchman).

BONE-CONDUCTION MICROPHONES

Bone-conduction microphones pick up the speech vibration signals that are transmitted through the skull and jaw, rather than as direct acoustic signals formed through the vocal system. As such, they are generally poor in high-frequency content and suffer from the same problems as throat microphones. However, under some specialized applications, such as covert surveillance, they can be regarded as suitable and effective transducers.

A further factor that affects speech signal-to-noise ratios in all types of microphone is the normal variation in speech output levels found in airborne and other communications. Some people talk more quietly than others, and there is, essentially, a Gaussian or normal distribution of speaker levels. Since the noise levels at the input are essentially constant in a given environment, louder speakers will produce higher signal-to-noise levels than quieter speakers. Also, the noise levels experienced at the ear have an effect on speaking levels. As the noise levels at the ear increase, so the talking levels increase; this phenomenon is known as the Lombard effect. In most aircraft communication systems, because the free-field pathway between the mouth and the ear, which controls speech output levels, is occluded by a helmet or headset, an artificial pathway is provided, feeding the speech signal through the communication system back to the ear. This is the side-tone signal, which can be adjusted to control voice output levels in most communication systems.

Measurements made during experimental flights in Royal Navy Merlin helicopters showed a variation in speech signal-to-noise ratios between speakers of between 3 dB and 29 dB, and this is considered typical of operational flight.

Input to the person

In aviation, aircrew personnel normally wear a headset or flying helmet that incorporates a communications system. Some pre-Second World War systems used an acoustic tube that fed directly to the ear of the aircrew, from one crew member's mouth direct to the crew member's ear. This was known as the Gosport tube. It worked, but not necessarily well: in order to 'turn up the volume', one had to shout louder. Some intermediate systems used a telephone with an acoustic tube to feed the signal to the pilot's ear (e.g. the Second World War type C and the 1960s Mk2 series flight helmets), but generally these were superseded by full electrical communications, in which each aircrew member had control of their input volume levels to the headset.

In principle, it should be possible to provide a satisfactory signal-to-noise ratio at the ear simply by turning up the gain of the communications system until the signal is loud enough to hear above the ambient noise. Several factors make this solution impractical. First, speech at or greater than 125 dB causes discomfort and pain. Second, listening to speech at sound-pressure levels even considerably less than 125 dB for any significant period of time poses a distinct threat of damage to the hearing. Third, physiological changes take place in the ear at high sound levels, and it is not clear that a given signal-to-noise ratio at a high noise level would produce the same intelligibility as that produced at more moderate levels. It is undesirable to present speech at levels much in excess of 100 dB. If a 15-dB ratio is required, then the ambient noise at the ear must not be greater than 85 dB. Thus, in general terms, if the ambient sound-pressure level inside the aircraft cabin is 115 dB, then the helmet or headset should provide an attenuation of at least 30 dB. By applying the same reasoning in more detail across each frequency band, the amount of attenuation required throughout the frequency spectrum may be defined.

The use of the helmet or headset to provide protection against high noise levels is commonplace. This protection allows speech and non-speech communications to be effective and the intelligibility of incoming messages to be at a high enough level to be operationally acceptable.

PHYSICAL NATURE OF SPEECH

Speech sounds are not steady or continuous through time. Although from a perceptual point of view speech is composed of phonemes, these phonemes do not correspond precisely to any physical pattern of sound or to the letters used in a word.

The word 'meaty' is written phonemically as /m/, /i/, /t/, /i/. The pattern of sound associated with a given phoneme depends on the age, sex and personal idiosyncrasies of the speaker and the location of the phonemes in the word. The /p/ in 'spoon' is physically very different from the /p/ in 'pan', and yet perceptually they are identical. The perceptual system is not, therefore, performing a simple decoding of the incoming signal but is performing a complicated pattern-recognition task in which many cues, including the context in which the sound occurs, are being utilized.

Each sound consists of various combinations of different frequencies. Some sounds, e.g. the 's' in 'sea', contain almost all the speech frequencies and approximate to white noise in which all frequencies are represented equally. Vowels consist of high-amplitude sounds. All vowels are voiced, i.e. the larynx is used in their production, as are some consonants, e.g. /b/. However, many consonants, e.g. /t/, are unvoiced and are of lower amplitude than vowel sounds; this has some consequence in the testing of equipment.

The energy content of speech is distributed widely. The dynamic range of male speech varies from about 52 dB for casual speech, to around 76 dB for loud speech, to 89 dB for shouting. The corresponding female figures are some 2–3 dB lower during casual speech, increasing to some 5–7 dB lower at shouting levels. The frequency spectrum of speech contains frequencies from around 100 Hz to above 10 kHz; however, the information content of speech is not distributed equally or so widely, which is a matter of primary importance in the design of communication systems. The way in which the information content of speech is distributed can be seen from the weighting constants in the articulation index (AI) calculation procedure (see Table 25.1); as an example, almost 73 per cent of the speech intelligibility is contained in frequencies of 1 kHz and above, and only 27 per cent is in frequencies below 1 kHz. Most communication systems for aircraft are specified with a flat frequency response from around 300 Hz to 3–4 kHz, with a gradual roll-off outside these frequencies; generally, this is wide enough to allow for good communications.

The amplitude of the speech often is not great enough for good intelligibility in a noise environment. This is due to a complicated phenomenon known as masking. For the purposes of this chapter, it is sufficient to state that it is difficult to comprehend quiet speech in a loud-noise environment. Many types of physical distortion and clipping of speech peaks can occur; in aircraft, various protective devices and communication systems are used to protect and preserve the speech. The effectiveness of these devices can be assessed only in terms of intelligibility.

SPEECH INTELLIGIBILITY

In most aircraft, aircrew members use an intercommunication system (intercom) to talk to each other, partly because noise levels may be high but mainly because normally the crew members are physically separated, sometimes by the length of the aircraft; this type of communication falls under the heading of 'aided communication'. Where crew members are in close proximity, either on the flight deck or where rear-crew systems operators are at a console, crew may talk face-to-face rather than over the intercom – this is known as 'unaided communication'.

Aided communication

In order to be able to quantify reliably the transmission and reception quality of a communication system, there are a number of tests that allow adequate levels of repeatability and a diagnostic capability. These have been developed over the years and consist of either word lists, e.g. the Harvard phonetically balanced (PB) list, or rhyming tests, e.g. the modified rhyme test (MRT) and the diagnostic rhyme test (DRT).

The most straightforward form of intelligibility test is one in which a single word is read to a listener. The listener writes down the word that they believe they have heard and the response is marked for correctness. This is the fundamental method used in the Harvard PB word lists, against which other tests are compared. The 50 word lists used in the Harvard PB test are intended to have a phonetic constitution similar to that of spoken English.

The Harvard PB word lists are, however, open to many sorts of error and need practice. To counteract these difficulties, intelligibility assessments can be made more easily by means of one of the forms of rhyme test. In these tests, the listener is provided with a multiple-choice answer sheet. Thus, the response alternatives given to the stimulus word 'hat' might be 'bat', 'cat', 'fat', 'rat', 'hat' and 'mat', from which the listener deletes the one that he or she hears. The response list generally contains words varying in only one phoneme from one another (in the example given here, a consonant phoneme).

Consonant phonemes are generally used in such tests, as vowel phonemes are, on the whole, louder and consequently not affected so readily by poor signal-to-noise ratio (the difference in decibels between the level of the signal and that of the masking signal).

In the USA, the test used most commonly for military communication systems is the MRT. This test, like the PB lists, consists of prepared lists of monosyllabic words. The listener selects the word perceived from a list of six words on a multiple-choice answer sheet. The difference between the six words is in only one consonant, and the test is useful for studying confusions between particular speech sounds. It also has the significant benefit of requiring short training times and lends itself to mechanized scoring. Other types of distortion, such as that produced by overdriving an inadequate transducer, may require a vowel test; suitable tests do exist.

A further type of two-choice intelligibility test is the DRT. This uses two rhyming words, with the initial consonants differing by a single attribute. The words in each pair are chosen so that a particular attribute of speech is present in one word but not in the other. Detailed analysis of the responses will indicate which parameter of a communication system will need to be improved. DRT tests are important in the assessment of narrow-band digital speech channels (secure speech transmissions), where plain speech is encoded, transmitted in scrambled digital form and decoded back into plain speech at the receiver's end. The DRT is used as the standard test for linear predictive coders (LPCs) in North Atlantic Treaty Organisation (NATO) standardization agreement (STANAG) 4198.

The intelligibility of a signal is affected not only by the masking noise in which the signal is heard (Figure 25.1) but also by the size of the vocabulary from which the signal is taken (e.g. digits compared with isolated words), the internal redundancy of the signal or words (e.g. totally nonredundant nonsense syllables fare poorly) and the context of the signal (e.g. isolated words compared with words in sentences). Some speech is intelligible at negative signal-to-noise ratios, i.e. when the average (long-term root mean square) level of the speech is less than that of the noise. An example may be drawn from Figure 25.1, where, at a signal-to-noise ratio of −12 dB, digit intelligibility is around 55 per cent, but for isolated words (where intelligent guesses are not so productive), an increase of around 15 dB in the signal to a signal-to-noise ratio of +3 dB is required in order to obtain a similar level of intelligibility. This is because the level of speech varies in time, and for 'very probable' words (drawn from a small vocabulary or where contextual information is given) enough information is still present above the ambient noise to provide the perceptual system with data on which to base identification.

Because of the poor quality of many aircraft communications systems, the speech used in aircraft is fairly redundant, so in any individual utterance, more speech sounds are present than are necessary for the unambiguous detection of a digit, letter or word. For example, instead of the letter 'I' (pronounced 'eye'), which contains only two vowel phonemes, the word 'India', which contains five phonemes, is used, with a consequently higher probability

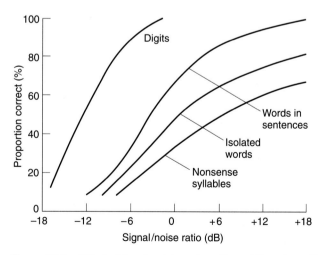

Figure 25.1 *Effect of the signal-to-noise ratio and the nature of the signal on its intelligibility. The intelligibility of the signal increases with signal-to-noise ratio, size of the vocabulary employed, internal redundancy and context of the signal.*

of recognition. However, the problem remains that any perceptual process relies to a very large extent on the experience of the listener; thus, if message A is probable but message B (which is acoustically similar) arrives, then B will be heard as A. This sort of mishearing has often had serious consequences, but it is best illustrated by the apocryphal story about the pilot who, during the takeoff run, noticed that his co-pilot was looking unhappy. 'Cheer up!' he said, whereupon the co-pilot lifted the undercarriage ('gear up'), to the general detriment of the aircraft and particular embarrassment of the aircrew.

The final test of the quality of any communications system must remain the intelligibility test. However, the inconvenience of using large numbers of people to test systems has led to the adoption of physical or objective methods of assessment by calculation. We have noted that although the energy of speech is distributed widely, the information content is not, i.e. although there are a large number of speech sounds in the part of the speech spectrum below, say, 300 Hz, these do not contribute a great deal to the intelligibility of the speech. It is generally correct to say that only 20 per cent of intelligibility is contained in 80 per cent of the energy of speech – the vowel sounds – while 80 per cent of the intelligibility is found in 20 per cent of the total energy – the consonants. Large numbers of experiments have been performed in an attempt to assess the relative contributions of different parts of the spectrum to intelligibility. As a result of these calculations, such as those presented in Table 25.1, a predictive and calculable method of assessing probable speech intelligibility has been developed. This method of dividing the speech and noise spectrum into a number of bands and assessing the contribution of each band to the overall sum is the Articulation Index (AI).

Depending on the relative accuracy required, the overall spectrum can be divided into a greater or lesser number of bands. Generally, it is preferable to use the larger number; in the example shown in Table 25.1, the spectrum is split into 15 bands, each one-third of an octave wide. For a smaller number of bands, octave bandwidths may be used. The signal-to-noise level in each band is multiplied by its weighting factor, which indicates its relative contribution to the overall speech intelligibility, and the resultant figures are summed to give the AI figure. This figure is then related to an intelligibility figure proper by use of the curves shown in Figure 25.2, which is similar to the approach given in Figure 25.1 in respect to changes in intelligibility due to contextual information, redundancy, size of vocabulary, etc.

Thus, a measure of subjective intelligibility may be obtained from direct physical measurement. The method must, however, be used with care, since it is subject to many caveats and qualifications, particularly if there is any trace of distortion in the speech signal. This AI method is used with aided communication systems, i.e. using an air-

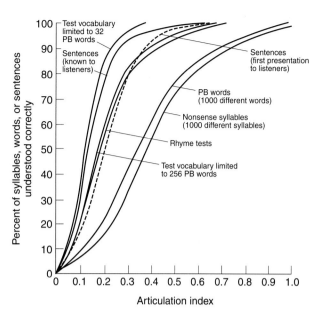

Figure 25.2 *Relationships between articulation index and intelligibility. These relationships vary with the type of material and the skill of the talkers and listeners.*

craft crew communication system in conjunction with headsets or flying helmets.

A form of automated, more sophisticated AI is used in the form of the speech transmission index (STI) or rapid speech transmission index (RASTI). STI is similar to AI, in that it determines specific signal-to-noise ratios in each frequency band and then weights and combines them in order to give an overall summed AI figure. In STI, however, the signal-to-noise ratio in each band is determined from the modulation transfer function (MTF) in that band, which is constructed from an artificial input test signal (representative of the temporal characteristics of running speech) and the interfering noise. The subsequent MTF is used to give an equivalent signal-to-noise ratio, and the weighted mean of these signal-to-noise ratios forms the basis of STI. Like AI, the STI output figures vary between 0 and 1.

RASTI has a similar approach, using the measurement of a MTF, but only two octave bands are employed (500 Hz, 2 kHz), which allows a rapid evaluation of STI within ten seconds.

All of these calculative methods are useful as they allow a rapid rating of communication systems on a scale from excellent to poor, but they are not yet sufficiently precise in order to measure subtle but often important differences between systems in the way that MRT or DRT can. Both subjective testing (MRT, DRT, PB, etc.) and objective calculative approaches (AI, STI, RASTI, etc.) have their merits, and their use is based on the principle of the appropriate test for both the particular operational circumstances and any limitations in testing time or cost.

Table 25.1 *Method of calculating the articulation index (AI) using the weighted and summed speech signal-to-noise ratios to enable an AI figure to be determined. The speech signal-to-noise ratio is taken at the output from the microphone. This AI figure is then related to Figure 25.2, which gives the level of intelligibility for particular types of text material (sentences, limited vocabularies, nonsense syllables, etc.)*

(a) Measured values

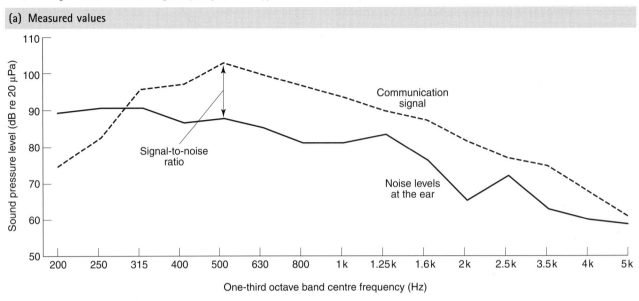

(b) Calculation of articulation index

Frequency (Hz)	Signal-to-noise ratio (A) (dB)	Weighting factor (B)	Product (A × B)
200	0	0.0004	0
250	0	0.0010	0
315	5	0.0010	0.0050
400	10	0.0014	0.0140
500	16	0.0014	0.0224
630	14	0.0020	0.0280
800	15	0.0020	0.0300
1000	12	0.0024	0.0288
1250	6	0.0030	0.0180
1600	11	0.0037	0.0407
2000	16	0.0037	0.0592
2500	6	0.0034	0.0204
3150	11	0.0034	0.0374
4000	7	0.0024	0.0168
5000	2	0.0020	0.0040
			AI = 0.3267

(c) Calculated intelligibility (from Figure 25.2)

AI = 0.33 = 85% intelligibility for sentences for first presentation to listeners
        = 94% intelligibility for sentences known to listeners

Non-aided face-to-face communication

In many aircraft and other vehicles, face-to-face communication is necessary without resort to an aided (intercom) system. In this case, a simpler method called speech interference level (SIL) is used to assess the suitability of the noise environment for communication. In this method, the cabin noise levels are measured in octave bands; the three bands centred on 500, 1000 and 2000 Hz are summed arithmetically and the average is taken. This average figure is compared with a set of figures that will indicate the level of communication possible. This method may be illustrated with the following example. It is useful to note that this method may be used over a wide range of transportation vehicles (buses, cars, etc.) as well as in the industrial environment.

The results of an octave analysis of noise levels on the flight-deck of a jet transport aircraft were as follows:

Octave band (frequency, Hz)	125	250	500	1000	2000	4000
Sound pressure (level, dB)	100	88	84	85	74	63

Speech interference level (dB) = (84 + 85 + 74)/3 = 81

The particular problem is to assess whether a pilot can talk to his or her co-pilot or engineer at a normal voice level while they are separated by a distance of 1.2 m.

Table 25.2 shows that at a separation distance of 1.2 m, the SIL would have to be 56 dB for normal speech effort, rising to 74 dB for a shouting voice. In this example, the pilot would be unable to talk to the crew, even using a shouting voice, and aided communications would be necessary. The cabin noise levels would have to be reduced to a level where an SIL of 56 dB could be obtained in order to allow communication.

The American National Standards Institute (ANSI 1977) specifies the SIL method for use in the USA. The European approach is to use the preferred speech interference level (PSIL) (International Organization for Standardization (ISO) 1974), which is identical in method of calculation but uses four octave bands centred on 500 Hz, 1 kHz, 2 kHz and 4 kHz. The ANSI method quotes separation distances between speakers 'for just reliable communication'; the ISO method is slightly more conservative, quoting differences for 'satisfactory conversation'. In practice, either method will give satisfactory predictions in all but marginal cases.

Secure speech systems

There is a final class of communication system that can suffer significantly from cockpit or aircraft environment noise, and this occurs in secure speech systems. In such systems, generally known as vocoder (voice-coder) systems, it is the effects of the noise on the coding of the speech signal, rather than the noise levels at the ear, that have the greatest effect on speech intelligibility. Vocoder systems work by the aircrew or operator speech from the normal oxygen mask microphone for fast jets, and from the standard noise-cancelling boom microphone for helicopters and transport/surveillance aircraft, and the coding of the pressure waveform. The waveform is then transmitted down the secure line or over the radio links in secure code form to the listener, where the waveform is decoded and then fed to the listener as clear speech. If there is no noise, e.g. as in an office environment, the system works well, as only the speech signal is encoded as the pressure waveform and decoding decodes only the correct signal. In a noisy environment, the encoded speech signal contains an amount of contaminating noise. The encoder does not have the capability to distinguish noise from speech and, therefore, encodes the whole speech-plus-noise signal. At the other end, the decoder treats this whole contaminated signal as a speech signal only and tries to make voicing sounds out of the whole signal, often with peculiar effects on the speech signal, which renders it unintelligible. This is predominantly so at low speech signal-to-noise ratios. Research into processing the speech signal at source to improve the speech signal-to-noise ratios is providing a partial alleviation solution.

As noted earlier, it is NATO practice to use DRT to test LPC secure-speech systems.

Machine-to-man and man-to-machine intelligibility

With regard to machine-to-man intelligibility, there are two types of signal, speech and non-speech. Speech is in its usual context, whether it is from recorded messages or from synthesized speech devices. Non-speech in this context means audio icons, such as a klaxon, horn or more sophisticated auditory warning such as those used in Merlin helicopters.

The speech signals, provided they are recorded, stored and replayed such that speech degradation is minimized,

Table 25.2 *Speech interference levels (SIL) of steady continuous noises at which reliable communication is barely possible. The values apply to male vocal effort and to a speaker and listener facing each other (subtract 5 dB for female voices)*

Separation distance (m)	Preferred speech interference level (dB)			
	Normal effort	Raised	Very loud	Shouting
0.15	74	80	86	92
0.3	68	74	80	86
0.6	62	68	74	80
1.2	56	62	68	74
1.8	52	58	64	70
3.7	46	52	58	64

Source: Beranek (1971).

can be treated as a normal speech signal obeying the dictates of normal intelligibility testing.

For non-speech signals, the required levels that must be transmitted to the ear to ensure 100 per cent probability of detection can be calculated. Figure 25.3 shows the approach, using a Lynx helicopter noise spectrum, measured under a Royal Air Force (RAF) Mk 4 helmet as a basis for the calculation. Other noise fields can be used, and calculations have been used for Tornado GR4 and other fixed-wing aircraft. From the noise levels at the ear, the auditory masked threshold is calculated. At a level 15 dB above that calculated threshold, a 100 per cent chance of detection of a signal is 'guaranteed'. Consequently, if a complex multi-frequency signal has frequency components that fall on that 100 per cent boundary, then the signal will be detected and the need to transmit auditory signals louder than necessary, on the basis that louder is better, can be prevented. If the signals are too loud, then the aircrew members are liable to spend the initial periods of an emergency trying to mute or cancel the signal; or if they let it continue, the high levels may interfere with the necessary emergency communication between crew. In Figure 25.3, an upper limit is added to the 100 per cent detection threshold in order to allow for the different noise levels experienced over a range of aircrew members' ears due to the normal variation in fit of the flying helmet and the different noise levels in different aircraft due to the operational status (e.g. flying with the windows open or the ramp down in a helicopter). Providing the frequency content warning signals is kept within that band, the listening task will have been optimized.

The use of man-to-machine communication has been in the research area for some 25 years or more and only recently has been incorporated into a production aircraft (the RAF Typhoon). This system allows the aircrew to speak directly to a machine; the machine recognizes the speech and acts on the command. In its simplest form, this is a method of switching by voice. The pilot can switch and interrogate systems by talking to the machine. A simple example of switching would be in selecting radio channels: instead of memorizing the radio frequency needed, selecting the individual frequencies on the channel selector switch and then communicating, the pilot can say 'Radio – Farnborough approach – go' and communication can be immediate. Similarly, the pilot can interrogate the aircraft systems by saying 'Check – bingo fuel – go' and the machine-to-man part of the system will tell the pilot how much fuel is left (and the range available, if it is programmed into the system). The recognition rates are well in to the 98 per cent level, which makes it similar to manual switching rates, and new algorithms are allowing close to 100 per cent recognition rates, even in the more extreme cockpit environments.

REDUCTION OF COCKPIT NOISE

Speech intelligibility invariably increases as the noise levels decrease, either from reduction in the working environment or by protecting the ear from the noise. Chapter 26 discusses in more detail the role of the helmet or headset in the reduction of cockpit and cabin noise levels at the aircrew ear, but a brief discussion is included in this chapter.

The primary purpose of any hearing protector is to prevent noise reaching the cochlea and subsequent transmission of the nerve firings from the cochlear output to the brain. In most cases, this can be achieved by occlusion of the ear canal, which prevents noise reaching the eardrum (tympanic membrane). This occlusion is achieved either from a circumaural earshell or by using an earplug, or by a combination of both. Most military earshells, as fitted to a flying helmet or headset, usually contain a telephone that allows communication with the aircrew from the intercom, radio or aircraft warning systems. With a passive earplug of the foam type (e.g. E-A-R®) or cylindrical plastic type (e.g. V51-R), a telephone is absent and communication is not possible, although specific versions (e.g. the communications ear plug, CEP) and some of newer active earplugs have a miniature telephone fitted that allows communications signals to be used as normal.

Helmets, headsets and earplugs

By reducing the noise level at the ear, the speech signal-to-noise ratios effectively increase, with the consequent

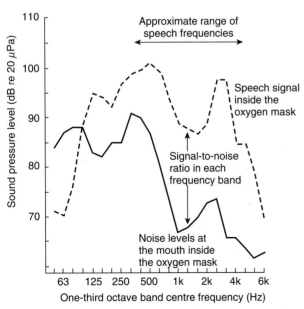

Figure 25.3 *Sound-pressure levels in the cavity of an oronasal oxygen mask due to transmission of noise from the cabin through the walls and valves of the mask and due to speech.*

increase in signal intelligibility. This is shown clearly in Figure 25.1 (p. 388). In many aircraft, the noise levels are such that a passive circumaural protector is effective enough to reduce the noise levels in order to allow effective communication. However, in higher-noise environments, passive attenuation alone may not suffice.

In higher-noise environments, the use of active noise reduction (ANR) can provide a useful reduction in noise levels. Although these reductions are used primarily to combat the risk of noise-induced hearing damage, the noise reduction from ANR can also improve speech and signal intelligibility.

In a series of experimental flying trials during an international collaboration programme between the UK, the USA and Australia, a number of helicopter sorties were flown and a number of aspects of speech intelligibility investigated, all related to the use of ANR. Four aspects were studied:

- Direct speech intelligibility using PB word lists and tested in accordance with military standard (MIL-STD) 1472.
- Subjective rating of communications clarity.
- Subjective rating of the attentional demand required in understanding the communications.
- Subjective rating of the perceived intelligibility.

In flights with the Royal Australian Navy Seahawk S-70-B, the PB word-list intelligibility improved from 83 per cent to 89 per cent. In the subjective ratings of clarity, attentional demand and perceived intelligibility, the ANR 'on' case improved all three to a statistically significant level. In a US trial with an OH58D, a noisy helicopter, and the EH-60, a surveillance helicopter, all the improvements in the ratings of perception were highly significant ($P < 0.002$). Also, in the OH58D, the experiments measuring the direct speech intelligibility gains showed a ten per cent improvement with a better passive helmet earshell and a further four per cent when using ANR. Thus, for speech intelligibility, the use of better acoustic protection, either passive or active, will improve communications. As the improvement is a direct function of the speech signal-to-noise ratio, the simpler passive improvements can be utilized for the less noisy range of aircraft; however, for noisier aircraft, active methods of noise reduction may be required.

Similarly, for non-speech signals such as passive or active sonar returns that are being interpreted by the sonar operator, reduced noise levels at the ear will increase the signal intelligibility. In two classified helicopter trials on operational sonar ranges during active sonar searches, the use of ANR significantly improved signal detectability, which in turn led to improved detection and classification thresholds at considerably increased ranges.

As discussed in Chapter 26, the communications signal can also have a deleterious affect on the ear, and high enough levels can result in a risk to hearing damage. This is because damage to the ear occurs in the cochlea, the part of the ear mechanism that translates the pressure signals into nerve signals, these signals being interpreted, later down the line – by the brain – as speech, noise, music, birdsong, etc. Thus, any form of pressure disturbance at the entrance to the ear can cause damage, irrespective of its artistic merit. High levels of speech or music alone, without any noise input, can cause damage.

In the aircraft environment, raising intercom levels will add the risk of damage posed by cockpit noise alone. Experimental measurements from operational sorties have shown the additional contribution to hearing damage risk caused by communications. By reducing the noise levels at the ear, in this case by ANR, the communications signals can also be reduced, maintaining intelligibility from the resultant constant signal-to-noise ratio. The overall risk from hearing damage is reduced, sometimes significantly – up to 9 dB(A) in operational Sea King helicopter trials.

COMMUNICATION IN CIVIL AIRCRAFT

In essence, there is little difference in the process of communication between a military transport or surveillance aircraft and its civil equivalent. Many of the military tankers and surveillance aircraft (e.g. E3D, Nimrod) are militarized versions of civil aircraft (Boeing 707, DH Comet) adapted for specific tasks in the armed forces. In most modern civil aircraft, especially those with two or three flight crew members, the captain and the co-pilot are the only communicators through the radio systems to air traffic control, and to the airfield controllers in the early and later parts of the flight. In the cockpit, the sources of noise are similar to the primary military noise sources – that of the boundary layer noise over the front nose of the aircraft, and a contribution from the cockpit conditioning. Many crew members wear a lightweight, abbreviated form of headset, most with little external noise rejection.

In a similar way to military crew, civilian aircrew members often wish to communicate with each other without going through the intercom. To do this, they push the headset off one ear and communicate face-to-face. This unaided form of communication can be assessed using the SIL or PSIL criteria described earlier.

In some earlier-generation airliners, the following figures were measured. In a Trident 1/1E at flight level (FL) 300 (i.e. 30 000 feet) (315 knots, mach (M) = 0.87), an SIL of 78 was calculated; at FL 200 (363 knots, M = 0.81), the figure rose to 81. For the Comet 4/4B at FL350 (235 knots, M = 0.74), the SIL was 72.5; at the lower FL240 (301 knots, M = 0.735), the figure increased to 78.5. If we assume that the crews were some 3 feet apart, the SIL for communication with a raised voice needs a SIL of 61 or below. Thus, in both of these aircraft, unaided communication would have been difficult, if not impossible.

CURRENTLY ACCEPTABLE FIGURES FOR SPEECH INTELLIGIBILITY

Regardless of whether communication systems are tested using subjective (PB, MRT, DRT, etc.) or objective (AI, STI, RASTI, etc.) methods, there have to be some criteria for acceptable levels of intelligibility.

In the UK, DEF STAN 00-25 Part 9: Voice Communication defines the minimum level of acceptability for AI as 'not less than 0.5'. For tests using DRT it states: 'The score shall be 85% or greater, desirably 90% or greater.' In the same DEF STAN, the figures for AI and their ratings are as in Table 25.3. For STI, similar figures are available (Table 25.4).

In the USA, the figures are defined in MIL-STD-1472F for both subjective (MRT, PB) and objective (AI) methods (Table 25.5).

Table 25.3 *Articulation index (AI) scores and ratings from DEF STAN 00-25 Part 9*

AI	Rating
< 0.3	Unsatisfactory
0.3–0.5	Acceptable
0.5–0.7	Good
> 0.7	Excellent

Table 25.4 *Speech transmission index (STI) scores and ratings from DEF STAN 00-25 Part 9*

STI	Rating
0–0.3	Bad
0.3–0.45	Poor
0.45–0.6	Fair
0.6–0.75	Good
> 0.75	Excellent

Table 25.5 *Phonetically balanced list (PB), modified rhyme test (MRT) and articulation index (AI) scores from MIL-STD-1472F*

Communication requirement	PB score (%)	MRT score (%)	AI score
Exceptionally high intelligibility: separate syllables understood	90	97	0.7
Normal acceptable intelligibility: about 98% of sentences heard correctly, single digits understood	75	91	0.5
Minimally acceptable intelligibility: limited standardized phrases understood, about 90% of sentences heard correctly (not acceptable for operational equipment)	43	75	0.3

REFERENCES

American National Standards Institute. For rating noise with respect to speech interference. ANSI S3.14. Washington, DC: American National Standards Institute, 1977.

Beranek LL. *Noise and Vibration Control.* New York: McGraw-Hill, 1971.

International Organization for Standardization. ISO TR 3352. Geneva: International Organization for Standardization, 1974. www.iso.org

FURTHER READING

American National Standards Institute. Methods for the calculation of the articulation index. ANSI S3.5. Washington, DC: American National Standards Institute, 1969.

American Standards Association. Measurement of monosyllabic word intelligibility. ASA S3.2. Washington, DC: American Standards Association, 1960.

Kryter KD. Physiological, psychological and social effects of noise. NASA reference publication 1115. Washington, DC: NASA, 1984.

26

Noise

GRAHAM M. ROOD AND SUSAN H. JAMES

INTRODUCTION

Noise may be defined as a sound that is unpleasant, distracting, unwarranted or in some other way undesirable. The definition is entirely subjective, and this reliance on humans as a measuring instrument recurs throughout most of the attempts to assess and quantify auditory effects.

The human hearing mechanism has a wide range and is fairly tolerant, but this tolerance is exceeded in many aircraft, with the following potential effects:

- Communications, both speech and other auditory signals, and inside the aircraft, air-to-air and air-to-ground, may be degraded.
- The sense of hearing may be damaged temporarily or permanently.
- Noise, acting as a stress, may interfere with the flying task.
- Noise may induce varying levels of fatigue.

This chapter deals primarily with the problem of noise within the aircraft. External noise is covered only briefly. The important, but different, problems of the effects on the environment are not covered but may be studied in the many books and papers on the subject.

PHYSICAL CHARACTERISTICS OF SOUND

Production of sound

Sound is any undulatory motion in an elastic medium (gaseous, liquid, solid) that is capable of producing the sensation of hearing. Normally, the medium is air. A simple sound may be produced by a piston vibrating in a tube (Figure 26.1). The movement of the piston produces variations of the pressure of the air in the tube, so that the molecules of air at any given point are alternately compressed and rarefied. A simple sound in which the pressure fluctuations follow a sinusoid is known as a pure tone. The velocity with which the waves of compression and rarefaction pass along the tube is the velocity of sound. The frequency of the sound is the number of times with which each complete cycle repeats itself in unit time, while the wavelength is the distance between two corresponding points in successive cycles (Figure 26.1). These quantities are related by the following expression:

$$\text{Wavelength} = \frac{\text{velocity of sound in the medium}}{\text{frequency}}$$

Sound pressure

In a pure tone, the sound pressure fluctuates, so that for half the time of a complete cycle it is above, and for the remainder of the time below, the prevailing atmospheric pressure. This average use can be specified in terms of the amplitude, which is the peak value of each half-cycle. Sound pressure is normally specified, however, as the average pressure throughout the cycle, notwithstanding the fact that the pressure is fluctuating about the prevailing atmospheric pressure. This average pressure is obtained from the squares of the values of the sound pressure at a large number of instants throughout one or more cycles (this eliminates the negative values). From this, one calculates the mean square and then the root mean square

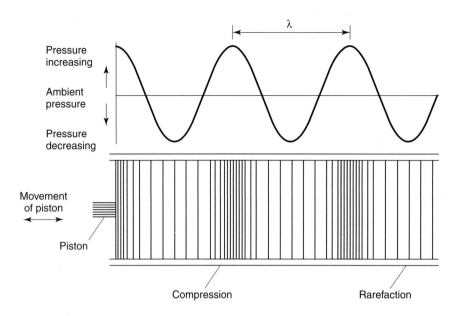

Figure 26.1   *Production of a simple sound by oscillation of a piston in a tube. The sinusoidal movement of the piston at the left-hand end of the tube produces regular compression and rarefaction of the gas immediately adjacent to it. These pressure fluctuations are transmitted through the gas in the tube. The distance between two consecutive peaks or troughs of pressure is the wavelength (λ) of the tone.*

(RMS) or 'effective' value. For pure tones, the RMS value is 0.707 of the amplitude of the wave. The standard unit of pressure used in measuring sound is the pascal (Pa).

The threshold of human hearing at a frequency of 1 kHz is a sound pressure of about $20\,\mu\text{Pa}$ ($2 \times 10^{-5}\,\text{N/m}^2$ or $2 \times 10^{-4}\,\mu\text{bar}$). This is a pressure of only 2×10^{-10} atmospheres. At the other end of the scale, a sound pressure of 200 Pa may be accommodated by the ear before the onset of pain. The ear is thus capable of responding over a very wide dynamic range, from 2×10^{-5} to 2×10^2 Pa (140 dB).

Sound pressure level

Since sound essentially comprises a series of pressure fluctuations, it follows that measurement of sound pressure level (SPL) involves measurement of an absolute pressure. The unit of SPL, however, is the decibel (dB), which is a dimensionless unit. The decibel is often associated uniquely with noise measurement, but it was borrowed originally from electrical communications engineering and represents a relative quantity, e.g. when used to measure noise, 94 dB refers to 94 dB above a reference quantity. This reference level is $20\,\mu\text{Pa}$ and is referred to as 0 dB, which is, in fact, about the weakest sound that can be heard by a person with good hearing in a very quiet location. The relationship between SPL and dB is as follows:

$$\text{SPL (in dB)} = 20 \log_{10} P/P_0$$

where P is the measured pressure and P_0 is reference pressure ($20\,\mu\text{Pa}$).

It is now possible to see that a doubling of pressure from the reference pressure of $20\,\mu\text{Pa}$, i.e. to $40\,\mu\text{Pa}$, may be described in decibels, thus:

$$\text{SPL (in dB)} = 20 \log_{10}(40/20) = 20 \log_{10}(2)$$

$$20 \times 0.3010 = 6\,\text{dB}$$

Thus, each increment of 6 dB represents a doubling of sound pressure. Similarly, a ten-fold increase in pressure to $200\,\mu\text{Pa}$ can be defined as follows:

$$\text{dB} = 20 \log_{10}(200/20) = 20 \log_{10} 10 = 20\,\text{dB}$$

Hence, it can be seen that as the decibel levels increase linearly, the actual SPLs increase logarithmically (6 dB twice, 12 dB four times, 18 dB eight times, etc.). This seemingly complicated logarithmic method is used because noise is nearly always related exclusively to human hearing or human response, and the human ear is a detector of unparalleled quality in relation to dynamic range. From the quietest sound that can be heard (the threshold of hearing) to the loudest sound that can be tolerated before the onset of pain (pain threshold), the range is more than one to ten million. The direct application of linear scales to the measurement of sound pressure would, therefore, lead to the use of very high and unwieldy numbers.

Conveniently, the response of the ear to sound stimuli is also logarithmic and not linear, i.e. the ear is at its most sensitive at low sound levels and responds progressively less sensitively as the sound level increases. It has been found, therefore, most practical to express acoustic parameters as a logarithmic ratio of the measured value to the standard value.

Use of the decibel scale thus reduces a dynamic range of SPLs of one to 10 000 000 to a more manageable range of 0 to 140 dB ($1\,\text{dB} = 20 \log_{10}7 = 140\,\text{dB}$). It is also useful because 1 dB is about the smallest value of significance, in that under normal circumstances a change of 1 dB may be just detectable by the human ear.

It is worth noting that 0 dB does not mean an absence of noise; it merely implies that the level in question is equal to the reference level. Thus, if the measured sound pressure level is 10 μPa, then the level in decibels would be

$$20 \log_{10} 10/20 = 20 \log_{10} 0.5 = 20 \times (-0.3010) = -6 \text{ dB}.$$

Hence, it can be seen clearly that negative decibel values are possible: it may not be possible to hear them, but it is possible to measure them with sensitive measuring devices.

A further point worthy of note, but not of prolonged explanation, is that if two sound sources having the same sound pressure level, say 70 dB, are measured together, then the overall sound pressure level (OASPL) will be not 140 dB but 73 dB. Doubling the number of sources raises the SPL by 3 dB, a further doubling (to four equal sound sources) raises the SPL by 6 dB to 76 dB, and so on. Conversely, any measure that reduces the measured decibel value by 3 dB signifies a reduction of no less than half in sound energy.

Similarly, if there are two sources at, say, 80 dB and 86 dB, then the overall level is only 1 dB up on the higher source, in this case 87 dB overall. It follows that if one source is 10 dB quieter than another source, it does not contribute significantly to the summed overall SPL. The absolute sound pressures and equivalent sound pressure levels for a number of noise environments are presented in Table 26.1.

Complex sounds and frequency analysis

A finite signal, regardless of its complexity, may be considered to be made up of a number of simple sine waves (Fourier series). The sine-wave components of a signal constitute the frequency spectrum. The frequency spectrum of a sine wave (Figure 26.2a) clearly consists of only one line, while that of more complicated but periodic waves consists of harmonically related discrete lines (Figure 26.2b), and that of statistically distributed signals, such as random noise, shows a continuous spectrum (Figure 26.2c). There is a subjective significance here: if two pure tones are played together, then they are heard as a chord rather than as a single sound, i.e. the ear appears to be performing some sort of Fourier analysis on the signal. The analogous effect does not prevail in the visual system: a red light mixed with a green light produces a perception of yellow light indistinguishable from that produced by a pure yellow light source.

The noises in real life that are usually measured, however, are rarely simple acoustic waves of single frequency (pure tones) but usually are a jumble of sounds that vary from a low-frequency rumble to a high-frequency screech. Human reaction to such sounds depends not only on the overall level but also on the composition of the noise in terms of frequency. To measure this composition, frequency analysis is carried out, which gives a curve showing how the sound energy is distributed over a range of frequencies (Figure 26.2c). The noise is separated electronically into its

Table 26.1 *Sound pressures and sound pressure levels of various sound environments*

Sound pressure (Pa)	Sound pressure level (dB)	Environment
200	140	Turbojet at 50 feet
20	120	Jet takeoff 500 feet
		Inside low-level fighter
		Large jet landing
		Inside helicopter
2	100	
2×10^{-1}	80	
		Street-corner traffic
		Normal speech at 3 feet
2×10^{-2}	60	
		Office
		Living-room
2×10^{-3}	40	
		Library
2×10^{-4}	20	
		Broadcasting studio
2×10^{-5}	0	Threshold of hearing at 1 kHz

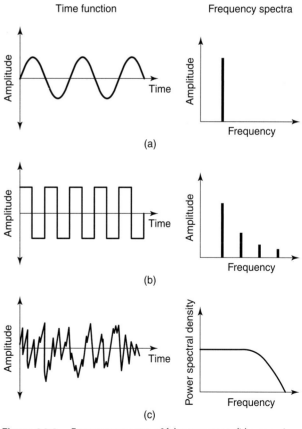

Figure 26.2 *Frequency spectra of (a) a pure tone, (b) a complex periodic and (c) a complex non-periodic signal.*

frequency bands, such as octave bands, each of which covers a two-to-one range of frequencies. Such analysis yields a level for each band, called, appropriately, band levels. For octave band analysis, these are called octave-band levels.

If a more detailed analysis is required, narrower bands are used. By splitting an octave band into three parts, one-third octave bands are produced, which represent to a much greater degree the way in which humans hear. In one-third octave bands, the bandwidth is about 23 per cent of the centre frequency.

For some purposes, however, e.g. for noise control, still narrower bands are necessary, and it is possible to use analysers with one-tenth octave bands (about seven per cent in width). Analysers with one per cent bandwidths are also available.

Finally, a point is reached at which the bandwidth is no longer a percentage of the band centre frequency but is actually 1 Hz wide. This is called the spectrum level.

Propagation of noise

Sound generated from a noise source does not remain at constant SPL as the distance from the source increases. The further the distance from the source, the lower the level. The energy in the sound wave is proportional to the area that the wave front occupies; thus, as the distance increases, the SPLs decrease.

There are essentially two types of noise source:

- A point source, in which the source is small compared with the measuring distance from that source. An analogy could be a loudspeaker in a field.
- A line source, which is a source, or series of sources, spread in a line that is longer than the measuring distance from it. For example, a train with a number of carriages emits noise that may be regarded as a line source. However, as the distance from the line source increases, it can be seen that the line source begins to approach a point source.

These two definitions are important, as the propagation of noise from a point source occurs with a spherical wave front and the SPLs decrease by 6 dB each time the distance from the source is doubled, while a line source has an attenuation of 3 dB per doubling of distance. As the distance increases, finally to a point where the line source may be regarded as a point source, then the attenuation of sound changes gradually from 3 dB to 6 dB at these points.

A reasonable analogy for visualizing point and line sources is the dropping of a stone or series of stones in a pond. A single stone will result in spherical propagation, while a series of stones, dropped in line, will result in line propagation, the result of a series of spherical propagations.

To this natural attenuation must be added the additional attenuations, or amplifications, due to atmospheric influences or contact with solid objects. Atmospheric influences include air absorption (including fog and rain), the effects of temperature gradients and wind, and changes in the product of air density and speed of sound. In addition to these small changes in attenuation must be added the effects of ground absorption, which differs for propagation over hard surfaces (e.g. concrete) or soft surfaces (e.g. vegetation) as on an airfield, due to obstructions such as walls, buildings, clumps of trees, etc., and the fact that at a point the total SPL may consist of a direct acoustic path plus a reflected path, which can be high or low, depending on the relative phases of the two sound waves.

Thus, it is clear that the noise measurement of, say, a jet aircraft running up on an airfield depends not only on the distance from the aircraft but also on the environmental conditions between the source and receiver and the prevailing meteorology conditions, and this may change from day to day and even from hour to hour. Single simple measurement is rarely enough to provide an adequate description of noise exposure under these conditions.

MECHANISM OF HEARING

The outer ear

The outer ear has long been regarded as unimportant in hearing, but it plays a part in localizing sound sources. For mammals with limited visual acuity, such as humans, it is (or was) essential to have a pinna presenting a wide mobile surface to enable both detection and localization of any danger sounds. The pinna in humans essentially is limited to the production of high-frequency reinforcement for directional effects in localization of sound. The process of monaural hearing allows detection, while binaural hearing enables spatial location. Unlike a horse, which has ten vestigial mobilizing muscles for its pinna or auricle, humans are limited to three and must compensate for this deficiency in aural mobility by making movements of the head and neck.

The beginning of the process of auditory transduction, however, can be said to start at the tympanic membrane, which vibrates in response to changes in air pressure in the auditory canal. The tympanic membrane has a certain resistance to movement or 'impedance'. The auditory canal, about 36 mm in length, performs significant 'matching' of this impedance to the air. This matching is somewhat frequency-dependent, being poor at frequencies below about 400 Hz.

The middle ear

The air-containing middle ear is vented to atmosphere via the Eustachian tube so that atmospheric pressure variations do not cause maintained pressure differences across the tympanic membrane. The important function of the middle car is that of impedance matching. Because the inner ear is filled with fluid while the eardrum is a membrane driven by changes of gas pressure, there is a large impedance difference caused by the difference of acoustical impedance in the two media (i.e. fluid and air). The specific acoustic resistance of air is approximately 42 acoustic ohms, while that of a small body of water is 9000 ohms. A loss of some 30 dB is apparent, which must be regained. Two processes in the middle ear affect this process: a leverage effect and a hydraulic effect. The ossicles provide a leverage ratio of only one to three to one, giving only a 2.3 dB gain, and it is left to the area ratio of

the tympanic membrane to the stapes base to provide the major gain path (Figure 26.3a). The malleus, connected to the tympanic membrane, experiences large excursions, but these are transformed to much smaller amplitude at the stapes, which is connected to the relatively much smaller area (compared with the tympanic membrane) of the oval window, generating much higher pressures suitable for driving the fluid-filled inner ear. The diameter of the tympanic membrane is approximately 9.5 mm, giving an area of 71 mm², only two-thirds (47 mm²) of this area being effective.

The area of the stapes base is in the region of 3.2 mm², giving an area ratio of 14.7, which provides 23 dB of gain. This combination of leverage and area ratios compensates

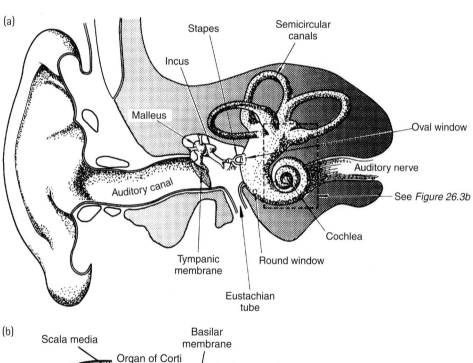

(a)

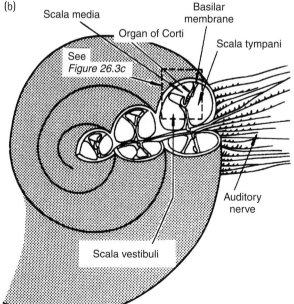

(b)

Figure 26.3   *(a) Diagram of the ear. (b) Cut-away diagram of the cochlea of the inner ear.*

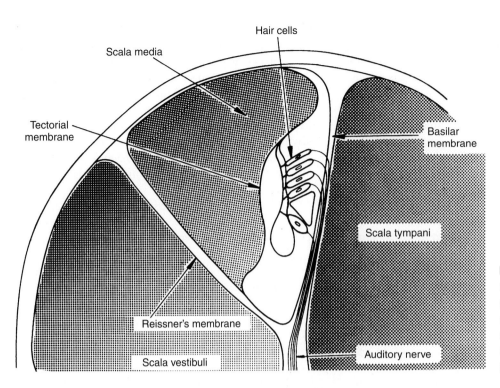

Figure 26.3c *Cross-section of the basilar membrane and the organ of Corti, the hair cells of which are stimulated by movement of the tectorial membrane relative to the basilar membrane.*

to a major extent for the losses due to impedance mismatch. The ossicles are not, therefore, acting as an amplifier, since no energy is gained in the process; they simply modify the nature of the vibration, in order to maximize the efficiency of the transfer of energy between outer and inner ear.

The other main function of the middle ear is that of protecting the inner ear against particularly large-amplitude vibrations (loud noises), which could be damaging. This is achieved in two ways, as follows:

- *Acoustic reflex:* this reflex changes the impedance of the middle ear in order to discriminate against large-amplitude, low-frequency vibrations. It works by contraction of the stapedius and tensor tympani muscles, which act on the bones in the middle ear. Although primarily a brainstem reflex, this response is affected by the state of the subject's attention.
- *Subluxation of the ossicles:* the articular portions of the malleus, incus and stapes move in and out of joint. The subluxation reduces the efficiency of the ossicles as a transmission system and protects the inner ear.

The inner ear

The functions of the outer and middle ear are to 'condition' the auditory signal arriving at the pinna in order to make it suitable for the inner ear, the function of which is to transduce this signal (which still consists of rapid pressure changes) into a neural code.

The cochlea is a coiled tube that is divided longitudinally into three main compartments: the scala vestibuli, scala tympani and scala media or cochlear duct (Figure 26.3b). The scala vestibuli and scala tympani contain perilymph and are in communication with one another as the cochlear partition does not completely divide the cochlea. The pressures are equalized via the orifice, the helicotrema, at the end of the cochlea furthest from the oval window. A structure called the basilar membrane (Figure 26.3c) performs a mechanical frequency analysis on the incoming signal. The membrane runs almost the length of the cochlea and is narrow at the basal (oval window) end of the cochlea and gradually widens towards the apex. Running along the basilar membrane are rows of hair cells. The short processes of hairs of these cells extend to touch the lower side of the tectorial membrane, a gelatinous shelf that overlies the basilar membrane. Movement of the basilar membrane relative to the tectorial membrane deforms the hairs. This deformation initiates the nerve impulse.

When the stapes causes pressure changes in the endolymph of the scala vestibuli (these are at the same frequency as the sound arriving at the ear and proportional in amplitude), a travelling wave is produced in the basilar membrane. This travelling wave appears initially as a bulge at the basal end of the membrane and over the course of the next 4 ms travels along the membrane, waxing and then waning. The point at which the maximum amplitude of vibration occurs on the basilar membrane depends on the frequency of the stimulating sound. Low tones produce maximum excitation at the basal end of the membrane and high tones at the apex. The information is relayed to the brain by the auditory maximum vibration on the membrane. The frequency of impulses in any fibre or collection of fibres corresponds to the frequency of the stimulating sound. This relationship holds for frequencies up to 3–4 kHz, the highest frequencies used in speech. Thus, there are two ways in which the frequency of a sound is indicated to the brain:

- the rate of firing in the auditory nerve
- the locus of maximum displacement of the basilar membrane.

SUBJECTIVE SENSATION

Loudness and noisiness

Objective or physical methods of measurement are defined in terms of SPL and frequency, while the corresponding subjective sensations (what we actually hear) are expressed in terms of loudness level (phons) and pitch, respectively. Loudness may be defined as the subjective magnitude of a sound, while pitch is the subjective sensation of frequency.

Since a sound at a particular frequency depends on the ear to translate its level into loudness, the response of the ear is of paramount importance in this translation. Unlike most hi-fi equipment the ear does not have a frequency response that is flat but one that varies with both frequency and level. Thus, the loudness of a sound depends not only on its SPL but also on its frequency. Figure 26.4 shows the pure-tone frequency response of the ear, taken from the

International Organization for Standardization (1961) R 226:1961 standard. These curves are known as the equal loudness contours, or phon curves. Each curve plotted has equal loudness. It can be seen that, for example, a loudness level of 50 phons requires an SPL of 50 dB at 1 kHz, while at lower frequencies, where the ear is less sensitive (e.g. 60 Hz), an SPL of 70 dB is required to maintain this loudness. Alternatively, at a higher frequency of 4 kHz (very close to where the ear is maximally sensitive), an SPL of only 44 dB is needed to maintain the loudness level of 50 phons.

The curves have been constructed from a number of psychoacoustic experiments in which large numbers of subjects judged loudness against the physical parameters of SPL and frequency, using a frequency of 1 kHz as a reference. Additionally, it can be seen clearly that as the SPLs rise, the response of the ear flattens. For example, at low levels, the difference on the 50-phon curve between 60 Hz and 1 kHz for equal loudness is 20 dB, while at the higher loudness level of 110 phons, the difference reduces to only 7 dB.

Loudness level is measured in phons, phons being the subjective sensation of SPL. The loudness of a pure tone of 1 kHz is said to have a value in phons equal to its SPL; this is simply how phons are defined.

During the psychoacoustic experiments, subjects were also asked to judge what represented a doubling of loudness, and this was judged as 10 phons. Thus, 60 phons is twice as loud as 50 phons. So, in terms of human response, loudness doubles with every 10-phon increment in stimulus. To some extent, this can be related to SPLs, since at 1 kHz an increase of 10 phons loudness level is the same as

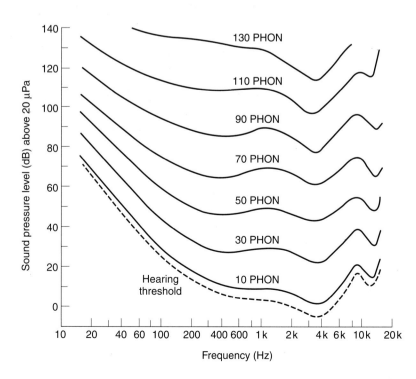

Figure 26.4 *Equal-loudness contours for pure tones at sound pressure levels of 10, 30, 50, 70, 90, 110 and 130 dB (phon). The dashed curve is the normal hearing threshold for pure tones.*

an increase of 10 dB. This is reasonably true across the frequency band generally, except at low frequencies, where the phon curves are spaced more closely and a lower decibel increase corresponds to a 10-phon increase.

While it is relatively easy to deduce how much louder a sound of 76 phons is than a 66-phon sound (10 phons, twice as loud), it is more difficult to deduce a difference of, say, 14 phons. Hence, another scale has been devised, known as the sone scale. This is a ratio scale in which the number of sones doubles as the loudness doubles: a sound of 6.4 sones is twice as loud as one of 3.2 sones.

To match the phon and sone scales, 1 sone is defined arbitrarily as equal to 40 phons. Thus, if 1 sone = 40 phons, then 2 sones = 50 phons, 4 sones = 60 phons, etc. Mathematically, this may be expressed as follows:

$$P = 40 + 33 \log_{10} S$$

where P is in phons and S is in sones.

Loudness expressed in phons is strictly called 'loudness level', whereas expressed in sones it is simply called 'loudness'. However, in many cases, these strict definitions are not adhered to and some care is required.

To calculate loudness or loudness level of a sound more complex than a pure tone, data must be available in the form of a sound spectrum, either in octave bands or one-third octave bands. The one-third octave band method was formulated by Zwicker (1960), while the octave-band method results from work by Stevens (1956). Often, the loudness levels calculated from Zwicker's method will be followed by the suffix GF or GD, meaning they were calculated from wither free-field frontal sound or diffuse field data, respectively. Stevens' method is valid only for diffuse fields and may be suffixed by OD (octave diffuse).

A further aspect of human sensation is the related concept of noisiness and annoyance. Like the equal-loudness (or phon) curves, similar curves may be constructed for noisiness (Figure 26.5), with noisiness being measured in noys. Comparison of the two types of curves shows that the noy contours dip more sharply between 2 kHz and 5 kHz, indicating that sounds in this frequency range do not have to have a very high SPL to be considered noisy.

The unit of noisiness, the noy, is the counterpart in noisiness of the sone in loudness. Perceived noise level (PNL), which is given the unit of perceived noise decibel (PNdB), is the counterpart of the loudness level in phons. Thus, where 40 phons = 1 sone, 40 PNdB = 1 noy. A doubling of noisiness to 2 noys = 50 PNdB, etc. PNL may be applied directly to aircraft external noise. In the USA, methods have been devised for evaluating the noisiness of aircraft using as a basis the equal-noisiness contours.

Although it is necessary to understand the concept of subjective loudness, the phon is seldom used in normal measurements of, for example, cockpit noise, which is usually quoted in decibel SPL, or dB(A).

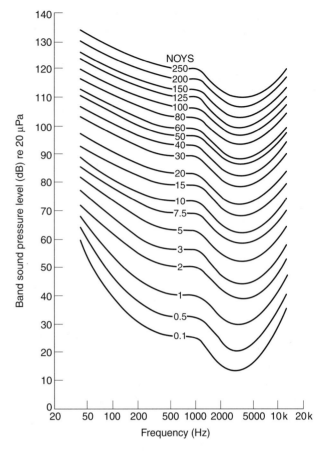

Figure 26.5   *Equal-noisiness contours (from Kryter 1970). The curves show equal impression of noisiness related to frequency and noise level. A pure tone of 50 Hz and 70 dB sound pressure level (SPL) is equally as noisy as a corresponding pure tone at 2 kHz but only 43 dB SPL, i.e. there is a 27-dB difference in level but they are equally noisy.*

From an inspection of the loudness curves, it might be natural (but not logical) to assume that the human hearing mechanism abruptly ceases to function below 20 Hz. As the system is predominantly an analogue system, this sharp cut-off is most unlikely. Research by workers at Salford University and the National Physical Laboratory has shown that human hearing extends down to below 2 Hz. The reason for the cut-off was due to the inability of the loudspeaker systems, at the time, to produce undistorted pure tones at the required levels below 20 Hz.

Measurement of noise

Physical measurement of noise and its relation to subjective impression is most important. Measurement is generally enabled by a sound-level meter, which measures the SPLs through a microphone, the microphone changing the SPLs measured to a voltage in a controlled manner, and these voltages being read on a voltmeter, usually calibrated in decibels. When measuring SPL, the instrument is set up such that the meter responds to all frequencies equally, i.e. no frequency weighting is involved. As has been shown previously, the ear does not respond to all frequencies equally, and if it is necessary to use a sound-level meter to provide an indication of human response to a noise field, then between the process of taking the voltage from the microphone and reading a level on the voltmeter, some frequency weighting must be included to take account of the response of the ear. Since the ear has a different frequency response with different SPLs, then, in theory at least, an infinite number of weighting curves would be required for each noise level. In practice, this is successfully reduced to three, which follow three of the equal-loudness contours.

For sounds that are judged 'not loud', the 40-phon contour was smoothed and used as the A weighting. For moderately loud sounds, the 70-phon contour was used as a basis for the B weighting. The C weighting was for 'loud' sounds and based on the 100-phon contour. These weightings are written as dB(A), dB(B) and dB(C), respectively. Figure 26.6 shows these weighting curves as well as the D weighting curve. The D weighting originated from the fact that dB(A) gave such a widely usable correlation of subjective response to physical measurement over a wide range of intensities and a wide range of human sensations that the 40-PNdB (1-noy) equal-noisiness contour was used in the D weighting as a simple correlate of noisiness. However, the D weighting has not shown itself to be sufficiently superior to the A weighting to be used generally, and the A weighting is now the most widely used method of correlating subjective impression and measured levels, even over the whole of the loudness range. Thus, B, C and D weightings are rarely used.

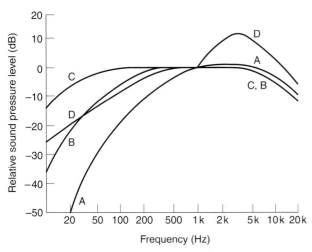

Figure 26.6   *A, B, C and D weighting scales for sound-level meters. The relative responses for the four characteristics at different frequencies are shown.*

Sound-level meters that have these weighting networks built into them may be used to give some indication of the frequency constitution of the noise being measured. Thus, if the measurement on the A scale is 70 dB(A) and on the C scale 77 dB(C), then it is clear from Figure 26.6 that the noise has a large low-frequency component.

NOISE AND AIRCRAFT

Noise generates problems both outside and inside aircraft. People who live near airfields understandably do not wish to be disturbed by the intrusion of aircraft noise into their homes. Ground crew working on aircraft do not wish to be deafened. Aircrew, naturally, would like a quiet working environment in which communication is not only possible but also easy. This section will concentrate on internal noise in the aircraft cockpit and cabin.

Noise sources

The sources of noise and, consequently, the associated internal noise fields differ with the type of aircraft. In military flying, the worst noise problems generally occur in high-performance jets and the helicopters. These are troublesome principally because of the high levels of internal noise, which not only cause difficulty with aircrew communications but also may, over a period, cause a degree of permanent hearing loss.

The major sources of internal noise in aircraft are:

- power sources, transmission systems, propellers and jet efflux
- interaction between the aircraft and the medium through which it flies (flow of air over aircraft surfaces)
- subsidiary noise arising from cabin-conditioning and -pressurizing systems, hydraulic systems, and communication equipment
- armament discharge.

Aircraft cockpit noise

Historically, noise levels in cockpits have always been high. Even in the early biplanes of the De Havilland DH4 type, communications were often a problem. In 1918, the German four-engined Staaken bomber had noise levels that were so high in its enclosed cockpit that the crew could communicate only through the use of an electric visual signalling system.

The problems continued into the Second World War. During that time, a series of more reliable noise measurements was made. Noise levels were high in many combat aircraft, and protection against these levels generally was low. The major sources from these piston-engined aircraft were from the open exhausts, the engine and the propeller(s). However, high levels of noise could be generated from other aircraft and engine systems, such as supercharger noise. Overall noise levels in two representative Second World War US Air Force aircraft, a General Motors FM-2 Wildcat and a Republic P-47D Thunderbolt, were in the region of 120–125 dB OASPL. The progression to the gas turbine engine removed the propeller and exhaust noise, and cabin noise levels were reduced. Thus, an early jet, the Bell P-59B Aircobra, had overall cabin noise levels of around 104 dB OASPL and the gradual movement of the engine(s) towards the rear of the aircraft or buried in the fuselage further helped the cockpit acoustic environment.

Fast jet aircraft

Beginning in the 1960s, the operational requirement to be able to fly fast and low has increased the problems due to internal cabin noise. Over the years, there have been gradual increases in cabin noise levels of fast jets during high-speed low-level flight, and it is now not uncommon for aircrew to be exposed to noise levels of between 115 and 120 dB when flying at operational speeds and heights – typically 420–480 knots at 250 feet.

The major source of noise in these cases is from the turbulent flow across the aircraft canopy and structure, and from the cabin-conditioning flows into the cockpit that are used for cooling, demisting and pressurization. The contribution from the boundary-layer turbulent flow depends essentially on the structure and shape of the canopy and its relation to the remaining aircraft structure, as well as the speed and height of the aircraft.

Additional sources are from cockpit-mounted equipment, in some aircraft from the engines, and from other mechanical/hydraulic systems within the aircraft structure, although generally these are of a secondary nature.

Figure 26.7a shows a typical fast-jet cabin-noise spectrum, and Figure 26.7b shows the extent of the decrease for the same aircraft in flight at high and low altitudes. As the aircraft climbs to altitude and the air density decreases, the

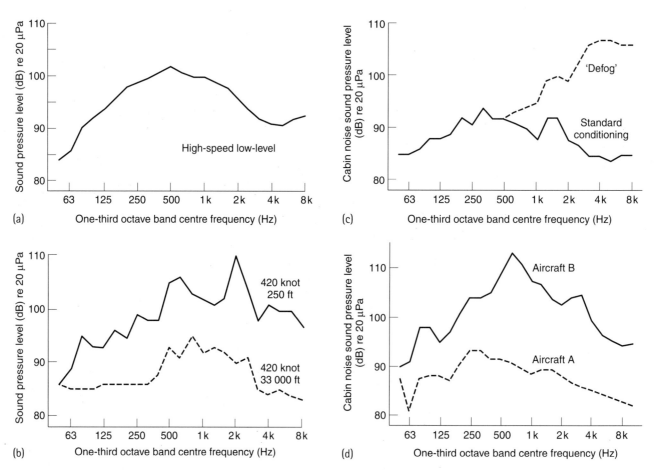

Figure 26.7 *(a) Typical cabin noise spectrum for a fast jet aircraft flying at high speed (450 knots) at low altitude (250 feet). Effects of (b) altitude of flight and (c) selection of defog on emergency demist on the cabin noise spectrum. (d) Cabin noise spectra of a 'quiet' (aircraft A) and less 'quiet' (aircraft B) fast jet aircraft flying at high speed (500 knots) at low level (500 feet).*

pressure fluctuations in the turbulent flow decrease in intensity and the contribution to the overall cabin noise level from the external aerodynamic sources is diminished. As the contribution from the external sources decreases, so the contribution from the cabin-conditioning source will increase and, depending on the quality of design of the conditioning system and the outlet sprays, may dominate the noise spectrum at higher altitudes, albeit at generally lower overall cabin noise level. However, some fast aircraft have poorly designed cabin-conditioning systems that result in no decreases in cabin noise as the aircraft operates at higher altitudes.

Normally, as air mass flow to the cabin-conditioning system increases, so the noise levels increase. In most aircraft, including even quiet examples, conditioning noise will dominate when it is necessary to use defog or emergency demist; in these cases (Figure 26.7c), substantial increases in high-frequency noise levels occur. Further differences occur between aircraft of the same type and, in multi-seat aircraft, between seat positions. Thus, noise levels may be different between the pilot and navigator positions, especially in tandem-seat aircraft, and it is commonly accepted that within aircraft types some aircraft are noisier than others.

Depending on the design, noise levels between different types of aircraft can vary greatly. The difference between a 'noisy' and 'quiet' aircraft operating at the same speed and height is depicted in Figure 26.7d to illustrate the range. While it is difficult, for many operational reasons, to design aircraft structures and transparent canopies to ensure low noise levels, it is considerably easier to design cabin-conditioning systems that do not contribute greatly to cabin noise.

Rotary-wing aircraft

Helicopters have a totally different noise spectrum, which essentially comprises of aerodynamically induced noise from the main and tail rotors and mechanically induced noise from the main gearbox and various transmission chains, all of which produce dominant narrow-band noise peaks. Consequently, the spectrum is built up from a combination of deterministic discrete and random broadband noise components. A typical spectrum for a single-rotor helicopter is shown in Figure 26.8, indicating the contributions from the rotor, gearbox and ancillaries. The rotor frequency is a product of the rotational speed of the rotor and the number of rotor blades; on most major single-rotor helicopters, it is around 20 Hz. The gearbox frequencies are related directly to the gear-meshing ratios of the power input/output gears and generally are in the higher frequency range around 400–600 Hz

For twin-rotor helicopters of the Chinook type, the rotor frequencies are generally lower, due partly to fewer

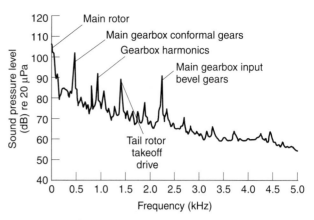

Figure 26.8 *Cabin noise spectrum of a helicopter with a single rotor (Lynx), showing the various aircraft components contributing to the cabin noise levels.*

rotor blades, and generate discrete noise at around 12 Hz at levels of up to 125 dB. In most cases, these levels of infrasonic noise will cause no problems, but some noise-induced symptoms may occur in a few people.

Owing to these high-level 'spikes' of noise from the various components, operational problems may occur when tasks involving listening for low-level signal returns are necessary, such as detecting or classifying sonar or electronic surveillance measures and electronic countermeasure returns. The high levels of discrete noise may cause frequencies above and below the dominant noise source, as well as at the particular source frequency, to go unheard. This phenomenon is known as auditory masking and is, very simply, the occlusion of one sound by another. It is possible to calculate the auditory threshold below which the detection of sounds is improbable; similarly, it is possible to show, using the human psychometric function, that 15 dB above this threshold, 100 per cent detection is possible. Thus, it is possible to predict the levels and frequencies of signals that may be detected and the probability of detection, which can be useful in the setting of warning signal levels in auditory warning or auditory information systems.

The external sound field of the helicopter is created predominantly by a combination of rotor noise and engine exhaust, which is at a maximum close to the exhaust outlets. This type of aircraft may be a noise nuisance to people on the ground, because it operates at low speed and low altitude and consequently remains within earshot for long periods.

Turbo-prop and piston-engined aircraft

Generally, the major source of noise in this type of aircraft is the propeller. In the same way as the helicopter, the dominant frequency is a function of the propeller rotational speed and the number of blades. As these aircraft fly at higher speeds than helicopters, there is a higher contribution from boundary layer noise, although it does not approach the levels generated by the jet transport types. The internal noise is generally at its highest levels in the plane of the propellers. Figure 26.9 is a narrow-band analysis of an RAF C130 Hercules aircraft, which shows clearly the dominant effect of the propeller noise.

Jet transport aircraft

Similar to fast military jets, the major contribution to passenger jet internal noise is from the boundary layer turbulent flow and from cabin conditioning. The noise spectrum is normally broadband, peaking at around 125 Hz, and varies down the length and across the width of the aircraft. Noise levels at the cabin side wall may be up to 6 dB higher than at the centre of the cabin. Noise also emanates from sources such as hydraulic and mechanical systems (e.g. flaps, slats), although generally these occur only during specific phases of flight (e.g. landing, takeoff).

Vertical takeoff and landing (VTOL), vertical/short takeoff and landing (VSTOL) and short takeoff and landing (STOL) aircraft

Aircraft of these types either are intended to take off or land vertically or have short takeoff and/or landing runs, or there may be a combination of both, e.g. short takeoff, vertical landing (STOVL).

The majority of STOL aircraft in current use are propeller-driven and utilize special wing designs such as high-aspect-ratio wings, slotted flaps and leading edge slots/slats to achieve lift coefficients that are high enough at slow speed to provide sufficient lift. A further group, aimed mainly at military use, utilize powered lift devices such as under-wing or over-wing blowing, augmentor wings and deflected slipstreams. Another technique is used in the Harrier type of aircraft, which utilizes vectored thrust alone to provide vertical transition during takeoff or landing (VTOL). Noise problems generally occur only during the landing or takeoff phase of flight, when the high lift or vectored thrust devices are in use. During all other phases of flight, the aircraft may be viewed as a standard aircraft of the appropriate type.

Aircraft external noise fields

The external sound field from a jet-powered aircraft is filled with distributed noise from the jet engine with some harmonic contribution from rotating parts of the engine. At high indicated air speeds in flight, aerodynamic noise can also contribute to the external sound field. The intensity of jet noise heard at any given distance from the aircraft varies with the listener's position with respect to the jet axis. Figure 26.10 shows the noise-level distribution around a single-jet aircraft for engine run-up on the ground. The highest noise is not directly in line with the jet but on the quarters.

Conventional turbojet engines produce thrust by heating a relatively small mass of air to a high temperature and thus accelerating it to a high velocity. This high-velocity air, mixing turbulently with the surrounding air, generates noise. The same amount of thrust can be produced, however, by imparting a lower velocity (and thereby causing less noise) to a larger mass of air. This occurs in jet engines with a high bypass ratio, where a cowled fan is fitted to the

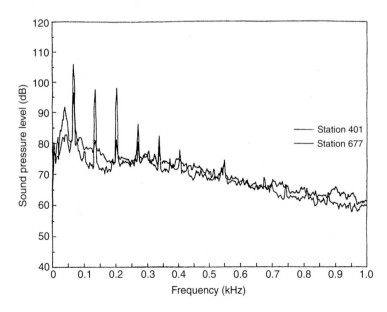

Figure 26.9 *Narrow-band analysis of RAF C130 Hercules aircraft.*

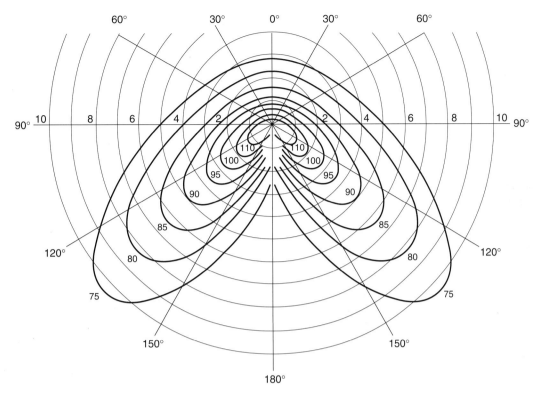

Figure 26.10 *Distribution of noise levels around a single-engined jet aircraft on ground run-up. The concentric circles indicate distance from the aircraft, the radii of the circles increasing from 1000 feet to 10 000 feet at intervals of 1000 feet. The long axis of the aircraft is indicated by the vertical 0–180-degree axis of the diagram. The heavy lines join points of equal perceived noise level (PNdB). The value of the perceived noise level is indicated for each contour by the number immediately below the contour. Note that the perceived noise level contours form lobes at an angle to the jet axis.*

front of the engine. The fan acts almost like a propeller to accelerate a large mass of air, only a fraction of which passes through the combustion chamber of the engine.

Reduction of cabin noise levels

The sound fields inside aircraft can vary from quiet to intensely noisy. There are certain engineering means of reducing the noise levels at source, but unless noise-control techniques are implemented at the design stage, reducing the noise at source by engineering means in a production aircraft has met with only limited success. Reduction of noise at the aircraft structure normally requires the addition of mass or bulk, both of which are generally unacceptable to the operator. Some possible ways of reducing cabin noise are as follows:

- *Increasing the canopy thickness:* this would undoubtedly help to reduce aerodynamic noise in strike aircraft, but it would also increase weight and possibly impede the ejection path.
- *Smoothing the boundary layer by removing unnecessary excrescences or by reshaping surfaces:* this is not an important problem in slow aircraft, and in fast aircraft it may be taken for granted that, because of aerodynamic considerations, all excrescences are necessary. Nevertheless, improvements occasionally have been brought about by this means.
- *Redesigning the conditioning system or reducing the air flow through the system:* in the past, the conditioning system has seldom been designed with noise in mind, and redesign may well be possible. It is also true that mass flows of air sometimes have been found to be in excess of that required and that a reduced flow has produced a reduction of cabin noise without affecting thermal conditioning.
- *Damping the walls of the cockpit:* this may be possible, again to reduce aerodynamic noise, but in fact the large amounts of avionic equipment already attached to the cockpit walls provide reasonable damping. It is certainly the case that damping could be, and is, used to quieten the interior of helicopters, in which structural vibrations are an important noise factor, but the weight penalty associated with providing full levels of damping is usually felt to be unacceptable, in particular for military operations, and compromises are made as to the quantity of damping, balancing

mass and volume of the damping materials against the levels of noise reduction.

Of course, a properly maintained aircraft is likely to be less noisy than a neglected one.

Protection of aircrew against noise

If, when all has been done to reduce the cabin noise levels at source, the noise levels are still too high, then other means must be found to protect the aircrew from these unacceptable levels. High noise levels will interfere with communications (see Chapter 25) and, if aircrew are exposed for enough time, may cause permanent hearing damage.

The primary way of protecting crew against noise is by use of the aircrew helmet or headset. In most military aircraft, the wearing of a helmet or headset is compulsory. The flying helmet provides a convenient attachment for the oxygen mask, protective visors, night-vision goggles, and helmet-mounted sights and displays. For noise protection, the helmet incorporates hearing protection in the form of earshells mounted inside the helmet.

HELMETS AND HEADSETS

Acoustically, an aircrew helmet consists of two parts, the shell and the earmuffs. The contribution of the shell to the overall attenuation of the helmet is small and consequently will be disregarded for the purposes of this chapter. Helmets and headsets are thus identical in that they attempt to protect the ear by placing around it a sound-proofed cavity that is sealed by some means to the head and that contains a transducer for transmission of speech and non-verbal signals. Some lightweight headsets produced for quiet environments are little more than transducers. Other headsets, which are really ear defenders with built-in transducers, provide very good attenuation. The earmuff is composed of four basic parts – the shell, the seal, the internal damping and the transducer. Similarly, the attenuation characteristics of the headset can be split into three distinct regions – low, medium and high frequencies.

At low frequencies, below 400 Hz, the attenuation of the earshell is controlled by movement of the earshell against the head. Thus, the important parameters of the earshell are the shell volume, the spring stiffness of the earshell seals and the air volume, and the fit of the earshell on the head. Increasing the volume of the shell will invariably increase low-frequency attenuation, but at the cost of increases in bulk. A doubling of volume will result in a general increase of low-frequency attenuation of the order of 6 dB maximum. A further doubling is needed (four times the original volume) to gain up to another 6 dB.

In the intermediate frequency range, from 400 Hz to around 2 kHz, it is the transmission loss of noise through the shell walls that is important; thus, the type and mass of shell material are the overriding factors. The greater the mass, the greater the attenuation, all other factors being equal.

Above 2 kHz, the noise field inside the earshells becomes considerably more complex, and it is the damping material within the shell that absorbs the high frequency noise. Typical materials are plastic foam or glass-wool. A change of material will change the attenuation characteristic.

A further factor that is rarely considered is the inclusion of any subsidiary structures within the earshell, such as telephones and structures or plates to contain the damping materials. Improper support of these devices can be highly detrimental to attenuation between, and sometimes above, 500 Hz and 2 kHz.

Transmission of sound to the inner ear occurs not only by airborne means down the ear canal to the auditory system but also by direct transmission through the body, generally through the skull and bony parts of the head, when it is described as bone conduction. Normally, the body-conducted or bone-conducted sound is negligible below 500 Hz. Bone-conduction transmission is greatest around 1–2 kHz, where the useful attenuation of conventional hearing protectors may be limited to around 45 dB. This is becoming more important, particularly for ground crew and deck crew, as military engines are becoming noisier due to their higher power outputs.

However, although it is possible to state those parameters that may, or may not, improve headset attenuation, headset design is a series of compromises, such as weight versus bulk versus subjective acceptability. As such, the optimum headset, although possible to design in general terms, may not be acceptable for normal use.

The importance of the noise attenuation provided by the aircrew helmet is not to be underestimated. This is a function that it is required to perform daily, while other functions, e.g. protecting the wearer against impact, may never be needed. Within the size and weight constraints placed on the helmet, the attenuation characteristic using conventional techniques is probably as good as it could be, given the currently available materials (Figure 26.11a).

Only a little attenuation is provided at low frequencies for the aforementioned reasons, but since the amount of information in speech is small at frequencies below 300 Hz, small gains in speech intelligibility can be made by reducing noise levels at these lower frequencies, apart from in very noisy aircraft. However, the noise levels under the flying helmet in a fast jet (Figure 26.11b) peak at around 250 Hz, and these high noise levels considerably increase the risk of hearing damage. Further reductions in noise levels are necessary at these lower frequencies, which, by passive means, are not practical and, in some cases, not possible.

The increasing use, however, of active noise-control techniques, generally described as active noise reduction

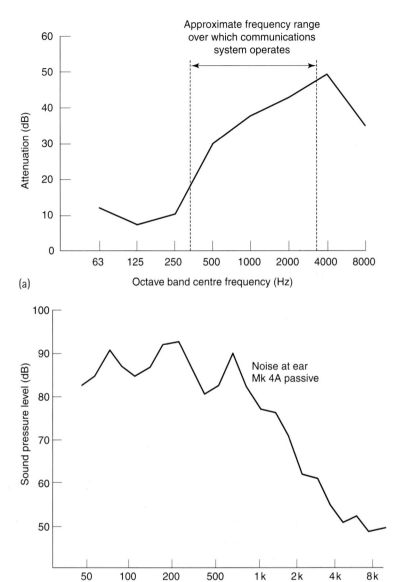

Figure 26.11 *(a) Attenuation of external noise provided by a modern protective helmet. Note that the attenuation is low at low frequencies. The approximate frequency range over which aircraft communication systems typically operate is also shown. (b) Noise levels at the ear under the helmet.*

(ANR), considerably increases the low-frequency attenuation that, without the attendant disadvantages of passive solutions, can be achieved. In simple terms, ANR is achieved by continuously sampling the noise in the earshell with a small microphone (Figure 26.12a). This signal is inverted in phase and then reintroduced into the shell by a telephone transducer, reducing the noise levels inside the earshell by destructive interference of the acoustic field. The increased helmet attenuation that can be achieved from the use of ANR is shown in Figure 26.12b. The reductions available from these analogue ANR systems are around 8–14 dB(A) and are different for fixed-wing, rotary-wing and transport aircraft due to the differences in the noise spectra for each of these aircraft. Results from flight trials in both fast jets (e.g. Harrier, Sea Harrier) and helicopters (e.g. Sea King, Lynx, Gazelle, UH60, UH1,

OH58D, AH64 Apache) confirm the validity of these results. This type of reduction, attained from the flick of a switch, significantly reduces the risk of noise-induced hearing impairment. Current ANR systems in the UK are fully compatible with current and future helmet design. Figure 26.13 shows a production ANR system contained within an existing UK helmet earshell with an insignificant increase in earshell mass.

The use of ANR brings noise levels at the aircrew ear in many operational aircraft down to a level at which hearing damage risk is within European and UK acceptable levels – at the time of writing 85 dB(A) – but this will be reduced in European Union (EU) countries in 2006 to a lower figure. There still remains a small risk at this 85 dB(A) level of around five per cent for those aircrew whose exposure does not exceed 85 dB(A), i.e. five pilots per 100 will suffer from

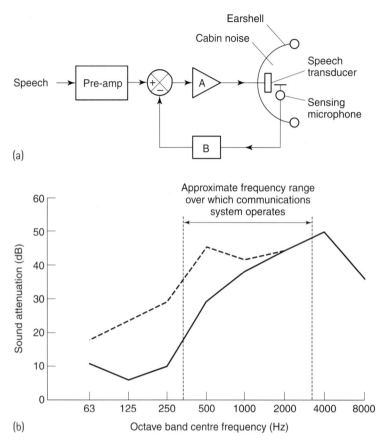

(a)

(b)

Figure 26.12   *(a) Schematic diagram of an active noise reduction system. The diagram shows how the noise inside the earshell is collected by the sensing microphone and fed back in a negative feedback loop via amplifier B, to be inverted in phase and fed through amplifier A back into the earshell via the speech transducer. The inverted phase noise from the feedback loop and the in-phase noise already in the earshell are mutually destructive, and the sound pressure levels in the earshell consequently are reduced. Since speech is also reduced in level, it is pre-amplified from its source and fed into the shell at an increased level, thus compensating for the active reduction of the speech levels. (b) Attenuation of external noise provided by a modern protective helmet is shown in the lower curve. Note that the acoustic attenuation is poor at low frequencies (below 250 Hz). The upper curve shows the extra acoustic attenuation afforded by a well-designed active noise reduction system, with increased protection from below 63 Hz up to 1 kHz.*

some form of socially unacceptable hearing loss. The level to which noise exposure will need to be reduced for a zero risk is in the region of 75 dB(A). Experimental work in the Ministry of Defence (MOD) research programmes at Farnborough is producing second-generation ANR systems that attain significantly higher levels of active attenuation; application of these techniques, as well as the development of active earplugs, are calculated to be able to reduce hearing damage risk in aircrew to close to zero risk levels.

EARPLUGS

Earplugs are an alternative to the conventional circumaural type of hearing protector and are defined as a hearing protector worn either within the external ear canal (aural)

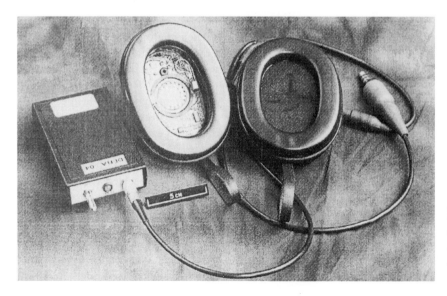

Figure 26.13   *Production active noise reduction system fitted to the earshell of an RAF aircrew helmet Mk 4 and Mk 10. The system requires only a 28-V aircraft supply to be fully operational.*

or in the concha against the external ear canal (supra-aural). There are several types, which follow the definitions of the European standard (draft) EN352-2. The categories are disposable, reusable, custom moulded and banded. For aircraft use, earplugs are often used under flying helmets to improve the overall attenuation. Although generally this helps to reduce the noise levels at the eardrum, the communications signal is also reduced in level, and raising the communication system output levels to maintain speech intelligibility may overload the communications system and induce distortion in the speech signal; therefore, it is not a generally recommended procedure to fit plugs and a helmet. Some earplugs include a transducer in the plug and introduce the speech signal directly into the ear canal, and this bypasses such problems.

There are some worries about the use of earplugs in fast jets, where explosive decompression is a possibility, and occlusion of the external ear canal may cause pressure differentials across the tympanic membrane between the Eustachian tube and the outer ear canal (see Figure 26.3 on p. 399 for visual explanation), which may be slow to equalize during explosive decompression, with the possibility of damage to the membrane.

For aircraft use in a harsh environment, there may be some comfort problems – depending, to a large extent, on the type of plug – and some potential for some interaction between the plug and the skin, particularly in hot environments, causing rashes. Ear plugs, however, do have good acoustic attenuation properties, particularly at low frequency, and do provide good levels of protection in appropriate circumstances.

ACTIVE EARPLUGS

In the past few years, there have been developments in the design and build of active earplugs. These earplugs work in a similar way to the helmet or headset ANR and provide similar active acoustic attenuation. They have some advantages, particularly when a device such as a nuclear, biological and chemical warfare hood needs to be worn under a flying helmet. The active plug allows a communication signal to be fed to the ear through the noise cancelling transducer (as with conventional earshell ANR). Transmission technology allows a wire-less connection between the headset and the earplug communication transducer.

Effects of high noise environments in military aviation

The principal effects of high noise levels in the aircraft cockpit and cabin are the risk of long-term hearing damage and the interference with the full range of aircraft communications. Hearing damage risk is a longer-term effect,

and communications interference can have an immediate effect on any aircraft sortie.

HEARING LOSS

When exposure to high noise levels ceases, a number of after effects may be manifest, which can be permanent or temporary. These effects include ringing in the ears (tinnitus), caused by continued firing in the auditory nerve (apparently a sort of irritative after-effect) and a partial deafness or reduced sensitivity to sound known as noise-induced temporary threshold shift (TTS). If exposure to loud noises is continued, then a permanent form of deafness, or permanent threshold shift (PTS), is manifested. Although permanent deafness is of more practical interest than TTS (TTS may, however, be important, for example to combat troops being discharged from a noisy troop-carrying aircraft), there is a relationship between the two quantities.

Permanent threshold shift

The risk to hearing damage from high noise levels was quantified in the late 1960s through a study of industrial workers exposed to a range of noise levels. The level of noise and the level of hearing loss was correlated. In the UK, the best correlation was with A-weighted noise energy. From this, the A-weighting and the allowances for time exposure (3 dB/doubling) were established. In the USA, a stronger industrial lobby prevented the level of 3 dB from being used, and a 5 dB level was chosen, making it far less stringent. The US military services used a compromise figure between the energy basis and the industrial figure and chose 4 dB. Science finally prevailed, and a level of 3 dB is now used worldwide. In the late 1960s, the figure of 90 dB(A) was chosen for continuous noise to represent an acceptable risk of damage, and this was the limit that should not be exceeded for a normal working lifetime. So, in practice, an L_{eq} (average noise level over an eight-hour period – an equivalent continuous noise level) of 90 dB(A) for an eight-hour working day should not be exceeded.

There remains, however, a finite risk at that level of some 12 per cent at 90 dB(A) and five per cent at 85 dB(A). To reach negligible risk, levels need to be reduced to an Leq of around 75 dB(A).

Over the years, industrial legislation has reduced the allowable limit to 85 dB(A) at the time of writing; this will be reduced further in the EU to 80 dB(A) in 2006, with an upper limit of 87 dB(A).

Since the Leq is a product of noise level and time, it is permissible to trade noise levels for decreases or increases in exposure time. This is implemented on an 'energy' basis;

for every doubling of noise level (3 dB(A)), the time exposure must be halved. Thus, if the allowable level is 85 dB(A) for an eight-hour exposure, then a level of 88 dB(A) can be allowed for only four hours and 91 dB(A) for two hours. Similarly, time exposures may be extended beyond eight hours if the levels are below 85 dB(A).

Temporary threshold shift

The degree of TTS is measured by subtracting the threshold data measured for an individual at a given time after a noise exposure from his resting (unexposed) threshold data. Since recovery of hearing after the exposure is fairly rapid, the time between the end of the exposure and the measurement of the hearing level is important. The frequency at which the maximum TTS is manifested is not necessarily that of the sound exposure. The maximum TTS generally occurs at a higher frequency than that of the sound that caused it (Figure 26.14). The greater degree of shift is found in the 3–6-kHz band. It is also this band that shows the greatest permanent loss due to continued exposure, in particular at 4 kHz. The magnitude of the TTS following exposure to a sound of a given pressure level is determined by the logarithm of the exposure time. When the length of the exposure is fixed, the magnitude of the TTS is determined by the SPL of the sound producing the TTS. The pressure level of the sound and the exposure time may be combined to describe the overall noise exposure or 'noise dose'. In a changing noise environment, this quantity is difficult to assess by independent measurements of SPL and duration of exposure; consequently, noise 'dose-meters' are available to give a direct readout of the integrated dose.

There is some evidence that there is a relationship between the TTS produced by a short exposure to a noise

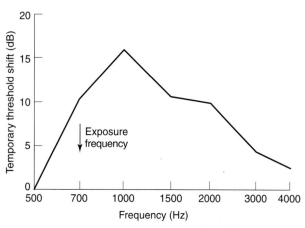

Figure 26.14 *Temporary threshold shift measured five minutes after the end of an exposure to a pure tone of 700 Hz for five minutes. The maximum shift occurred at a frequency of 1000 Hz.*

and the PTS brought about by continued exposure. It is suggested, for example, that if the TTS is measured two minutes after an eight-hour exposure, then this is equivalent in decibels to the ten-year PTS produced by exposure to the noise for eight hours per day. This is a statistical relationship that cannot be applied to the individual. TTS measured on a large number of individuals can be used, however, to make some predictions about the long-term hazards presented by the noise to that population.

ACCEPTABLE NOISE LEVELS

Acceptable noise depends largely on the reason for the need for acceptability. Acceptability for good speech communications is liable to be very different from that for the reduction of hearing damage risk. For instance, in aircraft cabin noise specifications, some compromises are made to the varying requirements, but generally, in both fixed- and rotary-wing aircraft, if the aircraft cabin noise meets the recommended levels, then the majority of criteria for acceptable noise levels will be satisfied.

For hearing damage alone, it is difficult to establish an 'acceptable' or 'safe' noise level, whether by retrospective or prospective means, because such a survey depends on a population that has been exposed to a reasonably constant source of noise for a long time. In a retrospective survey, some assumptions must be made about the original audiograms (which, almost certainly, will be unavailable). It is generally agreed that exposures to noises of less than 75–80 dB(A) produce no increase in deafness in a population. (A population becomes deafer as it grows older because of normal ageing processes – presbyacusis. When the effects of noise are referred to, what is meant is the increased incidence or level of deafness in a population, over that occurring by normal ageing.) Above this level, there is a relationship between the degree of PTS, the duration of the exposure and the SPL, and the frequency constitution of the noise.

The methods of calculating the hearing damage risk in specific conditions are simplified, but not degraded, by the requirements to measure the noise on the A weighting scale only.

Different daily exposures can be converted to a standard exposure by adjusting the effective sound pressure level, i.e. producing a 'loudness equivalent' (Leq), and thus the increased risk of deafness can be determined from a table (International Organization for Standardization 1999).

In industry, it is common practice for safety's sake to make the simple, easily supervised rule that all personnel should wear ear defenders whenever they work in an environment where the ambient noise is in excess of 85 dB(A). Military aircrew regularly wear the best ear protection available, and yet during normal operational flying they may be exposed to levels well in excess of 85 dB(A) despite protection. Early measurements in the 1970s in aircrew using the Mk 2/3 series of flying helmet, and in which acoustic attenuation was poor, showed a high incidence of hearing damage risk for many Royal Air Force, Royal Navy and Army Air Corps aircrew. The introduction of the Mk4 and Mk 10 helmets, with better acoustic attenuation, has reduced significantly the risk of hearing damage. Current measurements made under operational conditions for a number of aircraft (Harrier, Jaguar, Lynx, Hercules) generally show a reduced risk, but in noisier aircraft some risk still remains for a reasonable percentage of the aircrew.

Apart from the direct impingement of noise on the ear from cockpit or cabin noise causing a risk of hearing damage, another significant contributor to increased risk in aircraft operations is from the aircraft communications. Since the cochlea does not distinguish between noise, speech, music, etc. – this function is performed by higher centres in the brain – damage may occur not only by cabin noise but also by high communication levels or non-verbal signals. The noise dose may be measured at the ear directly by means of miniature microphones placed beneath the earmuff. This technique has shown that the contribution to the overall dose made by the communications signal is significant, and measurements in fixed-wing and rotary-wing aircraft show a contribution of between 6 and 10 dB(A), depending to a large extent on the time spent communicating. For instance, in a single-seat aircraft on a photo-reconnaissance mission, where there may be virtually no communication apart from during takeoff and landing, the communication contribution will be small. But in a two-seat jet or a multi seat helicopter, the inter-crew communication and communication with the outside world, particularly if a number of radio nets are in use, may raise the communications contribution to a significantly higher level. In general, it is possible to measure the noise emission at the ear of aircrew and, hence, to predict likely risk, but one cannot yet be certain whether the modern helmet worn properly in modern military aircraft sufficiently protects the hearing, as individual susceptibility to noise is a major factor. Final conclusions on this point can emerge only from the study of regular audiograms of aircrew and controls over a long period.

It is important to be aware that since individuals vary greatly in their susceptibility to hearing damage, there is no method for predicting individual risk of hearing damage. Current predictions are for groups of humans exposed to a given noise immission (a product of level and time of exposure) and will allow only prediction as to the percentage of the group that will suffer impairment, not the individuals within that group that will suffer. Personal audiograms, however, do allow an assessment of an individual's hearing loss directly and should be taken on a regular basis for aircrew, ground crew and others regularly exposed to high noise levels.

PSYCHOLOGICAL EFFECTS OF NOISE

Few people like noise. Aircrew operating noisy aircraft state that the noise causes fatigue, makes them irritated, and effectively increases their workload. They all regard it as some sort of flight safety hazard. It may be that these effects are direct consequences of the noise acting as a stressor, but this is unlikely. The effects that aircrew report probably arise from the increased difficulty in interpreting communications. Listening to speech is work in the sense that it is a form of information processing, i.e. it requires mental capacity and takes time.

Identification or response time to speech is related to the intelligibility of what is said. While intelligibility cannot, for practical reasons, be used as a convenient index of the workload generated by communications, response time can be.

Figure 26.15 shows the result of an experiment in which a subject was required to respond to a rapidly presented series of digits at various signal/noise ratios, both when the subject was concurrently performing a tracking task and when not. The time to respond to a list of digits is affected by the signal/noise ratio and by the addition of the other task, i.e. there is competition for the available mental

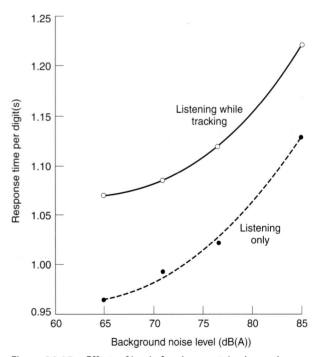

Figure 26.15 *Effects of level of environmental noise on time taken to respond to a rapidly presented series of digits. The higher the background noise, i.e. the lower the signal/noise ratio, the longer the response time. When the subject had to perform a tracking task as well as a listening task, the response time at a given signal/noise ratio was increased.*

capacity between the person's normal piloting activities and his or her communications processing requirements. This competition is aggravated by reduced intelligibility (increasing the noise level), and it should not be regarded as surprising that the result is fatigue and irritation produced by this effective increase in workload.

In the laboratory, noise may certainly be shown to act as a stressor, affecting the performance of tasks, producing 'narrowing of attention' as well as making other tasks (e.g. memorizing of some sort of material) more difficult, although it is not easy to design experiments that are free of extraneous influences. There are, however, a number of generalized statements that can be made on noise levels, the task involved and the individual characteristics of the operator.

For the noise field, the following parameters may affect task performance:

- Continuous noise with specific meaning to the task involved generally will not impair performance below 90 dB(A).
- Intermittent noise and impulsive noise generally are more disruptive than continuous noise at the same level.
- High-frequency components of noise generally have a more adverse affect on performance than the lower-frequency content.
- Noise tends to increase errors and variability rather than directly affect work rate.

It has been shown that greater performance decrements are attributable to noise when the task involves continuous operation or requires prolonged vigilance or two tasks are performed simultaneously compared with tasks that require simple repetition. In fact, in simple repetitive tasks, the overall performance may be enhanced by noise. Tasks that involve perception of auditory cues are, per se, most susceptible to noise impairment.

Where individual differences are concerned, identical levels of noise and exposure will affect different operators in (sometimes radically) different ways. Essentially, this will depend on the operator's previous experience in performing the task under conditions of noise, the levels of arousal and motivation, and generally the personality; introverts may be more affected than extroverts.

Other stressors, such as vibration, heat, hypoxia and loss of sleep, are known to interact with noise and result in synergistic effects, i.e. the combined effect is greater than the sum of the individual effects. An example is in the perception of ride quality in aircraft, where ride quality is assessed more severely under conditions of noise and vibration together than an assessment using the sum of the two individual stress contributors.

A further parameter is duration of exposure, since the adverse effects of noise appear to be cumulative, involving a large decrease in performance at the end of the task period – particularly important if the period of exposure is prolonged.

In many ways, defining the effects of noise on human performance is like trying to define annoyance. Both are a function of many parameters, human and environmental, and research results, generally available on a statistical basis, apply only to groups of people and not to individuals. The psychological effects of noise are weighted differently under different conditions. Much effort, ingenuity and skill may be needed to carry out tasks under adverse noise conditions. There are innumerable ways of completing a task, and even under ideal conditions humans vary in the way they approach and deal with each phase of the problem. Welford (1978) notes: 'Performance and workload appear, therefore, to depend upon the interaction of four factors: the demands of the task; the capacities of the performer; the strategies used to relate demands to capacities; and, when a range of strategies is available, skill in choosing the most efficient.' He goes on to look at each variable and, when discussing strategy, states: 'The precise strategy adopted on any one occasion for a particular task involves a synthesis of various generic strategies, all of which are necessary for the particular performance, but none of which is sufficient alone. This is true for familiar activities repeated on different occasions, and is even more true of the strategies adopted when tackling an entirely novel task.'

All of these problems point strongly to the wide range of difficulties in producing a general model of human performance, but there remains general agreement that high levels of noise in the crew compartment have a deleterious effect on performance, and this is supported by increasing anecdotal and empirical evidence drawn from comparisons of quieter combat aircraft, such as the Tornado, with less quiet aircraft.

REFERENCES

International Organization for Standardization. Normal equal loudness contours for pure tones and normal threshold of hearing under free field listening conditions. ISO R 226:1961. Geneva: International Organization for Standardization, 1961.

International Organization for Standardization. Assessment of occupational noise exposure for hearing conservation purposes. ISO R 1999. Geneva: International Organization for Standardization, 1999.

Kryter KD. *The Effect of Noise on Man*. New York: Academic Press, 1970.

Stevens SS. Calculation of the loudness of a complex noise. *Journal of the Acoustical Society of. America* 1956; **28**: 807–32.

Welford AT. Mental workload as a function of. demand, capacity, strategy and skill. *Ergonomics* 1978; **21**: 151–67.

Zwicker E. Ein Verfahren zur Berechnung der Lautstärke. *Acustica* 1960; **10**: 304–8.

FURTHER READING

American National Standards Institute. Definitions and procedures for computing the effective perceived noise level for flyover aircraft noise. ANSI S6.4 (1973). Washington, DC: American National Standards Institute, 1973.

American National Standards Institute. Method for the measurement of real ear protection of hearing protectors. ANSI S12.6 (1984)/ASA STD 1 (1975). Washington, DC: American National Standards Institute, 1984.

American National Standards Institute. Design response of weighting networks for acoustical measurements. ANSI SI.42 (1986). Washington, DC: American National Standards Institute, 1986.

Beranek LL. *Noise Reduction.* New York: McGraw-Hill, 1960.

Beranek LL. *Noise and Vibration Control.* New York: McGraw-Hill, 1971.

British Standards Institution. The relation between the sone scale of loudness and the phon scale of loudness level. BS 3045 (1958). London: British Standards Institution, 1958.

British Standards Institution. The normal threshold of hearing for fine tones by earphone listening. BS 2497 (1972). London: British Standards Institution. 1972.

British Standards Institution. BS 5108 (1974). Method of measurement of hearing protectors at threshold. BS 5108 (1974). London: British Standards Institution, 1974.

British Standards Institution. Estimating the risk of hearing handicap due to noise exposure. BS 5330 (1976). London: British Standards Institution, 1976.

British Standards Institution. Measurement of sound attenuation of hearing protectors. BS 5108 (1983)/ISO 4869 (1981). London: British Standards Institution, 1981.

Broch JP. *Acoustic Noise Measurement.* Naerum, Denmark: Bruel and Kjaer, 1971.

Burns W. *Noise and Man.* London: John Murray, 1973.

International Organization for Standardization. Expression of the physical and subjective magnitudes of sound or noise. ISO R 131 (1959). Geneva: International Organization for Standardization, 1959.

International Organization for Standardization. Assessment of noise with respect to community response. ISO R 1996 (1971). Geneva: International Organization for Standardization, 1971.

International Organization for Standardization. Guide to the measurement of airborne acoustical noise and evaluation of its effects on man. ISO 2204 (1973). Geneva: International Organization for Standardization, 1973.

International Organization for Standardization. Specification for precision sound level meters. IEC 179. Geneva: International Organization for Standardization, 1973.

International Organization for Standardization. Preferred frequencies for acoustical measurements. ISO R 266 (1975). Geneva: International Organization for Standardization, 1975.

Kryter KD. *Physiological, Psychological and Social Effects of Noise.* Washington, DC: National Aeronautics and Space Administration, 1984.

May DN. *Handbook of Noise Assessment.* New York: Van Nostrand Reinhold, 1978.

Miller RD. *Effects of Noise on People.* Washington, DC: US Environmental Protection Agency, 1971.

Peterson APG, Gross EE. *Handbook of Noise Measurement.* Concord: General Radio, 1972.

US Department of Defense. General specification for sound pressure levels in aircraft. MIL-S-8806B (1970). Washington, DC: US Department of Defense, 1970.

US Department of Defense. Acoustical noise limits in helicopters. MIL-STD-1294 (1981). Washington, DC: US Department of Defense, 1981.

Welch B, Welch AS. *Psychological Effects of Noise.* New York: Plenum Press, 1970.

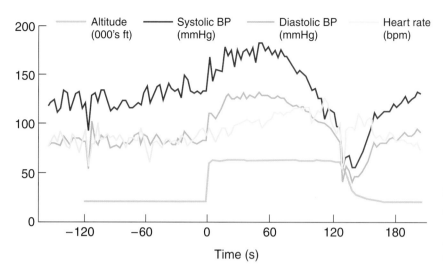

Figure 4.8 *A graph of blood pressure and heart rate during a rapid decompression which shows a PPB induced syncope. Time zero represents the moment of rapid decompression.*

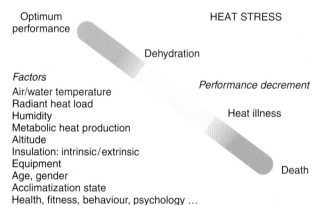

Optimum performance

Factors
Air/water temperature
Radiant heat load
Humidity
Metabolic heat production
Altitude
Insulation: intrinsic/extrinsic
Equipment
Age, gender
Acclimatization state
Health, fitness, behaviour, psychology …

HEAT STRESS

Dehydration

Performance decrement

Heat illness

Death

Figure 13.2 *Effects of heat on the body.*

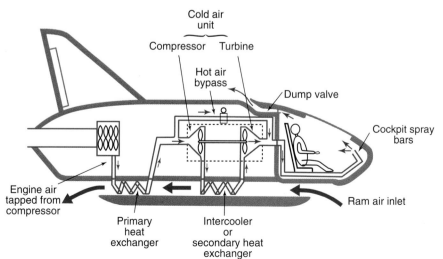

Figure 13.3 *Schematic diagram showing the arrangement of the main components of a typical environmental control system.*

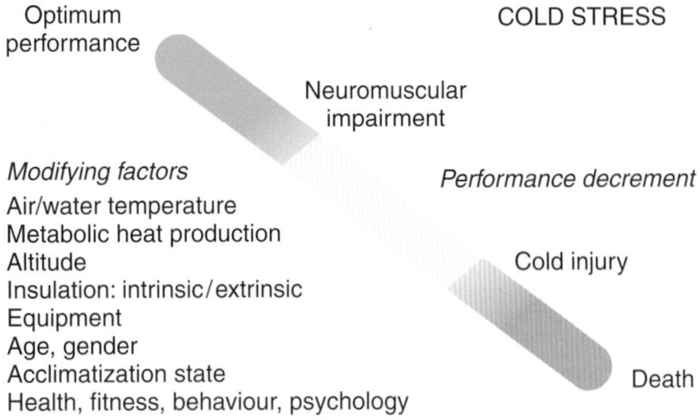

Optimum performance

COLD STRESS

Neuromuscular impairment

Modifying factors
Air/water temperature
Metabolic heat production
Altitude
Insulation: intrinsic/extrinsic
Equipment
Age, gender
Acclimatization state
Health, fitness, behaviour, psychology

Performance decrement

Cold injury

Death

Figure 13.5 *Effects of cold on the body.*

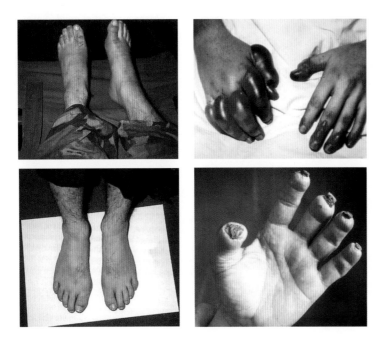

Figure 13.7 *Non-freezing and freezing cold injuries.*

Table 13.5 *Heat stress index (coloured numbers represent 'heat sensation')*

Relative humidity (%)	Air temperature (°C)										
	46.1 21.1	48.9 23.9	26.7	29.4	32.2	35	37.8	40.6	43.3	46.1	48.9
0	17.7	20.6	22.8	25.6	28.3	30.6	32.8	35	37.2	39.4	41.7
10	18.3	21.1	23.9	26.7	29.4	32.2	35	37.8	40.6	43.9	46.7
20	18.9	22.2	25	27.8	30.6	33.9	37.2	40.6	44.4	48.9	54.4
30	19.4	22.8	25.6	28.9	32.2	35.6	40	45	50.6	57.2	64.4
40	20	23.3	26.1	30	33.9	38.3	43.3	50.6	58.3	66.1	
50	20.6	23.9	27.2	31.1	35.6	41.7	48.9	57.2	65.6		
60	21.1	24.4	27.8	32.2	37.8	45.6	55.6	65			
70	21.1	25	29.4	33.9	41.1	51.1	62.2				
80	21.7	25.6	30	36.1	45	57.8					
90	21.7	26.1	31.1	38.9	50						
100	22.2	26.7	32.8	42.2							

32.2–40.6 °C: possibility of heat cramps during exercise.
40.6–54.4 °C: heat cramps or heat exhaustion likely; heat stroke possible.
54.4 °C +: heat stroke a definite risk.

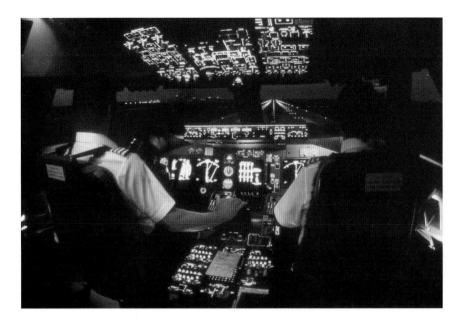

Figure 23.6 *Boeing 747-400 flight deck.*

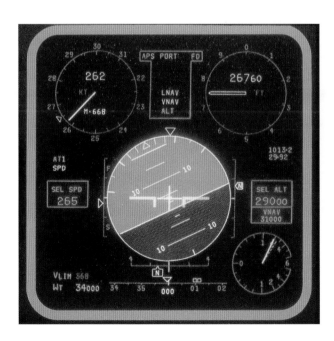

Figure 23.10 *Electronic instrument display.*

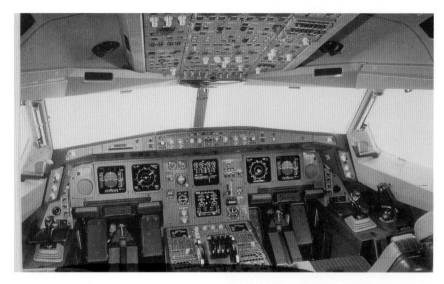

Figure 23.11 *Airbus flight deck.*

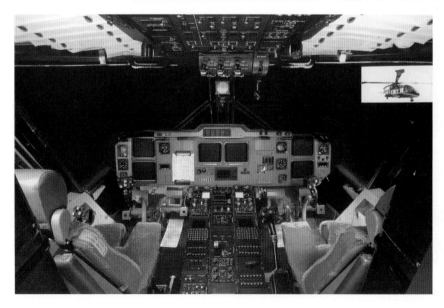

Figure 23.12 *EH 101 Merlin flight deck.*

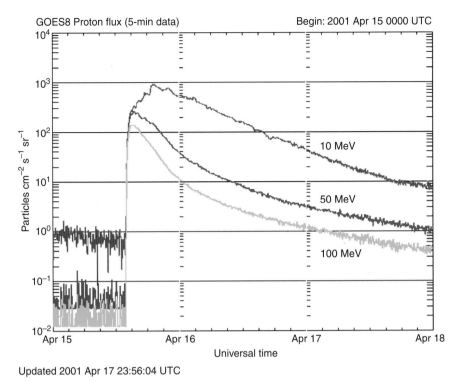

GOES8 Proton flux (5-min data)   Begin: 2001 Apr 15 0000 UTC

10 MeV

50 MeV

100 MeV

Updated 2001 Apr 17 23:56:04 UTC

Figure 27.3 *Proton flux for three energy intervals – E>10 MeV, E> 50 MeV and E> 100 MeV – measured by the GOES8 satellite during the 15 April 2001 event. Data provided by the National Oceanic and Atmospheric Administration (NPAA), Space Environment Center (SEC), Boulder, CO, USA.*

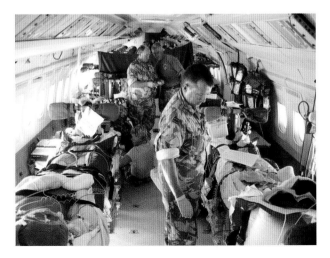

Figure 31.1 *Example of multipatient care.*

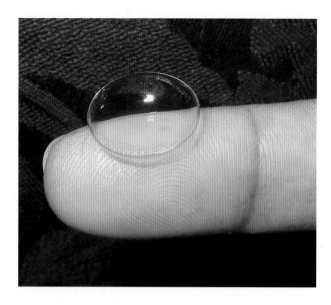

Figure 46.4   *Contact lens on finger.*

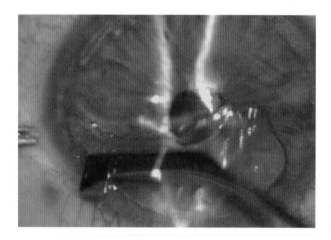

Figure 46.6   *Temporary removal of corneal epithelium during laser epithelial keratomileusis (LASEK).*

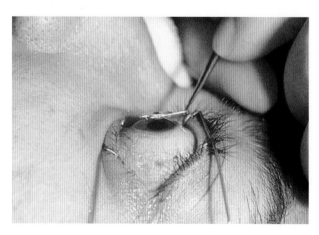

Figure 46.7   *Partial-thickness corneal laser in-situ keratomileusis (LASIK) flap before excimer laser treatment.*

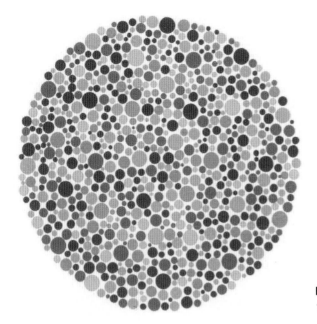

Figure 46.9 *Ishihara plate test card. The number '5' is read by red/green colour-normal people.*

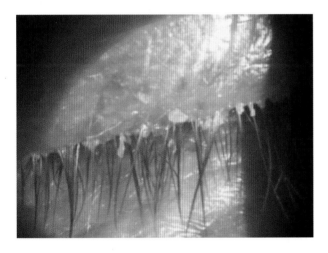

Figure 46.12 *Anterior blepharitis.*

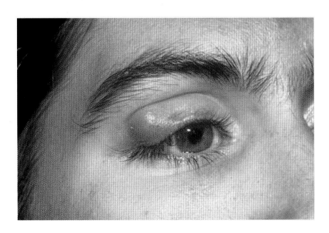

Figure 46.13 *Meibomian cyst (chalazion).*

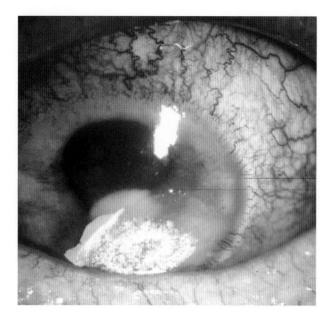

Figure 46.14 *Microbial keratitis in a wearer of soft contact lenses. The white precipitate is from the topical ofloxacin treatment.*

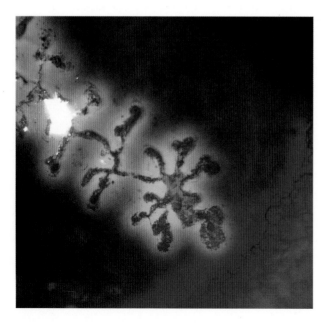

Figure 46.15 *Dendritic corneal ulcer.*

27

Aircrew and cosmic radiation

DENIS O'SULLIVAN AND DAZHUANG ZHOU

INTRODUCTION

Exposure to radiation is difficult to avoid on the Earth. As we go about our daily lives, several sources irradiate us, even at ground level. Most of us receive our greatest radiation dose from natural radiation. The main contribution comes from radon, a gas that is produced when uranium in soil and rocks undergoes radioactive decay. Radon decays to form short-lived radioactive particles. All of these stages involve human exposure to radiation. Radon accounts for approximately 50 per cent of the total dose received from natural sources. The unit of measurement is the becquerel (Bq), which is defined as one disintegration per second of radon atoms. The national average exposure in the home in the UK is 20 Bq per cubic metre of air, but levels can greatly exceed this value, depending on local geological conditions and the concentration of uranium. For instance, very high values have been recorded in Cornwall and in south-west Ireland. It is estimated that the lifetime risk of lung cancer from a lifetime of exposure to radon levels of 200 Bq/m^3 is about three per cent.

Another 40 per cent of the total radiation dose is a result of exposure to gamma radiation from the ground and buildings (14 per cent); from medical, dental and veterinary sources (14 per cent); and from the food and drink we consume (12 per cent). The next biggest contribution at sea level is from secondary cosmic radiation (10 per cent). People involved in the nuclear industry can receive additional radiation.

As discussed later, radiation dose is measured in units called sieverts (Sv); this unit takes into account the damage caused by a particular type of radiation. The millisievert (mSv) is one-thousandth of a sievert. In Britain and Ireland, the average radiation dose received from all natural sources at ground level is approximately 3 mSv per year. This is equivalent to about 150 times the dose received from a normal chest X-ray. The cosmic ray contribution is about 0.3 mSv per year and is relatively small due to the fact that it has its origin outside the Earth's environment and its intensity is reduced greatly by the shielding effect of the atmosphere. Its impact on radiation exposure of human beings becomes more significant as we travel upwards from the Earth's surface; at aircraft altitudes, it becomes the predominant radiation source.

COSMIC RADIATION

Cosmic rays were discovered by an Austrian physicist, Victor Hess. In 1911, Hess carried out experiments on board a balloon, reaching altitudes of up to 5 km in the atmosphere. Our knowledge of this galactic radiation, which comes from sources outside our solar system, is quite extensive due to several decades of research using high-altitude balloons and satellites. This radiation continually bombards the top of the Earth's atmosphere with equal intensity from all directions. Information on the direction of cosmic ray sources is lost completely due to scattering in interstellar magnetic fields. About 98 per cent of cosmic radiation is composed of nuclear particles; the remainder comprises electrons, positrons and antiprotons. Of the nuclei, approximately 87 per cent are protons (hydrogen), 12 per cent are helium and the remainder are heavier nuclei, representing all the elements of the periodic table. Measurement of the relative abundances of the heavier nuclei shows significant levels of elements such as lithium, beryllium and boron, which are very rare in the rest of the universe. It is now accepted that this is one of the many indications that cosmic rays travel through several g/cm² of interstellar matter from source to Earth and break up into lower-charged species, producing the light elements from carbon, nitrogen and oxygen. Relative to general abundances in the solar system, there are also greater abundances of secondary elements, such as fluorine, scandium, titanium, vanadium and chromium, in the cosmic radiation. All elements known in the periodic table up to and including the actinides are present in cosmic radiation, but the contribution of very heavy elements is very small and does not make any significant impact on radiation exposure in the Earth's atmosphere.

Galactic cosmic rays are believed to be produced mainly by acceleration of ambient interstellar matter to high energies by shockwaves from exploding supernovae. The energy of cosmic ray particles is usually given in units of kinetic energy per nucleon (eV/N), which allows a description of some features that are independent of the element in question. In the energy regions above about 1 GeV (10^9 eV) to 10^{14} eV/nucleon, the energy spectra of all species from protons up to the actinide elements appear to be represented by a single-power law:

$$N(E) \propto E^{-2.65 \pm 0.5}$$

where N is the number of particles and E is the kinetic energy per nulceon.

As cosmic rays impinge on the Earth's atmosphere, they lose energy through interactions with atoms of air and are slowed down. In order to penetrate right down to sea level, a proton needs to have an energy of ~2 GeV. Energy is used up in the production of new secondary particles such as neutrons, protons, kaons and pions. These secondary particles can repeat the same process, producing successive interactions and forming a cascade of particles down through the atmosphere, as shown in Figure 27.1. However, muons are produced by the decay of pions; because they are very weakly interacting, they can survive to sea level and are responsible for most of the cosmic ray component that we all experience from day to day. Further up in the atmosphere, in the region of 8000–17 000 m, where commercial aircraft fly, the radiation field is very complex, consisting of some of the original primary particles and secondary products, all travelling at speeds that are a significant fraction of the speed of light. The flux of particles reaches a maximum known as the Pfotzer maximum at approximately 20 km (65 000 feet) above sea level.

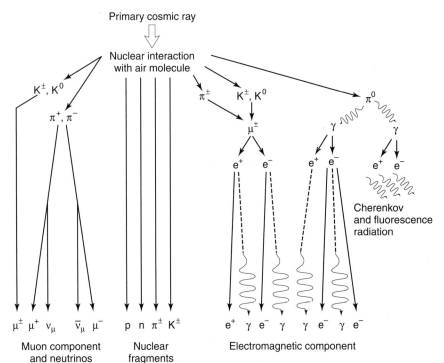

Figure 27.1 *Particle cascade produced by high-energy cosmic rays.*

Solar modulation of galactic cosmic rays

Galactic cosmic rays observed at Earth have been affected by their passage through the solar system. They interact with the outflowing solar wind, which is a plasma travelling into space from the solar corona. This ionized gas contains an embedded magnetic field, which causes a deceleration of the charged particles coming from outside the solar system. The effect of the solar modulation can be likened to the influence that an electric potential (heliocentric potential) ϕ centred on the sun would have against charged particles entering our solar system from outside. During a period of high solar activity, as indicated by increased numbers of sunspots on the sun's surface, the amount of matter ejected from the sun increases and the solar wind intensity increases. The effect on galactic cosmic rays rises during these occasions and the flux of particles observed at Earth diminishes. Solar modulation follows a 22-year activity cycle, as shown in Figure 27.2, which in turn consists of two 11-year cycles separated by reversal of the sun's magnetic field. Thus, cosmic ray intensity observed at Earth reaches a maximum every 11 years (quiet sun) followed by minimum intensity (active sun). The main effect at solar maximum is to sweep the lower-energy particles out of the Earth's environment and, thus, lower the total flux observed. Recently, solar maximum period peaked around 2000–02 and the next one is expected around 2011. Between these periods, solar activity will decrease to minimum in approximately 2006 and galactic cosmic ray intensity at Earth will increase. Thus, to summarize, when solar maximum arrives, more solar energetic particles are observed but the galactic component decreases. At solar minimum, fewer solar energetic particles are present and galactic component is greatest.

An important ground-based instrument for studying variations in the intensity in the interplanetary spectrum is the neutron monitor. Among the products of the interaction of the primary cosmic rays in the atmosphere are protons and neutrons. Since neutrons are not slowed down by ionization losses because they have zero charge, they can penetrate deeply into the atmosphere. Early work in recording neutron fluxes at ground level was pioneered by the late John Simpson and colleagues at the University of Chicago. By surrounding the monitor with a combination of lead sheets to increase the reaction rate and a moderating material such as paraffin to slow down the neutrons, a very efficient detector was developed. A network of neutron monitor stations was set up over a wide range of geomagnetic latitudes, starting in the 1950s. Some of these stations have been operating successfully since then and have been recording ground-level events (GLEs) associated with major solar events. These events are quite rare, occurring on average about once a year. High-latitude stations have a better chance of determining the source direction because of the combined effects of the Earth's magnetic field and the atmosphere. Neutron monitors contributed to the investigation of dose enhancement on board aircraft during the GLE of 15 April 2001 (Spurny and Datchev 2001).

SOLAR PARTICLE RADIATION

Energetic particles from the sun impinge on the Earth's atmosphere from time to time. Solar particle events produced by sudden release of energy in the solar atmosphere (solar flares) and coronal mass ejections (CMEs) can influence radiation levels deep into the atmosphere. In the former case, charged particles, including electrons, protons and heavier charged particles, escape from the sun and spiral around the interplanetary magnetic field lines, which expand into interplanetary space like the jet of a rotating garden hose. The Earth is connected to certain regions in the sun by these field lines. If the particle source area is not well connected to the Earth, then the flux of solar particles can make a significant contribution to the intensity at 10 MeV observed at the top of the atmosphere and compete with the galactic component. However, if the source region is well connected and produces high particle fluxes, then we have a so-called solar energetic particle event (SPE). These events can last for hours or even several days. SPEs are relatively rare and occur most often during the maximum phase of the 11-year solar cycle. They reach a peak of a few per year around solar maximum.

The mechanisms that produce SPEs within the sun and solar corona are poorly understood, although substantial progress has been made in recent years. There has been a significant change in our thinking regarding the source of

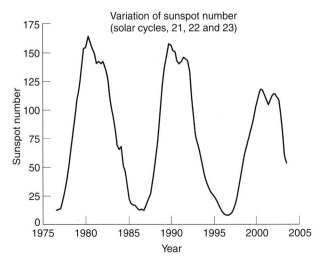

Figure 27.2 *Eleven-year cycle of solar activity.*

SPEs (Smart and Shea 1997). For nearly four decades, it was assumed that SPEs were produced by solar flares because of the sometimes large transient increases in the particle fluence rate found to be associated with them. A new process has been identified, such that the generation of very energetic particles is thought to be the result of acceleration associated with interplanetary shocks generated by fast coronal mass ejections (Reames 1995). About half of the SPEs observed at 1 astronomical unit (AU) (distance from Earth to sun) can be associated with specific solar flares, and the intensity–time profiles for many SPEs show that acceleration by interplanetary shocks has occurred.

So far, it has not been possible to predict SPEs. However, X-rays and other types of electromagnetic radiation are emitted during SPE events and travel at the speed of light and in straight lines, since they are not influenced by solar magnetic and geomagnetic fields. X-rays from the solar active region reach the Earth in approximately eight minutes. Times for energetic solar particles to reach Earth range from more than eight minutes for relativistic particles whose energies are greater than several hundred mega-electron-volts per nucleon, to hours for lower-energy (≤ 20 MeV/nucleon) particles. Thus, since lower-energy solar protons arrive at the Earth several hours later than X-rays, a brief warning signal is observable.

The intensities of solar protons observed near the Earth during SPEs have been the subject of regular investigations for several solar cycles. The proton flux spectra are measured by geostationary observational environment satellites (GOES). Several SPEs had total proton fluences in excess of 10^{10}/cm^2. An event observed in February 1956 had the spectrum with the largest fraction of high-energy particles of any extremely large SPE measured to date, with fluence of > 1-GeV protons in excess of 10^7/cm^2. This was followed by the November 1960 SPE, with a > 400-MeV proton spectrum in excess of 10^7/cm^2. Some of the largest SPEs on record occurred within three months in 1989. These events all resulted in doses in excess of 50 Gy in low-Earth orbit, the October 1989 SPE having a dose above 30 Gy. The largest SPEs are the most likely to result in both early and late health effects in space crew and aircrew and biological systems.

Of particular interest to the present discussion is the solar event of 15 April 2001. This is shown in Figure 27.3. The upper curve shows the flux of particles with energy greater than 10 MeV, the middle curve the flux of particles with energy greater than 50 MeV, and the lower curve the flux of particles with energy greater than 100 MeV. The particle intensities of all three groups rose by a factor of more than 1000 above the background levels seen early on 15 April. This produced a GLE that was observed at several neutron monitor locations on Earth. As discussed later, instruments on an aircraft en route from Europe to the USA succeeded in measuring the effect of this solar event on dose rate.

Having survived their passage through the interplanetary medium, cosmic ray particles face a further obstacle as they approach Earth. They are deflected by the Earth's magnetic field, and their ability to penetrate to the Earth depends on their momentum per unit charge, $(pc)/(Ze)$,

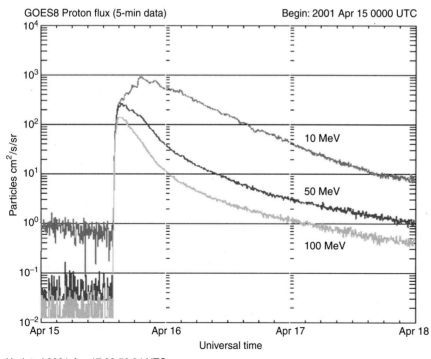

Figure 27.3 *Proton flux for three energy intervals – E > 10 MeV, E > 50 MeV and E > 100 MeV – measured by the GOES8 satellite during the 15 April 2001 event. Data provided by the National Oceanic and Atmospheric Administration (NPAA), Space Environment Center (SEC), Boulder, CO, USA. See also colour plate 27.3.*

known as rigidity (R). Particles below a certain cut-off rigidity, R_c, do not succeed and are deflected away. R_c has a maximum value at the Equator, where the cosmic ray particles move perpendicularly to the Earth's field lines. R_c is equal to zero at the magnetic poles, where the motion is parallel to the field lines. In order to penetrate at the Equator, a particle must have a kinetic energy value of ~17.6 GV (17.6 GeV per proton). This means that particle intensity will increase as one travels from the Equatorial region to the poles.

RADIATION FIELD AT AIRCRAFT ALTITUDE

Aircrew and passengers, while enjoying a certain amount of protection from the typical 100–300 g/cm^2 of air above them, are not as well shielded as people at ground level or as vulnerably exposed as astronauts. Aircrew and passengers travel in a radiation environment that is quite complicated and of sufficiently high level that the need for a major programme of investigation was recognized some years ago. Interest in the matter was motivated largely by three main developments. First, there was concern that the relative biological damage caused by neutrons may have been underestimated in the past. As we will see later, neutrons occur in significant numbers at aircraft altitudes, and it was agreed that a thorough study of this contribution to the radiation field was necessary. Second, there has been a tendency for aircraft to cruise at higher altitudes, thus increasing exposure to radiation. Third, the International Commission on Radiological Protection (ICRP) made a series of recommendations concerning exposure to cosmic rays. Following the ICRP guidelines, the European Council revised its Basic Safety Standards Directive (Directive 96/29/EURATOM) to include, for the first time, exposure to naturally occurring sources of ionizing radiation, including cosmic radiation, as a natural hazard. Since the beginning of solar cycle 23, starting around 1993, a number of investigations prompted by these considerations have greatly extended our knowledge of the components of the radiation field at aircraft altitudes as well as their dependence on latitude, altitude and stage of solar cycle. The problems involved in measuring cosmic radiation at high altitudes are much more complex than those encountered at sea level by, for example, the nuclear industry. The wide range of particles and energies (which can be thousands of times greater than at sea level) requires a very different approach. Several different detector systems have been adapted for use in aircraft, and much effort has gone into understanding their response characteristics in this complicated radiation environment.

Over the past decade, a number of European Union (EU)-supported projects have been undertaken. At the time of writing, the most recent project, DOSMAX (dosimetry of

aircrew exposure to radiation during solar maximum), is nearing completion as solar cycle 23 approaches its end. DOSMAX is a collaboration involving a number of major European research laboratories, including the National Radiological Protection Board (NRPB; the UK), the Physikalisch-Technische Bundesanstalt (PTB; Germany), the Austrian Research Centers in Seibersdorf (ARCS), the Institut de radioprotection et de sûreté nucléaire (IRSN; France), the Agenzia per la protezione dell'ambiente e per i servizi tecnici (APAT; Italy), the Swedish Radiation Protection Authority (SSI) and the Dublin Institute for Advanced Studies (DIAS; Ireland), which acts as overall coordinator. These have been joined at various stages by scientists at the Nuclear Physics Institute (NPI; Czech Republic), the National Research Center for Environment and Health (GSF; Germany), the European Centre for Particle Physics (CERN; Switzerland) and the University of Munich (Germany), allowing a wide range of expertise in cosmic radiation studies and radiation protection to be combined. Investigations have also been carried out by other groups in the USA, Canada and Europe.

Detection methods at aircraft altitude

Choice and development of instrumentation, both active and passive, is influenced by the fact that the radiation field is complex, varies with altitude, geomagnetic latitude and heliocentric potential, and has to be operated in aircraft. Passive detectors, which are analysed after flight and do not involve electronic components, are accepted by airlines without difficulty. Exposure of active detectors generally requires more detailed planning, and consideration of electromagnetic cleanliness is important in order that there is no interference with the aircraft's electronic systems. The main active detector used in recent years is the tissue-equivalent proportional counter (TEPC), which provides not only complete measurements of the cosmic ray field and associated total dose equivalents but also the micro-dosimetric distribution of the radiation as a function of energy deposited in the detector. Geiger-Müller counters and ionization chambers have also been used. The dosimetric telescope (dostel) (Beaujean *et al.* 1999), an instrument developed originally for space flight, based on two identical implanted planar silicon detectors, and designed to measure the energy deposited by charged particles, has also provided many data. Passive detectors such as nuclear-track detectors, neutron-bubble detectors, thermoluminescent detectors (TLDs) and bismuth-fission detectors are used for different ranges of linear energy transfer (LET). Several developments have improved our understanding of the response characteristics of these detectors, and several modifications have enhanced their performance in the complicated radiation field. A detailed description of some of these detection methods can be found in Lindborg *et al.* (2004).

CALIBRATION AND INTERCOMPARISON OF INSTRUMENTATION

In order to understand the output from cosmic ray detectors, it is necessary to know how the instrument responds to the energy deposited by various particles, such as protons, neutrons, electrons, gamma-rays, mesons and heavy nuclei, all of which are present in the radiation field at aircraft altitudes. Fortunately, there are now several facilities available throughout the world where radiation conditions at aircraft altitude can be simulated using neutron, photon, heavy-ion and other particle beams. A reference field for the calibration and inter-comparison of active and passive detectors in neutron fields has been operating at CERN since 1992. A beam of protons and pions with momentum of 120 GeV/c impinges on a copper target. The secondary particles produced as a result of nuclear interactions traverse a shield of either concrete or iron. With this arrangement, a neutron spectrum similar to that at aircraft altitudes is produced, and both active and passive instruments can be calibrated and compared. Most of the investigations of aircrew exposure to radiation have included this facility in their research programmes over the past decade. Calibrations in neutron fields are also carried out at the Université Catholique de Louvain (UCL; Louvain la Neuve, Belgium), PTB (Braunschweig, Germany), the Svedberg Laboratory (TSL; Uppsala, Sweden) and the iThemba Laboratory for Accelerator Based Sciences (South Africa). Each of these facilities provides neutrons of a particular energy range and fluence. For instance, the iThemba facility provides neutrons with energies up to 200 MeV and can cover the whole spectral range observed in the secondary cosmic radiation. A high-energy photon beam produced at PTB has been used to simulate the low-LET electron and photon field at flight altitudes. High-energy heavy ions such as carbon, neon and iron also play a role in calibration. Heavy-ion accelerators at Gesellschaft für Schwerionenforschung (GSI; Darmstadt, Germany), Brookhaven (the USA) and the Heavy Ion Medical Accelerator in Chiba (HIMAC; Japan) have provided essential calibration facilities for detectors that determine dose through the measurement of LET spectra at altitudes. The consistency and quality of data obtained in recent investigations of radiation exposure of aircrew and astronauts have been due largely to the availability of these beams.

DOSE AND RELATED QUANTITIES

The basic quantity of radiation dosimetry is dose D, or absorbed dose, which is the amount of energy absorbed per unit mass of material when exposed to radiation and is measured in joules/kilogram. The unit of absorbed dose is the gray (Gy):

$$1 \, \text{Gy} = 1 \, \text{J/kg}$$

The dose rate is then

$$D = \text{d}D/\text{d}T$$

Linear energy transfer

The concept of LET is of central importance to the interaction of radiation with matter, including human tissue. There have been many attempts to find a model that describes the deposition of energy in matter caused by the passage of charged particles. One of the most successful of these is the restricted energy loss (REL) model, which takes account of the damage done by secondary ionization produced by low-energy electrons (delta-rays). REL is the portion of total energy loss that produces delta-rays of energy less than some specified value, E_Δ, and only this part of energy loss is relevant to the damage process. The quantity $(\text{d}E/\text{d}X)_{E < E_\Delta}$ is known as the LET and is usually expressed in units of KeV/μm. LET depends on the material through which the charged particle is travelling. To emphasize this dependence, the quantity is written as, for example, in the case of water, LET (H_2O). Absorbed dose can be determined from a knowledge of the fluence of particles and their LET distribution.

Relative biological effectiveness

Early studies of the effect of identical doses of different types of radiation on biological systems showed that they produced different amounts of damage. This gave rise to the concept of relative biological effectiveness (RBE), which is defined as the ratio of the dose of a particular type of radiation to the dose of gamma-rays or X-rays that yield the same biological end point. In order to take into account the RBE of different types of radiation, the ICRP has recommended a number of quantities that are based on weighting absorbed dose. Dose equivalent is one of these. The unit of dose equivalent is the sievert (Sv).

The dose equivalent H is defined as

$$H(\text{LET}) = Q(\text{LET}) \times D(\text{LET})$$

where Q is a function of LET and is known as the quality factor. In ICRP publication no. 15 (ICRP 1973), Q is defined as in Table 27.1. Following further refinement of data in ICRP publication no. 60 (ICRP 1991), Q was redefined as in Table 27.2.

Table 27.1 *Radiation quality factor of International Commission on Radiological Protection (ICRP) publication no. 21*

LET$_\infty$ in water (KeV/μm)	Q (LET)
< 3.5	1
7	2
23	5
53	10
> 175	20

LET, linear energy transfer; Q, quality factor.

Table 27.2 *Radiation quality factor of International Commission on Radiological Protection (ICRP) publication no. 60*

LET$_\infty$ in water (KeV/μm)	Q (LET)
< 10	1
10–100	$(0.32 \times LET) - 2.2$
> 100	$300/LET^{0.5}$

LET, linear energy transfer; Q, quality factor.

For the purposes of international regulations with respect to dose control, the quantity effective dose is used. Effective dose is obtained by the use of absorbed dose, D, along with different weighting factors for organs and tissues. A further addition to these quantities is ambient dose equivalent $H^*(10)$, also defined in ICRP 60. In this chapter, all of these quantities are treated as generally equivalent.

Recommended exposure limits

Limits for annual exposure of the public and occupationally exposed workers to radiation have been proposed by the ICRP and by the US equivalent organization, the National Council on Radiation Protection and Measurements (NCRP). The ICRP classifies aircrew as radiation workers. It recommends an annual limit of 1 mSv/year (above natural background) for the general public and 20 mSv/year for occupationally exposed workers. The recommendations cover a wide range of situations, taking into account the organs involved, the age of the individual and cumulative factors. The European Council has introduced a Basic Safety Standards Directive, which includes exposure to cosmic radiation of aircrew and frequent travellers. The Joint Aviation Authority, which oversees the activities of civil airlines in 35 states, also introduced requirements in 2001. The main points of interest to air travel can be summarized as follows:

- Controls are not necessary for aircrew whose annual dose can be shown to be less than 1 mSv/year. This corresponds, for example, to approximately 200 hours'

flight time at 35 000 feet on typical north European-North American routes or 400 hours at the same height above the Equatorial region.
- Operators whose aircrew may receive an effective dose greater than 1 mSv per year should assess the maximum exposure likely to occur, using a suitable computer program.
- If the assessment above exceeds 6 mSv per year, then individual monitoring is recommended.
- If an aircrew member declares she is pregnant, then the operator must ensure that future exposures at altitude for that person should not be greater than 1 mSv during the remainder of pregnancy.
- Aircraft flying at altitudes greater than 49 000 feet (15 km) should carry an active radiation monitor to detect any short-term variations (due to increased solar activity) during flight.

COMPUTER MODELS FOR PREDICTING DOSES AT AIRCRAFT ALTITUDES

A number of computer programs have been developed for calculating dose rates and route doses at aircraft altitudes. The recent upsurge in interest in this field has resulted in some new approaches and improvements of older methods of calculation. The basic idea is to consider cosmic rays at the top of the Earth's atmosphere, and to use radiation transport equations and geomagnetic location to follow their path down through the atmosphere. Although differences exist between the various computer codes, the background physics to develop these codes are the same and are explained briefly here. High-energy primary radiation (GCR), dominated by protons from interstellar space enters our solar system, strikes the Earth's atmosphere, where it produces an avalanche of secondary particles: protons, neutrons, pions, muons, electrons, positrons and photons. We have seen that depending on their energy and charge, the GCR particles interact with the material of Earth's atmosphere, thereby losing energy and ultimately being absorbed in the Earth's atmosphere. The main difference between different computer codes is due to the use of different GCR models and/or solar modulation models.

One of the oldest of these codes is LUIN, developed by Keran O'Brien in 1971 and later updated (O'Brien *et al.* 1992). The LUIN code is an analytical model based on solving the Boltzmann equation. Solar modulation is modelled using a heliocentric potential based on ground neutron monitor data. Vertical cut-off rigidity is based on the work of Smart and Shea (1997). The output includes fluences of primary and secondary particle species, including neutrons, protons, electrons, positrons, pions, muons and photons, as a function of altitude, latitude and direction of zenith angle. These fluences are then converted to dose rates and effective dose rates. LUIN requires extensive computational facilities; for this reason, a smaller personal computer (PC)-based code called CARI, which uses a LUIN output base and details of date, altitude, origin and destination of a flight to interpolate the transport code results, was produced. At the time of writing, the latest version is CARI-6, developed at the Civil Aerospace Medical Institute of the Federal Aviation Administration (FAA). CARI-6 calculates the effective dose of galactic radiation received by an adult on an aircraft flying a great circle route (or a reasonable approximation) between any two airports in the world. The program takes into account changes in altitude and geographic location during the course of the flight. Based on the date of the flight, appropriate databases are used to account for effects of changes in the Earth's magnetic field and solar activity on galactic radiation levels. The program also calculates the effective dose rate from galactic radiation at any location in the atmosphere at altitudes up to 87 298 feet (26.6 km). CARI-6 calculates effective doses and dose rates back to January 1958. The CARI-6 transport code has been tested extensively against experimental measurements.

A second important code is EPCARD (European Program Package for the Calculation of Aviation Route Doses), developed by Schraube *et al.* (2002), which is based on the results of Monte Carlo radiation transport calculations and uses the most recent data on nuclear reaction probabilities in the atmosphere as well as the most recent information on the cosmic ray field at the top of the atmosphere. EPCARD makes it possible to calculate the dose exposure from all the components of penetrating cosmic radiation on any aviation route and for any flight profiles. Like CARI-6, the solar heliocentric potential is derived from ground-level neutron monitors, and the data of Smart and Shea (1997) are used to determine the effects of geomagnetic shielding. The resulting particle fluences are converted to dose quantity by conversion factors based on ICRP 60. The dose rate is expressed by $H^*(10)$ in EPCARD. At the time of writing, the latest version of EPCARD is 3.2. The data used in EPCARD are updated continually. The authors of EPCARD have maintained close liaison with an EU working group set up to harmonize experimental and calculated data on radiation exposure at flight altitudes. Table 27.3 is an example of dose equivalent rates ($H^*(10)$) calculated using EPCARD version 3.2 for several supersonic and subsonic locations.

Figure 27.4 shows the dose equivalent rates calculated using EPCARD version 3.2 for different flight altitudes (subsonic and supersonic) and different latitudes at solar minimum and maximum. The main points to notice are (i) the general increase in dose rates with latitude, (ii) the increase in dose rate with altitude for all cases, (iii) the larger dose rates at solar minimum for a given altitude, and (iv) the levelling off of dose rates as the altitude approaches the level of the Pfotzer maximum (approximately 20 km).

Several other codes are also in use, including FLUKA, AIR, FREE, SIEVERT and PC-AIR, all of which have greatly improved the ease of route-dose calculations in recent times. FLUKA is a multipurpose particle interaction and transport code that has been adapted for use in space and cosmic ray studies. For comparison with measured dose quantities, CARI-6 and EPCARD will be the main codes considered in this chapter.

In-flight data and comparison with computer-code predictions

Data collected in recent years at aircraft altitudes are now quite extensive, and scientists in Europe, the USA, Japan and other locations have contributed to the great store of information available. Some of these data have been published, and more are being prepared for major reports by international organizations that deal with radioprotection guidelines and standards. Here, we will discuss a number of sets of data that represent an overall picture of the present status of our knowledge in this field, with some emphasis on projects supported by the EU, which has been at the fore in encouraging research in this area. Figure 27.5 shows some of the routes investigated during solar cycle 23.

Table 27.3 *Sample of dose rates (H*(10)) calculated using EPCARD version 3.2*

Radiation component	Dose (μSv/h)				
	London–New York, 48° N 27° W, 54 000 feet, March 1995	Dublin–New York, 41° N 72° W, 36 000 feet, August 1993	Milan–Los Angeles, 51° N 0° W, 36 000 feet, January 1996	Milan–Tokyo, 57° N 112° E, 36 000 feet, June 1997	Rome–Rio de Janeiro, 13° N 2° W, 34 000 feet, November 1996
Neutrons	4.86	3.52	3.27	3.33	0.71
Protons + pions	1.92	0.86	0.81	0.77	0.18
Electrons	1.95	1.07	1.07	0.96	0.58
Muons	0.24	0.19	0.19	0.19	0.11
Photons	0.41	0.26	0.26	0.24	0.14
Total	9.38	5.90	5.60	5.49	1.72

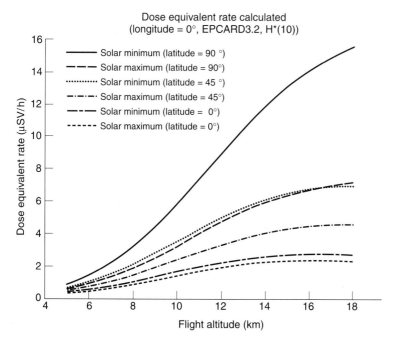

Figure 27.4 *Dose equivalent rates calculated by EPCARD version 3.2.*

Routes were determined mainly by the schedules of commercial airlines. Several airline companies, including Aer Lingus, British Airways, Austrian Airlines, Lufthansa, Scandinavian Airlines, Finnair, Alitalia, Air France and Czech Airlines, and the National Aeronautics and Space Administration (NASA) provided facilities for detector exposures at altitude, and their cooperation was a vital factor in the success of the investigation.

During the past decade, many types of detector have been used to assess the dose to which aircrew are subjected.

As explained earlier, this was to cover the wide range of radiation sources and energies involved. Because of the complexity of the field, there was also a strong element of confidence-building, as researchers dedicated themselves to understanding the response of their detectors, some designed or modified for the investigations. For measurements and monitoring, the instrument most likely to contribute for the foreseeable future is the tissue equivalent proportional counter (TEPC), since it covers the whole LET range and whose response is now better understood

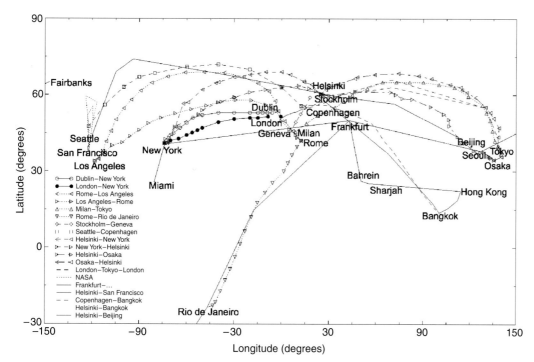

Figure 27.5 *Some of the flight routes investigated in the European Commission programme, 1993–2003.*

following the joint calibration and characterization studies carried out by many experimenters. However, we discuss here some typical results obtained by a variety of detector systems, including passive detectors. By including a number of recent investigations at aircraft altitude, it will be shown that the radiation dose experienced by aircrew is confined to within well-measured limits for both supersonic and subsonic aircraft, while embracing all variations in altitude, latitude and solar cycle, and that comparisons with values calculated by computer codes generally are quite good.

Figure 27.6 shows the dose equivalent measurements (Zhou et al. 2003) in microsieverts/hour for flights covering the period from 1993 to 2002 using the DIAS detector system, which is sensitive in the high LET region (O'Sullivan et al. 1999). For comparison, the calculated values of $H^*(10)$ using the EPCARD code are also displayed. The data cover the period of solar cycle 23. Each calculated value takes into account the appropriate heliocentric potential for that particular stage of the cycle. There is very good agreement (with ± 20 per cent) over the wide range of altitudes, latitudes and stages in the solar cycle. Measurements performed by DIAS over this period have also shown that the contribution of nuclei heavier than

protons (helium and beyond) to overall dose values is approximately 1.3 per cent at supersonic altitudes and only ~0.3 per cent at subsonic altitudes.

Table 27.4 shows data for Europe–Japan routes measured by the National Agency for Environmental Protection (ANPA; Italy) group between 1997 and 2002 (Curzio et al. 2001). Here, the total dose measured as $H^*(10)$ is compared with that predicted by EPCARD version 3 and with effective dose E estimated by CARI-6 and EPCARD version 3. Again, there is agreement within ± 25 per cent for all cases.

Using a Hawk tissue equivalent proportional counter TEPC (Far West Technology, Goleta, USA), the IRSN group (Bottollier-Depois et al. 2000) obtained a series of route measurements, as shown in Figure 27.7. Here, the average dose equivalent rate (μSv/h) and the radiation mean quality factor are contained within the circles, and the total dose equivalent is given for a round-trip (black rectangles). Note that with the exception of the Concorde flight between Paris and New York, all dose equivalent rates are less than 7 μ Sv/h.

A similar instrument was used by the Royal Military College of Canada (RMC) group (Lewis et al. 2002) to investigate dose values on a wide range of flight routes covering North and South America, Europe and New Zealand.

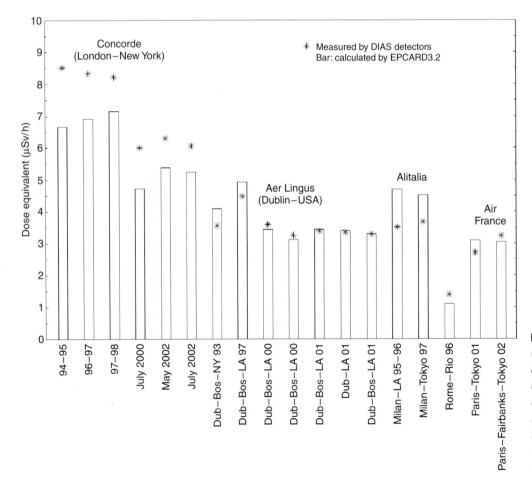

Figure 27.6

Comparison of measured and calculated dose equivalents for routes originating at Dublin, London, Milan, Rome and Paris. Bos, Boston; Dub, Dublin; LA, Los Angeles; Rio, Rio de Janeiro.

Table 27.4   *Measured and calculated doses on round-trips between Europe and Japan at different phases of the solar cycle*

Date	Round-trip	Flights (n)	Duration (h)	Measured $H^*(10)$ (μSv)	CARI-6 E (μSv)	EPCARD 3.0 (μSv)	
						$H^*(10)$	E
May 1997	Milan–Tokyo	8	21.5	104 ± 10	104 ± 14	108 ± 12	128 ± 16
May 2002	Paris–Fairbanks–Tokyo	1	28	130 ± 15	127	114	133
July 2002	Rome–Tokyo	1	22.3	104 ± 16	93	83	95

Measured values obtained by the RMC and the PTB were compared with those predicted by the LUIN and FLUKA codes. The experimental data were normalized to an altitude of 10.6 km (atmospheric depth h_0 = 243 g/cm^2). There was excellent agreement between the experimental measurements and the theoretical $H^*(10)$ code predictions, apart from a slight underestimate by the FLUKA code near the Equator.

The active on-board dose assessment system ACREM (aircrew radiation exposure monitoring) (Beck *et al.* 1999) also carried out many investigations on aircrew radiation exposure. Measurements obtained on a flight from Frankfurt to Chicago on 31 December 2000 on a Lufthansa A340 Airbus showed a total ambient dose of 44 μSv, in excellent agreement with values calculated from the LUIN code and EPCARD. Figure 27.8 shows a set of data obtained over a wide range of geomagnetic latitudes. Dose rates at the lowest latitudes are approximately three times less than those above 60 degrees latitude. It is also worth noting the levelling off that occurs around 60 degrees. The lack of symmetry in the plot centred around zero geomagnetic latitude is due to the fact that the axis of the Earth's magnetic field is displaced from the centre of the Earth, which leads to higher dose rates in the southern hemisphere than those in the northern hemisphere at the same geomagnetic latitude.

Table 27.5 shows a set of measurements obtained between 33 000 and 67 000 feet using a variety of passive and active detectors during the period 1993–98 (Bartlett *et al.* 2001). It includes the results of several studies carried out by an EU-funded project during the late 1990s. The close agreement obtained is an indication of the improvements in measurement techniques brought about by improved calibration facilities and detector development. For normal altitudes reached by subsonic aircraft, dose rates are less than 6 μSv/h; dose rates at higher levels are approximately twice this value.

The SSI (Stockholm) and University of Munich collaboration developed two types of TEPC for investigations on Scandinavian Airlines and Finnair routes (Kyllonen *et al.* 2001). The Sievert and AMIRA (active monitoring in mixed radiation fields) instruments are now contributing valuable data on these routes. Concentrating on the Helsinki, New York and San Francisco routes and the Bangkok–Copenhagen route, the group has shown excellent agreement of measured data with model predictions. The flights to and from San Francisco were performed during Forbush decreases. Again, excellent agreement was found with the predictions of CARI-6 and EPCARD and other models for all routes investigated. For instance, the total dose measured from Copenhagen to Bangkok was

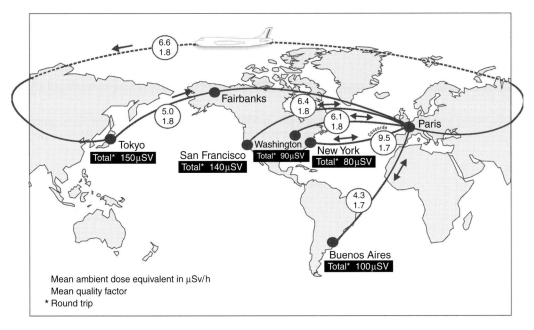

Figure 27.7   *Results obtained by the Institut de radioprotection et de sûreté nucléaire (IRSN) group.*

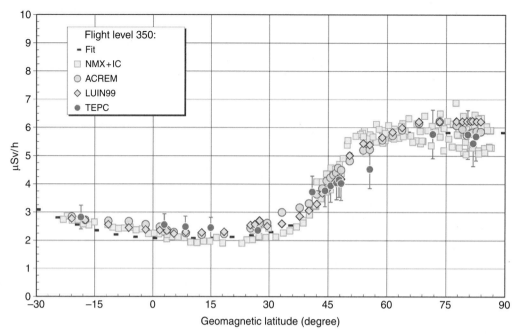

Figure 27.8   *Dose equivalent rate as a function of geomagnetic latitudes measured by the Aircrew Radiation Exposure Monitoring (ACREM) group.*

Table 27.5   *Measured ambient dose equivalent rates at latitudes of 40–60° N*

Altitude	Investigator	$H^*(10)$ rate (μSv/h)	
		Neutron	**Total**
10 km (33 000 feet)	ANPA passive (TLDs, bubble detectors, etched-track detectors, fission foils)	$2.9 \pm 0.3^*$	4.7 ± 0.5
	ANPA active (ionization chamber, extended-range rem meter)	2.8 ± 0.5	4.6 ± 0.6
10.6 km (35 000 feet)	DIAS (etched-track with full analysis)	3.2 ± 0.3	–
	USAAR (HANDITEPC)	3.5 ± 0.8	5.7 ± 0.8
	SSI (SIEVERT variance TEPC)	3.1 ± 0.3	5.1 ± 0.3
	NRPB (TLDs and etched-track)	3.8 ± 0.5	5.5 ± 0.5
16 km (53 000 feet)	NRPB	6.7 ± 0.4	11.0 ± 0.5
	DIAS	7.1 ± 0.6	–
	ANPA passive	6.1 ± 0.5	11.0 ± 0.5
20 km (67 000 feet)	NRPB	8.3 ± 0.8	12.7 ± 0.8
	NASA (multisphere spectrometer)	8.5	–

*One standard deviation on instrument reading, or standard deviation of the mean for repeated measurements.
ANPA, National Agency for Environmental Protection (Italy); DIAS, Dublin Institute for Advanced Studies; HANDITEPC, Homburg area neutron dosimeter tissue equivalent proportional counter; NRPB, National Radiological Protection Board; SSI, Swedish Radiation Protection Authority; TEPC, tissue-equivalent proportional counter; TLD, thermoluminescent detector; USAAR, University of Saarland.

approximately 22 μSv compared with an average of 26 μSv predicted by the model calculations.

The DOSTEL system (Beaujean *et al.* 1999), originally developed for space flight, based on two identical silicon detectors and designed to measure energy deposit of charged particles, has also been employed at aircraft altitudes. Measurements taken at atmospheric depths between 200 and 290 g/cm² (i.e. 11.9 km and 9.5 km) showed dose equivalent values of between approximately 8 μSv/h and

4 μSv/h at high latitudes and between 2.3 μSv/h and 1.5 μSv/h at low altitudes. These measurements agreed well with the results of studies by Schrewe (2000) using a TEPC for the same time period before solar maximum (1997–99).

By measuring dose rates for a complete solar cycle starting in 1992, it has been possible to estimate the variation in the galactic component between solar maximum and solar minimum. Overall, dose values decreased by approximately 25 per cent between solar minimum and maximum.

SPACE WEATHER EFFECTS

As mentioned earlier, transient solar effects produced by sudden releases of energy in solar flares and coronal mass ejections can be observed at commercial aircraft-cruising altitudes. Because these events are quite rare and are not predictable, the DOSMAX project set out to have active detectors deployed at altitude as frequently as possible during the period of maximum activity for solar cycle 23. This policy was successful and was rewarded with an excellent set of data collected on 15 April 2001 when GLE 60 occurred during a flight from Prague to New York (Spurny and Datchev 2001). A significant increase in dose rate was observed for over one hour. An estimate of the dose predicted by CARI-6 in the absence of solar activity was made. Although the impact of the solar event was shown to be appreciable over the period in question, and an increase in dose of approximately 20 μSv above the galactic cosmic ray contribution was recorded, the overall effect on the annual exposure of the aircrew was negligible. While solar particle events of greater intensity could occur in the future, it is unlikely that this source of radiation will present any major problems for aircrew while the present ranges of altitudes and subsonic aircraft are in use. A study by Lantos and Fuller (2003) concludes that of the 64 GLEs recorded so far, only 18 are likely to have caused a 30 μSv increase in effective dose, and only four would have contributed more than 1 mSv.

SUPERSONIC FLIGHT

Following the end of the Concorde service in October 2003, the world said farewell to commercial supersonic flight, at least for the foreseeable future. The joint British and French achievement that had attracted headlines for over three decades marked an important period in airline history. Unlike its ill-fated Russian counterpart, the TU-144, which crashed at the Le Bourget air show in 1973, Concorde enjoyed a level of prestige rarely seen in the world of commercial transportation. Although its high-altitude flight path (cruising at 17 km) exposed its passengers and crew to a higher radiation field than that experienced on subsonic aircraft, the shorter flight time more or less compensated, and the total dose received was similar for both types of journey.

There have been a number of other attempts to develop supersonic passenger airline services, but the future looks rather bleak. After the TU-144 was removed from service,

US and Russian aerospace researchers adapted it to become a flying supersonic research laboratory. The TU-144 was reconfigured to give a maximum cruising speed of Mach 2.3 (~2575 km/h). NASA and Boeing began to explore a next-generation supersonic aircraft called the High Speed Civil Transport, but the research collaboration was terminated following a decision that the concept was not economically feasible. Although a new design could call for higher cruising altitudes and increased radiation exposure in the region of the Pfotzer maximum (~20 km altitude), the development of commercial supersonic travel in the next few decades is uncertain and will not be an immediate concern for radiation protection.

CANCER RISK IN AIRLINE CABIN ATTENDANTS

Epidemiological investigations of cancer risk and other causes of death of aircrew in relation to occupational factors have been undertaken with increased interest over the past decade. Although the level of cancer risk following exposure to low-level radiation has been estimated from various radiobiological models and epidemiological studies of different populations, information on the particular circumstances of aircrew who work for long periods in this complicated field at altitude has been relatively scarce until recently. Statistical methods allow evaluation of the ratio of the risk of an exposed aircrew population and a non-exposed reference population. Account is taken of the differences between the two groups with respect to age, sex and other influencing factors. Because exposure of aircrew involves relatively low-level radiation and a long induction period, any study in this field requires significantly large samples. Relative risk is usually stated along with a confidence level to indicate statistical variation. A standardized incidence ratio (SIR) is defined as the number of cases of a particular phenomenon in the exposed group divided by the number of expected cases. The number of expected cases is determined from the reference population. Early studies on Canadian, British, Nordic and other aircrew provided little conclusive evidence for an increase in cancer risk attributable to cosmic radiation. Some of these investigations were hampered by small samples and inadequate control of reference populations. Results ranged from reports of elevated risk for several types of cancer to significantly decreased incidence rates. It is possible that aircrew members' lifestyles, socioeconomic status and recreational habits were not compensated for fully when comparisons were made with the general population.

Recent investigations of incidence of cancer among Nordic aircrew may throw new light on this subject. These studies have the advantage that the Nordic countries have a history of several decades of population-based registration of cancer, and the SIR can be considered very reliable. In a project involving 10 032 male airline pilots with an average follow-up period of 17 years, 466 cases of cancer were diagnosed compared with 456 expected (Pukkala *et al.* 2002). The authors conclude that overall, there is no marked increase in cancer risk attributable to cosmic radiation exposure. Increased SIR values were found for some specific cancers, including melanoma (2.3, 95 per cent confidence limit 1.7 to 3.0). It was also noted that the occurrence of prostate cancer increased with increasing the number of flight hours in long-distance aircraft. This phenomenon could, as the authors point out, be due to circadian (sleep/wake) hormonal disturbances. However, the authors do not exclude some influence of cosmic radiation in the cases of skin cancer.

An investigation of 2324 women and 632 men employed by SAS between 1957 and 1994 concluded that Swedish cabin crew had an overall cancer incidence similar to that of the general population (Linnersjo *et al.* 2003). The authors state that an increased incidence of malignant melanoma and non-melanoma skin cancer may be associated with exposure to ultraviolet radiation, either at work or as a result of recreational activities. However, female cabin crew had what was considered a non-significant increase of breast cancer (SIR 1.30). No clear link was found between length of employment or cumulative block hours and incidence of cancer.

A third report describes a study to determine whether length of employment as aircrew was related to breast cancer risk when adjusted for reproductive factors (Rafnsson *et al.* 2003). This study involved 1532 female cabin crew in Iceland. An odds ratio of 5.24 (95 per cent confidence limit 1.58 to 17.38) was found for those with five or more years of service before 1971 compared with those with less than five years' service before 1971, adjusted for age at first childbirth and length of service. This study is the first published case–control study of breast cancer among cabin attendants adjusting for individual reproductive factors. In previous investigations, these factors were not controlled directly. The authors express the view that the data are compatible with a long induction period between ionizing radiation and development of breast cancer. It is worth noting that the period involved was before the era of jet aircraft in the Icelandic case. A similar analysis of data collected from the era of jet aircraft, which fly at higher altitude and, consequently, are exposed to higher radiation doses, may throw some further light on this important topic.

CONCLUSIONS

Although the presence of cosmic radiation and its secondaries in the Earth's atmosphere has been shown for almost a century, it is only in recent years that a thorough under-

standing of its role as a potential hazard to aircrew and frequent travellers has been established. Where once large gaps existed in our knowledge and significant uncertainties concerning radiation exposure were commonplace, we now have experimental measurements on a global scale with which to determine dose as a function of altitude and latitude. Because of the complexity of the radiation field, several types of detector have been used. The effects of events on the sun have also been investigated in detail during one complete cycle between 1993 and 2004. Several computer codes have been developed to estimate dose values for any chosen flight route at any stage of solar cycle. These codes will be used in the future to determine route doses on a routine basis. Much of this work was motivated by the need to protect aircrew and frequent travellers, who are now included among those considered as 'radiation workers'. In this regard, the European Commission played an important role in encouraging both experimental and theoretical research undertaken over the past decade, following recommendations of the ICRP.

For the vast majority of aircrew, who clock up about 600 flight hours per annum, a total radiation exposure of more than 6 mSv per annum (the level beyond which individual monitoring is recommended) is unlikely at any stage in a solar cycle. We have seen that both experimental and theoretical estimates of dose equivalent confirm that for subsonic aircraft that cruise at approximately 12 km altitude or less, exposure to dose rates of $10\,\mu$ Sv/hr or greater is very rare. Where this level of exposure is likely to occur, it is possible to adjust rostering so that no individual receives more than 6 mSv per annum during a typical 600 flying hours. Exposure to cosmic radiation in Concorde, which cruised at approximately 17 km, could be greater than $10\,\mu$ Sv/hr, particularly at northern latitudes, but the reduced flight time compensated for this. Although increases in radiation dose may occur due to solar energetic particles during periods of increased solar activity, the incidence of significant increase is very rare, and in most cases investigated over the past four or five solar cycles, their contribution to annual dose rates experienced by aircrew is not a matter of serious concern.

Epidemiological investigations of cancer risks among aircrew suggest that there may be evidence for a long induction period between ionizing radiation and development of breast cancer, although further studies are required.

ACKNOWLEDGEMENTS

The authors wish to thank the staff of the many airlines and accelerator centres who made the collection and analysis of data possible. We are indebted to our colleagues in the DOSMAX collaboration for many years of joint scientific investigation and to the many other scientists who have contributed to the world database of cosmic rays at aviation altitudes. This chapter was written during the term of EU contract FIGM-CT-2000-00068, and we are very grateful for the financial support. Finally, a big thank you to Eileen Flood, who compiled the final document.

REFERENCES

Bartlett DT, Beck P, Bottollier-Depois J-F, *et al.* Investigation of radiation doses at aircraft altitudes during a complete solar cycle. Presented at SOLSPA: the Second Solar Cycle and Space Weather Euro Conference. Vico Equense, 24–29 September, 2001. ESA Publication SP-477.

Beaujean R, Kapp J, Reitz G. Radiation exposure in civil aircraft. *Radiation Protection Dosimetry* 1999; **85**: 287–90.

Beck P, Schrewe U, O'Brien K, Ambrosi P. ACREM. Aircrew exposure monitoring. Austrian Research Centers in Siebersdorf report OEFZS-008. Siebersdorf: Austrian Research Centers in Siebersdorf, 1999.

Bottollier-Depois JF, Chau Q, Bouisset P, *et al.* Assessing exposure to cosmic radiation during long-haul flights. *Radiation Research* 2000; **153**: 526–32.

Curzio G, Grillmaier RE, O'Sullivan D, *et al.* The Italian national survey of aircrew exposure. II. On board measurement and results. *Radiation Protection Dosimetry* 2001; **93**: 125–33.

International Commission on Radiological Protection. *Data for Protection against Ionising Radiation from External Sources: Supplement to ICRP Publication 15.* ICRP Publication 21. Oxford@ Pergamon Press, 1973.

International Commission on Radiological Protection. *Recommendations of the International Commission on Radiological Protection.* ICRP publication 60. Oxford: Pergamon Press, 1991.

Kyllonen J-K, Lindborg L, Samuelson G. Cosmic radiation measurements onboard aircraft with the variance method. *Radiation Protection Dosimetry* 2001; **93**: 197–205.

Lantos P, Fuller N. History of the solar flare radiation doses on-board aeroplanes using semi-empirical model and Concorde measurements. *Radiation Protection Dosimetry* 2003; **104**: 199–210.

Lewis BJ, Bennett GI, Green AR, *et al.* Galactic and solar radiation exposure to aircrew during a solar cycle. *Radiation Protection Dosimetry* 2002; **102**: 207–27.

Lindborg L, Bartlett DT, Beck P, *et al.* Cosmic radiation exposure of aircraft crew: compilation of measured and calculated data. Report of EURADOS working group 5. *Radiation Protection Dosimetry* 2004; **110**: 417–22.

Linnersjo A, Hammar N, Dammstrom BG, Johansson M, Eliasch H. Cancer incidence in airline cabin crew: experience from Sweden, *Occupational Environmental Medicine* 2003; **60**: 810–14.

O'Brien K, Friedberg W, Duke FE, *et al.* The exposure of aircraft crews to radiations of extraterrestrial origin. *Radiation Protection Dosimetry* 1992; **45**: 145–62.

O'Sullivan D, Zhou D, Heinrich W, *et al.* Cosmic rays and dosimetry at aviation altitudes. *Radiation Measurements* 1999; **31**: 579–84.

Pukkala E, Aspholm R, Auvinen A, *et al.* Incidence of cancer among Nordic airline pilots over five decades: occupational cohort study. *British Medical Journal* 2002; **325**: 567–71.

Rafnsson V, Sulem P, Tulinius H, Hrafnkelsson J. Breast cancer risk in airline cabin attendants: a nested case–control study in Iceland. *Occupational Environmental Medicine* 2003; **60**: 807–9.

Reames DV. Solar energetic particles: a paradigm shift. *Reviews in Geophysics* 1995; **33**: 585–9.

Schraube H, Leuthold G, Heinrich W, *et al.* EPCARD: European Program Package for the Calculation of Aviation Route Doses. User's Manual. GSF report 08/02. Neuherberg, Germany: GSF National Research Center, 2002.

Schrewe UJ. Global measurements of the radiation exposure of civil aircrew from 1997–1999. *Radiation Protection Dosimetry* 2000; **94**: 347–64.

Smart DF, Shea MA. Solar radiation. In: Trigg GL (ed.). *Encyclopaedia of Applied Physics.* New York: VCH Publishers, 1997; pp. 394–429.

Spurny F, Datchev T. Measurement in an aircraft during an intense solar flare, Ground Level Event 60, on the 15th April 2001. *Radiation Protection Dosimetry* 2001; **95**: 273–5.

Zhou D, O'Sullivan D, Xu B, Flood E. Cosmic ray measurements at aircraft altitudes and comparison with predictions of computer codes. *Advances in Space Research* 2003; **32**: 47–52.

FURTHER READING

Cosmic radiation and aircrew exposure: proceedings of an international conference, Dublin, Ireland, July 1–3, 1998. *Radiation Protection Dosimetry* 1999; **86**: 4.

28

Spatial disorientation in flight

ALAN J. BENSON AND J.R. ROLLIN STOTT

INTRODUCTION

Definition

Spatial disorientation is a term used to describe a variety of incidents occurring in flight in which the pilot fails to sense correctly the position, motion or attitude of the aircraft or of him- or herself within the fixed coordinate system provided by the surface of the Earth and the gravitational vertical. In addition, errors in perception by pilots of their position, motion or attitude with respect to their aircraft, or of their own aircraft relative to other aircraft, may also be embraced within a broader definition of spatial disorientation in flight.

Although spatial disorientation, according to the definition given above, includes errors in the perception of aircraft position, such incidents are described more accurately by the term 'geographic disorientation'. The determination of position with respect to fixed coordinates on the surface of the Earth is the task of aerial navigation and is one that uses different skills from those used in the perception of aircraft attitude and motion. For this reason, the topics of geographic orientation and disorientation are discussed elsewhere in this book.

The concept of situational awareness (SA) has gained currency since the early 1980s, although there is still some uncertainty about what should be included within the definition of the term. For some, it has become synonymous with the aviator's awareness of the aircraft's spatial orientation. However, more commonly, the term embraces an awareness not only of spatial orientation but also of other aspects of the current state of the aircraft and of the external environment. It also incorporates an element of anticipation of future events. There should be no ambiguity: a pilot who has an erroneous perception of aircraft orientation also incurs a loss of SA, but loss of SA can occur for many different reasons in the absence of any spatial disorientation.

In some countries, particularly the USA, the term 'vertigo' or 'aviator's vertigo' is synonymous with spatial disorientation, but as vertigo has the more specific meaning of 'a sensation of turning' or 'dizziness', it has been suggested that the use of the word 'vertigo' should be confined to this particular kind of sensory experience. A pilot with vertigo may well be suffering from spatial disorientation, but there are many incidents in which the pilot is spatially disoriented but does not have vertigo.

Incidence

Nearly all aircrew experience illusory sensations of aircraft attitude and motion or fail to detect changes in aircraft orientation at some time during their flying career. Such incidents are quite normal, for they are due, in general, to physiological limitations of sensory mechanisms. Human sense organs are functionally adapted to terrestrial life in a stable 1-g environment. It is, therefore, not surprising that in the aerial environment, in which the aviator is exposed to motion stimuli that differ in magnitude, frequency and direction from those experienced on the ground, errors in the perception of spatial orientation occur. The incidence and frequencies of spatial disorientation differ widely between aircrew and are as much influenced by the individual pilot's concept of the term as by the type of flying in which he or she is engaged. Some will say that they have never suffered from disorientation because they always knew the aircraft's correct orientation, usually by reference to aircraft instruments, even though they were experiencing erroneous sensations, i.e. illusions of spatial orientation. Others will say that they have some form of disorientation on almost every flight, although they, like their colleagues who ostensibly have never been disoriented, successfully resolve the perceptual conflict and maintain correct control of the aircraft.

Quantitative information on the incidence of spatial disorientation comes from questionnaire surveys of military pilots, although these have tended to concentrate on the illusions of spatial orientation rather than identifying those situations in which performance was degraded by spatial disorientation. A further problem associated with an illusion-based approach to disorientation is that it gives no indication of the likelihood that a given illusion will lead to a disorientation incident or accident. The illusion that an aircraft feels straight and level when it is not is probably the most frequent underlying cause of disorientation episodes, and yet this illusion hardly merits inclusion in any list of illusions of flight, as it is just too commonplace.

For example, in the Royal Netherlands Air Force, it was found that all of the 209 F5 and F16 pilots had been disoriented at some time or other in their flying careers, and 26 per cent had severe incidents with narrow escape from disaster. Data from a survey of 413 Indian Air Force pilots yielded lower figures: 75 per cent of fighter pilots, 64 per cent of transport pilots and only 55 per cent of helicopter pilots acknowledged that they had been disoriented. In contrast, surveys of helicopter pilots of the US Navy, the UK Royal Navy and the UK army yielded incidences of spatial disorientation of 91 per cent, 95 per cent and 90 per cent, respectively. Of the Royal Navy pilots, 61 per cent had been disoriented severely on one or more occasions, and situations in which both pilot and co-pilot were disoriented at the same time were reported in 21 per cent of the questionnaires. In the more recent UK army survey, 24 per cent of pilots had suffered severe disorientation, and both crew members were disoriented in 24 per cent of incidents, a figure that rose to 44 per cent for incidents occurring during flight with night-vision goggles (NVGs).

Spatial disorientation is also a significant problem in civil transport and general aviation (private) pilots, although the frequency with which illusory perception of attitude and motion occur is not known. Over the period 1982–96, only 1.1 per cent of the returns made by UK civil pilots in a confidential human factors incident reporting programme (CHIRP) described disorientation incidents. This figure is certainly an appreciable underestimate of the frequency with which disorientation is experienced by this pilot population, for they are unlikely to report common illusions or incidents in which control of the aircraft was not compromised. Private pilots also suffer from disorien-

tation, which, in this group, is a greater threat to flight safety than in the generally more experienced and better-trained military and civil transport pilots. Unfortunately, no data, other than anecdotal accounts, are available on the frequency with which spatial disorientation is experienced by general aviation pilots.

Information on the incidence of the many different types of perceptual disturbances, embraced by the definition of spatial disorientation, has been obtained solely from questionnaire studies of military pilots. Table 28.1 summarizes the findings of two such surveys. The table shows the percentage of pilots who reported having experienced particular illusions or perceptual problems 'sufficient to affect performance, situational awareness or workload – however slight that effect may be'. As in many earlier studies, the most widely experienced illusion was the 'the leans', a false perception of roll attitude when flying straight and level. However, the importance of these statistics is not in the precise percentage of pilots who reported a specific illusion but in the demonstration of the variety of illusions and conditions of flight in which spatial disorientation can occur. Unfortunately, it tells us little about which conditions carry the greatest hazard to flight safety.

OPERATIONAL SIGNIFICANCE

Orientation error accident

By far the most important consequence of spatial disorientation is the orientation error accident. If control of the aircraft is based on the pilot's erroneous perception of its attitude or flight trajectory, then, by definition, there is an error in the human–machine closed-loop system, which, if not corrected, will almost inevitably lead to impact with the ground. Fortunately, only a small fraction of the disorientation incidents experienced by aircrew end in disaster. Nevertheless, aircraft crash each year, and aircrew and passengers are killed because pilots fail to perceive correctly the orientation of their aircraft. This problem is not a new one: early in the history of powered flight, it was recognized that limitations of sensory function could lead to loss of control, particularly when external visual cues for spatial orientation were degraded, as, for example, when flying in cloud or at night. Yet, despite progressive improvements in aircraft instruments and displays, which should, and generally do, allow the pilot to maintain correct orientation in all conditions of flight, accidents still occur. The greater proportion of orientation error accidents are associated with flight in poor visibility, technically described as instrument meteorological conditions (IMC), when flight should be by reference to aircraft instruments (instrument flight rules, IFR), but accidents also occur in good visibility (visual meteorological condi-

Table 28.1   *Incidence of spatial disorientation*

Spatial disorientation incident	% reporting at least one incident	
	USAF	RAF
'Leans'	76	92
Loss of horizon due to atmospheric conditions	69	82
Undetected drift (helicopter pilots only)	90	55
Sloping horizon	66	75
Misleading altitude cues	50	79
Distraction	61	66
Tumbling sensation (Coriolis)	61	66
Night (black hole) approach	58	60
Loss of horizon due to sand/snow	33	56
Poor crew coordination	41	50
Graveyard spiral/spin	38	50
Autokinesis	37	43
False sensation of pitching up	44	34
Misjudgement of position – night	38	37
Elevator illusion	37	35
G-excess illusion	36	33
False sensation of pitching down	37	28
When using night-vision goggles	12	48
Roll-reversal error	23	31
Inability to read instruments clearly on recovery	22	29
False sensation of yaw	32	20
When using head-down displays	20	30
False sensation of inversion	23	18
Inappropriate use of the sun or ground lights as vertical cue	24	17
Instrument malfunction	13	24
Feeling of detachment (break-off)	11	17
Flicker vertigo	20	8
Problem interpreting head-up display	10	13
When using FLIR/targeting aids	9	11
When using aerial flare	10	10

FLIR, forward-looking infrared; RAF, Royal Air Force; USAF, US Air Force.
Data from 2582 USAF aviators (Matthews *et al.* 2003) and 752 RAF aircrew (Holmes *et al.* 2003). (Both papers in *RTO Symposium HFM-085, TP/42.*)

tions, VMC) and are due to the misinterpretation of external visual cues.

Orientation error poses a difficult problem of accident investigation. If the pilot is dead or is unable to remember what happened immediately before the accident, then the evidence that substantiates the identification of 'orientation error' as a prime cause of the accident is at best circumstantial and at worst conjectural. In many, and perhaps most, accidents in which disorientation is considered to be a primary cause, an element of uncertainty must remain. This is less when information on the aircraft's flight trajectory and the pilot's responses and control inputs is available from flight-data and cockpit-voice recorders and radar plots. However, even with such evidence, it is unlikely that there can be absolute certainty in ascribing the accident to an error in the pilot's perception of aircraft spatial disorientation.

Reports published over the past 40 years show the wide variation in the proportion of aircraft accidents that the

authors attributed to pilot disorientation. It ranges from 2.5 per cent in the Indian Air Force to 39 per cent of F16 accidents in the Netherlands Air Force. The mean incidence is 12.4 per cent, which is close to the 12 per cent reported in the study of 406 accidents in the Royal Air Force (RAF) over the period 1973–91. In the decade 1991–2000, spatial disorientation was considered to be a causal or major contributory factor in 20.2 per cent of class A mishaps in the US Air Force (USAF), with a fatality rate three times greater than in accidents in which spatial disorientation was not implicated.

Orientation error accidents are not confined to military aircraft. In the civil sector, it is the private flyer who is most at risk. US general aviation statistics for the period 1968–75 involving over 35 000 accidents identified spatial disorientation as a prime cause or contributory factor in 2.5 per cent of all accidents; 90 per cent of orientation error accidents were fatal. Indeed, it is in the category of fatal accidents that disorientation had greater prominence, for it was the third most important factor in this group and accounted for 16 per cent of all fatalities. Orientation error was associated closely with the second leading cause – continued visual traffic rules (VTR) flight into adverse weather – in which it was a cause or factor in 35.6 per cent of fatal accidents.

Dynamics of the orientation error accident

Just as the illusory perceptions embraced within the term 'spatial disorientation' are protean, so are the ways in which perceptual errors lead to loss of control and orientation error accidents. Figure 28.1 attempts to illustrate the dynamics of the disorientation accident. The reader's attention is drawn first to the classification of disorientation into two types. One covers those incidents in which pilots do not recognize that their perception of aircraft orientation is erroneous; this is type I or unrecognized spatial disorientation (USD). The other is type II or recognized spatial disorientation (RSD), in which the pilot is aware that they are having a problem in their perception of aircraft orientation, often with a conflict between what they feel is happening to the aircraft and what the flight instruments indicate. Some authors consider that those incidents in which pilots experience disorientation of an overwhelming intensity should be classified as type III or incapacitating spatial disorientation (ISD). We do not endorse the use of type III in the classification of disorientation because it is based not on the nature of the pilot's perception but on the behavioural consequences of the disordered perception. In those rare instances in which pilots are incapacitated by spatial disorientation, they are usually aware of their difficulties and are suffering from type II disorientation (RSD).

Unrecognized (type I) disorientation is the greater hazard to flight safety. Pilots who base their control of the aircraft on false cues may soon lose control and be left with insufficient time or altitude to regain control, even if they have the skill to re-establish orientation from instruments or other veridical cues. However, loss of control per se is not necessarily a feature of the orientation error accident, although control is inappropriate in all incidents. The pilot who flies the aircraft into the ground because of, say, an erroneous perception of pitch attitude on accelerating during a 'missed approach' manoeuvre, or because of an erroneous perception of ground clearance, has not lost control of the aircraft, for, given the sudden realization of an error, appropriate recovery action could be taken. Nevertheless, it is disturbing that many, and perhaps the majority, of orientation error accidents are due to type I disorientation, in which the pilot does not realize that he or she is disoriented.

In contrast, only a small fraction of type II (RSD) incidents lead to an aircraft accident. Commonly, the perceptual conflict is resolved and control of the aircraft is based on the correct interpretation of reliable, usually instrument, cues. Only rarely are the perceptual and motor functions of the pilot so impaired by the conflict – 'disorientation stress' is, perhaps, a better term – that control is jeopardized. The manner in which disorientation stress degrades performance is considered in some detail later in this chapter; suffice it is to say that it may lead to: (i) the acceptance of erroneous cues and their use in aircraft control, (ii) disturbance of motor function with inappropriate or inadequate control responses, and (iii) impairment of higher mental function, so that errors of judgement are made. Thus, infrequently, although not insignificantly, type II disorientation may, either of itself or in synergism with other stresses of the flight environment,

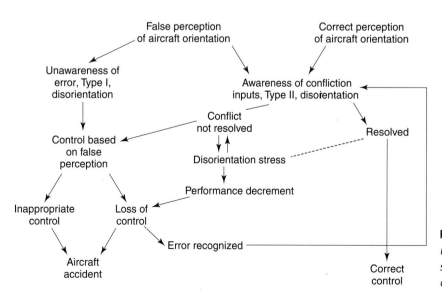

Figure 28.1 *Representation of how unrecognized (type I) and recognized (type II) spatial disorientation can affect the pilot's control of the aircraft.*

lead to a type I incident, with its attendant high probability of an aircraft accident. Disorientation stress can also bring about a complete breakdown in skilled behaviour, such that the pilot capitulates and gives up trying to resolve the sensory conflict. Incidents have also been described in which the pilot 'freezes' at the controls and is apparently incapable of making any corrective movement.

Anxiety reactions

Aircraft accidents and impairment of skilled performance are the principal operational consequences of spatial disorientation. Anxiety reactions, although relatively uncommon in relation to the frequency of occurrence of disorientation incidents, are also responsible for some morbidity in flying personnel. The interrelationship between perceptual disturbance and neurotic reaction is a close one, so when attempting to unravel aetiological mechanisms in an individual patient, it is often difficult to determine whether the disorientation was the manifestation of an anxiety reaction or whether the perceptual disturbance was the cause of the anxiety. In some aircrew, it is clear from the clinical history that the neurotic reaction is precipitated by an unusually intense disorientation or other illusory perception, such as 'break-off' (see later). Typically, the first incident is one that creates apprehension or even frank anxiety because it is outside the individual's previous experience. On subsequent flights, there is heightened introspection and attention to the abnormal sensations. Not surprisingly, disorientation recurs with increasing anxiety and apprehension. The pilot is trapped in a vicious circle, from which escape is likely to come only by admission of the disability and the acceptance of appropriate therapy.

In about 50 per cent of the few aircrew who come under medical care because of spatial disorientation, the perceptual disorder would appear to be the expression of an anxiety neurosis rather than the precipitant of mental ill health. Often, there is a pronounced phobic element, with symptoms occurring only in specific environmental conditions. If no treatment is given, then typically there is generalization of the anxiety, with loss of confidence and development of fear of flying reactions.

AETIOLOGY

Aircrew have described many different types of spatial disorientation that have occurred in different flight conditions and during different flight manoeuvres. Not surprisingly, the mechanisms underlying the disordered perceptions are commensurately varied. However, in an attempt to bring some order to the diversity of incidents

and causal factors, it is convenient to discuss aetiology under two main headings, even though they are not mutually exclusive: (i) when erroneous or inadequate sensory information is transmitted to the brain (an input error) and (ii) when there is an erroneous or inadequate perception of correct sensory information by the brain (a central error).

Input error

EXTERNAL VISUAL CUES

Disorientation is uncommon when pilots have well-defined and familiar external visual cues. However, when they attempt to fly when sight of the ground or the horizon is degraded by cloud, fog, snow, rain, smoke, dust or darkness, they may quickly become disoriented unless attention is given to the aircraft instruments. The period in which the ability to maintain control of an aircraft is retained without vision is quite short, typically about 60 seconds, even when the aircraft is in straight and level flight at the time vision is lost, and is shorter still if the aircraft is in a turn. In such circumstances, loss of control occurs because the non-visual receptors give either inadequate or erroneous information about the position, attitude and motion of the aircraft.

Even in good visibility, the external visual cues provided by ground texture can be poor and may be quite inadequate for the perception of altitude or, more accurately, height above ground level. Typically, difficulty is experienced when flying over featureless terrain, such as sand or snow, or over water when it lacks wave texture. The difficulty of estimating height when attempting to land on such surfaces, or of maintaining accurate ground clearance in a hovering helicopter, is well recognized by experienced aircrew. At night, the restricted area of ground illuminated by lights on the aircraft exacerbates the problem. The particular problems of the perception of orientation by external visual cues during that critical phase of flight – the approach and landing – are of special importance and merit more detailed analysis later in this chapter.

Erroneous, as opposed to inadequate, external visual cues less frequently disorientate aircrew, although there is no shortage of anecdotal reports of incidents in which the pilot was confused by atypical visual cues. The pilot who uses the top of a bank of clouds as a horizontal reference or the streamers of an auroral display as the vertical reference is, by definition, disoriented when these visual references do not accord with the true horizontal or vertical. The perceptual error can be ascribed to an error of expectancy. Cloud tops commonly are horizontal; therefore, there is a high conditional probability – a high expectancy – that a cloud top is horizontal. Accordingly, an error of perception occurs when the pilot uses a familiar cue that may not look atypical but does not accord with the usual rule. At lower altitudes, the trunks of conifers, which are commonly vertical, may give a false reference when, in response to prevailing wind or local topography, they grow at an angle inclined to the true vertical.

When flying at low level, a pilot tends to judge his or her height above the ground by the scale of objects in the field of view. This becomes more difficult when terrain features are largely absent, as when flying over water, desert or a snow-covered landscape. The pilot of a float-plane attempting to land on the glassy surface of a lake may be obliged to set up a descent rate of about 150 feet/min and wait until the aircraft touches down on the water rather than risk rounding out too soon or impacting the water at too high a descent rate. A similar approach may be required by a pilot when landing on snow. Trees can be unreliable features against which to judge height. Stunted trees and bushes may lead to an overgenerous estimate of ground clearance.

Flight in mountainous terrain may give rise to difficulties with height and distance estimation for lack of scale features. There can also be problems in certain lighting conditions, often with the sun low in the sky and directly behind the aircraft, when the distant terrain masks the contour of more imminent high ground that is lying in the flight path of the aircraft. These problems are exacerbated when the ground is snow-covered and ground textural features are lost. Similarly, a snow-covered ridge may become invisible against a background of uniform brightly lit cloud. Such conditions, known as 'whiteout', were a contributory factor in the crash of a DC10 aircraft on Mount Erebus in Antarctica in 1979.

Even in apparently clear visual conditions at ground level, with increasing altitude the horizon may become hazy and indistinct, possibly to the extent that the pilot describes him- or herself as flying in goldfish-bowl conditions. In the circumstance of deteriorating external vision, the pilot has to assess when the external visual cues are no longer sufficiently reliable and to make the decision to transfer to instruments.

When flying in thin cloud, the increased brightness of the cloud in the direction of the sun may give a false sense of what the pilot considers to be 'upward' and lead the pilot to bank the aircraft in that direction. Cloud may give rise to false horizons. A line of low cloud over the sea when viewed from a higher altitude may suggest a horizon that is below the true horizon and result in an inadvertent descent of the aircraft. The tops of clouds may often appear flat but are not necessarily horizontal and may lead a pilot, who assumes them to be so, to make an error in bank attitude.

Whereas the preceding examples are associated with errors in the perception of attitude, illusory perception of motion, called vection illusions, can also be generated by movement of external visual cues. Disorientation of this type is experienced mainly by helicopter pilots, who, on attempting to maintain an accurate hover at low altitude, may feel that their aircraft is moving when they look at the motion of waves on water or long grass generated by the ground effect of the rotor. Comparable illusions of vertical motion are produced by the downward movement of water droplets or snowflakes entrained in the downwash of the rotor. The moving shadow of helicopter rotor blades cast across the cockpit, or the backscatter of light from a rotating anti-collision light when flying in cloud, are two further situations in which illusory sensations of motion can be engendered by these vection stimuli. Disorientation produced by such visual stimuli, whether these are the essentially static sloping cloud bank or the dynamic moving shadow of a rotor blade, can be very powerful because the ambient visual system reacts in proportion to the area of retina stimulated. Hence, the larger the angle subtended at the eye by the static or moving stimulus, the more compelling the erroneous sensation.

VISUAL CUES FROM AIRCRAFT INSTRUMENTS

The primary stimulus for the development of flight instruments was the inability of humans to sense important variables such as airspeed, heading, altitude and attitude in those flight conditions where external cues were degraded by cloud, darkness, etc. Although every effort is made by designers and manufacturers to ensure the accuracy and reliability of primary flight instruments, on which the safety of aircraft and occupants depends when flying in IMC, defects do occur. Failure of an instrument is normally indicated by a warning flag, but incidents have occurred in which instruments have failed or the display jammed without indication of malfunction. The pilot fails to realize that control of the aircraft is based on an erroneous cue and is, by definition, disoriented, but he or she may not be aware of the hazardous situation unless the instrument malfunction is detected on cross-checking against other flight instruments.

Neither head-up nor the more conventional head-down instruments are immune from this type of fault. The problem is, however, usually more serious when failure of a head-up display occurs. The pilot has to transfer gaze from the head-up display to the head-down instruments; whatever external orientational cues that were visible are lost, and the pilot is temporarily 'unoriented' until the basic flight instruments are scanned and interpreted. In some modern aircraft, the pilot's task has been made the more difficult because the head-up presentation has been made the primary display of flight information (attitude, heading, air-speed, etc.) and the conventional instruments have been relegated to a standby role. Consequently, they are small and not positioned optimally within the cockpit. A large movement of the head and eyes is required in order to see them, and even when in sight they are not easy to read.

Dynamic limitations of instruments have also been implicated in a few aircraft accidents. Pressure-operated instruments, in particular, can be slow to respond and may only indicate correctly some four to five seconds after a sudden change in the displayed variable. Such a dynamic error in the vertical speed indicator (VSI) was regarded as a contributory cause of an accident in which an aircraft failed to climb away on a 'missed approach'. It was suggested that as the aircraft climbed away from the runaway, the VSI would have indicated too high a rate of climb and that, as the pilot pushed forward on the stick, several seconds would have elapsed before the instrument would have displayed the loss of altitude.

IMPAIRMENT OF VISION

The ability of the pilot to perceive the all-important visual cues, whether from the external visual world or the flight-deck instruments, can be degraded by factors that impair either the quality of the retinal image or the transduction of the image by the sensory cells of the retina. Unless the retinal image is reasonably stable and fixation of the eye relative to the observed object is preserved for 100 ms or so, then visual acuity is impaired. In flight, vibration is one of the common causes of destabilization of the retinal image and can, in certain circumstances, be of sufficient severity to prevent the pilot from reading the instruments. In helicopters, this problem occurs most commonly when maximum power is applied, such as at transition to the hover. In fixed-wing aircraft, the vibration that results from the aircraft entering buffet boundary at high altitude (as in a 'jet upset'-type incident) or from high-speed flight at low altitude in turbulence has prevented pilots from reading their instruments and thus potentiated the disorientation engendered by the concurrent changes in the force environment.

Vestibular nystagmus can also degrade vision when the vestibular response is inappropriate (Figure 18.13, page 303). These nystagmic eye movements impair the pilot's only reliable channel of information about aircraft orientation at the very time that false sensations are being evoked by erroneous vestibular signals. On initiating recovery from a spin, the pilot may have a strong sensation of turning in a direction opposite to that of the spin and be unable to see the instruments or even external cues with sufficient clarity to know, unambiguously, that the aircraft has ceased to gyrate. In addition to the nystagmus associated with the onset and recovery from high rates of angular motion, as in a roll or spin, comparable difficulties arise when the vestibular apparatus is stimulated by middle ear pressure change. The sudden and unexpected onset of pressure vertigo is a potent cause of disorientation where resolution of sensory conflict by reference to aircraft instruments is not aided by the concomitant nystagmus.

Laboratory experiments have shown that the period for which vision is degraded by inappropriate nystagmus is reduced when the brightness and contrast of the observed object are increased. Consequently, the advice to aircrew who find themselves in the unfortunate position of being unable to read the aircraft instruments because of nystagmus is to increase the level of illumination to the maximum available. Another factor influencing the period of visual impairment is the plane of the nystagmus. Nystagmus in yaw is suppressed more rapidly than in roll. Hence, during the recovery from a prolonged spin, nystagmus dies away more rapidly if the pilot tilts the head backward and tries to look at the horizon during the spin than if he or she bends the head forward and looks at the ground. On the other hand, if recovery from the spin has to be made by reference to instruments, then the movement of the head on transferring gaze from the horizon to the instrument panel can produce a cross-coupled stimulus, which is potentially more disorientating than when no head movement is made.

Vision can also be degraded by the nystagmus associated with the consumption of ethyl alcohol (ethanol). Experiments have shown that alcohol increases the duration and intensity of post-rotational nystagmus (e.g. on recovery from a spin) by attenuating the suppressive action of the fixation reflex (Figure 28.2). A blood alcohol concentration as low as 20 mg/100 ml has been shown to prolong the nystagmic response on stimulating the semicircular canals and to cause a significant impairment of visual performance. With substantially higher levels of blood alcohol, the nystagmus recorded while the subject tries to fixate is hardly of lower velocity or shorter duration

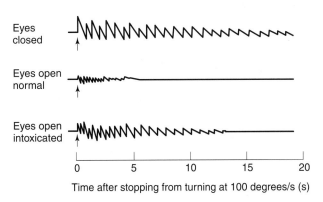

Figure 28.2 *Alterations of post-rotational eye movements by alcohol. The graphs show the nystagmus produced by recovery from sustained rotation at 100 degrees/second. In the dark, or with the eyes closed, the eye movements last for 30 seconds or more, but when the pilot fixates on objects inside or outside the aircraft the nystagmus is suppressed, although it is not abolished until about five seconds after the stimulus. Intoxication with ethyl alcohol reduces the effectiveness of the suppressive mechanism and, hence, prolongs the time for which vision is impaired by inappropriate nystagmus.*

than that recorded in the absence of fixation in a subject who has not taken alcohol.

In addition, alcohol can cause nystagmus and its associated vertigo by a direct effect on the labyrinth. It appears that on consumption of alcohol, it diffuses into the cupula and sets up a density difference between the cupula and the endolymph in which it lies. As a result, the receptors of the semicircular canals are stimulated by linear acceleration and, hence, the orientation of the head to gravity. This is manifested by the vertigo and nystagmus that occurs on moving from a sitting position to a lying posture with the head turned to one side. This positional response declines over a few hours after drinking alcohol but is then replaced by a new positional response with nystagmus and sensations of turning in the opposite direction to that experienced initially. Depending on the amount of alcohol consumed, this second phase of the positional response can remain for 48 hours or more. The implication for flying is that prolonged generous alcohol ingestion is not amenable to the 12-hour 'bottle-to-throttle' rule. Although alcohol may be cleared from the blood and cognition unimpaired after this time, it is sequestered in the endolymph for a longer period and may cause positional vertigo after a much longer interval. If flying involves high-G manoeuvres, then the increased G amplifies the effect of any density disparity and, thus, any consequent vertigo and nystagmus.

Impairment of vision by glare and dazzle or by the reduction in retinal blood flow with $+G_z$ acceleration has been reported as the primary cause of disorientation and loss of control in a number of aircraft accidents. The specific mechanisms in these derangements of retinal function are described in Chapter 8.

Cues from vestibular and other mechanoreceptors

INADEQUATE CUES

The failure of non-visual sensory systems to detect changes in attitude or motion of the aircraft is probably the most important single cause of orientation error accidents, although in accounts of disorientation incidents the absence of sensation is rarely reported; rather, it is the unexpected vertigo or other strong illusory sensation that is described. Vestibular and kinaesthetic receptors are all mechanoreceptors and transduce motion stimuli only when deformation or deflection occurs under the influence of inertial or reactive forces. In general, the sensory receptors and their associated central perceptual mechanisms respond only to change. We have no absolute sense of position or velocity within a spatial coordinate system, although we can sense changes in position and velocity by detecting the angular or linear acceleration associated with

the movement. Furthermore, information provided by the stimulated receptors can be integrated perceptually so that reasonably accurate assessments of the magnitude of the change in position can be made. However, the foregoing is true only for 'adequate' stimuli, i.e. stimuli that are substantially above the detection threshold and within the dynamic range of the sensory system.

In common with other sensory systems, detection thresholds for motion stimuli transduced by vestibular and kinaesthetic receptors have to be defined in terms of the intensity and the duration of action of the stimulus. For angular movements of short duration (i.e. not greater than about five seconds), the angular velocity must exceed a median value of 1.5 °/s (26 mrad/s) for motion in yaw and 2 °/s (35 mrad/s) for motion in pitch and roll. When a rotational movement is prolonged, then the angular acceleration is the more important parameter. The threshold for detection of a sustained (more than ten seconds) angular acceleration has a median value of 0.3 °/s² (5 mrad/s²) but, in common with other motion detection thresholds, the variation between subjects is large, being 0.05–2.2 °/s² (0.1–38 mrad/s²). Threshold as a function of the frequency of the angular stimulus is shown in Figure 18.12.

The detection of linear movement is determined principally by the magnitude of the change in linear velocity, i.e. the linear acceleration, although as the response of the otoliths and other mechanoreceptors (in skin, etc.) is determined partly by the rate of change of acceleration, i.e. jerk, the threshold of detection varies with the frequency spectrum of the linear motion stimulus. Thus, for vertical sinusoidal oscillation in the z-body axis, threshold falls from a mean value of 0.18 m/s² at 0.2 Hz to 0.05 m/s² at 2 Hz. Thresholds for detection of linear accelerations acting in the x and y body axes are approximately 50 per cent lower than those for the detection of z-axis stimuli. Threshold as a function of the frequency of sinusoidal acceleration is shown in Figure 18.11.

Changes in attitude in pitch and roll (i.e. rotation about the y-and x-axes) from the normal upright position (z-body axis aligned with gravity) can involve stimulation of both semicircular canal and otolithic receptors. If the movement is at an angular velocity greater than 1–2 °/s, then the motion is detected by the semicircular canals. If body tilt occurs at a slower rate, then detection is dependent on signals from the otoliths. Typically, an individual can set or determine bodily attitude with respect to the gravitational vertical with an accuracy of ± 2 degrees, but if the rate of movement is very slow (0.1 °/s), then body tilt of 10 ° or more can take place before deviation from verticality is detected.

It is important to recognize that these threshold values have largely been determined in laboratory experiments where the subjects' sole task was to detect the motion stimulus. In flight, the pilot's attention is rarely so restricted and, in addition, there is a gamut of other sensory stimuli.

These factors make it likely that on occasions, the magnitude (or time/intensity integral) of the stimulus associated with motion of the aircraft can be substantially greater than the quoted threshold value before a change in attitude or velocity is sensed by the pilot.

ERRONEOUS CUES

In this category lie many of the most commonly described disorientation incidents in which the pilot is presented with a perceptual conflict. Signals from vestibular and kinaesthetic receptors give rise to sensations of body, and hence aircraft, motion that do not accord with the correct perception of aircraft orientation obtained from instrument cues. As noted earlier in this chapter, the conflict is usually but not always resolved. The pilot may accept, for a number of reasons, the false vestibular information and initiate inappropriate control movements with dangerous consequences.

Erroneous vestibular and kinaesthetic cues occur in flight because the pilot is exposed to rotational and transitional motion stimuli that differ in respect of magnitude, direction or time course from those that humans experience on the ground and for which the receptor systems are functionally adapted. Illusions of angular motion and of attitude, engendered by false vestibular and kinaesthetic cues, may be classified broadly as follows: (i) false information from semicircular canal receptors on recovery from prolonged rotation (somatogyral illusions) and on moving the head during rotation (cross-coupled or Coriolis illusions) and (ii) false information from otoliths and kinaesthetic receptors during sustained acceleration (somatogravic illusions) and on moving the head in an atypical force environment (G-excess illusions). In addition, the semicircular canal receptors can be stimulated by changes in middle ear pressure during ascent and descent, so that erroneous sensations of turning (pressure vertigo) are produced without there being any angular motion of the aircraft.

Central errors

Disorientation due to the pilot's failure to make optimum use of reliable information about aircraft orientation can arise because of limitations of the brain mechanisms that mediate the perceptual process. In general, the limitations are not caused by disease but are normal behavioural responses to the physical and mental load imposed by the flying task.

CONING OF ATTENTION OR 'FASCINATION'

This occurs most commonly in the student pilot who, under the stress of attempting to perform a demanding and unfamiliar task, allows their attention to be confined to one aspect of the task. With experience and the acquisition of skill, the pilot learns to maintain a regular scan, so that all aspects of the aircraft's flight trajectory and systems are monitored adequately. However, even the experienced pilot, when presented with a high workload, when anxious or when unduly aroused, can lose efficiency. One aspect of this impairment of performance is a restriction of the field of attention. Thus, when flying by instruments, the pilot may fix attention on one instrument, e.g. airspeed, and fail to notice a potentially dangerous change in attitude or height. The absence of information from non-visual receptors at such a time is, of course, contributory to the disorientation that occurs with the coning of attention. This type of perceptual limitation occurs most commonly during instrument flight, but it is not unknown for a pilot in good VMC to become 'fascinated' during an attack manoeuvre on a ground target and to fail to perceive their height above the ground until dangerously late in the manoeuvre. Coning of attention should not be mistaken for coning of vision. While it is true that visual events outside the restricted area subtended by a particular instrument are not perceived, this cone of attention is not a solid angle of invariant size. The problem is not overcome by presenting more information within a smaller area, as in a head-up display, for it has been found that coning of attention still occurs, even though the angular subtense of the display is considerably less than that of basic flight instruments.

ERROR OF EXPECTANCY

The heuristic nature of the perceptual process was mentioned earlier, where it was pointed out that an individual's perception of a particular sensory event is based on past experience and, hence, on the conditional probability of a particular temporospatial pattern of sensory information being associated with that event. The example quoted was one in which the pilot levelled the wings of the aircraft with cloud tops that he or she thought were, and expected to be horizontal, but that were inclined to the horizontal. Other incidents have been described in which visual information is misinterpreted and gives rise to an illusory perception of attitude. The pilot flying over the sea on a dark night looks out of the aircraft and sees a number of points of light below, which are perceived as stars, because at night it is more likely for stars rather than lights on fishing boats to be seen. This misperception leads to another: stars should be above not below, and therefore the aircraft must be inverted. Without checking the attitude display, the pilot rolls the aircraft over in order to bring it to what is mistakenly thought to be the correct attitude. Errors in the perception of distance can occur when ground features are atypical. There have been a number of accidents in which the pilot has overestimated aircraft height above the ground or distance from the side of a mountain because the trees were unusually small. If, for example, the pilot, from past experience, expects birch trees to be 10–20 m tall, then his or her perception of distance from ground covered by stunted trees only 4–5 m high is likely to be in error by a factor of two or more.

During approach and landing, pilots use a variety of visual cues to judge their spatial orientation, which embraces variables such as distance from touchdown, glide slope angle, altitude and airspeed. The perceptual processes are complex and have to be learned by repeated practice. It is, therefore, not surprising that errors occur when the visual cues are atypical, are degraded or do not accord with expectancy. Modification of aerial perspective by atmospheric conditions that reduce visibility, such as fog, rain, smoke, haze or snow, can lead to overestimation of distance. In such conditions, the runway may appear to be further away than its true distance, and the pilot may also think that his or her height above the ground is greater than in fact it is. Conversely, when atmospheric attenuation is less than that which the pilot has commonly experienced (e.g. the clear bright conditions of a high-altitude airfield), then distances may be underestimated and therefore a high approach may be flown, necessitating an overshoot. This tendency to match perceptually what is seen with what experience has led the pilot to expect is also the most likely cause of misjudgement during the approach to runways whose dimensions differ from those with which the pilot is familiar. Thus, on an approach to a runway that is unusually wide, the pilot will tend to underestimate distance; conversely, a narrow runway can lead to an overestimation of distance from threshold and increase the probability of landing long or having to overshoot. Even more confusing are those runways that preserve the typical length/width ratio but are wider and longer, or narrower and shorter, than runways with which the pilot is more familiar. Other aspects of the local topography may also lead to errors. Featureless terrain, snow-covered ground or a smooth sea are examples of situations where there is a lack of visual texture and insufficient visual cues to allow any reliable perception of height. Sloping terrain also contributes to the false perception of height on the approach in much the same way as sloping runways. It has been found, for example, that ground that slopes up towards the runway or has a similar upward inclination beyond the runway is likely to cause the pilot to overestimate height and lead to a lower than normal descent and approach to landing.

Darkness degrades or eliminates many of the visual cues employed during daytime approach and landings. Most accidents during this phase of flight occur at night, and characteristically the pilot makes a low approach and lands short. At night, the pilot must rely on the limited visual cues provided by runway and approach lights; the perceptual task is made even more difficult if the approach is over water or terrain without lights, the so-called black-hole approach. In simulations of a black-hole situation, in which only runway and approach lights were visible, it was found that pilots overestimated their approach angle, on occasions by a factor of two, and made a low approach.

The particular danger of disorientation during this phase of flight lies in the narrow temporal and spatial limits within which the aircraft must be controlled. There is little time and little altitude for errors to be corrected, and a decision to execute a missed-approach procedure and to overshoot must be made quickly if an accident is to be avoided. The basic problem is summarized neatly by Perrone: 'Humans are not very good at judging the slant of long narrow rectangular surfaces. Pilots must learn to believe their instruments, not their eyes.'

Visual information that differs from expectancy is the cause of a number of other illusions experienced by aircrew. The 'lean-on-the-sun' illusion is a false perception of attitude that occurs when flying in cloud, particularly when close to the top of the cloud. Although the sun is not visible, the cloud is distinctly brighter in the direction of the sun than in the rest of an amorphous visual scene. In these circumstances, the pilot equates the brightest area of cloud with 'up' and the dark cloud below as 'down' and so acquires a false vertical reference. Thus, if the sun appears to the left of the flight path, the pilot may bank the aircraft to the left to preserve an apparent straight and level attitude; conversely, the pilot may feel that the aircraft is right-wing low when instruments indicate a wings-level attitude. Comparable illusions of pitch attitude have also occurred when flying in cloud on a heading towards the sun.

Expectancy also contributes to the perceptual errors engendered by inappropriate vestibular cues. Years of experience of movement and postural activity in a terrestrial environment lead to a high conditional probability that signals from the semicircular canals are an accurate representation of angular movement of the head and that otolithic signals represent the dynamic component of translational movement and the attitude of the head with respect to the force of gravity. Accordingly, when comparable signals are generated by these sense organs by atypical motion stimuli, there is no reason why the sensation or perception of motion engendered should differ from that which occurs when the receptors correctly transduce a typical stimulus. When the semicircular canals erroneously signal rotation, e.g. on recovery from a spin, the pilot, naturally, perceives rotation. Likewise, during sustained acceleration (or deceleration) in the line of flight where the resultant of the imposed acceleration and that of gravity deviates from the vertical, the perceptual process does not distinguish the resultant acceleration from that of gravity alone. Errors in the perception of attitude occur because of the high conditional probability that the sustained discharge from the otoliths represents the orientation of the head to the gravitational vertical rather than their response to a sustained acceleration other than that of gravity.

OTHER DISTURBANCES OF BRAIN FUNCTION

The coning of attention that occurs when an individual has to perform a demanding or emotionally stressful task is but one manifestation of the changes in brain function and behaviour that are associated with 'arousal' beyond an optimum level. The term 'arousal' in this context is used in a somewhat specialized way to identify a behavioural continuum – the arousal continuum – which ranges from drowsiness at one extreme to acute awareness, or even panic, at the other. Although the concept has its limitations, it is useful when one attempts to integrate the varied effects of physical and mental stress on behaviour and brain function.

One important effect of high arousal is that it causes 'regression', a term first used by Head to describe the reversion to a more firmly established, more primitive pattern of behaviour that he observed in flying personnel under stress during the First World War. In flight, this regression may be manifest as a breakdown of the more complex and more recently acquired skills, of which instrument flying is the prime example. When learning to fly by instruments, the pilot is trained to ignore vestibular and kinaesthetic sensations; indeed, the experienced pilot is frequently unaware of such potentially disorientating sensations, even though they may be accessible to introspection. However, when aroused, the pilot is more likely to attend to these endogenous vestibular signals and may even base control of the aircraft on such inappropriate cues, despite training to disregard them.

Associated with the loss of recently acquired skills is a diminution of cerebral competence. This term is used to describe the impairment of higher mental function with supra-optimal arousal. It embraces the decrement in perceptual integration, decision-making ability, cognitive function and supervisory activity that can occur in high arousal states. Again, it is when flying on instruments that such disturbances of brain function are most apparent. A few pilots who have been highly aroused by, for example, sudden and severe disorientation have reported that they were unable to interpret the cockpit instruments, even though they could be seen with clarity. In contrast, aircrew rarely have any difficulty in the interpretation of external visual cues unless vision is seriously degraded.

Although disorientation is more commonly a feature of behavioural states in which the level of arousal is high, in a few incidents it is the low level of arousal that is the prime aetiological factor. Arousal below the optimum also causes a diminution of cerebral competence and with it a greater probability of perceptual errors. In particular, when the pilot is drowsy or inattentive, he or she is more likely to fail to perceive motion cues and to make an ill-considered response to misinterpreted sensory information.

The level of arousal is far from being the only factor that modifies the process of perception, for this depends on the normal function of the central nervous system, which, in turn, depends on the maintenance of the chemical and physical milieu of the brain within relatively narrow limits. It would be inappropriate to detail here the many factors that, in flight, may interfere with brain function, as they range from the classic environmental stresses of flight, such as hypoxia, hypocapnia, high G and toxic agents, to the myriad clinical disorders that, albeit rarely, can impair cerebral competence and disorientate the pilot.

FALSE PERCEPTION OF ATTITUDE AND LINEAR MOTION

Somatogravic illusions

Errors in the perception of attitude can occur when the aviator is exposed to force environments that differ significantly from those experienced during normal activity on the surface of the Earth, where the force of gravity is a stable reference and is regarded as the vertical. The acceleration of gravity is the same physical phenomenon as a linear (or translational) acceleration, and hence the one is not easily distinguished from the other. When the imposed linear acceleration is of short duration or oscillatory, humans are able to separate, perceptually, the imposed motion from that of gravity. For example, the cyclical motion of walking or the motion of a swing are sensed with reasonable accuracy, but when the acceleration is sustained, as in a centrifuge or when an aircraft accelerates in response to an increase in thrust or a reduction of drag, the perceptual mechanism is unable to distinguish reliably the imposed acceleration from that of gravity. The two accelerations are combined, and the resultant becomes the reference acceleration, which is the perceived vertical. This occurs because there is a high expectancy that a sustained acceleration is gravity and, hence, the vertical.

The simplest example of an illusory perception of attitude, due to an atypical resultant acceleration (or force) vector, is the inability of the pilot to sense accurately, other than by visual cues, the angle of bank during a prolonged coordinated turn (Figure 28.3). Some information about bank angle comes from the semicircular canals that are stimulated by the angular motion in roll as the aircraft enters the turn, but they cease to contribute once a steady rate of turn and constant bank angle is established. In such a coordinated turn, the resultant of the force of gravity and the inertial force due to the radial (or centripetal) acceleration engendered by the curved flight path is normal to the

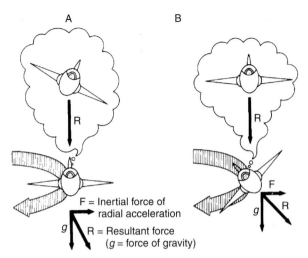

Figure 28.3 *False perception of attitude – the somatogravic illusion – in a turn. The pilot equates the sustained resultant (R) with the vertical. Hence, in a flat turn (A), the pilot may feel as if they are rolled out of the turn. In the more usual coordinated turn (B), the resultant is aligned with the pilot's z-axis and they have no sensation of being in a banked attitude.*

longitudinal and transverse axes of the aircraft and is aligned with the pilot's *z*-axis. The direction of action of this resultant force does not differ from that of gravity on the body when it is in a normal upright position in a 1-G environment. Apart from an increase in the magnitude of the *z*-axis acceleration, vestibular and kinaesthetic cues are not dissimilar to those in level flights, and so the pilot is

likely to feel that the aircraft is in a wings-level attitude. Conversely, in a flat turn, when the resultant vector is not normal to the transverse axis of the aircraft (Figure 28.3), the pilot may feel as if the aircraft is banked out of the turn.

These are examples of a group of illusions, termed somatogravic illusions, in which there is a false perception of attitude on exposure to a force vector that differs in direction and/or magnitude from the normal gravitational force. Of no less importance, from the viewpoint of flight safety, than the illusory perceptions of roll attitude described above are those somatogravic illusions in which there is an error in the perception of pitch attitude (Figure 28.4). Consider an aircraft on the runway threshold before takeoff. A typical takeoff run involves an acceleration of 0.25 G along the runway. If after takeoff the aircraft is put into a gentle climb, then this level of forward acceleration may continue for some time. In fact, at 0.25 G in the line of flight it would be a further 60 seconds before the aircraft reached 450 knots – a typical fast-jet airspeed in the cruise. In clear external visual conditions, a pilot should have no difficulty in maintaining an appropriate climb angle. If, however, the aircraft enters cloud, the pilot will have to transfer to instruments. Any attempt to continue the climb simply by the feel of the aircraft is likely to lead to an error in pitch attitude. In these circumstances, the pilot experiences the effect of two steady forces. Gravity pushes the pilot down into the seat, and the forward acceleration of the aircraft pushes the pilot back in the seat. The net effect of these two forces is a single force acting downwards and backwards that feels exactly like gravity. The pilot could only experience this pattern of forces from gravity alone if

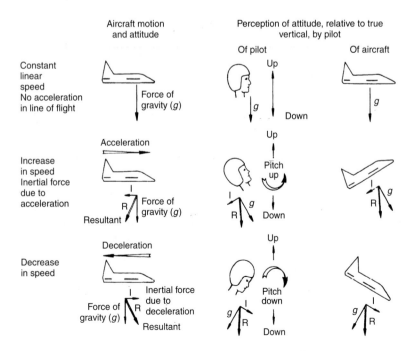

Figure 28.4 *Somatogravic illusions during linear acceleration in the line of flight give errors in the perception of pitch attitude.*

he or she and the seat were tilted backwards. A sense of backward tilt equates with a perception of nose-up attitude of the aircraft that is greater than it actually is. Furthermore, any adjustment that the pilot makes to the pitch attitude of the aircraft is unlikely to make much difference to the perceived sense of pitch-up. This is because a reduction in climb angle allows a greater proportion of the engine thrust to accelerate the aircraft in the line of flight and, hence, to add to the illusory sensation of pitch-up. Likewise, should the pilot increase the climb angle of the aircraft, there would be a reduced forward acceleration, since more of the thrust would be required for the climb. Consequently, any sensation associated with actual pitch change would be offset by a reduced illusory sensation of pitch-up and, thus, little change in perceived pitch attitude.

Because of the somatogravic effect, a fixed wing aircraft accelerating in the line of flight will tend to feel more nose-up than it actually is; correspondingly, a decelerating aircraft will tend to feel more nose-down. It does not matter how these accelerations and decelerations come about. The example cited above considers the forward acceleration of the aircraft that results from the level of engine thrust required for takeoff and climb-out. To take another example, if a pilot flying straight and level at constant speed inadvertently allows the nose to drop, the aircraft will begin to accelerate under the influence of gravity and it will feel more nose-up than it actually is. Until the aerodynamic drag increases and establishes a new constant airspeed, it may still feel as if the aircraft is in level flight, even though it is going downhill. In just the same way, if the pilot allows the nose to rise, the aircraft will decelerate, and it will feel more nose-down than it actually is – in fact, as if in level flight.

Although this manifestation of the somatogravic effect will occur in all aircraft types, it is of great relevance to glider pilots. Gliders are designed to have minimum levels of aerodynamic drag. An increased nose-down attitude allows the glider to accelerate and can lead to the build-up of excessive airspeed before the pilot becomes aware from the feel of the aircraft of a change in pitch attitude.

In addition to changes of heading, an aerobatic aircraft can generate a curved flight path in any direction, e.g. when flying a loop or a barrel roll. The result is that an aircraft can generate aerodynamically its own force environment, this being a combination of the force of gravity and the aerodynamic forces involved in the manoeuvre. For this reason, an aircraft can feel level when it is in a coordinated turn or when inverted at the top of a loop; it can be made to feel inverted when in fact it is upright if the pilot pushes the stick forward and initiates a vigorous bunt manoeuvre.

There are particular circumstances in flight when pilots have to remain very aware of possible errors of aircraft attitude arising from the somatogravic effect. Mention has already been made of takeoff into low cloud, where the transition from external vision to instruments must be anticipated and an appropriate rate of climb maintained. A similar situation occurs when a pilot intending to land the aircraft has, for some, reason to overshoot the runway and go around for a second approach (Figure 28.5). Poor weather conditions often may underlie the need to overshoot, and a pilot may be distracted by the other tasks involved in the manoeuvre and fail to establish a positive rate of climb. Low-level flight in a military aircraft may have to be aborted on account of deteriorating visual conditions, low cloud or failing light. This manoeuvre involves

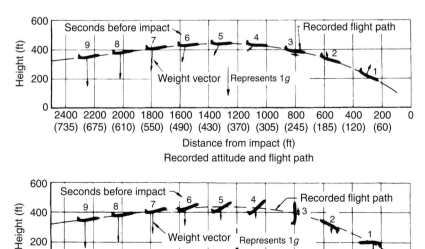

Figure 28.5 *Recorded flight path and calculated force (weight) vector of an aircraft (Vanguard G-APEE) that crashed after initiating an overshoot. The initial change in the direction of the force vector was caused by acceleration in the line of flight. Later, the curved flight path introduced a radial acceleration and was responsible for large changes in the direction and magnitude of the force vector. Over the relatively short timescale in which changes in the force environment occurred, it is unlikely that the illusory perception of attitude was as erroneous as indicated in the lower half of the figure, but illusions of the form shown have been reported during comparable bunt manoeuvres. (Distance from impact in m given in parentheses.)*

a rapid climb to a safe altitude with full thrust applied to the engines. The desire to correct for what feels like an excessive pitch angle has to be resisted in favour of what the aircraft instruments are saying.

Oculogravic illusions

The illusory perception of attitude engendered by a force vector that is not aligned with the gravitational vertical is not dependent on vision: it is an illusion of body orientation – hence the term 'somatogravic illusion' (from the Greek *soma*, body). Unfortunately, the term 'oculogravic' is often, albeit incorrectly, used to describe such illusions, but this adjective should be confined to the apparent movement and false localization of visual targets that may be produced by the same atypical force environments as evoke somatogravic illusions. Indeed, the oculogravic illusion is best regarded as a visual component of the somatogravic illusion. Thus, when an aircraft accelerates and there is a backward rotation of the resultant force vector (Figure 28.6), the pilot may experience a somatogravic illusion of a nose-up change in attitude, which may be accompanied by an apparent upward movement and displacement of objects within the visual field. Conversely, on deceleration, the visual world may appear to move downwards and to be displaced, until the force environment returns to the normal 1 g. This apparent movement and displacement of the visual scene, brought about by a change in the force environment (i.e. the oculogravic illusion), is considered not to be due primarily to eye movement but to processes within the brain that integrate retinal information with signals from the otoliths and other receptors stimulated by the linear accelerations.

The oculogravic illusion is rarely a problem when external visual cues are well defined, for the illusory movement affects all objects within the visual field so that there is no relative movement between objects in the external visual scene and the frame of reference provided by aircraft structures, e.g. cockpit canopy, instrument panel. In the presence of a resultant force vector that is not aligned with the gravitational vertical, the surface of the Earth may appear to be in a non-horizontal plane, but the position and attitude of the aircraft are not changed with respect to the external visual reference. At night, however, particularly when only a few stars or isolated lights are visible – conditions in which external visual cues are largely inadequate – the oculogravic illusion can be a significant cause of spatial disorientation. The apparent movement and transient displacement of light sources in the external visual scene can be interpreted by the aviator as a change in attitude of the aircraft. Alternatively, the apparent movement of an isolated light on the ground can lead to the misperception that the light is on another aircraft, which, if the pilot attempts to follow, could lead to disaster.

Visual illusions also occur when there is a change in the magnitude of the force vector without rotation of the vector. These were given the name elevator illusions because

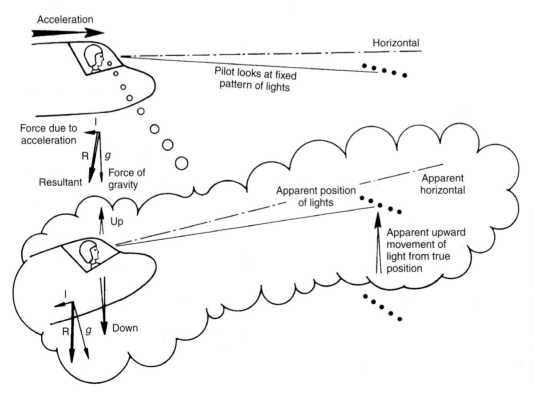

Figure 28.6
Oculogravic illusion. This is the visual component of the somatogravic illusion in which a change in the force environment causes apparent movement and false localization of observed objects.

they were first studied in lifts (elevators), although comparable changes in the force environment occur during flight through an up- or down-draught. With an increase in the magnitude in z-axis acceleration, such as occurs during vertical acceleration in the upward direction (up-draught), there is a correct sensation of upward movement, which is accompanied by an apparent upward motion and displacement of the visual scene. Conversely, when the force vector decreases, as during flight through a down-draught, there is an apparent downward movement and displacement of objects within the pilot's visual scene. These oculogravic illusions are relatively easily suppressed and are rarely noticed when flying with good external visual cues, but when external visual cues are sparse the apparent movement of an isolated light may be interpreted as a change in pitch attitude of the aircraft; an upward movement is perceived as pitch nose-down and the converse when there is a reduction in the magnitude of the aircraft's normal acceleration. The hazard from these errors in perception, as in other manifestations of the somatogravic and oculogravic illusions, is that control responses may be made by the pilot before the orientation of the aircraft is checked by reference to flight instruments.

Effect of head movement: 'G excess' illusions

It has long been recognized that erroneous sensations of angular motion are evoked when head movements are made in a turning aircraft, and it has been customary to attribute such illusions to cross-coupled stimulation of the semicircular canals. However, experiments carried out in high-performance aircraft where a large-radius coordinated turn was flown with a resultant acceleration of $2\,G_z$ but with a low rate of turn ($4\,°/s$), have shown that head movements in pitch, roll or yaw could induce false sensations of aircraft attitude. Commonly, subjects reported an illusory sensation of climb or dive on moving the head in pitch, although none of direction, magnitude of the illusion or evocative head movement was entirely consistent between individuals. These false sensations were not caused by cross-coupled stimulation of the semicircular canals because the plane of the apparent motion did not accord with such a mechanism and the rate of turn was so low. Rather, it is suggested that the sensations are the consequence of a transient and atypical stimulation of otolithic receptors, as their orientation to the abnormal force vector changes when the head is moved. Despite the lack of a clear-cut relationship between head movement and sensation, the illusory sensation experienced by some subjects can be powerful, particularly when the head is moved quickly; others find the sensations confusing and disorientating and yet difficult to describe precisely in terms of aircraft attitude and motion. Other experiments have shown that a forward head movement in pitch, made

during a pull-up from a dive, consistently evoked a sensation of tumbling forward in pitch. The illusion is not just an apparent change in attitude but contains an element of rotation in the plane of the head movement, despite the absence of any cross-coupled stimulus to the semicircular canals.

The leans

A pilot manoeuvring an aircraft when flying in cloud may return the aircraft to straight and level flight according to the attitude instruments only to be left with the sensation that the aircraft is flying with one wing low. This sensation may be so compelling that the pilot feels the need to tilt him- or herself in the seat to bring the head and trunk more in line with what he or she feels to be vertical – hence the name 'the leans'. Surveys of military pilots indicate that over 90 per cent have experienced the leans. However, the assertion that the leans is the most common illusion of flight is incorrect. The illusion that an aircraft is in level flight when it is in a banked turn is far more common – so common that pilots do not consider it to be an illusion but rather an everyday part of flying.

A sequence of events that may lead to the leans is illustrated in Figure 28.7. A pilot is flying without any external visual reference. An unperceived rightward bank leads the aircraft to enter a co-ordinated turn to the right. Having recognised this unintended aircraft attitude, the pilot rolls the aircraft to the left at a supra-threshold rate to restore level flight. Because the aircraft felt to be straight and level while in the turn there is a possibility that, following an abrupt roll to the left, the aircraft may feel to the pilot to be flying with the left wing low. Though instructors fly this sequence of manoeuvres in an attempt to demonstrate the leans to their student, they do not always succeed. Similarly, when pilots do develop the leans they are often unable to say what sequence of manoeuvres brought it about.

When a pilot has the leans, the sensation that he or she experiences is not the same as would be experienced if one wing were actually low, for then the aircraft would tend to enter a coordinated turn and, in consequence, feel level. It is possible for a pilot deliberately to reproduce the sensation of the leans if he or she banks the aircraft but then opposes its tendency to turn by applying opposite rudder. In general, however, if, in cloud, a pilot feels that he or she is flying with one wing low, then they probably have the leans.

For many pilots, the leans are a minor distraction, readily overcome by attention to correct instrument flying. The false sensation of bank may persist for many minutes and on occasions much longer; indeed, durations of over an hour have been reported. Control is maintained by instrument reference, but the continued sensory conflict can

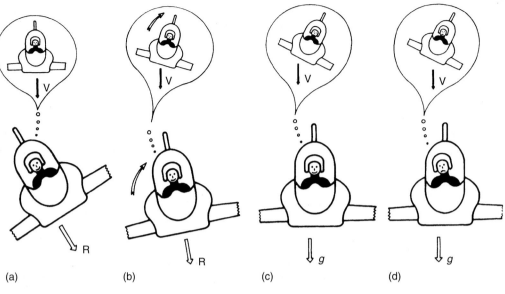

Figure 28.7
Diagrammatic representation of a cause of 'the leans'. R, resultant force vector, V, perceived vertical, g, force of gravity.

(a)
Aircraft in co-ordinated turn to right. Pilot feels that wings are level

(b)
Pilot rolls out of turn, feels that aircraft is banking to left

(c)
Aircraft in straight and level flight. Pilot feels left wing low

(d)
Pilot aligns head and trunk to perceived vertical and leans to right

drain the nervous energy of even the most experienced pilot. The reason why, on some occasions, the illusory sensation should be so persistent is not known, but, quite characteristically, the leans are dispelled as soon as the pilot has unambiguous external visual cues, such as a well-defined horizon or a clear sight of the ground. Here, then, is a demonstration of the greater strength of ambient visual cues over focal cues from instruments in determining spatial orientation in flight. Occasionally, while still in cloud, a pilot can cancel the leans by allowing the aircraft slowly to bank in the same direction as the sensation of the leans and then initiating an abrupt return to wings level. But, just as this sequence does not always produce the leans, so its inverse does not always dispel them.

In some circumstances, the leans can be a much more alarming experience. This is particularly so if the leans develops during air-to-air refuelling or in a pilot flying in close formation in the wing position. Such a pilot takes his or her attitude reference from the lead aircraft, and the task of maintaining correct separation is demanding enough without the intrusion of false sensations of aircraft attitude.

The physiology of the otolithic system has little to contribute to an understanding of the leans. In continuous straight and level flight, there is no reason why there should be spurious otolithic signals to indicate a tilt from the vertical. The problem must arise at the level of perception. The aircraft manoeuvres that provoke the leans are likely to have involved the sensory conflict of rotations in roll that are not accompanied by any corresponding sensa-

tion of tilt. It would seem that in these circumstances, the otolithic input to the perceptual model of what is vertical requires to be 're-zeroed' by visual means and that visual orientation information consciously acquired from the aircraft instruments is inadequate for this purpose.

The leans can also be caused by the misinterpretation of visual cues. The use of an erroneous horizontal reference, as in 'cloud leans', or the false localization of the vertical during flight in cloud because the brightest part of the cloud is regarded as up (the 'lean-on-the-sun' illusion) are described earlier in this chapter.

FALSE PERCEPTION OF ANGULAR MOTION: VERTIGO

Vertigo is defined as an illusory sensation of turning, but, as noted earlier, in aircrew jargon the term 'vertigo' is applied to any form of spatial disorientation, even when there is no illusory sensation of turning. Accordingly, the adjective 'somatogyral' will be applied to those incidents in which the aviator has an illusory perception of angular motion either of self or of self and aircraft. The term 'oculogyral' will be restricted to the visual illusions produced by angular motion stimuli, in the same manner as the terms 'oculogravic' and 'somatogravic' are used, respectively, to identify the visual and non-visual components of the illusions engendered by atypical force environments.

The somatogyral illusion

It was pointed out earlier that the semicircular canal receptors are stimulated only by angular accelerations and, hence, signal changes in angular velocity. Thus, during a prolonged turning manoeuvre at a constant angular speed, whether this be a coordinated turn, a sustained roll or a spin, these receptors give correct information only during the first few seconds of the manoeuvre (see Figure 18.6). Once a steady speed of rotation has been achieved, the signals from the semicircular canals, stimulated by the initial angular acceleration, die away progressively and fall below the threshold value after about 10–20 seconds. The time taken for the sensation of turning to die away depends on a number of factors: the speed of rotation, the axis of rotation, the nature of cues from other sensory receptors, and the extent to which the pilot is familiar with the motion stimuli (level of habituation). But for a typical spin, in which the aircraft may reach a rotational speed of 120–150 °/s (2–3 rad) in two to three seconds, it can be reckoned that most pilots will be unable to perceive rotation accurately by purely vestibular mechanisms after 15–30 seconds. They can, however, detect the continuation of the spin by the erratic pitching rolling and yawing movements that occur in most spinning aircraft and can determine the direction of the spin from the blurred image of the outside world as it swirls past the pilot's gaze. The task of maintaining an awareness of aircraft orientation is even more difficult during an inverted spin, partly because rolling and yawing movements do not appear to occur in the same sense as they do in an erect spin and partly because of the pilot's unfamiliarity with this configuration of flight.

In an erect or inverted spin, external visual cues and, more reliably, the turn indicator display allow the pilot to determine the direction of the spin and to initiate appropriate recovery action, but as soon as the aircraft begins to come out of the spin there is an angular acceleration in the opposite direction to that which occurred on entering the spin. The semicircular canals are stimulated again and evoke a sensation of turning in the opposite direction. This somatogyral illusion occurs at a time when the pilot has to decide when the rotational component of the spin has ceased in order to complete the recovery manoeuvre. The only reliable means of detecting the cessation of the spin is by reference either to instruments or to the appearance of the external visual scene. At this critical point, vision may be degraded by nystagmus that is as inappropriate as the concomitant sensation of turning. No matter how hard the pilot may try to 'see', it commonly takes several seconds for the eye movement to be suppressed sufficiently so that instruments can be read.

The presence of false sensations and impaired vision can have serious consequences during spin recovery. On the one hand, the pilot may feel that the spin has been neutralized before this has actually happened and subsequently get into difficulties on attempting to pull out. Alternatively, having recovered correctly, the pilot may feel that the aircraft is spinning in the opposite direction and may make inappropriate control movements to counteract this illusory spin. If this happens, then the aircraft can enter a spin in the original direction or even an inverted spin. This can give rise to an even more complex and confusing impression of motion, so that, finally, it might be impossible for the pilot to regain control of the aircraft.

Spinning provides an extreme example of rotational and post-rotational effects. More recently described is the post-rotational effect in roll that can be demonstrated following a roll manoeuvre from a banked attitude of 45 degrees, say left wing down, to the equivalent 45-degree attitude with right wing down. If a pilot immediately after making this manoeuvre is asked to close his or her eyes and attempt to maintain this banked attitude, the pilot will tend to overbank the aircraft in compensation for the perceived postrotational sensation in roll, which leads the pilot to think the aircraft is rolling back towards a wings-level attitude.

During turning manoeuvres in an aircraft, particularly when external visual conditions are degraded, pilots are taught to avoid making unnecessary head movements. The risk in these circumstances is in provoking false sensations from the cross-coupled or Coriolis effect (see Chapter 18). Cross-coupled sensations can be produced much more readily in a rotating chair on the ground than can be achieved in the aircraft. For this reason, demonstration of these sensations is a well-established feature of ground-based disorientation training. However, in flight, illusory sensations due to cross-coupling are less evident, either because the rate of rotation, e.g. during a change of heading, is usually much less than can be achieved on a rotating chair or because rotations that can be made at high rates, e.g. roll manoeuvres, are often not sustained for long periods. Nonetheless, even mild cross-coupled sensations induced by head movement during turning manoeuvres can be disconcerting to a pilot in circumstances where there is no stable external visual reference to countermand erroneous vestibular sensations.

The oculogyral illusion

Apart from the impairment of visual acuity caused by nystagmic eye movements, inappropriate signals from the semicircular canals have other effects on visual perception that can disorientate aircrew. These take the form of apparent motion and errors in the localization of the visual scene. At the beginning of rotation, such as a turn or roll, the vestibulo-ocular reflex stabilizes the retinal image of an Earth-fixed visual scene and allows it to be seen clearly. However, these eye movements are inappropriate for seeing objects within the aircraft, which, accordingly, can appear to move and be displaced in the same direction and in the same plane as the sensed turn. This effect is known as the oculogyral illusion. Even when there is no visual reference to the outside world, the apparent movement and displacement of the visual scene, relative to the observer, within the aircraft reinforces the veridical sensation of turning engendered by the semicircular canals. Conversely, on recovery from prolonged rotation, the oculogyral illusion takes the form of an apparent displacement and movement of the visual scene in the same direction as the erroneous sensation of turning (somatogyral illusion).

In laboratory experiments, it has been found that the detection threshold of angular motions is lower when the subject is provided with a discrete visual target and can perceive an oculogyral illusion than when in darkness and can report only on the detection of somatogyral sensation. In flight, the illusory perception of movement of an isolated light can thus be caused by quite liminal angular motion of the aircraft; the pilot perceives movement of the light but not of the aircraft. This error may in turn lead to a further misinterpretation, namely that the light is not fixed in space but is carried by another aircraft. Disorientation ensues if the pilot accepts this false cue and alters the flight path to join up with the illusory aircraft. Fortunately, the pilot usually becomes aware of the error before an accident occurs, although this type of incident, in common with other manifestations of spatial disorientation, can be a frightening experience.

Illusions due to cross-coupled (Coriolis) stimulation of the semicircular canals

Reference has already been made to the disorientation evoked by head movements in an abnormal force environment, but no less important are the illusory and apparently bizarre sensations that can be produced when angular movements of the head are made in an aircraft that is turning. These cross-coupled responses, due to the stimulation of the semicircular canals by the interaction of angular motion in two planes, can be analysed in terms of the Coriolis forces induced by the complex motion. However, it is conceptually much simpler to consider each canal as an angular velocity sensor and to analyse how the angular velocity in the plane of each canal changes with the head movement; this approach is followed in Chapter 18, where cross-coupled effects are described in some detail (pp. 297–300).

In flight, the disorientation produced by head movement in a turning or spinning aircraft is probably a combination of cross-coupled and 'G excess' illusions, for it is rare for the aircraft to execute a manoeuvre involving angular motion without there being an associated change in the force environment. The relative importance of canal and otolithic responses in the disorientation caused by head movement has yet to be resolved, but head move-

ments are undoubtedly a potent cause of perceptual errors in flight. The inappropriate sensations frequently have a sudden and unexpected onset and occur at a time when the pilot's attention is directed to some other aspect of the flying task. The classic situation is one in which the pilot, during a descending instrument turn, has to turn his or her head in order to operate controls on the side-consoles in the cockpit, such as the selection of a new radiofrequency. False vestibular sensations produced by head movement occur at the very time that the pilot has no reliable visual cues about the orientation of the aircraft, thereby increasing the probability that aircraft control will be based on these erroneous cues.

With the advent of super-manoeuvrable high-agility aircraft, it is possible that cross-coupled and 'G excess' illusions can be induced in the absence of head movement by the aviator. In conventional aircraft, aerodynamic limitations do not allow large and sustained changes in attitude to occur independently of the flight path. However, in high-agility aircraft with post-stall capability, vectored thrust or other technology, large and rapid changes in attitude can be achieved and sustained without significant alteration in the flight trajectory. This ability to achieve relatively large angular excursions, e.g. 90-degree change in angle of attack at rates of up to 50 °/s, has the potential to cause a cross-coupled stimulus to the semicircular canals as well as an adequate stimulus to the otolith organs if the flight trajectory has a significant angular velocity vector.

Flicker vertigo

Aircrew have described a number of sensory disturbances that can be attributed to a flickering visual stimulus. Such problems are more common in rotary-wing aircraft, where the shadow cast by the main rotor blades passes across the cockpit several times a second. Difficulties have also been experienced when light from a rotating anti-collision beacon illuminates the cockpit, either directly or by reflection from cloud or smoke. The principal complaint is irritation and distraction. Less frequently, there is a true disorientation in which the visual stimulus gives rise to a vection illusion characterized by a sensation of angular motion of the aircraft in the opposite direction to that of the moving shadow. Fortunately, there is usually little difficulty in determining the true orientation of the aircraft or helicopter, although there is a conflict to be resolved. An associated problem is one of nausea, which must be regarded as a form of visually induced motion sickness in which visual motion cues are not 'matched' by appropriate cues from other sensory receptors. Finally, there remains the possibility of disturbances of consciousness and the induction of epileptiform fits by a photic stimulus that flickers at a frequency close to a dominant rhythm (commonly 8–10 Hz of the alpha-waves) of the electroencephalogram (EEG). Fortunately, the incidence of flicker-induced epilepsy is very low in the population as a whole and is negligible in military aircrew.

Pressure (alternobaric) vertigo

Although somatogyral and oculogyral illusions are usually the consequence of stimulation of the semicircular canals by angular accelerations, it is well established that, in susceptible individuals, pressure change within the middle ear can evoke powerful and quite unexpected vertigo. Typically, this is of sudden onset and is related to the equilibration of middle-ear pressure as the pilot 'clears the ears' on ascent. It may also appear on descent, although usually in response to a voluntary Valsalva manoeuvre. The vertigo is often initially intense, with blurring of vision and apparent movement of the visual scene, but this is usually short-lived and dies away in 10–15 seconds, in much the same way as the vertigo produced by a sudden change in angular velocity. However, the symptoms are not always transient; some aircrew have reported a less intense vertigo that has persisted for many minutes. There is also considerable variability in the plane of the illusory sensation, although it is usually of a consistent and repeatable pattern in any one individual.

Surveys have shown that some 10–17 per cent of pilots have experienced pressure vertigo at some time or other during their flying careers. Symptoms are most likely to occur when there is some difficult in equilibrating middle ear pressure because of a 'stickiness' of the Eustachian tubes, usually due to mild congestion and inflammation brought about by a common cold or other infection of the upper respiratory tract. There are, however, a few individuals who suffer from pressure vertigo even in the absence of infection. Experiments in Sweden have shown that these individuals require a higher middle ear pressure (> 5.9 kPa above ambient) than the norm (4.3 kPa) in order to open the Eustachian tube and vent gas to ambient. On the other hand, not all individuals with high opening pressure suffer from pressure vertigo, and nor does the lack of Eustachian patency, as indicated by the Valsalva test, correlate well with susceptibility. In some subjects, the additional requirement for the induction of symptoms would appear to be an asymmetry in the opening pressures of the Eustachian tubes, such that one ear equilibrates at a low differential pressure and the other at a high tubal pressure.

The mechanism by which the sensory receptors of the vestibular apparatus are stimulated by changes in middle-ear pressure is still a matter for conjecture. The dominant symptom, vertigo, suggests strongly that it is the ampullary receptors of the semicircular canals, rather than the maculae, that are stimulated. Furthermore, the transient nature of the disturbance accords with the theory that the cupula is deflected when the overpressure in the middle ear is suddenly relieved on passive venting or when middle-ear pressure is raised transiently above ambient by a Valsalva manoeuvre. Overpressure in the middle ear may not be transmitted equally to the fluid systems of the inner ear by the round and oval windows, for the stapes footplate might be moved against the pressure gradient by the outward displacement of the tympanic membrane. With the sudden restoration of middle-ear pressure, there may be a movement of endolymph and perilymph that causes a displacement of the cupula of one or more of the semicircular canals of the affected ear. Unfortunately, little is known about the transient response of the hydrodynamic systems of the inner ear to large-amplitude pressure changes, and so it is difficult to explain why some individuals show an altered pattern of end-organ activity with such a stimulus and others do not.

Despite uncertainties about the mechanism of pressure vertigo and the nature of individual differences in susceptibility, there is little doubt that it can be a cause of severe and potentially dangerous spatial disorientation. Apart from the dangers of otic barotrauma, the increased probability of pressure vertigo is another reason why aircrew should not fly when suffering from an upper respiratory tract infection or other condition that impairs ventilation of the middle ear. Aircrew who continue to suffer from pressure vertigo in the absence of intercurrent infection should be referred to an otologist for investigation and treatment.

OPERATIONAL FACTORS

Disorientation in helicopter operations

Spatial disorientation is no less of a problem in helicopter operations than it is in fixed-wing aircraft. There are certain features of the way helicopters fly and the way in which they are operated that lead to specific types of disorientation. Helicopter operations generally are carried out at low level, and although this does not of itself increase the likelihood of disorientation, it may leave little time to recover from an unexpected aircraft attitude. Unlike a fixed-wing aircraft, a helicopter has no motive power in the longitudinal axis of the fuselage. In order to transition from the hover to forward flight, the nose of the helicopter is pitched down, so that a component of the lift provided by the main rotor now accelerates the aircraft in the forward direction. As ever, forward acceleration of an aircraft causes it to feel more pitched up than it really is. Initially, before significant aerodynamic drag builds up, the pitch-up sensation of forward acceleration exactly balances the actual pitch-down of the aircraft, so that it continues to feel level, just as it did in the hover. Likewise, in order to transition from forward flight into the hover, the pilot brings the nose of the aircraft up so that a component of the rotor lift now acts in the rearward direction and decelerates the aircraft. A decelerating aircraft feels more nose-down than it actually is, and this sensation exactly balances the effect of the actual nose-up tilt and again causes the aircraft to feel level. The situation is not significantly different in the roll axis. A helicopter tilted in roll will tend to side-slip with increasing lateral velocity and as a result will continue to feel level. In summary, a helicopter will tend to feel level whatever its true attitude.

In search-and-rescue operations, the helicopter pilot is often required to maintain an exact height and location when in the hover. This is not made any easier by the motion of waves when hovering over the sea or the wave effects on grass produced by the rotor downdraft. In these circumstances, close coordination between the pilot and the rear crew is often crucial. Landing on snow also poses problems. Lack of features on the surface of snow makes it difficult to detect a drift in position. In addition, if the snow is loose, the rotor down-draft may whip up the snow and unsight the pilot at a critical phase in the landing (whiteout). The same may occur when landing on dry, dusty terrain (brownout).

Maritime operations may require a helicopter pilot to take off and land on the deck of a ship. To land at night on a minimally lit ship is a highly demanding manoeuvre. As with the black-hole approach on land, the pattern of lights on the ship gives little sense of perspective until late in the approach, and the heading and glide-slope indication provided by the ship are essential aids. On takeoff from a ship, the pilot has to make a rapid and reliable transfer to instruments as he or she heads out over the side of the ship into a black hole.

Night operations are often carried out with the assistance of night-vision goggles or using images from a forward-looking infrared (FLIR) camera mounted on a swivel turret on the nose of the aircraft. By enhancing the visual environment, such devices should, potentially, reduce the likelihood of disorientation. However, they enable hazardous operations that would be impossible without their use but have limitations in the quality of the visual image they present to the pilot (see below).

Formation flying

When flying in close formation, the pilot of the number-two aircraft in the formation takes his or her orientation cues from the leader. The primary task is to maintain a fixed spatial relationship to the leader; in so doing, the pilot tends to lose awareness of their spatial orientation with respect to the outside world. The pilot of the lead aircraft has the major responsibility of maintaining spatial orientation on behalf of the formation and to ensure that his or her manoeuvres are sufficiently gentle to allow the number-two pilot to respond to them. Formation flying often continues despite cloud penetration, and the only differ-

ence may be that the aircraft fly closer to each other in order to maintain visual contact. In these circumstances, even greater concentration is required in order to maintain separation from the lead aircraft. If visual contact be lost and the number-two pilot is obliged to break away, the pilot may have great difficulty reorienting him- or herself relative to the real world through the aircraft instruments.

Aircrew reports indicate that formation flying in cloud is particularly conducive to producing the leans in the number-two aircraft. The sensation can be very disconcerting, and the task of staying with the lead aircraft becomes increasingly demanding. The alternative of breaking away from the formation means losing the orientation cue provided by the leader and having to use instruments, without necessarily alleviating the leans.

Night flying

Once clear of the runway, aircraft flying at night operate under instrument flight rules (IFR), which require pilots to hold a current instrument rating. At night, what remains visible to the pilot outside the aircraft depends on many factors, such as the presence of moonlight or ground lights from towns and cities and the prevailing weather conditions. However, even in apparently clear conditions, there may be no distinct horizon and, consequently, starlight and points of light on the ground may become confused. Lines of light, e.g. from road lighting or around a bay, may create false horizons. A particular instance of this can be experienced by a pilot approaching at an angle to an inhabited coastline. Because of the effect of perspective, the border between unlit sea and the lights onshore forms an oblique line across the cockpit canopy, which can be misinterpreted as horizontal and lead to an error in the perception of roll attitude. In the absence of a visual context, stationary isolated lights may appear to be in motion, which can lead to misinterpretation of their true nature. This phenomenon, known as autokinesis, is particularly evident when there are isolated flashing lights. The effect is probably the result of ocular drift occurring in the dark intervals between flashes, so that the next flash falls on an adjacent portion of the retina, which the brain interprets as movement of the light source.

Surveys of aircraft accidents attributable to disorientation have shown a greater incidence of spatial disorientation accidents at night, particularly when using night-vision aids. In military operations, there are important tactical advantages to be gained from the use of night-vision devices. However, the potential increase in safety that such devices might afford is outweighed by the increased hazard associated with the night-time operations that they enable. NVGs amplify the residual light to create a monochromatic image of the view ahead. However, they restrict the field of view to about 40 degrees and so deprive the pilot of important peripheral visual orientation cues. The image presented to the pilot is of lower resolution, and its single green colour leads to problems with depth perception. In helicopter operations, the spatial disorientation accidents associated with the use of NVGs have most frequently involved undetected drift or descent from the hover or controlled flight into terrain or water.

Other night-vision devices generate a visible image using the thermal radiation from ground features. Contrast within the image is determined by the amount of infrared radiation from different objects in the field of view. This does not remain constant over time, since it is dependent on the amount of previously absorbed solar radiation and the rate at which it is re-radiated during the night. More so than with daytime flying, the pilot has to exercise particular care during flight over featureless terrain when using these devices.

Dissociative sensations, the 'break-off phenomenon'

Apart from illusory perceptions of aircraft attitude and motion, aircrew report other incidents in which the disorientation takes the form of an altered perception of the pilot's own orientation with respect to the aircraft and to the ground. Typically, the perceptual disturbance is described by the aviator as a feeling of detachment, isolation or remoteness from their or immediate environment and the aircraft they are controlling. Less commonly, the sensory disturbance is more severe and takes the form of an 'outside-the-body experience', in which the pilot feels that he is outside the aircraft, or at least outside himself, and is watching himself fly the aircraft (to date, there is no report of female pilots experiencing these sensations). The term 'break-off phenomenon' was coined by Clark and Graybiel to identify this type of disordered perception, because one of the early descriptions came from a pilot who felt as if he had 'broken off from reality'. While accepting the descriptive utility of this term, it must be recognized that comparable sensory disturbance are seen in patients with psychiatric and organic disorders, when they are called dissociative sensations. However, the occurrence of such dissociative sensations in flight does not imply ipso facto that the pilot is psychiatrically ill.

The break-off phenomenon is primarily a sensory disturbance experienced by pilots of single-seat aircraft when flying at high altitudes (about 30 000 feet (10 000 m) and above) during monotonous phases of flight, such as level cruise on a constant heading. Although described originally as a problem of high-altitude flight in fixed-wing aircraft, dissociative sensations also occur at very much lower altitudes in helicopters. Symptoms have been reported at 500 feet (150 m) when flying over a featureless sea in hazy conditions, although more characteristically break-off is associated with flight at altitudes of 5000–10 000 feet (1500–3000 m), which can be classified as 'high' for a rotary-wing aircraft. The dissociative sensations are usually short-lived and often disappear spontaneously when the pilot directs their attention to some other aspect of the flying task, such as cockpit checks, a change of heading or a radio/telephony message. Less commonly, the pilot has to make a positive effort to redirect attention in order to dispel the illusion. On other occasions, break-off may persist until the pilot has a clear view of the ground or is close to clouds that give unambiguous relative motion cues and a reliable external visual reference.

The results of several surveys have shown that some 14–35 per cent of aircrew who have flown in a provocative environment (i.e. single seat, high altitude) have experienced dissociative sensations. For the majority, these have not been a cause for concern; indeed, some pilots find the sensation pleasurable and a contribution to the joy of flying. However, about one-third of the pilots who have experienced break-off find the altered perceptual state to be disturbing and anxiety-provoking. It is in this group of aircrew that break-off disrupts performance by engendering a high arousal state and by acting as the precipitant of an anxiety reaction. Specifically, such aircrew frequently have an increased awareness of changes in aircraft attitude and motion, with quantitative errors in perception; for example, five degrees of bank may feel like 30 degrees of bank. Some also have illusory perceptions of aircraft orientation, such as a false sensation of turn or roll when flying straight and level. These errors in the perception of aircraft orientation are often consistent and are associated with break-off whenever it occurs. Other aircrew do not suffer specific illusions of aircraft attitude and motion but have a feeling of instability, characteristically likened to the aircraft being balanced on a knife edge or as if on top of a pin. Furthermore, their anxiety is potentiated by the thought that the aircraft will topple from this unstable configuration and fall out of the sky.

Such unrealistic perceptions are commonly, although not necessarily, the manifestation of a neurotic reaction. However, they do emphasize the role of an unusual sensory experience, like break-off, in the genesis of neurotic reactions. In some cases there is a well-defined phobic element, as the occurrence of anxiety is related quite specifically to the flight conditions in which break-off first occurred, but in others there is generalization of the anxiety, with loss of confidence in flying ability and the development of the fear-of-flying syndrome. It must also be recognized that dissociative sensations may be the first symptom of a neurosis that develops because of other factors in the individual's work, social life or constitution. The elucidation of aetiology in an aircrew patient who comes under medical care because of dissociative sensations and anxiety neurosis can be difficult, and may, on occasion, perplex even the skilled psychiatrist.

PROPHYLAXIS

Spatial disorientation can have a deleterious effect on the safety of flight operations, on mission effectiveness and on the mental health of aircrew. Thus, every effort should be made to prevent the occurrence of perceptual errors, in particular those that lead to loss of control and aircraft accidents. 'Prevent' is perhaps too strong a word to use when considering disorders of perception caused by natural limitations of sensory function and the fallibility of the central perceptual mechanism, but sufficient is known about the aetiology of spatial disorientation in order to allow rational prophylactic measures to be developed. Many of the factors that lead to spatial disorientation have already been discussed. These will now be summarized under different headings in order to emphasize the methods, techniques and procedures that may be employed to prevent, or at least minimize, disorientation.

Aircraft factors

INSTRUMENTATION

Spatial disorientation is predominantly a problem of flight in IMC, and hence the quality of instrument displays is of vital importance if the pilot is to perceive, both correctly and quickly, the behaviour and orientation of the aircraft so that erroneous cues may be disregarded. Ideally, the instruments should provide cues that have the same visual strength as external cues in good visibility conditions, although to date such displays do not exist. Indeed, it is unlikely that flight-deck instruments will ever be as compelling as sight of the real world. Nevertheless, every effort should be made to provide the pilot with instruments that can be read quickly and unambiguously, both by day and by night. It is, of course, axiomatic that the instrumentation should be adequate for the manoeuvres and conditions in which the pilot has to fly the aircraft. The impropriety of attempting to fly in marginal weather conditions in an aircraft without an attitude display is obvious, but many accidents to light aircraft and some helicopters are attributable directly to the continuation of a flight, initially in VMC, into IMC in aircraft without appropriate instrument displays.

Instrument reliability is also of prime importance, for once this becomes suspect, the pilot may question the veracity of the display and hence take longer, or even fail, to resolve conflicting sensory cues. Likewise, a clear indication of malfunction is necessary if the perceptual load on the pilot is not to be increased by the display of erroneous information.

The use of head-up and helmet-mounted displays undoubtedly assists in the transfer from external visual to instrument cues and should reduce the possibility of disorientation at such times. Likewise, this type of display should reduce perceptual conflict in those flight situations where external visual cues are uncertain, even though the pilot is obliged by operational requirements to look outside the cockpit. However, if the head-up or helmet-mounted display has poor symbology or lacks accuracy, clarity or reliability, then it may contribute to disorientation by increasing arousal or by adding to perceptual conflict.

COCKPIT ERGONOMICS

The need to position ancillary instruments and controls so that the pilot does not have to make head movements during critical phases of flight has been discussed in the sections dealing with cross-coupled stimulation and 'G excess' illusions. It should also be recognized that aircrew equipment, such as a flying helmet, can obstruct the field of vision and require head movements to be made in order in order to see even the primary instrument display. The configuration of the cockpit canopy is also of significance. The lack of a well-defined aircraft frame of reference undoubtedly contributes to the development of the leans and break-off in those aircraft where the pilot is placed well forward and can see the wings or other parts of the aircraft only with difficulty. Likewise, the presence of a sloping edge to the canopy, augmented perhaps by an instrument panel in which the dials are not aligned with the transverse axis of the aircraft, does not assist the pilot to maintain a level attitude when using external visual cues.

OPERATIONAL FACTORS

Preventive measures in this broad area depend on the recognition of aircraft manoeuvres and flight environments that carry a high risk of disorientation. These factors cannot, of course, be considered in isolation and have to be evaluated in relation to the training and experience of the aircrew. For example, pilots without instrument flying experience will become disoriented if they attempt to fly in cloud or other poor-visibility conditions (IMC) where instrument flying is required, but those who are in instrument-flying practice are unlikely to suffer from potentially dangerous disorientation in similar flight conditions. Indeed, it is obvious that aircrew should only fly those aircraft, those manoeuvres and in those flight conditions that are commensurate with their training, experience and proficiency. Yet each year, many orientation error accidents occur, particularly among private flyers, because of a failure to comply with this fundamental rule. In part, the avoidance of potentially disorientating situations can be achieved by supervisory control, but of no less importance is awareness by the pilot of his or her own limitations and of the flight conditions and aircraft manoeuvres likely to induce spatial disorientation. The acquisition of such knowledge again depends on the training and the experience of the individual pilot.

The principal environmental factors and flight manoeuvres likely to produce or potentiate disorientation are summarised in Table 28.2.

Aircrew factors

It is now necessary to consider what prophylactic measures can be applied to the aircrew to reduce or, better, prevent spatial disorientation. Training and experience are clearly of paramount importance, but there are other behavioural and clinical factors that should not be overlooked.

SELECTION

Because of the large differences between individuals in their apparent susceptibility to disorientation in flight, it might be assumed that selection procedures could be employed to identify the disorientation-prone pilot. Individuals with gross disturbances of vestibular function due to clinical disorders, such as Ménière's disease or impairment of equilibratory function due to a central lesion, should be recognized at the initial medical examination from the clinical history or on examination. However, a more detailed clinical investigation of vestibular function, such as the use of precise rotational or positional tests, is unnecessary, for it has not been found to have predictive value. On the other hand, the response of the candidate to strong cross-coupled vestibular stimulation (head movements made when rotating at 180 °/s) has been found to correlate quite well with success in flying training. Students who reacted badly with the rapid development of autonomic symptoms after only a few head movements showed a significantly higher failure rate than those with a higher tolerance to the vestibular stimulus. However, this test is not specifically one of disorientation susceptibility, as it embraces those students who fail because of airsickness, those with poor air-work and those

Table 28.2   *Principal environmental factors and flight manoeuvres likely to produce or potentiate disorientation*

Factor	Nature of spatial disorientation
Flight environment	
Flight in IMC	Acceptance of erroneous vestibular/kinaesthetic cues especially on transfer from external visual to instrument cues
Night	Use of inadequate external visual cues
	Apparent motion of isolated lights due to the oculogravic and autokinetic illusions
	Ground/sky confusion
	Inadequate ground illumination preventing accurate perception of height and attitude for landing or maintenance of hover
High altitude	Dissociative sensations (break-off)
	False horizontal references
Flight over featureless terrain	Error in height perception
Flight manoeuvre	
Prolonged linear acceleration/deceleration	Somatogravic and oculogravic illusions
	'G excess' illusion with head movement
Prolonged angular motion	Turn not sensed
	Somatogyral and oculogyral illusions (particularly on recovery)
	Impairment of vision by nystagmus
	Cross-coupled (Coriolis) stimulation with head movement
Sub-threshold changes in attitude	Changes in attitude not sensed
	The leans
Workload	High arousal enhances disorientation and reduced ability to resolve conflict
Ascent	Pressure (alternobaric) vertigo
Cloud penetration	VMC/IMC transfer especially when flying in formation or on breaking formation
	Lean-on-the-sun illusion
Low altitude in helicopters and VSTOL aircraft	VMC/IMC transfer necessitated by flight into dust, smoke, snow, etc.
	Illusions of relative motion

IMC, instrument meteorological conditions; VMC, visual meteorological conditions; VSTOL, vertical/short takeoff and landing.

with difficulties in maintaining correct orientation in flight.

HEALTH

It is essential that any trained pilot who suffers a disorder affecting the vestibular and visual sensory systems should not be permitted to fly. There are many disease processes, although few common, that necessitate suspension from flying because they predispose the pilot to disorientation in flight. It is outside the scope of this chapter to discuss them in detail. Nevertheless, it is important to distinguish chronic disorders, such as Ménière's syndrome, where the disability is recurrent and unpredictable, from those that are acute, such labyrinthitis, where complete recovery is to be expected and suspension from flying is only temporary. Pressure vertigo is a specific disability that can be minimized by the restriction of flying of people suffering from upper respiratory tract infections (typically the common cold). Certain individuals may benefit from the limited use of decongestants, but if pressure vertigo is a recurrent problem, specialist advice is required.

Apart from the maintenance of physical health, the prevention of disorientation is also dependent on mental health. It is known that perceptual errors are more likely to occur when the pilot is anxious or has a high level of behavioural arousal because of endogenous or environmental factors. Likewise, the pilot who is preoccupied by problems of a social or domestic nature is also more susceptible. It is more difficult to recognize such psychiatric problems than the organic disorders mentioned in the preceding paragraphs, and even when they are identified, a high degree of judgement is required to decide whether a particular pilot is fit to fly. Specialist opinion can always be sought; nevertheless, it is the responsibility of the pilot's doctor to initially identify those aircrew whose safety in flight might be at risk because of mental ill health.

DRUGS

There is anecdotal evidence that self-medication with over-the-counter drugs increases susceptibility to spatial disorientation. It may be argued that any pharmacologically active substance that is a central depressant or in some other way impairs cognitive function is likely to increase the likelihood of the pilot experiencing an illusory perception or of impairing his or her ability to resolve correctly perceptual conflict. Thus, aircrew, and especially pilots, should not be permitted to fly when taking drugs that are known to adversely affect the central nervous system. In particular, aircrew should be made aware of the potential danger of flying after taking certain readily available medications, such as preparations to allay the symptoms of the common cold and of motion sickness, containing sedative antihistamines or scopolamine

(hyoscine). Ethyl alcohol also has a depressant effect on brain mechanisms and can cause or potentiate disorientation by its specific action on the vestibular system. The production of positional alcohol vertigo and nystagmus, and the diminution of the pilot's ability to suppress inappropriate vestibular nystagmus, are but two examples. Thus, alcohol, even in small quantities, jeopardizes flight safety on several counts and is likely to increase the pilot's susceptibility to disorientation long into the hangover period. The common regulation that flying should be avoided for at least 12 hours after having taken alcohol is probably too lenient. As noted earlier, in some circumstances, especially after heavy drinking, more than 12 hours is required for the blood alcohol to fall to a level where there is no impairment of piloting performance or disturbance of vestibular function.

TRAINING

Reference has already been made to the need for flying personnel to have not only an adequate knowledge of the aetiology and varied manifestations of spatial disorientation but also the skill to cope with the problem when it occurs in flight. The specific objectives of training may be summarized as follows: (i) to inform aircrew about those factors that contribute to effective spatial orientation in the flight environment; (ii) to familiarize them with the various conditions and flight operations that may lead to spatial disorientation; (iii) to inform about the differing manifestations of spatial disorientation and how to detect the onset or existence of spatial disorientation; (iv) to explain the mechanisms by which spatial disorientation is produced and to discuss normal limitations of sensory functions; and (v) to inform how disorientation may be overcome and to develop skill so that they can maintain correct control of the aircraft or quickly regain control when experiencing illusory sensations.

These training objectives are met in part by ground-school lectures and in part by experience in the air. It is most desirable that each student should have personally experienced some form of illusory perception, either in a ground-based familiarization device or in an aircraft, for this is the most certain way of convincing the individual that spatial disorientation is a potential problem to all aircrew and that he or she is not an exception. The equipment required for classroom demonstration of the physiological limitations of sensory function that are responsible for spatial disorientation in flight need not be complex. A modified bar stool, turned by hand, will suffice to familiarize the student pilot with the fallibility of semicircular canal mechanisms. A simple centrifuge allows the demonstration of somatogravic and oculogravic illusions as well. The possible benefits of a familiarization device having more than one degree of angular freedom are debatable, although it can be argued that time spent controlling what is in effect a dynamic flight simulator capable of generating illusory sensations could reduce susceptibility to spatial disorientation in actual flight.

Ground-based lectures and demonstrations undoubtedly play a part in the orientation training of aircrew, but it is in the flight environment itself that aircrew learn how to cope with the problem of disorientation. Illusory perceptions are much more likely to occur and to distract the pilot when they are, or should be, flying by instruments, and hence a high degree of proficiency at this type of flying must be acquired during training. The skill, once acquired, must be maintained by regular practice. One aspect of the maintenance of flying skill – much is to be achieved by consistent exposure to the flying task – is that the level of adaptation (or habituation) to the motion experienced in the flight environment is sustained. Aircrew who are in current flying practice, particularly of high-performance aircraft, are in general less aware of vestibular and kinaesthetic sensations than aircrew who have not had recent experience in comparable flight conditions.

The loss of skill associated with prolonged periods of ground duty is well recognized in service flying, and refresher training with some dual flying is commonly carried out before the pilot returns to operational duties. Yet, even after being grounded for only two weeks, some habituation is lost. Surveys have shown that pilots are much more likely to be aware of aircraft motion and to suffer disorientation on the first flight after a period of leave. Such problems can be ameliorated by the gradual re-introduction of stressful flight manoeuvres on return to flying duties.

Advice to aircrew

GENERAL

- No pilot has ever been able to fly an aeroplane by the seat of their pants: you are no exception.
- You don't have to be flying in cloud or at night to become disoriented, but it helps.
- When disoriented, your instruments are your lifeline.
- Never be tempted to think your instruments are not telling you the truth without an exceptionally good reason.
- Cross-check instruments in clear visual conditions to give you confidence in their reliability when you need them.
- Aim to make an early transition to instruments in poor visibility; once on instruments, stay on instruments until external cues are unambiguous.
- Do not unnecessarily mix flying by instruments with flying by external visual cues.
- Remain aware of the circumstances in which the feel of the aircraft can deceive you, e.g. takeoff into cloud or at night, overshoot, low-level abort.

- Be alert to manoeuvres in which small errors in aircraft attitude can have significant consequences, e.g. turns at low level.
- The allowable distraction time when in a turn is much shorter than when in straight and level flight.
- First, fly the aircraft. Many instances of disorientation arise from an excessive preoccupation with one aspect of the mission to the temporary exclusion of controlling the aircraft.
- The most dangerous forms of disorientation arise when you think nothing has changed when, in fact, it has.
- Ensure that you are fit to fly. Do not fly if you feel ill or cannot clear your ears.
- Take care with alcohol. Excessive alcohol may require longer than the 12-hour 'bottle-to-throttle' rule to clear from the system.
- Maintain a high proficiency and be in practice at flight in IMC.
- Avoid unnecessary manoeuvres of aircraft or head movements that are known to induce disorientation.
- Make your first flight after a period off flying a simple day VMC sortie.
- Leave your worries behind when you go flying; the aircraft needs your full attention.
- Remember: experience does not make you immune.

WHAT TO DO IF YOU EXPERIENCE DISORIENTING SENSATIONS IN FLIGHT

- You can dispel persistent minor disorientation, e.g. 'the leans', by making a positive effort to redirect attention to other aspects of the flying task. A quick shake of the head, provided the aircraft is straight and level, is effective for some pilots.
- When you are confronted suddenly by strong illusory sensations or have difficulties in establishing orientation and control of the aircraft:

  - Get on to instruments: check and cross-check and ensure good instrument illumination.
  - Maintain instrument reference and correct scan pattern; watch your height at all times.
  - Control the aircraft in such a way as to make the instruments display the desired flight configuration.
  - Do not attempt to mix flight by external visual reference with instrument flight until external visual cues are unambiguous.
  - Seek help if severe disorientation persists. Hand over to co-pilot (if present), call ground controller and other aircraft; check altimeter.
  - If control cannot be regained, abandon aircraft with safe ground clearance. Do not leave it too late.

- Remember: nearly all disorientation is a normal response to the unnatural environment of flight. If you have been alarmed by a flight incident, discuss it with colleagues, including your station medical officer. Your experience probably will not be as unusual as you think.

FURTHER READING

Previc FH, Ercoline WR, *Spatial Orientation in Aviation*. Reston, VA: American Institute of Astronautics and Aeronautics, 2004.

RTO Symposium. Spatial disorientation in military vehicles, causes, consequences and cures. Report no. HFM-085, TP/42. Neuilly-sur-Seine: NATO Research Technology Agency, 2003.

29

Motion sickness

ALAN J. BENSON AND J.R. ROLLIN STOTT

INTRODUCTION

Motion sickness is a condition characterized primarily by nausea, vomiting, pallor and cold sweating that occurs when a person is exposed to real or apparent motion stimuli with which he or she is unfamiliar and hence unadapted. Motion sickness is a generic term that embraces seasickness, airsickness, carsickness, swing-sickness, simulator-sickness, virtual-reality-sickness and space-sickness, all various forms of the malady named after the provocative environment or vehicle. Despite the diversity of the causal environment, the essential characteristics of the provocative stimulus and the response of the afflicted individual are common to all these conditions, hence the use of the general term. However, motion sickness is, in certain respects, a misnomer. First, symptoms characteristic of the condition can be evoked as much by the absence of expected motion as by the presence of unfamiliar motion; 'simulator-sickness' and 'cinerama-sickness' (see below) are examples of conditions where the evocative stimulus is visual motion in the absence of bodily motion. Second, the word 'sickness' carries the connotation of 'affected with disease' and tends to obscure the fact that motion sickness is a normal response of a healthy individual, without organic or functional disorder, when exposed for a sufficient length of time to unfamiliar motion of sufficient severity. Indeed, under severe stimulus conditions, it is the absence rather than the presence of symptoms that is indicative of true pathology, for only those individuals who lack a functional vestibular system are truly immune. It would be better to label the condition as 'motion maladaptation syndrome', for this term implies the fundamental nature of the disability.

SYMPTOMS AND SIGNS

The cardinal symptom of motion sickness is nausea. The cardinal signs are vomiting, pallor and sweating. Other responses are reported frequently, but in general these occur more variably. Typically, the development of motion sickness follows an orderly sequence, the timescale being determined primarily by the intensity of the stimulus and the susceptibility of the individual. The earliest symptom is, commonly, the unfamiliar sensation of epigastric discomfort, best described as 'stomach awareness'. Should the provocative motion continue, wellbeing usually deteriorates quite quickly, with the appearance of nausea of increasing severity. Concomitantly, circumoral or facial pallor may be observed, and the individual begins to sweat; this cold sweat is usually confined to those areas of skin where thermal sweating rather than emotive sweating occurs. With the rapid exacerbation of symptoms, the so-called 'avalanche phenomenon', there may be increased salivation, feelings of bodily warmth and a light-headedness.

By this stage, vomiting is not usually long delayed, although some individuals remain severely nauseated for long periods and do not obtain the relief, albeit transitory, that many report following emesis. If exposure to the motion continues, nausea typically increases in intensity and culminates in vomiting or retching. In more susceptible people, this cyclical pattern, with waxing and waning symptoms and recurrent vomiting, may last for several days. Those so afflicted are commonly severely anorexic, depressed and apathetic, incapable of carrying out allotted duties or caring for the safety of themselves or others. Their disability is also compounded by dehydration and disturbances of electrolyte balance brought about by repeated vomiting.

Associated symptoms and signs

Apart from the characteristic features of motion sickness – pallor, sweating, nausea and vomiting – other signs and symptoms are reported frequently, although more variably. In the early stages, increased salivation, belching and flatulence commonly are associated with the development of nausea. Hyperventilation is observed occasionally, while an alteration of respiratory rhythm by sighing and yawning not infrequently precedes the 'avalanche phenomenon'. Headache is another variable prodromal symptom; this is usually frontal in distribution, although complaints of tightness around the forehead or of a 'buzzing in the head' are not uncommon.

Drowsiness is an important and yet often ignored symptom commonly associated with exposure to unfamiliar motion, even if not necessarily an integral part of the motion sickness syndrome. Typically, feelings of lethargy and somnolence persist for many hours after withdrawal of the provocative motion stimulus and nausea has abated. However, in certain circumstances, a desire to sleep may be the only symptom evoked by exposure to motion, especially when the intensity of the stimulus is such that adaptation occurs without significant malaise. The soporific effect of a repetitive motion stimulus on infants has long been recognized. It may be that the drowsiness observed in adults exposed to appropriate motion is a manifestation of the same mechanism, although it must be acknowledged that somnolence in an individual who has suffered overt motion sickness is frequently of abnormal intensity and persistence.

Physiological correlates

Motion sickness is associated with measurable changes in physiological activity, primarily of the autonomic nervous system. Sudomotor activity can be recorded by changes in skin resistance or actual sweat production by means of a ventilated capsule. Pallor caused by vasoconstriction of cutaneous vessels is accompanied by vasodilation of deeper vessels and an increase in muscle blood flow. Techniques are available for the measurement of these alterations in superficial and deep vascular tone. Motility and tonus of the stomach and gut are decreased in motion sickness. Surface electrodes placed over the stomach allow an electrogastrogram (EGG) to be recorded, which, with the development of symptoms, shows a decrease in amplitude and increase in frequency of the EGG, termed tachygastria. There is an increased secretion of stress hormones. Most pronounced is the elevation of antidiuretic hormone

(ADH), which is responsible for the oliguria that accompanies motion sickness. Adrenocorticotrophic hormone (ACTH) and growth hormone (GH) are also raised.

OPERATIONAL SIGNIFICANCE

Motion sickness is a debilitating condition that has an adverse effect on performance. In the air, the loss of well-being is, at least, a distraction that interferes with the aviator's ability to devote his or her undivided attention to the task in hand. At the other extreme, flying personnel can be prostrated by sickness and be completely unable to perform their allotted duties. Severe sickness in trained flying personnel is unusual, but it is a recurrent if not frequent problem in non-pilot aircrew, such as navigators and air electronic operators, who are exposed to provocative flight environments. More commonly, airsickness is a problem during flight training. Vomiting interferes directly with the student's ability to control the aircraft and may require the instructor to modify or abort the sortie. When sickness is not overt, the student may suffer in silence. Performance in flight may be impaired and be attributed by the flying instructor to a fundamental lack of skill. In either circumstance, the student may feel humiliated and disgraced by the sickness, which can be construed as a personal weakness or constitutional defect. Continued introspection with increasing anxiety and loss of confidence can further impair progress and may strengthen the instructor's opinion about the student's lack of aptitude.

Simulator-sickness

Since the first report of symptoms resembling those of motion sickness by pilots who flew helicopter simulators, there have been a number of studies of what has come to be known as 'simulator-sickness'. Some of the symptoms experienced by people flying aircraft simulators are typically those of motion sickness, notably stomach awareness, nausea, dizziness, sweating and drowsiness. Severe nausea, vomiting and retching are, however, rare. In addition, other symptoms commonly are reported that are not typical of motion sickness, namely eyestrain, blurred vision, difficulty in focusing, headache and difficulty in concentrating. Whereas the early reports of simulator-sickness came from a fixed-base simulator having a distorted display of the external visual scene, subsequently symptoms have been experienced by pilots flying many different types of simulator. Typically, these had wide external scene visual displays, and many had motion systems providing whole-body motion cues.

Symptoms of simulator-sickness are rarely of sufficient severity to necessitate the abandonment of a sortie, but they can lead to the development of a negative attitude towards the validity of the simulation. In addition to the symptoms experienced during simulated flight, a number of post-exposure effects have been described, including disturbances of postural control, illusory sensations of motion, visual flashbacks, disorientation and dizziness. Typically, these sensory and motor disturbances rarely last more than 12 hours, but delayed effects occurring a week or more after a simulated flight have been reported. These post-exposure disturbances could, it is postulated, be a hazard to flight safety if the aviator were to fly a real aircraft immediately after a simulated flight, so in many centres there are constraints on the activities of aircrew following flights in the simulator.

Virtual reality

Virtual-reality systems may be regarded as a particular type of visual simulation in which a device worn on the head of the observer displays a computer-generated image of the external scene, typically without a frame of reference such as is provided by the canopy and instruments in a flight simulator. Movement of the image occurs in response to movement of the subject's head or to commands made by the subject to explore and move through the simulated environment. The quality of the visual display in most contemporary systems has deficiencies with regard to resolution, geometric distortion and delay in the updating of the visual display. These factors, coupled with the dissociation between the visual display of motion as the observer 'moves' through the virtual environment and the lack of concomitant somatic cues, are considered to be important aetiological factors in the genesis of visual-reality-sickness. Post-exposure effects, similar to those occurring after flight-simulator sorties, have been reported following 'immersion' in virtual-reality systems.

Passengers

Airsickness in passengers is also of operational significance when passengers are required to carry out duties immediately after landing or on leaving the aircraft. Usually, however, the affected passenger has an opportunity to recuperate on arrival before being required to carry out demanding mental or physical tasks. Paratroops are likely to suffer more. In the critical phase of the mission, the aircraft cannot fly at high altitude, above the weather, and hence the occupants may be exposed to the provocative motion of flight through turbulent air. Although anecdotal and circumstantial evidence implies that the airsick soldier or paratrooper is a less effective fighter than one who has not suffered from this disability, it must be acknowledged

that the postulated decrement in performance has yet to be quantified.

Space motion sickness

Approximately 70 per cent of the men and women who have flown in space vehicles have experienced symptoms similar to those of terrestrial motion sickness. The signs and symptoms of space-sickness usually appear within the first few hours in the weightless (or, more precisely, microgravity) environment and frequently are precipitated by head and body movements within the vehicle. The severity of symptoms can range from mild malaise and associated anorexia to severe nausea with repeated vomiting. Characteristically, there is a progressive decline in the intensity of symptoms with continued exposure to the atypical force environment, and most astronauts have adapted and are symptom-free by the third or fourth day in space.

Despite the high motivation and extensive training of space-flight crews, space-sickness impairs working efficiency during the first few days in flight. Provocative head and body movements are restricted or made more slowly, vomiting interrupts the performance of tasks, and the loss of wellbeing causes a general degradation of performance. Thus, space-sickness is primarily an operational problem during short space flights, such as those of the space shuttle, in which the operational effectiveness of crew members may be impaired for a substantial proportion of the time in weightlessness. Vomiting within the pressure suit that must be worn during extra-vehicular activity (EVA) is potentially lethal. It is, therefore, essential that work outside the spacecraft is performed only by astronauts who either are not susceptible to space-sickness or have recovered from this disability.

Seasickness

In aviation medicine, seasickness cannot be ignored, for it is a potentially serious problem to the unfortunate few who have to abandon their aircraft on or above the sea. The motion of a life-raft is a highly provocative stimulus, and all but the very resistant succumb in rough seas. Even moderate seas induce symptoms in a relatively short period. In the survival situation, sickness erodes the individual's will to survive; furthermore, it reduces the ability and the will to take positive action to aid survival. In addition to these behavioural consequences, dehydration and electrolyte disturbances brought about by continued vomiting can degrade an individual's capacity to withstand the privation, exposure and other stresses imposed by a hostile marine environment.

AETIOLOGY

An adequate theory of the causation of motion sickness must embrace the fact that this disability can be induced not only by motion in which the individual experiences changing linear and angular accelerations but also by purely visual stimuli without a changing force environment. Furthermore, it should account for the phenomenon of adaptation to the provocative motion as well as the sickness (*mal de débarquement*) that can occur when an individual returns to a normal motion environment after having adapted to an atypical one. Undoubtedly, the vestibular apparatus plays a significant role in the genesis of motion sickness, for it has been known for more than a century that those without vestibular function do not get motion sickness. Nevertheless, the theory that motion sickness is due to vestibular 'overstimulation' alone does not account for the fact that fairly strong motion stimuli (e.g. vertical oscillation at frequencies above 0.5–1 Hz) may not induce sickness, and yet weaker stimuli (e.g. head movement during turns) are highly provocative. Nor does it account for the visually induced forms of motion sickness (as in some flight simulators) or the phenomenon of adaptation.

A more acceptable hypothesis is that motion sickness is the response of the organism to discordant sensory information provided by those receptor systems that transduce the motion stimuli. The sensory conflict or neural mis-match hypothesis gained wide acceptance following the publication of studies by Reason (Reason and Brand 1975). In essence, the neural mismatch hypothesis states that in all situations where motion sickness is induced, not only is there a conflict between the signals from the eyes, the vestibular apparatus and the other receptors stimulated by the motion, but also these signals are at variance with those that the central nervous system expects to receive. An essential feature of the neural mismatch hypothesis is that the presence of a sustained mismatch signal has two effects: (i) it causes a rearrangement of the internal model and (ii) it evokes the sequence of neural and hormonal responses that constitute the motion sickness syndrome. There is clearly benefit in the modification of sensory and motor responses that accompany the updating of the internal model, for this allows the individual to function more effectively in the novel motion environment.

A diagrammatic representation of the functional components and processes currently embraced by the neural mismatch hypothesis is given in Figure 29.1. Active or passive motion of the body is detected principally by the eyes and the vestibular apparatus, although changes in the body's orientation to gravity and imposed linear accelerations also stimulate mechanoreceptors in the skin, muscles, capsules of joints and other tissues. All these sense organs send information to the central nervous system, where, it is postulated, there is a neural centre that acts as a comparator of signals from the receptors and of 'expected' signals provided by the internal model. The output of this

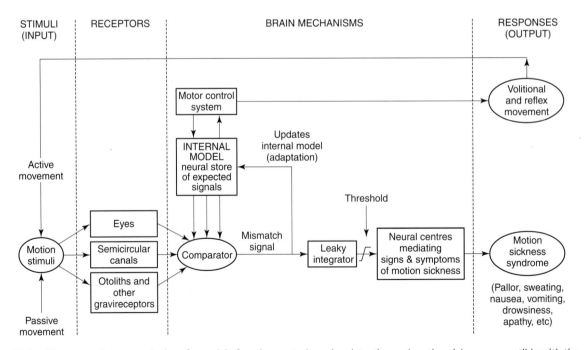

Figure 29.1 *Diagrammatic representation of a model of motion control, motion detection and motion sickness compatible with the neural mismatch hypothesis. Reproduced from Benson AJ. Motion sickness. In: Dix MR, Hood JD (eds). Vertigo. Chichester: John Wiley & Sons, 1984; pp. 391–426 by kind permission of John Wiley & Sons.*

comparator is the mismatch signal that, as noted above, updates the internal model and activates the neural centres and pathways mediating the signs and symptoms of motion sickness.

To explain the relatively slow development of symptoms on exposure to provocative motion, it is necessary to postulate the presence in the mediating pathway of a mechanism that accumulates the mismatch signal while at the same time allowing it to leak away slowly. In addition to this leaky integrator (the hydraulic analogy is a bucket with a hole in it), there must also be a threshold function in the mediating pathway, for it is known that adaptation to motion can occur, particularly if the stimulus is not intense, without the individual becoming motion sick. A threshold, or even several different threshold functions, is required to account for the large individual differences in susceptibility and the order in which the various signs and symptoms develop on exposure to provocative motion.

The manner in which the mismatch signal is likely to change on transfer from one motion environment to another is represented in Figure 29.2. In the normal, familiar environment, inputs from the sensory receptors are in accord with those of the internal model, but on initial exposure to unfamiliar motion there is a large mismatch signal. This decays slowly, probably with an exponential trajectory, as the internal model is updated until there is no longer a mismatch between the information from the sensory receptors and that which is 'expected' by the internal model. At this stage, the individual may be considered to have adapted to the atypical motion environment, and the signs and symptoms of motion sickness will have disappeared. On return to the familiar, or to some other, motion environment, a mismatch occurs initially because the internal model is no longer appropriate, and motion sick-

ness may recur (*mal de débarquement*). The internal model has to be modified to make it compatible again with the sensory input. In general, this phase of adaptation proceeds more quickly than the initial adaptation to the atypical environment, because the correlations established by long experience are retrieved more easily than new ones are acquired. By the same argument, should the individual return to the atypical environment, adaptation is likely to be a more rapid process than on first exposure, because the internal model can be rearranged with the aid of retained stimulus patterns acquired during previous exposures to the atypical environment. If transfer from one specific motion environment to another is frequent, then a stage is reached when the internal model can be modified quite rapidly, so that the mismatch signal is short-lived or of insufficient intensity or duration to engender motion sickness.

The sensory conflict theory aims to explain the types of motion that give rise to motion sickness. However, it has nothing to say about why such motion should give rise to nausea and vomiting or, indeed, any symptoms at all. The response of nausea and vomiting in a person exposed to abnormal motion appears to serve no useful purpose. A puzzling feature of the physiology of motion sickness is the output of pituitary stress hormones that accompanies the development of nausea. It is as if an abnormal motion environment evokes the declaration of a physiological state of emergency. Another feature of motion sickness is that many other animals will vomit when exposed to motion environments that make humans sick. Even fish have been observed to vomit when exposed to certain types of motion. Neither these creatures nor humans can have evolved this vomiting mechanism as a purposeful response to motion environments that they could never have encountered in their evolutionary past.

The capacity to vomit undoubtedly has survival value if it serves to eliminate toxic substances that an animal may have ingested. In what we call 'motion sickness', we may have stumbled upon one mechanism that the body uses to recognize the effects of potentially harmful neurotoxic substances and initiate vomiting. This theory suggests that the brain has evolved to use the constancy of the gravitational environment and the stability of the visual world as a form of self-calibration. A failure to encounter the expected interrelationships between sensory information derived from vision, the semicircular canals and the otoliths is interpreted as a malfunction of the brain itself, which could have been brought about by an ingested neurotoxin. Vomiting in these circumstances is an appropriate response to eliminate any toxic substances that may remain in the gut. It can now be seen as an unfortunate coincidence that, in the recent few seconds of evolutionary time, humans have developed modes of transport that generate sensory patterns that the brain has evolved to recognize as inconsistent.

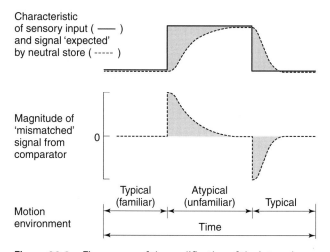

Figure 29.2 *Time course of the modification of the internal model on exposure to a new (atypical) motion environment and on return to the normal (typical) environment.*

Provocative stimuli

Implicit in the neural mismatch hypothesis of motion sickness is the idea that in all motion environments where sickness is induced, there is dissonance between the incoming sensory signals and those 'expected' by the neural store. There are two sensory systems of relevance: the visual system and the vestibular system. The latter is divided further into the angular acceleration receptors – the ampullary receptors – of the semicircular canals and the linear acceleration or force environment receptor system of the utricular and saccular maculae – the otolith organs, as they are more commonly called. Other mechanoreceptors are also stimulated by changes in the force environment, but in general they act synergistically with the otolithic receptors and need not, in the present context, be considered separately.

Two main types of motion cue mismatch can be specified according to the sensory system involved: visual–vestibular mismatch and canal–otolith mismatch. In each of these, two types of conflict can occur: type 1 conflict, in which both systems concurrently signal contradictory or uncorrelated information, and type 2 conflict, in which one system signals information in the absence of the expected signal from the other system. Examples of these different types of mismatch are summarized in Table 29.1, and the characteristic features are explained below.

VISUAL–VESTIBULAR CONFLICT

Type 1

In this condition, both the eyes and the vestibular receptors simultaneously signal motion but of an unrelated or incompatible kind. Cues in the two modalities do not accord with expectation based on previous experience. A prime example in the aerial environment is the sickness provoked on viewing ground or aerial targets through binoculars from a moving aircraft. Direct observation of the passing landscape from side or rear windows of a vehicle that is changing direction or speed also causes sickness, without the exaggerated apparent motion of the visual field introduced by the use of an unstabilized optical device. Likewise, attempting to read a handheld map or text in a moving vehicle can be highly provocative, because visual and vestibular motion cues are uncorrelated. In addition, the requirement to scan and maintain fixation on the visual material considerably potentiates the induction of sickness. Certain flight simulators, in which there is both a motion base and a visual display of the external scene (visual flight attachment), have been found to cause sickness during simulated flight manoeuvres that would not have been provocative in actual flight. Disparities, often of a rather subtle kind, between the visual cues of motion and those engendered by the moving cockpit of the simulator are thought to be responsible for the problem. Simulator-sickness is, however, more likely to occur in simulators that have a realistic visual display of large angular subtence but no cockpit motion, and the conflict is of type 2 rather than type 1.

Type 2

In this category, there are two kinds of conflict: one occurs when there are visual cues without the expected and normally correlated vestibular signals – type 2(i) – and the other when the vestibular cues are not accompanied by the expected visual cues – type 2(ii). The induction of sickness in a type 2(i) situation is important, perhaps more in rela-

Table 29.1 *Classification of motion cue mismatch*

Type	Identification of motion cue mismatch engendering motion sickness		
	Visual(A)–vestibular (B) mismatch		Canal(A)–otolith (B) mismatch
Type 1 (A) and (B) simultaneously signal contradictory information	(i) Reading handheld map or text in turbulent flight	(i) Cross-coupled (Coriolis) stimulation; head movement during rotation about another axis	
	(ii) Inspection through binoculars of ground or aerial targets from moving aircraft	(ii) Head movements in abnormal force environment, which may be stable (e.g. hyper- or hypo-gravity) or fluctuating (e.g. linear oscillation)	
Type 2 (i) (A) signals without expected (B) signal	(i) 'Simulator-sickness'; piloting of fixed-base simulator with moving external visual display	(i) 'Space-sickness'; head movement in weightless environment	
		(ii) Pressure (alternobaric) vertigo	
Type 2 (ii) (B) signals without expected (A) signal	(i) Looking inside aircraft when exposed to motion	(i) Low-frequency (< 0.5 Hz) linear oscillation	
		(ii) Rotation about non-vertical axis	

tion to theories of motion sickness as in an operational context, because sickness is caused purely by the perceived motion of visual images without physical motion of the observer and, hence, without stimulation of vestibular receptors. Such visually induced motion sickness is a problem in some fixed-base simulators fitted with a display of the external visual world, which moves in accord with the computed attitude and flight path of the aircraft. In simulator-sickness, the principal mismatch is between the visual input and the absence of those signals from semicircular canals, otoliths and other mechanoreceptors, which the pilot expects to accompany the flight manoeuvre executed in the simulator.

The argument that simulator-sickness is due to the unfulfilled expectations of vestibular and somatosensory inputs is supported by the finding that pilots with considerable experience of the real aircraft are more susceptible to this disorder than those with little or no previous experience of actual flight in the aircraft being simulated. This difference presumably reflects the greater entrenchment of the association between specific visual and vestibular cues in the former group than in the latter and, hence, the greater severity of the conflict when they are confronted with the 'rearranged' sensory inputs in the simulator. Sickness is usually less when the simulator cabin is given some motion, even though the linear and angular accelerations experienced by the pilot are but a caricature of the real motion of the aircraft. Sickness may be exacerbated, however, if there is not good concordance between the physical motion of the simulator and that of the visual display, especially in the temporal relationship between visual and vestibular motion cues. The sickness ('cinerama sickness' or 'Imax® sickness') that can be induced by viewing a motion picture shot from a moving vehicle (e.g. from a helicopter manoeuvring at low level) and displayed on a large screen is another example of the same type of visual–vestibular mismatch.

With a type 2(ii) conflict, there is an absence of the expected visual signal when the vestibular receptors are stimulated by the motion of the vehicle. This kind of conflict is present in all modes of passive transport where the passenger lacks a clear view of the visual scene outside the vehicle. In the air, for example, the linear and angular accelerations associated with flight in turbulence are signalled by vestibular receptors, but there is no correlated visual information when the individual looks at aircraft instrument displays or indeed any part of the interior of the aircraft that moves with them and hence provides a relatively stable visual input. It is well known that the incidence of sickness is lower when one has a clear view of the outside world than when vision is confined to the cabin or structure with which one moves. Thus, pilots typically suffer less sickness than navigators, except when the pilot becomes a passenger and is deprived of familiar external visual cues.

It should be recognized clearly that motion sickness can occur in many situations when the individual experiencing motion has their eyes closed and the basic mismatch is of the intravestibular kind (see below). However, the nature of the visual input can materially augment or decrease the intensity of the conflict and, in less severe motion environments, can determine whether the person does or does not become sick.

INTRAVESTIBULAR CONFLICT

During natural postural and locomotor activity in a stable 1-g environment, a correlated pattern of vestibular activity is established. For example, angular movement of the head in pitch and roll is associated with the concomitant stimulation both of the vertical semicircular canals and of the otolith organs, as the position of the head with respect to the gravitational acceleration changes. On the other hand, rotation of the head in yaw about a vertical axis is not accompanied by an alteration in the signals from the otoliths. This normal, established association between semicircular canal and otolith organ information is disturbed by certain volitional and yet natural head movements when made in an abnormal motion or force environment as well as by atypical passive motion itself.

Type 1

In this situation, both canals and otoliths signal contradictory information when the head is moved, either voluntarily or passively, in the presence of some other angular motion or an abnormal force environment. Cross-coupled (or Coriolis) stimulation of the semicircular canals occurs when an individual who is being rotated about a particular axis moves their head other than in the plane of the imposed rotation. One configuration of canals is taken out of the plane of rotation and they are stimulated by the apparent reduction in rotational speed. Concomitantly, another set of orthogonal canals is brought into the plane of rotation, and they receive a stimulus equivalent to an increase in the rate of turn. The result of this cross-coupled stimulus is to produce an erroneous signal of turn about an axis that accords neither with that of the imposed rotation nor with the axis in which the voluntary head movement is made. (A more detailed description of cross-coupled stimulation of the semicircular canals is given on p. 297 of Chapter 16.) Furthermore, the signal from the stimulated canals persists after the movement has been completed, for the deflected cupulae commonly take ten seconds or more to return to their neutral positions. During this time, the otoliths correctly sense the true attitude of the head with respect to gravity, and hence there is a mismatch between the otolith signal and that from the canals. This is a potent form of stimulation for inducing sickness to which all individuals with an intact vestibular system may succumb, provided the speed of rotation is high enough and the head movements are of sufficient amplitude and are made repetitively for long enough.

Head movements made in an abnormal force environment also cause sickness, although in this situation the canals, as they are essentially insensitive to linear acceleration, correctly transduce the angular movement of the head while the otoliths give inappropriate and hence conflicting information. In an abnormal force environment, any head movement that alters the orientation of the head with respect to the force vector will be associated with atypical signals from the otoliths. There will be a mismatch between the signals from the semicircular canals, which correctly transduce the head movement, and those from the otolith organs, which will not accord with the signals 'expected' by the neural store.

Type 2(i)

There are a number of situations and conditions occurring in aerospace flight in which motion sickness is induced by stimulation of the semicircular canals in the absence of expected and correlated signals from the otolith organs and other gravireceptors. Space-sickness is one example. In the weightless environment of space flight, angular movements of the head are transduced correctly by the semicircular canals but the otoliths do not signal the change in orientation of the head in pitch and roll as they do on Earth. Whereas most voluntary head and body movements can be provocative on initial exposure to weightlessness, the finding that head movements in pitch and roll are the most nauseogenic strengthen the argument that space-sickness is caused by a canalo-otolith mismatch. With head movements having high angular accelerations and velocity, there is likely to be atypical stimulation of otolithic receptors, and the mismatch is of type 1. A type II conflict is present when the head is moved slowly at rates that stimulate the semicircular canals but not the otoliths.

Another problem, common to divers and aircrew, is pressure or alternobaric vertigo (see p. 451 in Chapter 28). In this condition, asymmetric stimulation of semicircular canals is brought about, without apparent involvement of the otoliths by changes in ambient pressure. The vertigo is usually transient, and motion sickness is not a common feature, although in some individuals the stimulus can be quite intense and may engender nausea but rarely vomiting. Atypical stimulation of the semicircular canals without disturbance of otolithic function is seen in a number of other pathological and toxic states in which vertigo and nystagmus are accompanied by the signs and symptoms of motion sickness. Specific mention should be made of the positional vertigo associated with the consumption of ethyl alcohol (positional alcohol nystagmus) and benign paroxysmal vertigo. Both of these conditions cause symptoms on the ground, but in flight they can be intensified by linear accelerations greater than 1 g produced by high-rate turns and other flight manoeuvres.

Type 2(ii)

The converse to the type 2(i) canal–otolith mismatch occurs when the otolith signal is not accompanied by the expected signal from the semicircular canals. Provided the individual does not move the head, sustained rotation at a steady speed about a vertical axis does not cause sickness, because once the effect of the initial velocity change has died away neither the semicircular canals nor the otoliths signal rotation. However, when the axis of rotation is not vertical or, in the worst case, when it is horizontal (as in a barbecue-spit), there is a mismatch between canal and otolithic signals. The otoliths are stimulated by the continued reorientation of the body to the force vector and signal rotation, but the canals fail to signal rotation, as rotation is at a constant speed and there is no angular acceleration stimulus. Sustained rolling manoeuvres in level flight are associated with this kind of intravestibular mismatch, although in general the period of exposure is brief and is usually executed by pilots who have acquired some adaptive immunity.

Much more significant is the motion sickness induced by linear oscillation, typically the heaving motion of a ship or the repetitive linear accelerations experienced in an aircraft flying through turbulence and vertical gusts. In such a motion environment, the force vector (i.e. the resultant of the gravitational force and that due to the imposed linear acceleration) is changing continuously in magnitude and direction without the expected correlated signal from the semicircular canals. Furthermore, when the oscillation is of low frequency (< 0.5 Hz), there is a phase error in the signalling of the linear motion by the otoliths, which can be in conflict with the transduction of the changing force by pressure receptors in the skin or with visual information.

In a number of experiments carried out on four-pole swings, vertical oscillators and modified lifts, it has been shown that the incidence of sickness increases as the frequency of oscillation falls (Figure 29.3). This clearly defined laboratory relationship between the frequency of the stimulus and sickness rate accords with observations made in flight. Aircraft whose modal frequency of oscillation in response to gust perturbation is high (0.8–0.9 Hz), as when flying through turbulence, tend to produce less sickness and less impairment of performance than an aircraft that responds at a lower frequency (0.4 Hz). Similarly, a large motorcar with a soft underdamped suspension and low natural frequency is likely to cause more sickness in passengers than a car with a stiffer suspension and a more rapid dynamic response to perturbations from the road or the driver.

NEURAL CENTRES AND PATHWAYS

The principal neural structures and pathways that can be implicated in the genesis of motion sickness are summa-

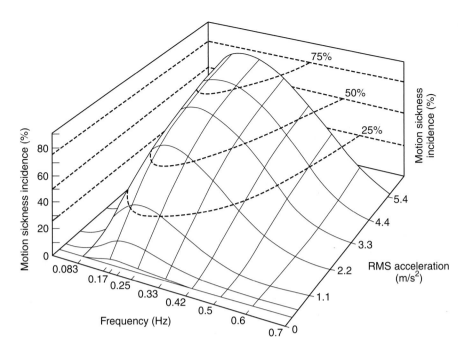

Figure 29.3 *Incidence of motion sickness as a function of frequency and acceleration, evoked by two-hour exposure to vertical (z-body axis) sinusoidal oscillation. After McCauley ME, Royal JW, Wylie CD, et al. Motion sickness incidence: exploratory studies of habituation, pitch and roll and the refinement of a mathematical model. Technical report no. 1729-2. Goleta, CA: Human Factors Research, 1976. RMS, root mean square.*

rized in Figure 29.4. There is good evidence that the vestibular apparatus and, hence, the vestibular nuclei and their central projections to the cerebellum have to be intact for motion sickness to be induced. Removal of the entire cerebellum confers immunity to swing-sickness in the dog, although it is less certain which part of the cerebellum is essential. Previously, the nodulus and uvula were considered to be critical structures, but it has been shown that ablation of these structures does not prevent vestibularly induced vomiting in cats. Convergence of vestibular,

visual, kinaesthetic and cerebellar afferents occurs at the level of the vestibular nuclei, so the comparison of actual and expected motion cues could take place within these brainstem nuclei. It is, however, more likely that the cerebellum is the locus of both the comparator and the internal model. The cerebellum receives the necessary afferent signals about body motion from retinal, vestibular, kinaesthetic and somatosensory receptors; in addition, the cerebellum is known to be an important integrative centre in the control of motor activity and movement.

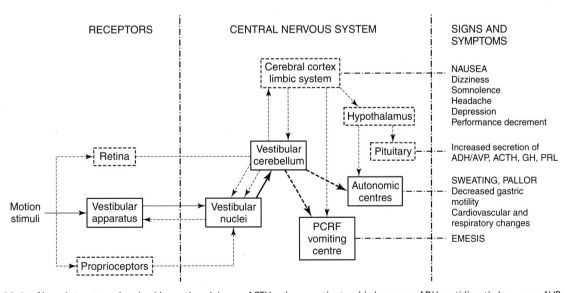

Figure 29.4 *Neural structures involved in motion sickness. ACTH, adrenocorticotrophic hormone; ADH, antidiuretic hormone; AVP, arginine vasopressin; GH, growth hormone; PCRF, parvicellular reticular formation; PRL, prolactin. Thick arrows and lined boxes indicate essential components in the mediation of motion sickness, thin arrows and dashed line boxes indicate components implicated in motion sickness, but which are probably not always significant.*

The way in which the cerebellum, or some other neural centre, initiates the sequence of sensory and autonomic responses that characterize the motion sickness syndrome remains a matter for speculation. The slow development of the syndrome and the persistence of signs and symptoms after the withdrawal of provocative stimuli suggests that there is some neurohumoral mechanism. The identity of neurotransmitters or the possible accumulation of a substance within the cerebrospinal fluid that stimulates the vomiting centre in the medulla oblongata has yet to be determined. It would appear that a neuronal centre, close to the area postrema at the level of the calamus scriptorius, is a vital element coupling higher centres to the neuroanatomically ill-defined vomiting centre in the region of the parvicellular reticular formation (PCRF) in the medulla. Modification of the activity of hypothalamic nuclei is manifest by the increased secretion of antidiuretic and other pituitary hormones that accompany motion sickness. However, neither hypophysectomy nor partial destruction of the hypothalamus prevents the development of motion sickness in dogs. Indeed, decerebrate dogs and, anecdotally, decerebrate humans are not immune.

INCIDENCE

Motion sickness is a normal response to an unfamiliar motion environment, but there are very considerable differences between individuals in their susceptibility to the condition. Nevertheless, provided the motion stimulus is of sufficient intensity and duration, only those people without a functioning vestibular system are truly immune. The incidence of sickness in a particular motion environment is governed by a number of factors, notably the physical characteristics of the stimulus (i.e. its frequency, intensity, duration and direction), the intrinsic susceptibility of the individual, the nature of the task performed and other environmental factors (e.g. odour).

The incidence of airsickness ranges from a fraction of one per cent in large civil transport aircraft to 100 per cent during hurricane-penetration flights. In military aviation, airsickness is most manifest during flying training, where the disability at least impairs training and at worst leads to attrition with all its economic and social consequences. A survey of the incidence of air sickness in Royal Air Force (RAF) trainee pilots, based on instructor reports, revealed that 39 per cent of students suffered from airsickness at some time during training, usually in the early stages, and that in 15 per cent of students it was sufficiently severe to lead to disruption or abandonment of the flight. An extensive review of the problem in US Navy flight officers being trained to perform various non-pilot duties (navigators, radar operators, etc.) produced a mean incidence of airsickness of 13.5 per cent of all flights. This was associated with vomiting on 5.9 per cent of flights and led to a performance decrement (as assessed by both instructor and student) on 7.3 per cent of flights. Some 59–63 per cent of students experienced symptoms on their first flight, 55–83 per cent were sick on more than one flight, and 15–30 per cent were never airsick. (The ranges quoted reflect the differing incidences in the several categories and stages of training.)

Typically, airsickness is most troublesome during initial training flights. Thereafter, the incidence of sickness falls as the student becomes adapted to the motion of the aircraft, but it often rises again when aerobatic and high-G manoeuvres are introduced in the training programme. Much can be done to ease the student's problem, by the instructor grading the flight manoeuvres during the first few hours of instruction. The initial demonstration of general handling should not be a test of the student's resistance (or susceptibility) to airsickness. The induction of symptoms early in training does not accelerate adaptation; indeed, it may impede this process by engendering anxiety and eroding the student's confidence in his or her ability to be a successful pilot. Once trained to an operational standard, it is rare for pilots to suffer from airsickness, although they sometimes experience symptoms when they are passengers and not in control of the aircraft. Non-pilot aircrew, in particular navigators, in high-performance aircraft and those working within the body of maritime reconnaissance aircraft may, however, continue to be troubled by airsickness. The proportion so afflicted is low, but anecdotally there are a few aircrew members who continue to vomit on nearly every flight and yet stoically and effectively carry out their operational duties.

Troops being transported by air are very much at risk. Paratroops, in particular, are likely to be exposed to provocative motion during low-level approaches to dropping zones. In-flight studies have revealed sickness rates as high as 75 per cent, although an incidence of ten per cent is perhaps more typical. Paratroops rarely fly with sufficient frequency to allow substantial adaptation to occur; furthermore, in flight they are usually closeted in the fuselage without sight of the ground or other external visual reference.

The incidence of seasickness is no less variable than that of airsickness, although in terms of the number of people affected it is much more common, as the motion is generally more severe and more prolonged than in other forms of transportation. The motion of life-rafts can be the most provocative, for in rough seas all but the very resistant succumb; an incidence of 99 per cent has been reported. Even moderate seas induce symptoms relatively quickly. For example, in a life-raft trial, 55 per cent of subjects had vomited and only 24 per cent were symptom-free after exposure for one hour to artificial wave motion.

Space-sickness, like other types of motion sickness, varies in severity and frequency. Symptoms were not reported by early US astronauts who flew in the small Mercury and Gemini spacecraft, but in the large vehicles where astronauts and cosmonauts could move about, many experienced symptoms. An analysis of the incidence of space sickness among 85 shuttle astronauts revealed that 67 per cent had symptoms, which were severe in 13 per cent. The data suggest that the incidence of sickness was less, symptoms were less severe and adaptation to weightlessness was more rapid in astronauts who had previous experience of space flight.

Prediction of incidence

Despite the many factors that play a part in the aetiology of motion sickness, the few quantitative studies that have been carried out, both in the laboratory and in the field, have yielded reasonably concordant data from which a procedure for predicting the incidence of motion sickness has been developed. In essence, calculation of the effective stimulus dose (motion sickness dose value, MSV) to which the incidence of vomiting is related linearly (Figure 29.5) takes into account three factors: (i) the intensity of the periodic motion, (ii) the frequency spectrum of the motion, and (iii) the duration of exposure.

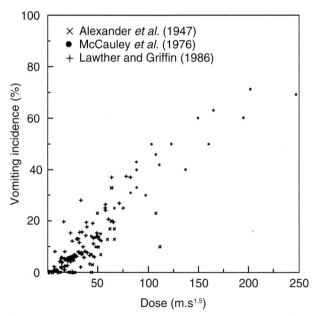

Figure 29.5 *Relationship between incidence of vomiting and stimulus dose, calculated by the procedure described in the text. Alexander* et al. *and McCauley* et al. *provoked sickness by vertical oscillation. Lawther and Griffin used data from ships' passengers on six-hour voyages. Reproduced from Lawther A, Griffin MJ. Prediction of the incidence of motion sickness from the magnitude, frequency and duration of vertical oscillation.* Journal of the Acoustical Society of America *1987; **82**: 957–66 by kind permission of the authors and the publishers.*

Expressed mathematically, the stimulus dose (MSDV) is as follows:

$$MSDV = aW_{(f)}t^{0.5}$$

where a is the mean square (rms) heave acceleration in m/s^2, $W_{(f)}$ is a frequency weighting factor and t is the duration of exposure in seconds.

The frequency weighting $W_{(f)}$ is achieved by a filter having characteristics similar to the frequency dependence shown in Figure 29.3 (p. 467). The greatest weight is given to frequency components in the octave 0.125–0.250 Hz, frequencies above and below this band being progressively attenuated.

Prediction of the percentage incidence of vomiting (V) in the population is given as follows:

$$V = K \times MSDV$$

where K is a factor estimated at 1/3 for the general population for vertical (heave) oscillatory motion acting in the head–foot z-body axis.

The findings of experiments in which body orientation to gravity and to stimulus direction were varied systematically suggest that for a given intensity of low-frequency linear oscillation, the incidence of sickness is higher (i) when the stimulus acts in the x-body axis (anterior–posterior) rather than the z-body axis (head–foot) and (ii) when the individual is upright rather than supine.

Susceptibility

The considerable variability between subjects in their response to provocative motion is an important feature of motion sickness. The broad dispersion of susceptibility is illustrated in Figure 29.6, which shows the number of subjects who developed well-defined signs and symptoms as a function of the intensity of the cross-coupled (Coriolis) stimulus to which they were exposed. The distribution is even more asymmetric than implied by the figure, for the measure of stimulus intensity is non-linear function of the speed of rotation, which was increased incrementally throughout the test until definite signs and symptoms were elicited. Individual differences in the rate at which the subjects adapted to the stimulus also influence the shape of the histogram. Those having a low tolerance to the stimulus had little time to adapt, whereas those who were less sensitive were able to make a larger number of head movements and hence had a greater opportunity to adapt to the stimulus. The high-tolerance tail of the distribution embraces the fortunate few who probably have low intrinsic susceptibility and are fast adapters.

An adult's susceptibility to motion sickness appears to be a relatively stable and enduring characteristic, for there

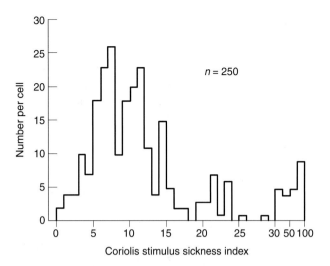

Figure 29.6 *Distribution of susceptibility to cross-coupled (Coriolis) stimulation in 250 normal subjects. Reproduced from Miller EF and Graybiel A. The semicircular canals as a primary etiological factor in motion sickness. In: Proceedings of the 4th Symposium on the Role of the Vestibular Organs in NASA. Space Exploration SP-187. Washington, DC: NASA, 1970; pp. 69–82, by kind permission of the authors and the publishers.*

is evidence that those who are sensitive to one type of provocative motion are likely to succumb when exposed to another. Susceptibility to space-sickness is, however, an exception to this general rule, for no significant correlation has been established, despite considerable effort to do so, between astronauts' responses to provocative stimuli, both on the ground and in aircraft, and their malaise in orbital flight.

Susceptibility changes with age. Motion sickness is rare before the age of two years, but susceptibility increases rapidly to reach a peak between the ages of 3 and 12 years. Over the next decade, there is a progressive increase in tolerance, which continues, albeit more slowly, with increasing age. This reduction in susceptibility with age has been recorded for both seasickness and airsickness. However, elderly people are not immune: 22 per cent of people suffering from seasickness on a Channel Islands ferry were over the age of 59 years. Females are more susceptible than males of the same age to motion sickness, in a ratio of approximately 1.7 to one.

In a group of men or women of the same age, large differences in susceptibility exist that reflect a basic characteristic of the individual. At least three factors can be recognized that contribute to inter-subject variability in susceptibility. One of these factors is 'receptivity', a term that refers to the way in which the individual processes the stimulus within the nervous system. It is suggested that people who have high inherent responsiveness transduce the sensory stimulus more effectively and hence have a

more intense mismatch signal and a higher susceptibility to motion. Another factor is adaptability, which describes the rate at which the individual adapts to an atypical motion environment. Those who adapt slowly suffer more severe symptoms and require a longer period for adjustment to the motion than the fast 'adaptor'.

Concepts of receptivity and adaptability permit explanation of how an individual will react on first exposure to an unfamiliar motion environment. But there remains one more factor – the manner in which adaptation is retained between exposures to the provocative motion. Poor retention of adaptation is illustrated by an aircrew member, typically a navigator, who is troubled by motion sickness when flights are separated by several days of ground duty but is symptom-free when able to fly regularly with not more than one or two days on the ground between flights. The aviator with better retention is not so afflicted: having adapted to the provocative motion of a particular flight environment, he or she remains symptom-free, even when flights are quite spasmodic.

These factors – receptivity, adaptability and retentivity – all influence susceptibility (Figure 29.7) but are not of equal importance when one attempts to assess whether airsickness is likely to be a problem to a particular aviator or potential aviator. Evidence of high receptivity implies that sickness will occur on initial exposure to unfamiliar motion; but, if the individual is a fast adaptor and has good retention of adaptation, then airsickness is unlikely to be a persistent problem. On the other hand, a person with low adaptability and poor retention is likely to continue to be afflicted by sickness when exposed to provocative motion. Knowledge of these constitutional factors can thus be an aid in the prediction of both motion sickness susceptibility

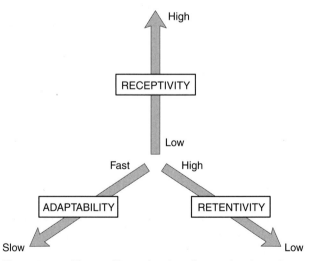

Figure 29.7 *Diagram illustrating three factors that determine motion sickness susceptibility, once allowance is made for the age and sex of the individual. The susceptibility to motion sickness increases with the length of the arrow.*

and the likely benefit to a particular individual of desensitization therapy (see below).

In addition to the perceptual factors described above, there is another psychological (or behavioural) factor that influences susceptibility, namely the nature of mental activity during exposure to the provocative motion. Laboratory studies and observation aboard ships and aircraft have shown that people who concentrate their attention and mental effort on a task are less likely to become sick than those who are not so occupied. When one relaxes and has more time for introspection, or has to report bodily sensations, then the appearance of symptoms and also signs of motion sickness is not delayed for so long. The mechanism underlying the role of cognitive processes in the aetiology of motion sickness is not understood. Nevertheless, if aircrew and passengers can be kept occupied by tasks that take their minds off the state of their stomachs, then the incidence of sickness is likely to be decreased.

The similarity of the cardinal signs and symptoms of motion sickness with those engendered by fear and anxiety has fostered the opinion in a number of authors that such psychogenic factors are of prime importance in the aetiology of motion sickness. The weight of evidence favours the conclusion that the physical characteristics of the motion stimulus and dimensions of personality other than anxiety traits are the principal factors determining the incidence of motion sickness; fear and anxiety are of only secondary importance. Nevertheless, significant correlations have been found in a number of studies between susceptibility and several personality characteristics. The most consistent finding was a relationship between neuroticism and susceptibility; in addition, however, susceptible subjects tended to score higher on measures of introversion and anxiety and had more medical and emotional problems than non-susceptible people.

Anxiety can be considered as both a potentiator of susceptibility and a consequence of motion sickness. Anxiety per se can also produce symptoms that are essentially indistinguishable from those evoked by provocative motion. The differentiation of fear sickness from motion sickness is relatively straightforward when nausea and vomiting occur in the absence of provocative motion. Examples are the student pilot who develops symptoms after a certain time in the air, irrespective of the intensity of the motion stimuli experienced, or the passenger who becomes sick as soon as he or she steps aboard the aircraft. On the other hand, when symptoms are produced consistently by certain flight manoeuvres, such as aerobatics, it is much more difficult to determine whether the symptoms are the expression of a neurotic reaction or are a 'normal' response to discordant motion cues. Typically, flying personnel with airsickness report a diminution in the severity of symptoms with repeated exposure to the provocative motion. The individual with anxiety characteristically does not show such adaptation; indeed, symptoms may become worse on successive flights, particularly when there is a strong phobic element to the neurotic reaction or when a conditioned behavioural response becomes established. However, when the severity of symptoms remains relatively constant on repeated exposure to the provocative motion, then it is difficult to determine whether the airsickness is caused by low adaptability and poor retentivity or whether it is the manifestation of a neurotic reaction.

PREVENTION

Behavioural measures

Passengers in an aircraft can minimize motion cue conflict by restriction of head movement, which may be achieved, for example, by pressing the head firmly against the seat or other available support. If space permits, they should lie down on the back or at least adopt a reclined position, as this posture has been shown in laboratory trials to reduce the incidence of motion sickness by approximately 20 per cent. Visual–vestibular conflict is decreased by closing the eyes, unless of course the passenger has a clear view of the horizon or other stable visual reference outside the aircraft. Attempting to read a book, although a desirable means of occupying the mind and diverting attention from a lack of wellbeing, is a task that commonly accentuates discordant visual cues and is rarely helpful. Aircrew are not usually able to lie down and close their eyes when engaged on operational duties, but they can still organize their activity so that unnecessary movements are not made. In particular, head movements should be reduced to a minimum, although not to the extent that either scan or lookout are impaired. Where possible, discordant visual cues should be minimized, as noted above. When aids to vision are employed for target recognition (e.g. use of binoculars or other targeting devices for the identification of ground targets), sickness is reduced and visual acuity enhanced if the optical image is stabilized.

Adaptation

The most potent therapeutic measure, at least in the long term, is adaptation to the provocative motion. This is nature's own cure and is the preferred method of preventing sickness, particularly for aircrew, who should not fly under the influence of anti-motion sickness drugs. The basic philosophy governing the acquisition and maintenance of protective adaptation is that aircrew should be introduced gradually to the provocative motions of the flight environment, and that adaptation, once achieved, should be maintained by regular and repeated exposure to the motion stimuli. Student pilots and those returning to flying after ground duties should have a graded introduction to the more stressful flight manoeuvres, so that adaptation may be acquired, preferably without severe malaise.

The wide differences between aircrew, both in initial susceptibility and rate of adaptation, make it difficult to set down firm guidelines. Nevertheless, instructors should be advised to grade the duration of exposure and intensity of provocative motion stimuli in a manner that is commensurate with the tolerance of the aircrew under training. The maintenance of protective adaptation is best assured by regular flying duties, although factors such as interindividual differences in the retention of adaptation, variations in weather conditions and operational roles preclude temporal definition of the word 'regular'. Some aircrew members are troubled by motion sickness if two to three days elapse between flights; others with better 'retentivity' may not be more susceptible, even after several weeks on the ground.

'Desensitization therapy'

Despite the high incidence of airsickness during the initial phases of flight training, most aircrew adapt with repeated exposure to the provocative motion of flight, sometimes aided by a short course of an anti-motion sickness drug. There is, however, a small percentage (estimated at about five per cent) of aircrew who fail to develop sufficient protective adaptation and in whom continued sickness may necessitate suspension from flight training or, more rarely, operational duties. Most of the aircrew with what may be called 'intractable airsickness' can be helped by a programme of treatment of a type initiated in the RAF by Dobie in 1974. In its current form, this 'desensitization therapy' involves first a three-week period of twice-daily exposure to either cross-coupled (Coriolis) stimulation of progressively increasing intensity or low-frequency motion on a vertical oscillator or lateral swing. The ground-based phase of therapy is followed by 10–15 hours of dual flying in which there is incremental exposure to progressively more provocative flight manoeuvres. All return to flying duties following this treatment, and in less than ten per cent does a recurrence of airsickness lead to a suspension from flight training.

The desensitization programme outlined above places considerable emphasis on exposure and adaptation to physical motion stimuli. There is, nevertheless, a psychotherapeutic element in so far as the 'patient' is reassured that airsickness is a normal response and that it is not the manifestation of a personal weakness or lack of moral fibre. Furthermore, as treatment progresses, the person is made aware of his or her increasing tolerance, which serves to allay any anxiety that may have existed about their ability to cope with provocative motion in the flight environment.

In the US Air Force, the desensitization therapy employs biofeedback and relaxation techniques in addition to passive Coriolis stimulation. The underlying concept is that by learning to control autonomic responses and allay anxiety evoked by motion stimuli, susceptibility to motion sickness will be decreased and the rate at which protective adaptation is acquired will be enhanced. Biofeedback and relaxation techniques coupled with supportive psychotherapy were effective in returning some 40 per cent of referred aircrew to flying duties. In contrast, when these behavioural techniques were combined with 20 sessions of incremental Coriolis stimulation and were followed by five 'reorientation' flights, 85 per cent of the aircrew were returned to flying duties.

Selection

A variety of techniques is available for assessing an individual's susceptibility to motion sickness. Most widely used is some form of cross-coupled (Coriolis) stimulation, but tests in which there is visual–vestibular mismatch (the visual–vestibular interaction test) or stimulation of the otoliths (e.g. tilted-axis rotation, parabolic flight, linear oscillation) also have been employed. In an extensive longitudinal study of US Navy flying personnel, significant correlations were found between the incidence of airsickness during flight training and the student's responses to cross-coupled stimulation and to visual–vestibular conflict. Motion sickness questionnaire data also correlated highly with susceptibility to sickness in flight. It should be noted, however, that in this study, the questionnaire was administered after the personnel had been accepted into the navy. Questions about previous history of motion sickness presented during the pre-entry medical are not answered with objective honesty. For example, in the RAF, it was found that only 3.6 per cent of potential aircrew admitted to having suffered from motion sickness before selection; subsequently, when the same questions were posed in a confidential questionnaire to the same group during aircrew training, 59 per cent gave affirmative responses.

Because of the essential role of the vestibular system in the aetiology of motion sickness, attempts have been made to relate indices of vestibular function to susceptibility. Most of these studies have failed to show any correlation, although one did find a higher frequency of labyrinthine imbalance (on caloric testing) in a group suffering from chronic seasickness than in the control group.

As discussed earlier, susceptibility is associated with certain dimensions of personality (neuroticism, anxiety, introversion), but the correlations, although significant, are relatively weak. They are not high enough for the results of provocative-test and motion-sickness questionnaire scores to be used as selection determinants, for they do not reliably identify those individuals in whom sickness will be a continuing problem during flight training or subsequent operational duties. Whereas correlations have been established between data from various laboratory tests and susceptibility to motion sickness in a number of terrestrial environments, no consistent relationship has yet been found between such measures and susceptibility to space-sickness, despite considerable research efforts.

Aircraft factors

Although it is known that the incidence of motion sickness increases as the frequency of oscillation decreases, this fact apparently has not been considered by aircraft designers or others concerned with aircraft dynamics. An aircraft that responds to a gust perturbation by low-frequency (< 0.5 Hz) movement is clearly less desirable from the airsickness viewpoint for long-duration sorties at low level or for 'hurricane hunter'-type operations than an aircraft with a higher characteristic frequency. In some aircraft, low-frequency oscillation, usually of a 'Dutch roll' type, is induced by the autopilot control system. A reduction in the incidence of airsickness, particularly in passengers and non-flight-deck aircrew of such aircraft, can be achieved by improvement of control dynamics.

Other relevant aspects of aircraft design concern the postural stability of the aircrew or passenger within the aircraft. Thus, restraint harnesses, the provision of head support and seat design in general all play a part. The arrangement of instruments and displays can also contribute to a reduction in the incidence of air sickness, as can the siting of workstations within the aircraft. Such factors are of particular concern to non-flight-deck aircrew, who should, whenever possible, be seated close to the centre of gravity of the aircraft. Furthermore, they should be provided with displays and controls that do not require large-amplitude head movements to be made in the course of normal operations.

Environmental factors such as heat and unpleasant odours are usually overemphasized in the aetiology of motion sickness, although it must be acknowledged that comfort is enhanced and sickness perhaps less likely if they are controlled adequately. A feeling of warmth is a common feature of motion sickness, so it is not surprising that fresh air or a cooling breeze can lead to symptomatic improvement. However, the belief that a hot oppressive atmosphere increases susceptibility, although understandable, has not been supported by several objective studies.

Medication

Over the years, many medicinal remedies have been proposed for the prevention of motion sickness. The number of drugs that has been tested is large, but relatively few are effective (Table 29.2), and none can completely prevent the development of signs and symptoms in everyone in all provocative motion environments. The protection afforded by differing doses of one of the most effective drugs, scopolamine, is shown in Figure 29.8. If the motion is relatively mild and only ten per cent of the unmedicated population suffer from sickness, then use of the drug can increase protection so that all but two per cent of the population are not sick. When the motion is of such severity and duration that 50 per cent are sick when no drug is given, then a large dose (1 mg) of scopolamine still leaves eight per cent of the population unprotected. In life-rafts, sickness rates approaching 100 per cent have been reported, so it is not surprising that a significant proportion of the occupants will still suffer from seasickness, even when the dose of drug given is sufficient to cause side effects.

None of the drugs of proven efficacy in the prophylaxis of motion sickness is entirely specific, and all have side

Table 29.2 *Adult dosages and duration of action of anti-motion-sickness drugs*

Drug	Route	Adult dose	Time of onset	Duration of action (h)
Hyoscine hydrobromide (scopolamine) (Kwells®)	Oral	0.3–0.6 mg	30 min	4
Hyoscine hydrobromide	Injection	0.1–0.2 mg	15 min	4
Hyoscine hydrobromide (Scopoderm TTS®)	Patch	One	6–8 h	72
Promethazine hydrochloride (Phenergan®)	Oral	25–50 mg	2 h	15
Promethazine hydrochloride	Injection	25 mg	15 min	15
Dimenhydrinate (Dramamine®)	Oral	50–100 mg	2 h	8
Dimenhydrinate	Injection	50 mg	15 min	8
Cyclizine hydrochloride (Marzine®)	Oral	50 mg	2 h	6
Cyclizine lactate (Valoid®)	Injection	50 mg	15 min	6
Meclizine (Sea-legs®)	Oral	25–50 mg	2 h	8
Cinnarizine (Stugeron®)	Oral	15–30 mg	4 h	8

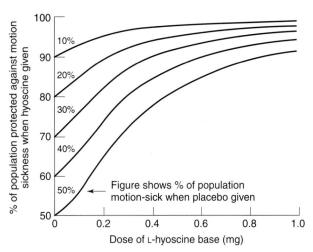

Figure 29.8 *Protection against motion sickness afforded by scopolamine, at five levels of 'placebo sickness'. Note the logarithmic shape of the curves and the lack of complete (100 per cent) protection, even with a large dose of the drug. After Brand JJ, Perry WLM. Drugs used in motion sickness.* Pharmaceutical Review *1966; 18: 895–924.*

effects. The antihistamines (e.g. promethazine, dimenhydrinate) and scopolamine, an anticholinergic, are also central depressants and can cause impairment of performance. Scopolamine at all therapeutic doses has been shown to cause a performance decrement on tasks requiring continuous attention and memory storage for new information, but only at doses greater than 0.8 mg does it interfere with performance of a pursuit-tracking task. Promethazine 25 mg has also been shown to impair psychomotor performance. Other side effects of scopolamine, notably blurred vision, sedation, dizziness and dry mouth, may also contribute to performance decrement. There is, thus, good reason for the general rule that anti-motion sickness drugs should not be taken by aircrew, and under no circumstances should they be taken by a pilot when required to fly. There is a place for the administration of prophylactic drugs to susceptible student aircrew, particularly during the early stages of flying training when accompanied by an instructor. However, there is evidence to suggest that scopolamine, although allaying symptoms, does interfere with the acquisition of protective adaptation. This is one reason why the continued use of anti-motion-sickness drugs by aircrew is to be deprecated; furthermore, such a pharmacological crutch is not compatible with operational duties.

No such restrictions apply to the use of drugs by passengers for the alleviation of motion sickness. Paratroops and other personnel who must operate at peak efficiency on leaving the aircraft or at the end of a flight are a possible exception, although the putative performance decrement attributable to motion sickness and that due to drug side effects is a dilemma to be assessed only with detailed

knowledge of all facets of the operational situation. The choice of prophylactic drug depends in part on the foreseen duration of exposure to provocative motion and in part on differences between individuals, in both the efficacy of a particular drug and the severity of side effects. Therefore, if in practice one drug is not effective or not well tolerated, then it is justifiable to give another drug or combination of drugs.

Where the therapeutic objective is to provide short-term protection, oral scopolamine (0.3–0.6 mg) is the drug of choice. This acts within 0.5–1 hours and provides protection for about four hours. Side effects can be troublesome and tend to be accentuated if repeated administration (at four- to six-hour intervals) is required for more prolonged prophylaxis. With the development of transdermal drug-transport techniques, it is now possible to provide a loading dose of 200 µg scopolamine and its controlled release at 10 µg/h for up to 60 hours by means of a patch placed behind the ear (transdermal therapeutic system, TTS). The protection afforded by TTS is reported to be comparable with that achieved by oral scopolamine, but there does appear to be greater inter-subject variability in both the efficacy and the incidence of side effects than found with repeated oral administration of the drug. When scopolamine is administered transdermally, peak blood levels are not reached until 8–12 hours after application of the patch, and so it is necessary to anticipate a requirement for prophylaxis by at least six hours. The antihistamines promethazine and meclizine when taken by mouth are absorbed more slowly than scopolamine and are not effective until about two hours after administration, but they provide protection for at least 12 hours. Other drugs in the same group, such as cyclizine, dimenhydrinate and cinnarizine, are absorbed at about the same rate, although their duration of action is shorter, at about six hours.

The demonstration that dexamphetamine increases tolerance to cross-coupled stimulation led to an evaluation of the use of this analeptic in combination with established anti-motion sickness drugs. It was found that there was a synergistic increase in prophylactic potency and a decrease in the sedation that is a common side effect of scopolamine and the antihistamines. Ephedrine is almost as effective as dexamphetamine in enhancing the efficacy of the anti-motion sickness drugs and should be used in preference to amphetamine when prescription of this potentially addictive drug is contraindicated. Assessment of therapeutic potency in both laboratory and field trials has indicated that the combination of scopolamine (0.3 mg) with ephedrine sulphate (25 mg) or dexamphetamine sulphate (5 mg) is most effective for short-term (four hours) protection. In situations requiring more sustained prophylaxis, the combination of promethazine hydrochloride (25 mg) with ephedrine sulphate (25 mg) is recommended.

Management of vomiting

Vomiting that is severe and repeated can lead to dehydration and loss of electrolytes. If this occurs in a survival situation (e.g. on a life-raft), it may cause breakdown in morale, loss of interest in surroundings, and a loss of ability to cooperate with rescue attempts. In such cases, attention should be given to the following:

- Maintenance of intake of fluids and electrolytes.
- Use of drugs: these must be given parenterally; if given by mouth, they may not be absorbed or may be returned with the vomit. The following preparations are recommended: intramuscular injection of scopolamine hydrobromide 0.1–0.2 mg, or cyclizine lactate 50 mg, or promethazine hydrochloride 25–50 mg.
- Supportive measures: make the patient lie down, attend to general comfort and give reassurance.

REFERENCES

Benson A. Motion sickness. In: Dix MR, Hood JD (eds). *Vertigo.* Chichester: John Wiley & Sons, 1984; pp. 391–426.

Brand JJ, Perry WLM. Drugs used in motion sickness. *Pharmaceutical Review* 1966; **18**: 895–924.

Lawther A, Griffin MJ. Prediction of the incidence of motion sickness from the magnitude, frequency and duration of vertical oscillation. *Journal of the Acoustical Society of America* 1987; **82**: 957–66.

McCauley ME, Royal JW, Wylie CD, *et al.* Motion sickness incidence: explanatory studies of habituation, pitch and roll and the refinement of a mathematical model. Technical report no. 1729–2. Goleta, CA: Human Factors Research, 1976.

Miller EF, Graybiel A. The semicircular canals as a primary etiological factor in motion sickness. In: Proceedings of the 4th Symposium on the Role of the Vestibular Organs in NASA. Space Exploration SP-187. Washington, DC: NASA, 1970; pp. 69–82.

Reason JT, Brand JJ. *Motion Sickness.* London: Academic Press, 1975.

FURTHER READING

Benson AJ. Motion sickness: significance in aerospace operations and prophylaxis. Lecture series 175. Neuilly-sur-Seine: AGARD/NATO, 1991.

Crampton GH. *Motion and Space Sickness.* Boca Raton, FL: CRC Press, 1990.

Griffin MJ. Motion sickness. In: *Handbook of Human Vibration.* London: Academic Press, 1990; pp. 271–92.

Mitchelson F. Pharmacological agents affecting emesis: a review. Parts 1 and 2. *Drugs* 1992; **43**: 295–313, 443–63.

30

Passenger safety in transport aircraft

HELEN MUIR AND LAUREN J. THOMAS

BACKGROUND

Since the first powered flight of Orville and Wilbur Wright in 1903, the development of airframes capable of carrying large numbers of people over extended distances has to be regarded as one of the major achievements of the twentieth century. The current aircraft fleet includes planes that carry over 400 passengers, and aircraft carrying up to 880 passengers are in the latter stages of development. As a consequence, a large percentage of people in the developed world, and a smaller percentage in the developing world, are able to travel frequently, at relatively lost cost, for the purposes of business and leisure.

The aviation industry has achieved a remarkable safety record, making it currently the safest form of mass transportation in the world today. Since the introduction of commercial jet transportation in the 1950s, there have been tremendous improvements. Within a period between 1951 and 2001, the hull-loss accident rate has reduced from 28 per one million departures to 1.5 per one million departures (Boeing Commercial Airplanes 1989).

There is an average of one fatality for every 12.5 million passengers carried by UK airlines. This makes it four times safer than rail travel and 20 times safer than travelling by car, with 3500 people being killed each year in the UK in road accidents (Begg 2003). However, the public perception of the relative safety of air travel is vastly different from the actual statistics. Indeed, one study showed that for civil aircraft accidents in the period 1983–2000, the overall survivability rate was 95.7 per cent (National Transportation Safety Board 2001). This decrease has been achieved only by continuous and concerted efforts from all members of the industry, including the airframe manufacturers, the people responsible for operating and maintaining the aircraft, air traffic control and airports, and the associated regulatory authorities. Unfortunately, the public perception of survivability in air accidents is significantly less. This may stem partly from the fact that accidents involving multiple deaths attract major media attention. Ironically, if the accidents in which the majority or all of the passengers survive were given greater media attention, then it would be easier to persuade passengers that the majority of aircraft accidents are survivable and that it is therefore worthwhile taking steps to help themselves in an emergency and to pay attention to safety information.

The behaviour of passengers and their impact on emergency evacuations has also come under scrutiny. It is believed that with a comprehensive understanding of passenger behaviour in highly stressful and disorientating conditions, steps could be taken to improve the probability that all passengers will successfully evacuate the airframe and survive in the event of an emergency.

ACCIDENTS AND PASSENGER SURVIVABILITY

From the perspective of human behaviour and survival, aircraft may be regarded as boxes with a limited number of small exits and high seating density. In order to understand the factors influencing passenger safety, it is necessary to determine the causes of fatalities in accidents. These can be classified broadly into three groups: impact fatalities, fire fatalities, and terrorism.

The purpose for identifying these categories is that once the contributors to passenger fatalities are understood, then it is possible to determine the steps that can be taken to improve the probability of passengers surviving in future accidents.

Impact fatalities

In some accidents, when the airframe hits the ground the forces are so great that either the human frame cannot withstand the pressure or, more frequently, passengers die as a result of the injuries sustained from being thrown against solid structures within the cabin. In this event, the injuries involve fractures to limbs, the head or parts of the body cavity.

An example of such an accident was the one that occurred in the UK at Kegworth in 1989 (Air Accidents Investigation Branch 1990). In this accident, the aircraft crashed on to the M1 motorway as a consequence of the pilots' mistakenly shutting down the only functioning engine. Many fatalities occurred as a consequence of the initial impact, and further fatalities occurred when, shortly after the airframe had come to a halt, the seat track broke away from the floor and further passengers were crushed fatally as the seats cascaded into each other.

Fire fatalities

The second group of accidents comprises those in which a fire is involved. Airframes carry large quantities of kerosene fuel, which is highly inflammable. In a large percentage of accidents, a fire occurs; in this event, there is typically a maximum of two minutes between the first spark and the conditions in the cabin becoming non-survivable due to the presence of smoke and toxic fumes. In these situations, passengers are required to evacuate the airframe rapidly. Although the majority of fatalities occur as a result of the inhalation of smoke and toxic fumes, other injuries include thermal injuries, burns and fractures. There have been instances of passengers breaking arms falling from a wing and passengers breaking ankles by jumping out of an exit that did not have a slide. In the National Transportation Safety Board (1985) study, older passengers statistically were no more likely to sustain injury than younger passengers. Nevertheless, they believed that their condition and age hindered their evacuation. In many but not all of the cases studied, behaviour included passengers pushing or being pushed, passengers climbing over seats, and disputes among passengers. In some of these cases, seats were broken and the cabin was damaged by the behaviour of the passengers. In contrast, in other cases, the behaviour was reported to have been orderly.

An example of an accident in the UK where non-orderly behaviour occurred and passengers tragically died as a consequence was the accident that happened in 1985 at Manchester Airport (Air Accidents Investigation Branch 1985). In this accident involving a 737 aircraft with 155 passengers on board, one of the engines caught fire on takeoff and smoke and toxic fumes rapidly entered the cabin. Although a period of more than two minutes was available for evacuation, with half the exits to the plane open and in operation, 55 passengers failed to evacuate the aircraft before they were overcome by the smoke and toxic fumes.

This and similar accidents caused major concern to safety professions. Before any new passenger aircraft is certificated to fly, the manufacturer is required to perform a test to demonstrate that it is possible to evacuate all of the passengers in 90 seconds or less using half of the available exits. This test had been performed successfully on the 737 aircraft on a number of occasions. The question asked after the accident at Manchester was why, when it had been possible to evacuate all of the passengers through half of the exits in a test, was it not possible to do so in an accident?

Terrorism

Although the overall number of passengers who have lost their lives as a consequence of some act of terrorism is relatively low, these accidents are starting to form a distinct category. They include the accident that happened at Lockerbie in the UK in 1988 (Air Accident Investigation Branch 1988) in which a passenger boarded an aircraft carrying sufficient explosives to destroy the airframe and all the passengers. Other examples include the Canada Air accident in 1984 in which the captain flew the aircraft into the sea beside Nova Scotia, in what was believed to be a suicide attempt, with the loss of all crew and passengers. In this category, the fatalities that occurred on the four planes involved in the 11 September 2001 attack on the Twin Towers in the USA must also be included. A response to this event has been the introduction of air marshals on many transport aircraft.

Accident analysis

Although no two accidents are ever the same, it is possible to learn from the similarities and differences between the causes of the accidents, their locations, the environmental conditions present, and the types of passengers on board and their responses to the emergency. From the information gained from investigations into accidents, it is possible to build up a picture of the factors influencing survival.

There were many similarities between the accident at Manchester in 1985 (Air Accidents Investigation Branch 1985) and the accident that occurred at Calgary, Canada, in 1984 (ICAO 1984), in that they were both caused by an engine fire at takeoff. However, they differed in one important respect, namely that at Manchester there were 55 fatalities whereas at Calgary everyone survived. We know that in some aircraft accidents, everyone files out of the plane in a rapid but orderly manner, e.g. in the evacuation of a British Airways 747 at Los Angeles in 1987 following a bomb scare (Civil Aviation Authority 1991). In other accidents, however, the orderly process breaks down, and confusion in the cabin can lead to blockages in the aisles and at exits, with a consequent loss of life (Air Accidents Investigation Branch 1985). There has been a lack of understanding about the circumstances in which these behaviours occur. The frequency with which passengers panic, freeze, give up and get crushed by other people has never been documented fully. Many questions remain unanswered about the behaviour of people in emergencies, including the important question of why in some accidents the passengers evacuate in an orderly manner but in others their behaviour is disorderly.

From the reports of a number of accidents, it is possible to build up a picture of the exits typically used by passengers who survive an emergency when there is smoke and fire and the behaviour is disorderly. The information in Figure 30.1, for example, indicates that:

- some passengers exit by their nearest door, as would be expected
- other passengers do not exit by their nearest available door but travel for considerable distances along the cabin, e.g. from the rear of the cabin to the forward exits
- other passengers apparently close to exits do not survive.

It is suggested that one of the primary reasons for the differences in behaviour between the orderly and disorderly situations arises from the motivation of individual passengers (Muir *et al.* 1990a). In some accidents, as in aircraft certification evacuations, all of the passengers assume that the objective is to get everyone out of the aircraft as quickly as possible, and therefore they all work collaboratively. In other emergencies, however, the motivation of individual passengers may be very different, especially in

the presence of smoke and fire. In a situation where an immediate threat to life is perceived, rather than all passengers being motivated to help each other, the main objective that will govern their behaviour will be survival for themselves and, in some instances, members of their family. In this situation, when the primary survival instinct takes over, people do not work collaboratively. The evacuation can become disorganized, with some individuals competing to get through the exits. The behaviour observed in the accidents at Manchester (Air Accidents Investigation Branch 1985) and Los Angeles (Civil Aviation Authority 1991) supports this interpretation.

ACCIDENT SURVIVAL AND SAFETY IMPROVEMENTS

From a review of the information available from accidents it is possible to identify the major factors which influence the probability of survival and some of the safety improvements which could be made as a consequence. These include the following:

Crashworthiness and occupant protection

This includes not only the strength of the components of the airframe to withstand the crash impact but also the strength of components within the cabin. For example, as a consequence of the fatalities and injuries sustained by the passengers in the Kegworth accident (Air Accidents Investigation Branch 1990), the regulatory authorities revised the standard for seat strength to require that all seats had to be capable of withstanding a force of up to 16 g (Federal Aviation Administration (FAA) federal aviation regulation (FAR) 25.562). More recently, it has become a requirement that inflatable airbags are fitted within bulkheads in order to reduce the probability of injuries caused to passengers sitting facing a bulkhead. Seatbelts have been a requirement for all passengers and crew for many years, but recently the potential benefits of seatbelts with three-point harnesses have been suggested.

■ Fatality   ⊠ Unoccupied seat   ⊘ Air cabin staff

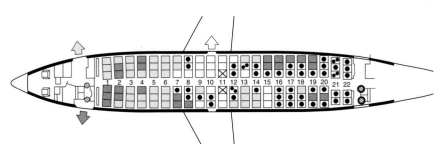

Figure 30.1 *Simulation of survivor escape door and seating fatalities. The shading of the seats corresponds with the shading of the exits showing where each surviving occupant exited. Three exits (one in the middle and two at the rear of the plane) are not shown because they were not available for use due to the fire at the rear and along one side of the airframe.*

Fire protection

Fire is a major hazard in aircraft accidents. Following the accident at Manchester in 1985 (Air Accidents Investigation Branch 1985), new regulations were introduced that required fire-blocking materials to be used in seats and smoke detectors to be installed in toilet cubicles. Major programmes of research into the potential benefits to passengers of smoke hoods and cabin water-mist systems were undertaken, although these have not been introduced.

Interior configuration

The configuration of the seats, monuments and services within the cabin can all influence not only the injuries that can be sustained by passengers but also the speed at which passengers can evacuate the airframe. Another factor is the location of exits and the space adjacent to the exits for both passengers and cabin crew.

There is some evidence from the video recordings taken during the evacuation certification of new airframes that bigger cabin-crew members are not able to stay within the minimum assist space while helping passengers to evacuate, which consequently can reduce the rate at which passengers are able to evacuate the airframe.

Following the accident at Manchester in 1985, the regulatory authorities introduced a requirement for a maximum distance of 60 feet between exits (FAR 25.807) to limit the distance that passengers would be required to travel in order to leave the aircraft. Regulations were also introduced in which additional space adjacent to the type III exit was required (Civil Aviation Authority 1986).

Crew performance

The usual maximum number of passengers per flight attendant is 50. However, Scandinavian Airlines flies with one flight attendant per 30 passengers, and indeed many other operators fly with more than the minimum number of flight attendants. It should be recognized, however, that operators that fly with additional crew usually do so for reasons of service as well as safety.

The information from both accidents and research indicates that a major influence on the behaviour of passengers in an emergency is the performance of the crew. Research has shown, for example, that one assertive cabin crew member can evacuate the passengers more quickly than two non-assertive cabin crew members; 'assertiveness' involved strong and active physical and verbal commands (Muir and Cobbett 1995). In the accidents where a successful rapid evacuation of all the passengers is achieved, the cabin crew will have managed to control the passengers (despite a fire and the presence of smoke in the cabin) and prevented disorderly behaviour from occurring (National Transportation Safety Board 1996).

Evacuation aids

Following the accident at Manchester in 1985, the regulatory authorities introduced new requirements for operators to provide floor-proximity lighting and fluorescent exit signs to assist passengers to evacuate the aircraft in the event of their vision being restricted by the presence of smoke (Muir et al. 1990b). Research has also been undertaken into the possibility of introducing directional noise to assist passengers to locate operational exits when conditions in the cabin have become visually degraded (Rutherford and Withington 1998). Directional noise systems have been introduced on ships and in tunnels in order to assist evacuation (Greene and Friedrich 2003).

Safety information

The regulations (US Department of Transportation 1974) require that passenger-carrying aeroplane operators must ensure that all passengers are briefed orally by the appropriate crew member before takeoff. This briefing should include restrictions on smoking, the location of the emergency exits, the use of safety belts and when to use them, and the location and use of any required flotation means. In addition, each passenger-carrying operator must provide a safety card in a convenient location for use by each passenger. This card supplements the oral briefing and should contain diagrams of, and methods of operating, the emergency exits, and other instructions necessary for the use of emergency equipment.

Passenger performance in an evacuation depends on how well they have prepared for such an eventuality. A large part of this preparedness is their knowledge of exit location and operation, information that is normally provided either by the oral briefing or by the safety card. There is a considerable body of evidence that suggests that passengers do not pay attention to this safety information. For example, an National Transportation Safety Board safety study (National Transportation Safety Board 2000) examined 46 evacuations, sending questionnaires to all passengers involved. Of 457 passengers who returned questionnaires, 54 per cent reported that they had not watched the entire briefing because they had seen it before. Of 431 passengers who answered the question relating to the safety card, 68 per cent said that they had not read it.

Furthermore, even those passengers who do read the safety card many not necessarily understand it. In a recent study, 36 pictorial diagrams chosen randomly from 50 safety cards were presented to 113 people. Of these 36 diagrams, 20 were understood by less than 50 per cent of people tested (Caird *et al.* 1997). As a result, the National Transportation Safety Board has recommended that the FAA requires minimum comprehension testing standards for safety briefing cards. Until this comes into effect, the guidance provided in FAA advisory circular 121-24B provides suggestions on how to motivate passengers to pay attention to safety briefings and how best to present this critical information.

RESEARCH INTO PASSENGER EVACUATION BEHAVIOUR

Since passenger behaviour in accidents has been shown to have a significant influence on survival rates (Air Accidents Investigation Branch 1985; Civil Aviation Authority 1991), major programmes of research have been undertaken. An initial objective was to determine whether it was possible to produce experimentally a simulation of the behaviour that was known to occur in emergencies when passengers rushed towards exits and the behaviour in the cabin became disorderly.

The challenge facing the designers of any research, in which the objective includes the evaluation of safety systems for use in an emergency (whether from aircraft, public-transport vehicles, buildings, etc.), is to determine a satisfactory trade-off between the realism required and the potential physical or mental risk to the participants.

For both ethical and practical reasons, it is not possible to put volunteers into a situation of fear and threat for the purposes of research. For instance, it would not be acceptable to take a group of volunteers on a flight and then tell them that an emergency has occurred and video their behaviour. However, a technique used in laboratory work in behavioural science is to offer an incentive payment to subjects. This is done in an attempt to influence the motivation and performance of individuals, either individually or in groups.

An extensive experimental programme was conducted in which an incentive payment system was developed in order to introduce an element of competition (Muir *et al.* 1990a). A series of evacuation exercises were performed in which an additional payment was made to the first half of the subjects to leave the aircraft. Volunteers recruited from the public were paid £10 attendance fee to perform four emergency evacuations from an aircraft, with a £5 bonus paid to the first half of the volunteers to exit the aircraft on each evacuation. No previous research had been reported in which bonus payments had been made to groups of subjects performing a strenuous physical task; therefore, the decision to give £5 to 50 per cent of the participants was

based on findings from laboratory research. The experiment was then replicated without the use of bonus payments in order that a comparison could be made between the influence of highly motivated behaviour and orderly behaviour on evacuation rates.

In order to introduce as much realism as possible, evacuations took place from an aircraft parked on an airfield. On boarding the aircraft, volunteers were met by members of the research team trained and dressed as cabin staff. Following a standard pre-flight briefing, volunteers heard the noise of the engine start up, taxi down the runway and finally the sound of an aborted takeoff, followed by the voice of the captain telling them to undo their seat belts and get out. The exits to be used were opened by the 'cabin staff', i.e. members of the research team. Volunteers were recruited from the public to take part in a series of four evacuations. Their behaviour and evacuation times were recorded using video cameras mounted inside and around the exits from the cabin.

It was found from these tests not only that the differences between the evacuation times in actual accidents and the times when the aircraft was tested for certification could be understood, but also that the features of the cabin layout that caused blockages and congestion when passenger behaviour was disorganized could be identified. A subsequent programme of testing enabled recommendations to be made for minimum distances between bulkheads and distances between seat rows adjacent to exits. The results from the test programme showed clearly that if sufficient space is available for passengers, even when the evacuation is disorderly, the speed of the evacuation will be increased. The programme was repeated in conditions of non-toxic smoke in the cabin. This showed that although the presence of smoke slows down the speed of passenger movement, what is of most help to passengers in this situation is the availability of tactile cues and the route to the exit having regular and predictable features that can be identified. A sudden gap between seats, or nothing to grasp hold of, leads to hesitation and congestion, with a consequent increase in the length of time it takes passengers to evacuate. All of these results have implications for other modes. A similar study in the rail industry using bonus payments to passengers also highlighted the dangers of narrow passageways just before exits and problems with carriage furniture (e.g. seat tables) causing congestion.

PASSENGER RESPONSES IN AN ACCIDENT

In any potential emergency situation, an individual will initially try to identify the nature and extent of the problem or the source of the threat. However, the actual situation and an individual's perception of the situation are not always exactly the same. What we perceive and how we respond to that perception will be influenced by:

- what we are expecting
- what we have experienced in the past
- the expected consequences from the situation.

For example, because of our previous experiences of speed limits on motorways, these are frequently ignored. By contrast, a warning of fire on an aircraft certainly would not be ignored.

In a crisis, passengers can experience any of the reactions described below:

Fear

Fear is the primary response when survival is threatened. The two reactions to fear are fight and flight. We know that either of these responses can occur in an accident. This response causes our physiology to change in order to enable us to fight or flee the threat more efficiently than when our physiology is in its normal state. In other words, we have enhanced physical performance. Indeed, there have been instances where passengers in accidents have performed physical tasks that they would not have been able to achieve in normal circumstances (Civil Aviation Authority 1991).

Anxiety

Anxiety is a response experienced by the majority of passengers in an emergency situation. This is due to the fact that the situation is frequently perceived as potentially life-threatening. In this situation, passengers are required to make a series of novel and difficult responses, and it is hardly surprising that the optimum performance does not always occur. In an airframe emergency situation, simple tasks such as unfastening the lap-belt become more difficult for passengers; in fact, sometimes passengers revert to the actions that would release a car seatbelt. The implications of this for an emergency are that if we are to fight the threat, the instructions and any equipment must be simple and intuitive. If we are to escape quickly, the route must be clear and there must be sufficient space in the event of a rush of passengers.

Disorientation

Disorientation can be experienced as a result of factors such as a reduction in visibility caused by dense black smoke or the vehicle having come to rest on its side or at some strange angle. The disorientation will not only increase levels of anxiety among passengers but also may cause them to enter areas of the vehicle from which there is no escape. It is important, therefore, that in the design of vehicles, consideration should be given to features that could assist passengers to maintain their situational awareness as they move through the vehicle, especially in the event of smoke being present.

Depersonalization

People who have encountered life-threatening events often say that the passage of time slows while mental activity increases. For some people, detaching themselves from the actual situation and acting as an 'observer' means that they feel better and are able to think and respond effectively.

Panic

Panic may be defined as uncontrollable and irrational behaviour. In practice, it is believed that true instances of panic among passengers involved in accidents are relatively rare. When the behaviour of passengers in emergencies is studied in detail and their changing perceptions of the situation as the accident develops are followed, the behaviour exhibited usually can be interpreted as a series of rational responses. For instance, it cannot be considered to be inappropriate for people to put enormous energy and drive into escaping from fire. In the train collision that occurred in 1996 at Watford South, UK, where many of the passengers sustained serious injuries, the time spent by passengers screaming and shouting was brief. One survivor reported that in his part of the train, passengers, including those who were injured, rapidly became calm (Health and Safety Executive 1998).

Behavioural inaction

Behavioural inaction is a term used to describe the behaviour of passengers who, after an accident has occurred, seem to 'freeze' in their seats and remain immobile. The evidence from accidents across modes seems to indicate that there are many more instances of behavioural inaction than of panic. The analysis of four disasters led Allerton (1964) to conclude that between 10 and 25 per cent of people did little or nothing to escape from danger. A number of passengers on a taxiing Boeing 747 at Tenerife in 1977 (Civil Aviation Authority 1977) were judged by their fellow passengers to make little attempt to escape from the burning aircraft.

Affiliative behaviour

Affiliative behaviour involves movement towards the familiar. In an accident, movement towards the familiar occurs frequently. Passengers' attachment to their hand luggage has often been observed, with many passengers insisting on taking their personal belongings with them when undertaking an emergency evacuation. It seems the perceived value of the contents outweighs the increased risk they believe they will encounter.

Focused attention

In normal circumstances, humans selectively take in information from all around. In any situation in which they have clearly identified a task that they are highly motivated to achieve (such as escaping from an aircraft that is on fire), they are able to focus all of their attention on this primary task and ignore all other sensory inputs. This process can be highly adaptive, but there can be occasions when important information can be missed.

The extent to which some of these reactions and behaviours occur (together with the performances of the crew) will be a major determinant of the occurrence of orderly or disorderly behaviour.

PASSENGER SAFETY AND FUTURE VERY-LARGE TRANSPORT AIRCRAFT

The challenge for the development of future very-large transport aircraft (VLTAs) will be to ensure that with passenger loads above 400, together with cabin interiors that will include innovative features such as twin decks or

blended wings involving up to six aisles, the standards of safety can be maintained (Figure 30.2).

For airframes with twin decks, it is currently assumed that in an emergency passengers on the upper and lower decks will evacuate down slides from each of the decks and that the stairs will not be used. This implies that a large number of passengers will be evacuating down slides from a height of 8 m. Although assertive cabin crew probably will ensure that passengers do jump on to slides from this height, it will be important to ensure that with such large numbers of passengers, multiple injuries are not sustained due to congestion at the bottom of the slides.

For blended-wing airframes (Figure 30.3), it will be important to ensure that passengers are briefed with sufficient information in order to ensure that they are aware of their location in such a complex cabin and of their route to their nearest exits, especially if there is smoke in the cabin in the event of a fire.

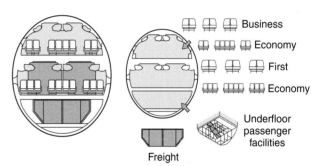

Figure 30.2 *Future very-large transport aircraft: twin deck.*

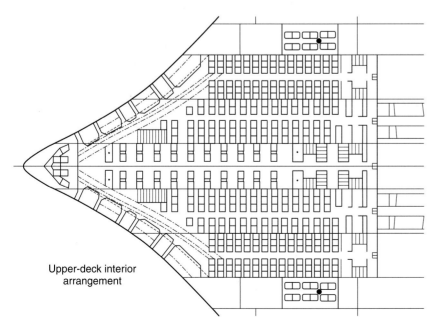

Figure 30.3 *Blended-wing airframe.*

CONCLUSIONS

Individual passenger survival

The factors that influence whether an individual passenger survives an accident include:

- the accuracy of their perception of the sources and level of threat
- their level of education and frequency of flying
- their knowledge of the vehicle and the safety procedures
- their situational awareness of their location within the vehicle, and their proximity and routes to available exits or safe locations
- the behaviour and characteristics of other passengers, including their knowledge, culture, age and gender
- their personal characteristics, such as age, gender and culture.

Enhanced occupant survivability

In order to enable passengers to behave optimally to assist their survival in the event of an accident, the manufacturers and operators of air transport vehicles should endeavour to ensure that:

- the crashworthiness of the airframe and interior cabin configuration are such that injuries due to crash impact are kept to a minimum
- the design of the interior of the vehicle is such that there is sufficient space adjacent to exits and between bulkheads to ensure that serious congestion will not occur, even when passengers are rushing through the vehicle in a disorganized manner
- the routes to available exits or safe havens are signed clearly
- the procedures for operating exits or other equipment that may be used by passengers or crew in an emergency are relatively simple to use and are designed to follow intuitive principles
- the emergency procedures and training of the cabin crew will ensure that they are able to control the passengers in order to ensure optimal use of all available exits
- information or knowledge required for use by passengers in an emergency is specific and unambiguous and can be fully understood and remembered, and furthermore all passengers know that they have a high probability of surviving an accident and that their knowledge of the safety information will significantly improve their chances of survival

- when tests on any new vehicle are conducted to evaluate the vehicle design and procedures for use in an emergency, consideration is given to the full range of passenger reactions and behaviours, as these can influence the probability of all of the passengers successfully surviving in the event of an accident.

In summary, from our learning from accidents and the knowledge of how passengers behave in emergencies, the industry has made changes that have improved the probability of passengers surviving accidents. The challenge will be to ensure that in the future, as airframes increase in size and passenger loads rise, the impressive level of safety that has been achieved is maintained.

REFERENCES

Air Accidents Investigation Branch. Report on the accident to Boeing 737-236 Series 1 G-BGJL at Manchester International Airport on 22 August 1985. Aircraft accident report 8/88. Aldershot: Air Accidents Investigation Branch, 1985.

Air Accidents Investigation Branch. Report on the accident to Boeing 747-121, N739PA at Lockerbie, Dumfriesshire, Scotland on 21 December 1988. Aircraft accident report no. 2/90 (EW/C1094). Aldershot: Air Accidents Investigation Branch, 1988.

Air Accidents Investigation Branch. Report on the accident to Boeing 737-400 G-ONME near Kegworth, Leicester in January 1989. Aircraft accident report 4/90. Aldershot: Air Accidents Investigation Branch, 1990.

Allerton CW. Mass casualty care and human behaviour. *Medical Annals of the District of Columbia* 1964; **33**: 206–8.

Begg D. Transport safety and integration: putting the two together. 14th Westminster lecture. London: Parliamentary Advisory Council for Transport Safety, 2003.

Boeing Commercial Airplanes. *World Travel Demand and Airplane Supply Requirements*. Seattle: Boeing Commercial Airplanes, 1989

Caird JK, Wheat B, McIntosh KR, Dewar RE. The comprehensibility of airline safety card pictorials. In: *Proceedings of the Human Factors and Ergonomics Society 41st Annual Meeting*. Santa Monica, CA: Human Factors Society, 1997; pp. 801–5.

Civil Aviation Authority. World airline accident summary CAP 479, Report of accident to Boeing 747 at Tenerife on 27 March 1977. London: Civil Aviation Authority, 1977.

Civil Aviation Authority. Access to and opening of type III and type IV emergency exits. Airworthiness notice 709. London: Civil Aviation Authority, 1986.

Civil Aviation Authority. World airline accident summary CAP 479. Report on the accident to Boeing 737-N388US at Los Angeles Airport on 1 February 1991. London: Civil Aviation Authority, 1991.

Greene G, Friedrich P. Very large transport aircraft (VLTA) emergency requirements research evacuation study (VERRES): a project summary. Joint Aviation Authorities research paper 2003/1. Hoofddorp, the Netherlands: Joint Aviation Authorities, 2003.

Health and Safety Executive. *Railway Accident at Watford*. Sudbury: HSE Books, 1998.

ICAO. Summary 1984-2. Report on the accident to Boeing 737 C-GQPW at Calgary Airport on 22nd March 1984. Montreal: ICAO, 1984.

Muir HC, Cobbett AM. Cabin crew behaviour in emergency evacuations. Civil Aviation Authority/Federal Aviation Administration paper DOT/FAA/CT-95/16. London: Civil Aviation Authority, 1995.

Muir H, Marrison C, Evans A. Aircraft evacuations: the effects of passengers' motivation and cabin configuration adjacent to the exit. Civil Aviation Authority paper 89019. London: Civil Aviation Authority, 1990a.

Muir HC, Marrison C, Evans A. Aircraft evacuations: preliminary investigation of the effect of non-toxic smoke and cabin configuration adjacent to the exit. Civil Aviation Authority Paper 90013. London: Civil Aviation Authority, 1990b.

National Transportation Safety Board. Airline passenger safety education: a review of methods used to present safety information. NTSB/SS-85/09, PB85-917014. Washington, DC: National Transportation Safety Board, 1985.

National Transportation Safety Board. Report on the accident to Boeing 747-131 N93119 at New York on 17th July 1996. Washington, DC: National Transportation Safety Board, 1996.

National Transportation Safety Board. Emergency evacuation of commercial airplanes. NTSB/SS-00/01, PB2000-917002. Washington, DC: National Transportation Safety Board, 2000.

National Transportation Safety Board. Survivability of accidents involving Part 121 US air carrier operations, 1983 through 2000. NTSB/SR-01/01, PB2001-917001. Washington, DC: National Transportation Safety Board, 2001.

Rutherford P, Withington DJ. Sound location for aiding emergency egress. *Fire Safety Engineering* 1998; 5: 14–17.

US Department of Transportation. Federal Aviation Regulations part 121: operating requirements. Washington, DC: US Department of Transportation, 1974.

31

Patient transport by air-logistic considerations

NEIL MCGUIRE

INTRODUCTION

The increasing sophistication and cost of healthcare has meant that in many countries there has been rationalization of services. This has resulted in centralization of resources and an increased need to move patients to gain access to them. The increasing mobility of our populations and the ready access to air travel has also resulted in a requirement to consider the needs of the patient who has become ill outside their own country. Chapter 56 outlines the general principles of aeromedical evacuation and Chapter 57 deals specifically with clinical issues related to the critically ill. This chapter covers the logistic issues involved in moving patients by air.

In order to assess dependency and priority for transfer, patients must be classified. For illustration, the North Atlantic Treaty Organization (NATO) classification (Table 31.1) will be used in this chapter. These definitions are not absolute and represent a continuum of dependency. With this in mind, careful assessment is required to ensure, for example, that patients who are dependency 3 or 4 are not likely to deteriorate due to the effects of flight. If they change to a higher category, then different care is required. Changes such as this must be anticipated, as team composition and equipment cannot be altered easily during the mission.

In the UK, there are tens of thousands of patient transfers and thousands of critical-care transfers every year; most are by road. Movement by air should be considered

Table 31.1 *North Atlantic Treaty Organization (NATO) classification of patient dependency*

Dependency	Definition
1	Patients who require intensive support, e.g. ventilation, monitoring of central venous pressure, cardiac monitoring. They may be unconscious or under general anaesthesia.
2	Patients who, although not requiring intensive support, require regular, frequent monitoring and whose condition may deteriorate in flight, e.g. patient with combination of oxygen therapy, one or more intravenous infusions and multiple drains and catheters.
3	Patients whose condition is not expected to deteriorate during flight but who require nursing care, e.g. simple oxygen therapy, intravenous infusion or urinary catheter.
4	Patients who do not require nursing attention in flight but who might need assistance with mobility or bodily functions.

if terrain is difficult, roads are congested or unreliable, or if the journey is likely to be over two hours in duration. The timing is not absolute and depends on many factors, but issues such as patient stability, equipment capability, consumable supplies, oxygen supply and staff fatigue should be considered.

For critical-care transfers in particular, the initial premise must be to avoid them if at all possible. If the transfer cannot be avoided, it should never be undertaken lightly. Only appropriately trained personnel should be used. They should have equipment that can deliver care to the same standard offered in the fixed hospital environment (see below). It must be remembered that the journey begins as soon as the patient leaves a secure environment (piped gas supplies, mains power, immediate assistance) and ends only when a secure environment is reached again.

Where air transfer is deemed appropriate, the choice of rotary-wing or fixed-wing aircraft needs to be considered. Rotary-wing aircraft are more suitable for shorter transfers (when the choice is limited only by which vehicle and not by patient factors). Rotary-wing aircraft are inherently smaller, are less stable, have short ranges and present a more hostile environment. Small fixed-wing aircraft may also have these problems, and it should not be assumed that they can be pressurized to attenuate the effects of altitude. Larger fixed-wing aircraft tend to be more comfortable, have greater ranges, can be pressurized and usually have a less hostile environment, although some transport aircraft may present serious environmental hazards as the patient may be accommodated in a cargo area. These factors are discussed in more detail below.

For the military medical services, there is a constant need to provide medical support for military operations. These include peacekeeping, humanitarian missions and combat operations. All of these have led to the requirement to repatriate injured and sick service personnel. The UK military medical doctrine is focused on providing care from the point of wounding, through the evacuation chain and back to the healthcare system that will provide definitive care and rehabilitation. Implicit is continuous, progressive, proactive care.

Humanitarian operations following natural disaster or war where there has been destruction of medical infrastructure may also require the evacuation of patients. Loss or absence of medical care facilities in a community presents a dilemma to outside attendant medical personnel. On the one hand there is a duty of care to the sick and injured, but on the other hand there is the need to avoid altering the level of care that normally would be available in a country. If this occurs, then when the aid is withdrawn, a medical vacuum is created due to the inappropriate raising of expectations. This may be very damaging to national recovery.

In war, it must also be remembered that the articles of the Geneva Convention maintain that there is a duty of care to countries by an occupying power. This leads to a legal and moral obligation to offer aid. If infrastructure is damaged in the initial period following the cessation of hostilities, then there may be a need to evacuate patients to treat them appropriately. For example, this occurred following the military operations in Kosovo and in the Gulf conflict.

MILITARY TRANSFERS

Doctrine for the British Defence Medical Services (DMS) sets out the requirements for the UK military medical services and also gives guidance on the standards that are to be adhered to for patient care. It also defines the roles of each of the services in the provision of care. The Royal Air Force Medical Service (RAFMS) is responsible for the care of all patients transported by air.

The majority of armed services will have doctrine and policy for air evacuation of casualties. These may differ from those of the UK, which is used in this chapter for illustration of principle.

The RAFMS remit is to ensure that patients are transferred from the operational area as soon as is practical. This allows medical assets to be maximally effective by freeing their resources and allowing them to deal with any new or developing situation. Field units have a number of choke points that restrict their activity by blocking patient flow. These are shown in Table 31.2. Any restriction at these points will compromise capability. They need to be cleared within 48 hours if at all possible, as delay beyond this has both logistic and clinical consequences (see below). The most demanding areas on resources are those involved in the provision of critical care.

Deployed medical facilities have limited staff and resources. They often rely on long and, at times, tenuous logistic chains. In some circumstances, the flow of fresh troops and ammunition may have a higher priority than medical supplies. Likewise, following major disasters or intensive war fighting, the overwhelming number of patients also impairs capability.

Table 31.2   *Choke points in field medical facilities*

Area	Limitations
Reception	Administrative personnel
Triage	Specialist medical and nursing personnel
Resuscitation	Specialist personnel (anaesthetic, emergency medicine), equipment, consumables, resuscitation bays
Operating room	Specialist personnel (anaesthetic, surgical), equipment, consumables, operating tables
Postoperative recovery	Specialist personnel (recovery practitioner), equipment, consumables, recovery bays
High dependency	Specialist personnel (critical care), equipment, consumables, bed spaces
Intensive care	Specialist personnel (critical care), equipment, consumables, bed spaces

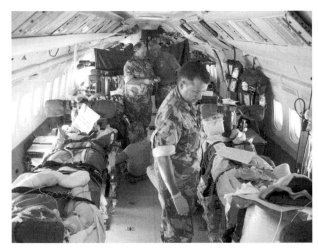

Figure 31.1   *Example of multipatient care. See also colour plate 31.1.*

The very nature of field units means they have limitations in capability in terms of expertise, equipment and holding facilities. They are usually in very austere locations. By transferring patients away, assets are freed and there is the opportunity to rest and prepare for the next, usually unpredictable, influx of patients.

Transfer team composition

To direct the correct resources, patients are classified according to NATO standard agreements (STANAGS). STANAGS also provide guidelines for the composition of aeromedical crews, and these vary according to the dependency level of the patients being carried. For example, the RAFMS utilizes critical-care air-support teams (CCASTs) to care for critically ill patients who are being transferred. A similar concept is used by the US military, which has critical-care air-transport teams (CCATTs), but the team composition and roles are different in the two systems. The CCAST assumption is that a single team can provide care for a critically ill patient for up to 24 hours. This care provision may have to be completely independent of any local or transfer resources. It is capable of being delivered in a wide range of environments, from close support to forward military operations, through a variety of tactical and strategic settings. It is also able to utilize almost any form of transport, whether land- or air-based.

The standards and policy for the care of patients moved by the RAFMS are the ultimate responsibility of the director general medical services, Royal Air Force (DGMS (RAF)). This person is advised by the deputy director aviation medicine (DDAvMed). For critically ill patients, the consultant adviser in anaesthetics, who is also the specialist adviser in aeromedical evacuation, is consulted. Policy is then implemented by the deputy adviser chief of staff medical operations (DACOS Med Ops). Day-to-day con-

trol of aeromedical missions is the responsibility of staff officer aeromed (SO2 A3 Aeromed). Finally, missions are undertaken through tactical medical wing and aeromedical evacuation squadron teams. These include the CCAST teams for critical-care missions.

CIVILIAN TRANSFERS

In the UK, the National Health Service (NHS) has a standard classification of patients (Table 31.3). These are used in the organization and provision of healthcare services. This system cannot be used for prioritizing transfers, as it relies on the ready availability of hospital specialty services. In the UK, therefore, the standards of care for transfers are advised upon by professional bodies such as the Intensive Care Society (1997, 2002) and the Association of Anaesthetists of Great Britain and Northern Ireland (1996).

In the UK, there is a distinction between the provision of care for adults and children. This has occurred partly due to the even more specialized requirements of neonates and very young children. At the time of writing, the provision of care for children is much better organized and usually performed to a considerably higher standard than for adults.

Ideally, the provision of services should depend on the requirements of each area. Although there may be generalizations that may be applied to this service provision, each system should be tailored to the particular region and country in which it operates. The underlying principles

Table 31.3   *National Health Service (NHS) standard classification of patients (based on Department of Health. Comprehensive critical care: a review of adult critical care services. London: Department of Health, 2000)*

Level	Definition
0	Patients whose needs can be met through normal ward care in an acute hospital.
1	Patients at risk of the condition deteriorating and patients recently relocated from higher levels of care and whose needs can be met on an acute ward with additional advice and support from the critical-care team.
2	Patients requiring more detailed observation or intervention including support for a single failing organ system or postoperative care and patients 'stepping down' from higher levels of care.
3	Patients requiring advanced respiratory support alone or basic respiratory support together with support of at least two organ systems. This includes all complex patients requiring support for multiorgan failure.

should remain the same, namely patient-focused services, providing the highest quality of care that at least mirrors the standard in fixed facilities. In many areas, this is not the case, and much work needs to be done.

The RAFMS has different standards than those of the UK civilian professional bodies with regard to transfer of patients, particularly those who are critically ill. These differences are borne out of operational considerations and factors such as mission duration and diverse environments encountered. For critically ill patients, this results in a consultant-based service supported by larger and more diverse teams. The relative merits of the differences between the military and civilian systems will not be dealt with in this chapter, as the underlying principles are the same, i.e. to provide the highest standard of care for all patients.

REQUIREMENTS FOR TRANSFER

All transfers subject patients to risk. Any risks must be weighed in the light of a number of considerations, not all of which may be patient-focused. The clinical situation should be the major factor when deciding on the relative merits of remaining in a location or transferring. Exceptions are found particularly in the military environment (Table 31.4). Generally, however, a patient should be transferred only to gain access to essential facilities that are not available locally or to prevent the patient from being exposed to greater risk by remaining where they are. For example, a patient may be in a facility that does not provide adequate care for their condition. This may result in increased and continuing risk of unacceptable morbidity and mortality. Likewise, there may be a risk that this treatment may result in inadequate basis for rehabilitation. None of these can be justified in normal circumstances, and the decision to move is weighted heavily in favour of transfer. Similarly, if a patient is being cared for in a facility with appropriate levels of clinical care, then normally it would not be justified to move the patient from a clinical

perspective, but other influences may justify the risk to the patient during transfer, including the patient being treated in an area where there is continuing risk due to war or a major disaster such as flood or earthquake.

Patients and their relatives also have expectations of levels of care. In the military setting, an expectation of service personnel to have an equivalent level of care that might be expected in the home country is implicit in doctrine. Inadequate care with no prospect of transfer to better facilities also impinges on the political arena and could influence national support for a military campaign.

In the civilian setting, people generally wish to be treated close to home and their relatives. In the case of critically ill patients, where the risk of mortality is higher, this consideration assumes a greater importance. This factor may influence the decision to transfer within the national setting as well as at an international level.

There may be economic considerations that alter the balance of whether to transfer, or not, in either direction. It may be expensive to keep a patient in a hospital abroad, and an insurance company may press for repatriation. Conversely, the cost of transfer may be prohibitive for an uninsured individual. In addition, internal transfer of patients may be required to make the best use of available resources such as critical-care beds and centralized specialist services.

For the military, the tempo of operations or success of the enemy may make the transfer of any patients impossible. It may also restrict the availability of air assets or the ability to fly at certain times. As stated above, it may also not be at the highest priority at certain times. If, however, this is not addressed as soon as practical, then it will prove false economy, as the effects on morale and political impact will become apparent rapidly.

Prevailing climatic conditions may interfere with air operations and may make transfer to the air point of departure (APOD) difficult or impossible. Likewise, access to the APOD may be restricted by the same natural disaster that led to the casualties in the first instance. It may also be that ambulances or rotary-wing assets are otherwise occupied or unserviceable.

Table 31.4. *Factors influencing the decision to transfer patients*

Factor	Example
Place of safety vs transfer	Already in well-equipped facility but requires long-term care
Access to care unavailable locally	Advanced imaging, treatment, expertise
Patient expectation	National level of care
Risk	If patient remains in location, option of transfer will be lost
Clinical	Unstable, inadequate resources or expertise for complex transfer
Political	Obligation, humanitarian
Diplomatic	Permission refused or timescale too short
Economic	Expense of transfer vs not transferring, use of critical-care bed
Operational	Hostile activity, unavailable assets
Environmental	Weather, fire, flood, earthquake
Logistic	Unavailable transport, infrastructure (roads, bridges)

There will be times when it is logistically impossible to link up assets to enable the safe transfer of the patient. It may not be possible to obtain the diplomatic permissions to overfly certain areas or refuel. Added to this, diplomatic considerations may deny access to the military of other nations, or the need to obtain visas for teams collecting patients may cause delay or make a mission unviable.

The balance of risk in some circumstances may be influenced by the welfare of the many outweighing the risk to the few. This is a major influence in the mass-casualty situation, where resources are overwhelmed by sheer numbers of sick or injured people. In these cases, decisions must be made that may not be in the best interests of the most unwell patients but are in the interests of the greater number of individuals. Problems may arise subsequently when these decisions are exposed to the scrutiny of the survivors.

GENERAL TRANSFER CONSIDERATIONS

Organization

To ensure that patients are transferred safely and in a timely manner, taking into consideration all the factors highlighted above, an effective organization needs to be in place. Proper coordination of the mission is essential in order to avoid added risk to the patient. Organizations vary, and there is a contrast between the military and civilian systems.

Civilian organizations are operationally smaller and do not have access to the resources available to the military. This means that usually they can deal with only small numbers of patients and do not have the surge capability allowed for by military organizations. More often than not, civilian organizations are businesses that are required to be profitable; as would be expected, this influences the nature of the organization. Some are charitable organizations and, as a result, have access to greater resources.

Ideally, such an organization would be based around a central control room that is run continuously by mission controllers. It would have a number of control desks to receive calls from any location, whether national or international. The control room would be supervised by a resident doctor who assists the controllers with additional medical advice and coordinates the movement of patients according to medical priority. They would have access to small aircraft such as the Hawker Siddeley HS 125 and occasionally larger aircraft such as the Canadair CL 604 Challenger aircraft for missions. The HS 125 could carry up to two stretcher patients, while the Challenger could have up to four stretchers. For critical-care purposes, one patient in the HS 125, and a maximum of two people in the Challenger, is optimal. Aircraft types can be adapted specifically for the aeromedical role, and larger organiza-

tions do indeed do this. This allows for full intensive-care provision during flight and maximum provisions for the attending medical and nursing staff.

Adapting aircraft for purpose, or purpose-building aircraft, has advantages and disadvantages. Advantages include potential avoidance of difficulties with flight clearance of equipment, as this should have been undertaken at the planning stage. Proper space for the patient and integral restraints are fitted, and piped gases and electrical supplies can be made available. Specific fittings for restraining equipment are incorporated, and unnecessary seating and equipment can be excluded.

Disadvantages include total loss of capability if the aircraft is unserviceable for whatever reason. Loss of aircraft auxiliary power may compromise patient maintenance if insufficient back-up is included, and this may be compounded by plumbed-in equipment being difficult to access to change batteries or access emergency gas supplies. Dedicated aircraft also remove flexibility from the mission, as the team are confined to one aircraft. This rules out, for example, advance assessment and preparation by predeploying the team to the patient location. Also, this system often requires additional equipment to ensure the ability to collect patients from their locations. In some systems, the team is tied completely to its aircraft. The team members rely on the patient being delivered to them at the APOD. This latter situation is fraught with risk for the patient, particularly critically ill patients, for reasons that become apparent below and in Chapter 57.

Team composition

The team composition should reflect the level of care required to support the patient. This will vary from a nurse caring for one or more patients of lower dependency, to a full critical-care team for the highest-dependency patients. Medical personnel with differing qualifications and skill levels will also be required to augment this care. STANAGS provides guidance for the level of nursing and medical care required for categories and numbers of patients cared for. These are broad guidelines and represent the minimum standard applicable. They may not be appropriate if the healthcare system of the receiving country exceeds them. Critical-care teams are dealt with in Chapter 57.

PRE-FLIGHT PREPARATION

Information

Before a patient transfer can be considered, information relating to the patient's condition needs to be collected. This is important for all patients, but particularly for those who are critically ill. In the latter case, the decision to attempt the transfer will rely heavily on this information, but it should be considered that in most peacetime scenarios the primary aim of an aeromedical mission is to assess.

Following this assessment, the final decision on whether to move the patient should be made. Just because a mission has been planned as if a patient move were to occur does not mean that it will occur. There are many examples where the pressure is to move the patient but it is not in the best interests of the patient. In these circumstances, the experienced transfer physician must make the most appropriate decision, on behalf of his or her patient, having carefully weighed up all the relevant information.

In the interests of patient confidentiality, names may be substituted by a number code, so that it is possible to communicate effectively about a patient's condition without identifying them. This should be routine, but it is of particular importance to the military. Identifying personnel inappropriately may be distressing to relatives if they have not been informed formally, and in extreme circumstances it may be information of value to an enemy. The most important information required is shown in Table 31.5.

The use of secure communications assists in the transfer of information, but with care and experience most information can be passed effectively without compromise during non-secure communication. Ideally, the physician caring for the patient should communicate directly with the specialist physician undertaking the transfer. However, this is not always possible; for example, language, world time zones and differing working practices of different health organizations and countries may make person-to-person medical contact impractical. In these circumstances, the use of trained intermediaries may be acceptable, but this also is often difficult to organize. In the case of large multinational corporations and countries with large numbers of workers from another country for whom they are responsible, specific agents may be employed to liaise in the case of medical emergencies. The RAFMS concept of the deployed air evacuation liaison officer (AELO) and air evacuation coordinating officer (AECO) does much to assist in the collection of the information required. In addition, the military system of sending preformatted signals also aids in the processing and transmission of data. The AELO is responsible for interfacing with deployed field units and the aeromedical

Table 31.5 *Patient identification and essential data*

Information	Notes
Name	May be substituted for a unique identifier
Age	Additional identifier
Medical condition	Trauma, infection, contagious
Scoring for severity of condition	TISS, APACHE II, GCS
Requirement for transfer	Access to greater level of care, terminal, rehabilitation
History of present illness	Duration, increased risk of complications
Past medical history	Any other relevant illnesses influencing transfer
Previous medications	Indication of underlying relevant pathology
Present medications	Antimicrobials, inotropes
Allergies	Avoidance of therapies may be necessary
Course of illness	Deteriorating, complications, improving
Present observations	Indicate risk of immediate transfer
Recent blood tests	Assist in risk assessment
Arterial blood gases	Improving, deteriorating, severity of illness
Oxygen requirements	Sea-level requirement, incipient respiratory failure
Results of investigations	X-rays, CT scan, MRI
Ventilatory parameters	Severity of pulmonary compromise
Supporting equipment	Ventilator, syringe drivers
Current circumstances	Stable or not, prognosis
Information given to relatives	Nature, latest update
Timescale for evacuation	Priority, urgency
Additional equipment for transfer	Pacemaker, haemofiltration before transfer
Additional treatment for transfer	Escharotomy, tracheostomy, vascular access
Location	Hospital, proximity to APOD, transport problems
Clearances required	Visas, landing permission for medical flight, overfly
Local transport arrangements	Reliability, availability, restrictions
Point of contact	Available

APACHE II, acute physiology and chronic health evaluation; APOD, air point of departure; CT, computed tomography; GCS, Glasgow coma scale; MRI magnetic resonance imaging; TISS, therapeutic intervention scoring system.

authorities, and the AECO provides additional medical input locally. No system is infallible, and the final decision to transfer rests with the transferring physician.

The overall scenario of the transfer should be considered in the context of the timescales involved. The question of 'what if?' should always be addressed with reference to the patient's initial condition, likely progress, potential complications, mission timings, transport problems and route deviations. All should have a contingency plan in terms of alternative treatments, resources and options. The longer and further the mission, the more critical these issues become. It is often the case that a mission appears to the financiers to represent a high degree of overkill, but to the experienced aeromedical team the mission is the result of planning and clinical prudence.

Patient preparation

The patient should be seen and assessed by the team that is to perform the transfer, as the team will be responsible from the point of collection to the point of delivery at the receiving hospital. The aim is to attenuate all of the effects of the transfer and maintain stability at worst and improve the patient's condition at best. Preparation is both logistic and clinical.

CLINICAL CONSIDERATIONS

Clinical preparation of patients should be logical and thorough. The assessment should begin with a detailed history, particularly of recent events. This is followed by a thorough examination. A useful approach to examination is to adopt the principles of the Acute Trauma Life Support® system used by the American College of Surgeons. Using this ABC (airway, breathing, circulation) system, it is straightforward to address the patient's needs logically. As a general principle, all actions required to safeguard the patient and ensure stability should be undertaken before the patient is moved.

With most conditions, there are windows of opportunity for lower-risk transfer to occur, and whenever possible these should be used. For example, trauma patients who have been initially resuscitated and stabilized are usually best moved at 24–48 hours before they develop complications such as acute lung injury (ALI) or renal impairment. Patients presenting with a presumptive diagnosis of pancreatitis may appear relatively well initially but can deteriorate rapidly by developing systemic inflammatory response syndrome (SIRS), ALI, coagulopathy and renal dysfunction.

For some patients, the window of opportunity is later. For example, patients who have undergone bowel surgery normally would not be flown until ileus has resolved. Similarly, following thoracic surgery, where adequate

drainage of residual pneumothorax cannot be assured, delay is indicated. Post-myocardial infarction, the period of highest risk of arrhythmia is avoided. Each case is considered individually to minimize risk. In some conditions, the use of sea-level cabin altitude attenuates risk (see below).

Airway and respiratory system

The first consideration is to assess and secure the airway. If there is any doubt over whether it will remain secure once the move has commenced, a definitive airway must be provided by endotracheal intubation.

Patients who have had thoracic trauma with rib fractures often give rise to difficulties. The identified number of fractured ribs is a poor indicator of the level of trauma or the extent of pulmonary injury. Over the hours following what may be seem to be a minor injury, ventilation may deteriorate and hypoxia develop. This is usually assumed to be related to the pain of fractures and increased analgesia is prescribed. The actual underlying problem is shunting of blood through contused lung compounded by the more obvious mechanical impairment. The extent of the compromise is masked initially by supplemental oxygen.

Providing supplemental oxygen then leads to a false impression of the adequacy of pulmonary function. Some patients who appear normal or only mildly compromised may be much worse than they seem. For example, a patient with severe respiratory failure may have an adequate partial pressure of oxygen in arterial blood (Pa_{O_2}) even on only a fraction of inspired oxygen (Fi_{O_2}) of 0.35 (Table 31.6). It is possible to work out what the expected Pa_{O_2} should be using the simplified alveolar gas equation:

$$Pa_{O_2} > = Fi_{O_2}(P_B - P_{H_2O}) - (Pa_{CO_2}/RQ) + F$$

where P_B is barometric pressure, P_{H_2O} is partial pressure of water vapour, Pa_{CO_2} is partial pressure of arterial carbon dioxide, RQ is the respiratory quotient (normally taken as 0.8) and F is a small correction factor when air is breathed.

Normally,

$$Pa_{O_2} = 0.21(100 - 6) - 5.3/0.8 = 13$$

Table 31.6 *Predicted and actual Pa_{O_2} and different values of inspired oxygen*

Fi_{O_2}	Predicted		Respiratory failure	
	Pa_{O_2}	Sp_{O_2}	Pa_{O_2}	Sp_{O_2}
0.21	12	98	4	60+
0.24	15	100	5	75
0.28	19	100	7	85
0.35	25	100	8.3	92
0.4	30	100	10	95
0.6	50	100	17	100

Fi_{O_2}, fraction of inspired oxygen; Pa_{O_2}, partial pressure of oxygen in arterial blood; Sp_{O_2}, arterial oxyhaemoglobin saturation.

Pa_{O_2} is normally 2–3 kPa lower due to one to four per cent pure shunt.

As a useful approximation, Pa_{O_2} should be around 8–12 kPa below FI_{O_2}.

These circumstances may also occur in patients with chemical pneumonitis due to aspiration, smoke inhalation, airway burns, fat embolism, near-drowning or blast injury. These injuries are often underestimated, and the potential for acute deterioration during transfer is high, with pulmonary oedema and severe hypoxia rapidly developing in the first 24–48 hours post-injury.

The head-up posture is the most appropriate for almost all patients. This reduces the effect of abdominal contents on diaphragmatic excursion, attenuates the atelectatic influences on the lung, and reduces the likelihood of gastric reflux regurgitation and inhalation. This is one of the manoeuvres used routinely in the intensive care unit (ICU) to help to reduce the incidence of ventilator-associated pneumonia (VAP). An exception to this rule is the spontaneously breathing patient with a spinal cord injury and in whom airway reflexes are intact. If it is deemed appropriate to allow the patient to be transferred without assisted ventilation, then respiratory function is better if the patient is supine. It must be emphasized that these patients are at high risk of developing respiratory and ventilatory problems, and this course of management must be undertaken with this knowledge.

Cardiovascular system

The effects of flight on the cardiovascular system may be marked and will vary according to the phase of the flight, with near-opposite forces applying during takeoff and landing. Sudden changes in aircraft attitude at these times and during banking, and vertical forces during turbulence, may interfere with cardiovascular function to a lesser or greater extent. Factors that influence these effects are the cardiac output and the vascular resistance. These in turn depend on the fluid status of the patient, the general tone and responsiveness of the circulation, and myocardial contractility and rhythm. More information is provided in Chapter 57.

Gastrointestinal tract

The gastrointestinal tract is often overlooked as a potential source of problems during transfers. It may, however, be the origin of further morbidity. It may be obstructed and lead to nausea, vomiting or reflux and VAP in the unconscious patient. It may interfere with ventilation. It may also be a source of occult or overt bleeding. It may also contribute to the development of sepsis or severe sepsis and multiorgan failure (MOF) due to the translocation of bacteria or bacterial toxins.

Hepatic function

Impairment of hepatic function may be minor. Mildly deranged hepatic function may have little effect on the patient during transfer, although there may be a greater tendency to nausea and vomiting in flight. In greater derangement with jaundice, clotting may be affected. In patients with more severe hepatic failure, ascites may impair respiratory function sufficiently to require remedial action. Other issues are dealt with in Chapter 57.

Renal function

Impaired renal function is common in sick patients. Mild impairment in the ambulant or critically ill patient is seldom a cause for concern and simply indicates the severity of the underlying condition or gives clues to the likely development of further complications. Uraemia increases the likelihood of nausea and vomiting. In marked renal impairment or renal failure, it may be necessary to provide renal replacement therapy.

Renal replacement is provided to control fluid balance, acid–base balance and electrolytes. In the air-transfer environment, provision of support has been only to the level of addressing fluid balance (Stevens et al. 1986). The ability to control acid–base balance and electrolytes requires sophisticated equipment, which will not function correctly in the air given the nature of weight-activated controls. Such equipment usually is bulky, requires mains power and uses large quantities of fluid in the process. For this reason, patients who have physiobiochemical derangements associated with renal impairment require renal replacement before transfer, with a period of stabilization post-treatment. Even if the measured parameters are acceptable, treatment in the immediate period before transfer is advisable in patients who are known to be dependent on this therapy. If this is not available locally, then renal support must be provided by the aeromedical team in order to ensure optimization before the patient is moved.

Fluid balance

In all aeromedical missions, adequate fluids must be carried to allow for maintenance, replacement of losses (including insensible) and potential resuscitation requirements. Patients with high gastrointestinal losses from nasogastric tubes, drains or fistulae must have these replaced with isotonic fluid. Burns patients will require these fluids plus a consideration given to colloids and blood. Patients who have had recent trauma will have occult losses of blood and fluid as well as those that are obvious.

All critically ill patients may require blood or blood products (fresh frozen plasma, platelets, cryoprecipitate) during the course of their illness. This is more likely during the initial phase or during a later deterioration following a complicating episode of sepsis. The development of disseminated intravascular coagulation is a serious problem that should be addressed before a transfer is contemplated.

Central nervous system

Head injury and spinal cord injury are the most common problems of the central nervous system disorder encountered in patients requiring aeromedical evacuation. These injuries may be in isolation or may be accompanied by multi-trauma. Although it is correct to focus on immediately life-threatening conditions, these neurological injuries must not be neglected, as they represent a significant cause of post-incident instability, morbidity and impediment to rehabilitation. It is, therefore, important to understand the potential difficulties that these conditions pose during aeromedical evacuation, as they cannot be ignored during transfer.

A patients with a Glasgow coma scale (GCS) of 8 or less should be intubated and ventilated (Association of Anaesthetists of Great Britain and Northern Ireland 1996). This will require the correct use of drugs to induce anaesthesia, because failure to do so will have serious consequences (see Chapter 57).

Spinal cord injuries following trauma may lead to neurological deficit. This will vary according to the severity of the injury and the level at which it occurs. The clinical picture also varies with the time post-injury. The higher the level and the more severe the injury, the more marked the effects become. Likewise other spinal injuries are accompanied by consequences often overlooked or, more worryingly, ignored by those who undertake patient transfers. These are dealt with in greater detail in Chapter 57.

Trauma and burns

Trauma and burns patients may be fluid-depleted and cardiovascularly compromised. These patients require resuscitation and stabilization before transfer is contemplated. Disseminated intravascular coagulation, other clotting disorders, and organ damage or failure may be additional complicating factors.

The use of inflatable type splints is not appropriate in these patients due to the changes in air pressure and their effects over extended periods. Properly applied traction splints may be invaluable in aiding pain management, but pressure points from their application or elasticated bandages may lead to problems with limb perfusion or skin integrity.

Burned patients may require escharotomy of the limbs or torso. This should be carried out before transfer, in order to avoid complications in flight. Dressing changes should have been undertaken before transfer, with sufficient time elapsed to allow for restabilization, as many patients become unstable due to the inflammatory insult of the procedure. Anaesthesia and surgery immediately before transfer are always high relative contraindications to flight, but particularly so in these patients.

The use of vacuum mattresses should be considered in all patients to provide the necessary support and restraint. This is even more important in trauma patients, who may have occult injury undetected in the field environment. In addition, this type of mattress allows for rapid carriage of the patient out of danger, should an emergency occur on the aircraft, while minimizing the potential for further injury.

Difficult patients

Some patients present the aeromedical team with particular difficulties (Table 31.7). For example, a patient with otitis media and Eustachian tube insufficiency will be unable to equalize pressures in the middle ear and will experience severe pain during altitude changes, particularly on descent. This may lead to tympanic membrane rupture and haemorrhage. Likewise, if pressures cannot be equalized in air-filled sinuses, severe pain and haemorrhage may result.

A patient with recent myocardial infarction (within 24 hours) is prone to acute arrhythmia and, as a consequence, may have a cardiac arrest. In the hospital setting or in the air, it may be possible to correct the arrhythmia, but if the attending aeromedical team is inappropriate, a subsequent arrest may not be dealt with optimally. In flight, the cardiac arrest team cannot be summoned to augment the team.

In the case of acute surgical haemorrhage, recourse to the blood bank or surgical team will not be possible during transfer, and thus a condition that could lead to this eventuality is a relative contraindication to flight.

Acute trauma patients may have unstable fractures, external fixators and complex fluid-balance issues as well as the potential to develop further critical complications, regardless of the care they have received. In light of this, they may be physically difficult to move and secure. They may also react adversely to changes in posture and to the effects of acceleration and deceleration.

Most of the problems associated with these patients are relative contraindications to transfer and relate to unavail-

Table 31.7 *Relative contraindications to transfer and patients presenting particular difficulties during transfer*

- Otitis media, sinusitis
- Myocardial infarction
- Cardiac failure
- Intracerebral haemorrhage
- Air-insufflation examinations
- Wired mandible
- Pregnancy over 36 weeks/bleeding in pregnancy
- Recent thoracic or abdominal surgery
- Gastrointestinal haemorrhage
- Severe anaemia
- Contagious disease
- Head injury
- Fractured skull
- Acute haemorrhage
- Burns
- High spinal-cord transection
- Unstable spinal fractures
- Multiple trauma
- Unstable sepsis with or without multiple organ failure

ability of expertise or resources, but some are related purely to the complexity of the underlying illness or condition. We cannot consider every scenario in this chapter, but it is hoped that the examples above show that the thought process of considering potential outcomes and options must be conducted for every patient.

Therapeutics

Patients may require therapeutic agents such as antimicrobials, anticoagulants and drugs to aid in the prevention of gastrointestinal haemorrhage (H_2 receptor blockers, proton-pump inhibitors). These drugs may all be at therapeutic levels before transfer, but during a prolonged transfer further administration will be required.

Drugs carried by the team should allow the continuation of established regimens; alternatively, appropriate supplies may be uplifted with the patient. The latter is not recommended in the case of field units, as it may deprive an isolated location of resources. Drugs must also be carried to cover any emergency situation that might reasonably be predicted, including unexpected delays and diversions. Oxygen is included in this consideration.

Consideration should be given to the use of prophylaxis for deep venous thrombosis. It should be exceptional for this not to be used, and justification for this action should be recorded in the patient chart. For trauma patients and other patients in whom complex coagulation issues prevent the use of prophylaxis, consideration should be given to the use of inferior vena cava filters if they are available.

Management during transfer

Patients who are stable should be maintained in that state by as little interference with their management as possible. Unstable patients should be stabilized before moving, unless there is no other option and remaining in the location would compromise them further. In these circumstances, the aeromedical team must be prepared and able to continue efforts to stabilize while transferring.

In the event of an emergency, the team must be able to provide adequate resuscitation for all reasonably predicted eventualities. The incidence of untoward events will vary with each patient, but the potential for a particular scenario may be predicted and action considered in advance of such an occurrence. Each scenario needs to be viewed logically in sequence and taken through to the most extreme potential conclusion – the 'worst-case scenario'. The risk of this occurring and the overall effect on patient outcome need to be weighed against the resources in terms of personnel and equipment that would be required to deal with it.

Having been through this process, it is then possible to make more informed decisions on the requirements for a given mission. Returning to the example of a patient who has had a myocardial infarction (and who is most at risk of developing life-threatening arrhythmia within the first 24–48 hours of the event), it is necessary to deal with the potential for cardiac arrest. This requires cardiopulmonary resuscitation, including defibrillation, intubation and ventilation. Even if resuscitation is successful, not all patients wake immediately and may require more prolonged critical-care support.

The team, therefore, must be equipped to provide this support should such an event occur. In the immediate post-myocardial infarction scenario, the decision to provide a full critical-care team therefore is simplified. As the time from the initial event extends, the decisions about team composition and equipment become more difficult. This is because use of full critical-care teams and their equipment is resource intensive-and concomitantly more expensive. It is necessary to engage the experienced clinician in these decisions so that the transition from a patient deemed to be at high risk to one walking on to the aircraft carrying their own luggage is considered properly and appropriate mission-tailoring occurs.

This exercise should be repeated for all patients and all scenarios in the preparation for a mission.

EQUIPMENT

Aircraft authorities such as the Civil Aviation Authority (CAA) have regulations that deal with the carriage of equipment in addition to that integral to the aircraft. These regulations also cover equipment that is not related to, and potentially may interfere with, aircraft function. At present, restrictions relating to medical equipment are such that carry-on equipment is largely exempt. This is of interest, as usually restrictions are placed on the operation of handheld portable electrical equipment during takeoff and landing. For example, critical-care equipment is required to be functional at all stages of the flight, and the potential outputs from screens, transformers and other electrical items integral to the equipment may be significant. It has been recognized that laptop computers may interfere with navigation systems – and all of the medical support equipment has screens and contains computer processors.

For this reason, where the aircraft authorities of military aircraft used are within NATO, for example, there are tight controls related to the potential for electromagnetic interference. These controls are embodied in the STANAGS that lay out in detail the levels of electrical and magnetic outputs that are acceptable within different aircraft types. There are also regulations pertaining to materials used in construction of equipment and to power supplies. This is important in the case of portable equipment, as some types of internal battery, for example, may explode under certain conditions (Table 31.8).

It is also important to be aware of the effects that aircraft systems, particularly communications and navigation equipment, may have on the equipment being used to care

Table 31.8 *Standards relevant to aeromedical equipment*

Number	Title
DEF STAN 00-13	Requirements for the achievement of testability in electronic and allied equipment
DEF STAN 00-18 Pt4	Avionic data-transmission interface systems
DEF STAN 00-35	Environmental handbook for defence materiel
DEF STAN 00-40	Reliability and maintenance
QSTAG 362	Guide to chemical environmental contaminants and corrosion affecting the design of military materiel
DEF STAN 05-123	Technical procedures for the procurement of aircraft, weapon and electronic systems
DEF STAN 00-970	Design requirements for service aircraft
DEF STAN 16-1	Oxygen: liquid and gaseous (breathing) for aircraft systems
DEF STAN 59-41	Electromagnetic compatibility
DEF STAN 61-3	Generic specification for batteries, non-rechargeable, primary
DEF STAN 61-5	Electrical power systems below 650 V
DEF STAN 61-9	Generic specification for batteries, rechargeable, secondary
DEF STAN 61-17	The requirements for the selection of batteries for service equipment
DEF STAN 66-31	Basic requirements and tests for proprietary electronic and electrical test equipment
STANAG 2872	Medical design requirements
STANAG 2905	Basic voltage and current characteristics of electro-medical equipment
BS EN 60068 PT2	Environmental testing: test methods
BS 2G 239	Specification for primary active lithium batteries for use in aircraft
BS 3G 100	Environmental testing of all equipment used in aircraft
BS 2011	Environmental testing
BS 5724	Medical electrical equipment
IEC 513	Fundamental aspects of safety standards for medical electrical equipment
IEC 601	Medical electrical equipment
ISO 10079/1	Medical suction equipment
RTCA/DO-160	Environmental conditions and test procedures for airborne equipment
EUROCA ED-14	Environmental conditions and test procedures for airborne equipment
MDD 93/42/EEC	European Union medical device directive
CEN/TC 239/WG5 N 42	Air, water and difficult-terrain ambulances; medical devices for continuity of patient care

for the patient. Life-vital equipment such as ventilators must function normally at all times without interruption. For this reason, all UK aeromedical equipment used is subject to the Special Purpose Medical Equipment (SPAME) testing programme. This programme was commenced in the 1980s to ensure that all medical equipment carried on RAF aircraft was compliant with STANAGS and was not subject to interference by aircraft systems. It also addressed the other issues related to the overall survivability of equipment in the aircraft-transfer environment. Examples of the parameters tested are given in Table 31.9. These were used to construct a generic specification of equipment to be used to care for patients in the air. As a result of this, when new equipment is being considered for purchase, the general performance characteristics are available so that the most cost-effective equipment may be purchased while providing all of the functions for optimal care. It also provides manufacturers with the opportunity to view what is expected of equipment when considering future development.

The air-transfer market is seen by manufacturers as small compared with the fixed hospital environment, and many have been slow to realize that their products can also be used in the general patient-transfer field, which is a much larger market. This has reduced the development of

transfer equipment suitable for more than very short times. With increasing technological advances and miniaturization, it is now possible to produce equipment for fixed environments that are also perfectly capable of providing full function in the transfer environment.

There are absolute requirements to test to parameters such as the effects of sudden or explosive decompression and the effects of changes in gravity in a simulated aircraft environment. In certain special circumstances, there still have to be compromises. For example, a test to assess the waterproof characteristics of a given piece of equipment is acceptable if resistance to liquid splash is considered. Immersing equipment completely is taking the test to an inappropriate level, as the cost of producing equipment to this standard would be prohibitive and unnecessary.

Tests must also consider other aspects of the environment to which the aeromedical equipment may be subjected, before it is used for the care of the patient. For example, extremes of heat and cold may be encountered at different phases of a given transfer. During these phases, the equipment must continue to function and provide the patient with appropriate support.

To illustrate this, consider a mission that commences in the early morning in the mountains at a field unit, where the temperature overnight has dropped to −10° C.

Table 31.9 *Equipment test parameters*

Test parameter	Reference	Notes
Electromagnetic compatibility	DEF-STAN 59-41 Part 3	All tests to supplements of this DEF-STAN
Conducted emissions	DCE01, supplement A	Conducted emissions on primary power lines, 20–150 Hz
Radiated susceptibility	DRS02, supplement V, E	Susceptibility environment of 10 V/m in range MHz–10 GHz
Conducted susceptibility (low frequency)	DCS01, supplement G	Primary power lines over range 20 Hz–50 kHz
Conducted susceptibility (high frequency)	DCS02, supplement H	Range 2–400 MHz, maximum cable bundle current of 100 mA
Electrostatic discharge	DCS10, supplement R	Should be protected against effects of static electricity
Shock, drop and topple survivability	BS EN 60068 PT2-31	Survive and be fully functioning after half-sine shocks of 30 g_n in each mutually perpendicular direction; function after being dropped on face or corner
Altitude		No deterioration in function at altitudes up to 10 000 feet (69.59 kPa pressure equivalent)
Sudden decompression	DEF STAN 00-35	Reduce pressure from 1 atm to partial pressure equating to 10 000 feet (69.59 kPa); settle for 10 min; reduce pressure exponentially to 20 000 feet (46.5 kPa); return to ambient 1 atm pressure within 15 min; no loss of function to occur
Explosive decompression		Explosive decompression at altitude of 40 000 feet (18.67 kPa); rapid descent to 10 000 feet (69.59 kPa); aircraft unaffected
Vibration		In plane of use, exposed to vibration in all axes; maintain function in ASD levels: ASD level 0.02 g^2/Hz over range 10–500 Hz, reducing to ± 6 dB/octave 500–2000 Hz
Acceleration (crash conditions)		If mounted or restrained, harness attachments and any back-up structure should have same standard strength as aircraft to meet standard of proof acceleration without disintegration of component parts of fittings: forward, $-9(g_n)$; other directions, $6(g_n)$*
Humidity	Environmental tests to current edition of EUROCAE ED-14 and/or RTCA/DO-160	No performance degradation with temperature cycling; test at 95% humidity, but allowed to fall no lower than 85% on cooling
Mould growth	British Standard 2001, part 2.1J	Should not support mould growth
Salt corrosion	BS EN 60068 PT2-52	Similar standard for aircraft cabin instrumentation
Fluid contamination	BS 3G 100 part 2 sub-section 3.12 and Q Stag 362	Should not be affected by fluid contamination
Waterproofness	BS2011, part 2.1R	Protected against spray or seepage
Temperature		Operate in range −10 to +50 °C; storage conditions may exceed these limits
Sand and dustproofing		Steps made to protect
Requirements of aircraft design and technical authorities: aircraft electrical and mechanical interface requirements	BS 3G100, part 3 and CEN/TC 239/WG5 N 42	
Other regulations		1997–98 edition of International Civil Aviation Organization's Technical Instructions for the Safe Transport of Dangerous Goods by Air; Air Navigation (Dangerous Goods) Regulations modified to reflect this (amended 2002)

*g_n is the standard sea-level acceleration due to gravity (9.807 m/s^2).
ASD, acceleration spectral density.

Equipment accompanies the patient from the heated environment of the field unit at 20° C to the external environment and into a cold short-haul tactical fixed-wing aircraft. This flies to a staging unit, where at midday the outside temperature is 45° C and the ambulance internal temperature is 51° C. There is then a transfer to another fixed-wing aircraft, which flies to a mainland location where the temperature is 2° C. This example does not discuss the changes in humidity that may accompany the temperature changes. It is, therefore, imperative that consideration of such environmental changes is incorporated into the overall programme of procuring aeromedical equipment.

General considerations

Equipment may be categorized according to function, type or role. From an engineering perspective, it may be mechanical or electrical, or both. This has implications for the carriage on aircraft (see below). The general characteristics of ideal transfer equipment are listed in Table 31.10.

From the perspective of patient care, equipment either is directly supportive to the patient, i.e. life-vital, or may be accessory to aid in care. Other equipment allows patient care to be carried out safely or allows equipment to func-

tion. These categorizations can also be subdivided into capital and disposable equipment. Capital equipment includes life-vital machines such as ventilators, cardiac pacemakers, intra-aortic balloon pumps, left ventricular assist devices and extracorporeal membrane oxygenators. Accessory capital equipment for patient care includes devices such as syringe drivers, volumetric pumps, suction apparatus and patient-warming blankets.

Accessory equipment supporting the overall transfer includes items such as stretchers, stretcher frames and backrests, restraining harnesses, electrical inverters and portable lighting. These pieces of equipment allow safe restraint of the patient while aiding and enhancing the environment for more straightforward patient care.

Connection to aircraft power supplies

If equipment is connected to aircraft power supplies, more rigorous testing is required, as the potential for adverse effects is much greater. This is increased further by the use of inverters or transformers, which convert the aircraft alternating current from 115 V and 400 Hz. For this reason, and if the supply is compromised, self-sufficiency is desirable. The cost of testing equipment may be as much as

Table 31.10 *Main characteristics of ideal transfer equipment*

Characteristic	Note
Type	Suitable for all patient clinical requirements; equivalent to fixed-facility equipment
Weight	Lightweight, readily portable
Fixation	Can be fixed securely to required standard
Size	Small enough to facilitate space requirements but displays large enough to be readily visible
Shape	Low centre of gravity; easily fixed, held and moved
Simplicity of operation	Easily manipulated controls (in all conditions); readily recognizable modes and settings
Intuitive controls	Menu-led, with expected parameters available immediately
Consumables	User-friendly, interchangeable, universal connections
Failsafe	Loss of function reverts to least hazardous condition possible
Function indication	Normal function indicated
Abnormal function	Identified promptly and appropriately, both visually and audibly (may be modified for military use)
Failure	Indicates failure visually and audibly, with reversion to failsafe mode
Rugged	Able to meet or exceed standards and survive environment
Reliability	High reliability, low failure risk
Functional	Has all required functions for equipment type
Interfaces	Data collection and transmission, remote alarms
Power supplies	Multiple, independent
Mains power supply	Worldwide voltage- and frequency-capable
Aircraft power supply	Able to use aircraft auxiliary power supply
Battery power supply	Exchangeable internal battery, external connection
Back-up battery	Internal battery for total external power failure
Medical gases	Low consumption, multiple types, ambient as failsafe
Equipment characteristics	Maintain all functions in all environments
STANAGS/DEF STAN/IEC/ISO	Complies with all relevant regulations and standards
Generic specification	Preferably complies with generic specification to avoid unnecessary training
Training programme	Comes complete with full training package

DEF STAN, defence standard; IEC, International Engineering Consortium; ISO, International Standardization Organization; STANAGS, North Atlantic Treaty Organization (NATO) Standard Agreements.

£20 000 per item; this can be reduced if connection to the aircraft is not required.

Internal batteries supplying equipment should be accessible for replacement or should be able to be backed up by external batteries, but preferably both options should be available. This allows for uninterrupted or acceptable interruption of supply while remaining independent of the aircraft should that supply fail or be unavailable during patient transfer to an alternative vehicle.

Packaging for transfer

Equipment requires secure packaging and should resist breaking up during gravitational forces expected during flight or an accident according to the relevant safety standards. This applies to the outward journey to collect the patient as well as during the transfer. Likewise, drugs need to be stored so that they are not degraded beyond the point where they are effective for the return journey. Medical gases present a particular problem, and specific regulations apply to their carriage in the air. Finally, disposable items must be packaged to maintain their integrity and avoid contamination.

Maintenance

Equipment needs to be maintained to the highest standard and requires the application of, or even the exceeding of, the most rigorous schedule recommended by the manufacturer. Ideally, equipment should have been serviced, but at the least it must have had appropriate pre-use checks before departure on the mission. The team undertaking the mission should be responsible for these checks. Having ownership of any subsequent issues or failures focuses the mind considerably.

Given the nature of the environment, it is often impossible to rely on the normal clues to change in clinical condition and to the normal function of equipment. To maintain the patient's safely, equipment used to transfer patients must fulfil a number of requirements. Not all equipment currently available to transfer patients fits the profile well. This is because it is usually designed for short intra-hospital or inter-hospital transfers, and many of the considerations for long transfers in difficult circumstances are overlooked or ignored.

MONITORING

All patients being transferred require monitoring. Critically ill patients require monitoring of more parameters, and these need to be monitored continuously by an experienced clinical operator. Monitoring is divided broadly into two categories: monitoring of the patient and monitoring of monitor-machine function. Patient parameters that are required for routine monitoring of the unconscious patient are determined by guidelines from professional bodies (Association of Anaesthetists of Great Britain and Northern Ireland 2000), as are those required for transfer.

All monitoring that would be available to the patient in the hospital setting should be available during transfer. This is particularly important during the extended transfers undertaken in international repatriation. Examples of patient-monitored and machine-monitored parameters are given in Tables 31.11 and 31.12, respectively. Machine-

Table 31.11   *Examples of patient-monitored parameters*

- Electrocardiograph
- Non-invasive blood pressure
- Invasive blood pressure
- Central venous pressure
- Intracranial pressure
- End-tidal carbon dioxide concentration
- Oxygen saturation
- Neuromuscular block
- Temperature
- Tidal volume
- Respiratory frequency
- Inspiratory pressures (mean, peak, plateau, PEEP)

PEEP, positive end-expiratory pressure.

Table 31.12   *Examples of machine-monitored parameters*

Multifunction monitor	Ventilator	Volumetric pump	Syringe driver	Suction apparatus
ECG connections	Oxygen pressure	Delivered pressure	Pressure	Suction pressure
Artefact report	Inspired oxygen level	Rate of delivery	Rate of delivery	Battery status
Defibrillator power selected	Air pressure	Volume delivered	Volume delivered	Charging status
Mains power	Normal function or malfunction	Infusion volume set	Syringe near-empty	Mains power
Battery status	Turbine function	Air in IV line	Battery status	
Mode (manual, auto)	Battery status	Battery status		
Malfunction indication	Power supply			

ECG, electrocardiogram; IV, intravenous.

monitored parameters depend on the type and function of the machine.

During flights, whenever possible it should be considered that patient care is progressive and proactive, as it is in the hospital environment. Continuity of care is essential in order to reduce morbidity and mortality. The concept of a chain of care is applicable to all patients, and inadequate care early in the episode cannot be compensated for by the application of a higher standard later. Resulting morbidity from this circumstance may be deemed to be due to negligence.

Oxygen is a pollutant in the aircraft environment – the less that is passed into the cabin, the better. If oxygen supplies are compromised, then using oxygen as a driving gas is wasteful. If the supply fails, it is useful to have a ventilator that can continue to function using entrained air, as at least this contains 21 per cent oxygen.

AEROMEDICAL CONSIDERATIONS

Altitude

In the normal individual, at sea level there are changes in gas exchange associated merely with changing posture from standing to sitting or lying positions. The effects are greatest on oxygen and, theoretically, could result in hypoxia. These changes are associated with the postural effects on functional residual capacity, anatomical dead space and pulmonary blood flow. Age-related changes in closing volumes are also a factor. Normally, these effects of posture are compensated for by changes in ventilation and perfusion to reduce the potential for hypoxia. However, when pulmonary pathology is superimposed on these normal changes, problems can arise.

At sea level, it may be possible to compensate for some of these pathological changes by treatment of underlying pathology, resuscitation, ventilatory strategies and circulatory support. With increasing altitude, the effects of falling barometric pressure exacerbate the problems, as reducing inspired oxygen leads to a fall in alveolar oxygen tension and the overall gradient driving the oxygen cascade (Table 31.13). It may then be impossible to compensate despite

Table 31.13   *Oxygen cascade*

	Pressure	
	(kPa)	(mmHg)
Inspired	21.3	160
Alveolar	13.7	103
Arterial	13.3	100
Capillary	6.8	51
Mitochondrial	0.13–1.3	1–10

Table 31.14   *Patient oxygen requirements*

- In theory, require about 10% above sea-level requirements to maintain Pa_{O_2}
- In practice, changes in pulmonary blood flow and functional residual capacity usually mean that more is required
- Problems are accentuated in critically ill patients and change with different phases of transfer

using the manoeuvres outlined above. Rough guidelines for patient oxygen requirements are given in Table 31.14.

To overcome these respiratory limitations, sea-level cabin altitude may be required, but this is unusual and the request for this facility is most likely to be required for other reasons (see below). Using sea-level cabin altitude is not without consequence. The normal cruising cabin altitude for pressurized aircraft is 1830–2400 m (6000–8000 feet). This is chosen to provide a given differential pressure across the cabin wall of about 62 kPa (9 psi). This allows the aircraft to fly at up to around 10 700 m (35 000 feet). At this altitude, air is less dense and resistance to flight is reduced. Engines are more efficient and fuel consumption is reduced.

Flying at sea-level cabin altitude requires a lower overall altitude to ensure the differential across the cabin wall. This increases fuel consumption due to increased air density. To cover the same distance, more fuel must be carried, which in turn increases the weight of the aircraft, which consumes more fuel to carry it. This can result in an overall increase in fuel cost of up to 40 per cent for a given journey. This is not a viable option for a commercial carrier and will have significant effects on the cost of a private air ambulance mission, which in turn is passed on to the customer. Reluctance to use this manoeuvre for financial reasons could compromise patient safety.

When using rotary-wing aircraft, the effect of altitude may be dismissed as inconsequential due to the relatively low altitudes that these aircraft fly at. There are circumstances when a transfer commences at a coastal region and during the journey the aircraft flies over increasingly higher terrain. While the altitude above ground may not change significantly, the altitude above sea level might change. Apart from the absolute effect on inspired oxygen, the other concerns regarding altitude then become relevant.

Consequent on the fall in barometric pressure, there is also an increase in volume according to Boyle's law:

$$\text{Pressure} \times \text{volume} = \text{constant}$$

At 1800 m (approximately 6000 feet), gas at sea level will have increased in volume by about 20 per cent. This volume change affects all air-filled cavities in the patient, whether present normally or as a consequence of pathology. Sudden changes are of greatest consequence, due to the presence of relatively poorly diffusible nitrogen, but

Table 31.15 *Potential consequences of volume changes within sequestrated air**

Area affected	Potential consequence
Skull (middle ear, sinuses, CSF)	Pain, tympanic membrane rupture, haemorrhage, raised intracranial pressure
Chest (pulmonary, pleural, pericardial)	Pneumothorax, tension pneumothorax, pneumomediastinum, pneumopericardium
Abdomen (peritoneum, bowel, stomach)	Pain, intra-abdominal hypertension, acute gastric dilation, gastrointestinal reflux, perforation, loss of integrity of surgical repair or anastomosis, acute haemorrhage
Circulation (bends)	Rupture of pulmonary vasculature, neurological deficit, circulatory insufficiency
Equipment (endotracheal tube cuff, intravenous lines, catheter balloons)	Cuff rupture, loss of ventilation, air embolism, failure of infusions

*Suspicion of trauma or following investigations that may, or normally do, introduce air should give rise to the appropriate investigations and precautions. CSF, cerebrospinal fluid.

slower changes may also be problematic if there is not enough time for equilibration.

Air-containing cavities of concern are listed in Table 31.15. The consequences of expanding gas depend on the system affected (see above). While Eustachian tube insufficiency may occur in conscious patients if there is obstruction, patients with general incapacity or unconsciousness may also experience tympanic barotrauma.

As well as the patient, equipment that contains, or has the potential to contain, air has to be considered. Endotracheal tube cuffs, intravenous lines containing fluids, and balloons on catheters all present a potential hazard to the patient. Monitoring and support equipment also comprise items such as touch-control pads, which contain air and may be vulnerable to pressure change. The equipment itself is not usually air-tight, but transport containers may be and may have to be vented.

Temperature

In some patients, hypothermic tendency may be balanced by the pyretic influences of acute sepsis. In others, active cooling is required, but this is less likely as the overall balance in the air environment is towards hypothermia. Even within fixed medical facilities where conditions are good, this problem occurs. During transfer, unless adequate precautions are taken, it is even more likely to be a problem. The patient is most vulnerable during the phases of embarkation and disembarkation. The final transfer to and from the aircraft is not usually directly via a vehicle, and during the manual transfer exposure to the environment usually occurs.

Once in the aircraft, the problem may continue, as in the case of rotary-wing aircraft where heating or cooling is usually poor. While aircraft are being prepared for flight, and during customs and emigration formalities, doors are open and temperature control of the environment is compromised. These influences vary widely depending on the airfield location and the ambient conditions.

Noise

Noise is a particular problem of aircraft transfers and poses hazards to the patient and the attending staff from a number of perspectives. It is a greater problem in rotary-wing and small aircraft, but larger military aircraft used primarily for freight have little or no soundproofing. Of immediate significance is the disorientation caused by the lack of normal feedback from familiar sounds in the patient care environment. These include sound of equipment functioning normally and abnormal sounds, such as that of a disconnected ventilator, monitor sounds and alarm warnings.

The ability to communicate with the patient, their relatives and colleagues also poses problems. The awake patient normally receives continuous reassurance, with explanation of the situation and during procedures. Even in sedated patient this is important. Relatives travelling with the patient also need to be updated and reassured regularly. Routine monitoring, taking observations, planning and providing care are essential components of patient safety, and all rely on adequate communication.

In rapidly changing circumstances and emergencies, it is even more essential to have adequate communications. Lack of coordinated effort in these situations can compromise patient safety. In some circumstances, the safety of the aircraft and flight crew may be compromised, such as during use of the defibrillator, if the flight crew are not warned. In aircraft emergencies, poor communication with the aeromedical team will compromise care and potentially endanger the patient and the team.

Finally, noise may present a health and safety issue that may affect both the patient and the attendant team. The intensity and frequency may give rise to long-term hearing impairment if exposure is of sufficient duration. In critically ill patients who are unable to respond, auditory protection must be provided as a routine. In addition, noise may contribute to motion sickness in susceptible individuals. Noise also degrades performance and affects behaviour.

Movement and vibration

Motion in general and vibration inherent in aircraft are other factors that intrude on the aeromedical environment. As with noise, smaller aircraft, military aircraft and rotary-wing aircraft are more susceptible to these factors. Military aircraft in operational areas are also more likely to fly in unpredictable patterns. The most sustained effects are during takeoff and landing, when the forces change rapidly as the direction of motion alters. There are also the effects of acceleration or deceleration. During air turbulence, similar effects may be seen. Patients, attending staff and equipment are all affected by movement and vibration. The patient may be made more uncomfortable, and the effects of trauma aggravated, by movement and vibration. Motion sickness may be induced in both patients and staff. Staff affected in this way may be unable to perform their role of providing patient care. Critically ill patients may be acutely sensitive to movements of this type, with acute cardiovascular or ventilatory instability being induced.

The overall function of equipment that is not designed specifically to be used in this environment must also be considered. Batteries and attachments may be dislodged and render the equipment ineffective. Even simple manoeuvres such as the timing of gravity-controlled infusions may be impossible. In the case of a critically ill patient, all infusions, except on occasions with acute fluid resuscitation, must be controlled by infusion devices, as they may be life-vital in this context.

The ability to undertake clinical monitoring, such as manually measuring the patient's pulse or blood pressure, may be precluded. Monitors may become unreliable. Accurate monitoring of cardiac activity or recording an interpretable electrocardiograph may be impossible. Pulse oximetry may be interfered with; this, added to the inherent difficulties of pulse oximetry in critically ill patients, may make this monitoring of no value. Alarms may be activated inappropriately, and reliance on their outputs inevitably must be reduced.

Motion and vibration are also health and safety considerations. There are regulations controlling the restraint and resistance of equipment to structural failure when subjected to gravitational forces, as discussed above. The displacement of equipment in normal flight or during a crash may lead to serious injury of the patient or others on the aircraft. It may also cause malfunction or equipment failure, despite the reassurance of the drop test, which all medical equipment should have passed before being accepted into service by standards applied by bodies such as the European Union.

Visibility

The limitations of space and lighting within the aircraft environment may impair visibility. As with other environ-

mental considerations, some aircraft provide better conditions than others. Reduced visibility makes normal clinical observations such as patient colour and visualization of respiratory pattern difficult or unreliable. It may be difficult to see certain types of display on monitors due to low light levels and the positioning of the monitor.

It is customary to reduce lighting levels during takeoff and landing in all aircraft at night. In the confines of rotary-wing aircraft and small fixed-wing aircraft, low lighting may be required at all phases of night flight to avoid degrading aircrew visual acuity. When the human eye has compensated for night vision, exposure to light may impair this for more than 20 minutes. In the military setting, there may be periods of tactical red lighting or no light when the use of image-intensifier equipment is used.

General aircraft environment

Routinely considered aspects of the air environment have been discussed above, but there are additional hazards within the environment. There is the potential for exposure to various oils and lubricants, and there is altered humidity in the controlled atmosphere. Avoidance of these is more straightforward for the patient, but the attendant medical staff members need to be aware of them. There are also trip hazards and the potential for falls from open doors, which may occur during loading and unloading of the aircraft. Awkward lifting of the patient, stretcher and equipment may lead to injury. An awareness of external hazards such as aircraft exhausts, propellers, jet engines and rotor blades is necessary. Sudden effects of aircraft manoeuvring, turbulence, acceleration and deceleration pose potential hazards to attendants when caring for the patient. Actions in the event of emergency require training and coordination if death or injury are to be avoided.

Communication

Due to the factors discussed above, communication between staff, the patient and their relatives is potentially difficult in the air. It is important that all aspects of the patient transfer be discussed in detail before the move. If the patient can be informed, then any risks must be outlined and the proposed course of the mission and any actions to be taken indicated. If this is not possible, then the patient's relatives may need to be informed of the broad mission objectives and any attendant risks (see below).

Before departure for the mission, or when the patient has been assessed, it may be deemed necessary to consult with specialists in given areas of medicine or surgery. When doing this, it must be remembered that although there may be many specialists in these areas, very few have experience of the requirements for transfer of the patient by air in general, and even fewer have experience of care of the critically ill in flight. In this specialist circumstance, advice must be subject to the additional considerations of the flight environment. There are occasions when it may be acceptable to watch and wait in the static hospital environment, but this would be unacceptable for prolonged transfer, and temporizing or definitive action should be undertaken before the move in all but exceptional circumstances; some examples are given in Table 31.16. Most relate to the unavailability of immediate resources or specialist input when transferring.

It is important to communicate to the organizing or coordinating authority any changes in the patient's condition or requirements for the receiving airfield before departure, because in flight communication to base is not straightforward. There may be occasions when the patient's condition changes unexpectedly during the flight. In these circumstances, limited options are available (see below). Communicating via radio to a ground station with a landline patch occasionally is feasible, but the development of satellite communication should aid communication between the aircraft and the destination hospital in due course (see below).

ETHICAL AND LEGAL CONSIDERATIONS

Discussion of the patient's medical condition and explanations of treatment options often take place between criti-cal-care physicians and the patient's immediate relatives. Normally, this information is confidential between the patient and their doctor. Any disclosure of information to anyone else is a breach of this legal requirement. In talking to relatives, it is with the understanding that there is no obligation to do so, and the issue of patient confidentiality must be borne in mind when considering what is necessary to aid understanding and the risk of betraying confidence. It is, however, prudent to address issues where patient safety is potentially compromised with an explanation of risk reduction and the overall justification for the transfer in broad terms. This may avoid subsequent litigation should all not proceed as planned.

Some problems arise due to cultural differences that raise ethical issues. In some countries, for example, the diagnosis of brainstem death is not sought or recognized. For a transfer team, a patient with a serious neurological injury may fit the criteria for testing in their own country and would be pronounced legally dead if those tests were performed. It has been customary to treat these patients as was the case in the country that they were being repatriated from, in order to avoid the issue of transferring a ventilated dead person. This poses serious issues clinically, as these patients are extremely unstable and are very difficult to move.

Within the team, the physician and nurse carry independent legal responsibility for the patient, even though the physician ultimately may be responsible for patient care. They are answerable to their professional bodies and are required to be current in their practice according to the requirements of those bodies. They are also subject to the

Table 31.16 *Resource availability and influence on patient transfer*

Condition	Problem	Resource implication
Acute colitis	Ileus and bowel distension could lead to perforation and SIRS or acute uncontrolled haemorrhage	Immediate surgery, massive transfusion
Acute coronary syndrome	Acute arrhythmia, cardiac arrest, cardiogenic shock	Acute interventional cardiology
Burns	Respiratory obstruction, ventilatory insufficiency, limb ischaemia	Intubation and ventilation, escharotomy
Disseminated intravascular coagulation	Bleeding and consumption of clotting factors	Requirement for platelets and other blood products
Fracture with vascular compromise	Acute limb ischaemia	Stabilization of limb, vascular surgery
Gastrointestinal haemorrhage	Continued bleeding	Need for surgery, massive transfusion
Inflammatory aortic aneurysm	Leak	Immediate surgery ± transfusion
Haemopneumothorax	Tension pneumothorax, haemorrhage	Drainage ± thoracic surgery
Head injury with low GCS	Raised ICP, compromised airway, ventilatory failure	Surgery, airway control, ventilation
Limb trauma	Compartment syndrome	Surgery
Premature labour	Delivery of premature infant	Obstetric and paediatric care
Respiratory failure	Acute decompensation	Ventilatory support
Thrombocytopenia of unknown aetiology	Haemorrhage	Blood and haematological advice

GSC, Glasgow coma scale; ICP, intracranial pressure; SIRS, systemic inflammatory response syndrome.

guidelines and standards of those professional bodies, as they represent the standards against which they will be judged should problems arise while the patient is in their care. In the UK, peer review remains the current method of judgement, rather than it resting with the judiciary (*Bolam* v. *Friern Barnet Hospital Committee* [1957]). It is, therefore, important that professional currency includes training and currency in the care of patients during transfer.

TRAINING

Aeromedical teams require training to the highest standard to be able to function in the hostile air environment (Table 31.17). It is implicit that the entry level of this training is the qualifications demanded by professional bodies to undertake whatever specialist patient care is required. Having satisfied these requirements, nursing and medical personnel must be current in their clinical practice and satisfy these professional bodies' requirements for currency.

Table 31.17 *Training for aeromedical evacuation*

- Physiology of patient transfer
- Transport of the critically ill
- Transport of the critically ill by air
- Patient ventilation
- Invasive monitoring (anatomy, analysis)
- Infectious diseases
- Air-transit isolator
- Equipment
- Resuscitation of unprepared patients
- Aircraft safety
- Health and safety at work
- Fitness to fly
- Hypobaric and hyperbaric medical considerations
- Law and ethics
- Aviation medicine update
- RAF concept of operations
- Workshops and practical experience
- Use of monitors, ventilators and other equipment
- Invasive monitoring techniques
- Patient transfers within the hospital environment
- Inter-hospital transfers
- Safety
- Dunker drills
- Smoke egress training
- Transfer simulator training
- Annual fitness
- Aircraft familiarization
- Joint exercises with aircraft and support helicopters
- Winch training
- Military training

RAF, Royal Air Force.

This includes clinical education and professional development.

Teams must be trained in transfer medicine and be current in that practice. For those not actively engaged in regular air experience, currency is maintained in the less hostile environments of intra- and inter-hospital transfers. It is unlikely that a practitioner can function optimally and offer the required patient care in the air if they are preoccupied with anxiety about their clinical practice. This must be second nature if they are not to be distracted by the aircraft environment. This is even more important in military situations, where the added pressure of concerns for personal safety may be superadded.

It is often assumed, erroneously, that entry-level clinical practice is adequate. In these circumstances, undue pressure will be applied to poorly prepared inappropriate personnel in the most demanding and isolated situations. It is also unfortunate that many personnel in this situation do not understand their limitations until serious problems arise. When faced with difficulty, they are unable to rely on peer support and additional resources as they would in the hospital environment. The most concerning individuals do not even know what they do not know.

To complete clinical training, each item of equipment must be understood fully. This reduces the likelihood of underestimating battery life, misunderstanding capability and accepting limitations that may add risk to the patient or negate previous progress. It also does much to reduce inappropriate mode selection and ignorance of alarm indications, which are common user errors. As an example, the SPAME training course has been designed to address these issues and has proved successful in educating all team members in the normal function and idiosyncrasies of equipment used in critical-care aeromedicine for the RAFMS.

Often neglected are the remaining elements of training, including as aircraft safety, dunker drills for rotary-wing escape in water, smoke drills and training specific for aircraft types. Education should also include aspects of aviation medicine, specific effects of flight on both normal and abnormal physiology, and legal and ethical issues. Support personnel must be included in this training. Although they are not involved directly in patient care, they are within a clinical environment during an aeromedical mission. They may help in the physical movement of patients on and off the aircraft, and they may have responsibilities for setting up and maintaining the clinical environment within the aircraft. As such, they require clinical awareness training.

Exposure to the secure clinical environment of the base hospital serves a number of purposes, including understanding patient needs and avoiding inadvertently compromising the patient during activities in which they may be assisting, e.g. understanding why disconnecting oxygen from a ventilator may have adverse effects even if it does ease the complication of lifting the patient on to an ambulance trolley.

Additionally, familiarization of non-medical personnel with the clinical environment reduces their stress. This, in turn, facilitates their ability to perform their roles without distraction. It also serves to highlight personnel who may be unsuitable for the role. Lastly, it converts willing volunteers into educated hands who may prove invaluable in an emergency situation.

SUMMARY

Aeromedical evacuation is a complex and demanding undertaking. To ensure minimal risk to patients, it requires a robust organization, meticulous planning and highly trained personnel. Personnel must be supported with appropriate resources and equipment to offer the required standard of care. These provisions should be met regardless of the patient's condition and, with few exceptions, missions should be entirely patient-focused.

REFERENCES

Association of Anaesthetists of Great Britain and Northern Ireland. Recommendations for the transfer of patients with acute head injuries to neurosurgical units. London: Association of Anaesthetists of Great Britain and Northern Ireland, 1996.

Association of Anaesthetists of Great Britain and Northern Ireland. Recommendations for standards of monitoring during anaesthesia and recovery. London: Association of Anaesthetists of Great Britain and Northern Ireland, 2000.

Department of Health. Comprehensive critical care: a review of adult critical care services. London: Department of Health, 2000.

Intensive Care Society. Guidelines for the transport of the critically ill adult. London: Intensive Care Society, 1997.

Intensive Care Society. Guidelines for the transport of the critically ill adult. London: Intensive Care Society, 2002.

Stevens PE, Bloodworth LL, Rainford DJ. High altitude haemofiltration. *British Medical Journal (Clinical Research Edition)* 1986; **292**: 1354.

32

Accident investigation

IAN R. HILL AND S. ANTHONY CULLEN

INTRODUCTION

Aviation is controlled by a complex web of national and international laws and agreements, which are intended to facilitate smooth, trouble-free air travel to the highest standards. Although these objectives are achieved in many parts of the world, others fail and the system for reporting transgressions is flawed. Balancing technical, humanitarian, political, legal and commercial activities is not easy, and considerable pressures can be exerted upon investigators. To some degree, aviation has made difficulties for itself, because it has been loathe to publicize poor safety standards. The 41 countries of the European Civil Aviation Conference carry out safety checks on airlines but do not publicize the names of those found wanting (*Flight International* 2000).

INTERNATIONAL LAWS AND TREATIES

The standards and recommended practices for aircraft accident inquiries were first adopted in 1951 pursuant to Article 37 of the Convention on International Civil Aviation and were designated as Annex 13 to the Convention. Article 26 imposes an obligation on the state in which an aircraft accident occurs to institute an inquiry in accordance with the procedure laid down by the International Civil Aviation Organization (ICAO). Subsequent meetings of the assembly directed efforts towards a procedure to make available promptly the reports of aircraft accident investigations, particularly when large transport aircraft were involved. The contracting states were urged to provide timely notification of all

aircraft accidents to the state of manufacture of the aircraft and the state in which the aircraft is registered.

Annex 13 defines an accident. This states, in part, that an accident is an occurrence associated with the operation of an aircraft that takes place between the time any person boards the aircraft with the intention of flight until such time as all such people have disembarked, in which a person is fatally or seriously injured as a result of being in the aircraft, or by being in direct contact with any part of the aircraft, including parts that have become detached from the aircraft, or by direct exposure to jet blast. Excluded from this definition are deaths from natural causes, self-inflicted injuries, injuries inflicted by other people and injuries to stowaways hiding outside the areas normally available to the passengers or crew.

It is stated clearly that the sole objective of the investigation is the prevention of accidents and incidents and not to apportion blame or liability. It places an obligation on the state in which the accident occurs to preserve the evidence and maintain safe custody of the aircraft and its contents. It requires the state of occurrence to notify the states of registry, operation, design and manufacture of the aircraft and the ICAO when the accident involves an aircraft whose maximum mass is greater than 2250 kg. These states have the right to appoint accredited representatives to the inquiry. They have the duty to provide information about the aircraft, its crew and any other relevant information pertaining to the inquiry. The state of occurrence may delegate the whole or part of the conduct of the investigation to one of the other concerned states. Annex 13 to the Convention defines in detail the responsibilities of all concerned and the format of the reports and their distribution. The extent to which the agreement is honoured varies. There have been instances in which the host nation has failed to cooperate fully, and despite criticism those states have refused to abide by the rules, thus compromising the interests of flight safety. Unfortunately, they cannot be brought before any tribunal.

The ICAO (1970) *Manual of Aircraft Accident Investigation* states:

The pathological evidence is an essential part of the technical investigation and the Investigator-in-Charge must ensure that investigative information is not sacrificed to meet sociological and legal desires for rapid identification and disposal of bodies. To this end, he should, if possible, obtain the services of a pathologist familiar with aircraft accident investigation and who is capable of coordinating the two interdependent functions of investigation and identification.

Civil accidents in the UK

The regulation of aircraft accident investigation is embodied in the Civil Aviation Acts of 1949, 1980 and 1982, which give the inspectors of accidents the authority to conduct their investigations. The detailed regulations are found in the Civil Aviation (Investigation of Air Accidents) Regulations 1996. Among other things, these state:

The fundamental purpose of investigating accidents under these regulations shall be to determine the circumstances and causes of the accident with a view to the preservation of life and the avoidance of accidents in the future; it is not the purpose to apportion blame or liability.

The Air Accident Investigation Branch (AAIB) of the Department of Transport employs the Inspectors of Air Accidents. The statutes that define the procedures to be followed in aircraft accident investigation and the powers of the Inspectors of Air Accidents are found in the Civil Aviation (Investigation of Air Accidents) Regulations 1996 and the Air Navigation (Investigations of Air Accidents Involving Civil and Military Aircraft or Installations) Regulations 1986. These regulations define accidents and incidents, and these are summarized in the Air Accident Investigation Branch Memorandum on the Investigation of Civil Air Accidents. The report prepared by the inspector is submitted by the Chief Inspector to the Secretary of State, who has no authority to alter its contents. It is the Chief Inspector of Accidents and not the Secretary of State who decides whether an investigation is to be carried out. Regulations allow for a review of the report if this is required. When there is a particularly serious accident with many fatalities, the Secretary of State may order a public enquiry. In this case, the Lord Chancellor in England will appoint a commissioner, who conducts the enquiry. Technical assessors will assist the commissioner. The AAIB investigation will continue, and the inspectors from that organization and others will be called as witnesses to the public enquiry. A public enquiry is seen to alleviate public anxiety and to remove all suspicion of a cover-up by any government department.

Before a report is submitted to the Secretary of State, the inspector conducting the investigation is obliged to notify everyone whose reputation is, in the inspector's opinion, likely to be affected adversely by the report, inviting them to make representations. Such people may obtain legal advice and representation before responding. The inspector is required to consider all the points put to him or her and, if necessary, to amend the report. If the participant is still unhappy, he or she may ask for a review board, which the Secretary of State is not permitted to refuse. A Queen's Counsel normally chairs a review board with two technical assessors. The board reports to the Secretary of State, who orders both the inspector's report and the review board's report to be published, usually within the same cover.

CORONER OR PROCURATOR FISCAL

Fatal accidents come under the jurisdiction of the coroner in whose area the accident occurs. The coroner will appoint an appropriately qualified pathologist to perform the autopsies on his or her behalf (Coroner's Rules 1984). As early as 1955, the Home Office realized the importance of having an appropriate pathologist perform the autopsies. They issued a circular to all coroners, suggesting that in the event of a flying accident involving loss of life, the coroner having jurisdiction might invite the Royal Air Force (RAF) Department of Aviation Pathology to attend the autopsy. In 1971, the Home Office issued a further circular to coroners, suggesting that they may wish to consider asking an RAF pathologist to perform the post-mortem examinations. The pathologist will liaise with the AAIB so that the AAIB may include the pathologist's evidence in the report. Coroners have the right to impound evidence relating to the death being investigated. In an aircraft accident, this can include the aircraft wreckage, flight data recorder and all the navigation and technical records of the flight. The inspectors of accidents also have the legal right to impound the same evidence. Theoretically, there could be a conflict of interests. However, the roles of the coroner's and the AAIB's inquiries are complementary, and there is rarely conflict between the two.

In Scotland, the judicial office of coroner does not exist, and the procurator fiscal, whose office covers a small part of the coroner's duties, is a part of the Lord Advocate's department. The procurator fiscal applies to the Sheriff Court for permission to order an autopsy in many cases where such an investigation is the normal practice in England. However, the procurator fiscal may accept multiple injuries as a cause of death deduced solely from an external examination of the victim. In the past, it has proved difficult to persuade a procurator fiscal of the need for a full post-mortem examination following aircraft accidents. This is particularly true of passengers who may have died in an aircraft crash. The procurator fiscal will look into the matter of fatal aviation accidents and will, if he or she considers appropriate, raise the matter at a fatal accident inquiry in the Sheriff Court.

Witness statements given to the procurator fiscal are not comparable to those taken by the police in England and Wales. They are given in confidence and thus may not be used in any subsequent proceedings and consequently will not be passed to the coroners if the body is returned to England or Wales. The relevance of this lies in whether the coroner will need to hold an inquest if the procurator fiscal decides that it is not necessary to hold a public inquiry under the Fatal Accidents and Sudden Death Inquiry (Scotland) Act 1976. Once the matter has been resolved in Scotland, the Scottish Office will supply a synopsis of the case plus a post-mortem report (Levine and Pyke 1999).

Laws in other countries

In the USA, each state has its own laws regarding accidental deaths. As a rule, the next of kin of the fatality must give permission for an autopsy. The exception to this is when public interest outweighs the rights of the family members. In aviation accidents, there is a federal interest because of the federal regulations exercised through the Federal Aviation Administration, which controls aviation in the USA. The federal interest was formalized by the Federal Aviation Act of 1958, which gave the federal government power to promulgate regulations governing reports of accidents involving civil aircraft. They were also empowered to make recommendations designed to prevent future accidents.

The importance of post-mortem examination was recognized in an amendment to the Federal Aviation Act enacted in 1962, which provided:

In the case of any fatal accident, the Board is authorized to examine the remains of any deceased person aboard the aircraft at the time of the accident, who dies as a result of the accident, and to conduct autopsies or such other tests thereof as may be necessary to the investigation of the accident; provided that to the extent consistent with the needs of the accident investigation, provisions of local law protecting religious beliefs with respect to autopsies shall be observed.

The 'Board' in this legislation was the Civil Aeronautics Board, but this authority was transferred to the National Transportation Safety Board (NTSB) under the Department of Transportation Act of 1966.

The individual states do, however, have a legitimate interest in aircraft accident fatalities. The 1962 amendment to the Federal Aviation Act does not require that autopsies be obtained, but it authorizes the NTSB investigator to request them. The state coroner or medical examiner has different reasons for requiring an autopsy. Some states authorize the coroner to obtain autopsies only in cases of people who have died by unlawful means. This conflict of authority may give rise to potential conflict and confusion, as some state officials may be unaware of the federal legislation.

In continental Europe the law in most countries is based on the Napoleonic Code. The role of the investigating magistrate or chief of police is similar to that of the coroner, in that he or she is concerned mainly with finding out who has died and ensuring that there are no criminal aspects to the case. Some authorities require no more than a list of those on board the aircraft and, if the number of bodies agrees, they are willing to accept that those named on the manifest have all died. The investigating magistrate in these countries has the right to the wreckage, flight data recorder and other records. Many countries have a system by which the officials from the aircraft accident investigation organization, such as the Bureau d'Enquete d'Accident in France, are recognized formally by the examining magistrate. This enables the professional investigators to have access to the wreckage of the aircraft and its records in their search for a cause of the accident. Unfortunately, this system does not apply in all countries. In some countries, the law positively hinders accident investigation. In Greece, for example, the law requires that a body be released to the next of kin for burial as soon as it is identified. Despite the importance of post-mortem examination, this law does not permit the authorities to allow an autopsy before it is released.

Military accidents

In the UK, a military board of inquiry whose role is analogous to that of the AAIB investigates RAF accidents. They derive their authority from the Air Force Act 1955 and the Board of Inquiry Rules. Accidents to Royal Navy and British Army aircraft are investigated in a similar manner, with authority from the equivalent acts of parliament relating to those services. The board has a president who is a serving officer, normally an aircrew officer who has current or recent experience on the aircraft type involved. Junior members will include an engineering officer who is current on, or familiar with, the aircraft type. The board may call upon the AAIB for help if it deems it necessary. Mixed military and civil accidents are covered by the Air Navigation (Investigation of Air Accidents involving Civil and Military Aircraft or Installations) Regulations 1986. Accidents with fatalities come under the jurisdiction of the coroner or procurator fiscal unless they solely involve fatalities from countries other than the UK; in this case, the provision of the Visiting Forces Act 1953 allows the authorities of visiting forces to hold inquiries into the death of members of that force. Military boards of inquiry always assist the coroner in his or her inquiries into the fatalities.

In the USA, statutes authorize the military authorities to conduct autopsies on people fatally injured on board military aircraft when the accident occurs on a military reservation where there is sole military jurisdiction. However, the importance of post-mortem examination is recognized, and regulations require autopsy examinations no matter where death occurred. Military commanders are given the power to direct the performance of autopsies of aircraft accident fatalities involving military personnel. The US armed forces have a medical examiner's office located in Washington, DC, with a staff of fully trained forensic pathologists who investigate all fatal US military aircraft accidents.

Armed forces of most countries have similar authorities to investigate accidents involving their aircraft.

Conclusion

Although laws and agreements cover accident investigations, there is still considerable potential for hindrance, some of which rests in the criminal law of the host nation and what has been described as the compensation culture. Although investigators may be intent upon finding causes without apportioning blame, others have different motives. The fact that a pilot's disregard for the rules has been shown to be the most common primary cause of civil approach and landing accidents exemplifies the problem (Learmont 1998). In the USA, pilots and airlines have expressed anxiety about the use of flight operational quality assurance data by the FAA, despite the latter's assurances that it would be used only in exceptional cases in enforcement actions (Lopez 2000).

Safety in aviation is, in part, a matter of learning from what has gone wrong. Impediments to accident investigation, including publishing all of the findings, are inimical to safety. The ICAO has been more proactive in recent years, and individual countries have acted against states and airlines found to be wanting. Nevertheless, there are still failures. The concept that it is unwise to compete commercially on safety grounds is still believed because it implies that industry standards are questionable. There is no organization that is 'charged with creating the awareness that is essential' (*Flight International* 2003). Investigators must have a free hand unimpeded by misinterpretations of the legal framework of accident investigation, and their findings must be publicized if safety is to improve. The fact that 'Airlines operating into European airports are often crewed by pilots with invalid licences, have emergency exits blocked by seats and fly with unsecured cargo in the hold, leaking hydraulics and worn out tyres' (Learmont 2000) is unacceptable. However, creating a balance between safety and legal sanctions, which may induce reticence in potential witnesses, is not easy.

INVESTIGATION OF AIRCRAFT ACCIDENTS

There are three broad areas that need to be explored to explain the breakdown in the interface between humans, machine and environment. These are human, aircraft and operational factors. Although these are defined relatively broadly, interactive experience has shown that in all but the smallest accidents, the number of 'groups' will need to be expanded. The areas of interest and responsibility of the various groups are as follows:

- The *operations group* elicits all the facts about the history of the flight, the flight path, the crew experience and the flying procedures. The group also interviews any surviving crew members.
- The *air traffic control group* examines all the air traffic control records, including the voice communication tapes. The group interviews the personnel involved and examines the navigation aids and other equipment that might be relevant.
- The *weather group* compiles all the meteorological data and obtains aftercasts of the weather at the time and location of the accident. The group also examines the adequacy of the meteorological forecasts and briefings.
- The *witness group* obtains statements from all who may have seen or heard some part of the flight or who have any knowledge concerning the flight. The group obtains signed statements from witnesses, including the survivors of the accident. Information concerning the observed positions, height and behaviour of the aircraft is obtained. The location of the witnesses can be plotted on a suitable map of the area in order to aid reconstruction.
- The *flight recorder group* will locate and secure the flight data recorder and cockpit voice recorder and arrange for their readout. The voice recorder provides a continuous record of the last 30 minutes of cockpit communications and sound. Its information can be correlated with the flight data recorder to help in reconstructing the accident sequence. It may give information about the crew, which may be analysed by a psychologist and give vital clues to the operational inspectors.
- The *structures group* locates and identifies the aircraft wreckage and plots it on a wreckage distribution chart. The group determines the aircraft's configuration at impact and the structural integrity of all the mechanical controls. This may involve a reconstruction of the aircraft particularly in cases of collision, structural failure and in-flight fire or explosion.
- The *power plants group* investigates the engines, including the fuel and oil, propellers and controls. The group's work is carried out with the structures group

in locating and plotting the aircraft wreckage. The group is also concerned with the effectiveness of the engine fire extinguisher systems.

- The *systems group* examines the condition and capability of all the aircraft systems and components, such as hydraulics, pneumatics, electrical systems and electronics, radio communication and navigation equipment, air-conditioning, pressurization, ice and rain protection, cabin fire extinguishers and oxygen. The group will record the positions of all controls and switches.

- The *maintenance records group* reviews the maintenance history of the aircraft with an emphasis on any recent repairs or modifications that might have bearing on the accident. The group also examines any flight documents recovered.

- The *human factors group* is responsible for all of the aeromedical aspects of the crew's performance, including physical, physiological and psychological elements. The group is concerned with the possibility of crew incapacitation. Evacuation and design factors that may have a bearing on survival are examined, together with the crashworthiness of the aircraft. An examination of the injuries sustained by the fatalities may contribute to the resolution of the aircraft's mode of impact. The group works closely with the local authorities in the matter of body recovery, identification and subsequent post-mortem examinations.

- The *evacuation, search, rescue and fire-fighting group* investigates the circumstances, performance and equipment of these aspects of the accident.

A senior operations investigator is normally designated as the investigator in charge. He or she will arrange for frequent meetings of the various groups involved in the investigation. The areas of responsibility overlap, and it is vital that no group works in isolation. The pathologist may be a member or head of the human factors group, and he or she must learn of any developments in the investigation that might have a bearing on his or her work. In turn, the pathologist can report any of his or her findings that could provide a lead for members of other groups. Without frequent meetings, the investigation may lose its impetus. This may lead to duplication of effort, the pursuit of false leads and failure to recognize vital evidence. This in turn may lead to an inadequate investigation.

Other experts

A specialist in aviation medicine should study the medical records of the flight crew, record visual and auditory acuity, and look for any condition that could have led to incapacitation in flight or to deterioration in fitness and performance. Such information should be correlated with the pathological findings. However, it must be appreciated that many functional abnormalities, such as epilepsy, are not demonstrable at autopsy. Close cooperation with the operations group is essential, as some general problems may have an aeromedical component. For example, a problem with the pressurization system may indicate the need to eliminate hypoxia as a factor in the accident.

A medical examination, preferably by an aviation medical specialist, should be made on surviving flight crew members to find out whether any physical, physiological or psychological factors in the operating crew had a bearing on the circumstances of the accident. Such interviews are likely to be harrowing to those being questioned and should be properly planned and coordinated through the operational investigators, who will also wish to interview the surviving aircrew. It may be appropriate for blood and/or urine samples to be taken for analysis, both for the presence of therapeutic substances and to help to determine whether any abnormal state such as hypoglycaemia may have been present. Before taking such specimens, the investigator should ensure that there are no local legal contraindications. He should have the consent of the subject and explain the purpose of the tests.

A detailed record should be made of injuries to all occupants with an assessment of their cause. The findings must be collated with their seat position, location in the aircraft and adjacent environment so that preventive action such as redesign may be considered. If the aircraft has been evacuated in the presence of fire or a similar hazard, such as a ditching, then a full account of each person's escape is a valuable contribution to an assessment of factors influencing success or failure. As the aim of accident investigation is prevention, attention should also be given to the behavioural effects of the accident on the flight crew before they are allowed to return to flying duties. The adverse effects of any accident on the rescuers should not be forgotten, and debriefing sessions may be needed to prevent post-traumatic stress disorder.

An aviation psychologist may be needed to carry out an investigation of the background of the flight deck crew. This has been called a 'psychological autopsy' (Yanowitch *et al.* 1972) and includes matters such as motivation for flying, general intelligence, emotional stability, character and behaviour. Information from friends, relatives, supervisors, instructors and others may provide information about the recent activities and attitudes of the flight crew and their personal circumstances and flying habits. These psychological variables have not always been given the appropriate degree of attention. Elements of perception, judgement, decision, morale, motivation, ageing, fatigue and incapacitation may be intangible but are, nevertheless, important.

Special attention should be paid to the possible impairment of aircrew fitness and performance. Errors and impairment of performance may occur during normal operations or, more commonly, when emergencies or other unexpected conditions develop. These include errors of perception, which may be related to auditory, visual, tactile or postural stimuli. There may be errors of judgement and interpretation that could involve poor judgement of distances, misinterpretation of instruments, confusion of instructions, sensory illusions and disorientation. Errors of reaction may occur related to timing and coordination of neuromuscular performance and technique in the operation of controls. Contributing causes of these errors and performance deficits may lie in such areas as attitude and motivation, emotional effect and perseverance. Fatigue is likely to exaggerate all these factors.

The RAF Inspectorate of Flight Safety provides expert help to military boards of inquiry in the UK. Other countries have similar bodies. They have experience in accident investigation, are familiar with the operation of the type of aircraft involved in the accident, and will be aware of previous accidents similar to that under investigation.

The support of many other specialists may be needed during the conduct of an investigation. Armament specialists are needed if the accident involved ejection seats and will also ensure that they are safe. Advice may also be needed on other explosives such as life-saving flares and ordnance. Environmental health and protection officers will be needed in most accidents. Aircraft incorporate hazardous materials, including heavy metals and carbon fibre; they may carry dangerous cargoes such as organophosphorus insecticides for crop-spraying and in every accident fuel spillage may be a problem. The safety of the salvage crew must also be borne in mind, particularly in the case of cargo such as organophosphorus insecticides. The police may be needed to investigate suspected sabotage or other acts of criminal or wilful damage. The specialist knowledge and advice of the aircraft manufacturer is vital, though it is important that any suspect aircraft components are examined by independent experts.

Action at the scene

The police and emergency services will be the first at the scene of a disaster. Their first concern will be the saving of life. If this is impossible, then effective investigation aimed at saving lives in the future assumes major importance. Planning and training ensure that the emergency services are aware of their contribution to successful investigation. However, there is usually public pressure for a speedy disposal of the fatal casualties and restoration to their next of kin. Investigation can impede this process, and cooperation between the police and the accident investigators is essential. A team of doctors who are not involved in caring for the injured will be needed in order to certify formally the fact of death. At the scene, the main contributions of

the police to the investigation are the maintenance of the security of the area and the preservation of evidence, particularly the distribution of the bodies and the aircraft wreckage. Security includes security from both bystanders and the presence of well-intentioned officials.

It is important to ascertain whether the aircraft is carrying any hazardous freight before further action is taken. Photographs should be taken as soon as possible after the accident occurs and before the wreckage is moved or disturbed. Efforts should be made to preserve or record evidence of an ephemeral nature such as ice and soot deposits. If possible, photographs of the bodies should be taken before removal. However, there is considerable public pressure to remove the dead bodies as soon as possible and, in general, the lack of such photographs has not impeded the investigation, provided the location of each body in the wreckage is known. Mapping the locations of the fatalities is more important. This is best achieved with a system of staking and labelling. This is normally the responsibility of the police. However, it is important that they are made aware of any potential hazards and matters of health and safety. They may need to obtain advice from environmental health officers and consultants in communicable disease control. All personnel involved in the recovery procedures should be provided with appropriate protective clothing.

Once death has been confirmed, a uniquely numbered label should be attached securely to the body. Most disaster kits contain preprinted labels in triplicate for this purpose. The bodies should not be undressed or searched at the scene; nor should any property be removed from them or their clothing. The recovery teams will then place the body or remains into a body bag and fix identically numbered labels to both the bag and the location from which it was removed. The location markers could be stakes or free-standing markers. Pin-on labels are used when fatalities are retained in their seats. It is sometimes useful for the pathologist to view the bodies in situ, but this is not normally possible. Parts of bodies should be treated in a similar manner to whole bodies. Once the coroner has given permission to remove the bodies they may be moved from the site, but a strict procedure is needed to avoid cross-contamination and to preserve the evidence. The bodies should then be taken to a holding area close to the accident site before being taken to the temporary mortuary. Ideally, this holding area should be under cover and out of public view. It should be accessible to vehicles and be secure. This holding area serves as a collection point and as a checking point to ensure that labelling of body bags is complete. Refrigerated lorries may also attend the holding area to allow appropriate storage and phased and orderly transfer of the bodies to the temporary mortuary. The body bags remain sealed throughout their time in the holding area.

Accident investigators and police are now able to make detailed maps of the scene. This can be done when the bodies have been removed and the site is free and may be some days after the accident. The preparation of these maps can provide valuable information for the investigation. In one case with a suspected fire in the air, the body plot showed that the burnt bodies had been burnt on the ground in the post-crash fire after impact.

Mortuary organization

In the UK, the responsibility for providing support to coroners under the Coroners Act 1988 lies with the county council in shire areas and the borough council in metropolitan areas. These also have emergency planning responsibilities under the Civil Defence (General Local Authority Functions) Regulations 1993. Although these regulations do not specify detailed requirements to plan for temporary mortuaries, the regulations and Home Office (1992) guidance promote the concept of integrated emergency management. These councils therefore should identify suitable premises for use as a temporary mortuary in an emergency. Ideally, one mortuary would be identified for each coroner's district. Each site identified as suitable for a temporary mortuary should be capable of being equipped and fully operational in no more than 24 hours. The costs incurred fall on the local authority responsible for funding the coroner's service.

All the bodies from a major disaster should be taken to a single mortuary. This facilitates the difficult task of identification, avoids the unnecessary duplication of personnel, and minimizes the burden on the communications system, which inevitably will be under great strain. In major disasters, the use of a hospital mortuary is not appropriate. If there are live casualties as well as fatalities, the hospital approach roads should not be encumbered by vehicles bringing the dead to the mortuary. Additionally, the arrival of a large number of bodies at a hospital mortuary would hinder the day-to-day activities and overwhelm the capacity of the mortuary, necessitating the use of a second or third mortuary. Many of the bodies from a major disaster may be severely burned or mutilated, and a hospital mortuary is not suitable for large numbers of such cases. A public mortuary is similarly unsuitable because the capacity is likely to be overwhelmed by the arrival of a large number of bodies. A specifically designated temporary mortuary is the best solution for such a disaster. Ideally, buildings for use as a temporary mortuary should have been selected before a disaster occurs.

The fundamental requirement for a temporary mortuary is a large floor space at ground level in a sheltered building. It should be of sufficient size to allow all the investigations to be carried out efficiently on an open-plan design. We have successfully used tents when such a building was not available. The key requirements are security and privacy. Easy road access is essential to facilitate the transport of bodies to and from the mortuary. If an aircraft hangar is used, it may be possible to drive into the hangar.

Adequate space and facilities for clerical work will be needed. The mortuary will need to be in constant and direct contact with the police, particularly their casualty bureau. Telephones and facsimile machines should be included in the communication system. Adequate light, heat, ventilation, water supply, drainage and sewerage will be needed, together with power for electric saws and radiological equipment. However, often it is possible to improvise. As far as is practicable, the recommendations of the Health Services Advisory Committee (1991) on safe practice in the mortuary and post-mortem room should be followed. The responsibility for the health and safety aspects of the operation of the temporary mortuary rests with the designated supervising pathologist, who will liaise with the environmental health officer, consultants in communicable disease control and others who may give useful advice.

Many personnel from a variety of backgrounds will be required during the investigation, including pathologists, mortuary technicians, clerks, photographers, police, forensic odontologists and, perhaps most important of all, personnel to move bodies within the mortuary. The mortuary should be divided into a reception area for bodies as they are received, where the documentation may be initiated. Another area for external examination, unclothing and photography will be required; dental examination may take place here. Autopsy facilities will be required, as will areas for special investigations, such as radiology and fingerprinting. Finally, an area should be set aside for the embalming and encoffining of the bodies. Because embalming results in the production of fumes, this should be done in a separate room. It is useful to have a secure room for the storage of specimens and property removed from the fatalities. There are many publications listing the equipment that should be available in the temporary mortuary (Royal College of Pathologists 1990; Association of Chief Police Officers 1997). If possible, trolleys should be provided, which can act as autopsy tables and also be used to move bodies within the mortuary area. Every person in the mortuary must wear protective clothing. In many accidents, particularly those in which sabotage or explosions are thought to play a part, radiology will be required. Special facilities will be needed for this purpose.

In addition to the facilities that will be needed at the temporary mortuary, additional facilities will be required to complete the investigations. These include a toxicology laboratory with appropriate personnel, a histology laboratory and, occasionally, a serology laboratory and even a DNA analysis laboratory. In many countries, including the UK and the USA, specialized aviation toxicology laboratories are available, but in others the assistance of the local forensic medicine organization will have to be invoked. Under these circumstances, the nature of the work and investigation will have to be explained to them.

In major disasters, the provision of refrigeration is a great advantage, because this removes the need for haste in the investigation, which subsequently may lead to evidence being overlooked or destroyed. Portable refrigeration in the form of refrigerated lorries may well provide an answer to this problem. It is advisable to advise the provider of any refrigerated lorry to obscure their company name from the side of the lorry in order to avoid the problem of press photographs damaging the company's trading position.

As part of the disaster plan, the coroner or procurator fiscal in conjunction with the police will have nominated a pathologist with appropriate experience to act as the supervising pathologist. He or she will be responsible for the planning of the mortuary facilities, identifying the equipment needed and organizing the mortuary once it has been activated. The mortuary will be commissioned when it is known that any disaster is of such a size as to require special arrangements. To maintain security, it is important that all personnel who may need access to the mortuary have some readily identifiable security pass or badge.

Some authorities (Royal College of Pathologists 1990) recommend that each body be given a mortuary number on arrival at the temporary mortuary. However, each body will already have a label bearing the recovery number, and clearly there is room for confusion unless the two labels are obviously distinct, perhaps of different colours. The experience of the RAF Department of Aviation Pathology, which has used this system and an alternative system that uses the scene number alone, suggests that confusion is eliminated if only one numbering system is used. In this case, the scene number would be appropriate, and it is then possible to dispense with the use of mortuary numbers.

On arrival, each body or part of a body will be logged in a register. If separate mortuary numbers are used, they will be included in the register alongside the scene number. A document case containing appropriate documents is allocated to each body or part. It is helpful if this is transparent and waterproof. It should have a checklist of procedures to be followed that can be signed or initialled by the appropriate person once the action is complete. Every document should bear the body number. The documents contained in the case will include a list of property collected and a card detailing the clothing. It is useful to have a separate card to which clean samples of identifiable clothing can be fixed, as these may be useful in subsequent identification. Other documents in the case include a chart for depicting injuries, a post-mortem examination form, a dental chart and a form detailing the specimens collected for toxicology and histology.

The International Criminal Police Organisation (INTERPOL) has a disaster victim identification form that many authorities advocate using. This form is excellent for the identification of single unknown bodies, but it is very cumbersome to use and less than ideal for use in a major disas-

ter. We have devised forms that are considered to be easier to use. The Metropolitan Police has adapted our forms, and these are used in all major disasters in the UK. Figure 32.1 shows the plan for the management of a disaster.

The autopsy

Before undertaking the autopsy examination, the body must be undressed and searched. The findings must be recorded accurately, as they may contribute to the investigation. Tears may match cockpit projections and bloodstains may indicate the direction of forces. Controls may leave imprints on gloves and shoes. This may be helpful in the case of dual controls when there is doubt as to who was flying the aircraft at the moment of impact. If incapacitation of the pilot is suspected, such evidence may help to eliminate this possibility. Photography before and during the autopsy is often very helpful.

The post-mortem protocol is the standard one and merits no further description. As all aviators have regular med-

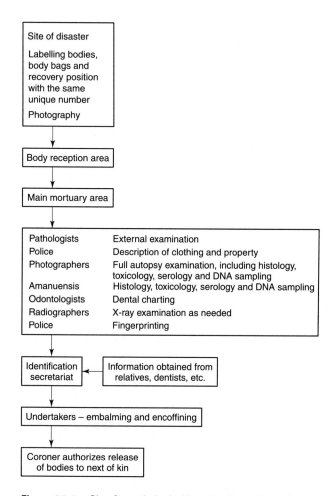

Figure 32.1 *Plan for pathological investigations of a major disaster.*

ical examinations, it is helpful to have obtained the information from their medical records before embarking on the autopsy; however, this is frequently impracticable. Such evidence may include a limitation for spectacles on the licence, and this may prompt a search of the scene for evidence that they were worn. Details of distinguishing marks and scars helpful in identification may also be noted on the medical records.

The following list details the minimal requirements for post-mortem examinations based on investigative, medicolegal and sociological needs:

- Identification and complete examination of the operating crew on the flight deck or in the cockpit.
- Full external examination of all fatal casualties.
- Identification of cabin attendants and comparison with passengers.
- Minimal internal autopsy on all passengers and cabin crew to include:
  - establishment of the cause of death
  - discovery of major disease likely to influence life expectancy
  - assessment of deceleration injury to:
    (a) cardiovascular system, liver and diaphragm
    (b) head, sternum, spine and pelvis.
- Selection of blood specimens from all casualties for carboxyhaemoglobin studies.
- Collection of lung specimens from all casualties for estimation of mode of death.

The pathologist must interpret his or her findings with caution. The head of the human factors group and the investigator-in-charge must ensure that the pathological findings are taken as part of the investigation as a whole and are correlated fully with evidence adduced within the group and by other groups. Experience has shown that this is facilitated and maximum advantage gained if the pathologist attends the periodic briefings by the investigator-in-charge.

Multiple samples for toxicology need to be taken into appropriate containers. The quality of the analysis depends on the quality of the specimens (Forrest 1993). If there are several victims, then it is useful to have an assistant to undertake the labelling. Samples from all major organs should be taken for histology. We have found that the retention of the pilot's whole heart is a wise precaution, as occasionally it is necessary to return to it if there are abnormal findings. However, recent events and changes in the law mean that permission from the coroner has to be obtained before any tissues are removed and that the family must be informed about all sampling. They may at the completion of the investigation demand the return of the samples for appropriate disposal (Human Tissue Act 2004, Coroners' Rules 2005).

Radiological examination may be very important. The discovery of embedded particles or foreign bodies from an explosion is clearly vital. However, availability and cost may limit the use of such facilities.

Trauma accounts for most of the autopsy findings. The sometimes tedious task of describing all the injuries may prove valuable in the assessment of the forces suffered by the victims or the sequence of the injuries.

IDENTIFICATION

Identification is the responsibility of the coroner, procurator fiscal or other legal authority in charge of the investigation, who may devolve the technical process to a team including pathologists, police officers and dentists. Their job is to match observations made in the mortuary with information provided by relatives and friends. It is a task that cannot be rushed, despite outside pressures, if mistakes are not to be made. Identification is fundamental to the investigation and reconstruction of an accident and for legal and sociological reasons. The bereaved have to be satisfied that all that can be done has been done and that they can make suitable arrangements for disposal of the body.

Detailed ante-mortem information listing the physical appearance, clothing, medical and dental histories, and any belongings such as jewellery that they may have with them is sought from family and friends. Approaches to doctors and dentists may have to be made to provide detailed records, such as dental charts and radiographs. This information should be gathered as soon as possible, preferably when contact is first made. However, this is contingent upon the reaction of the relative or friend at the time. If questioning is causing too much distress, then another approach may have to be made later. This decision has to be made cautiously, because repeated intrusions exacerbate distress and may make the bereaved believe that events are worse than they are.

In the mortuary, a full description of every victim has to be made, including names and sizes of clothing. This has to be done in much greater detail than in an autopsy for suspicious death. Clothing, documents and belongings must be carefully bagged and noted, listing every single item. In the case of jewellery, the description must be exhaustive. Similarly, birthmarks, defects, scars, tattoos and the like must be documented carefully and photographed.

Once the ante-mortem information has been collected and the post-mortem observations have been made, comparisons can be started. In practice, this tends to be ongoing. It may be helpful to divide the population into males and females, adults and children. Further subdivision can be made to look at those with outstanding features, such as complex dental bridges and tattoos. This helps to speed up

Table 32.1 *Example of identification chart (may be modified to suit requirements)*

Body number	Name	Clothing	Personal appearance	Jewellery/ belongings	Dental	Medical	Tattoos	Fingerprints	Form of disposal
123	Jones	✔	–	–	✔	✔	–	–	Burial
124	–	–	–	–	–	–	–	–	–
125	Brown	–	–	✔	–	–	✔	✔	Cremation

the process and in a big accident helps to make the task seem less daunting.

A chart should be created, as in Table 32.1. The first column gives the body number. In the next column is space for the name. The other columns should contain headings of all the criteria being matched. Computer programmes have been written that facilitate this task.

Once a post-mortem finding has been shown to match an ante-mortem description, this should be recorded. When all, or as many as possible, of the features have been analysed for a body, ticks can be placed in the appropriate columns on the chart. If the lead investigator for this phase of the process has been convinced that the identity has been proved, then the person's name can be entered on the chart.

In highly destructive accidents, and in accidents where there are separate body parts, DNA analysis will be necessary. Only in this way can the body parts be matched with accuracy.

On rare occasions, it may be necessary to resort to exclusion. This can be done only when it is certain that the passenger manifest is accurate. Essentially, it involves distinguishing a small number of individuals from one another based on flimsy data; it is a last resort.

Once the team is sure that it has made all of the identifications, these can be related to the coroner or other official for his approval. Only then can the names be released. It is at this stage that relatives can be shown the bodies in a chapel of rest, if they so wish. This is the only reliable method of visual identification. Asking relatives to parade around many dead bodies in search of their own relative is inhuman and unreliable. Relatives and friends may also be able to visually confirm clothing and belongings.

Ideally, all bodies should be X-rayed, as this can be useful in identification by revealing various prostheses. This is mandatory if there is suspicion of a terrorist attack. It may reveal evidence of previous injury or surgery, as well as firing devices, detonators and explosive particles. In an explosion, these have to be put in special bags and handed to the appropriate exhibits officer or forensic scientist, who will look for evidence of explosive residue together with other appropriate analyses.

REFERENCES

Association of Chief Police Officers. *Emergency Procedures Manual.* London: Association of Chief Police Officers, 1997.

Coroners Rules. London: HM Stationery Office, 2005.

Flight International. Left unsaid. *Flight International* 2000; 6 June: 3.

Flight International. Mutual assistance. *Flight International* 2003; 14 January: 3.

Forrest ARW. Obtaining samples at post mortem examination for toxicological and biochemical analysis. *Journal of Clinical Pathology* 1993; **46**: 292–6.

Health Services Advisory Committee. *Safe Working and the Prevention of Infection in the Mortuary and Post Mortem Room.* London: HM Stationery Office, 1991.

Home Office. *Dealing with Disaster.* London: HM Stationery Office, 1992.

Human Tissue Act 2004. Chapter 30.

International Civil Aviation Organization. *Manual of Aircraft Accident Investigation*, 4th edn. Cheltenham: Civil Aviation Authority, 1970.

Learmont D. Rule breaking revealed as most deadly factor in air accidents. *Flight International* 1998; 25 November: 8.

Learmont D. Safety inspections reveal extent of danger airlines. *Flight International* 2000; 6 June: 9.

Levine M, Pyke J. *Levine on Coroner's Courts.* London: Sweet & Maxwell, 1999.

Lopez R. FAA prepares to rule on safety data sharing. *Flight International* 2000; 11 June: 8.

Royal College of Pathologists. *Deaths in Major Disasters: the Pathologist's Role.* London: Royal College of Pathologists, 1990.

Yanowitch RE, Mohler SR, Nichols EA. Psychosocial reconstruction inventory: a postdictal instrument in aircraft accident reconstruction. *Aerospace Medicine* 1972; **43**: 551–4.

FURTHER READING

International Civil Aviation Organization. *Annex 13: Aircraft Accident Investigation.* Cheltenham: Civil Aviation Authority, 1994.

33

Aviation pathology and toxicology

S. ANTHONY CULLEN AND IAN R. HILL

INTRODUCTION

In 1962, Mason defined aviation accident pathology as 'the comprehensive study of aviation fatalities whereby the medical history of the casualty and the findings at autopsy can be correlated with the environmental factors, the structural or other damage to the aircraft and the use or abuse of equipment so that a complete picture of the accident may be formed'. This definition cannot be bettered today. The original definition was applied particularly to military aircraft accidents. Stevens (1970) expressed the objectives of aviation pathology in relation to civil aviation. He suggested that each investigation should aim to find any medical evidence that might reveal:

1 Natural disease or abnormality such as could cause impaired function in the operating crew and provide, therefore:

   a. a possible medical cause for the accident, or
   b. a probable medical cause for the accident

2 A possible or probable non-medical cause for the accident
3 The probable events in the aircraft prior to the accident, or
4 The probable events at impact and immediately after the accident, particularly insofar as these are related to the questions of survivability and escape.

Detailed post-mortem examination of the bodies of fatalities is the main source of pathological evidence. The findings at autopsy are correlated with the medical histories of the people involved, the histological and toxicological investigation, and the evidence from examination of the victims' clothing and the aircraft wreckage. It is vital that the pathologist's evidence is interpreted in conjunction with the evidence found by the operational and engineering investigators. The investigation of an aircraft accident is a collaborative effort, and it is important that no member of the team hinders another.

DISEASE IN THE OPERATING CREW

The discovery of organic disease during the post-mortem examination of a pilot presents the accident investigator with a number of problems. The investigator wishes to know whether the disease caused the accident, whether it contributed to the cause of the accident, or whether its discovery is entirely coincidental. The difficulty is compounded, as the normal pathological sequence of events following an acute episode of disease may be cut short by the accident. The familiar morbid anatomical changes then will not be present. In order to solve this problem, the pathologist will need to know the prevalence of the disease in the pilot population. Disease may cause accidents by incapacitating the pilot, and the circumstances surrounding the crash may give valuable clues as to the likelihood of such an event. A pilot may become subtly impaired by virtue of their disease. The problem facing the accident investigator is the reverse of that facing the clinician. The clinician elicits the symptoms and signs from the patient and tries to deduce the underlying pathology. The accident investigator has discovered the underlying pathology and tries to determine what symptoms the pilot may have had and how they may have affected his or her ability to fly the aircraft properly.

Heart disease

In order to determine the prevalence of coronary atheroma, the coronary arteries from 1188 pilots were evaluated to discover the extent of the coronary artery disease present. Arteries in which the lumen area was reduced by less than 20 per cent were classified as having no coronary artery disease. Those with a reduction of area of 20–50 per cent were judged to have mild disease. Moderate disease required a reduction in area of 51–70 per cent, while severe disease required a reduction greater than this.

Using this method of evaluation, the results of the study of all pilots are shown in Table 33.1 and Figure 33.1.

Evidence of previous ischaemic damage was seen in 43 of the 1000 pilots in whom histological examination of the heart was undertaken. This presents similar problems to the discovery of coronary artery atheroma, namely what

role did the heart disease play in the causation of the accident?

Coronary artery atheroma causing a reduction in the area of the lumen of greater that 50 per cent was seen in just under 20 per cent of the pilots examined. The frequency of this finding makes the interpretation of its significance all the more difficult. Over the period of this study, four pilots (ages 39, 62, 52 and 54 years) were examined who had died in their aircraft but whose death did not precipitate an accident. Three of these were commercial aircraft that were landed by the co-pilot; the fourth was a light aircraft that was landed by the passenger, who was 'talked down' by a check pilot. In only one of these fatalities was there any evidence of an acute change: a 54-year-old pilot had evidence of a recent thrombus. The problem that these cases illustrate is the difficulty in interpreting the discovery of coronary artery disease in a pilot who was involved in an accident. In common with the investigation of any sudden death, it is the circumstances surrounding the death that determine the interpretation of the findings if no acute change is discovered.

In the study, four other pilots (ages 67, 66, 64 and 52 years) were involved in aircraft accidents, but the degree of injury was so trivial that death was ascribed to their severe coronary artery disease. Two of these had acute changes. One case had haemorrhage into an atheromatous plaque, and another had evidence of contraction-band necrosis in his myocardium, suggesting reperfusion of a recent infarct. Three of these pilots were flying gliders at the time that their collapse precipitated the accident.

In ten accidents, the presence of coronary artery atheroma was deemed to be the cause of, or a major contributory factor in, the accident. The coronary artery disease in a further ten pilots was thought possibly to have contributed to the cause of the accident. Not surprisingly, the ages of the pilots was relevant: the average age of those dying in their aircraft was 57 years; those whose disease was a probable cause of the accident averaged 53.7 years; and

Table 33.1   *Occurrence of coronary artery disease in pilots*

| Age (years) | Total | Coronary artery disease | | | |
		None	Mild	Moderate	Severe
17–20	50	48	2	0	0
21–25	157	128	21	5	3
26–30	204	156	29	10	9
31–35	183	121	37	17	8
36–40	178	103	41	25	9
41–45	116	59	29	16	12
46–50	110	39	33	21	17
51–55	83	34	19	19	11
56–60	53	15	16	11	11
61+	54	20	9	5	20
Total	1188	723	236	129	100

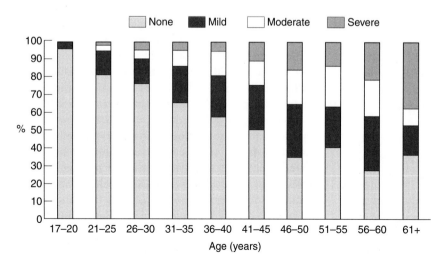

Figure 33.1   *Occurrence of coronary artery disease in 1188 pilots.*

those in whom the disease was thought to be a possible cause averaged 51.9 years. Table 33.2 summarizes the relationship of coronary artery disease with cause of accident. Coronary artery disease was thought to be the cause of the accident in 1.3 per cent of cases and a possible factor in a further 1.3 per cent.

Arrhythmia is the most common cause of sudden cardiac death and may be the first symptom of coronary artery disease (Toff *et al.* 1988). Arrhythmia has been regarded as incompatible with flying duties, but it has been accepted that single isolated cases of atrial fibrillation with no underlying cardiac abnormality may be licensed after certain conditions have been met. In one study, paroxysmal atrial fibrillation was found to have a prevalence of 0.024 per cent, while persistent atrial fibrillation had a prevalence of 0.018 per cent (Busby and Davis 1976). The pathologist is faced with the difficulty in demonstrating morbid anatomical changes that may cause atrial fibrillation. This problem is compounded by the damage to the heart that often accompanies aviation deaths. Only two accidents investigated by our department were ascribed to incapacitation caused by atrial fibrillation.

The presence of collections of non-specific inflammatory cells in the interstitial tissues of the myocardium is termed focal myocarditis. This has a variety of causes, of which viral infection is one of the most common. Protozoal and bacterial infections and drug reactions are other causes. The clinical picture varies from the patient being asymptomatic to a short clinical course with cardiac failure, arrhythmias and death. Many years ago, it was thought to be an important cause of sudden death in obscure or difficult cases. A study of the prevalence of focal myocarditis in deaths from trauma suggested that it might be as high as five per cent of British males between the ages of 18 and 50 years (Stevens and Underwood-Ground 1970). In a study in our department, focal myocarditis was found in 41 of the 1028 hearts studied histologically.

The discovery of focal myocarditis presents the investigator with a problem. Is the myocarditis entirely coincidental, or did it cause sudden collapse or death? Clearly, foci of inflammation situated in the conducting system may cause a sudden arrhythmia. However, a similar picture is seen in acute rejection following cardiac transplantation. This appearance is seen in 16 per cent of cardiac biopsies following transplant. In only two cases investigated by our department was the presence of focal myocarditis thought to have precipitated an acute cardiac collapse. Given that a wide range of viruses may cause cardiac damage, the discovery of focal myocarditis occasionally has been used as a marker of viral infection, particularly when other evidence of infection has been present.

There are few studies on the causes of in-flight incapacitation without accident because of double crewing. In the few studies that exist, neurological problems are among the common causes of loss of consciousness (McCormick and Lyons 1991; Martin-Saint-Laurent *et al.* 1990). Assuming that in-flight incidents are surrogates for accidents, one would expect neurological conditions to account for a significant number of aviation accidents. However, this is not the case, and in our department there were only ten accidents in which a neurological condition was discovered to have been present in the pilot. The lack of an anatomical basis for many neurological diseases coupled with the frequency with which the brain is severely traumatized must be the explanation for this. The ten cases in our study comprised four of epilepsy, two of migraine, two with a chromophobe adenoma of the pituitary, one with acute encephalitis, and one with a cerebellar arteriovenous malformation. Two of the cases of epilepsy were a sequel of trauma to the head. Of the ten cases with neurological conditions, only two were thought to have caused or contributed to the cause of the accident. Four of the ten cases possibly could have contributed to the accident, and four were deemed to be entirely coincidental findings.

Suicide

Ungs (1994) stated that pilots rarely crash aircraft to commit suicide. He found ten cases of intentional suicide in the period 1979–89 and 20 cases in which suicide was a possibility but not determined. This represents a very small proportion of the 5929 general aviation accidents during this period. However, Mäulen and Faust (1990) estimate that approximately two to three per cent of all fatal air accidents may be attributed to suicide, and in many other accidents there were grounds for inferring that self-destructive or suicidal behaviour was involved. Our department has investigated 475 general aviation accidents. In nine of these, it is certain that the victims took their own lives, as they had indicated this intention in written or verbal mes-

Table 33.2   *Coronary artery disease in pilots*

Type of flying and age range	Died		Probable cause of accident		Possible cause of accident	
	n	Age range (years)	*n*	Age range (years)	*n*	Age range (years)
Commercial	3	39–54	3 (1.9%)	47–51	2 (1.3%)	52–57
General aviation	2	52–62	4 (0.9%)	44–67	3 (0.6%)	36–73
Glider/micro-light	3	64–67	3 (2.1%)	43–65	5 (3.4%)	35–66

sages. Coroners do not record suicide verdicts unless there is positive evidence of suicidal intent. In seven other cases, it seemed highly likely that the pilots took their own lives but the coroner did not record suicide verdicts. This series suggests that suicide contributes to about two per cent of fatal general aviation accidents.

It is generally believed that overall rates of suicide in the general population are two to three times higher than those actually reported. The main reasons for this are the legal constraints placed on coroners and reluctance by doctors to record suicide as a cause of death. Studies in the USA suggest that this is equally true for aviation suicides. The problem is compounded in aviation, as the circumstances and findings in suicidal and accidental aircraft crashes are often nearly identical. Only careful investigation of the psychological problems encountered by the victim can help to elucidate this problem. This has been termed a 'psychological autopsy'.

The introduction of this chapter describes the problems facing a pathologist investigating a fatal aircraft accident. Despite these difficulties, it is possible to attribute the medical condition discovered in the pilot as a probable or possible cause or contributory factor in the cause of an accident. Table 33.3 shows the number of accidents in which the medical condition was thought likely to be a cause, or a major contributory factor in the cause, of an accident. Table 33.4 shows the number of accidents in which the condition possibly contributed to the cause of the accident. In each table, 'other' includes gliders and micro-light aircraft.

It can be seen from these tables that medical conditions in the pilot are an infrequent cause or contributory factor in fatal accidents. The differences in the percentage of medical causes between the various categories of flying might, at first, be thought to be due to the differing standards of the medical examinations applied to the various categories of pilots. However, this proved not to be the case, and, like the prevalence of coronary artery disease, the main reason for these differences was found to be the age of the pilots involved in each type of flying.

The UK rate of medical causes for fatal general aviation accidents is comparable to that reported from the USA (Booze 1989). It is difficult to see how this low rate may be reduced still further. Perhaps one might consider having an age bar above which pilots must fly as or with a co-pilot. It is unlikely that such a restriction would be placed on general aviation and glider pilots, as it would be seen to interfere with an individual's right to practise their sport. Most commercial pilots already fly in double-crewed aircraft, and older military pilots do not fly solo aircraft.

INJURY CAUSATION

Injuries in transport accidents are caused by the reaction between the individual and the environment created during all phases of the crash sequence. Thus, because there may be a wide range of potentially injurious situations, even in relatively simple accidents, causation tends to be a complex affair. The injury finally seen may be the result of more than one impact, and although Locard's principle states that every contact leaves a trace, these traces may not be discernable. Unlike other areas of medicine, but in common with other areas of safety design, randomized controlled trials cannot be used to provide evidence (Rivora et al. 2000).

Table 33.3   *Medical conditions as probable cause or contributory cause of accidents*

Category	Number	Cardiovascular	Suicide	Other	Total
Military	514	1 (0.2%)	0	1 (0.2%)	2 (0.4%)
Commercial	154	3 (1.9%)	0	0	3 (1.9%)
General	475	5 (1.0%)	9 (1.9%)	0	14 (2.9%)
Other	216	7 (3.2%)	2 (0.9%)	1 (0.4%)	10 (4.6%)
Mixed	9	0	0	0	0
Total	1368	16 (1.2%)	11 (0.8%)	1 (0.07%)	29 (2.1%)

Table 33.4   *Medical conditions as possible cause or contributory cause of accidents*

Category	Number	Cardiovascular	Suicide	Other	Total
Military	514	0	0	1 (0.2%)	1 (0.2%)
Commercial	154	2 (1.3%)	0	0	2 (1.3%)
General	475	4 (0.8%)	0	4 (0.8%)	8 (1.7%)
Other	216	7 (3.2%)	0	1 (0.4%)	8 (3.7%)
Mixed	9	0	0	0	0
Total	1368	13 (0.9%)	0	6 (0.4%)	19 (1.4%)

Evidence must come from the careful analysis of accidents, and investigators must always bear in mind that the unexpected can occur and that this may explain why the aeroplane crashed (Detlef *et al.* 1999). Similarly, if injuries are to be prevented, then detailed information is needed about how they were caused. Proposals for improved safety must be evidence-based if they are to prove effective; if not, and changes to a design are made that fail to afford greater protection, then flight safety suffers.

Basis of injury causation

Injuries occur when a stimulus that is big enough to exceed the tolerance of the tissues is applied to the body. Although a considerable amount of work has been done in an attempt to define what each tissue will withstand, the immense variability has precluded finite definition in all situations. Thus, all that we have are broadly based criteria. This aspect of the subject and the problems related to accelerations are considered in Chapters 10–12.

Arguably, the easiest way of looking at the problem of injury causation is to consider the way in which an aircraft's structure behaves in a crash and how this may affect the body. The crash sequence may begin some way before the primary impact. If the aeroplane suffers control problems, then it may be subjected to a variety of movements, which may be violent, such as may occur in turbulence. Thus, people and the contents of the aeroplane may be thrown about. Once ground impact occurs, there will be further excursions, all of which are potentially injurious; these will continue until the aircraft finally comes to rest. Other factors that have to be considered are fire, water, and fuel and other materials either carried on the aeroplane or present at the crash site.

Traditionally, the causes of injuries can be mechanical, chemical, thermal or thermonuclear. It is unlikely that the last will be present in any appreciable quantities in an aircraft accident, except in highly unusual circumstances, and it will not be dealt with here. Mechanical causes are by far the greatest problem, even when there is a fire. The type of injury produced can be classified broadly into blunt and sharp trauma. This is an important differentiation that is often confused, thereby compromising diagnosis. Blunt trauma is caused by relatively broad surfaces, resulting in lacerations, bruises, grazes, fractures and the like. Sharp objects such as glass, pieces of metal and knives produce incised wounds. Typically, these are deeper than their length; because they can penetrate deeply, they may cause damage to deep structures, giving rise to complications such as peritonitis. It is also important to describe correctly the type of injury, so that attempts can be made to identify its cause.

The timing of injuries is much more difficult. Because they are caused over a short period, any changes that might be used to estimate the time since infliction will not have taken place. Dating bruises and injuries is more an art than a science, since all of the colour changes seen in bruising taken place over a highly variable period. A bruise may take three weeks to go through all of the colour changes, but this can happen over 72 hours. Thus, it is not easy to say whether an injury is ante-mortem, cum-mortem or immediately post-mortem. It may be necessary to take pieces of tissue and study them histologically. The relevance of this lies in the need to try to establish whether any injuries were caused before the aircraft crashed and whether this had any relevance to the cause of the accident. At one extreme, Detlef *et al.* (1999) found a bullet wound in a pilot and in a passenger, which undoubtedly caused the accident.

Given that the dynamics of an accident can be highly variable, and that there will be individual variations in responses to impact trauma based on the person's health and restraint and combined with the nature of the accident, it is helpful to have some guide as to how the injuries may be caused. The ways in which this can happen may be classified as in Table 33.5.

Table 33.5   *Methods of injury causation*

- Being subjected to violent pre-impact movement
- Crushing within a collapsing airframe
- Entrapment within the wreckage
- Being struck by loose objects
- Injuries associated with escape
- Environmental factors

VIOLENT PRE-IMPACT MOVEMENTS

Injuries caused thus may not be distinguishable from impact injuries. However, they do occur in turbulence, when bruises, limb and spinal fractures, and head injuries may occur. It may not be possible to differentiate these from crash injuries. However, like all other injuries, they should be photographed with a scale, so that attempts can be made to match them with the aircraft structure. The importance and relevance of doing this will depend on the circumstances of the accident and may not be practicable in instances where there are a large number of victims.

CRUSHING WITHIN A COLLAPSING AIRFRAME

Varying degrees of collapse can occur in any intensity of crash, but usually there has to be a substantial degree of damage, and that requires a moderately intense impact. The amount of airframe damage produced is, of course, variable. When substantial crushing occurs in a low-velocity impact, it indicates that the structural strength of the airframe is inadequate. This may be a problem with some gliders, which seem to break up comparatively easily. However, there is a paradox here, as the intensity of injury produced is often less than in other types of aircraft. This indicates that if the airframe breaks up around the occupant, then it can be protective, as the majority of forces are dispersed away from the body.

In its typical form, crushing is a feature of high-velocity impacts, in which there is intense structural deformation. It is associated with severe injuries, notably amputations and crushing of the body between parts of the airframe. Perineal splitting, which is usually accompanied by varying degrees of sacroiliac joint injury, with or without visceral herniation, indicates a high vertical loading.

ENTRAPMENT WITHIN THE WRECKAGE

This occurs in two ways, as a result of widely different circumstances. In a deforming but not very intense impact, the hull may twist, making exits inoperable. This may be accompanied by fire, which can stop people using exits. In these circumstances, traumatic injuries may be minimal, usually comprising soft-tissue bruising and at the most extreme limb fractures and concussion. Deaths resulting from asphyxia and burning may be seen if people cannot get out, even in the absence of mechanical trauma.

Structural collapse may pin passengers and crew members in their seats or cause injuries that prevent escape. As well as severe limb injuries, there may be widespread limb lacerations, more severe injuries to the torso, and almost certainly severe head injuries. Death may occur because of the injuries themselves, because of complications resulting from the injuries either alone or due in part to delay in rescue and treatment, and because of fire.

ABSENCE OR FAILURE OF RESTRAINT

To a certain extent, the injuries seen here may be similar, but they occur at different intensities of impact. Absence of restraint is associated with a high rate of ejection through gaps in the aircraft. On the way out, contact may produce severe lacerations and/or impact injuries. Further phases of injury may occur when the body lands and if it hits objects before doing so. Limbs may be torn off, long wide lacerations may be seen, and typically there are severe head injuries. Ejection increases the mortality rate by as much as six times.

Failure of restraint may occur in the harness itself, at its attachments, or at the seat, or the floor may fail. Combinations of these may also occur. Seat failure occurs either because the vertical load is too great or because the horizontal forces overstress the mountings. The pattern of injuries produced is different in the two types of failure, but because of the high forces involved, it may not be easy to distinguish them in some accidents.

If the vertical forces are high, then failure may occur only at the seat legs, or there may be disruption of the floor. In each case, the legs will be fractured, particularly the tibiae and fibulae, and there may be ankle and foot injuries,

partly as a result of entrapment but also because of the transmission of impact forces through the foot. The pattern seen will depend on the position of the limbs. If they are flat on the floor, then the appearances may simulate a hard landing on the feet, with calcaneal fractures. Entrapment of the foot will cause fracture and displacement of the more anterior parts of the foot. Breakage of the floor may be associated with lacerations caused by the jagged edges of the metal. There may also be penetration of the legs and the body by displaced spars. More intense forces can cause limb amputations. When the seat collapses forwards, the appearance of injuries is similar to that seen when entrapment within the wreckage occurs.

In all of these situations, there is a high incidence of injuries to the head, thorax, pelvis and abdomen, in descending order of frequency. Visceral ruptures are seen frequently; commonly, they are very severe, often amounting to total disruption of the organ.

INJURIES ASSOCIATED WITH ESCAPE

Ejection at altitude may be associated with hypoxia and/or cold injuries as well as those injuries discussed earlier. In civilian aircraft, these are usually associated with falling from the aeroplane. Fractures, sprains and bruises, usually of the limbs, predominate. Lacerations may occur if there is any jagged metal in the vicinity. Flash burns and blast injuries are also seen. Occasionally, aviation fuel and hydraulic fluid produce chemical burns. If the aircraft has ditched, then drowning may occur. There may also be cold injuries if there is exposure to high altitude. In this situation, the limbs may be twisted around one another, clothing may be torn off, and there may be petechial haemorrhages.

EXPLOSIVE DECOMPRESSION

By itself, this is seldom fatal, being well-tolerated. The classic injury is rupture of the eardrum without fracture of the base of the skull.

PATTERNS OF INJURY

The pattern of injuries recorded in fatalities and survivors can be an important aid to the investigation by indicating what happened in the accident. Analyses of this type, especially in major accidents, are not easy because of the numbers of people involved, and it may be necessary to use an injury scoring system such as the abbreviated injury scale (AIS). This will not work alone in all cases, because it may be sensible to look at other findings, such as loss of clothing, tumbling and hypoxia. The individual scores combined with other findings can then be looked at in relation to the seating portions of the victims. This will reveal patterns and variations more easily than by using lists of injuries alone.

Variations may occur between people seated close to each other and those located in different parts of the same aeroplane. This may mean that an individual variant was elsewhere in the aeroplane when it crashed, as he or she was subjected to different accident forces while in their seat. These findings have to be considered in the light of the accident as a whole. It is the area where the interests of the pathologist and the other accident investigators meet. All of the observations must be considered in relation to the wreckage analysis, but individual variations warrant special attention.

The value of collating data like these is not restricted to the analysis of an individual accident. It is also of great importance in comparing and contrasting different accidents. Recurring patterns of injury may indicate a failure of safety design that is dangerous to the individual. It may also identify an unexpected safety issue.

Injury patterns may be useful in helping to understand how the accident occurred or what happened during the crash sequence. Some indications of the types of pattern that may be seen have been given above. They may be difficult to detect. It is quite conceivable that when a group of pathologists is working together, they may get subsets of the victims, which can give different conceptions of the accident. This emphasizes the need to look at the whole population and to compare this with the evidence afforded by other accidents.

Essentially, investigators are asking: do the injury patterns fit the observed features of the crash, and if not why not? Does this mean that there is something in the rest of the study that has been missed, or are we looking at a new situation? If it is the latter, does that mean that there is a new set of safety implications, and what are they? The 'odd one out' may indicate that he or she was either the victim or the perpetrator of an act of sabotage. Evidence of unusual injuries in one victim or a group of victims may indicate the detonation of an explosive device in the vicinity. If this is mooted, then the advice of explosives experts must be sought. Any such diagnosis will depend on the demonstration of explosive residues in or on the body, together with explosive injuries and circumstantial evidence.

It is not unusual for injuries from more than one injury cause to coexist; consequently, it can be difficult to decide upon the exact sequence of events. As well as a degree of rigidity of the airframe, the following factors may influence the pattern and severity of injuries:

- Helicopter rotors put big lateral loads on the fuselage, which have to be withstood.
- Light aircraft have fewer spars than airliners because they are smaller, and thus their absorptive area is less and they behave as more rigid structures.
- Light aircraft have a much smaller area between the cockpit and the cabin, and thus the differences

between the crew and passenger impact loadings may be minimal.

- The arrangement of the seating, the number and weight of the occupants, their mass relative to the floor, and the stiffness all have effects.

All of these factors play a part in influencing the way in which the aircraft breaks up, and how and what types of injuries are produced. They can have just as potent an influence as the type of impact. As an aeroplane slides along the ground on its belly, earth and other objects may be scooped up and piled up in front of it. Rigid structures may fracture, push the aircraft away, and/or tear pieces out of it, rupturing the cabin and fuel lines and tearing out seats.

Anything that moves along with the airframe acquires its velocity. Those things that are not cast off are carried forwards, and their added weight has to be supported by the forward bulkhead, collapse of which induces floor failure. If the forward drag is very high, then the forepart of the aeroplane will slow down, but the rear part retains its momentum; consequently, if it is high enough, then it will fold the rear of the aeroplane over on itself. In this situation, the impact forces to which the occupants are subjected will be very complex. Those in the forepart will suffer severe forward forces, decreasing towards the point of fold-over. Here, there will be high crushing forces. In the rear part, horizontal and rotational forces will be experienced. It is easy to see that the pattern of injuries so produced will be extremely variable.

When an aeroplane dives into the ground, the rate of deceleration on impact is high. The intensity depends on the impact speed and the stopping distance. Up to an angle of 40 degrees, there is a gradual increase in longitudinal acceleration for constant impact speeds; thereafter, the aircraft behaves as if the impact were vertical. The tendency here is for complete detachment of seats, with impaction of them and their occupants in the forepart of the aeroplane. Moderately high impact angles are also associated with the production of transverse loadings, which adds to the severity of impact for the occupant.

Even in a simple accident, there is the ever-present possibility that the victims will be subjected to more than one direction of impact, especially if they are wearing lap-belts. The potential for injury is, therefore, very high, and in severe accidents it is not surprising that there should be a high incidence of severe and even fatal injuries. People do survive these accidents, however, and so it is important to try to define what constitutes a survivable accident.

The suggestion that 'luck' may be a factor has, quite rightly, been abhorred. It may be that the choice of seat is fortuitous, but in terms of crash dynamics and biodynamics this is irrelevant – although the victim might not think so. Extraneous factors such as starvation, climate and terrain are, for similar reasons, irrelevant, despite the fact that they can have a potent effect on ultimate survival. Judged like this, survivability would seem to be a graded phenomenon, and worldwide accident experiences support this view. However, the majority of survivors do seem to sustain very little injury.

The fact that people with minor injuries sit alongside those with severe injuries, and that a few centimetres can mean the difference between living and dying, suggests that other factors are at play. For example, in the Denver DC-8 accident of 1961, the Rome Boeing 707 accident of 1962 and the Salt Lake City Boeing 727 accident of 1965, those people who sat nearest to the exits showed the best survival patterns. In other crashes, people have died because they chose to go to inoperable exits some way from their seats.

It is argued by some authors that to classify an accident as being survivable because some people live is dangerous. It is difficult to gauge how much truth there is in this. It is obvious that different intensities of impact force can be generated in the same crash. Where people sitting next to each other show different patterns of survivability, then this must indicate a failure of crashworthiness. A survivable accident may, therefore, be defined as one in which there is room for the occupant to exist and the impact forces generated and transmitted to the individual are tolerable.

Thus, every accident has to be considered on its own merits. It may be implied that non-survivable areas in the same accident should be judged based on whether they represent regions in which crashworthiness has failed and that the whole aircraft may, therefore, by suspect. Also, it underlines the need for designers to use the level at which major injuries occur as a criterion of desirable impact strength.

One feature that is particularly dangerous for pilots is the control column. This is of variable shape, being referred to by names such as 'yoke' and 'spectacle frame'. It may break easily, producing disabling or fatal injuries. Military pilots use a stick that is designed carefully to carry out many functions and such that it is not in a position to do a lot of damage. It is true that hand injuries may occur and that these can be very severe, but they are not likely to be life-threatening, although they ultimately disable if the thumb is lost. Traditionally, it has been argued that injuries to the web space between the thumb and forefinger in a pilot's hand is evidence of him or her being in control. This diagnosis must be approached cautiously, because such an injury may be caused in other ways, such as putting the hand up against the fascia of the instrument panel.

CAUSES OF DEATH

In an aviation accident, most people will die from the effects of mechanical trauma; others will succumb to fire and environmental factors. Fires kill either by burning or because of the effects of noxious fumes, which cause chemical asphyxia.

If the aircraft ditches or breaks up in the air and people fall into water, some of them may drown. This is often a difficult diagnosis and depends to a degree on the exclusion of other causes of death, such as injuries.

Where there is exposure to extremes of temperature, heat exhaustion or hypothermia may kill some people who otherwise would have survived. The effects of temperature are dealt with in Chapters 14 and 15.

Some people may die of natural causes such as myocardial infarction. The neurological effects of traumatic events in people who have severe heart disease have been well documented in the literature.

In all these cases, the diagnostic difficulties are profound and can have serious medicolegal effects. The possibility that a potential survivor has died may raise questions about the efficacy of any rescue operation. Such deaths may also indicate elements of neglect by other survivors. Accordingly, any such death may need special investigation and careful discussion with the coroner and police.

TOXICOLOGY

The toxicological investigation of tissue and fluid specimens from air accident victims requires a careful examination for the presence of prescription, over-the-counter and illicit drugs, substances of social use and abuse, environmental contaminants and toxins, as well as the detection and discrimination of artefactual changes such as the production of ethanol due to post-mortem fermentation. Ideally, the range of tests will be broad and the sensitivity at the therapeutic and subtherapeutic level. Since in many instances physical trauma is severe, toxicological examination may provide the only evidence of the existence of disease states that could produce subtle or sudden incapacitation, such as hypertension and epilepsy.

If possible, a central reference laboratory that has developed methods specific for air accident investigation as opposed to general forensic testing should carry out the examinations. A variety of tissues and fluids are required for successful testing. Due to the high impact forces involved, fluids often are not available, but adequate quantities of blood from two separate sites, sterile urine from an intact bladder, bile and vitreous humour should be obtained if possible.

The tests commonly performed on blood include qualitative and quantitative analyses for:

- ethyl alcohol
- other alcohols, solvents, fuels, hydraulic fluids, etc.
- carbon monoxide

- hydrogen cyanide
- delta-9-tetrahydrocannabinol (THC) and metabolites (marijuana)

and:

- gas chromatography–mass spectroscopy (GC–MS) screen and quantitation for drugs and metabolites, including illicit, prescribed and over-the-counter drugs
- GC–MS screen and quantitation of pesticides and herbicides
- enzyme-multiplied immunoassay technique (EMIT) analyses of drugs.

The tests commonly performed on urine include qualitative and quantitative analyses for:

- ethyl alcohol
- other alcohols and solvents

and:

- GC–MS screen for drugs and metabolites, including illicit, prescribed and over-the-counter drugs
- GC–MS screen for pesticides, herbicides, etc.
- EMIT screen for illicit drugs.

Tests commonly performed on liver and other tissue fluid extracts are as for blood tests.

Table 33.6 indicates the optimum sample sizes required by most laboratories.

Specimens should be uncontaminated if possible and preserved as indicated in Table 33.6. Prevention of bacterial or fungal growth is especially important in the examination for the presence of ethyl alcohol.

If possible, samples should be obtained from all accident victims. Specimens from passengers may serve as controls for samples obtained from flight crew and provide valuable evidence of, for example, the presence of fermentation-producing ethanol. Fire patterns may be discerned through the detection of distribution patterns in the levels of hydrogen cyanide or carbon monoxide in cabin attendants and passengers. Carbon monoxide in flight crew may suggest a causal contamination problem due possibly to faulty heat exchangers.

Victims of crop-spraying accidents should be screened for the presence of pesticides or herbicides and the inhibition of cholinesterase. Accident investigators should be warned of the dangers of contamination when investigating agricultural accidents and should be given adequate protective suits and equipment. They should also be tested if they experience symptoms.

Analytical methods

Because of the problems caused by the variable quality of specimens, it is important that robust methods of analysis are used. Headspace gas chromatography is used for ethanol analysis and screening for volatile compounds. Carbon monoxide may be measured by spectrophotometry using a CO-Oximeter (Instrumentation Laboratories (UK) Limited, Warrington, UK), but with contaminated samples or decomposed blood, gas chromatography or derivative spectrophotometry is required (Mayes 1993). Cyanide is separated from acidified blood by Conway diffusion and analysis is undertaken by colorimetry or gas chromatography.

A drug screen is undertaken on blood, urine or liver tissue using immunoassay and gas chromatography. Any drugs that are discovered are confirmed using gas chromatography with a flame-ionization or nitrogen/phosphorus detector. Mass-selective detection is essential in order to confirm the identity of some drugs. Appropriate internal and external quality-assurance programmes are essential.

Alcohol

POST-MORTEM PRODUCTION OF ALCOHOL

The problem of the production of alcohol in putrefying tissue has been investigated for many years. In a study from our department in 1968, it was shown that many organisms commonly found in the body at post-mortem examination were capable of the production of alcohol in blood. The production of alcohol in urine by bacteria was found

Table 33.6 *Samples for toxicological analysis*

Specimen	1% fluoride/oxalate preservative	EDTA anticoagulant	Plain, no preservative	Frozen
Blood	2 ml from two clean sites	5 ml	10 ml	–
Urine	2 ml	–	Remainder	–
Bile	2 ml	–	Remainder	–
Vitreous humour	2 ml	–	–	–
Stomach contents	–	–	All	–
Liver	–	–	–	100 g
Lung	–	–	–	100 g

EDTA, ethylenediaminetetraacetic acid.

to be unlikely to occur. It was also demonstrated that sodium fluoride at a concentration of not less than 10 mg/ml inhibited alcohol formation. Following an underground train disaster in London in 1975, Corry (1978) undertook an extensive review of the subject. She found that ethanol levels up to 150 mg/dl could be produced by putrefaction. This production of ethanol could occur within a relatively short time, especially when temperatures were elevated. The obvious signs of putrefaction may be evident in these cases.

A US study of nearly 1000 victims of aircraft accidents found that eight per cent had ethanol levels above 40 mg/dl. Of these, 27 per cent were from the post-mortem production of alcohol (Canfield *et al.* 1993). In 45 per cent, no conclusion could be reached regarding the origin of the alcohol. The authors reported one victim with a blood alcohol of more than 300 mg/dl.

This problem is best overcome by taking adequate samples in an appropriate preservative. Blood should be taken from at least two peripheral veins; urine and vitreous humour also should be taken. When urine is not available, bile is a suitable alternative. The levels of alcohol found in the samples analysed should be concordant. If they are not, then post-mortem production should be suspected. The samples may be cultured in order to demonstrate the presence of microorganisms capable of producing alcohol. Any organisms that are grown can be cultured in glucose broth to prove that they do produce alcohol. The simple technique of leaving the sample at room temperature for a week and repeating the analysis may help in resolving this problem. If alcohol-producing organisms are present, then the alcohol level normally will have increased in the intervening period.

When ethanol is produced by microbial action, higher alcohols are also produced. The presence of peaks of propanol and butanol in the chromatogram will suggest the possibility of bacterial production. It has been suggested that the ratio of 5-hydroxytryptophal (5-HTOL) to 5-hydroxyindoleacetic acid (5-HIAA) in the urine may be used as a marker of recent alcohol consumption. The rationale behind this marker is that the normal oxidative deamination of serotonin to 5-HIAA is disturbed after alcohol consumption, leading to the formation of a minor metabolite, 5-HTOL. The 5-HTOL is normally less than one per cent of the 5-HIAA levels, but recent ingestion of alcohol increases this proportion. We have no experience with this technique, but it is possible that it could become a tool in the investigation of problem cases.

Even when appropriate samples are taken, the interpretation of post-mortem alcohol analyses may be difficult and sometimes inconclusive.

ALCOHOL AND PILOT PERFORMANCE

The intoxicating effects of alcohol have been known for thousands of years. The dangers of drinking and driving are now so well known that it may be considered self-evident that drinking and flying are also incompatible. Aviators operate complex machines in three dimensions and, therefore, slight or subtle errors on the part of the pilot are potentially more serious than for the intoxicated car driver. There have been many studies on the effects of alcohol on pilot performance, but only one has studied the effects on pilots flying real aircraft. The pilots were accompanied by a qualified flying instructor and were tested at various blood alcohol levels (40, 80 and 120 mg/dl). None of the blood alcohol levels was compatible with flight safety, and all pilots showed an increase in procedural errors compared with their performance in the alcohol-free state. Not surprisingly, this study has never been repeated, but simulator studies have confirmed the findings.

The performance of pilots has been shown to be impaired with blood alcohol levels as low as 11 mg/dl. It has also been shown that the number and severity of the errors rises in proportion to the level of alcohol in the blood. Cook (1997) lists a number of adverse effects on the performance of aircrew tasks that may be attributable to alcohol (Table 33.7).

POST-ALCOHOL IMPAIRMENT

Many people are aware that their performance is impaired after their blood alcohol might be expected to have returned to zero following heavy consumption of alcohol. This is known colloquially as a hangover and more cor-

Table 33.7 *Adverse effects on pilot performance attributable to alcohol*

Blood alcohol (mg/dl)	Impaired task performance
10–30	Terrain separation Aircraft descent Performance during angular acceleration With or without dim lighting
30–50	Management of heavy workload Tracking radio signals Target tracking Airport traffic control vectoring Flight coordination and configuration Traffic observation and avoidance Complex coordination Short-term memory Reaction time Performance during linear acceleration (5 G_z)
50–120	Progressively larger and more consistent impairment of all the above Oculovestibular function Performance during linear acceleration (3 G_z)

From Cook (1997).

rectly as post-alcohol impairment. However, it is difficult to find an objective measurement of this state that could be used in the investigation of aviation fatalities. A number of studies have shown measurable impairment of simulator performance as long as 14 hours after a peak alcohol level of 100 mg/dl. Post alcohol-impairment is potentially capable of causing aircraft accidents after the pilot is, according to most regulations, considered fit to fly. The mechanism for post-alcohol impairment may relate to the histotoxic hypoxic effect of alcohol. It has been suggested that alcohol is a histotoxic hypoxic agent and that it may be possible that, after alcohol is no longer detectable, there is residual impairment of oxygen metabolism, perhaps of the cytochrome oxidase system.

Another way in which alcohol may affect performance after it is no longer detectable in the blood is through a phenomenon known as positional alcohol nystagmus. This is a manifestation of labyrinthine involvement and may occur without external stimulation such as angular rotation. Positional alcohol nystagmus may be manifest 34 hours after alcohol stimulation, long after alcohol is no longer measurable in the blood. Positional alcohol nystagmus could cause impairment with dangerous implications for a pilot. It has been shown that increased gravitational forces could provoke positional alcohol nystagmus up to 48 hours after ingestion. This was due not to a toxic effect of alcohol on the labyrinth but to a physical phenomenon. Alcohol alters the specific gravity of the endolymph, which may cause or contribute to abnormal vestibular function. Positional alcohol nystagmus may have serious significance for a pilot who may be subject to disorientating conditions of poor visual reference. The true extent to which positional alcohol nystagmus affects a pilot's performance and contributes to accidents is still unclear.

REGULATIONS RELATING TO ALCOHOL AND AVIATION

The Federal Aviation Regulations in the USA state that no person may operate an aircraft within eight hours of having consumed alcohol, while under the influence of alcohol or with a blood alcohol content of 0.04 per cent (40 mg/dl) or greater. In many other countries, the regulations are less specific. For instance, in the UK, the regulations state that 'a person shall not, when acting as a member of the crew of any aircraft, be under the influence of drink or a drug to such an extent as to impair his capacity so to act' (Air Navigation Order (no. 2) 1995). Pilots are advised that they should not fly for at least eight hours after drinking small amounts of alcohol. They are also informed of the effects on the inner ear and the increased susceptibility to disorientation and motion sickness. They are told 'it would be prudent for a pilot to abstain from alcohol for at least 24 hours before flying'. If this advice was taken, then nobody flying an aircraft should have any detectable alcohol in his or her blood. The Joint Aviation Authorities, the European aviation authority, have ruled that it is illegal to act as a member of a flight crew with a blood alcohol greater than 20 mg/dl. This level has been introduced into British law.

Findings in aviation accidents

In our department, ethanol has been measured in all air-crew fatalities since the early 1960s. Because of the destruction involved in accidents, blood has not been always available. In these circumstances, attempts are made to use urine, vitreous humour, bile or other suitable fluids for the analysis. Early cases were analysed using dichromate reduction methods or enzymatic techniques. Gas-chromatographic methods were introduced in the late 1960s.

Alcohol has been discovered in the blood of ten per cent of pilots from fatal accidents. A small number of pilots whose blood alcohol was less than 8 mg/dl or whose blood was not available for analysis had urine alcohol levels between 10 and 40 mg/dl. In no case was the urine alcohol found to be greater than 40 mg/dl without alcohol being discovered in the blood. Table 33.8 shows the levels of alcohol discovered in pilots.

The number of analyses that were ascribed positively to ante-mortem ingestion was slightly less than 30 per cent of the total. For levels above 40 mg/dl, nearly 70 per cent were ascribed to ingestion. These findings are in broad agreement with those in the USA (Canfield et al. 1993), where 27 per cent of alcohol measurements over 40 mg/dl were due to post-mortem alcohol production. Where doubt existed in these analyses, the cases were classified with the artefacts.

Table 33.8 *Alcohol discovered in pilots*

Blood alcohol (mg/dl)	Urine alcohol (mg/dl)	% of cases where alcohol found	% of positive alcohols due to artefact	% of positive alcohols due to ingestion
< 8	10–40	13.4	7.1	6.2
8–19		39.3	36.6	5.4
20–39		19.7	15.2	3.6
40–79		11.6	7.1	2.7
80–150		8.9	2.7	6.2
> 151		7.1	1.8	5.4

A number of cases showed alcohol in the urine when little or none was present in the blood. The presence of alcohol in the urine usually indicates ante-mortem ingestion, as there is not normally an appropriate substrate from which the microorganisms can produce alcohol. However, in severe putrefaction in the pelvic area, alcohol may diffuse into the urine from the surrounding tissues. Ten per cent of the bodies in which a raised urine alcohol was deemed to be due to artefact had been recovered from the sea. It seems that the anaerobic conditions encountered, coupled with the delay in the recovery of the body, facilitate the diffusion of alcohol into the urine from adjacent putrefying tissue.

In 3.7 per cent of general aviation accidents, the pilots had a blood alcohol level greater than 20 mg/dl. In some of the accidents, there were two pilots on board of whom both had blood alcohol levels over 20 mg/dl. In the USA, Canfield et al. (2001) report alcohol levels greater than 40 mg/dl in seven per cent of 1683 fatal civil aircraft accidents between 1994 and 1998. Three per cent of our cases had levels greater than 40 mg/dl. The discovery of any evidence of ante-mortem ingestion of alcohol by pilots means that they have ignored the 'eight-hour rule'.

One unusual finding in this study was that six pilots had clearly been drinking and flying – concurrently rather consecutively! Evidence for this was the discovery of bottles of spirits in the cockpit and, in some cases, discovery of alcohol in the stomach. The blood alcohol levels in these cases ranged from 135 mg/dl to 325 mg/dl. Two of these cases had a history that might lead to the conclusion that the crash was deliberate. These have been included in the discussion of suicide. However, the behaviour of the other pilots was so reckless as to suggest that self-destruction may have been a deliberate or subconscious reason for the crash.

In two other cases, the passenger seated alongside the pilot had raised blood alcohol levels (139 mg/dl and 116 mg/dl). While there was no suggestion in either case that these passengers may have interfered with the pilot's flying, the possibility that this could happen must be considered.

Alcohol may be a factor in three to four per cent of general aviation accidents in the UK. Despite the reduction in the rate of alcohol-related accidents from the 16 per cent of 20 years ago, it is important that efforts to educate pilots about the dangers of flying after alcohol consumption are not relaxed. It is important that pilots are told that blood alcohol levels may still be raised the day after an evening's heavy drinking. Only by education can this cause of accidents be eliminated.

Carbon monoxide and cyanide

Carbon monoxide and cyanide are found in fire atmospheres, and carbon monoxide is produced during incomplete combustion. Carbon monoxide binds to haemoglobin to form carboxyhaemoglobin. Carbon monoxide has an affinity for haemoglobin about 200 times higher than that of oxygen, and so a comparatively low level of carbon monoxide in the inhaled air will produce a comparatively high level of carboxyhaemoglobin. This may give rise to tissue hypoxia.

The concentration of carbon monoxide in the blood is expressed as the percentage of haemoglobin saturated with carbon monoxide. A small amount, usually less than one per cent, is produced during haem catabolism. This may rise to five per cent in haemolytic anaemia. Increases in carboxyhaemoglobin are almost always the result of inhalation of smoke from fires, including cigarette smoke, vehicle exhaust fumes and poorly maintained heating appliances. Carboxyhaemoglobin has a half-life of four to five hours and is eliminated through the lungs. The half-life can be reduced to about one hour by breathing pure oxygen and still further by breathing hyperbaric oxygen.

The spectrophotometric method of measurement depends on the comparison of carboxyhaemoglobin to reduced haemoglobin. Any oxyhaemoglobin that is present is reduced before analysis. Very low levels of haemoglobin in the fluids analysed increase the likelihood of an artificially raised carboxyhaemoglobin. With aged or putrefied post-mortem blood, the resistance of some of the haemoglobin pigments to conversion to reduced haemoglobin may invalidate these methods. In these circumstances, gas chromatography is the only reliable method.

Gas-chromatographic methods depend on the release of carbon monoxide from lysed blood using a releasing agent. The carbon monoxide is released into the headspace, where it is measured using a gas chromatograph with a thermal conductivity or flame ionization detector. The volume of carbon monoxide that would be released from a fully saturated specimen can then be measured directly or calculated from the haemoglobin or iron content of the sample.

Concentrations of carboxyhaemoglobin in non-smokers may be as high as three per cent, while smokers may achieve levels up to ten per cent (Mayes 1993). Thus, ten per cent saturation is a useful cut-off to separate those who have inhaled toxic atmospheres from those who have not. Carbon monoxide displaces oxygen from haemoglobin and also shifts the oxygen dissociation curve to the left, resulting in a reduced ability of haemoglobin to release oxygen. The fatal threshold for fire deaths has been taken as 50 per cent, but fatalities occur with saturations ranging from 10 to 90 per cent. In these circumstances, it is clear that the mode of death cannot always be ascribed to hypoxia. Under conditions of high carbon monoxide concentration in inhaled air, the toxic effect of carbon monoxide may operate at the cellular level by inhibiting the cytochrome systems.

Hydrogen cyanide disrupts mitochondrial electron transfer and inhibits cytochrome oxidase, affecting cellular respiration. Low concentrations may be found in the blood of normal people as a result of normal metabolism or smoking. Hydrogen cyanide is liberated by fires with high temperatures and may exert a very rapid incapacitating effect. Measurement of cyanide in the blood depends on the release of gaseous hydrogen cyanide following acidification, which is measured using gas chromatography or colorimetry. A considerable delay between death and post-mortem examination may lead to significant loss of cyanide from the blood by a number of mechanisms. These losses may continue in the laboratory but can be minimized by storage in a deep freezer. The formation of cyanide by the metabolism of microorganisms can be prevented by preservation with 1% sodium fluoride. In the bodies of people who have not inhaled combustion products, the cyanide levels discovered are usually less than 0.22 mg/l. In deaths that have occurred during fires, the levels are greater than 2.7 mg/l.

Fire was associated with the accident in 25.3 per cent of our cases. However, the rates of fire varied widely with the different types of flying. Passenger-carrying aircraft had the highest rate of post-crash fires, with 55.3 per cent of accidents being followed by fire. The comparable rates for other types of flying were as follows: helicopters 31.3 per cent, military fast jet aircraft 29.1 per cent, and light fixed-wing aircraft 27.2 per cent. In those accidents without fire, only ten per cent of victims had measured carboxyhaemoglobin levels greater than one per cent. The levels achieved are shown in Table 33.9.

In cases with levels greater than ten per cent, it was deemed that 62.5 per cent were due to artefact on account of the poor quality of the samples. Some dated from before the advent of gas chromatography and others were dilute, with very low haemoglobin levels. The genuine levels pointed to defective exhaust systems and, in one case, a perforated cockpit heater.

Thirty per cent of the crew of aircraft crashes that were followed by fire had carboxyhaemoglobin levels greater than one per cent. Most had died of their injuries and did not have raised levels. The findings are shown in Table 33.10.

When the cases included in Table 33.10 are limited to those in which the cause of death was attributed to the fire, seven per cent remain. These findings are detailed in Table 33.11.

Aircraft fires are particularly intense, and the cockpit integrity may be maintained until the fire has destroyed it. Victims trapped in aircraft fires frequently die of thermal injury or anoxia resulting from the consumption of oxygen by the fire. Half the cases of crew dying of the fire had carboxyhaemoglobin levels less than ten per cent.

Drugs of abuse

With the worldwide increase in the use of drugs of abuse, it is essential that pilots and other crew be examined for their presence following a fatal accident. Blood or urine should be screened using immunoassay. Any positive results should be confirmed using gas chromatography and mass-selective detection. Only in this way can cross-reactions be eliminated. For instance, pholcodine gives a positive reaction for opiates in the screening test. When the presence of an illicit drug has been confirmed, it should, if possible, be quantitated in both blood and urine.

In our department, screening is undertaken to detect the presence of the following drugs of abuse:

- barbiturates
- cocaine

Table 33.9 *Distribution of carboxyhaemoglobin levels greater than one per cent in accidents without fire*

Carboxyhaemoglobin level (%)	% of cases
1.1–2.0	41.6
2.1–3.0	19.5
3.1–4.0	13.3
4.1–5.0	9.9
5.1–6.0	4.8
6.1–7.0	4.8
7.1–8.0	1.4
8.1–9.0	1.0
9.1–10.0	1.0
> 10	2.7

Table 33.10 *Distribution of carboxyhaemoglobin levels greater than one per cent in crew of accidents with fire*

Carboxyhaemoglobin level (%)	% of cases
< 5.0	69.1
5.1–10.0	18.2
10.1–15.0	7.6
15.1–20.0	1.4
20.1–30.0	3.3
> 30	0.4

Table 33.11 *Distribution of carboxyhaemoglobin levels in aircrew dying of burning in accidents with fire*

Carboxyhaemoglobin level (%)	% of cases
< 5.0	31.2
5.1–10.0	18.8
10.1–15.0	27.1
15.1–20.0	6.2
20.1–30.0	14.6
> 30	2.1

- phencyclidine
- methadone
- benzodiazepines
- opiates
- amphetamines
- cannabinoids
- lysergic acid diethylamide (LSD).

In an analysis of the findings in the USA, Canfield *et al.* (2001) examined 1683 fatal aviation accidents. Controlled drugs were found on 138 occasions. Some of these were positive for more than one type of drug, and 159 drugs were detected. The major drugs listed are shown in Table 33.12.

People take drugs in order to induce a state of euphoria or to heighten their sensations. The drugs act as stimulants or depressants or may alter the individual's perception of their environment. Any of these effects are incompatible with aviation, as they may have a profound influence on a pilot's ability to fly his or her aircraft properly. Flying under the influence of drugs is expressly forbidden by the Air Navigation Order (ANO (no. 2) 1995). The psychoactive drugs that are abused can be divided into five classes.

- psychedelics and hallucinogens, including cannabis, LSD and substituted amphetamines
- stimulants and convulsants, such as cocaine, amphetamines and clinical antidepressants
- sedatives and hypnotics, including barbiturates and benzodiazepines
- narcotic analgesics, such as opium and heroin
- antipsychotic agents, such as the phenothiazines.

CANNABIS (MARIJUANA)

Cannabis is neither a stimulant nor a depressant. It can be regarded as a psychedelic drug. It impairs cognitive process in the working memory. It also affects divided attention and perceptual motor performance involving tasks such as fine motor performance and target tracking. Simpler motor skills are not affected. Impairment is therefore likely in the complex environment of aviation. Pilots were studied in a flight simulator after taking a moderate social dose of marijuana (Leirer *et al.* 1991). There was evidence of

Table 33.12 *Controlled drugs found in aviation accidents in the USA, 1994–98*

Drug	n	%
Marijuana	43	31.2
Benzodiazepines	33	23.9
Codeine/morphine	17	12.3
Cocaine	13	9.4
Barbiturates	9	6.5
Synthetic opiates	6	4.3
Amphetamines	6	4.3

impaired performance of flying tasks up to 24 hours after smoking the marijuana. The user was unaware of the effects of the drug. The drug dose, the delay between taking the drug and flying, the age of the pilot, and the complexity of the task all affect the pilot's performance. Importantly, these variables produced cumulative effects.

A problem that arises with cannabis is the interpretation of the concentrations discovered in the urine or blood. The concentration in the blood or serum is much lower than the tissue concentration, and after smoking the cannabis is released from the tissue and excreted in the urine. This release may be slow, and cannabis may be detected in the urine up to three weeks after it was taken and long after it had any effect on performance. The active ingredient of cannabis is THC. However, this is metabolized in the liver to 11-hydroxy-THC and then to THC-carboxylic acid. The former is active but the acid is not. Research to evaluate the significance of all of the metabolites in intoxication is being undertaken at a number of laboratories, but it has not yet proved possible to use any measurement as an index of intoxication in the same way that the blood alcohol level is used to measure intoxication due to alcohol.

Cannabis is commonly smoked with tobacco in cigarettes known as reefers. In the absence of any objective measure of intoxication, we have used the concentrations of carbon monoxide and nicotine and its metabolites as an indication of recent smoking. While nicotine and carbon monoxide are raised after smoking conventional cigarettes, we have taken increases in these compounds, when they accompany raised levels of cannabis metabolites, to indicate recent cannabis ingestion.

OTHER DRUGS OF ABUSE

The pharmacological effects of other drugs of abuse are well known. They have been found rarely in pilots involved in accidents in the UK. Of the 523 general aviation pilots in our study, only eight had controlled drugs discovered on toxicological examination: four cannabis, three amphetamines and one barbiturates. The British experience does not mirror the US findings (see Table 33.12). However, it is likely that the increasing use of recreational drugs will mean that more of these cases will occur in the future.

PRESCRIPTION-ONLY AND OVER-THE-COUNTER DRUGS

Prescription-only and over-the-counter drugs are being detected with increasing frequency. Canfield *et al.* (2001) report that over a five-year period, such drugs were detected in 32.1 per cent of the 1683 pilots tested, compared with 17.2 per cent over the previous five-year period. Prescription-only drugs were found in 14 per cent and over-the-counter drugs in 18 per cent. Drugs were detected about twice as often in private pilots when compared with commercial pilots. The most common drugs found are listed in Table 33.13.

Table 33.13 *Most common drugs found in fatal US aviation accidents*

Drug detected	No. of times detected
Salicylates	114
Pseudoephedrine	84
Phenylpropanolamine	82
Paracetamol	81
Diphenhydramine	54
Ephedrine	47
Chlorpheniramine	44
Benzodiazepines	33

The UK tends to lag behind the USA, and in this series drugs were found in three per cent of the pilots tested. The division between the various groups of pilots is not surprising: 1.6 per cent of military pilots tested positively for these categories of drugs, compared with 1.7 per cent of commercial pilots, 4.6 per cent of private pilots and 6.2 per cent of glider or micro-light pilots. The pattern of drugs detected in the UK is similar to the US experience, the most common being analgesics followed by decongestants, antihistamines and benzodiazepines.

The detection of any drug raises two important questions. Did the drug cause or contribute to the cause of the accident, or is its discovery entirely coincidental? The corollary is did the disease for which the drug is being taken cause or contribute to the cause of the accident, or is it entirely coincidental? These questions can be very difficult to answer. A particular problem is faced by the discovery of first-generation antihistamines, which may cause drowsiness and impair the pilot's ability to fly his or her aircraft properly. They are frequently taken for colds and upper respiratory tract infections, which may, because of their effect on the ear, give rise to an increased tendency to disorientation.

CROP-SPRAYING ACCIDENTS

The aerial application of insecticides, weed-control chemicals, defoliants and fertilizers is common. Many chemicals used for these purposes are highly toxic and can cause illness and death. Aircraft accidents have occurred because of impairment caused by exposure to these substances. To understand the problems that may arise from crop spraying, it is essential to understand the toxic potential of the various chemicals used.

Organophosphorus insecticides are toxic to both insects and humans by their inhibition of acetylcholinesterase enzymes within the nervous system. They have toxic effects on the central nervous system. Early symptoms of poisoning include giddiness, restlessness, blurred vision and respiratory depression. Death may follow. Plasma cholinesterase measurements are useful as indicators of exposure. Carbamate insecticides may cause similar signs and symptoms, but the effect does not last as long. Red-cell cholinesterase measurements may be used to assess the extent of the exposure. Chlorinated insecticides such as dieldrin and dichlorodiphenyltrichloroethane (DDT) are rarely used nowadays because of their toxicity on the central nervous system. Chlorinated herbicides have low toxicity for humans, as shown by the use by the USA of the herbicide Agent Orange during the Vietnam war. Nitrophenols produce thirst, excessive sweating, euphoria and fatigue. They have no antidote. The toxicity of paraquat is well known.

Agricultural pilots in countries of the former Soviet Union are required to maintain a logbook that records the specific chemicals used during crop-spraying and the duration of the exposure. These records are valuable should the pilot develop symptoms that may be due to exposure to the chemicals used. In only one of the eight crop-spraying accidents investigated by our department was a reduced level of cholinesterase discovered in the pilot. The chemical involved, demeton-S-methyl, was also demonstrated in the pilot's blood. The cause of the accident was unexplained, but it seemed possible that incapacitation could have played a part in its causation. Three of the salvage workers became ill because of the toxic effects of the chemical. It is important that rescuers and salvage workers are made aware of the potential harmful effects of agricultural chemicals to which they may be exposed when they are dealing with the aftermath of an accident involving a crop-spraying aircraft.

Causes of accidents

Aviation accidents rarely have single causes. Usually, they are caused by a combination of factors, each of which on its own would not cause an accident. In attempting to classify the causes of aircraft accidents, it is common practice to use the initial or main cause of the accident. If this is done, then human factors become the single most important cause of accidents.

An analysis of commercial jet accidents over a ten-year period (1988–97) showed that 70 per cent of the accidents with known causes were due to flight crew factors, compared with ten per cent for aircraft factors and six per cent for maintenance factors. Another analysis of all aircraft accidents from a database including general aviation recorded human error as a cause in 47 per cent of accidents. The bulk of the human-error accidents were due to crew errors. These human errors include failure to monitor instruments and errors of judgement. Pilot incapacitation was thought to be a main cause in only one per cent of accidents.

The cost of commercial aircraft hull and liability losses runs at about US$1.5 billion each year. General aviation losses are difficult to quantify but must be large. In the USA, about 350 general aviation aircraft are lost each year in fatal accidents. The cost of the aircraft alone must account for at least US$35 million. The losses in human life are similarly large.

Aviation pathology has two goals. The first is to identify the cause of an aircraft accident and to try to remove similar causes in order to prevent future accidents. However, accidents are going to occur despite our best efforts, and so the second aim is to identify the causes of death in accidents, to relate these to the safety equipment provided and hopefully to prevent future fatalities by modifying this equipment. The pathological investigation of accidents must always address these two aims.

REFERENCES

Booze CF. Sudden in-flight incapacitation in general aviation. *Aviation, Space, and Environmental Medicine* 1989; **60**: 332–5.

Busby DE, Davis AW. Paroxysmal and chronic atrial fibrillation and airman certification. *Aviation, Space, and Environmental Medicine* 1976; **47**: 185–6.

Canfield DV, Kupiec T, Huffine E. Post-mortem alcohol production in fatal aircraft accidents. *Journal of Forensic Sciences* 1993; **38**: 914–17.

Canfield DV, Hordinsky J, Millett DP, Endecott B, Smith D. Drugs and alcohol found in fatal civil aviation accidents between 1994 and 1998. *Aviation, Space, and Environmental Medicine* 2001; **72**: 120–24.

Cook CHC. Alcohol and flying. *Addiction* 1997; **92**: 539–55.

Corry JEL. Possible sources of ethanol ante- and post-mortem: its relationship to the biochemistry and microbiology of decomposition. *Journal of Applied Microbiology* 1978; **44**: 1–56.

Detlef G, Ast F-W, Tröger HD, Kleeman WJ. Unexpected findings in the investigation of an airplane crash. *Forensic Science International* 1999; **104**: 189–94.

Leirer VO, Yesavage JA, Morrow DG. Marijuana carry-over effects on aircraft pilot performance. *Aviation, Space, and Environmental Medicine* 1991; **62**: 221–7.

McCormick TJ, Lyons TJ. Medical causes of in-flight incapacitation: USAF experience 1978–1987. *Aviation, Space, and Environmental Medicine* 1991; **62**: 884–7.

Martin-Saint-Laurent A, Lavernhe J, Casano G, Simkoff A. Clinical aspects of in-flight incapacitations in commercial aviation. *Aviation, Space, and Environmental Medicine* 1990; **61**: 256–60.

Mason JK. *Aviation Accident Pathology*. London: Butterworths, 1962.

Mäulen B, Faust, V. Suizid mit dem Flugzeug. *Münchener Medizinische Wochenschrift* 1990; **132**: 572–4.

Mayes RW. Measurement of carbon monoxide and cyanide in blood. *Journal of Clinical Pathology* 1993; **46**: 982–8.

Rivora P, Thompson DC, Thompson RS. Bicycle helmets: it's time to use them. *British Medical Journal* 2000; **321**: 1035–6.

Stevens PJ. *Fatal Civil Aircraft Accidents*. Bristol: John Wright, 1970.

Stevens PJ, Underwood-Ground KEA. Occurrence and significance of myocarditis in trauma. *Aerospace Medicine* 1970; **41**: 776–80.

Toff WD, Joy M, Camm AJ. Exercise induced arrhythmia. *European Heart Journal* 1988; **9** (suppl. G): 119–26.

Ungs TJ. Suicide by use of aircraft in the United States, 1979–1989. *Aviation, Space, and Environmental Medicine* 1994; **65**: 953–6.

34

Aircraft hygiene

MICHAEL J. KELLY

INTRODUCTION

It is less than 100 years since commercial aviation began, and yet flying has become so much a part of everyday life that few people boarding an aircraft belonging to any international airline would ever consider that the aircraft could be a vehicle of infection. However, infection can arise in many ways. It can be food-borne, waterborne or transmitted by flying insects or rodents, and it may be encouraged by the incorrect handling and disposal of waste. Of these, food-borne illness is the most important, if only by virtue of the large quantities of food that have to be provided on aircraft daily on a worldwide basis.

IN-FLIGHT CATERING

In-flight catering is usually supplied by contractors who operate custom-built premises situated on, or adjacent to, airports. They are often companies whose main business is in-flight catering and who will supply any type of food, ranging from simple beverages and biscuits to six-course dinners. The menu is normally chosen by the airline, which takes into account the food available locally and the ability of the caterer to produce food to acceptable culinary and hygienic standards.

It could be said that from the hygiene point of view, airline catering is its own worst enemy. Since competition between airlines often relates to standards of service, there is considerable pressure to produce haute cuisine from those parts of the world least able to supply it, in terms not only of culinary expertise but also of hygiene.

Nevertheless, the record of in-flight catering over the years has been good, with the number of recorded incidents of illness related to the consumption of airline food being small in relation to the millions of meals served annually on aircraft worldwide.

Flight catering units differ considerably in terms of size, daily output and facilities, but the basic requirements are the same for all of them. These include the need to provide a flow pattern for food and equipment through the premises, which will separate raw products from cooked products and clean from dirty equipment, together with an environment that provides hard surfaces that can be well-maintained and are cleaned easily. A potable water system must be provided, allied to an efficient drainage and waste-disposal system. Hygienic handling and processing of foodstuffs utilizing modern methods of control are essential if safe food is to be produced. Modern methods follow the principles of hazard analysis and critical control points (HACCP). This system, designed originally in the 1960s for the National Aeronautics and Space Administration (NASA) space programme, requires that the caterer identifies hazards associated with the handling of food. These fall into three basic groups: bacterial survival, bacterial growth, and contamination of the product by physical or chemical means. The system makes use of a flow diagram of food and equipment from point of entry into the building through to the dispatch of food to the aircraft.

From this flowchart, each step in the operation can be defined. Hazards can be identified along with the controls needed to reduce or eliminate them. A decision must also be made as to whether the control in place at that point is critical to the safety of the food. The control is designated as critical if no subsequent step in the operation will either remove the hazard completely or reduce it to a level that will not cause a problem to the ultimate consumer. For example, cooking raw food to pasteurization temperature is critical for the removal of heat-sensitive organisms such as *Salmonella* spp., since if the cooked item is going to be used as a cold meal ingredient there will be no control subsequent to the cooking that would remove the organism. Similarly, the rapid cooling of food after cooking has taken place will greatly reduce the possibility of heat-resistant organisms such as *Clostridium perfringens* proliferating to an extent that will cause subsequent food poisoning.

Once the controls have been identified, critical limits must be put in place for each of them, e.g. it may be decided that a pasteurization temperature of 72°C for 15 seconds is desirable for the cooking of some meat products. Similarly, upper limits for cold-food handling may be defined, e.g. 15°C for not more than 45 minutes.

Measurements must then be taken for each batch of food passing through the system in order to ensure that the critical limits are being complied with. These measurements must be recorded and should be verified on a regular basis by the management team within the kitchen.

Training of all food-handling staff in the principles of food safety, and in particular HACCP, is essential in the promotion of safety of the prepared product. In theory the use of a HACCP programme should be fairly simple, but in practice it can be a difficult system to install and to operate consistently and correctly. This may be due in part to the conditions in which the catering premises are situated. In developing countries, there may be endemic diseases and lack of basic services and modern equipment essential for safe food production. Some problems are simply the result of poor management. The introduction of HACCP in the flight catering industry has required a change in culture. The HACCP system is designed to record those temperatures, for example, that are correct and within preset parameters, and to ensure that, when the parameters are not being met, the records reflect this accurately so that corrective action can be taken, not only with the individual product on the day in question but also with the entire system. This ensures that hazards that have been identified are eliminated where necessary by a change in the method of production.

Food handlers, including chefs, normally are not used to writing down the results of their actions, particularly if the measurements that they are taking are obviously in breach of the preset parameters. It is essential, therefore, that the training of the staff involved highlights the need for accuracy while at the same time ensuring that they do not feel that they will become scapegoats in instances when the parameters are breached.

To ensure that standards are maintained, it is necessary for all flight catering units to be audited regularly. This should be carried out using a recognized audit procedure such as that of the International Standards Organization (ISO). The audit will include auditing systems and procedures in use within the premises via a 'paper' exercise, and checking methods of internal auditing, monitoring practices, processes, temperature control and use of equipment. All or part of the premises must be inspected to ascertain whether the theory espoused by the management is in fact being carried out in the food-handling areas. The records required to establish that a flight kitchen complies with a good HACCP programme include the specification of raw material requirements to external suppliers; the monitoring of raw materials delivered to the kitchen with respect to quality, quantity, date-coding and temperature to prevent receipt of any substandard raw material; the daily monitoring of temperatures in cold rooms, refrigerators and deep-freeze units; the measurement of core temperature attained in the cooking of high-risk food items such as poultry; the temperature attained by food passed through the blast-chilling equipment after cooking, and the time taken to reach that temperature; maintenance of the chill chain through the kitchen and on to the aircraft; a written cleaning schedule showing areas and items to be cleaned, with the frequency of cleaning and methods to be used and the name of the person responsible for ensuring that the necessary work has been completed to a correct standard; medical screening records of food handlers; and the level of training attained by each food handler.

Changes in the flight catering industry in recent years have meant that in many kitchens, a large number of the meals produced are not cooked within the premises but are purchased ready prepared from outside suppliers. In such instances, it is essential that the external supplier also operates a recognizable and verifiable food-safety programme of the HACCP type in order that the provenance and safety of the food can be guaranteed from its initial handling as a raw product through to delivery as a ready-to-eat (RTE) item at the flight catering unit. In such cases, the flight kitchen has become an assembly unit rather than a manufacturer, but nonetheless it carries responsibility for the safety of the product that is being offered to the airline. The audit of the flight kitchen in this case would include a verification of the auditing of the initial manufacturer of the product.

On completion of the audit of the flight kitchen, it may be necessary to adopt recommendations for improvement. These should be agreed with the unit management at a debriefing session, and specified timescales for completion of remedial work should be agreed at this time. If the audit is particularly poor, and assuming that catering must be provided, then it may be necessary to change the catering arrangement. Often, the best solution is to design a new menu to eliminate high-risk food items, such as shellfish, cold meats and egg mayonnaise, and it may be possible to supply frozen RTE items from another kitchen. Once the recommendations for improvement have been adopted and samples of food have been examined microbiologically and found to be satisfactory, then a full unrestricted menu may be reinstated. However, continued vigilance is essential in order to ensure that standards do not lapse.

Food handling in airline catering is no different from that in any other form of catering and demands hygienic working practices and temperature control of the food through its production, storage and distribution chain. To avoid growth of food-poisoning organisms, cold meals should be stored at temperatures below 10°C and hot meals above 63°C if maintained hot from point of cooking to service. Alternatively, hot meals can be blast-chilled to a temperature below 5°C and then handled as a cold meal before being reheated in the aircraft oven just before service. The cold chain must be continued from the flight kitchen to the aircraft and followed up on board by the storage of food at temperatures ranging from 2 to 7°C until served. Ovens in the aircraft should be able to raise the temperature of chilled meals to at least 72°C.

With modern refrigeration equipment, temperature control within the flight kitchen should pose few problems. Transportation to the aircraft may, however, pose some difficulties, particularly in hot climates, and it may be necessary to use refrigerated lorries or to refrigerate the aircraft trolleys by using solid carbon dioxide (dry ice) as slabs or pellets loaded into the aircraft with them. Hot meals may be delivered to the aircraft either as preheated items for smaller aircraft that do not have ovens or as chilled items to be reheated in electric convection ovens on board. Safe transportation of preheated foods may be jeopardized if the aircraft departure time is delayed once the food has been loaded, even though such food normally is stored in polyurethane boxes, which help to maintain the temperature.

Microbiological examination of samples of food from flight kitchens should be used as a verification of the HACCP programmes in use. Samples should be taken initially from the end product and then, where necessary, from raw materials or from products during processing and handling. Caterers should be encouraged to set up their own microbiological testing programmes rather than to rely on their customer airlines to carry out such assessments.

WATER SUPPLIES

Drinking water on a modern aircraft is stored in stainless-steel or reinforced fibre-glass tanks built into the aircraft structure and from which the water is fed by gravity or pumped to the galleys, sink taps, wash hand basins and drinking points. The water is supplied via a fill point on the belly of the aircraft and is fed either directly from the main airport water supply by hose pipe or, more often, via a self-propelled tanker.

To avoid infection by contaminated water, it is essential that the water supply comes from an uncontaminated source and is suitable for drinking purposes. It is essential that the water supply point is maintained in a sanitary condition; to ensure this, it should be kept covered and locked to avoid uncontrolled use for other purposes. The drinking point should be labelled 'for aircraft drinking water use only'.

Although the main water supply at the airport may be potable and suitable for drinking use, the transfer of water from the main supply to the aircraft gives rise to a possible risk of contamination. It is important, therefore, that the water supply is treated using a suitable chemical such as chlorine. This may be used in the form of sodium hypochlorite (bleach) or, more commonly, in the form of a combined chemical such as chloramine-T or chlorine dioxide. Chloramine-T is more stable than chlorine, is completely tasteless at the manufacturer's recommended-use concentration (16 mg/l, equivalent to 4 ppm available chlorine due to the chemical makeup of the product), and has been used for many years by a number of major airlines.

Chlorine dioxide has two advantages: it will destroy the biofilm that builds up on the inside of the water tanks of both the aircraft and the water tankers, and it is effective against *Cryptosporidium*.

Recent changes have seen the introduction of hydrogen peroxide combined with silver as an alternative to chlorine-based products. The combination of hydrogen peroxide and silver ions destroys bacteria, viruses and fungi but has no effect on the environment, since the breakdown products are simply oxygen and water, the silver – usually present as a coating on the internal surface of the treatment vessel – remaining unchanged.

Whatever system is used, it must be readily detectable in the water system by means of a simple check procedure.

Water servicing normally will be carried out by ramp service staff and should follow a detailed written code of practice. This requires the regular and recorded sterilization of the water bowsers, aircraft tanks and pipe lines. Regular microbiological checks of the water at the fill point, in the water tankers and from aircraft should be carried out, with corrective action being taken when necessary.

DISPOSAL OF WASTE

Aircraft waste falls into four categories, namely food waste, dry waste, clinical waste and human waste. Food waste leaves the aircraft on the meal trays or in waste-food garbage trolleys and is delivered to the flight catering unit, where it is stripped and disposed of in the way in which local regulations demand, e.g. by incineration or disposal in deep landfill sites. During transportation to the catering unit and subsequent disposal, it must be sealed to avoid attracting pests. Dry waste (paper, rubbish, etc.) deposited in the passenger cabin during the flight is collected by the aircraft cleaners at the end of each flight sector, placed in polythene sacks, and disposed of through the normal airport waste-disposal system. Clinical waste is handled via identified biohazard bags, which are sealed, removed by the aircraft cleaners, and disposed of safely and correctly via contracted companies. Sharps are disposed of in sharps boxes provided on the aircraft either in the medical bag or in locked containers fitted in the toilets, with correct disposal being provided by contracted companies.

Human waste is contained in tanks on board the aircraft. Aircraft toilets come in two types. In older aircraft, the toilets are self-contained, with a large holding tank directly below the toilet, operating in much the same manner as a chemical toilet in a caravan. Flushing is provided by recirculating the liquid contents after filtration of the solids. The toilets are serviced at each stop, with the tanks being emptied, flushed and refilled to a predetermined level with a mixture of water and a chemical. The chemical is aromatic and coloured to disguise the toilet contents. It must also be an effective bactericide capable of killing pathogenic organisms within 15 minutes at 18–20°C and remaining effective at maximum dilution in a fully loaded toilet.

More modern aircraft have vacuum toilets in which the holding tanks are situated in the tail of the aircraft. Flushing is carried out by making use of the pressure differential outside the aircraft. The flush handle on the toilet operates a valve via which a vacuum is created and the toilet contents are sucked down a pipe to the holding tank at the rear. A small quantity of water is added to the toilet bowl during the flushing process, mainly as an aesthetic exercise. The toilet is constructed of stainless-steel, often with a non-stick Teflon™-coated surface.

Waste is emptied from the aircraft into waste-disposal tankers. These discharge the contents into the airport drainage system, usually at a disposal block provided with wash-down facilities and a macerator or coarse screen to remove solids. Care has to be taken in the handling of toilet waste and of the toilet and component parts. Strict controls must be enforced to ensure that customers, staff and any others are not exposed to any risk. It is also essential to ensure that staff members engaged in the handling of toilet waste do not handle aircraft drinking-water supplies during the same shift.

PEST CONTROL

Aircraft can harbour and carry numerous pests, including insects such as mosquitoes and cockroaches and rats and mice, which may be both disease-carrying and dangerous to the fabric of the aircraft. Control of such pests is essential in order to protect public health and to ensure passenger confidence. The transmission of illness by insects carried on board aircraft has long been recognized as a problem and is dealt with by the disinsection of aircraft, as laid down in the International Health Regulations 1969, published and amended by the World Health Organization (WHO 1969). Article 90(a) of these regulations states:

> Every aircraft leaving an airport situated in an area where transmission of malaria or other mosquito borne disease is occurring, or where insecticide resistant mosquito vectors of disease are present, or where a vector species is present that has been eradicated in the area where the airport of destination of the aircraft is situated shall be disinsected in accordance with Article 26, using the methods recommended by the Organization. States concerned shall accept disinsecting of aircraft by the approved method carried out in flight.

Recommendations for the disinsecting of aircraft are contained in Annexe VI of the second annotated edition of the regulations published (World Health Organization 1974) and were amended in 1977, 1979 and 1985 to add new insecticides and provide new disinsecting procedures. The recommendations detail the specifications for the aerosols to be used. Two methods of disinsection are currently in use by airlines. 'Blocks away' is a method of disinsecting the passenger cabin, and all other accessible interior spaces of the aircraft, except the flight deck, by spraying the cabin airspace of the aircraft after the doors have been secured following embarkation of passengers and before takeoff. The method uses hand-operated aerosol single-use dispensers containing the knockdown insecticide d-phenothrin, which are discharged by the flight attendants. When activated, the discharge valve locks in the open position and the aerosol will continue to discharge its contents even if the flight attendant removes his or her finger from the activating trigger. The aerosol cans should be serially numbered for ease of reference and should be retained for inspection by the port health authority at the airport of arrival, if required.

Disinsection is carried out by crew members walking slowly down the aisle of the aircraft discharging the aerosol into the space above the passengers' heads, towards the cabin ceiling and locker area. Passengers must be advised that spraying is to take place. The ventilation system to the aircraft cabins should be switched off so that the spray is not sucked directly out of the cabin. The aerosol must be dispensed uniformly throughout the aircraft, as required by WHO International Health Regulations requirements at a rate of 35 g of formulation per 100 m³ (10 g/1000 cubic feet) of enclosed space. This method is limited in its effectiveness, as not all areas of the aircraft are exposed to the insecticide. The flight deck, cargo hold and external areas such as the wheel wells must be sprayed by ground personnel before departure of the aircraft, with the used cans also being retained for inspection by the port health authority.

An alternative to 'blocks away' disinsection is the application of residual insecticide film, carried out as part of an engineering procedure at the base airport of the airline in question. This is designed to provide a film of insecticide covering all the internal surfaces of the aircraft, thus ensuring that any insect landing on a treated surface will subsequently die. The residual insecticide used is permethrin. The procedure is detailed by the WHO and is based on discussions held in Geneva in November 1984 and subsequently published in the *Epidemiological Record* (8 November 1985). The procedure is aimed at producing an even deposit of $0.5\,g/m^2$ of permethrin on carpets and $0.2\,g/m^2$ on other internal surfaces. Aircraft that have been treated previously can be treated again with $0.2\,g/m^2$ on carpets and other surfaces. A fluorescent dye such as photine 14 BS is added to the mixture to enable identification of treated areas. The insecticide is applied using a compression spray that delivers about 300 litres of air per minute at a pressure of 690 kPa (100 psi). A single operator using this equipment could treat a Boeing 747 aircraft in about two hours. Electrically sensitive areas such as the flight deck can also be treated using 2% permethrin. To carry out the process effectively, the delivery output of the spray has to be maintained to cover an area of surface in the required time.

Before treatment, the aircraft has to be prepared by opening and clearing all storage areas and closing all window blinds. Carpet covers must be removed. All surfaces of the passenger, crew and cargo compartments are sprayed, including toilets, galleys and wall areas behind curtains. Both sides of doors and locker lids are sprayed at the end of the operation, and the carpets are then resprayed. After spraying, the air-conditioning must be operated for at least an hour to clear the air of volatile components. Mirrors and other surfaces may have to be cleaned. The aircraft must be resprayed at intervals not exceeding eight weeks, but a weekly treatment schedule has to be adopted for interior areas subject to regular cleaning, and any area receiving deep cleansing has to be given a supplementary spray. After treatment, a certificate of residual disinsection is issued and carried on board as part of the aircraft paperwork. This method is comparatively costly and time-consuming, but individual customers may vary their requirements within the scope of the International Health Regulations.

Rodents such as rats and mice may gain access to aircraft in many parts of the world, either directly from infested terminal buildings or from the cargo. Rodents can be the carriers of many diseases, including rabies, so their presence on an aircraft, or their accidental importation into any country, cannot be tolerated. Rodents present an air safety hazard, as they have a predilection for the plastic coating of the many cables running through the aircraft. They may also be crushed in the moving parts on an aircraft. If there is evidence or reasonable suspicion that rodents are present, the aircraft should be taken out of service and disinfested as soon as possible. Disinfestation can be achieved by fumigation using methyl bromide, applied at a dose of 230 g per $30\,m^3$ of airspace in the aircraft for a period of four hours. Following fumigation, the aircraft must be ventilated fully to ensure dispersal of the methyl bromide fumigant. The effectiveness of ventilation must be checked using Draeger tubes to ensure the complete absence of fumigant in all areas of the aircraft. Methyl bromide is heavier than air and, therefore, will sink naturally into the lower areas of the aircraft, such as cargo holds and avionics bay, so care must be taken to ensure that all such areas are ventilated completely. Methyl bromide is not detectable by smell and normally contains added picrin to aid in the detection of the gas. Picrin, however, is damaging to the aircraft fabric, and therefore methyl bromide used for aircraft fumigation must be free of picrin. Fumigation is a dangerous process and should be carried out only by authorised experts. Treatment must follow established practice to ensure the safety of everybody involved, the care of the aircraft fabric, and the subsequent safety of staff and passengers.

CLEANING AND DISINFECTION

Cleaning of an aircraft can be either transit cleaning or deep cleaning and depends on the length of time available. Transit cleaning is carried out when time is short, such as in domestic or short intercity journeys where speed of turn-round is important and when as little as 35 minutes may be allocated for aircraft to arrive, offload the incoming passengers, de-cater the galley, re-cater for the outgoing flight, and board the oncoming passengers. In such instances, it may be possible only to clear the visible rubbish out of the main cabin area, brush down the seats, check the seat-back pockets and quickly sweep the main cabin carpet. The galley area will be given a wipe down after the residual catering has been offloaded and a final clean of the work surfaces and floor area will be completed in the few moments after the new catering has been embarked and before the passengers board. The toilet areas will be cleaned and restocked. Even a turn-round time of 1.5 hours may be insufficient to do little more, due to the size of the aircraft and the presence of passengers remaining on board during transit stops on intercontinental flights. More detailed cleaning is carried out at terminating stations, where the aircraft may be on the ground for periods in excess of four hours, and during maintenance, when, with the aircraft in a hangar and with component parts stripped from it, deep cleaning can take place.

Routine cleaning of cabins, galleys and toilet areas must include disinfection, which is usually provided by a chemical sanitizer contained in a hand-operated spray bottle. All cleaning and disinfectant materials used on board an aircraft must comply with the Aerospace Material Specification (AMS) 1452 of the Society of Automotive Engineers to ensure that they do not have a deleterious effect on the fabric of the aircraft. This need for a non-damaging disinfectant restricts those that can be used on aircraft; the most commonly used is a quaternary ammonium compound, or 'quat'. These are used widely in the food industry but suffer the disadvantage of being readily neutralized when in contact with dirty conditions.

To prevent cross-contamination risks when cleaning the aircraft, it is essential that the cleaners are divided into three groups, with one group responsible for the cleaning of the toilets and associated facilities, the second responsible for the main cabin, including the dropdown tables, and the third responsible for the galleys. Cleaning should be carried out according to a preset practice. Identification of the teams involved in each area can be facilitated by the use of different-coloured cleaning cloths. With toilet cleaning, it is essential that the programme includes the cleaning and disinfecting of all 'touch surfaces', such as door handles, locks, flushing mechanisms and taps.

Occasionally, an airline may, inadvertently, carry a passenger who is suffering from an infectious disease. In such instances, the port health authority may ask for a full disinfection of the aircraft to ensure that any risk of contamination from the passenger concerned has been removed. This must be carried out using a disinfectant suitable for use against the infectious disease concerned and that also complies with the Aerospace Material Specification (AMS). This can be applied to the interior of the aircraft by either a fine-mist fogging process or by a coarse-mist application by hand-operated backpack spray. It is likely, however, that by the time the airline has been notified by the port health authority of a requirement for disinfection, the aircraft will have completed a number of flying sectors and is likely to have been cleaned many times.

REFERENCES

World Health Organization. *International Health Regulations*. Geneva: World Health Organization, 1969.

World Health Organization. *International Health Regulations*, 2nd annotated edn. Geneva: World Health Organization, 1974.

FURTHER READING

Association of Port Health Authorities in the UK. *Code of Practice: Dealing with Infectious Disease on Aircraft*. Runcorn, UK: Association of Port Health Authorities in the UK, 1995. www.apha.org.uk

Burslem CD, Kelly MJ, Preston FS. Food poisoning: a major threat to airline operations. *Journal of Society of Occupational Medicine* 1990; **40**: 97–100.

International Travel Catering Association and International Inflight Food Service Association. *ITCA/IFSA World Food Safety Guidelines*. Godalming, UK: International Travel Catering Association and the International Inflight Food Service Association, 2003. www.ifcanet.com

Kelly M. Control of infection in an international airline. *Journal of Society of Occupational Medicine* 1983; **43**: 91–4.

Kelly M. Food hygiene as part of a total quality management programme. *UK Quality* 1993; **December**.

35

Naval air operations

ADRIAN BAKER AND MARK GROOM

INTRODUCTION

The military use of aircraft at sea has followed closely the development of powered flight itself. Both the UK Royal Navy and the US Navy commenced studies within five years of the Wright brothers' first flight. Eugene Ely performed the first successful takeoff from a ship on 14 November 1910, when he flew a Curtiss pusher from a ramp constructed over the forecastle of the USS Birmingham at anchor off Norfolk, Virginia. The underpowered aircraft dipped, its wing sponsons contacted the water, and the propeller tips splintered. After recovering from contact with the water, Ely flew to a successful landing ashore. On 18 January 1911, Ely performed the first successful landing-on, aboard the USS Pennsylvania at anchor off San Francisco, with the aircraft slowed by engaging a series of transverse ropes weighted by sandbags.

Operations from a warship under way were even more taxing, but on 2 May 1912 Lieutenant C.R. Sampson, Royal Navy, flew an S27 Box Kite from a ramp over the forward turret and bow of *HMS Hibernia*. The first landing-on under way was performed by Lieutenant Commander Durnford aboard *HMS Furious* in 1917. Operational imperatives and experience during the First World War forced development of dedicated carrier vessels; the first full-length flush-deck aircraft carrier, *HMS Argus*, entered service in September 1918. The first purpose-built aircraft carrier, *HMS Hermes*, was laid down in January 1918, launched in September 1919 and commissioned in July 1923.

In the inter-war years, the aircraft carrier was subject to relative neglect by the Royal Navy, which viewed aircraft as a means to spot and slow enemy capital ships in order to enable their destruction by the big-gun battleships. In contrast, the United States Navy viewed carrier-borne aviation as a strike arm in its own right and developed ships and aircraft accordingly. However, the Royal Navy demonstrated decisive use of carrier aviation in the attack on the Italian fleet in harbour at Taranto on 11 November 1940. On a larger scale, but ultimately with less success, this action was repeated by the Imperial Japanese Navy at Pearl Harbour on 7 December 1941. Six months later, on 4 June 1942, the Battle of Midway was fought entirely between carrier battle groups, the US and Japanese fleets never within visual range of each other. By the end of the Second World War, the aircraft carrier battle group had become the dominant force at sea.

After the Second World War, a number of technical developments led to a rapid increase in aircraft carrier capability. The first was the introduction of jet aircraft, first trialled aboard *HMS Ocean* in 1945. Increased operating weights and launch speeds led to the development of the steam catapult, in which steam from the ship's boiler was used to propel a shuttle down a track and accelerate the aircraft to launch velocity. Introduction of a flight deck angled at 10.5 degrees to port allowed an aircraft that missed the arrester wires on landing to go around, rather than engage a barrier or damage aircraft parked on deck. Higher approach speeds meant that the pilot had less time to react to signals from a deck landing control officer and modify the approach. The mirror landing sight consisting of a light projected on to a gyroscopically stabilized mirror enabled pilots to compare their approach against a datum. When on the correct approach path, the pilot sees a white light; with any deviation in vertical or horizontal plane, a different colour is presented. The landing sight has since been refined further by use of Fresnel lenses and, more recently, laser projectors.

The development of the helicopter from 1945 onwards enabled vertical takeoff and landing operations from small platforms. Low-powered early helicopters could lift little useful payload, but their utility for recovery of ditched aircrew was demonstrated by 1947, and the helicopter has performed the 'plane guard' function during carrier flight operations ever since. As improvements in engine power permitted development of larger helicopters with greater payload, the helicopter became the preferred platform for sea-based antisubmarine warfare (ASW), aided by the ability to hover while deploying a dipping sonar. Mass use of transport helicopters in an assault role from the sea – vertical envelopment – was first demonstrated during the landing of 45 Commando Royal Marines at Port Said from HMS Ocean in November 1956. Following this, the Royal Navy and others converted aircraft carriers to the commando carrier or landing platform helicopter (LPH) role. As with the introduction of fixed-wing aircraft a generation earlier, new warships were increasingly designed around the helicopter rather than modified to operate them, the first specifically designed frigates and destroyers entering service in the early 1960s.

PRESENT–DAY PLATFORMS

The USA is the major operator of large-deck aircraft carriers. Its current Nimitz class vessels provide a capability for power projection with global reach. Nuclear propulsion provides considerable endurance, limited only by the need to resupply food for the crew and fuel for the aircraft. The ships displace 90 000 tons and have an overall length of 360 m and a total usable flight-deck area of 18 200 m². This size permits the operation of a mixed air group of 85 aircraft, including three fixed-wing strike squadrons, two air-defence squadrons, electronic warfare and airborne early-warning (AEW) aircraft. Four steam catapults – two on the bow and two on the angled flight deck – accelerate aircraft to 160 knots in 100 m. Three transverse arrestor wires at the rear of the angled deck stop recovering aircraft in a similar distance. France has a single 45 000-ton vessel nuclear-powered catapult and arrester-wire-equipped vessel operating a similar but proportionately smaller air group.

The UK operates three Invincible class vessels, each displacing 20 000 tons and with an overall length of 210 m. They were designed to operate ASW helicopters with a secondary capability for operating vertical/short takeoff and landing (VSTOL) aircraft to enable engagement of aircraft providing targeting information for ship-launched missiles. With geopolitical developments and a perceived diminution in the submarine threat, they now operate a mixed air group of 18 aircraft and can operate 24 at overload. An airborne surveillance and command (ASaC) capability is provided by a search-radar-equipped Sea King helicopter variant. For fixed-wing operations, there is a 170-m runway ending at the bow in a 50-m ski ramp with a 12-degree exit angle. The embarked vectored nozzle Harrier aircraft commence their takeoff run with the nozzles directed aft and then transition to vertically directed nozzles as airspeed builds. This enables operation at higher all-up weights and in sea-state, weather and wind-over-deck conditions that would preclude operations by conventionally launched aircraft. Aircraft recover by coming to the hover alongside to port and then translating to a vertical landing towards the rear of the deck. This mode of operation and smaller ski-ramp-equipped carriers have been adopted by the Italian, Spanish and Thai navies.

Outwardly similar in appearance to the traditional aircraft carrier, current US LPHs are 270 m long and displace some 40 000 tons. US practice is to embark around 30 light and medium lift-support helicopters, attack helicopters and six VSTOL aircraft as the mixed air component of a marine air ground task force. The VSTOL aircraft operate from the forward area of the deck and the helicopters from further aft.

Most navies operate smaller general-purpose vessels in which the embarked helicopter provides a significant proportion of overall capability. Indeed, most naval vessels over 1000 tons provide at least a deck for helicopter operations if not the hangar to enable their maintenance. These decks typically have a single helicopter operating spot. The role of the embarked helicopter has evolved; originally employed in utility and ASW duties, developments in air-launched anti-ship missiles have resulted in increased use against surface targets. With the emergence of greater threat from very small surface vessels and suicide attacks from small boats, the helicopter is the most effective platform for assessment and neutralization.

AEROMEDICAL CONSIDERATIONS

Maritime environment

The maritime environment is characterized by a number of challenges to the safe and effective conduct of flying operations. In addition, there may be no diversion airfield within range in the event of adverse weather or technical difficulty. Ambient temperatures can be at either extreme of human thermal comfort. Lighting conditions range from high illumination and solar glare, with the attendant risks to vision, to low light levels and reduced visual contrast at night and in haze. The absence of fixed features makes unaided navigation and maintenance of height difficult. Precession effects due to rotor downwash on water impede station-keeping in the hover.

In the event of forced landing on, or entry into, water, immersion can result in cold shock, arrhythmia and muscular incoordination, affecting breathing and ability to swim and float before loss of body heat results in hypothermia. Brief incapacitations due to minor head injury with minimal consequence on land can be fatal due to drowning. Ditched helicopters tend to invert due to their high centre of mass and then sink rapidly, with adverse consequences for occupants. Trapping due to snagging of equipment and harness and distortion of the airframe are then compounded by disorientation. Rapid sinking to depth will result in the body becoming neutrally buoyant and less likely to rise to the surface. For personnel who fly frequently over water, military and civilian operators conduct helicopter underwater escape training. In this, a mock-up of a helicopter cabin is lowered into water and inverted in a graduated series of exercises under both lit and dark conditions, with safety divers in attendance. The small but finite risk of the training is outweighed by its operational benefit. To enhance chances of escape, current life-preservers include a small compressed-air bottle – the short-term air supply system (STASS). This can provide sufficient air to effect escape, but being a compressed gas system it has an attendant risk of pulmonary barotrauma on ascent. Aircrew require training in its use, and those with a forced expiratory volume in one second (FEV_1)/forced vital capacity (FVC) ratio of less than 70 per cent should be considered unfit for 'wet STASS' training. A newer system consisting of a rebreather bag is under development, which will reduce the risk of barotrauma and be suitable for use by untrained individuals.

Should escape attempts prove unsuccessful, the recovery of bodies for forensic examination can be extremely difficult, although commercial organizations can recover a craft of 2 m diameter lost at a depth of 4500 m. Unless recovered quickly, post-mortem effects of immersion and the activities of marine fauna result in difficulty in interpretation of soft-tissue findings.

On successful escape from a ditched aircraft, or successful entry into water on abandonment, the survival priorities of protection followed by location are pre-eminent. An inflatable life-preserver is required to maintain buoyancy and is fitted with a face shield to reduce ingestion of water. Layered aircrew equipment assemblies (AEA) with a relatively impermeable immersion coverall is required to delay onset of hypothermia. Further protection is afforded by individual or multi-person inflatable rafts, which provide further insulation and shelter. Location is aided by the use of high-visibility materials in life-preservers and rafts, with a radio beacon for longer-range detection.

A person floating in water is subject to hydrostatic squeeze on the vascular system, resulting in central shift of the circulating blood volume. When this squeeze is removed, peripheral pooling will occur, with resultant orthostatic hypotension. Historically, this was the cause of post-rescue collapse and, indeed, death. The standard rescue technique now features the use of a double-lift strop, with one loop under the axillae and one under the knees, to winch the individual from the water in a horizontal position. The survivor is then evacuated as a stretcher case until he or she has been assessed fully.

Shipboard environment

The environment aboard ship has a number of hazards of its own, ranging from physical through chemical, biological, psychological and social. The ship is a platform on a moving mass of water and, as a result, subject to movement. Larger vessels are inherently more stable, but any vessel can be subject to sudden or unpredictable motion resulting in movement of unsecured objects, including personnel and even aircraft ranged on deck. In vessels of mass up to 10 000 tons, the ship's movement can prove nauseogenic.

Slips, trips and falls on ladders and in passageways are not uncommon. Ships contain unfamiliar obstructions for the unwary or inexperienced. During a six-month carrier deployment, 335 injuries occurred on the flight deck, in the hangar and in the gym; of these, 36 per cent resulted in duty days lost (Krentz et al. 1997). Injuries from flight-deck recreation were less frequent than work-related accidents but accounted for a greater loss of duty days. Despite the size of current aircraft carriers, deck crews are far closer to operating aircraft than would be the case at airfields on land. The proximity of fast-moving aircraft and rotor tips requires constant vigilance and a high degree of situational awareness for safe incident-free operations.

Apart from mechanical hazards, other physical features include constant noise of varying intensity, from the noise of the sea itself to constantly running ship machinery. Activities of personnel on deck, such as dragging chains or lashings, and aircraft engine noise can constitute nuisance, distraction or frank hazard, both directly to hearing and by disruption of sleep. Noise levels on a carrier deck average 109 dB A over a working day of 12 hours (Rovig et al. 2004). Peak noise levels during launch reach 150 dB A. At this level, temporary threshold shifts and permanent damage occur with very short exposures, and a single launch exceeds statutory 24-hour limits. Active noise-reduction headphones are being developed for the next-generation deck-crew helmets and offer the possibility of 48-dB attenuation. Chemical hazards include fuels and lubricants.

The relatively high population density aboard ship results in rapid transmission of minor infectious disease such as upper respiratory tract infection on leaving harbour. More serious outbreaks such as gastroenteritis due to Norwalk virus can result in a high percentage of a ship's company being affected (Corwin *et al.* 1999), with clear effect on operational capability. However, once the outbreak has run its course, the shipboard environment is far cleaner than most shoreside forward operating bases.

Psychological and social hazards are closely mixed. An individual can be isolated and lonely and yet, conversely, without privacy. Colleagues are impossible to avoid. With deployments lasting for extended periods, individuals may consider themselves unable to influence their situation at home and be subject to uncertainty as a result. The pressure to maintain the tempo of operations can result in higher workloads on smaller teams, particularly for air-engineering personnel. At other times, there can be an absence of stimulation, requiring significant motivation to overcome. Finally, the relative austerity of shipboard medical facilities, and naval operating areas remote from major hospitals, limits therapeutic options and influences decision-making on fitness for task.

FLYING OPERATIONS

Fixed-wing aircraft

On launch from a catapult-equipped carrier, the aircraft accelerates to over 160 knots in just 100 m in 2.5 seconds, with a peak acceleration of $+5\,G_x$. The energy delivered to the individual is sufficient to have an effect on cardiac rhythm. Cardioversion of atrial fibrillation has been reported in a patient evacuated by catapult launched aircraft (Bohnker *et al.* 1993), and cardiac arrhythmias of uncertain significance may be induced. During the catapult stroke, low-frequency seat and pilot vibration can reach a peak acceleration of $6\text{–}8\,G_z$ (Smith 2004), with helmet rotation of 20 degree in pitch causing undesirable loss of helmet-mounted display image. The G_x acceleration results in potential somatogravic illusion, in which the aircraft is perceived as being five degrees nose-up compared with the gravitational vertical. This illusion can persist for 30 seconds into flight (Cohen 1976) and has been implicated in post-launch crashes, particularly at night. To mitigate this, some aircraft types are launched pilot-hands-off.

Flight over water is characterized by a paucity of visual features, unless there is cloud in the sky, ships on the water or visible coastline. Fixation on a single point such as a ship in an otherwise featureless field can result in autokinetic illusions, with a potential for disorientation, particularly at night. Break-off phenomena have been reported in single-pilot operations at higher altitudes. Once thought to affect fixed-wing aviators exclusively, this is also recognized in higher-altitude single-pilot helicopters.

Arguably, recovery and landing pose the greatest physiological and psychological challenges to the naval aviator. Workload is high, with increased heart rate, autonomic activity and glucocorticoid production. There is limited time in which to make critical adjustments to approach. Touchdown occurs with a sink rate of 4–7 m/s, depending on aircraft type, accuracy of approach and sea state. Failure to engage arrester wires requires instant application of full throttle to effect a bump-and-go and avoid entry into water. Successful engagement of the wire results in the aircraft slowing to a stop in 100 m, with resultant $-G_x$ and potential forward-pitched somatogravic illusion.

Accident rates have been analysed against aviators' experience and currency (Burowsky *et al.* 1981). Accident liability correlates with lifetime carrier experience, with the highest rates associated with minimal carrier experience. Accident rates among inexperienced carrier aviators are lower if a large number of landings have been conducted in the previous seven days. Conversely, there is a significant correlation between night carrier landing performance and the speed with which an aviator can shift gaze between near and far targets; these speeds slow with age (Morris and Temme 1989). Corrected refracted error causes no diminution in night carrier landing scores (Still and Temme 1992).

The recovery and landing of short takeoff and vertical landing (STOVL) aircraft have other features. These aircraft have the advantage of being able to 'stop then land', reducing the dangers associated with arrested landings. However, there is limited hover endurance at the end of a sortie, and with both present and proposed aircraft having single engines there is the risk of engine failure during a critical phase. Ejection seats for such aircraft must operate under conditions of high sink rate and thus exert high loads on lumbar vertebrae. The F35B Joint Strike Fighter will land on lift from the directional nozzle at the rear and a link-driven fan immediately behind the cockpit. Failure of the link will result in immediate nose-down pitch at a very high rate, and an automatic ejection system is being considered.

Rotary-wing aircraft

Much naval helicopter flying is from smaller warships of destroyer or frigate type and around 5000-tons displacement. Takeoff and landing are conducted from small platforms with limited clearance between the rotor disc and the ship's superstructure. The landing platform is subject to comparatively greater motion than a carrier flight deck, increasing the risk of tip strikes. Chains and lashings are needed to ensure that the helicopter remains on deck during higher sea states, which in turn requires exposed, at-risk deck-crew members to remove them before flight. Unsecured helicopters and crew have been lost overboard due to the ship's motion and flying operations requiring that guard rails were lowered. In a survey of Royal Navy pilots (Steele-Perkins and Evans 1978), 45 per cent of those questioned reported they had misjudged altitude after taking off. Sudden entry into darkness during night takeoff from a floodlit deck necessitates urgent transfer on to instruments. The introduction of night-vision devices has resulted in changes to procedures and refitting of flight-deck illumination to reduce disorientation by point-source lights.

Apart from specific ship's delivery service sorties, naval helicopter operations usually involve long sortie times conducting ASW, above-surface warfare (ASuW) and ASaC patrols. Visual search missions may be flown with doors open, exposing crews to cold due to wind chill. Although newer aircraft types offer significant improvements, crews are still exposed to noise and vibration. Relatively cramped conditions and the adoption of unnatural postures result in musculoskeletal morbidity. ASW helicopters hover 15 degrees nose up, three degrees port wing down 'in the dip' while deploying sonar, resulting in rear-facing crew members hanging out of their seats in their straps. Station-keeping while in the hover over water is made more difficult by the vection illusion induced by the effect of rotor downwash.

During approach to the ship, the absence of fixed points can make unaided assessment of ground speed and altitude difficult. Although the ship should assist by assuming an into-wind heading, tactical and navigational constraints may preclude this, necessitating approach on a suboptimal heading. To minimize the effects of turbulent airflow around the superstructure, approaches are commonly made from astern on a heading at 30 degrees to the ship's heading. This in turn results in a navigational problem for the pilot, who must find good visual references to maintain both position and situational awareness. On matching speed with the ship and being cleared into land, the pilot needs to correct for the effect of wind around the ship, which might draw the helicopter towards the superstructure, and judge and time the landing to coincide with minimum motion of the deck. UK helicopters then engage a harpoon in a deck grid to keep the aircraft on deck while deck crews apply safety lashings.

Driven by the need to improve the information presented to a pilot while landing, and a move to reduce the total numbers of personnel at risk on deck, helicopter visual approach systems have been developed. These provide a gyro-stabilized horizon reference, a lit horizontal bar above the hangar, a stabilized slope indicator and deck-edge lighting to improve the visual cues available.

FUTURE DEVELOPMENTS

Steam catapults are only five per cent efficient and the launch is not smooth or subject to feedback control. This risks injury to the aircrew and increases airframe fatigue. Some 600 kg of steam is required for each launch. This and the catapult braking system generate lubricant and metal residue-contaminated brake water, discharge of which is prohibited within 12 nautical miles of a coastline. Electromagnetic aircraft launch systems under development offer the possibility of greater efficiency and energy density, delivering 120 mJ compared with the steam catapult's 95 mJ, and thus enabling launch at higher all-up weights with smoother acceleration. This smoother acceleration will be less challenging to the aircrew.

Increasingly capable unmanned aerial vehicles and unmanned combat air vehicles are being operated from ships and controlled from afloat. The US Navy is considering the use of flight simulators at sea in order to help maintain currency on long deployments. In both cases, the operator is presented with visual information, which may be confounded by vestibular information resulting from the ship's movement and could possibly lead to motion adaptation syndrome. In tests using a personal computer (PC)-based flight simulator afloat, participants reported no nausea but showed a decrease in dynamic visual acuity (Muth and Lawson 2003). The study suggests that simulators could be used aboard but that they should be located near the ship's centre of motion and be used when motion is not provocative.

REFERENCES

Bohnker BK, Feeks EF, McEwen G. Catapult launch associated cardioversion of atrial fibrillation. *Aviation, Space, and Environmental Medicine* 1993; **64**: 939–40.

Burowsky MS, Gaynor J, Barrett G, Beck A. Relationships between U.S. Navy carrier landing accidents and flight experience parameters. *Aviation, Space, and Environmental Medicine* 1981; **52**: 109–11.

Cohen MM. Disorientating effects of aircraft catapult launchings. II. Visual and postural contributions. *Aviation, Space, and Environmental Medicine* 1976; **47**: 39–41.

Corwin AL, Sonderquist R, Edwards M, *et al.* Shipboard impact of probable Norwalk virus outbreak from coastal Japan. *American Journal of Tropical Medicine and Hygiene* 1999; **61**: 898–903.

Krentz MJ, Li G, Baker SP. At work and play in a hazardous environment: injuries aboard a deployed U.S. Navy aircraft carrier. *Aviation, Space, and Environmental Medicine* 1997; **68**: 51–5.

Morris M, Temme LA. The time required for U.S. Navy fighter pilots to shift gaze and identify near and far targets. *Aviation, Space, and Environmental Medicine* 1989; **60**: 1085–9.

Muth ER, Lawson B. Using flight simulators aboard ships: human side effects of an optimum scenario with smooth seas. *Aviation, Space, and Environmental Medicine* 2003; **74**: 497–505.

Rovig GW, Bohnker BK, Page JC. Hearing health risk in a population of aircraft carrier flight deck personnel. *Military Medicine* 2004; **169**: 429–32.

Smith SD. Cockpit seat and pilot helmet vibration during flight operations on aircraft carriers. *Aviation, Space, and Environmental Medicine* 2004; **75**: 247–54.

Steele-Perkins AP, Evans DA. Disorientation in naval helicopter pilots. In: AGARD/NATO (eds). *Operational Helicopter Aviation Medicine.* CP255, 48, 1-5; Neuilly-sur-Seine: AGARD/NATO, 1978: pp. 1-5.

Still DL, Temme LA. Eyeglass use by U.S. Navy jet pilots: effects on night carrier landing performance. *Aviation, Space, and Environmental Medicine* 1992; **63**: 273-5.

FURTHER READING

Royal Navy. www.royal-navy.mod.uk

United States Navy. www.navy.mil

PART III

Clinical aviation medicine

36

International regulation of medical standards

ANTHONY D.B. EVANS

INTRODUCTION

It is an expectation of affluent society that certain aspects of daily life, such as health, education, safety, security and the environment, will be maintained at a high standard and continue to improve with time. Public transport is expected to be safe, and perhaps the greatest demands in this area are reserved for commercial flight operations. Flight safety or, more accurately, risk reduction is achieved in many ways, and a complex set of rules has developed to ensure that air travel does not pose an unacceptable risk to society, given that zero risk is not possible. This chapter will explore the aeromedical practitioner's contribution to flight safety. It will concentrate mainly on aspects that are of relevance to commercial pilots, but it will also cover some of the requirements for military aviation and private pilots.

ACCIDENT RATES

The overall risk of air travel can be measured crudely by the fatal accident rate, a fatal accident being defined as one in which one or more people are killed. The fatal accident rate per one million flights has been falling over the past 40 years, due to the industry's continuing efforts to create an efficient air-transport system using modern, reliable technology and a regulatory framework designed to ensure certain minimum standards (Figure 36.1). The main

technological advances that have contributed to the improvement in flight safety are the increasing use of jet engines, the use of flight simulators for pilot training, and more accurate navigation systems. The best safety figures are for passenger-carrying large jet aircraft: worldwide fatal accident rates for freight, ferry and positioning flights, i.e. flights with no passengers, are eight times higher than for passenger flights (UK Civil Aviation Authority 1998). The worldwide fatal accident rate for turbo-propeller aircraft is about three times greater than for jet aircraft (UK Civil Aviation Authority 2000).

For long-distance journeys, the speed of air transport makes it the preferred mode of travel. When compared with other modes on a fatality-per-kilometre basis, air is the safest means of travel. Figures for aircraft registered in the UK indicate that air travel is 40 times safer than travel by rail and 300 times safer than travel by car (Table 36.1). However, there is a strong correlation between the efficiency of a country's economy (e.g. the gross national product) and achieved safety levels. Local socioeconomic factors ultimately determine acceptable levels of flight safety in each part of the world, and useful comparisons therefore can be made only using operational data from nations with similar socioeconomic conditions (Figure 36.2).

Measurement of accident rates

Various methods are used to present aircraft accident rates. Commonly used indices are fatal accidents per one million

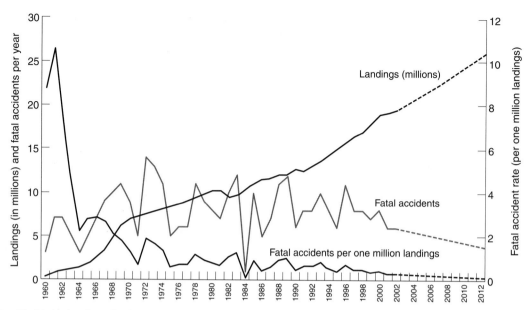

Figure 36.1 *Worldwide landings, fatal accidents and fatal accident rate in Western-built jets, 1960–2002. Trend lines 2003–12 assume a three per cent annual increase in landings. Source: Airclaims Ltd, world airfleet database. www.airclaims.co.uk*

Table 36.1 *Average number of passengers killed per one billion passenger-kilometres, by mode, 1992–2001*

Mode of transport	Passengers killed/one billion passenger-kilometres
Air	0.01
Water	0.3
Rail	0.4
Bus or coach	0.4
Van	1.2
Car	3.0
Pedal cycle	42
Pedestrian	58
Two-wheeled motor vehicle	111

Source: UK Department for Transport. Transport statistics for Great Britain, 2003. www.dft.gov.uk/stellent/groups/dft_transstats/documents/page/dft_transstats_025211.pdf

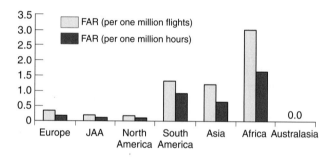

	FAR (per one million flights)	FAR (per one million hours)
Europe	0.34	0.18
JAA	0.20	0.11
North America	0.20	0.11
South America	1.33	0.93
Asia	1.24	0.65
Africa	3.05	1.67
Australasia	0.00	0.00

Figure 36.2 *Worldwide Western-built jet fatal accident rate (FAR) by operator region, 1993–2002. Europe, all European states; JAA, full Joint Aviation Authorities member states (primarily European Union). Source: UK Civil Aviation Authority, Strategic, Safety and Analysis Department, Gatwick, UK, personal communication.*

landings (flights) or per one million hours flown (see Figures 36.1 and 36.2). Another method is the number of fatalities per one billion passenger-kilometres travelled (passenger-kilometres = number of passengers × distance travelled) (see Table 36.1). Each has advantages and disadvantages. When assessing the relative risk of travel between different modes of transport and between different airlines, care must be taken to ensure that like is compared with like, particularly as there is no standardized method of recording statistics. For example, a long-haul airline may have a good record in comparison with a short-haul operator when based on fatal accidents per one million flight hours; however, because accidents tend to occur more frequently at the beginning and end of flights, the former may have a poorer record based on fatal accidents per one million flights.

Fatal accident rate per year

Airline scheduled traffic generally is increasing, although there was a dip in 2001–02. During 1993–2000, worldwide passenger-kilometres increased each year on average by 5.8 per cent. However, in 2001 and 2002, growth was −2.9 per cent and +0.4 per cent, respectively, making predictions for the next decade difficult (International Civil Aviation Organization 2002). Nevertheless, it can be anticipated that aviation will continue to expand in the medium to long term; if a growth rate of three per cent per annum is assumed, then a continuous reduction in the number of fatal accidents per one million flights is necessary to ensure that the number of fatal accidents per year does not increase (Figure 36.1).

FRAMEWORK FOR REGULATORY ACTIVITY OF CIVIL AVIATION

Chicago Convention

In 2002, airlines carried 1.6 billion passengers on international and domestic flights (International Civil Aviation Organization 2002). The safety regulation of this large industry dates back to the Second World War, when there was rapid development of both aircraft technical standards and networks of passenger and freight services. Political questions were raised concerning the right of airlines registered in one country to fly through the airspace of another, and with the practicalities regarding the maintenance of navigation facilities, particularly if located in sparsely populated areas or in non-technologically advanced states. To address such issues, the government of the USA invited 55 neutral and allied states to meet in Chicago in 1944; 52 states attended. The outcome, after five weeks of deliberations, was the Convention on International Civil Aviation, commonly known as the Chicago Convention. A total of 189 contracting states have now signed the Chicago Convention, thereby agreeing to abide by its requirements and automatically becoming members of the International Civil Aviation Organization (ICAO).

International Civil Aviation Organization

The ICAO was created to promote the safe and orderly development of civil aviation. A specialized agency of the United Nations, it sets international standards and recommended practices (SARPS) necessary for safety, security, efficiency and regularity of air transport and serves as the medium for cooperation in all fields of civil aviation among its 189 contracting states. It is responsible for updating the 18 annexes of the Chicago Convention.

Standards and recommended practices

Annex 1 of the Chicago Convention deals with personnel licensing, and Chapter 6 of this annex is devoted to medical aspects. As with other annexes, Annex 1 contains SARPS, which together are called the 'provisions' and underpin the regulation of civil aviation medicine practice throughout the world. An ICAO standard is defined as a specification 'recognized as necessary for the safety or regularity of international air navigation and to which Contracting States will conform in accordance with the Convention'. An example of a standard applicable to all classes of medical certificate is that an 'applicant shall have no established medical history or clinical diagnosis of ... epilepsy' (International Civil Aviation Organization 2001).

A standard is therefore mandatory; if a state is unable or unwilling to comply, it must notify ICAO, thereby 'filing a difference'. ICAO publishes a list of such differences; other states may, if they wish, refuse permission for airlines regulated by the non-compliant state to overfly or land in their territory. In practice, although many differences have been filed, this rarely occurs, with the exception of those concerning pilot age limits, a subject that attracts the single largest number of differences: many states permit airline captains over 60 years of age to continue operating, even though the ICAO limit is 60 years. (The Joint Aviation Authorities (JAA) specify an upper age limit of 65 years for both captains and co-pilots.) Several states exercise their right under the Chicago Convention to exclude 'over-60' captains from their airspace, including France and the USA. Issues regarding the ageing pilot are addressed in Chapter 53.

A recommended practice is defined as any specification 'recognized as desirable in the interests of safety, regularity or efficiency of international air navigation, and to which contracting states will endeavour to conform'. It is therefore not mandatory to comply with a recommendation or to notify any non-compliance to ICAO. An example is the ICAO recommendation that co-pilots should not operate when over 60 years of age. As with captains, some states choose not to impose this restriction. The provisions of Annex 1 permit this, without reference to ICAO and, unlike captains, contracting states cannot prevent co-pilots of any age operating in their airspace, since the Chicago Convention does not have a mandatory (a standard) upper age limit for co-pilots.

Accredited medical conclusion and flexibility

Although the SARPS specified in Annex 1, Chapter 6, provide useful information for the assessment of medical fitness of pilots, they cannot cover every circumstance that an aviation medical examiner, or a licensing authority, is likely to encounter. In some places, the standards themselves are open to interpretation, e.g. 'The systolic and diastolic blood pressures shall be within normal limits.' In other circumstances, a particular medical condition may not be mentioned in the SARPS, and the assessor has to determine whether a particular medical problem could, in the words of ICAO, 'render [an] applicant likely to become suddenly unable either to operate an aircraft safely or to perform assigned duties safely' and issue or withhold a medical certificate as appropriate.

There exists a special procedure for assessing cases where a medical standard is not achieved but which may nevertheless permit a certificate to be issued in an individual case. This involves obtaining 'accredited medical conclusion' and applying 'flexibility'. Accredited medical conclusion is defined as the 'conclusion reached by one or more medical experts acceptable to the Licensing Authority for the purposes of the case concerned, in consultation with flight operations or other experts as necessary' (International Civil Aviation Organization 2001). The licensing authority is synonymous with regulatory authority. In the UK, this is the Civil Aviation Authority (CAA); in the USA, it is the Federal Aviation Administration (FAA).

If accredited medical conclusion indicates that an individual applicant's failure to meet any standard is not likely to jeopardize flight safety, then a fit assessment may still be made. In reaching such a conclusion, relevant ability, skill and experience must be considered and the licence endorsed with any necessary limitations required to protect flight safety, i.e. 'flexibility' can be applied and no 'difference' needs to be filed with ICAO.

An example is the assessment of a professional pilot who loses sight in one eye. An ICAO standard is that the visual acuity shall be at least 6/9 in each eye, and a pilot with no sight in one eye cannot achieve this. However, some regulatory authorities, after due consideration of the individual circumstances, which may involve a practical flight test, may consider such applicants to have a sufficiently low risk to permit medical certification. In such cases, the ICAO flexibility standard can be used to aid decision-making. It reads as follows (International Civil Aviation Organization 2001):

If the Medical Standards prescribed in Chapter 6 for a particular licence are not met, the appropriate medical assessment [certificate] shall not be issued or renewed unless the following conditions are fulfilled:

a) Accredited Medical Conclusion indicates that in special circumstances the applicant's failure to meet any requirement, whether numerical or otherwise, is such that exercise of the privileges of the licence applied for is not likely to jeopardise flight safety;
b) relevant ability, skill and experience of the applicant

and operational conditions have been given due consideration; and

c) the licence is endorsed with any special limitation or limitations when the safe performance of the licence holder's duties is dependent on compliance with such limitation or limitations.

Its application may be illustrated by an example. Accredited medical conclusion in an ophthalmic case will usually involve a medical officer employed by the licensing authority in consultation with one or more consultant ophthalmologists, who will between them reach an assessment on future risk to flight safety. If judged 'acceptable', a medical certificate may be issued, but may include a limitation permitting a professional pilot to fly only in multi-pilot aircraft. Further, with respect to paragraph (b) above, although continued certification may be regarded as acceptable in an experienced pilot, it might not be considered so in an applicant embarking on a flying career and whose lack of operational experience is an additional flight safety risk in addition to his or her cardiac problem.

This flexibility, which permits applicants to be certificated when outside ICAO standards, can undoubtedly benefit individual pilots who develop medical problems, but it has led to wide variability in the application of SARPS throughout the world. In the case of a pilot, or a potential pilot, who has no sight in one eye, depending on his or her licensing authority he or she may be refused all further medical certification (following the ICAO standard), issued a certificate that permits multi-pilot operations only (such as in JAA member states), or issued a certificate without operational limitation (such as in the USA).

It is worth noting that the flexibility standard of ICAO applies only to Chapter 6 (medical provisions) of Annex 1. Such a standard does not feature in any other part of the ICAO provisions, in recognition of the particular difficulty in the medical field of applying rigid rules across different member states. Age limits for pilots do not appear in Chapter 6 (they are found in Chapter 2), so the flexibility standard cannot be applied; a state wishing to allow captains over 60 years of age to operate must file a difference with ICAO, thereby allowing other states to refuse permission for such pilots to operate in their airspace.

The fact that flexibility can be applied to the medical provisions and the variable interpretation in their application encourages a pilot who has been refused medical certification by his or her national authority to seek one that is more liberal in an attempt to obtain, or maintain, his or her licence. The pilot may be successful in this search and can then fly quite legally in aircraft registered in the state that has granted him or her a medical certificate, into the airspace of the country that previously refused such a certificate. Clearly, such 'medical tourism' is not an ideal situation, and the JAA attempted to solve it by taking a different approach with respect to flexibility.

Joint Aviation Authorities

The European JAA's work commenced in 1970 when it was known as the Joint Airworthiness Authorities, producing common type certification requirements for large aeroplanes and their engines, in order to reduce duplication of effort by individual states in approving new aviation hardware. Its name was subsequently changed (to the Joint Aviation Authorities) and its airworthiness work expanded to cover the certification of other aircraft types and components (e.g. light aircraft, helicopters, auxiliary power units, propellers). Maintenance, operations and flight crew licensing (incorporating medical requirements) now fall under the JAA umbrella. The JAA formulates the joint aviation requirements (JARs), the rules concerning civil aviation that are intended to apply in all JAA member states (39 countries). Unfortunately, however, implementation has been problematic in the field of licensing and medical certification.

Joint Aviation Requirements: Flight Crew Licensing Part 3 (Medical)

ICAO Annex 1 was chosen by the JAA to provide the basic structure for a set of common medical standards. The medical committee is a subcommittee (the Licensing Sub-Sectorial Team) of the flight crew licensing committee (the Licensing Sectorial Team). The medical standards document is the Joint Aviation Requirements: Flight Crew Licensing, Part 3 (Medical). Parts 1 and 2 are concerned with the licensing requirements (skill, technical knowledge) of pilots of aeroplanes and helicopters, respectively. Part 4 refers to flight engineers.

When the JARs were written at the beginning of the 1990s, there was no equivalent to the ICAO medical flexibility standard. There are theoretical advantages to this approach. It means that if an individual has a medical problem, then he or she will be investigated in a standard way (laid down in the JARs) and, if certain criteria are met, a medical certificate can be issued. If they are not, a certificate must be refused. Since it is an agreed procedure, the investigation process should be the same in whatever JAA member state the pilot chooses to be investigated, and the aeromedical decision should be the same. Because the procedure is designed to be identical throughout JAA member states, a certificate issued in one state is intended to be valid for operating aircraft registered in another state without further assessment. This commonality applies not only to medical certification but also to the licence, so transfer of pilots between countries and airlines should be easier under the JAA system.

The JAA intended that all full JAA member states would implement the licensing (including medical) JARs at the same time, in 1999. Only two states were ready to do so in that year – Denmark and the UK. Therefore, the desired 'level playing field' of common standards did not occur, as only these two countries had achieved 'mutual recognition' of licences, i.e. had been approved by Central JAA in Hoofddorp, the Netherlands, to issue valid JAA licences. Once mutual recognition is achieved, other mutually recognized member states are obliged to accept a state's licence as meeting all licensing requirements. At the time of writing, 21 JAA member states have become mutually recognized out of the 33 that are currently eligible; only 'full' (as opposed to 'candidate') JAA member states are eligible for mutual recognition. Class of JAA membership is defined by political criteria.

The main reason for the tardy response of JAA member states in adopting the JARs is that since they are not underpinned by any legally binding convention (such as the Chicago Convention of ICAO), there is no legal obligation on states to comply with them. States have agreed only to give their 'best endeavours' to apply the requirements. In order to provide a legal basis to the JARs, national law must be changed in each individual state, which takes time. A further difficulty is that if a state does not want to apply part of the JAR (such as a maximum age limit of 65 years for professional pilots, or the requirement for chest X-rays at initial class 1 examination), then it is not obliged to do so (if such requirements are not included in the ICAO standards). However, despite these difficulties, as more states voluntarily implement the JARs and become mutually recognized, pilots are starting to move more freely around JAA member states.

A problem that became apparent once the JARs were implemented concerned the lack of flexibility in aeromedical decision-making for those states that were applying them. After JAR implementation and mutual recognition by Central JAA, a pilot or potential pilot with a medical condition that was previously acceptable (perhaps under the ICAO flexibility standard) had to be refused JAR certification if he or she was outside the appropriate requirement, even though the pilot might be regarded as safe to operate by the assessing member state's medical department (national, non-JAR 'grandfather rights' were permitted for those already holding licences).

It became clear that some form of flexibility was necessary for those pilots who were regarded as fit to fly but who were outside the JAR. In 2003, the JAA recognized this by means of a limitation called a 'deviation'. A pilot whose medical condition deviates from that prescribed in the JAR may have a JAR medical certificate issued as a deviation. Such a certificate limits the pilot to operating only aircraft registered by the state granting the deviation. If the pilot is fit in accordance with ICAO SARPS (which, of course, include the flexibility standard), then no territorial limits need be applied, but the normal JAR privilege of acceptability to operate aircraft registered in other mutually recognized JAA member states cannot apply unless that other state agrees to this, on an individual basis.

The difficulty of balancing the needs of harmonization (consistency) and yet allowing a degree of flexibility in an individual case illustrates the fundamental dilemma for those formulating international aeromedical policies and guidelines.

European Aviation Safety Agency

The lack of any Europe-wide legal basis for the JARs has led to a further development in aviation regulation, the establishment of the European Aviation Safety Agency (EASA). Based in Cologne, Germany, the EASA has already taken over the JAA's role of certificating new aircraft as they come on to the market, and it is anticipated that rule-making in the field of personnel licensing, including medical certification, will become part of the EASA task in 2007. From the routine medical certification viewpoint, little is likely to change, since the EASA is not intended to be involved in day-to-day medical decision-making or appeals against such decisions. The main difference will be that, unlike the JARs, the rules set will be underpinned by a European directive, which is legally binding on European Union (EU) member states. Fortunately, the concern that rigid rules would be formulated by the EASA seems unfounded, as medical flexibility is likely to be permitted. The full relationship of the EASA with the ICAO (only individual states can become members of the ICAO) and the status of current JAA member states that are not members of the EU is yet to be determined.

Federal Aviation Administration

About half of all scheduled passenger, freight and mail traffic is accounted for by airlines of the USA (International Civil Aviation Organization 2002). The FAA regulates civil aviation activities in the USA, and its aeromedical certification division in Oklahoma receives 460 000 pilot medical report forms annually (compared with about 50 000 in the UK) (Federal Aviation Administration 2003).

Compared with the JAA, the FAA is regarded as a more liberal regulator. For example, the FAA approves a number of different colour-vision tests, including the 24-plate Ishihara test, the (only) screening test employed by the JAR. To pass this, an FAA applicant (for any class of medical certificate) is required to identify correctly nine of the first 15 plates; a JAA applicant has to identify all 15 plates correctly. The FAA requires no audiograms to be under- taken by any class of applicant – a spoken-voice test is adequate for screening purposes. For class 1 applicants (and private pilots holding an instrument rating), the JAA requires five-yearly audiograms until the age of 40 years, and then two-yearly. There is no FAA requirement for an ECG in airline co-pilots of any age. With the JAA, however, the ECG periodicity for co-pilots is the same as for captains: an ECG is undertaken at initial examination and then every five years until age 30 years, and then with increasing periodicity with age, reaching every six months at age 50 plus. The FAA accepts the use of warfarin (if well controlled) in professional pilots, but this is not permitted by the JAA.

Although there are important differences in licensing practises between the JAA and FAA, there is little apparent difference in accident rates, either for all causes (see Figure 36.2, p. 550) or for medical causes, although no directly comparable data exist for the latter. However, this may not be surprising, since such differences in medical standards are not likely to affect overall accident statistics when the large majority of pilots are operating multi-pilot aircraft and have no medical deficiency, the situation for the professional pilot population in most developed countries (Mitchell and Evans 2004).

IN-FLIGHT INCAPACITATION

The purpose of aeromedical examinations is to identify and exclude those who have an unacceptably increased risk of incapacitation during the relevant period of certification subsequent to the examination. Episodes of intercurrent illness that may lead to incapacitation are deemed to be self-regulatory, in that an ICAO standard requires of a pilot that they will not exercise the privileges of their licence if they are aware of any medical condition that might be a flight safety hazard. However, for any illness other than minor self-limiting conditions, formal assessment by, or at least guidelines from, a specialist in aviation medicine is required before a licence holder returns to duty. In-flight incapacitation is defined by the ICAO as 'any condition which affects the health of the licence holder during the performance of his duties associated with the privileges of his licence and renders him incapable of performing those duties' (International Civil Aviation Organization 1985).

In-flight incapacitation can occur in any pilot of any age, although the frequency from particular causes is normally related to the age-specific incidence in the general population. In-flight incapacitation may be of physical or mental origin. A study in 1991 revealed that 29 per cent of airline pilots had experienced at least one such incident during their career (Green and James 1991). The majority of incapacitations are caused by gastrointestinal symptoms, almost all of which are caused by self-limiting minor illnesses (Table 36.2).

Incapacitations may present suddenly or slowly. Here is an example of the latter (International Civil Aviation Organization 1985):

> Shortly after reaching cruise, I experienced severe abdominal pains, which soon rendered me incapable of operating a safe flight. I turned command over to the first officer and put the second officer in the first officer's seat, while I lay in great pain on the cockpit floor.

This may be regarded as a 'typical' incapacitation, which happens slowly and represents only a small risk to flight safety, since control of the aircraft is maintained and a coordinated handover of control can be effected. Rarely (and, therefore, unexpectedly) the pilot may collapse suddenly at the controls (Air Accidents Investigation Branch 1999):

> The first officer removed the checklist from its stowage and tried to read it. Although at this stage she looked normal, she was unable to read the check list sensibly and uttered what the commander described as 'gibberish'. After a few seconds, she suddenly twisted violently in her seat and her body went rigid, causing her to apply a significant amount of rudder, the effect of which was felt by those in the passenger cabin.

Both of these examples may be classed as 'obvious' incapacitations, in that it was clear to the crew that an incapacitation had occurred. 'Subtle' incapacitation, on the other hand, can present difficulties in identification. A pilot who has suffered a heart attack may continue to sit upright, with hands on the controls and with open eyes, and yet make no further useful control inputs. A subtle incapacitation occurred to the captain of a McDonnell Douglas DC10 on the approach to an airport in North America (National Transportation Safety Board 1987):

> Immediately after the hard landing, the captain was observed by the co-pilot and flight engineer to be incapacitated. The co-pilot took control of the airplane and guided it onto a high speed taxiway. The captain was found to have died of a myocardial infarction.

It is perhaps fortunate that the DC10 aircraft has a relatively high nose-up attitude on approach, such that the main wheels contact the ground first (before the nose wheel), even without any input from the pilot.

Incapacitation due to physical causes is usually relatively easy to detect and deal with. Mental incapacitation, however, is often subtle and may not be sustained, and the affected pilot may not agree that he or she is incapacitated. It can be defined as a pilot who is mentally disoriented, mentally unwell or obstinate, while physically able and vocally responsive, and yet whose behaviour represents a risk to flight safety (International Civil Aviation Organization 1985).

Mental incapacitation may be due to a number of causes, e.g. organic brain disease, psychiatric illness, extreme anxiety, or flying under the influence of drugs or alcohol. An example follows (International Civil Aviation Organization 1985):

> On two occasions, we descended through our assigned altitude. I was the non-flying pilot and made all the call outs ... On both occasions, in addition to the required call outs, I informed the handling pilot that we were descending through our assigned altitude. His corrections were slow and on one occasion we went 400 feet below, and on the other, 500 feet below the assigned altitude. In addition, his airspeed and heading control were not precise ...

It is easy to see the difficulties that mental incapacitation might entail if incapacitation occurs in a captain who refuses to accept he or she has a problem and demands that their commands are followed, especially if the first officer is inexperienced or unassertive. In 1982, a co-pilot failed to report his captain for carrying out an unnecessary 70-degree banked turn in a McDonnell Douglas DC8 (a four-engine jet airliner). The following day, at 164 feet on the approach, the same captain retarded all four thrust levers and selected

Table 36.2 *Causes of incapacitation in airline pilots*

Rank (1967)	Rank (1987)	Condition	1967		1987	
			n	(%)	*n*	(%)
1	1	Uncontrolled bowel action	450	23	336	19
2/3/4	2/3/4	Other gastrointestinal symptoms	1042	54	950	54
5	5	Earache/blocked ear	153	8	186	7
6	6	Faintness/general weakness	120	6	124	7
7	7	Headache, including migraine	118	6	109	6
8	8	Vertigo/disorientation	68	3	63	4

From Buley (1969) and Green and James (1991).

reverse thrust on two engines. The aircraft crashed short of the runway, with the loss of 24 lives. It was discovered later that the pilot was suffering from schizophrenia (Aircraft Accident Investigation Commission 1983).

PRACTICAL DECISION-MAKING IN AEROMEDICAL CERTIFICATION

It is fortunate that most airline operations are undertaken with two pilots, since this provides a remarkably effective fail-safe advantage should one become incapacitated. It also enables some pilots who become unfit for solo flying (demanding the lowest medical incapacitation risk) to continue their career in two-pilot operations. A pilot who has made a good recovery from a myocardial infarction will have a statistically increased risk of incapacitation compared with his or her age-matched peer group but may be permitted under the ICAO flexibility standard to continue flying, with the limitation (in some parts of the world, such as the JAA member states) that they fly 'as or with qualified co-pilot only'. This has enabled many professional aircrew personnel who have developed a medical problem to continue their careers in two-pilot operations.

Until the agreement of the Chicago Convention, different medical standards for civilian pilots were determined by individual states and were based largely on military experience. These tended to be relatively restrictive, with the examiner, quite reasonably, erring on the side of caution when faced with a condition whose prognosis was not predictable with accuracy. However, nowadays, many applicants with a previously unacceptable medical history can be classified into different risk groups, thus enabling some relatively low-risk individuals to continue operating when previously the condition would have been automatically disqualifying.

In a number of common conditions, there is sufficient knowledge of incapacitation on which to base a reasonably objective decision with respect to future risk. Objectivity has the great advantages of facilitating consistency of decision-making and enabling audit of past decisions, so that standards can be developed and refined more easily. However, it is only during the past 20 years that serious attempts have been made to determine an objective standard by which to judge medical fitness for flying.

Objective risk assessment

In 1973, Anderson presented a paper at the 44th Annual Scientific Meeting of the Aerospace Medical Association drawing on both his experience as senior consultant to the Civil Aviation Medicine Service of Canada and his engineering knowledge concerning the airworthiness require-

ments of airliners. At that time, the requirement for mechanical reliability was that a catastrophe (defined as an event involving the loss of an aircraft and/or fatalities) should not occur for airworthiness reasons more often then one in 10^7 (ten million) flying hours. An occurrence of this frequency could be regarded as 'extremely remote'. It was apparent to Anderson that the risk of pilot 'failure' could be assessed in a similar way and could provide a method of determining, for the first time, an objective method of assessing medical fitness.

This idea was taken up by the UK CAA, which, in 1982, convened the first of four cardiological workshops to refine the concept of risk assessment with respect to cardiovascular disease in pilots (Joy and Bennett 1984). At that time, the fatal accident rate for large jet transport aircraft in the UK was somewhat greater than 0.2 per one million flying hours. This was the all-cause rate, including weather, engine failure, aircraft system failure and pilot error. For the purpose of assessing medical risk, a target fatal accident rate was set at 0.1 fatal accidents per one million flying hours (0.1 in 10^6 or one in 10^7 flying hours), approximately half the rate at that time.

Having chosen one in 10^7 as the all-cause target fatal accident rate, the contribution from aeromedical causes to the overall operational risk that could be regarded as acceptable remained to be decided. It was felt that the flight-deck crew could be viewed in the same way as an aircraft system, and that no single system should contribute more than ten per cent to the total risk. Crew failure (pilot error plus incapacitation), when treated in the same way as any other system failure, should, therefore, result in a fatal accident no more often than one in 100 million flying hours. Finally, it was felt that medical incapacitation should account for only a small proportion (ten per cent) of the overall risk of crew failure, accepting that human error will comprise the majority of crew failures. Medical incapacitation should, therefore, cause a fatal accident no more often than one in 1000 million flying hours (Figure 36.3).

Acceptable risk in two-pilot operations: the one per cent rule

Cardiovascular disease (comprising mainly coronary heart attacks and strokes), although not the only cause of sudden incapacity in pilots, is the cause that is most amenable to a relatively accurate individual risk assessment by a licensing authority or aeromedical examiner. Decisions made by a licensing authority concerning cardiovascular disease are numerically likely to be the most important in the professional pilot community, thereby having the greatest impact on flight safety. For these reasons, such disease has been afforded a great deal of attention.

A cardiovascular mortality rate of one in 10^9 hours (equivalent to an annual cardiovascular mortality rate of

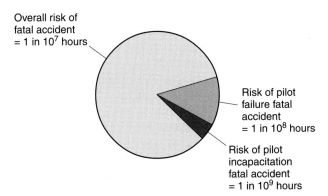

Overall risk of fatal accident = 1 in 10^7 hours

Risk of pilot failure fatal accident = 1 in 10^8 hours

Risk of pilot incapacitation fatal accident = 1 in 10^9 hours

Figure 36.3 *Medical incapacitation as a proportion of all-cause fatal accident risk.*

Table 36.3 *England and Wales mortality (2002) from coronary heart disease and cerebrovascular disease by age group and sex: rate per 100 000 population*

Age (years)	Coronary heart disease (ICD-10 120–25)		Cerebrovascular disease (ICD-10 160–69)	
	Male	Female	Male	Female
20–24	0.0	0.5	0.8	0.6
25–29	1.3	0.5	1.0	0.6
30–34	4.1	1.3	2.1	1.9
35–39	11.4	2.3	3.8	3.7
40–44	30.8	5.9	7.8	6.9
45–49	63.9	14.4	14.9	13.8
50–54	104.9	21.6	20.1	17.4
55–59	193.7	44.2	36.4	24.9
60–64	307.5	100.4	64.1	44.1
65–69	496.7	198.3	123.0	86.5
70–74	742.2	395.7	229.1	201.0
75–79	1041.3	746.3	413.9	470.2
80–84	1389.6	1275.9	670.7	981.9

ICD-10, *International Classification of Diseases*, 10th revision. Geneva: World Health Organization, 1990. Data from UK National Statistics, www.statistics.gov.uk.

one per 100 000 population) is, on average, not achievable at any age for a European male, except perhaps for those in their early 20s. Mortality from coronary heart disease and cerebrovascular disease, the main contributors to cardiovascular mortality, are given in Table 36.3 for England and Wales.

In order to achieve this very low level of risk, two-pilot operations are necessary to provide a fail-safe system in the event of one pilot's incapacitation. A simulator study indicated that subsequent to pilot incapacitation at a critical part of the flight (takeoff and initial climb, approach and landing; Figure 36.4) the second pilot would take over successfully on 399 occasions out of 400 such events (Chapman 1984). It was felt that this was probably optimistic for routine operations, where anticipation of a significant failure (aircraft or pilot) is likely to be less acute

than in the atmosphere associated with a simulator check. Taking this into account, it was assumed that a trained pilot should be able to take over safely on 99 occasions out of 100 (Bennett 1988).

Stated another way, one incapacitation per 100 occurring at a critical period of the flight could be expected to result in a fatal accident. Therefore, a second pilot on the flight deck reduces the risk of any such incapacitation at a

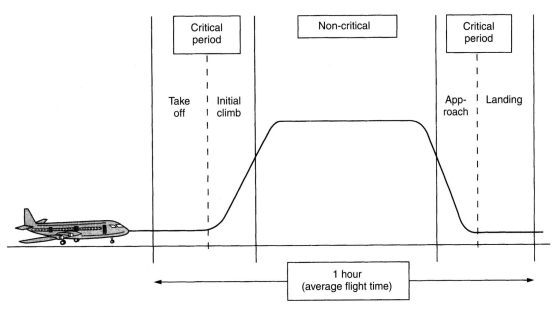

Critical period

Non-critical

Critical period

Take off | Initial climb

App-roach | Landing

1 hour (average flight time)

Figure 36.4 *Critical and non-critical phases of flight with respect to medical incapacitation.*

critical period causing a fatal accident by a factor of 100. Further, if it is assumed that

- the critical portions of flight represent ten per cent of total flight time (assumed to be approximately one hour)
- incapacitations occur randomly during flight, and
- the second pilot safely takes over control on all incapacitations occurring outside the critical portions of flight

then only one in ten incapacitation events during flight has the potential to result in a fatal accident (those occurring at a critical part of the flight), and in only one in 100 such events will the second pilot fail to take over safely. As one-tenth of one-hundredth is one-thousandth, it can be assumed that, on average, only one in 1000 pilot incapacitations occurring during a flight of one hour will cause a fatal accident.

As stated previously, the target fatal accident rate from medical causes is one in 10^9 flying hours. If airliners were flown by one pilot, this would be an 'acceptable' risk of pilot medical incapacitation, but it cannot be achieved for cardiovascular disease for males in England and Wales in their mid-20s or older. However, since at least two pilots invariably are required to operate large aircraft, an incapacitation rate greater than one in 10^9 flying hours is acceptable for an individual pilot operating such (two-pilot) aircraft. In two-pilot aircraft, only one in 1000 in-flight incapacitations is anticipated to result in a fatal accident, so the acceptable risk for a pilot can be increased by a factor of 1000 from one incapacitation in 10^9 hours to one in 10^6 hours.

Since there are 8760 hours in a year, approximating to 10 000 (10^4) hours, an incapacitation rate of one in 10^6 hours is equivalent to a rate of one per cent in 10^4 hours, or one per cent per annum (Figure 36.5). This is known as the one per cent rule and forms the basis of aeromedical decision-making in several countries. It has been adopted as guidance by the JAA for this purpose.

Applying the one per cent rule

In order to ensure that no individual with an incapacitation risk of over one per cent per annum operates as a pilot, it is essential that the risk of incapacitation for various medical conditions and at different ages is known.

An incapacitation rate of 1 in 10^6 hours is approximately equivalent to a rate of 1% per year

$\begin{cases} \text{1 in } 10^6 \text{ hours} \\ = 0.01 \text{ in } 10^4 \text{ hours} \\ = 1/100 \text{ in } 10^4 \text{ hours} \\ = 1\% \text{ in } 10^4 \text{ hours} \\ = 1\% \text{ in 1 year} \end{cases}$

Figure 36.5 *Derivation of one per cent in one year.*

Cardiovascular mortality rates (primarily coronary heart disease and cerebrovascular disease) are well documented and increase exponentially with age, reaching, for males in England and Wales, one per cent per annum (approximating to a cardiovascular mortality rate of 1000 per 100 000) at 70–74 years of age (see Table 36.3).

There are marked differences in mortality rates between different nationalities (Levi *et al.* 2002; Rayner and Peterson 2001). Death rates from coronary heart disease and strokes are falling in most northern and western European countries, as they are in the USA, but they are rising in most central and eastern European states. However, a common finding is an increase in mortality of approximately 100-fold between the ages of 30 and 65 years and a lower rate in females. However, currently no formal difference in medical certification policy applies to females as compared with males.

The one per cent rule has provided a very useful objective standard against which to assess the medical fitness of professional pilots. It has been found that despite its weaknesses, it represents methodology that at present cannot be replaced. However, several points have been raised concerning its use, which are addressed below.

CARDIOVASCULAR MORTALITY RATES DO NOT NECESSARILY CORRESPOND TO INCAPACITATION RATES

For licensing authorities, whether a pilot dies from a particular disease is not an important flight safety issue. More important is an assessment of the pilot's risk of becoming incapacitated during flight and whether that incapacitation will occur suddenly or slowly, the former posing a much greater risk to flight safety. As coronary heart attacks have statistically the greatest likelihood (along with neurological disease, especially seizures) of causing a sudden incapacity, and because accurate data concerning the risk of incapacitation in the professional pilot population are not available, existing general-population data have been applied to this group to assess the risk.

Tunstall-Pedoe (1984) reviewed the data from a study of a population in the Tower Hamlets area of London and found the coronary heart attack rate in males aged 55–64 years to be 2.3 times that of the same cause mortality rate for this group, indicating the majority who suffer a heart attack do not immediately die as a consequence. If this group comprised pilots, they could suffer incapacitating symptoms but not appear in the cardiovascular mortality statistics for that age group. Cardiovascular mortality statistics alone therefore underestimate the actual number of heart attacks, each one potentially incapacitating.

On the other hand Tunstall-Pedoe also reported that of those suffering an infarct, about 50 per cent have a history of conditions, such as insulin-treated diabetes, that normally would exclude a professional pilot from flying. Therefore, although they may eventually contribute to the cardiovascular mortality statistics, they do not pose a flight safety risk because these pilots would be taken off flying duties before they could suffer in-flight incapacity. Further, Tunstall-Pedoe estimates that 30–50 per cent of heart attacks are not likely to be immediately incapacitating, and pilots suffering such an event are likely to be removed from flying duties after their first cardiac event.

So, although the raw cardiovascular mortality statistics underestimate the total number of cardiovascular events in the general population, many of those dying from the disease would already have been assessed unfit for flying duties. Tunstall-Pedoe therefore concludes that the general-population cardiovascular mortality statistics give an approximation to the cardiovascular incapacitation rate for professional pilots.

CARDIOVASCULAR INCAPACITATION IS NOT CAUSED ONLY BY CORONARY HEART ATTACKS

Serious cardiac arrhythmias from causes other than coronary artery disease can cause sudden incapacitation. However, these are not as common as coronary artery disease as a cause of incapacitation. The other common cause of sudden cardiovascular incapacitation is stroke, but this is comparatively uncommon in the age range of airline pilots, i.e. up to age 65 years (see Table 36.3). The most common potential cause of a sudden cardiovascular incapacity therefore is coronary heart disease.

PROFESSIONAL PILOTS ARE IN SOCIAL CLASS 1

People in the higher social classes in Europe and North America have a lower cardiovascular risk than the general population. It seems that professional pilots live longer than the general population (Irvine and Davies 1992). Using general-population data will therefore tend towards a cautious outcome if used in aeromedical certification decisions.

SUDDEN INCAPACITATION DOES NOT OCCUR DUE TO CARDIOVASCULAR DISEASE ALONE

An International Air Transport Association (IATA) study documented epileptiform seizures and syncope in addition to cardiovascular disease as the causes of sudden incapacita-

Table 36.4 *Sudden incapacitations in airline pilots: 36 000 pilots at risk over a ten-year period*

Cause	n
Acute myocardial ischaemia	10
Epileptiform seizures	7
Syncope	6
Cerebral haemorrhage	3
Total	26

From Bennett (1984).

tion in 36 000 pilots followed for ten years (Table 36.4). Some degree of underreporting is likely; however, if taken at face value, and assuming the pilots were flying 600 hours per year, these 26 events represent a rate of sudden incapacitation of about one in every ten million flying hours. In this series, no accident resulted – an expected outcome since having a second pilot on the flight deck reduces the chance that an incapacitation will cause a fatal accident by a factor of 1000. Even taking other causes of risk into account, it would appear from this study that the average pilot has a risk of sudden incapacitation of less than one per cent per annum (one in 10^6 hours). The study is from a period when coronary heart disease in England and Wales was more prevalent than today: the mortality rate per 100 000 from coronary heart disease (previously termed ischaemic heart disease) for males aged 60–64 years was 926 in 1979 and 307 in 2002, a remarkable reduction. The trends in England and Wales for coronary heart disease/ischaemic heart disease in males are given in Table 36.5.

A survey of all types of incapacitations in UK airline pilots over the ten-year period 1990–99 found an incidence of 127 such events, but only 20 were 'serious', i.e. resulting in loss of consciousness or inability to contribute to the flight operation for a prolonged period (Evans 2002). Two of the serious events were of cardiac origin (both resulted in in-flight death) and four were neurological (including two seizures). Most of the other events were due to gastro-intestinal upset, which, although 'serious', did not occur suddenly. If all serious incapacitations in this study are regarded as 'sudden' (an incorrect, pessimistic assumption), then the 20 recorded incidents occurred during 19.3 million flight hours, representing a rate of approximately one in one million hours. It has been argued above that 1000 in-flight incapacitations will occur before a fatal accident occurs; therefore, if the observed rate is one in 10^6 hours, then the

Table 36.5 *Trends in coronary heart disease mortality (previously known as ischaemic heart disease) in England and Wales for males aged 60–64 years*

Year	Mortality (/100 000 population)
1979	926
1993	592
1994	537
1995	512
1996	481
1997	442
1998	424
1999	383
2000	361
2001	349
2002	307

From UK National Statistics (www.statistics.gov.uk) and Tunstall-Pedoe (1988).

target of one in 10^9 (1000 times lower) should be achieved. The UK has been applying a one per cent limit for incapacitation risk to cardiovascular disease and other diseases for more than two decades, so it would appear that this approach has been justified, and cautious, in terms of the number of incapacitations actually observed.

THE ONE PER CENT RULE MAY BE TOO RESTRICTIVE

The one per cent rule has proved to be useful over the years, but some have claimed it is too restrictive. This argument maintains that if the maximum acceptable risk for an individual is capped at 1% per annum, then the average risk of incapacitation for the whole pilot population must be less than this, probably below 0.1 per cent per annum (1 in 10^7 hours) since 0.1% per annum is the approximate cardiovascular mortality rate for males in England and Wales at age 50 years, and the average age of the pilot population is under 50. The addition of a second pilot reduces the risk by a factor of 1,000. So one might expect, on average, a medical-cause fatal accident rate of less than one in 10^{10} flying hours in two-pilot operations i.e. at least 10 times lower than the target rate of 1 in 10^9 hours.

This argument has merit if the risk assessment is considered per one million flight hours rather than per individual flight. If, in a cohort of 10 000 pilots, each flying 500 hours per year, one has a high risk of incapacitation, say ten per cent per annum, and the remaining 9999 have an average risk of 0.1 per cent per annum (this is not a realistic scenario, but it illustrates the point), then the overall decrease in flight safety, i.e. the additional risk per one million flying hours because of the 'unfit' pilot, is insignificant.

However, for each individual flight that the 'unfit' pilot operates as the handling pilot, the risk is increased (by a factor of 100) compared with those operated by an average crew. Nevertheless, the risk per one-hour flight is still exceedingly small, the chance of a fatal accident during such a flight being increased from one in 10^{10} to one in 10^8 (100 million).

ONLY SUDDEN INCAPACITY IS TAKEN INTO ACCOUNT

The analysis of risk and derivation of the one per cent rule assumes that an incapacitation that occurs slowly or during a non-critical portion of flight is inconsequential for flight safety, but this is probably unrealistic. Gastrointestinal illness is the most common cause of in-flight incapacitation, but it rarely causes a serious flight safety problem because it occurs slowly. However, the reduction in experience and absence of crew monitoring on the flight deck caused by the loss of one crew member clearly does affect flight safety detrimentally for the remainder of the flight – but it is difficult to quantify by how much. It is difficult to regulate for gastrointestinal illness, and the main responsibility lies with the airlines

themselves in terms of flight crew education in preventive hygiene measures and with the aircrew to follow the advice given. Mental incapacitation from psychiatric illness normally does not occur suddenly, but it represents a clear and important risk to flight safety, again which is hard to quantify in terms of risk of incapacitation.

FLIGHTS, ON AVERAGE, LAST FOR MORE THAN ONE HOUR

The average flight time is increasing. In 2000 for UK airline operations the average flight time was 2.3 hours, compared with 1.65 hours in 1983, a reflection of improved technology allowing aircraft to stay airborne for increasingly long periods (UK Civil Aviation Authority 2002). In the derivation of the one per cent rule, it was assumed that flights lasted one hour on average. Since the critical periods for incapacity are at the beginning and end of a flight, longer sectors are beneficial to safety with respect to the risk of medical cause accidents. Note that although statistics refer to 'flight time', what is actually recorded is 'block time', i.e. chock to chock, so the figures include a proportion of time spent taxiing before takeoff and after landing. If the one per cent rule was derived today, using a flight time of two hours instead of one hour, then an acceptable risk of two per cent per annum would be derived (Mitchell and Evans 2004). At least one licensing authority of a major ICAO Contracting State currently uses two per cent as its risk limit.

A CRITICAL PERIOD OF THREE MINUTES AT THE BEGINNING AND END OF A FLIGHT IS TOO LONG

Modern aircraft have improved performance and sophisticated autopilots, which may mean that three minutes is too long a period to be assumed 'critical'. Another way of looking at the critical period is to take a height (rather than a time period after takeoff or before landing) below which a safe handover is not guaranteed. It has been argued that 1500 feet is reasonable, as this is taken by the Joint Research Centre (European Commission) European Co-ordination Centre for Aviation Incident Reporting Systems (ECCAIRS) as defining the transition from the takeoff/initial climb phases to the climb phase, and from the descent/holding phases to the approach phase (European Co-ordination Centre for Aviation Incident Reporting Systems 2005). If this is accepted, while keeping all other assumptions the same as in the original derivation, the critical period is reduced from six to four minutes per flight, and a one per cent rule would be too conservative (Mitchell and Evans 2004).

MODERN AIRCRAFT ARE EASIER TO FLY

In a study carried out in the 1980s, it was found that 399 incapacitations out of 400 that occurred in a simulator during a critical flight phase were handled safely by the crew (Chapman 1984). Modern airliners are probably easier to fly single-handed and are more forgiving of mistakes, the most modern airliners protection devices preventing certain pilot inputs likely to jeopardize flight safety. The assumption that one incapacitation out of 99 would result in a fatal accident may, therefore, be pessimistic. Although plausible, this has yet to be demonstrated in an up-to-date simulator study.

Statistical uncertainties

Although it is possible to derive an acceptable objective risk using assumptions as outlined above, human performance and medical illness often are not easy to analyse statistically. Psychiatric illness is probably the most difficult to assess objectively and is more likely than physical illness to lead to subtle incapacitation. Another risk that is difficult to quantify is the possibility of the incapacitation of one pilot causing that of the other, e.g. incapacitation in one pilot might conceivably lead to a surge of catecholamine release in the other sufficient to provoke asymptomatic arrhythmia. This is currently regarded as unlikely, but accurate data are not available. However, the most common time of day for cardiovascular death is the early hours of the morning, when catecholamine effects from external events are absent (ISIS-2 1988).

Further, if two pilots each have an incapacitation risk of one per cent per annum (one in 10^6 hours), then the risk of a double incapacitation in one hour is one in $10^6 \times 10^6$, which is one in 10^{12} hours, a figure that may be discounted as insignificant. Put another way, an aeromedical assessment could be incorrect in a pilot by a factor of 1000 and thus could permit an individual to fly who in fact has an incapacitation risk of not one in 10^6 hours but one in 10^3 hours. If the other crew member has a risk of one in 10^6 hours, then the crew, in terms of the risk of a double incapacitation during a one-hour flight, would still achieve the target medical-cause fatal accident rate of one in 10^9 hours, since the double incapacitation risk would then become one in $10^6 \times 10^3$, i.e. one in 10^9 (the target rate, as outlined in the one per cent rule, above). An error of three orders of magnitude is exceedingly unlikely, since an incapacitation risk of one in 10^3 is equivalent to an incapacitation every 36.5 days (one-tenth of a year), and it is highly unlikely that an error of this degree in assessing risk would be made by a licensing authority.

As more medical data become available, objective risk assessments will be refined. Currently under consideration, and already introduced by one licensing authority, is the use of a cardiovascular risk evaluation based on allocating points for various risk factors, including age, sex, blood pressure and blood cholesterol level. Pilots whose total points exceed a certain value would be subjected to further testing, such as an exercise ECG.

Polymorphic risk

Polymorphic (absolute) risk is the sum of separate, lesser single risks, each known as an attributable risk. The one per cent rule has tended to be used in the context of determining whether an attributable risk, e.g. cardiovascular risk, is acceptable for medical certification. It has been argued that a pilot with a single medical problem, such as successfully treated single-vessel coronary disease (an attributable risk), may fall within the acceptable risk of a future event to continue flying, but if he or she also has diabetes (also an attributable risk) controlled by diet, then the total (polymorphic) risk may be above the acceptable threshold. For two-pilot operations, with their greatly increased safety margins when compared with single-pilot operations, concentrating on the most important single attributable risk may be acceptable when reaching an aeromedical decision on certification. However, for single-pilot operations, more attention should be given to polymorphic risk, since single-pilot flights are critically disadvantaged in the event of an incapacity (Chamberlain 1999).

Age is an important attributable risk. A disease that might be acceptable in a young person may not be acceptable in an older pilot. The effect of age is particularly important in pilots engaged in aerial work, such as flying instruction, where there are no age limits and the activity is usually undertaken in small aircraft with only one pilot. In fact, the JARs demand a cardiological examination and exercise ECG for professional pilots at 65 years and then four-yearly. Although this method of risk assessment is not very sophisticated, since it is based only on age, it does indicate the willingness of licensing authorities to take risk factors into account in setting regulatory policy.

OVERVIEW OF REGULATORY MEDICAL REQUIREMENTS

The dilemma facing the writer of aeromedical policies and guidelines is to make the requirements sufficiently prescriptive to ensure, if possible, consistent decision-making and yet to enable regulatory authorities to exercise flexibility to deal with individual cases on an individual basis. The ICAO recognizes that medical expertise, treatment and investigation facilities vary greatly throughout the world. Also, the view of different licensing authorities concerning what is an acceptable risk varies from state to state, as illustrated above with the example of how a case of myocardial infarction may be assessed, by the application, or not, of the ICAO flexibility standard.

The ICAO has largely succeeded in forming a set of medical standards that has worldwide application, because it has concentrated on writing minimum standards and permitting flexibility. Most authorities can agree on minimum standards, as long as in their state they can impose higher standards and additional examinations or investigations if they wish (and many do). At the other end of the spectrum, for those states that feel that even the minimum standards are too demanding, there is the option of 'filing a difference' or, in an individual case, applying the flexibility standard. Although this has resulted in heterogeneous medical standards throughout the world, the system has been successful in facilitating international air-transport operations, whilst minimizing the number of medically related fatal accidents. This is, however, not due only to the application of regulations, since airlines themselves have a keen interest in promoting safe operations for commercial reasons. In the past, large airlines, often state-owned and accounting for most international traffic, set higher medical requirements for their personnel than the licensing authority demanded, particularly on recruitment, although the various disability discrimination and human rights legal constraints now in place have tended to reduce the differences in recent years.

It is likely that significant differences in medical requirements will continue to exist among ICAO contracting states. There are a number of reasons for this. In some states, military examiners undertake civilian pilot assessments, and their natural tendency may be towards a relatively restrictive policy, more in keeping with the requirements for military personnel. If there is little consultation between industry representatives and the licensing authority, then aeromedical decisions are likely to be more restrictive; if the licensing authority and/or the medical care system is not well funded, then it will be difficult to apply flexibility, since expertise and relatively sophisticated investigations may be necessary to stratify pilots into a lower-risk category.

A belief that stricter medical standards and a greater number of routine examinations and investigations than the minimum set by the ICAO will result in an increased level of flight safety is a factor in many states. This view can be challenged and is discussed below. Further, the incidence of disease in the general (and flight crew) population varies throughout the world. It is reasonable for countries with a high incidence of, for example, diabetes or tuberculosis to incorporate additional measures to detect such potential problems. It is known that the prevalence of heart disease varies from country to country as well as over time (Levi *et al.* 2002; Rayner 2000). Such diverse prevalence of disease clearly will result in heterogeneous medical requirements for medical certification.

One reason for the small number of medically related fatal accidents is that the two-pilot flight deck is relatively forgiving of pilot incapacitation. In the derivation of the one per cent rule above, it was calculated that there would on average be 1000 in-flight sudden incapacitations for each fatal accident. On long-range flights, there are often three or even four pilots, and so there is a further in-built safety factor should one become unwell. The situation for single-pilot operations is, of course, very different. Any incapacitation with only one pilot aboard is very serious and even a slowly developing event that would not be difficult to contain in a multi-pilot aircraft can be problematic. However, single-pilot operations tend to be of short duration and occur within easy reach of a diversion airfield. Further, the aircraft flown are relatively small and carry few passengers, and the public seems to have a greater tolerance of fatal accidents involving small commercial aircraft (and therefore fewer deaths) than those involving large aircraft. There are, however, relatively few accidents per year in this category, because the number of hours flown is small in comparison with those flown by larger aircraft. The higher accident rate in small aircraft is not, in the main, due to reasons of medical incapacitation but rather, as with accidents in other categories, due to pilot error, when there is no other crew member to assist in the decision-making process and in monitoring the flight path.

Single-pilot public-transport operations tend to utilize relatively unsophisticated aircraft, often having piston engines and simple avionics, compared with large jet airliners. The overall accident rate can, therefore, be expected to be greater, for technical reasons, than for the latter group of aircraft. It may, therefore, be acceptable to have a greater medical-cause fatal accident rate for such operations. The ideal situation is for all public-transport aircraft operations to require two pilots, but this is not possible, because some are not certificated from an airworthiness viewpoint to operate other than single crew, and to require two pilots would make some operations financially unviable.

One way to reduce the medical risk is to permit only pilots without any known medical problems to operate as single pilots. This is the reason for the JAA adding an 'as or with co-pilot only' limitation to some pilots who have had a serious medical event, such as a myocardial infarction. Although such pilots may be investigated and found to have a relatively low risk of recurrence, statistically the risk is still increased when compared with their peer groups. There is an argument that pilots who are considered for a return to flying after a cardiac event might, on average, be safer than their peer groups, because they are investigated fully. There are, however, few data to support this assumption.

ICAO has recognised the safety benefit of having a second pilot in its standards. In November 2005 the relevant Annex 1 standard was changed to allow airline captains to continue with an annual medical examination when aged over 40 years, i.e. the same as for the under 40s, but only if they are operating in a multi-pilot flight deck. Previously, such pilots were obliged to undertake a six-monthly examination when over 40. On the other hand, for pilots engaged in single-crew commerical air transport operations carrying passengers, the annual examination increases to six-monthly for those over 40 years.

Evidence from fatal accident reports over more than 20 years indicates that licensing authorities may have overregulated for physical disease, especially cardiovascular disease, but paid insufficient attention to less easily quantifiable psychiatric illnesses. For two decades, the most common cause of premature retirement of airline pilots in the UK, as in most countries, has been cardiovascular disease, amounting to 40–50 per cent of the total of all cases. And yet, globally, in the same time period, there has not been a recorded fatal accident in a two-pilot airline operation caused by cardiovascular incapacitation (Evans 2001, 2003).

Airline accidents are well investigated. Since they occur mainly in large aircraft with monitoring equipment such as flight-data and cockpit-voice recorders, it is likely that a physical incapacitation contributing to the cause would be discovered. On the other hand, there have been many recorded physical incapacitations in two-pilot aircraft, including sudden cardiac deaths and seizures, that have not resulted in an adverse outcome for the flight involved. Two points are apparent from this. First, sudden (and, indeed, slow) incapacitation cannot be prevented in flight crew. The techniques for discovering cardiac or neurological disease in asymptomatic pilots are insufficiently sensitive to predict accurately those who are likely to succumb in the next 6 or 12 months, and so it is likely that many, if not most, incapacitations will occur in pilots who have no known medical problem. Second, as there is no apparent difference in medical-cause accidents between countries with very restrictive medical requirements and those with a more liberal approach, it seems that the mandatory incapacitation training in two-pilot aircraft is normally adequate to mitigate the flight safety risk of an in-flight physical incapacity.

Since 1980, the only recorded fatal accident in an aircraft over 5700 kg in which physical incapacitation played a part was caused partially by vomiting in a co-pilot when the captain flew the aircraft into terrain and it was assumed that the co-pilot was not monitoring the flight profile properly (Evans 2003). However, there have been several fatal accidents since 1980 in two-pilot operations when the inappropriate use of drugs or alcohol has been implicated in the accident, or when suicidal intent of the pilot has been proven or suspected.

Although at first it seems that the removal of pilots from the flight deck because of stringent medical standards might appear to be beneficial to flight safety, the opposite may also be the case. There is some evidence that experienced, older pilots, i.e. those more prone to degen-erative disease such as a cardiac-related illness, are safer pilots than their younger counterparts, especially those aged below 60 years (Broach et al. 2004a,b). If this is the case, then since the majority of accidents are caused by human error, medically retiring experienced pilots by the application of stringent standards may be increasing the accident risk. This possibility should, at least, be considered when assessing the fitness or otherwise of experienced professional pilots.

CLASSES OF CIVIL AVIATION MEDICAL CERTIFICATE

Different medical requirements apply to the various classes of medical certificate. The ICAO standard for some licence categories are as follows, together with the periodicity of routine renewal examinations:

- Class 1
  - Airline transport and commercial pilot (aeroplane and helicopter): 12 months (6 months after age 40 years for those engaged in single-crew commercial air transport operations carrying passengers)
  - Flight engineer: 12 months

- Class 2
  - Private pilot (aeroplane and helicopter), glider and balloon pilot: 60 months (24 months after age 40)

It is *recommended* that an annual examination be undertaken for those over 50 years.

It can be seen that the most frequent medical examinations apply to those having the greatest influence over flight safety, i.e. professional flight crew. Whereas an annual medical is required for most professional pilots, for private pilots the standard requires only a 5-year medical for private pilots under 40 years, and 2-yearly over 40.

The same principle applies to the ICAO medical criteria for fitness, in that those which are most demanding apply to professional flight crew. It would be inconsistent to apply the same standards to all licence holders, since the regulations in other areas vary with the type of operation undertaken. For example, a private pilot will normally fly a single-engine aircraft capable of carrying only a small number of passengers (or perhaps none). Compared with an airliner, the aircraft will be maintained and inspected to a lower level of safety, the instruments will be less sophisticated and the airspace in which he or she flies, at much lower speeds, is likely to be less congested. Given that the overall operation of a private flight is conducted to less rigorous flight safety requirements, it is reasonable to accept a lower level of medical fitness in the private pilot than the professional.

AUTHORIZED MEDICAL EXAMINERS

There are two common methods of administration regarding medical examinations for pilots. The first is a centralized system, whereby the applicant can attend only one place for examination, where facilities and trained staff are concentrated. Often, this will be associated with a hospital so that any investigations can be undertaken easily and quickly. It may be run by civilian or military personnel. The second system is decentralized, whereby a network of authorized (or 'designated') medical examiners (AMEs) carry out the examinations and forward a report to the licensing authority with the result. In this system, any investigations are carried out locally. There are variations between these systems, and some states undertake the initial class 1 medical examination centrally with later examinations being undertaken by an AME. The ICAO does not indicate a preference for any particular system, but it requires as a standard that 'medical examiners shall have received training in aviation medicine' (International Civil Aviation Organization 2001). It also requires that they 'shall have practical knowledge and experience of the conditions in which the holders of licences and ratings carry out their duties'.

LICENCE VERSUS MEDICAL CERTIFICATE

Much confusion exists concerning the terms 'licence' and 'medical certificate'. This is partly because the ICAO requires only a medical assessment, and no mention of a medical certificate is made. Some contracting states do not issue medical certificates but indicate on the licence that the appropriate medical standard has been reached. In these states, a new licence may be issued each time a medical examination is passed. However, other states do issue a certificate, which is attached to the licence and without which the licence is invalid. Whichever system is in place, it is incorrect to speak of a 'class 1 licence'; the licence and medical certificate (or assessment) are separate entities, and one is of no operational value without the other.

Medical certificate refusal

Medical certificate refusal by a licensing authority or AME is not uncommon. In the majority of cases, the 'unfit' assessment is temporary and once recovery has occurred a certificate can be re-issued. However, there are situations when it is not possible to quickly return a pilot to flying, and he or she may remain unfit for several months or more.

Most authorities keep records of long-term refusal of certification; that of the UK for 2001 is shown in Table 36.6. Over the past 30 years, the rate of such refusals per 1000 pilots has reduced: in 1975 the CAA records indicate that 65 pilots lost their class 1 medical certificates, compared with 61 in 2001, despite the increase in number of professional pilots flying. However, the single most common reason for termination of career on medical grounds has been ascribed consistently to cardiovascular disease, a tendency seen in many countries, reflecting not only the high prevalence of such disease that has existed but also the opportunity, compared with some other diseases, for detecting pilots at increased risk. It is notable that the percentage of all pilots assessed as long-term unfit for cardiovascular reasons in 1975 was 63.1 per cent, compared with 36.1 per cent in 2001, a downward trend first noticed in the 1980s, which is probably related to the UK trend in cardiovascular mortality and morbidity seen over the past two decades, as well as improved risk stratification.

In comparing the common causes of in-flight incapacitation (see Table 36.2, p. 553) with those of long-term medical certificate refusal (see Table 36.6), it will be seen that they are dissimilar. This is because the most frequent cause of incapacitation occurs slowly (i.e. gastrointestinal disease), and yet it is the potential to cause sudden incapacity (see Table 36.4, p. 557) that is of greatest concern to the licensing authority.

Insurance companies often ask the licensing authority how long a pilot is likely to be unfit for work. In some cases there may be little doubt, but in others the decision is not clear-cut. It may be argued that a licensing authority has no mandate to answer this question, since it has no bearing on flight safety: once a decision of unfitness is made, the pilot stops flying and flight safety is protected. Nevertheless, if the pilot holds a medical-cause loss-of-licence insurance, then the pilot's insurance company will want to know for

Table 36.6 *Causes of long-term unfit assessments in UK professional pilots, 2001*

Primary cause	n	% of total	Average age (years)
Cardiovascular	22	36.1	54
Neurological	11	18.0	48
Psychiatric	5	8.2	50
Diabetes	4	6.6	45
Otorhinolaryngological	4	6.6	53
Neoplasm	3	4.9	47
Musculoskeletal/orthopaedic	4	6.6	50
Cerebrovascular	2	3.3	55
Ophthalmological	2	3.3	38
Gastrointestinal	2	3.3	57
Immunology/allergy	1	1.6	57
Genitourinary	1	1.6	58
Total	61		

Source: UK Civil Aviation Authority Medical Department.

how long the pilot will be unfit for duty, and the medical department of the licensing authority is likely to be in the best position to assess this. One European company will not pay out unless the unfit assessment is likely to last for at least three years. This decision may not be simple, particularly when an unfit assessment is based on symptoms reported by the pilot, e.g. back pain or tinnitus, which may vary over time. Licensing authorities handle this problem in different ways, but it is rare for a permanently unfit assessment to be made, and often an insurance company will have to determine itself, using its own medical advisers, whether to pay out on a loss-of-licence insurance request.

AIRLINE MEDICAL REQUIREMENTS

Airline medical requirements for pilots may differ from those of a licensing authority, especially at the recruitment stage. This is because the untrained potential pilot requires a substantial training investment. Airlines prepared to make such an investment will demand reassurance that a trainee will not fail training due to a medical reason and that the potential pilot has the best chance of returning a reasonable length of service. The excess of applicants over available places for sponsored training ensures that applicants with any significant medical history are likely to be rejected.

The licensing authority requires only confirmation that an applicant for a medical certificate will remain fit for certification for the period of validity of the certificate. Certain stable medical conditions that are unlikely to deteriorate in the near future may, therefore, be acceptable to the regulator but unacceptable to an airline.

Smaller airlines sponsor fewer pilots through initial training, relying on ex-military personnel, pilots who have paid for their own training, and pilots who have been trained by other operators. In these cases, where training costs are less, the medical standards for pilot entry into the airline are often less exacting, and holding a class 1 medical certificate may be sufficient.

The selection criteria that airlines might apply to pilot applicants may also differ, depending on the supply and demand of aircrew in the job market. An expanding airline and a shortage of pilots may make a medical limitation acceptable if the alternative is to not operate some services.

REQUIREMENTS FOR MILITARY AIRCREW

This section concerns military requirements and compares them with civil flying. The underlying principles of assessing the medical fitness of military personnel to operate are considered, and reference to standards in the UK and other states is made for illustrative purposes.

In most countries, civil aviation licensing authorities have no jurisdiction over aircraft on the military register. Furthermore, the medical standards set for commercial aviation aircrew in order to ensure flight and passenger safety are not always sufficient to satisfy the demands of military operations. Militaries have therefore developed separate standards and regulatory systems to meet their needs.

The role of any aeromedical examiner, military or civil, is to assess the risk of human failure, for medical reasons, in a given task. However, since the task of a military pilot is different in many respects from that of an airline pilot, so the criteria for medical fitness are different. When compared with a military pilot, an airline pilot works in a highly predictable environment. Indeed, each flight on a particular route is operated in a manner as similar as possible to others on the same route. Strict adherence to standard operating procedures and predetermined flight plans is part and parcel of the work of airline pilots, and written (computer-generated on many modern airliners) procedures are available to deal with not only normal operations but also with the majority of emergency situations that a pilot might encounter. Unlike military fast-jet operations, it is unusual for quick reactions to an emergency to be desirable in an airline pilot; instead, what is typically required is a measured analysis of the problem, discussion with the crew, formulation of a plan, and a timely undertaking of the agreed course of action. Compared with military combat pilots, there are few physiological stresses associated with work on the airline pilot's flight deck, which is generally a relatively quiet, comfortable and low-G environment. Much routine flying is undertaken using sophisticated autopilots, and a single flight can be as long as 18 hours.

Fast-jet crew are expected to be able to operate to their physiological limits, both in the air and, if necessary, on the ground. The pilot may be operating entirely alone. The cockpit is likely to be relatively noisy and cramped, occasionally subject to high-G (positive and negative) manoeuvres, and with little flying undertaken on autopilot, although a single sortie is not likely to last more than two hours. Other types of military flying (helicopter, transport) are not so stressful from a physiological viewpoint, but all may be subject to enemy action and subsequent escape-and-evasion activities, which do not normally need to be taken into account for civil operations. Modern warfare can also involve exposure to nuclear, biological and chemical weapons, protection from which, while necessary, imposes further challenges, particularly in terms of increased respiratory effort (due to increased resistance of the chemical defence respirator) as well as thermal regulation and restriction of movement. Helmet-mounted displays, including night-vision goggles, are becoming more common and impose stresses on the cervical spine and associated musculature, particularly when under G loads. The medical tests to be considered for military flying are summarized in Table 36.7.

In order to recruit personnel who can be deployed in as wide a range of military roles as possible, in circumstances where even healthy individuals may not be able to withstand the physiological stresses of training and combat it is likely that a minor medical problem will result in rejection at selection, particularly as the cost of training a military pilot in any capacity is high. However, a military pilot who is already trained represents a valuable asset, and some conditions that are unsuitable for solo fast-jet flying may be acceptable for helicopter or multi-pilot operations.

Initial and periodic medical examinations

The greater emphasis on evidence-based medicine since the last edition of this book was published (1999) has resulted in important changes to the content of the periodic medical examinations (PMEs) for UK military aircrew. In the UK, recruits at selection undertake a battery of tests (Table 36.8). The routine electroencephalogram (EEG) on selection was abandoned by the UK in 2004.

A review of the costs and benefits of extensive blood testing, i.e. similar to those required on selection, every five years from age 30 has resulted in the requirements being reduced to those shown in Table 36.8 (Curry 2003).

A number of military pilots continue to fly after the age of 60 years, mainly in the role of providing air-experience flights in light aircraft to young people who are considering military flying as a career. Based on the increasing risk of cardiovascular pathology with increasing age, at age 60

in addition to the routine requirements, pilots undergo a review with a consultant physician who has aviation medicine experience, including an exercise ECG and a myocardial perfusion scan. Thereafter, an annual exercise ECG is required.

Colour vision is a topic under debate in the military, as in civilian aviation. Since 2003, the UK has required its pilots on selection to pass the Ishihara test and be assessed as colour perception standard 2 (CP2). Having failed the Ishihara test, it is no longer possible to be assessed as 'colour-safe' (CP3) by passing a lantern test. This is because of the increased use of colour in the modern cockpit. Blue/yellow testing is also under consideration, but its importance is uncertain, and a recent Royal Air Force (RAF) study showed that such deficiency is uncommon in middle-aged males (Marshall 2002).

Photorefractive keratectomy (PRK) has been accepted in the US Air Force, but other types of refractive surgery are not. In the UK (in 2004), any type of refractive surgery is prohibited, but this policy is under review (in most ICAO contracting states, refractive surgery is acceptable for civilian flying, as long as the result is satisfactory). Refractive surgery can result in a loss of contrast sensitivity, which is not easily detected or measured objectively by conventional tests. There is debate as to whether contrast sensitivity should be assessed in aircrew, but it is unknown how important any reduction might be in military (or civil) operations. Military personnel may need to operate in circumstances where visual contrast is degraded by equipment, e.g. using night-vision aids, hence the particular concern about reduced contrast acuity from refractive surgery. Some forms of refractive surgery, e.g. laser in situ keratomileusis (LASIK), have a potential for complications

Table 36.7 *Tests to consider in the assessment of medical fitness*

Timing	Test (blood tests after 10–h fast)
Aircrew selection	Full blood count: Hb, PCV, MCV, MCHC, WBC, platelets, ESR Sickle screen for disease and trait Total protein, albumin, uric acid, creatinine, calcium, glucose, cholesterol, triglycerides Liver function: bilirubin, alkaline phosphatase, AST, ALT and γ-GTP TSH ECG, EEG and chest radiograph
Age 30 years; 5-yearly thereafter	Full blood count, ESR Creatinine, uric acid, glucose Cholesterol and triglycerides Liver function TSH
Ages 25 and 30 years; 2-yearly to 40 years; annually to age 50 years; 6-monthly thereafter	ECG

ALT, alanine aminotransferase; AST, aspartate aminotransferase; ECG, electrocardiogram; EEG, electroencephalogram; ESR, erythrocyte sedimentation rate; γ-GTP, gamma-glutamyltranspeptidase; Hb, haemoglobin; MCV, mean corpuscular volume; MCHC, mean corpuscular haemoglobin concentration; PCV, packed cell volume; TSH, thyroid-stimulating hormone; WBC, white blood count. Adapted with permission from Hopkirk (1984).

Table 36.8 *Requirements for special tests at periodic medical examination for all three UK military services*

Timing	Test (blood tests after 10-h fast)
Aircrew selection	Hb, PCV, MCV, MCHC, WBC and platelets Total protein, albumin, uric acid, creatinine, calcium, glucose, cholesterol, triglycerides, alkaline phosphatase, SGOT, SGPT, γ-GTP, bilirubin, ESR, C-reactive protein or plasma viscosity
Aircrew selection, age 25 and 30 years; every 2 years to age 40 years; annually to 50 years; 6-monthly thereafter	Chest radiograph (on selection only) ECG
Age 40 years	Lipid profile, thyroid function tests, fasting blood sugar
Age 60 years	Consultant review, exercise ECG, cardiac perfusion scan
Age > 60 years	Annual exercise ECG

ECG, electrocardiogram; ESR, erythrocyte sedimentation rate; γ-GTP, gamma-glutamyltranspeptidase; Hb, haemoglobin; MCV, mean corpuscular volume; MCHC, mean corpuscular haemoglobin concentration; PCV, packed cell volume; SGOT, serum glutamic oxaloacetic transaminase; SGPT, serum glutamic pyruvic transaminase; WBC, white blood count.

when the person is subject to high-G events or wind blast at up to 400 knots on ejection.

Setting and monitoring of military medical standards

All three armed forces in the UK operate aircraft and require pilots to meet the same entry standards (there are slight differences in vision requirements). After deployment, there can be a degree of flexibility in assessing deterioration in health, depending on the operational role. There may be an opportunity for redeployment to other, less medically demanding duties, e.g. from fast-jet to multi-pilot transport operations. Occasionally, a fast-jet pilot with a medical problem may be able to return to flying with a G limitation, e.g. 3.5 G, which permits simple aerobatics but not the most demanding combat operations. Military forces are likely to have an assessment protocol that classifies personnel with respect to their medical fitness. In the UK, RAF and army personnel are graded according to the following: fitness to fly (A), fitness for ground duties (G), and fitness to operate in particular climatic zones (Z). At entry, potential pilots need to meet A1, G1, Z1 standards. An example of the different categories is given in Table 36.9. The Royal Navy uses a different classification, but for a similar purpose.

Unlike civil aviation, where the ICAO sets the minimum medical standards, there is (not surprisingly) no such global harmonization of military medical standards. However, allied forces have formed agreements, and countries in the North Atlantic Treaty Organization (NATO) have a set of standardized NATO agreements (STANAGS), the medical aspects of which are compiled by an aeromedical panel. These mandate minimum medical standards within NATO, the aim being to achieve interoperability of NATO

Table 36.9 *Aeromedical categories for the UK Royal Air Force and Army*

Category	Description
A1	Fit for full flying duty
A2	Fit for full flying duty, but eye and/or ear standards below A1
A3	Fit for flying duties with specified temporary or permanent flying duty limitations
A4	Fit for aviation ground crew duties and 'fit passenger flying duties'

forces wherever possible. Under a STANAG arrangement, the host nation accepts the standards of the deploying nation. However, if a medical problem develops during the period of detachment, then the host nation's medical standards are applied to deal with it.

Australia and New Zealand, along with the NATO countries of the UK, the USA and Canada, have formed the Air Standardization Coordinating Committee (ASCC). This was formed in 1948 to ensure that member nations were able to fight side by side as air personnel in joint and combined operations. It has a number of working parties (WPs); WP61 is concerned with aerospace medicine, life support and aircrew systems. The ASCC produces three types of publication: air standards, advisory publications and information publications.

ACKNOWLEDGEMENTS

The author wishes to thank Air Commodore Bill Coker for his assistance in writing the section on requirements for military aircrew.

All ICAO material is used with the kind permission of ICAO.

REFERENCES

Aircraft Accident Investigation Commission. Aircraft accident investigation report on Japan Air Lines DC-8-61 at Tokyo International Airport on 9 February 1982. Tokyo: Aircraft Accident Investigation Commission, Ministry of Transport, Japan, 1983.

Air Accidents Investigation Branch. London: Air Accidents Investigation Branch, UK Department for Transport, 1999. AAIB Bulletin no: 5/99 Ref EN/G00/01/06 Category 1.1. www.dft.gov.uk/stellent/groups/dft_aviation/documents/sectionhomepage/dft_aviation_page.hcsp

Anderson IH. Prediction of the high risk airline pilot. Presented at the 44th Annual Scientific Meeting of the Aerospace Medical Association, Las Vegas, 7–10 May, 1973.

Bennett G. Aviation accident risk and aircrew licensing. *European Heart Journal* 1984; **5** (suppl. A): 9–13.

Bennett G. Pilot incapacitation and aircraft accidents. *European Heart Journal* 1988; **9** (suppl. G), 21–4.

Broach D, Joseph KM, Schroeder DJ. Pilot age and accident rates. Report 3: an analysis of professional air transport pilot rates by age. Oklahoma City: Civil Aerospace Medical Institute 2003a. www.cami.jccbi.gov/aam-400A/AGE60/60_index.html

Broach D, Joseph KM, Schroeder DJ. Pilot age and accident rates. Report 4: an analysis of professional ATP and commercial pilot accident rates by age. Oklahoma City: Civil Aerospace Medical Institute 2003b. www.cami.jccbi.gov/aam-400A/AGE60/60_index.html

Buley LE. Incidence, causes and results of airline pilot incapacitation while on duty. *Aerospace Medicine* 1969; **40**: 64–70.

Chamberlain D. Attributable and absolute (polymorphic) risk in aviation certification: developing the 1% rule. *European Heart Journal* 1999; **1** (suppl. D): D19–24.

Chapman PJC. The consequences of in-flight incapacitation in civil aviation. *Aviation, Space, and Environmental Medicine* 1984; **55**: 497–500.

Curry IP. Routine blood testing of British Army pilots. *Aviation, Space, and Environmental Medicine* 2003; **74**: 332–6.

European Co-ordination Centre for Aviation Incident Reporting Systems. ECCAIRS4. Data definition standard. ECCAIRS, 2005. http://eccairs-www.jrc.it/Support/Downloads/Files/Documentation/Release40Taxonomy/R4CDEventPhases.pdf

Evans ADB. Long term unfit assessments in UK professional aircrew. Presented at the International Congress of Aviation and Space Medicine, Geneva, 19th September, 2001.

Evans ADB. Presentation: in-flight incapacitation in United Kingdom public transport operations: incidence and causes 1990–1999. *Aviation, Space, and Environmental Medicine* 2002; **73**: 242.

Evans ADB. Presentation: medical factors in fatal accidents during multi-pilot operations 1980–2000. *Aviation, Space, and Environmental Medicine* 2003; **74**: 396.

Federal Aviation Administration. Guide for aviation medical examiners. Washington, DC: Federal Aviation Administration, 2003. www.faa.gov/avr/aam/game/version_2/03amemanual/home/home.htm

Green R, James MR. International Federation of Airline Pilots Associations in-flight incapacitation survey. *Aviation, Space, and Environmental Medicine* 1991; **62**: 1068–72.

Hopkirk JAC. The management of common respiratory disease in aviation medicine. *British Journal of Aviation Medicine* 1984; **2**: 10–15.

International Civil Aviation Organization. *Manual of Civil Aviation Medicine*. Montreal: International Civil Aviation Organization, 1985; pp. II-2-1-6.

International Civil Aviation Organization. Annex 1 to the Convention on International Civil Aviation 2001, 9th edn. Montreal: International Civil Aviation Organization, 2001.

International Civil Aviation Organization. Annual Report of the Council. 9814. Montreal: International Civil Aviation Organization, 2002.

Irvine D, Davies DM. The mortality of British Airways pilots, 1966–89: a proportional mortality study. *Aviation, Space, and Environmental Medicine* 1992; **63**: 276–9.

ISIS-2 (Second International Study of Infarct Survival) Collaborative Group. Randomised trial of intravenous streptokinase, oral aspirin, both, or neither among 17,187 cases of suspected acute myocardial infarction. *Lancet* 1988; **2**: 349–60.

Joy M, Bennett G (eds). The first United Kingdom workshop in aviation cardiology. *European Heart Journal* 1984; **5** (suppl. A).

Levi F, Lucchini F, Negri E, La Vecchia C. Trends in mortality from cardiovascular and cerebrovascular diseases in Europe and other areas of the world. *Heart* 2002; **88**: 119–24.

Marshall DNF. Colour perception changes in the working population. Thesis for membership of the Faculty of Occupational Medicine. London: Royal College of Physicians, 2002.

Mitchell SJ, Evans AD. Flight safety and medical incapacitation risk of airline pilots. *Aviation, Space, and Environmental Medicine* 2004; **75**: 260–68.

National Transportation Safety Board. Accident database and synopses. McDonnell Douglas DC-10-10. Registration N121AA, 21 November 1987. www.ntsb.gov/aviation/aviation.htm

Rayner M, Peterson S. *European Cardiovascular Disease Statistics*. London: British Heart Foundation, 2000. www.heartstats.org

Tunstall-Pedoe H. Risk of a coronary heart attack in the normal population and how it might be modified in fliers. *European Heart Journal* 1984; **5** (suppl. A): 43–9.

Tunstall-Pedoe H. Acceptable cardiovascular risk in aircrew. *European Heart Journal* 1988; **9** (suppl. G): 9–11.

UK Civil Aviation Authority. *Global Fatal Accident Review 1980–1996*. CAP 681. Cheltenham: UK Civil Aviation Authority, 1998.

UK Civil Aviation Authority. *Aviation Safety Review 1990–1999*. CAP 701. Cheltenham: UK Civil Aviation Authority, 2000.

UK Civil Aviation Authority. UK airline financial tables: 2002. Total scheduled and non-scheduled services. Cheltenham: UK Civil Aviation Authority, 2000. www.caa.co.uk/docs/80/aln_financial/2002_2003/table_09_total_scheduled_and_non_scheduled_services_operating_and_traffic_statistics_for_the_financial_%20years_of_reporting_airlines.pdf

FURTHER READING

Joy M (ed.). First European workshop in aviation cardiology. *European Heart Journal* 1992; **13** (suppl. H).

Peterson S, Peto V, Rayner M. *Coronary Heart Disease Statistics*. London: British Heart Foundation, 2003.

37

Cardiovascular disease

MICHAEL JOY

INTRODUCTION

Historical considerations

Medical scrutiny of flyers originated in the First World War and was dominated by attention to the special senses vision and balance. Diabetes disqualified and high blood pressure, when it was found, was disallowed. Those with heart murmurs were likely to be excluded. Medical fitness of the professional licence-holder initially was the responsibility of the Royal Air Force (RAF) in the UK. General practitioners (GPs) assessed the fitness of private flyers, and the military set its own standard with a focus on applied physiology. The International Civil Aviation Organization (ICAO) International Standards and Recommended Practices (ISARPs) for personnel licensing were first adopted by the council of the ICAO in 1948 as Annex I to the Chicago Convention of 1944 (International Civil Aviation Organization 2001). These standards are legally binding on the signatory nations, although a statutory instrument is usually required (i.e. the Air Navigation Order in the UK) to give them the force of law. States are empowered to increase but not diminish them. Many states have now separated regulation in the civilian environment from the military in recognition of the somewhat different operational environment (see Chapter 36).

International Civil Aviation Organization

The relevant ICAO standard promulgated in the ISARPs Annex 1, Chapter 6, Personnel Licensing 6.3.2.5 states: 'The applicant shall not possess any abnormality of the heart ... which is likely to interfere with the safe exercise of the applicant's licence.' This standard, presently under revision, is minimal and runs to two five-line paragraphs, each with three brief qualifying statements. The word 'likely' needs interpretation in the aviation environment. In common usage, it implies a probability. With aviation accidents fortunately rare, but with incapacitation of a crew member more common, individual regulatory authorities have interpreted 'likely' as 'any increased risk of'.

All states are signatories to the Convention on International Civil Aviation and are required to comply with the standards or, if not, to file a 'difference'. Recertification outside the ICAO requirements is reliant upon the so-called 'waiver' clause 1.2.4.8, which permits recertification subject to 'accredited medical conclusion', provided that this 'is not likely to jeopardize flight safety'.

The European Joint Aviation Authorities (JAA), as part of the process of European harmonization, first promulgated Joint Aviation Requirements (JAR) FCL Part 3 Medical in 1998 with an expanded standard, which, with its associated appendices, but not the related guidance material, is binding. Although this approach is helpful to states relatively less experienced in aviation certification, it became clear during drafting that use of the imperative rather than the conditional and subjunctive forms of grammatical construction were likely to give rise to loss of flexibility. This risked unfairness to aircrew touched by the process and was unnecessary given the prevailing safety climate. Fortunately, member states agreed to devolve difficult decision-making to the individual national regulatory agencies. Commencing in 2006, the responsibilities of the JAA will be taken over by the European Aviation Safety Authority (EASA). For the time being the medical requirements will remain the same.

Levels of operation

The ICAO (2001) recognizes three levels of medical assessment (including Air Traffic Control Officers (ATCO)). The JAA (1998) has two levels – class 1 for professional pilots of all categories and class 2 for private or recreational pilots. There is no explicit standard for glider pilots (apart from instructors), who are regulated nationally by the individual associations, and air traffic controllers, the standards for whom have not yet been agreed. At the time of writing, the UK applies the class 1 standard to air traffic controllers, albeit at a different frequency of examination interval. In the UK, class 3 remains as a 'grandfather' certificate for those not achieving the JAA class 2 standard. In this chapter, reference will be made to 'full' or 'unrestricted' class 1 (professional) certification, with 'restricted' certification referring to the class 1 certificate with an operational multi-crew limitation (OML) thereon. In general terms, the class 2 (private pilot) medical standard is equivalent to the restricted class 1 requirement. Finally, some nations have a sport flying licence, the medical standard for which in the UK is based on the fitness requirements for a vocational driving licence; i.e. the National Private Pilot's licence (NPPL).

The UK cardiological experience

In 1978, the UK Civil Aviation Authority (CAA) set up its medical advisory panel, attended by a number of (mainly cardiological) specialists. As there was a perceived need for adequate scientific data to assist in making decisions more even, scientific and fair, the UK and European Workshops in Aviation Cardiology were conceived (Joy 1992, 1999; Joy and Bennett 1984, 1988). The focus of these workshops was the epidemiology, natural history and outcome of most of the commonly encountered cardiological problems. From them, a methodology evolved that was coherent with the human–machine interface in regulatory terms. The pilot was identified as one component in a continuum, the failure of any part of which would lead to an erosion of safety, with the ultimate potential for catastrophic outcome. Accidents are commonly the result of failure of a series of events, none of which in isolation needs to have been catastrophic. The workshops formed the basis of the first and second drafts of the JAR FCL Part 3 Medical in cardiology. However, even during the drafting process, it became clear that it was impossible to write an explicit, all-embracing standard, and the application of the 'JAR Med' has given rise to some difficulty.

Determination of the limits of certification

Responsibility in the regulatory process needs definition. The cardiologist is required to identify the probability of a cardiovascular event in a given individual over a defined period, but it is for the certificatory authority to set a cut-off point of the cursor that denies certification. In general terms, the following questions need to be satisfied (Joy 1989):

- What is the operational exposure? This may be expressed in terms of number of hours flown, number of departures, or number of passenger-kilometres travelled.
- What is the fatal/non-fatal accident rate expressed in the same units? Accidents are often expressed per one million hours flown or per one million departures, but they can also be expressed per unit of time, usually one year.
- What is the medical (cardiological) contribution to this accident experience, and is it acceptable? Such data may be difficult to come by with certainty in the single-crew situation: the finding of a cardiac abnormality in the context of an otherwise unexplained accident does not necessarily imply cause and effect.
- What level of routine medical assessment is appropriate, what is its sensitivity, and is it cost-beneficial, bearing in mind the parallels with regular airframe/engine review? What additional investigations can reasonably be requested?
- Should there be a target event rate beyond which the calculated risk of cardiovascular happenstance leads to an automatic denial of certification to fly? Without such a defined standard, there is the risk of unevenness and of lack of objectivity and of fairness.

Aviation and cardiovascular risk

Aviation is involved with risk of event. Airframes are 'lifed', and engines have a time before overhaul (TBO). This proscription attempts to reduce the possibility of failure to a predetermined target level in the interests of safety. The same applies to the pilot, and to his or her heart. At a young age, the probability of a cardiovascular event is very remote. In the three decades from age 30–34 to 70–74 years, male cardiovascular mortality increases by two orders of magnitude, but there are mitigating circumstances – older pilots have fewer accidents. In accidents attributable to incapacitation of the pilot, there are important differences in levels of operation, both civil and military. In those aircraft in which there is only one crew member, the (cardiovascular) event rate will equal the accident rate. In multi-crew operations, a cardiovascular event, like an engine failure, should be containable in all but the most adverse circumstances. There is a strong case, therefore, to demand a higher standard of fitness in single-crew operators.

During the 1960s, civil air-transportation accidents in which cardiovascular incapacitation was a contributory factor occurred on a worldwide basis at the rate of approximately one every 18 months, culminating in the loss of the HS Trident 1 G-ARPI near London Heathrow in 1972 (Department of Trade and Industry 1973). However, there were major training and operational differences at that time, and less was understood about the multifactorial nature of accident pathology. In the some half-billion multi-crew jet hours flown since 1974 the ICAO training requirement for the recognition of incapacitation of a colleague, hull loss from cardiovascular causes has been all but eliminated. There have, however, been a small number of significant incidents, and aircrew cardiovascular deaths continue to occur while pilots are on duty, varying at a rate of one to four per annum worldwide.

The early accident experience led to a number of working party reports by certain cardiologists (American College of Cardiology 1966, 1975; Cardiology Committee of the Royal College of Physicians of London 1978), none of which was either commissioned or adopted by the relevant certificatory agency. The recommendations were empirically based at a time when routine resting electrocardiography (ECG) had only recently been introduced for certain categories of licence. It was concluded that exercise ECG, still in its early days, might be helpful in the detection of coronary artery disease. A better understanding of probability theory in populations with a low prevalence of disease denied acceptance of this suggestion at the special cardiovascular study group at the ICAO in Montreal in 1980.

Cardiovascular causes of incapacitation

Incapacitation due to cardiovascular disease may be slow or abrupt in onset, and subtle or complete in its manifestation. The coronary syndromes, being capricious in presentation and bearing long-term implications in terms of outcome, are not infrequent in aircrew. Acute cardiovascular events such as stroke, aortic rupture and myocardial infarction, with or without ventricular fibrillation, may cause complete incapacitation, while the pain of acute myocardial ischaemia may be disabling. Non-lethal cardiac arrhythmias may be sufficiently subtle to cause distraction without the aircrew member being fully aware as to what is absorbing his or her attention. In the single-crew environment, such events have a high probability of a catastrophic outcome. Fortunately, the very large database on natural history and the impact of intervention in coronary artery disease has permitted the development of algorithms of management that assist safe, fair and evidence-based decisions.

Specific issues in cardiology

This discussion of specific issues in cardiology in relation to certification will represent the European interpretation of the ICAO ISARPs by the JAA. This chapter is not intended as a primer in clinical cardiology but as guidance material for licensing authorities, authorized medical examiners (AMEs) and others seeking to investigate and manage cardiological problems in aviators. From time to time, the author expresses opinions that are his own and may or may not reflect current regulatory practice. The topics are discussed in greater depth elsewhere (Joy 1989, 1996; Joy and Broustet 1996).

Epidemiological considerations

Cardiovascular disease, the prevalence of which has declined significantly over the past 20 years in Western nations, remains an important cause of premature death and disability (Petersen et al. 2003). It is also a substantial contributor to the cost of healthcare. In the aviation certificatory environment (in the West), common problems include the consequences of the vascular risk factors (hypertension, hyperlipidaemia, diabetes, smoking) presenting as coronary artery disease and its consequences, the disorders of cardiac rhythm and conduction, and myocardial disease.

Atherosclerotic disease of the great vessels (i.e. the aorta) and the medium-sized vessels (i.e. the coronary and cerebral arteries) is insidious in onset, often having an origin in early adulthood. It has a trajectory of many years' duration and may present abruptly with some cerebrovascular or myocardial catastrophe. In Europe, there is a north–south gradient, death from coronary heart disease being three times more common in the north than in the southern 'olive belt'. There is also an east–west gradient: heart-attack rates in Western Europe are generally lower than those in

Eastern Europe. The dietary, environmental and genetic factors involved have been demonstrated in the INTER-HEART study to be shared worldwide by both sexes in all regions (Yusuf *et al.* 2004).

Historically, some emerging nations have experienced low heart-attack rates, but this no longer applies to prosperous South Asians, who, both locally and following emigration, demonstrate rates that are generally some 50–60 per cent higher than those observed in the West (Patel and Bhopal 2003). Numerous factors, including inherited metabolic anomalies, e.g. increased prevalence of insulin resistance, are involved. Japan, sharing with some other countries in the Far East commendably low mean national levels of plasma cholesterol and some of the lowest heart-attack rates in the world, is showing some signs of increase in the prevalence of coronary artery disease. Japanese people who emigrate to the USA tend, like other migrant populations, to assume the risk of their country of adoption. This global burden is reflected unevenly in the aviation environment.

Vascular risk factors

Vascular risk factors predict coronary artery disease, and coronary artery disease predicts coronary events. The presence of coronary artery disease, in general, predicts an adverse outcome. The presence of one or more vascular risk factors implies a greater probability of event in an individual without identifying whether or when it might occur. It remains what has been called the 'prevention paradox' – that the greatest number of events will be seen in those individuals with a near-normal vascular risk profile on account of their far greater numbers. Predictions on the probability of an event should be over a defined period – usually a year – and based on data from an age- and sex-matched control population. There is now also considerable experience in civil and military aviation worldwide, most notably in the USA.

The one per cent rule

Tunstall-Pedoe (1984) made a seminal contribution to the first UK Workshop by suggesting that there was symmetry between the cardiovascular event rate in aircrew and the accident rate of aircraft. From this beginning, and over the course of the subsequent workshops emerged what has become known as the 'one per cent rule'. This is a mathematical model of accident probability based on the epidemiology of coronary artery disease. It is best applied to the coronary syndromes and not to one of the more capricious problems such as atrial fibrillation. It affirms that provided the predicted cardiovascular mortality of an individual is not exceeded (in a Western male aged 65 years, this is approxi-

mately one per cent annum), then the probability of an accident to a multi-crew aircraft from cardiovascular incapacitation of the pilot should be 'very remote', i.e. one $< 10^9$ flying hours. In spite of the rule being predicated on the basis of mortality, confusion continues in distinguishing this from the non-fatal event rate. Every coronary death will be clustered with perhaps three to four non-fatal comorbid events, but the population will be factored as some of the comorbid events will have brought about the removal of higher-risk pilots from the aviation scene.

The one per cent rule has been overinterpreted and is only one of several means of defining regulatory cut-off points. The rule has been reviewed comprehensively by Mitchell and Evans (2004), who found that it may be unnecessarily rigorous in the light of both experience and progress in aviation. They concluded that a two per cent cut-off point is justified. The rule is discussed in greater depth in Chapter 36.

HISTORY AND MEDICAL EXAMINATION

There is some variation worldwide in the implementation of the ICAO requirements. Most national certificatory agencies require the routine review of pilots to be carried out by practitioners with some familiarity and/or training in the field of aviation medicine. Such physicians (Authorised Medical Examiners (AMEs)) are usually family doctors without special training or experience in cardiology. In some countries, e.g. France, the scrutiny of professional pilots is carried out in one of a small number of designated centres. In the UK, there is no such restriction, although a large number of examinations are carried out by a small number of practitioners. Almost universally, a standardized format is used to record factors such as age, past and family history, weight, blood pressure, smoking habit, drug administration, and clinical observations, such as changes in the fundus occuli and heart murmurs. Increasingly, these forms are being computerized and transmitted online. Certain regulatory agencies, including the JAA, also require routine measurement of the serum cholesterol. A few require routine exercise ECG (see below), and, it is a requirement of some employers.

Resting electrocardiography

Regular 12-lead resting ECG is required in the routine scrutiny of aircrew, depending on age and level of certification. In practice, there is some divergence between ICAO signatories. In the USA, there is no routine requirement for class 2 or class 3 holders. The JAA requires a recording at first issue of a class 1 certificate, at five-yearly intervals until age 30 years, two-yearly until age 40 years, annually until age 50 years, and six-monthly thereafter. This may be reduced following the promulgation of the new ICAO Standard. The class 2 (private pilot) holder does not need to undergo ECG until the first examination after the fortieth birthday, every second year thereafter until age 50 years, annually until the sixty-fifth birthday, and then every six months. Sport flying licences as a rule do not require routine ECG, and this is the case in the UK.

It was not until 1965 that routine ECG examination of pilots was first required. Minor anomalies are quite common, requiring comparison with earlier recordings in at least 10–15 per cent. Two per cent of US Air Force and three per cent of UK civilian and RAF personnel demonstrated abnormality of the ST segment and/or T wave on routine scrutiny. In UK civilians, 18 per cent of 103 people in one study responded abnormally to exercise (Joy and Trump 1981).

The resting ECG is an insensitive tool for the detection of presymptomatic coronary artery disease although it does identify a small number of people who have suffered a silent myocardial infarction. In one ten-year period, 72 'silent' myocardial infarctions were detected in 48 633 aircrew screened at the US School of Aerospace Medicine (Hickman *et al.* 1996). Twenty-five per cent of those suffering such events in the Framingham study did not experience symptoms that they recognized as significant (Kannel *et al.* 1970), and 50 per cent of those dying suddenly do so without premonitory symptoms (Doyle *et al.* 1976). As the risk of further cardiovascular events is increased substantially following myocardial infarction, the identification of minor anomalies should provoke further and fuller review. Sometimes ECG changes are variable, but the misconception that a stable 'abnormal' recording is necessarily acceptable should not be tolerated. A recording demonstrating a pattern of myocardial infarction remains predictive of outcome, even if it does not change. A resting ECG, however, is rather better at detecting disturbances of rhythm and conduction.

Recording the resting electrocardiogram

A resting ECG should be recorded with the subject at rest in a warm environment. The skin should be prepared with spirit or abrasive, or both. The position of the limb electrodes is not important, but those on the chest must be placed accurately. Leads V1 and V2 should be placed in the fourth intercostal spaces on either side of the sternum. Lead V4 is placed at the position of the apex of the normal heart – the fifth intercostal space in the mid-clavicular line. Lead V3 is placed midway between V2 and V4. Leads V5 and V6 are placed at the same level as V4 in the anterior and mid-axillary lines, respectively (Figure 37.1).

The preferred instrument should record at least three channels simultaneously and be optimally filtered and

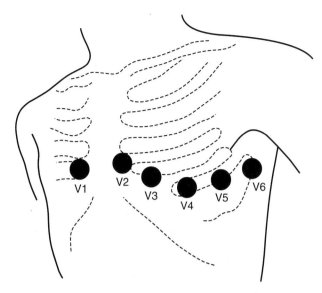

Figure 37.1 *Electrode positions of the chest leads used for the standard 12-lead electrocardiogram (ECG). The limb leads are placed on the right and left arms and right and left legs. The right leg is an indifferent electrode. During exercise, the limb leads are positioned on the shoulders and the iliac crests on each side. This gives a slightly different readout, and these positions should not be used for making standard recordings.*

damped. On such a machine, the length of a recording is 12 seconds at the standard speed (25 mm/s) and is presented on a single sheet of A4 paper. Some recording techniques use thermosensitive paper, which needs special care when archiving. A further 24 seconds of rhythm strip using an inferior, anterior and lateral lead such as II, V1 and V6 should be recorded. If a q wave is present in III, then a recording during inspiration should be included. If the q wave is less than 40 ms wide and disappears with inspiration, then it is probably innocent. A normal ECG is illustrated in figure 37.1.

Interpretation of the resting ECG is required to be by 'specialists acceptable to the AMS (Aero-medical Section)' under JAR FCL 3.130 (d). The intention is that approved scrutinizers should be involved. Since promulgation of this requirement, computer formatting and reporting have become widespread, questioning the need for specialist interpretation of large numbers of mainly normal ECGs. Nevertheless, an experienced interpreter is likely to be more sensitive and more accurate than a computer working to a preset profile, perhaps for no reason other than he or she can factor in experience and probability bias. None of the presently available commercial programmes are approved for the task. In practice, although the computer programmes tend to err on the side of caution, they underreport, as may scrutinizers due to lack of experience or fatigue. In safety terms, the difference is not likely to be measurable, although delegation of the responsibility for processing the reports raises issues of process account-ability and proper audit.

Exercise electrocardiography

There is no general requirement for exercise ECG in the ICAO ISARPs or the JAR Med. Specifically, 'exercise elec-trocardiography is required only when indicated in compli-ance with ...'. Some airlines require the investigation either routinely or before employment. The same approach in general terms applies to the military, although some air-forces require fast-jet pilots to undergo such investigation.

When exercise recordings are carried out, often to clarify some minor ECG anomaly, a standardized protocol such as the Bruce treadmill protocol or equivalent should be employed. The Bruce protocol is not the only one available (Table 37.1), but it is the most widely used. It suffers from a shortcoming that it does not present the same challenge to anthropomorphically different individuals in terms of height and weight.

The ECG should utilize the 12 standard leads, displaying at least three simultaneously, and be optimally filtered and damped. The limb leads should be placed on the shoulders and the lower trunk. Recordings should be made at rest in the erect and lying positions, and after hyperventilation for ten seconds. A 12-second recording should be made for each of the resting observations, for each minute of exer-cise, and for each ten minutes of recovery. Not infrequently, diagnostic changes are seen only in the recovery phase.

The subject should be exercised to symptom limitation and be expected to complete at least three stages – nine minutes – of the protocol or achieve an oxygen uptake equivalent to 11 metabolic equivalents (METs), 1 MET being the resting oxygen requirement of a 70-kg 40-year-old male (3.5 ml/min/kg). The age-predicted maximum heart rate is calculated by subtracting the age in years from 220 (beats/min). The test is most sensitive when taken to symptom limitation rather than any percentage of the age-predicted maximum. The reason for discontinuing the test should be recorded, together with the presence or absence of any symptoms.

In some countries, bicycle ergometry is still employed widely. This suffers from the relative disadvantage that the subject does not have to bear their own weight and there is no imperative to maintain speed. Furthermore, many peo-ple are not used to riding a bicycle. The bicycle protocol nearest to the Bruce treadmill protocol is the 20-W proto-col. The subject is seated and the workload increased from zero by 20 W every minute to the same symptom/heart-rate endpoints. The test is neither completely sensitive – it does not detect non-flow-limiting lesions – nor completely specific – it may falsely suggest its presence. Thus:

- *Sensitivity* = true positives/(true positives + false negatives). It reflects the percentage of all patients with coronary disease with an abnormal test.
- *Specificity* = true negatives/(false positives + true negatives). It reflects the percentage of negative tests in subjects without coronary disease.
- *Positive predictive accuracy* = true positives/(true positives + false positives). It reflects the percentage of abnormal responses in subjects with coronary disease.
- *Negative predictive accuracy* = true negatives/(true negatives + false negatives). It reflects the percentage of negative responses in subjects without coronary disease.

Interpretation of exercise ECG data has been reviewed widely. There remains an obsession with interpretation of the ST segment, the depression (or elevation) of which is measured at 60 ms after the J point, the junction of the S wave and the ST segment. Its pattern needs to be exam-ined closely at rest and in the early stages of exercise, dur-ing the recording, and especially during the early stages of recovery. It is at its most sensitive and specific when the resting ECG is normal and at its least when it is abnormal, e.g. in left bundle branch block. Often, 2 mm of plane ST segment depression is regarded as 'positive' (i.e. for coro-nary artery disease), but this is a confusing term as it may not be present. The skilled interpreter will be more influ-enced by the walking time, symptoms (if any) and pattern of change rather than numerical values. Some examples of abnormal exercise ECG responses are illustrated in Figure A37.2 (p. 600).

Table 37.1 *Standard treadmill protocols*

Stage	Bruce		Sheffield		Naughton		Ellestad	
	mph	%	mph	%	mph	%	mph	%
1	1.7	10.0	1.7	0.0	1.0	0.0	1.7	10.0
2	2.5	12.0	1.7	5.0	2.0	0.0	3.0	10.0
3	3.4	14.0	1.7	10.0	2.0	0.0	4.0	10.0
4	4.2	16.0	2.5	12.0	2.0	3.5	5.0	10.0
5	5.0	18.0	3.4	14.0	2.0	7.0	5.0	15.0
6	5.5	20.0	4.2	16.0	2.0	10.5	6.0	15.0
7	6.0	22.0	5.0	18.0	2.0	14.0	–	–

Ventricular function is a good predictor of outcome, and its surrogate the exercise walking time reflects this. A walking time better than ten minutes using the standard Bruce treadmill is associated with an annual event rate of < one per cent, even if the ECG response is not completely normal. This predictive capability also applies following myocardial infarction, coronary surgery, angioplasty and coronary stenting (Broustet *et al.* 1991; Dubach *et al.* 1989; Legrand *et al.* 1997; Mark *et al.* 1991).

The argument against routine ECG scrutiny of aircrew is as follows and depends on the Bayesian theory of conditional probability:

- In an average middle-aged pilot, the prevalence of significant coronary artery disease may be only one to two per cent.
- The exercise ECG is only 60–70 per cent sensitive, i.e. it detects only this percentage of those subjects with coronary artery disease – the true positives.
- If 1000 pilots underwent such a study, the 10–20 (one to two per cent) might have the disease, but only 6–14 (60–70 per cent of one to two per cent) would be detected.
- With 95 per cent specificity of the test (at best, and it may be much lower than this), five per cent (perhaps 50 pilots) would have diagnostic changes but no disease, i.e. would be false positives.
- The false-positive responders to exercise could thus outnumber the true-positive responders by a factor of up to seven or more.

This effect was demonstrated by McHenry *et al.* (1984) in healthy policemen with a mean age similar to the pilot population (38 years) in which 916 men were followed up with serial exercise ECG for between 8 and 15 years (mean 12.7 years). Twenty-three had an initially abnormal exercise response and 38 converted to an abnormal response during the follow-up period. There were nine coronary events in the first group and 12 in the second. In the much larger normally responding group, there were 44 events. The positive predictive accuracy was 25.3 per cent, but there was only one sudden death in the initially abnormal group. There were seven sudden deaths in the much larger 'normal' group.

Middle-aged males in the Seattle Heart Watch programme (Bruce and Fisher 1987) who had more than one abnormal exercise ECG response in the presence of vascular risk factor(s) had an annual coronary event rate greater than five per cent. By comparison, the risk of an event was only 0.22 per cent if there were no vascular risk factors and the exercise recording was normal. If there was one abnormal recording and no vascular risk factor present, then the risk of an event was 0.42 per cent per annum. Under such circumstances, the finding of a normal exercise ECG identifies a group in whom the risk of event is acceptably less than one per cent per annum.

The American College of Cardiology (ACC)/American Heart Association (AHA) guidelines (Gibbons *et al.* 1997) state that in patients with suspected coronary artery disease with a low (or high) pre-test probability of its presence, exercise ECG is less appropriate than if the probability is intermediate. This is based on greatest value in terms of diagnostic outcome: low-risk subjects are likely to have a normal response and high-risk subjects the reverse. Morise (2000) reviewed the ACC/AHA guidelines in a study of 5103 patients with symptoms suggestive of angina pectoris in whom the overall sensitivity of the investigation was 70 per cent and specificity 66 per cent. There was a progressive increase in positive predictive value – 21 per cent, 62 per cent and 92 per cent for low, intermediate and high pretest probability, respectively – and a fall in the negative predictive value – 94 per cent, 72 per cent and 28 per cent, respectively. Although this group does not represent closely the pilot population in terms of prevalence of disease, it emphasizes the usefulness of exercise ECG in returning aircrew to flying when the probability of coronary artery disease is low (i.e. lack of symptoms, unremarkable vascular risk burden (including age), non-specific ECG changes) due to the high negative predictive value.

Further investigation should be carried out when the probability of abnormality is high (i.e. symptoms, significant vascular risk (including age), possibly significant ECG changes, known coronary artery disease), irrespective of the result of the test. With the intermediate group, exercise evaluation alone may be insufficient, as some authors have noted a statistically significant difference between the pre-/post-test predictive values ($P < 0.0001$) and a significant false-negative rate that would not sit easily in the regulatory environment.

Although aviation used to be an almost exclusively male preserve, increasing numbers of females recruited over the past three decades have brought the need for investigation for coronary artery disease in a group in which its prevalence, overall, is low. One meta-analysis of exercise testing for coronary artery disease in women revealed an overall sensitivity of 61 per cent and a specificity of 70 per cent, comparable to males but of limited value, due to the high number of both positive and false-negative results (Kwok *et al.* 1999). Additional guidance should be sought, depending on the clinical situation.

Myocardial scintigraphy

Routine resting ECG anomalies are initially best assessed in a subject with a low probability of coronary artery disease by exercise ECG. When an exercise recording is equivocal or abnormal, and the probability of coronary artery disease is intermediate or high, then further evaluation will be clinically indicated. Of the techniques available, stress echocardiography is the least invasive. Using exercise or a beta-agonist such as dobutamine to increase myocardial oxygen requirement, stress echocardiography demonstrates ventricular-wall motion abnormality in the presence of myocardial ischaemia in response to stress. The technique is limited to comparatively few centres in the UK.

A more widely available investigation is myocardial scintigraphy. The largest experience with myocardial perfusion imaging (MPI) has been obtained with thallium-201, a radionuclide with a half-life of 72 hours and that decays to mercury-201. The standard dose is 80 MBq; approximately four per cent is cleared in the first pass through the coronary circulation. The radiation dose is quite high and is equivalent to 18 mSv, exceeding the radiation dose received during coronary angiography by a factor of two to three. It behaves as potassium in the exercising myocardium, being taken up by the myocardial cells via a sodium–potassium adenosine triphosphatase (ATPase)-dependent mechanism. Exercise is now being supplanted by pharmacological agents, commonly adenosine, as the means of myocardial stress (by maximal vasodilation), the heart rate response being limited. Imaging takes place following maximum stress and three hours later to permit redistribution of the isotope. Other stressor agents include dipyridamole and dobutamine. Other radionuclides such as technetium-99m-2-methoxy-isobutyl-isonitrile (MIBI) provide better resolution for a smaller radiation burden.

The power of scintigraphy in the prediction of outcome has been established and surpasses exercise ECG in spite of its incomplete specificity and sensitivity. The exercise ECG can be expected to be of the order of 68 per cent sensitive and 77 per cent specific in a hospital population; thallium scanning is a few percentage points better on both counts. Both modalities depend crucially on the prevalence of coronary disease in the population being studied. Brown (1991) reviewed the outcome of 3573 patients with angiographic coronary artery disease and a normal myocardial perfusion scan (MPS). The incidence of death or myocardial infarction was 0.9 per cent per annum over a mean of 28 months. More recently, Hachamovitch et al. (2003) reviewed the outcome of 7376 consecutive patients with a normal exercise or adenosine MPS. Unsurprisingly, hard events (cardiac death, myocardial infarction) were more common with increasing age, male gender, diabetes and known coronary artery disease, but the highest event rate was only 1.4–1.8 per cent per annum over the two-year study period.

The incremental prognostic value of sequential investigation of patients suspected of suffering from coronary artery disease has also been evaluated. The addition of exercise ECG to the clinical examination and resting ECG adds significant predictive power, while the addition of MPS improves it further. The hierarchical prognostic gain from adding exercise ECG, exercise single photon-emission computed tomography (SPECT) thallium-201 imaging and coronary angiography was reviewed by Iskandrian et al. (1993). They found that imaging quadrupled the prognostic power but coronary angiography provided no additional improvement.

Scintigraphy is an expensive investigation with a significant radiation burden. It is neither completely sensitive nor completely specific. It is, however, otherwise non-invasive. From the certificatory point of view, it may be indicated as the investigation of election when, for example, evidence of satisfactory revascularization is being sought following coronary surgery/angioplasty/stenting. The JAA now accepts the investigation for this purpose. As the primary investigation in the presence of an abnormal exercise ECG, it will give an indication of prognosis but only indirect evidence on the coronary anatomy. This may be inadequate from the clinical point of view. The recommendation to perform the investigation depends on both the clinical and the certificatory situations.

Electron–beam tomography

Electron-beam tomography (EBT) is a comparatively new radiographic technique that detects calcium in the coronary arteries, the 'score' correlating with the presence of atheromatous disease. Its value in determining prognosis is under evaluation. The American College of Cardiology consensus conference recorded a 70 per cent predictive accuracy for the technique but a lower specificity (O'Rourke et al. 2000). It was felt not to be indicated for diagnostic purposes and is not required for certificatory purposes. If an aircrew member undergoes the investigation for whatever reason, and the result suggests the possibility of coronary artery disease, then further investigation is indicated using available techniques.

Coronary angiography

Coronary angiography has long been regarded as the gold standard in the assessment of prognosis in coronary artery disease. If other tests have not been reassuringly negative during an assessment, then this investigation may be warranted in the certificatory environment. It cannot be demanded, although certification may not be possible without it. It carries a very small risk of death – less than one in 5000 in healthy individuals, with a slightly higher risk of vascular damage to the vessel of entry or due to stripping of the intima of the coronary artery. The latter may provoke a myocardial infarction. In private flyers, the procedure is difficult to justify, except at the insistence of the individual.

There is an assumption that a normal coronary angiogram showing no evidence of obstructive coronary artery disease together with a normal contrast ventriculogram bears a low risk of future event. From the certificatory point of view this is probably correct, but there remains a small group of people who have abnormal exercise ECG responses without clinical or other explanation. In these people, the tendency to regard them as fit based only on their coronary anatomy should be regarded with caution, as they may subsequently demonstrate a myocardial abnormality. Follow-up therefore is advisable.

CORONARY ARTERY DISEASE

Coronary artery disease remains a significant cause of premature death. Death from coronary artery disease is falling in the West, but elsewhere the trend is less favourable or may even be reversed. In the UK, nearly 40 per cent of the population die from cardiovascular disease. One in four men and one in six women die from coronary artery disease. Ten per cent of the population die from stroke (Petersen *et al.* 2003). One-third of cardiovascular deaths in males and one-quarter in women are premature (< age 75 years).

Of those presenting with a new coronary syndrome, one-sixth will present as sudden cardiac death (SCD) without recognizable premonitory symptoms; two-fifths will present with angina pectoris and two-fifths with myocardial infarction. The residue will suffer an unstable ischaemic syndrome. Of the third that die within 28 days following acute myocardial infarction, about half will do so within 15 minutes of the onset of symptoms, 60 per cent being dead at one hour and 70 per cent within 24 hours. As the average pilot spends some eight to ten per cent of his or her life on duty, the possibility of some manifestation at work is to be expected. Although in safety terms incapacitation, either complete or subtle, will be at greatest risk of occurrence at the time of the index event, the risk of fatal event is still increased substantially in the days and weeks that follow. With the exponential increase in cardiovascular events that occur with increasing age, older pilots will be at greatest risk of an event, particularly if other risk factors such as hypertension, hyperlipidaemia, smoking, insulin resistance and/or a family history are present.

Most of the coronary syndromes are attributable to obstruction of the vessels with atheroma. This lipid-rich material, which accumulates at sites of vascular injury, may be present in early adulthood and progress very slowly. These atheromatous foci are known as plaques and contain 'foamy macrophages' – cells of monocytic origin, smooth-muscle cells and lipids in the form of cholesterol, fatty acids and lipoproteins. There is significant variation in the composition of the plaques, their state of development and their behaviour in individuals. Their behaviour may also be modified by medication. Thrombosis occurs in association with plaque rupture, tripping the clotting cycle via several different mechanisms. The subsequent sequence of events depends on the morphology of the plaque, its site in the coronary artery, the extent of the related thrombus and the presence or absence of a collateral circulation. Flow varies as the fourth power of the radius, and symptoms may not be present until one or more major epicardial arteries are occluded by 50–70 per cent of the luminal diameter.

If the thrombotic event is minimal and the plaque not large, there may be no symptoms. Or, a change in symptoms such as angina pectoris may occur, which may then become unstable. If the vessel is occluded, infarction of the myocardium subtended by the vessel will occur unless an adequate collateral circulation is present. As collateral formation is most common when near-obstruction has been long-standing, such an outcome is less likely to apply to aviators, who must not only be asymptomatic but also pass routine medical surveillance. From these pathophysiological processes, the coronary syndromes of stable and unstable angina pectoris and myocardial infarction are seen.

Angina pectoris

The pain or discomfort that is angina pectoris is one of the more familiar symptoms in medicine. Yet the diagnosis is sometimes made casually, with little thought for the consequences for the patient. Its characteristics – crushing central pain or discomfort, commonly but not exclusively radiating to the left arm, which may also be present on the right, in the back or in the throat, and brought on by exertion – should make its identification possible. Unless presenting as an unstable syndrome or during myocardial infarction, angina is of brief duration (< 2–3 minutes) and likely to be associated with exercise, especially first thing in the morning, in the cold or after a meal.

The severity of angina pectoris correlates poorly with the extent of coronary artery disease present. An inactive subject may have no symptoms in spite of significant three-vessel obstruction, or a branch vessel obstruction may give rise to symptoms in an active individual. Although meaningless, as risk stratification with a fair degree of precision is possible, crude mortality in angina pectoris is of the order of four per cent per annum. 'Chest pain ?cause' is a familiar cardiological default diagnosis, which underscores the difficulty sometimes experienced in the diagnosis of chest pain.

Angina pectoris may also occur in the presence of normal coronary arteries as Prinzmetal or variant angina. There is a diurnal pattern, often occurring in the early morning. Other, non-coronary explanations for angina include hypertrophic or dilated cardiomyopathy, aortic stenosis, severe hypertension and anaemia. Such diagnoses should not have passed unnoticed in an otherwise healthy aviator. The diagnosis of angina pectoris from whatever cause, whether treated or not, disbars from all classes of licence to fly, both civil and military.

Chest pain ?cause

'Chest pain ?cause' is a common cardiological diagnosis in outpatient clinics, implying that although there may be symptoms, full evaluation does not lead to a cardiovascular explanation. Although such a diagnosis is rare in aircrew the presence of obstructive coronary artery disease needs to be excluded, often by exercise ECG. Any recurrent symptoms should be pursued in view of their potential as a cause of subtle incapacitation. In the presence of normal coronary arteries, it carries a normal prognosis.

Minor coronary artery disease

Coronary angiography has predictive power in terms of future cardiovascular events. It is noteworthy that of 347 patients who presented with chest pain in one study but who had normal coronary arteries, only two (0.6 per cent) died from coronary artery disease over the following ten years. Those with obstruction of < 30 per cent had a two per cent mortality; in those with obstruction of > 30 per cent but < 50 per cent, the ten-year mortality was 16 per cent. The Coronary Artery Surgery Study (CASS) registry data gave a 96 per cent seven-year survival for the 3136 patients with normal coronary arteries or arteries that were stenosed only minimally. The long-term study of the natural history of 1487 flyers with 'normal' vessels and vessels with 'luminal irregularity' from the US Air Force demonstrated no events in either group at five years (Zarr *et al.* 2004). Between five and ten years, the event rate was 0.1 per cent per annum in the first group and 0.56 per cent per annum in the second group. The event rate for 'minimal or non-occlusive coronary disease of < 50 per cent' was 1.2 per cent over the second five-year period.

In the absence of disqualifying symptoms or other contraindication, aircrew with normal coronary arteries or with only minor irregularities may be permitted full certification to fly, subject to regular review. Stenosis > 30 per cent in any major vessel should predicate a restriction to multi-crew operation, while stenosis > 50 per cent is disbarring, especially if involving the left main or left anterior descending vessels.

Moderate and severe coronary artery disease

It is conventional to describe the coronary circulation as consisting of three arteries – the right main vessel and the two branches of the left main vessel, i.e. the anterior descending and circumflex branches. There is, however, significant individual variation in the size, relative importance and physiological balance of the vessels. The early Cleveland Clinic data demonstrated a five-year survival of 83 per cent in patients with at least 'moderate' single-vessel disease, falling to 62 per cent and 48 per cent at 10 and 15 years, respectively (Bruschke *et al.* 1972). This is poor by any standard, and such a high event rate is not tolerable in the context of aviation. But much has changed over the past 30 years: not only has there been a general decline in the prevalence of coronary artery disease, but also there is overwhelming evidence that brisk intervention against vascular risk factors (hyperlipidaemia, hypertension, smoking, diabetes) significantly improves outcome in terms of reduction of a major adverse cardiac event (MACE) and stroke.

Sudden cardiac death (SCD)

Two-thirds of sudden deaths are attributable to the cardiovascular system with a population incidence of approximately one per 1000 population per year (Priori *et al.* 2001). The majority of such events in middle years and later are due to coronary artery disease. Increased left ventricular muscle mass is a powerful predictor, as are hypertension, hyperlipidaemia, smoking, diabetes mellitus and a family history (male death < age 55 years, female death < age 60 years). In the Framingham study, electrocardiographic left ventricular hypertrophy was associated with a five-year mortality of 33 per cent in males and 21 per cent in females. Left ventricular hypertrophy bears a relative risk independent of the presence or absence of hypertension similar to that of coronary artery disease. It is often ignored by regulators. Other causes of sudden cardiac death include hypertrophic cardiomyopathy, right ventricular cardiomyopathy, dilated cardiomyopathy, ischaemic left ventricular dysfunction, ion channelopathies, catecholaminergic polymorphic ventricular tachycardia, aortic stenosis, possibly mitral leaflet prolapse, anomalous origin of the coronary arteries, myocardial bridging, Wolff–Parkinson–White syndrome, atrioventricular (AV) conduction disturbances, myocarditis and certain medication. Many of these causes are rare, and their disposal in the aviation context is beyond the scope of this chapter; others are covered below.

RECERTIFICATION IN THE PRESENCE OF KNOWN CORONARY ARTERY DISEASE

Myocardial infarction

Myocardial infarction disqualifies from certification to fly either civil or military aircraft. Predictors of an adverse outcome after myocardial infarction include previous history of the same, reduced ejection fraction, angina pectoris, smoking (current or ex-), history of hypertension, systolic hypertension, diabetes, increased heart rate and reduced effort tolerance (Yap *et al.* 2000). The best-risk subject, by comparison, will be asymptomatic, non-diabetic and normotensive, with a normal ejection fraction and with coronary artery disease restricted to the vessel subtending the infarction (which should, preferably, be patent). It is likely that subjects with single-vessel disease subtending a completed infarction will be most suitable for eventual certification, although in one study of 262 patients with a mean age of 52.3 years, there was no difference in five- and ten-year survival, regardless of whether the infarct-related artery was patent (Imamura *et al.* 1997). At 96.9 per cent versus 93.8 per cent for five-year survival, and 90.7 per cent versus 92.7 per cent for ten-year survival, for patent and non-patent vessels, respectively, such outcomes in an asymptomatic individual are likely to be satisfactory for certificatory purposes but only if the ejection fraction is normal. The ten-year survivals are 94.8 per cent, 90.6 per cent and 74.8 per cent with ejection fractions > 60 per cent, < 60 per cent but > 40 per cent, and < 40 per cent, respectively.

It is well established that left ventricular function powerfully predicts both cardiovascular events and outcome. Data from the Cleveland Clinic first demonstrated five-year survival with single-vessel disease at 89 per cent and 77 per cent in the absence and presence, respectively, of wall-motion abnormality. CASS registry data revealed six-year survival in two-vessel disease spanning 49–88 per cent, the best outcome being predicted by normal left ventricular function. CASS registry data further confirmed the excellent outcome in males without ventricular damage who had undergone coronary artery bypass grafting (CABG) (Chaitman *et al.* 1986). Survival was significantly better than their Framingham peers. Reduction in left ventricular function rendered the prognosis less favourable, mild to moderate impairment function being associated with a significantly poorer outcome at five years.

Revascularization of the myocardium

CORONARY ARTERY BYPASS GRAFTING

The long-term outcome following CABG is now well established, although proof of benefit over medical treatment depends largely on the outcome of three studies set up 25 years ago. Subsequent developments include more generalized use of arterial conduits, including the internal mammary arteries, and radial artery as a graft in addition to, or instead of, saphenous vein grafts. These have been demonstrated to have enhanced late patency. Off-pump grafting and minimally invasive off-pump bypass (mini-

mally invasive direct coronary artery bypass, MIDCAB) have less morbidity, but long-term outcome has yet to be determined.

There are important differences between CABG and percutaneous transluminal coronary angioplasty (PTCA) in terms of early and late morbidity. One meta-analysis contrasting outcome of the two techniques identified mortality and non-fatal myocardial infarction at 10.1 per cent versus 9.8 per cent at 2.7 years, but the additional intervention rate in the first year was 33.7 per cent in the PTCA group, ten times that in the CABG group (Pocock *et al.* 1995). Surgery bore a prolonged period of rehabilitation, while PTCA was burdened by repeated late hospitalization. This was in the pre-drug-eluting stent era, but the surgical results speak for themselves.

Graft attrition occurs steadily, and 10 per cent, 20 per cent and 40 per cent of saphenous grafts would have been occluded by one, five and ten years, respectively, in the pre-statin era. Early recurrence of symptoms is likely to be due to graft attrition, and late recurrence to progression of disease in the native circulation. Aggressive lipid management improves the outcome. The robust performance of the internal mammary artery conduit is well known. Loop *et al.* (1986) first demonstrated a 93 per cent ten-year survival in patients in whom an internal mammary artery conduit was implanted into the left anterior descending coronary artery. The ejection fraction was an important predictor of outcome.

Coronary artery bypass grafting has a low risk of MACE once rehabilitation has taken place. Actuarial survival following saphenous vein bypass grafting in one group of 428 patients with a mean age of 52.6 years at 5, 10 and 15 years was 94.2 per cent, 82.4 per cent and 63 per cent, respectively. This was in the pre-statin era. The cumulative probability of event-free survival for cardiac death, acute myocardial infarction, re-intervention and angina pectoris at 5, 10 and 15 years was, respectively, 97.8 per cent, 90.1 per cent and 74.4 per cent; 98.5 per cent, 89.0 per cent and 77.4 per cent; 97.0 per cent, 83.0 per cent and 62.1 per cent; and 77.8 per cent, 52.1 per cent and 26.8 per cent. Left ventricular function and the number of vessels involved were independently predictive of survival in this study (Bypass Angioplasty Revascularization Investigation (BARI) 1996). These figures are reassuring for the first quinquennium only in certificatory terms.

PERCUTANEOUS TRANSLUMINAL CORONARY ANGIOPLASTY AND INTRACORONARY STENTING

PTCA has been established for over two decades. The technique has the advantage that an early return to full activity is usual but with the disadvantage that the subsequent trajectory is often not unblemished. The original technique employed a balloon inserted via a guide-wire which was inflated across the obstructing lesion. More recently, the insertion of a stent – a small wire basket – has been shown to improve the prognosis, while more recently still, stent performance has been enhanced by the elution of drugs from its surface, although long-term data are not yet available.

In the context of aviation, recertification requires both freedom from symptoms and complete revascularization. PTCA is good for the former but less easy to achieve for the latter. In the BARI (1996) trial, complete revascularization in the presence of multi-vessel coronary artery disease was achieved in only 57 per cent of PTCA patients but in 91 per cent of those undergoing CABG. In contrast to the results of surgery, no survival advantage over medical treatment has been demonstrated for PTCA. Indeed, in one study, the group treated with high-dose (80 mg) atorvastatin had a 36 per cent lower event rate than the PTCA group (Pitt et al. 1999). Diabetic patients did significantly worse with PTCA than with CABG in terms of survival (65.5 per cent versus 80.6 per cent at five years) in the BARI study, while the Coronary Angioplasty versus Bypass Revascularization Investigation (CABRI 1995) study confirmed a more favourable surgical outcome. Likewise, saphenous vein graft angioplasty has a poor outcome. In the Arterial Revascularization Therapy Study (ARTS), the MACE difference between surgery and angioplasty (on average 30–40 per cent) was reduced to 14 per cent with stenting at one year – still not impressive in the context of aviation (Serruys et al. 2001). Some 70 per cent of lesions undergoing the percutaneous approach are now stented.

It is still comparatively early to be confident that the early hopes for drug-eluting stents will be sustained. In a systematic review of their performance, 14 trials were meta-analysed (Hilla et al. 2004). The authors concluded that the data were limited in terms of patient numbers, length of outcome and methodology of assessment. Event rates were lower for both paclitaxel- and strolimus-eluting stents, but there was no significant improvement in rates of death or non-fatal myocardial infarction when compared with the bare metal stent. Current guidelines by the National Institute for Clinical Excellence (NICE) state that 'stents should be used routinely where percutaneous coronary intervention (PCI) is the clinically appropriate procedure'.

In the context of aviation, a very low post-intervention event rate is needed before certification can be considered. The standard, its appendix and the guidance material to the JAR FCL Part 3 (Medical) permit angioplasty without suggesting that only single lesions in a native vessel are appropriate targets, whilst graft angioplasty and angioplasty in diabetic patients should not be acceptable due to the high subsequent event rate. Furthermore, in multi-vessel disease, the technique is relatively unable to obtain 'full' revascularization. Angioplasty and stenting are not yet acceptable for return to flying duties in the UK military.

Intervention against vascular risk factors

There is now massive evidence that intervention against the major vascular risk factors – hypertension, hypercholesterolaemia, smoking and diabetes – is associated with a significant reduction in fatal and non-fatal cardiovascular events. This holds good in both primary and secondary prevention, across a broad age range and in the presence of multiple risk factors (ALLHAT Collaborative Research Group 2002; De-Backer et al. 2003; Downs et al. 1998; Heart Protection Study Collaborative Group 2002; Long-Term Intervention with Pravastatin Group in Ischaemic Disease (LIPID) Study Group 1998; Pedersen 1994; Sever et al. 2003; West of Scotland Coronary Prevention Study Group 1995). With such convincing evidence, the requirement that a reduction in the presence of risk factors should be undertaken in the presence of known coronary artery disease represents best clinical practice.

An applicant may regain a class 1 medical certificate to fly as/with a suitably qualified co-pilot (OML) in the presence of known coronary artery disease provided that:

- he or she is asymptomatic and requires no anti-anginal medication
- vascular risk factors have been addressed, including smoking cessation, lipid lowering (with a statin, unless contraindicated), treatment of hypertension (with an angiotensin-converting enzyme inhibitor, ACEI) and administration of aspirin. Subjects with an abnormality of glucose metabolism demand special scrutiny and management
- left ventricular function is normal (> 50 per cent) as measured by echocardiography (Simpson's rule), multiple-gated acquisition (MUGA) study, or contrast ventriculography
- exercise ECG to stage IV of the Bruce treadmill protocol can be achieved without evidence of myocardial ischaemia, significant rhythm disturbance or symptoms
- coronary angiography carried out at or around the time of the index event demonstrates less than 50 per cent stenosis in any major untreated vessel or in any venous/arterial graft remote from any infarction
- Holter monitoring, if indicated, shows no significant rhythm disturbance
- MPS shows no evidence of a reversible defect. A small fixed defect is permissible, provided the ejection fraction is within the normal range no sooner than six months after the index event
- a class 1 certificate is restricted with an OML. Unrestricted class 2 certification may be permissible
- annual follow-up by a cardiologist with exercise ECG and review of vascular risk factor status can be arranged. Further investigation may be required, if indicated.

In the military in the UK, due to the different demands, myocardial infarction precludes further flying duties.

RATE AND RHYTHM DISTURBANCES

The human heart beats some 100 000 times a day and in health remains remarkably regular. An increase in the heart rate – a tachycardia – is present when the rate is > 100 beats/min and a bradycardia when the rate is < 50 beats/min. A sinus bradycardia in a subject of aircrew age is rarely of importance and may reflect only physical fitness. A sinus tachycardia in an otherwise fit individual may suggest anxiety, and although most aircrew become used to routine scrutiny, others continue to demonstrate an alarm reaction that may also be associated with so-called 'white-coat hypertension'. Rhythm and conduction disturbances continue to form the single largest problem group referred to the UK Medical Advisory Panel and together they form some of the more difficult problems encountered in aviation cardiology.

Atrial and ventricular premature beats

The routine aircrew ECG should be recorded on a three-channel system. With a three-lead presentation, the recording will last 12 seconds on a page of A4 size; further rhythm 'strips' are unlikely to be longer than another 12 seconds. If an isolated atrial or ventricular premature contraction is recorded, then it may be a coincidence; if more than one is present, then it is more likely that such events are sufficiently frequent to justify review. With increasing age the probability of rhythm disturbance increases. As a rule, a single atrial or ventricular premature beat is not of prognostic importance and is likely to pass unnoticed. Anxiety, excessive tea, coffee or alcohol, or smoking may be the explanation; if the subject becomes symptomatic, anxiety may contribute to their continuation. Frequent atrial ectopy may predict atrial fibrillation.

More complex rhythm disturbances including frequent ventricular premature complexes, with or without multiformity or multifocality, couplets and salvoes may not be of prognostic importance in the otherwise normal heart. In the aviation environment cardiological assessment with echocardiography, Holter monitoring and exercise ECG is nevertheless required. As a general rule, ventricular premature complexes with a density of < 200 per hour are acceptable if the non-invasive investigations are satisfactory. As complexity increases, even in an asymptomatic and otherwise normal individual, it is likely that a multi-crew endorsement will have to be applied in view of our inability to predict outcome (Campbell 1992).

Sino-atrial disease (sick sinus syndrome; brady-tachy syndrome)

Sino-atrial disease (evidenced by sinus pauses, sino-atrial block and paroxysmal atrial tachy-arrhythmia from a variety of causes) is not commonly seen in subjects of pilot age. The sino-atrial node and atrial myocardium are primarily affected, although the AV node and more distal conducting tissue may also be involved. There is a tendency towards excessive bradycardia, especially at night, when sinus arrest may occur. Pauses of > 2.5 seconds are likely to be abnormal if the subject is in sinus rhythm. Characteristic salvoes of atrial and/or junctional complexes followed by prolonged sinus node recovery time are a feature. There is an increased risk of thromboembolic stroke. There is overlap with 'athlete's heart', which tends to be associated with excessive vagal inhibitory activity and which is not uncommon in younger pilots.

Patients with sino-atrial disease may remain relatively or completely free of symptoms for many years or may become symptomatic quite rapidly. For this reason, regular review with exercise ECG (seeking chronotropic incompetence – an attenuated exercise heart-rate response) and Holter monitoring is justified. Echocardiography should confirm the continuing structural integrity of the heart. Restriction to multi-crew operation is likely, unless the disturbance is no more than minor and the pilot is asymptomatic. Once symptoms occur, certification to fly should be denied.

Atrial tachy-arrhythmia

The abrupt onset of rhythm disturbances may be both alarming and distracting and is a cause of incapacitation, subtle or complete. If the rate is very rapid, then systemic hypotension may occur and lead to altered consciousness. If there is structural abnormality of the heart, such as myocardial hypertrophy with associated impairment of diastolic function, then the disturbance may be tolerated poorly. With increased atrial or ventricular internal diameters, the risk of thromboembolic stroke increases. The disturbance, underlying structural abnormality (or non-structural cause) and outcome all need to be considered in the context of certification.

Atrial fibrillation

Atrial fibrillation is the most common rhythm disturbance causing intermittent or persisting symptoms. It is often associated with structural abnormality of the heart and has as its basis continuous wave fronts of depolarization arising mainly in the left atrium. It has a prevalence in the population of 0.4 per cent < age of 60 years, two to four per cent > 60 years and ten per cent > 80 years. It may be associated with cardiovascular disease, there may be an extra-cardiac cause, or it may be 'lone', without obvious pathology. Common causes of atrial fibrillation are shown in Table 37.2.

The clinical management of atrial fibrillation involves identification of cause with reversion to sinus rhythm, if possible, either pharmacologically or by DC shock. Management is directed towards the maintenance of sinus rhythm or regulation of the heart rate (European Atrial Fibrillation Consensus Conference 2003). Anticoagulation may be required. The same applies to the aviation environment once other disqualifying conditions such as valvular heart disease have been excluded.

The following presentations of atrial fibrillation are seen:

- *Single episode* with a defined cause, e.g. a vomiting episode.
- *Paroxysmal* atrial fibrillation, defined as more than one self-terminating episode, usually of < 24 hours' duration.
- *Persistent* atrial fibrillation, in which the return to sinus rhythm occurs only following therapeutic intervention. The duration is more than seven days.
- *Permanent* atrial fibrillation, in which a return to sinus rhythm cannot be accomplished or has not been attempted. The duration is > 12 months.

The condition commonly comes to light in one of two ways in the aviation scene: either the rhythm is uncovered by ECG at routine examination, or, the aviator presents with symptoms. In general, pharmacological cardioversion with an agent such as flecainide is most likely to be successful in the first few hours after the onset of the episode. A DC shock may be needed. Overall, 50–80 per cent will return to sinus rhythm by such means, depending on the presence or absence of other pathology and the duration of the attack. All attempts at cardioversion require anticoagulation with warfarin and the maintenance of the international normalized ratio (INR) at 2.5–3.0 for one month, before and after, unless undertaken within 24 hours or the left atrial appendage is demonstrably free of thrombus at transoesophageal echocardiography (TOE). Before attempting cardioversion, the thyroid-stimulating

hormone (TSH) level should be measured and thyrotoxicosis treated if necessary. Likewise, the liver function tests (LFTs) and mean corpuscular volume (MCV) should be checked to review potential alcohol abuse. After one year about 50 per cent are likely to have relapsed at least once; a minority (< 25 per cent) will maintain sinus rhythm at three years.

Recertification requires:

- normotension
- sinus rhythm
- normal TSH, LFTs and MCV
- no history of transient ischaemic attack (TIA)
- absence of risk factors for recurrence and/or for thromboembolic stroke, including age over 65 years, hypertension, diabetes, left ventricular hypertrophy, valvular heart disease and previous TIA (predicating need for warfarin)
- normal cavity and structural dimensions of the heart, normal valves and normal Doppler flows on echocardiography. The left atrial internal diameter should be < 4.5 cm
- exercise walking time to be normal (more than ten minutes). In atrial fibrillation, the maximum heart rate should be < 230 beats per minute and the longest pause < 3.5 seconds
- three Holter recordings over two to three months to have shown no evidence of atrial fibrillation in arbitrarily three to five consecutive complexes
- restriction of the licence with a multi-crew (OML) limitation. After an event-free period of two years, the restriction may be removed, subject to review.

Subjects of pilot age fulfilling the above should not require anticoagulation with warfarin, which itself is disqualifying, although aspirin/clopidogrel may be recommended. These are rigorous standards, which will be achieved by only a minority. In the event of default, further consideration will include satisfactory answers to the following:

- Is the thromboembolic rate acceptable without warfarin?
- Are there symptoms at any time, i.e. on switching rhythm, and if so are they minimal?

Table 37.2 *Common causes of atrial fibrillation*

Atrial fibrillation with cardiovascular disease	Atrial fibrillation with extra–cardiac disease	Lone atrial fibrillation
Hypertension	Infection	
Coronary artery disease	Alcohol abuse	
Valvular heart disease	Thyrotoxicosis	
Myocardial disease	Electrolyte disturbance	
Congenital heart disease	Pulmonary disease	
Cardiac surgery (recent and remote)	Pericarditis	

- Is the heart rate controlled well at rest and on exercise?
- Is an approved /non-approved drug being taken?

Products that are permitted include:

- digoxin (mainly of value in controlling resting heart rate in the established condition)
- beta-blocking agents, usually atenolol or bisoprolol, which may to help preserve sinus rhythm and reduce the heart rate in atrial fibrillation. Sotalol also has some class III effects (as well as some pro-arrhythmic effects)
- verapamil (class IV), which may help to preserve sinus rhythm and control the heart rate
- diltiazem, both alone and combined with the foregoing (but not beta-blockade) is helpful in rate management.

None of these products is particularly effective and in the long term atrial fibrillation will become established. Their side-effect profiles generally are not high.

Products not permitted include the following:

- Class Ia anti-arrhythmic agents, such as:

  - quinidine (excessive risk of torsades de pointes and sudden cardiac death (SCD))
  - disopyramide (excessive anticholinergic side effects)
  - procainamide (lupus-like syndrome and occasionally agranulocytosis).

- Class Ib drugs (e.g. mexiletine) which are ineffective in atrial rhythm disturbances,
- Class Ic agents (flecainide, propafenone) which are effective in bringing about the restoration of sinus rhythm and its maintenance but which have undesirable effects such as tremor and persistence of vision. Both may provoke atrial flutter in a minority (five per cent).
- The most effective class III drug, amiodarone, which has a high-side effect profile and thus cannot be considered. The most common side effect, photosensitization, is less important than the disturbance of sleep and sedation that it may cause. Patients receiving this drug develop corneal micro-deposits, which may give a halo effect around lights at night.
- Class III drugs – moricizine, dofetilide and ibutilide.

Neither flecainide nor propafenone is permitted in flyers although the UK CAA has approved flecainide at a dose of 50 mg twice daily on an individual basis occasionally. Amiodarone is barred on account of its side effects and likely coexisting pathology although a small number of flight engineers have been certificated while using it.

The certification of civilian aircrew with paroxysmal or chronic atrial fibrillation requires a non-invasive work-up, including echocardiography, exercise ECG and regular Holter assessment. Lone atrial fibrillation only is permitted in view of the excess risk of TIA with underlying pathology such as valvular heart disease. The condition precludes all flying in the UK military.

WARFARIN AND ANTICOAGULATION IN ATRIAL FIBRILLATION

Five major primary stroke-prevention trials have identified the following risk factors for thromboembolic stroke (Verrheugt and Antman 2004):

- males over 65 years of age
- hypertension (systolic blood pressure > 160 mmHg)
- diabetes mellitus
- previous TIA
- left ventricular fractional shortening < 25 per cent
- females > 75 years of age
- left atrial internal diameter > 2.5 cm/m^2.

About a third of subjects in atrial fibrillation will be at a low (less than one per cent) risk of an event per annum. Pilots satisfying the criteria above may be certificated with a restriction (class 1 OML). Aspirin reduces the risk by about 20 per cent and should be given if it is tolerable. Studies are under way to determine whether higher-risk subjects are protected with aspirin and clopidogrel and by a direct thrombin inhibitor, ximelagatran, which does not need the INR to be checked regularly. Warfarin is associated with an excess risk of bleeding of one per cent per annum for a 70 per cent reduction of stroke risk. It is not permitted in European aviators at present.

Atrial flutter

Atrial flutter presents special problems. It originates in the right atrium as a continuous re-entry circuit often around a ridge called the crista terminalis. Its rate approximates 300 beats/min. Rates of 150 beats/min are commonly encountered with two-to-one AV conduction while the risk remains for one-to-one conduction at 300 beats/min to occur. Symptoms may be troublesome due to abrupt rate change. For these reasons it is incompatible with flying status.

The introduction of radio frequency ablation of the flutter circuit has revolutionized treatment. If the flutter circuit has been ablated successfully with no recurrence of the arrhythmia for three months and the following protocol can be fulfilled, a class 1 OML certificate may be issued subject to cardiological follow-up:

- exercise ECG to four stages of the Bruce protocol is normal
- echocardiography shows a structurally normal heart

- absence of atrial flutter on Holter monitoring (evidence of atrial fibrillation will need further review)
- electrophysiological study shows bidirectional isthmus block.

An unrestricted certificate may be considered after two years.

Atrioventricular nodal re-entry tachycardia

Atrioventricular nodal re-entry is the most common single cause of regular narrow complex tachycardia accounting for some 50 per cent of all. It is caused by a micro re-entry circuit with two pathways, one fast and one with decremental conduction. It often has a rate of about 200 beats/min, sufficient to cause breathlessness, chest discomfort and sometimes polyuria due to the release of atrial natriuretic peptide. As the disturbances tend to recur throughout life and cannot reliably be suppressed completely, the condition is incompatible with certification to fly. An exception may be the subject who has undergone slow pathway modification and in whom the rhythm cannot be induced on electrophysiological study (cf. Atrial flutter, above).

Atrioventricular re-entry tachycardia

Atrioventricular re-entry tachycardias are caused by an extranodal fast-conducting pathway that 'pre-excites' the ventricle. This is known as the Kent bundle, although other variations (i.e. Maheim with a nodofascicular pathway) are also seen. The eponymous term, Wolff–Parkinson–White (WPW) pattern, implying the appearance only of the characteristic configuration of the ECG, is often applied. If there is a tachycardia, the term 'syndrome' is applied. In a study of 238 military aviators of mean age 34.3 years, 17.6 per cent were symptomatic and 82.4 per cent were not (Fitzsimmons et al. 2001). Fifteen per cent of pilots with the pattern only developed the syndrome over a mean of 22 years. The characteristic appearance of the QRS complex with a slurred inscription of the R wave (the 'delta' wave) and a short PR interval (but normal PT interval) is seen in about 1.6 per 1000 routine resting ECGs. It is more common in men than women. The prevalence of atrioventricular re-entry tachycardia varies between 5 and 90 per cent in hospital patients with the WPW pattern due to the phenomenon of ascertainment bias. If there is prograde (orthodromic) conduction through the slow nodal pathway with retrograde conduction via the fast accessory pathway, then the QRS complex will be narrow. If there is prograde conduction via the accessory pathway with retrograde (antidromic) conduction via the slow nodal pathway, the QRS complex will be broad. The appearance of the delta wave may be intermittent, implying that it is refractory part of the time. This is usually associated with a longer effective refractory period (ERF; 300–500 ms) and the term 'safe' is applied, suggesting a low risk of rapid atrioventricular re-entry tachycardia. This implies the absence of ability to conduct at very fast rates in atrial fibrillation in which total anomalous conduction may occur via the accessory pathway (Toff and Camm 1992).

Although many subjects with pre-excitation never experience an episode of tachycardia and in an unknown number the pathway is concealed, the possibility of a re-entry tachycardia with abrupt onset at a rapid rate, or of atrial fibrillation with anomalous conduction, gives rise to certificatory difficulties. Atrial fibrillation with very rapid conduction may provoke ventricular fibrillation and sudden cardiac death, but the risk is very low (Toff and Camm 1992). There is also an association with other anomalies such as hypertrophic myopathy and Ebstein's syndrome.

On first presentation with the ECG pattern an aviator should be made unfit. Provided there is no history of arrhythmia, and an echocardiogram, exercise ECG and 24-hour ambulatory ECG recording are within normal limits, an OML certificate may be given. It is helpful if, at least part of the time, the accessory pathway is refractory. For an unrestricted certificate, an electrophysiological study is required demonstrating no inducible re-entry tachycardia and an antegrade ERF greater than 300 ms. If the subject has a history of re-entrant tachy-arrhythmia, certification is possible only following the demonstration of ablation of the accessory pathway. This may be accomplished by an adenosine challenge.

ATRIOVENTRICULAR CONDUCTION DISTURBANCES

First-degree atrioventricular block

First degree atrioventricular block is present if the PR interval exceeds 210 ms. It is present in at least one per cent of asymptomatic aircrew applicants. In the absence of bundle branch disturbance, the condition is very likely to be benign assuming the interval shortens on exercise. Occasionally, very long PR intervals are seen of up to 400 ms; these, too, seem to be benign, provided the QRS width is normal and the interval shortens on exercise and following atropine. It is sometimes associated with Mobitz type I atrioventricular block (decremental atrioventricular conduction), which should be of short periodicity and occur only at night in young adults. The additional presence of a bundle branch disturbance, particularly if the mean frontal QRS axis is abnormal, raises the possibility of distal conducting tissue disease. In the absence of such a complication an aviator may be certificated without restriction.

Second-degree atrioventricular block

Second-degree atrioventricular block is much less common than the first-degree form. It was seen in only 0.003 per cent of the 122 043 aviator ECGs reviewed by Hiss and Lamb (1962). Short periodicity (i.e. 2 : 3 and 3 : 4) Mobitz type I atrioventricular block in which the PR interval progressively prolongs until there is a non-conducted P wave is sometimes seen during sleep in normal young, especially athletic individuals. It appears to carry no special risk and represents delayed conduction at the level of the atrioventricular node which is of vagal origin. The coexistence of a bundle branch disturbance will raise the possibility of distal conducting tissue (His–Purkinje) disease. Type I atrioventricular block is very uncommon during the day and that, or the presence of an abnormality of electrical axis or of a conduction block, should provoke investigation with 24-hour ambulatory monitoring and an exercise recording. Further follow-up is necessary.

Mobitz type II and 2 : 1 atrioventricular blocks more commonly, although not exclusively, represent delay in the His–Purkinje network and carry a risk of progression to complete atrioventricular block with risk of syncope. Such abnormalities should lead to a denial of certification.

Third-degree (complete) atrioventricular heart block

Complete (third-degree) heart block disbars from all levels of certification to fly. Provided that there is no other disqualifying pathology and an endocardial pacemaker has been inserted (see pp. 586–587), then limited certification may be possible.

Congenital complete atrioventricular block is rare. Although survival to middle years and beyond is the rule, there is an excess risk of sudden cardiac death. Although there is limited experience in North America in military personnel with the anomaly, such individuals should be considered unfit for all forms of certification to fly.

INTRAVENTRICULAR CONDUCTION DISTURBANCES

Right bundle branch block

Incomplete right bundle branch block is a common anomaly that carries a normal prognosis in otherwise normal subjects. No special precautions are needed. If there is sig-nificant right axis deviation, then the possibility of a secundum atrial septal defect should be considered. Complete right bundle branch block is present in 0.2 per cent of pilot applicants. It is characterized by a QRS width greater than 120 ms, with significant S waves in S1, V5 and V6. There will be an rSR pattern in V1 and V2. Established complete right bundle branch block appears to carry no adverse risk in asymptomatic males of aircrew age. Even if it is newly acquired, there is no evidence of an increased risk of cardiovascular event unless the result of anteroseptal infarction. On first presentation, applicants should undergo cardiological review with:

- satisfactory exercise ECG response (at least three stages of the Bruce protocol)
- Holter monitoring – no significant rhythm or conduction disturbance
- echocardiography – no structural or functional abnormality of the heart
- if indicated, only electrophysiological study and/or coronary angiography
- licence restriction to class 1 OML. Satisfactory cardiological review at 12 months will usually permit unrestricted certification.

Left bundle branch block

Incomplete left bundle branch block is an ECG definition when the standard criteria for left bundle branch block are satisfied (absent q wave in I, aVL, V5 and V6; absent r'; in V1, with or without secondary T wave changes) but the QRS complex width is < 120 ms. The distinction is arbitrary.

Complete left bundle branch block has had a malign reputation, partly on account of its association with coronary artery disease in older subjects in whom the incidence may be as high as 25–50 per cent. It is one-tenth as common as right bundle branch block. Newly acquired left bundle branch block in one study observed a risk ratio for sudden cardiac death of ten to one above the age of 45 years (Rabkin et al. 1980). Notwithstanding, stable complete left bundle branch block appears to carry little excess risk of cardiovascular event in the otherwise normal heart and may, following the application of the above protocol and exclusion of a myocardial infarction, conducting tissue or coronary abnormality, be consistent with multi-crew operation. Return to restricted military flying duties may also be permitted. Coronary angiography or pharmacological stress myocardial perfusion imaging (MPI) is needed to exclude the possibility of coronary artery disease.

Hemi-blocks

Left anterior and left posterior (fascicular) hemi-blocks in the absence of other abnormalities appear to carry no excess risk of cardiovascular event. The prevalence of the former increases from 0.5 per cent at age 30 years to five per cent at age 60 years (Hickman *et al.* 1996). At first presentation, and by implication at the initial issue of a licence, cardiological review with exercise ECG and/or echocardiography is justified. Data are scant in relation to the significance of acquired left anterior and posterior hemi-block. The emergence of a change in axis on routine scrutiny justifies review.

ION CHANNELOPATHIES

The ion channelopathies form a rare group of inherited disorders of the sodium and potassium channels that regulate cardiac repolarization. Over 250 mutations involving six different genes have been identified. They are transmitted as autosomal dominants with incomplete penetrance and expression. They are associated with ventricular tachycardia – torsades de pointes and sudden cardiac death – commonly in the first two or three decades of life.

Brugada syndrome is transmitted autosomal dominantly with incomplete penetrance. It appears to be linked to the *SCN5A* gene, which encodes the sodium channel. Its prevalence has been reported as being between five and 66 per 100 000 (Wilde *et al.* 2002), but it is more common in the Far East and in Japan where the prevalence may be as high as 146 per 100 000. It is characterized by a male preponderance of eight or nine to one. The ECG anomaly is characteristic of the syndrome and tends to vacillate. In the type 1 form, there is coved upward ST segment elevation with a J wave amplitude >0.2 mV followed by an inverted T wave in V1 and V2. Less striking abnormalities are seen in types 2 and 3. The tendency to mimic right bundle branch aberration and its variability may give rise to interpretative difficulties. The QT interval may be normal or slightly prolonged. It is rare in the pilot population, having a prevalence of 0.08 per cent in 16 988 French Air Force personnel (Perrier *et al.* 2003) which was increased by a further 0.05 per cent following challenge with ajmaline. Of 334 Brugada phenotypes in one study, the pattern was recognized in 71 subjects following resuscitation after a cardiac arrest, in 73 subjects following a syncopal event and was recorded in a further 190 asymptomatic individuals.

Long QT syndrome (LQTS) may be congenital or acquired. It is characterized by an abnormality of myocardial repolarization. In the congenital form, it used to be known as the Romano–Ward syndrome or, if associated with nerve deafness, as the Jervell and Lange–Neilsen syndrome. Six different genotypes and three different phenotypes (LQT1, 2, 3) have been identified (Xhang *et al.* 2000). In all, there is an increased risk of syncope, ventricular tachycardia and sudden cardiac death. The T waves are bizarre and the QT interval often significantly prolonged (>550 ms; normal <440 ms in males, <460 ms in females). Outcome is related to the length of the QTc (the QT interval corrected by division of the QT interval by the RR interval expressed in seconds – Bazett's formula), the genotype, and the presence or absence of complex ventricular rhythm disturbances including the characteristic torsades de pointes tachycardia. Acquired prolongation of the QT interval can occur in electrolyte disturbance (hypocalcaemia, hypomagnesaemia), metabolic disturbance (myxoedema) and drug administration (including quinidine, amiodarone, sotalol, phenothiazines and tricyclics, erythromycin, quinine, chloroquine, ketanserin, cisapride, terfenadine, tacrolimus and probucol).

One of the problems with both syndromes is the overlap with the normal ECG (Joy 2004). Fifty per cent of LQT carriers are asymptomatic although up to four per cent may die suddenly. The LQT3 phenotype is the most lethal and LQT1 the least. A QTc >500 ms powerfully predicts an unfavourable outcome and such people should not be certificated (Priori *et al.* 2003). In the absence of genotyping likely candidates for retention of certification (i.e. not initial applicants) with either syndrome will:

- be asymptomatic
- have no family history of sudden cardiac death (SCD)
- have minimal ECG features
- have no evidence of complex ventricular rhythm disturbance on regular Holter monitoring.

Initial issue of a certificate in the future may require genotyping. If the condition is confirmed certification is likely to be denied. LQT1 and LQT2 phenotypes in females and LQT3 phenotype in males are adverse findings.

ENDOCARDIAL PACEMAKING

Conditions requiring the implantation of an endocardial pacemaker are uncommon in people of aircrew age, and coexisting pathology or congenital abnormality are likely to disbar from flying duty. Anti-tachycardia devices and implantable defibrillators are disbarring. Essentially the subject should:

- have no other disqualifying condition including unsuppressed atrial or ventricular rhythm disturbance
- have a bipolar system
- have a normal echocardiogram, Holter recording and satisfactory exercise ECG
- not be pacemaker-dependent (however defined)

- be restricted to class 1 OML/class 2
- undergo regular cardiological/pacemaker review.

A pacemaker precludes all forms of military flying in the UK.

HEART MURMURS AND VALVULAR HEART DISEASE

Innocent murmurs

Heart murmurs are very common, particularly in the young and the svelte. Most are innocent flow murmurs, which, by definition, will be brief and early systolic. Although a harsher murmur is more likely to be of significance, it may still be unimportant and reflect turbulence in the left and/or right ventricular outflow tracts. In older people, this may reflect thickening (sclerosis) of the aortic valve. Pan-systolic, late systolic or continuous murmurs are always abnormal. When any murmur is found at the initial examination for the issuance of a licence, a cardiological opinion should be sought. Usually a single consultation with or without echocardiography, will be sufficient to identify the few people in whom further review is justified. The remainder can be reassured. A previously unidentified murmur discovered in later years should also be reviewed.

Aortic valve disease

Bicuspid aortic valve is one of the most common congenital cardiac malformations and affects at least one per cent of the population. A significant percentage of subjects with such an anomaly will progress in later years to aortic stenosis and/or regurgitation. For this reason at least biennial review is required. It may be associated with aortic root disease which, when present, needs to be followed closely and eventually will disbar on account of risk of dissection and/or rupture. It may also be associated with patent ductus arteriosus or coarctation of the aorta. Any increase in the aortic root diameter needs ongoing echocardiographic follow-up; if the root diameter is > 5.0 cm, the certificate will need to be withdrawn. There is a small but finite risk of endocarditis which underscores the need for antibiotic cover for dental and urinary tract manipulation. As an isolated finding, following cardiological review, bicuspid aortic valve may be consistent with unrestricted certification to fly.

Many aircrew developing aortic stenosis are likely to have a bicuspid valve, although calcification of a tricuspid valve is more common with age. Isolated rheumatic involvement is rare in western countries. Mild aortic stenosis (< 30 mmHg, peak to peak) may be acceptable for unrestricted certification, but stenosis > 30 but

< 40 mmHg will restrict to multi-crew operation subject to annual cardiological review and Doppler echocardiograph. Attributable symptoms will disbar. Any increase in left ventricular wall thickness (> 1.1 cm) or history of cerebral embolic event will also be disqualifying. Gradients < 20 mmHg, peak to peak, allow restricted flying in the UK military.

Aortic regurgitation if mild or moderate is tolerated well over many years, the exception being if it is associated with root disease. Mild non-rheumatic aortic regurgitation (arbitrarily < 1/6) unassociated with root disease or other potentially disqualifying condition may be permissible for unrestricted certification to fly. There should be no significant increase in the systolic diameter of the heart (arbitrarily < 4.1 cm) and none of the diastolic diameter (> 6.2 cm) measured on echocardiography. There should be no significant arrhythmia and the effort performance should be normal. An aortic root diameter > 5 cm will disqualify. Significant increase in the end-systolic (> 4.4 cm) and/or end-diastolic (> 6.5 cm) diameters of the left ventricle, with or without evidence of impairment of systolic/diastolic function will also disqualify. Annual cardiological follow-up with echocardiography is required.

Mitral valve disease

Once diagnosed, rheumatic mitral stenosis/regurgitation, unless minimal with the subject in sinus rhythm, disbars from all forms of certification to fly. This is due to the excess risk of incapacitation secondary to the unpredictable onset of atrial fibrillation and a significant risk of cerebral embolism. The onset of atrial fibrillation, if the rate is rapid, may be associated with syncope or pulmonary oedema. Non-rheumatic mitral regurgitation is usually due to prolapse of either or both leaflets of the valve. When caused by rupture of the chordae or ischaemic injury to the papillary musculature it disbars from certification to fly.

Mitral leaflet prolapse is a common condition affecting up to five per cent of males and eight per cent of females, but definitions vary. It has been associated with a tendency to atrial and/or ventricular rhythm disturbances and atypical chest pain. There is a very small risk of cerebral embolus, sudden death and endocarditis (all < 0.02 per cent per annum) and also of chordal rupture (Webb-Peploe 1992). Thickening or significant redundancy of the valve leaflets is associated with a higher embolic risk and needs special consideration.

Isolated mid-systolic click needs no special precaution other than occasional cardiological review. Minor regurgitation (arbitrarily < 1/6) in the presence of a pan- or late systolic murmur, normal left ventricular dimensions on echocardiography and no other potentially disqualifying abnormality may be consistent with unrestricted certification but requires close cardiological review with early restriction if there is any change, especially in the end-diastolic diameter of the heart. A left ventricular end-diastolic diameter > 6.2 cm should disbar from all classes of certification. Annual cardiological review will be with echocardiography and 24-hour ambulatory monitoring. Exercise ECG may also be indicated. Precautions need to be taken against the risk of endocarditis in the context of dental or urinary tract manipulation.

Definite mitral valve prolapse is incompatible with recruitment to military flying duties. If discovered during a military flying career, then minor prolapse with a normal ECG and no symptoms is compatible with full flying duties. However, if more marked, then restriction to multi-crew, unfit acceleration $> +2.5\,G_z$ and unfit pressure breathing will be applied. Severe mitral valve prolapse is incompatible with any form of military flying duties.

Valvular surgery

In a review of the long-term outcome of prosthetic heart valve insertion over a 15-year period, survival was better ($P < 0.02$) with a mechanical prosthesis than with a tissue prosthesis; bleeding rates were higher with mechanical valves in the aortic (but not mitral) position and replacement rates were higher with bioprosthetic valves (Rahimtoola 2003). Bleeding rates were about 2.5 per cent per annum for mechanical valves and 0.9–2 per cent for porcine valves in the aortic position. In the mitral position, the rates were the same.

Late mortality is of the order of 66–79 per cent survival at 15 years following aortic valve replacement and 79–81 per cent following mitral valve replacement. Risk factors for a poorer outcome include greater age, left ventricular dysfunction, higher New York Heart Association (NYHA) functional class, coronary disease/surgery, hypertension, renal failure and lung disease. Bioprosthetic valves, including homograft prostheses, in the aortic position in patients under 40 years of age have a structural deterioration rate of 60 per cent at ten years and 90 per cent at 15 years.

With modern mechanical valves the thromboembolic risk in patients taking anticoagulants is similar to that of the bioprosthetic valves without anticoagulants, but the additional haemorrhagic risk has to be born in the former. Bioprosthetic valves start to deteriorate at five years in the mitral position and at eight years in the aortic position, deterioration being more rapid in younger subjects. There appear to be no important performance differences between the stented and stentless porcine valves in one review (Rahimtoola 2003). The Carpentier–Edwards porcine xenograft (Parker 1988) has an embolic risk approximating to one per cent per annum and in the absence of history of cerebral embolism is normally managed with aspirin alone.

Aortic valve replacement with the unmounted aortic homograft valve performs most favourably in terms of the risk of thromboembolism (assuming sinus rhythm) but its survival may be shorter than that of the porcine valve, particularly in younger individuals. In the certification of subjects of professional aircrew age it is likely that a mechanical valve will be recommended on the grounds of its long-term performance and this will disbar from certification to fly under the present requirements.

Mitral valve repair due to prolapse of either or both cusps has a survival of 88 per cent at eight years in one review (Totaro et al. 1999) with a 93 per cent freedom from thromboembolic events at six years (Perier et al. 1997). The majority maintained NYHA class I status as well as sinus rhythm.

Recertification may be considered in the best-risk subjects who have undergone aortic valve replacement/mitral valve repair at least six months previously and who:

- are free of symptoms
- are in sinus rhythm and not requiring treatment with warfarin
- have no significant left ventricular hypertrophy on echocardiography (> 1.3 cm, septum and free wall) or dilation (> 6.2 cm end diastole/4.1 cm end systole), nor dilation of the aortic root (> 4.5 cm)
- have no abnormality of wall motion on echocardiography (except that due to left bundle branch block)
- have no significant (ungrafted) coronary artery disease
- have no significant rhythm disturbance on Holter monitoring
- are restricted to fly on multi-crew operations only
- are able to undergo annual cardiological review.

In the case of aortic valve replacement, a cadaver homograft or possibly a Carpentier–Edwards/Hancock porcine xenograft, only, may be considered. Following mitral valve repair, only subjects who are in sinus rhythm and who have had the left atrial appendage amputated may be considered for certification. Mitral valve replacement is disbarring, and any history of thromboembolism will be disqualifying. Precautions are needed for the antibiotic cover of dental and urinary tract procedures.

PERICARDITIS, MYOCARDITIS AND ENDOCARDITIS

Pericarditis

Pericarditis involves the fibrous sac in which the heart lies and has a number of pathological causes of which acute benign aseptic pericarditis is the condition most likely to be encountered in aircrew. It is also the condition most likely to be associated with full recovery and eventual unrestricted certification to fly. Identifiable causes of pericarditis include the following:

- idiopathic (acute benign aseptic)
- viral: Coxsackie B, echovirus 8, Epstein–Barr virus, varicella, mumps
- bacterial: *Staphylococcus*, *Pneumococcus*, *Meningococcus*, *Gonococcus*
- mycobacterial: tuberculosis
- filamentous bacterial: actinomyces, nocardia
- fungal: candidiasis, *Histoplasma*
- protozoal: *Toxoplasma*, *Entamoeba*
- immunological: Dressler, rheumatoid arthritis, systemic lupus erythematosus, scleroderma, polyarteritis
- neoplastic
- traumatic
- metabolic
- post-irradiation.

Acute benign aseptic pericarditis is a self-limiting illness. It is often associated with a systemic disturbance resembling influenza, a friction rub and characteristic mid-sternal discomfort which may be worsened by inspiration. It is commonly relieved by bending forward. It is sometimes misdiagnosed as a coronary syndrome. Spontaneous recovery is to be expected with supportive treatment such as aspirin. The identification of a viral infective agent may or may not be possible. The characteristic ECG changes seen are concave ST segment elevation, with later diffuse ST–T changes which may be persistent and raise the possibility of myocardial involvement – so-called myopericarditis. This justifies subsequent monitoring until there is confidence that myocardial function remains unimpaired.

Three to six months should elapse before restricted certification is permitted which is contingent upon the subject being asymptomatic with a normal echocardiogram, 24-hour ambulatory ECG and exercise ECG. Follow-up for at least two years is required. Coronary angiography/stress thallium MPI may be needed to resolve doubt surrounding non-invasive investigations. Relapse following idiopathic pericarditis is not uncommon, particularly in the first year. The pain may be quite disabling and an aviator is not fit for duty during such an episode. The certification of aircrew following pericarditis attributable to other pathologies will depend on the completeness of resolution, clinical stability and expected long-term outcome.

Constrictive pericarditis may follow a number of infections or may be idiopathic. Fatigue, breathlessness and fluid retention are late clinical features, which, when evident, disbar from all forms of certification to fly. Following pericardectomy, recertification will be possible only subject to essentially normal ventricular function and demonstrated electrical stability.

Myocarditis

Acute viral myocarditis may merge seamlessly into dilated cardiomyopathy. About one-third of patients with a recent diagnosis of dilated cardiomyopathy are likely to have a history of febrile illness. Virus myocarditis is more frequent than is diagnosed and may be present in one in 20 patients with viraemia. Characteristically, there is a systemic upset which is associated with evidence of impaired ventricular function and disturbance of rhythm and/or conduction. There may be an associated myalgia. Most cases recover spontaneously although the possibility of the development of late cardiomyopathy is present.

Viruses are not the only agents responsible for myocarditis. A large number of pathogens, metabolic abnormalities, toxins and other causes have been described. The most common is ethyl alcohol. Acute alcoholic intoxication reduces myocardial function and predisposes to atrial and ventricular rhythm disturbance, the most important of which is atrial fibrillation. Other toxins include carbon monoxide, halogenated hydrocarbons, insect or snake bites and cocaine. One cause of occult myocardial damage, both acutely and long-term, is an anthracycline given in childhood for treatment of lymphoma and other neoplastic conditions (see Chapter 44). There may be an initial myocarditis followed years later by the insidious development of a cardiomyopathy (Steinherz *et al.* 1995). Unfortunately, the resting ECG is insensitive in the detection of the subtle abnormalities of function in this group of patients, who appear to have a potentially vulnerable myocardium. Likewise, the echocardiogram may be unhelpful, but nuclear techniques may be more sensitive.

Following an episode of myocarditis, full investigation should include echocardiography, exercise ECG and repeated 24-hour ambulatory monitoring to search for complex ventricular rhythm disturbances and atrial fibrillation. The echocardiogram should have returned to normal (i.e. have no evidence of rhythm or conduction disturbance) and should be repeated in regular follow-up. This should include repeated Holter monitoring. Any evidence of increasing (left) ventricular internal diameter and reduction of systolic (and/or diastolic) function will likely lead to the withdrawal of certification.

Endocarditis

Endocarditis has an overall mortality of six per cent although the presence of a virulent organism and/or involvement of a prosthetic valve can elevate this ten-fold. Causes of death include sepsis, valve failure giving rise to heart failure, and mycotic aneurysm. The acute illness disbars from all forms of certification to fly. Treatment involves at least six weeks of antibiotic therapy, and recovery to full health may take weeks longer, with a risk of relapse for several months. Once a patient has suffered an episode of endocarditis recertification depends on good residual function of the heart as judged by standard non-invasive techniques. The risk of further re-infection with recurrence of endocarditis is increased. Such patients require special precautions with dental and urinary tract surgery.

Outcome is influenced favourably if renal and myocardial function are normal after an attack and there has been no systemic embolism. Involvement of the mitral or aortic valve, if it does not lead to significant regurgitation, may leave a sterile vegetation that provides a nidus for cerebral embolism and re-infection. There are several reports that post-discharge survival is reduced; for these reasons, restricted certification only is the likely outcome following recovery.

CARDIOMYOPATHY

Cardiomyopathy is a heart-muscle disorder not associated with coronary heart disease, valvular heart disease, hypertension or congenital abnormality. If the ventricle is dilated with predominantly systolic dysfunction (it may also demonstrate secondary diastolic dysfunction) the term 'dilated cardiomyopathy' is appended. If it is inappropriately hypertrophied, sometimes grossly, and asymmetrically in the absence of provocative circumstance, the term 'hypertrophic cardiomyopathy' (HCM) is used. Systolic function normally is preserved in this case, but diastolic function is likely to be impaired. If the ventricle is stiffened due to infiltration by, for example, amyloidosis, sarcoidosis or a glycosphingolipid (Fabry's disease), the term 'restrictive cardiomyopathy' is more appropriate although hypertrophy may also be present as will both systolic and diastolic dysfunction.

Hypertrophic cardiomyopathy

HCM has a prevalence of about one in 500 adults. Most adults with the condition have inherited it as an autosomal dominant characteristic, and about 60 per cent have one of over 100 mutations involving 11 genes that encode the contractile proteins. It is marked by the diversity of its phenotypes and has a fairly specific histological appearance, which includes disarray of the myocytes with bizarre forms. An otherwise inexplicable wall diameter greater than 1.5 cm is sufficient to make the diagnosis, with characteristic asymmetry of the interventricular septum, although this is not always the case. About 25 per cent will have sub(aortic) valve obstruction caused by the hypertrophied septum. About one to two per cent die each year, 50 per cent suddenly and usually due to ventricular

arrhythmia. Stroke is also a cause of death in these people (Priori et al. 2001).

Although often asymptomatic, the patient with established HCM may suffer breathlessness (50 per cent); a smaller percentage will also suffer syncope at some point. The condition is likely to present in aviators with an abnormal resting ECG, changes ranging from diffuse ST–T abnormalities through QS waves in the inferior or high septal leads (the so-called pseudo-infarct pattern with a discordant QRST angle), or significant and widespread voltage increase with deep symmetrical T wave inversion. It may also present as a sustained ejection systolic murmur reflecting at least 'physiological' obstruction in the left ventricular outflow tract together with a third or fourth heart sound. Mitral regurgitation may be present due to distorted architecture. The association of systolic anterior motion of the mitral valve (SAM) with (asymmetric) septal hypertrophy (ASH) and premature closure of the aortic valve on M mode echocardiography is more or less pathognomonic of the condition.

The natural history of the condition complicates certification. Outcome may be genetically determined but progress can be very slow and the condition benign. Risk factors for SCD include previous cardiac event, family history of sudden death, ventricular tachycardia on ambulatory monitoring, abnormal blood pressure response (a fall) on exercise ECG, interventricular septum > 3 cm and sub-aortic gradient > 30 mmHg. Half of the sudden deaths occurring in young male athletes under 35 years of age are due to the condition. Atrial fibrillation, especially if paroxysmal and uncontrolled, may prove incapacitating and also worsens the prognosis (McKenna and Behr 2002). Continuing certification requires the absence of these risk factors.

The athlete's heart

Endurance training (running, swimming, bicycling) is associated with end-diastolic dilation of the left ventricle with an increased ejection fraction, while power work (lifting) is associated with hypertrophy. In the former both the left ventricle muscle mass and the end-diastolic diameter are related to lean body mass. Apart from the exercise history the ECG is helpful. Both athletes and subjects with HCM will have increased voltages but the latter will often show left axis deviation and a wide QRST angle. Sometimes they will also show QS waves in the inferior or anteroseptal leads while the athlete's heart is likely to demonstrate right axis deviation with no more than minor repolarization change in the ST–T segment.

The echocardiogram in the athlete will show a normal left atrial diameter (< 4 cm); in people with HCM, it will be > 4.5 cm. Likewise, the interventricular septum will be < 1.5 cm and > 1.5 cm and the left ventricular end-diastolic diameter in the athlete and > 1 .5 cm and < 5.5 cm respectively in HCM. Provided the subject can complete at least three stages of the Bruce treadmill protocol without symptoms, electrical instability or a fall in the blood pressure (which may be predictive of SCD), there is no ventricular tachycardia (defined as three or more consecutive ventricular complexes) whether sustained or not, there is no family history of related SCD, and the interventricular septum is < 2.5 cm, then an aviator may be considered for restricted certification to fly, subject to regular review. A history of atrial fibrillation, whether paroxysmal or sustained, is disqualifying.

Restrictive cardiomyopathy

Restrictive cardiomyopathy is a rare disorder characterized by normal or near-normal dimensions of the heart, sometimes with normal systolic function, but with failure of diastolic function due to increased stiffness of the myocardium. The causes include infiltrative conditions such as amyloidosis and sarcoidosis, storage diseases such as haemosiderosis and haemochromatosis, and endomyocardial disease, including fibrosis, the eosinophilic syndromes, carcinoid syndrome and radiation damage.

The majority of patients with a restrictive myocardial defect will be unfit for any form of certification to fly. Amyloidosis of the heart has a very poor prognosis by way of rapid deterioration of function complicated by rhythm disturbance. Haemochromatosis that is controlled well by venesection in a patient with normal glucose tolerance, normal echocardiogram, normal exercise ECG and normal ambulatory ECG may be considered for restricted certification, subject to regular review. Those with transfusion-dependent anaemias will be unfit. Eosinophilic heart disease is equally problematic; this has been reviewed by Webb-Peploe (1988).

Dilated cardiomyopathy

The causes of dilated cardiomyopathy are various, with up to 40 per cent being familial and transmitted predominantly by an autosomal dominant gene. The prognosis has improved strikingly over the past two decades, and mortality is now about 20 per cent at five years. Thirty per cent will die suddenly, many from a malignant tachy-arrhythmia, this outcome not being restricted to severe disease (Priori *et al.* 2001). In one study, nearly 50 per cent of 673 people with dilated cardiomyopathy were labelled idiopathic, while a further 12 per cent were considered to have myocarditis and only three per cent were considered to be due to alcohol (Kasper *et al.* 1996). An earlier study suggested that alcohol was responsible in up to one-third of cases.

The cause of death in dilated cardiomyopathy may be divided more or less equally into those perishing from pump failure and suffering a sudden arrhythmic event. The presence of high-grade ventricular rhythm disturbances is both common and predictive of outcome. In view of the generally poor prognosis, the diagnosis of dilated cardiomyopathy is inconsistent with any form of certification to fly. It is possible that mild global reduction in left ventricular systolic function (ejection fraction > 50 per cent) that is stable arbitrarily for a period of at least six months and with no evidence of electrical instability may be considered for restricted certification subject to close follow-up with echocardiography and Holter monitoring.

One group that bears special consideration are those who received an anthracycline, often in childhood for malignant disease, as described above. There is some evidence of a dose relationship in the incidence of subsequent myocardial abnormality; in one study of long-term survivors (median 8.9 years) of malignant bone disease aged between 10 and 45 years (mean 17.8 years), the incidence of cardiac abnormalities increased with length of follow-up (Postma *et al.* 1996). These investigators recommended life-long cardiological follow-up. Evans and Cooke (2003) have recommended cardiological review for all individuals seeking initial issue or follow-up certification to fly.

Sarcoidosis

Sarcoidosis presents special problems in certification due to its ubiquity and its occasional involvement of the heart. It is commonly a self-limiting condition seen in young adults with the extent of systemic involvement being largely unknown. There is often no significant systemic illness, and presentation may be fortuitous with bilateral hilar lymphadenopathy on routine chest X-ray. Or there may be erythema nodosum, malaise, arthralgia, iridocyclitis, respiratory symptoms or other constitutional upset. In those with systemic involvement, five per cent will also have cardiac involvement. Its aetiology is not understood, but a genetically determined sensitivity to pine pollen or an infective agent may be involved.

Involvement of the heart is associated with a poor prognosis and a significant risk of sudden death; half of those diagnosed with the condition during life die from the disease (Fleming 1994). Cardiac involvement may exist without concomitant involvement of other systems. Sudden death may be due to malignant ventricular rhythm disturbance or granulomatous involvement of the conducting system. Dilation of the ventricles due to patchy involvement of the myocardium may lead to the development of a dilated or restrictive cardiomyopathy. There are no characteristic ECG features although Holter monitoring may be premonitory of rhythm and conduction disturbance. Echocardiography may show patchy or generalized hypokinesia, especially if the basal myocardium is affected, with ventricular dilation and reduction of the ejection fraction. Deposits thicker than 3 mm may be detected non-invasively. Myocardial scintigraphy is inconclusive but magnetic resonance imaging (MRI) scanning may demonstrate localized high-intensity lesions with gadolinium enhancement. Raised plasma angiotensin-converting enzyme (ACE) activity is not diagnostic but may give an indication of active disease. A scalene node biopsy will confirm systemic sarcoidosis if present, but myocardial biopsy is often unhelpful due to the patchy nature of the disease.

The diagnosis of sarcoidosis (sometimes by way of the chance discovery of bilateral hilar lymphadenopathy) requires that the pilot should temporarily be made unfit. Satisfactory assessment for the restoration of restricted class I certification should attempt to establish that the disease is inactive and include:

- no increase in hilar lymphadenopathy on serial chest radiography
- stable gas transfer factor
- no evidence of active disease elsewhere (including scalene node biopsy)
- normal resting and exercise ECG (to at least nine minutes of the Bruce protocol)
- no significant rhythm or conduction disturbance on Holter monitoring
- normal echocardiogram.

Thallium stress MPI, transoesophageal echocardiography and/or MRI scanning will be required in the event of abnormality.

Restricted certification may be permitted subject to six-monthly cardiological follow-up for two years. Minimum re-investigation should include echocardiography and Holter monitoring. Full certification may be considered no sooner than two years after the initial observation, subject to regular follow-up. Any evidence of systemic involvement (except erythema nodosum) requires permanent restriction to multi-crew operation. Evidence of involvement of the heart is permanently disbarring for all licences.

Right ventricular cardiomyopathy

Right ventricular cardiomyopathy (previously arrhythmogenic right ventricular dysplasia) is characterized by dilation of the right ventricle with regional or global replacement of the myocardium with fibro-fatty tissue. It may also involve the left ventricle. It may account for up to 25 per cent of SCD in young adults (Priori *et al.* 2001) and is transmitted as an autosomal dominant gene with incomplete penetrance in at least 30 per cent. The characteristic ECG pattern is one of QRS prolongation with T wave inversion in V1–V3. Epsilon waves may also be present. Monomorphic ventricular rhythm disturbances with left bundle branch block and right-axis deviation, including sustained ventricular tachycardia, commonly are seen. An early sign may be minor T wave changes in the right ventricular leads. Exercise-induced ventricular tachycardia and SCDs are common. A family history has an uncertain predictive value but early presentation (< age 20 years) is likely to be an adverse factor. Syncope is an adverse event but QT dispersion, Holter monitoring, exercise ECG and programmed electrical stimulation are not reliable predictors of ventricular tachycardia.

Although right ventricular outflow tract tachycardia should prompt the search for dysplasia, the isolated rhythm disturbance may be benign in young adults. However, our ability to disentangle those with 'innocent' (and, perforce, asymptomatic) ventricular tachycardia from those with a potentially malignant outcome is not yet secure. For these reasons, right ventricular dilation in this context disbars from all forms of certification to fly.

CONGENITAL HEART DISEASE

Improvements in diagnostic and interventional techniques in the management of congenital heart disease have led to the emergence of the specialty of grown-up congenital heart disease (GUCH). A patient with such an anomaly on achieving adulthood naturally expects to lead as normal a life as possible which includes following employment and pursuing hobbies and pastimes, some of which will have defined fitness requirements. These pursuits are not confined to aviation but include activities such as diving, vocational driving and motor-racing.

In general terms the principles applied to other cardiovascular problems are equally applicable to GUCH, the defining requirement being that the risk of sudden or subtle incapacitation does not exceed that appropriate to the age of the individual. As we learn more about the long-term outcomes of these conditions it is increasingly possible to make certificatory recommendations that are both safe and fair, although an individual may not remain fit for a conventional career span. At present only those who have a normal, or almost normal, event-free outlook with or without surgery can be considered. Many forms of congenital heart disease are not consistent with flying status and cardiological review with appropriate, usually non-invasive, investigation and follow-up is mandatory in those accepted.

Atrial septal defect

Atrial septal defect is one of the most common congenital anomalies of the heart accounting for one-quarter of all.

Three-quarters are ostium secundum defects, one-fifth are ostium primum defects and one in 20 are sinus venosus defects. The life expectancy with all but small (pulmonary/systemic flow ratio $< 1.5 : 1$) uncorrected secundum defects is not normal with an increasing risk of atrial rhythm disturbances, including flutter and fibrillation, from the fourth decade and the eventual onset of right-sided heart failure in the sixth and seventh decades. Early (age < 24 years) closure of the defect carries a very low operative mortality and normal life expectancy, but later closure is associated with a poorer outcome – increasingly poor as the age of intervention rises – due to atrial fibrillation, thromboembolism and the onset of right heart failure. The use of clam-shell and angel-wing devices is accepted and may encourage the closure of smaller defects although long-term outcome data are not yet available. Small or early-corrected secundum defects are consistent with unrestricted certification, subject to occasional review. Any departure from this requirement implies restriction or denial.

Ostium primum defects present additional problems to those outlined above because the mitral valve and conducting system may be involved. Such involvement significantly worsens the outcome and applicants with this condition can be considered only for restricted certification. Regular review is required. Mitral regurgitation should be minimal and there should be no significant disturbance of rhythm or conduction. Sinus venosus defects bear the problem that significant rhythm disturbances are frequent both before and after correction. These need to be excluded before certification can be considered. Life-long periodic ambulatory ECG monitoring is required.

Ventricular septal defect

Isolated ventricular septal defect accounts for about one-third of congenital heart defects. Small (pulmonary/systemic flow ratio $< 1.5 : 1$) defects either close spontaneously or remain stable lifelong. There is no increased risk of sudden or subtle incapacitation, although there is a small risk of endocarditis and appropriate measures should be taken for its prophylaxis. Such candidates should be fit for unrestricted certification. Closure in childhood likewise carries a good outcome – five per cent mortality at 25 years (Morris and Menashe 1991), but larger defects that have undergone closure do not appear to have a normal life expectancy with an 82 per cent 30-year survival compared with 97 per cent in age-matched controls (Murphy *et al.* 1989). Age at surgery and the presence of pulmonary vascular change are predictors of survival. Applicants with such defects should undergo full cardiological review and may not be certifiable.

Pulmonary stenosis

Pulmonary valvular stenosis accounts for one in ten subjects with congenital heart disease. Stenosis of the infundibulum of the right ventricle and of the supravalvular region are much less common. The former may be present as a fibro-muscular ring or as concentric hypertrophy in an otherwise normal heart with an intact interventricular septum. Valvular stenosis may also be present. Supravalvular stenosis may be associated with multiple stenosis of the pulmonary trunk and its branches.

Mild degrees of pulmonary valvular stenosis (< 30 mmHg) are consistent with unrestricted certification. Following surgery, 25-year survival is five per cent – not quite normal – but discretion may be exercised in 'best-risk' subjects, judged by non-invasive and invasive means (Morris and Menashe 1991). Supravalvular stenosis is likely to disbar from all forms of certification to fly.

Aortic stenosis

Aortic stenosis has been reviewed above. Abnormalities of the aortic valve or the aortic outflow tract requiring surgery in childhood carry a relatively poor prognosis, the 25-year mortality being 17 per cent (Morris and Menashe 1991). Nevertheless, in one small study there were no late deaths in the 16-year period following resection of isolated discrete subaortic stenosis. This condition is unlikely to be acceptable for certification to fly.

Coarctation of the aorta

Coarctation of the aorta may be diagnosed in childhood or the diagnosis may be delayed until later years. In terms of outcome the difference is significant. In about one-third of patients a bicuspid aortic valve will also be present. Early intervention is important (Cohen *et al.* 1989). The 20-year survival of patients aged 14 years or younger at the time of operation was 91 per cent compared with an 84 per cent survival of those in whom surgery was delayed. The best outcome was in those operated on under the age of nine years. Age at operation predicted subsequent hypertension which was also associated with an increased risk of sudden death, myocardial infarction, stroke and aortic dissection.

Unrestricted certification can be considered in normotensive subjects who underwent correction of the anomaly below the age of 12–14 years. Continuous subsequent review is required to monitor the blood pressure. Echocardiographic follow-up should be determined by the presence or absence of a bicuspid aortic valve. Ascending aortic dilation should deny certification. Treated hypertension following late closure should deny unrestricted certification.

Tetralogy of Fallot

The tetralogy of Fallot – ventricular septal defect, pulmonary stenosis (which protects the pulmonary circulation), overriding aorta and right ventricular hypertrophy – is classically the only cyanotic congenital heart condition that is consistent with survival into adult life. Such survivors do not have a normal life expectancy and late closure (> 12 years) carries a less favourable outlook than early closure. In one study, the 32-year actuarial survival was 86 per cent overall compared with 96 per cent for an age- and sex-matched control population (Murphy *et al.* 1993); for patients operated on before the age of 12 years, the figure was 92 per cent – still not normal. An increased frequency of complex rhythm disturbances has been noted (Cullen *et al.* 1994) as has a higher than expected incidence of late SCD. The former do not appear to predict the latter reliably. In one study, the 25 year mortality was five per cent higher than predicted.

It is possible that in early years (< 40 years of age), the best-risks subjects can be considered for unrestricted certification but our present inability to identify later risk indicates that the tetralogy of Fallot is incompatible with unrestricted certification in the long term. Initial unrestricted certification should be confined to people operated on before the age of 12 years who have no evidence of residual right ventricular hypertrophy, significant pulmonary regurgitation or complex ventricular rhythm disturbance, subject to regular monitoring by a cardiologist.

Patent ductus arteriosus

Patent ductus arteriosus is usually recognized early in life and closed surgically. In one review, the 25-year mortality was less than one per cent, with no late deaths. There is an association with bicuspid aortic valve, subaortic stenosis, pulmonary stenosis and aortic root disease. In the absence of such complications, an applicant should be able to expect unrestricted certification. Complicating pathology requires further consideration and review.

Many congenital heart conditions are now consistent with long-term survival. Only those with the most favourable outcomes will be acceptable but as new data become available the certificatory position will require further updating.

DISEASE OF THE GREAT VESSELS

Aortic aneurysm describes dilation of the aorta. In one-sixth of cases this will involve more than one segment. Most commonly involving the abdomen, one-quarter of subjects with a thoracic aneurysm will also have involvement of the ascending segment. The condition is four times more common in men > age of 55 years than in women, the prevalence in this age group being three per cent (Pressler and McNamara 1985). Increasing age, atheromatous degeneration of the wall, hypertension and familial factors are all involved in the pathogenesis of abdominal aortic aneurysm. Aneurysms < 4.0 cm in size have a two-year risk of rupture of < two per cent, but with aneurysms > 5 cm in size the risk is 22 per cent. One, five- and ten-year survival rates following surgical repair in one large series were 93, 63 and 40 per cent respectively in an older mean age group than the pilot population, attrition being due to concomitant vascular complications. In another study, 5-, 10- and 15-year survival was 71, 38 and 16 per cent respectively in the absence of coronary artery disease in a population with a mean age of 69.8 years (Mukai *et al.* 2002). Coexistent coronary artery disease reduced survival further. Hypertension significantly impairs outcome both before and after treatment.

Thoracic aneurysms show less age-related increase in incidence, the descending, ascending and arch portions being involved in that order. Aneurysm of the ascending aorta most frequently shows cystic median degeneration with increasing prevalence of atheromatous disease further down. Occasional causes are giant-cell arteritis and syphilis. In younger patients, the inherited disorders of collagen will be more important. As with abdominal aneurysms, a luminal diameter > 5.0 cm is associated with a significantly increased risk of rupture. Surgery carries a five to ten per cent mortality and significant morbidity.

Marfan's syndrome

Marfan's syndrome is transmitted as a dominant gene with variable expression. It is one of several conditions marked by an inherited abnormality of the extracellular matrix, including the Ehlers–Danlos syndrome. It is a mutant form in about a sixth of cases. Its prevalence in the population may be as high as one per 10 000. At times its variability makes it difficult to diagnose with confidence although the causative gene has now been identified. In a report from the Cleveland Clinic males outnumbered females by a ratio of two to one. Three-fifths and two-fifths, respectively had a diastolic murmur and/or cardiomegaly on presentation; follow-up was a mean of 99 months. Thirty-one of the 81 patients died at a mean age of 35 (range 3–63) years, 87 per cent from cardiovascular cause. Even after surgery the survival is not good – 75 per cent at five years and 56 per cent at ten years (Svennson *et al.* 1989). Survival following surgery for non-Marfan cystic median necrosis of the aorta is equally bleak, at 57 per cent at five years (Marsalese *et al.* 1990). Increased ascending aortic diameter predicts the onset of aortic regurgitation but less reliably of dissection.

Pilots in whom the diagnosis of aortic aneurysm has been queried require evaluation with transthoracic echocardiography MRI/magnetic resonance angiography (MRA) and, if indicated, aortography. A luminal diameter > 4.0 cm but < 5.0 cm should lead to restriction of the class 1 certificate, whilst a diameter > 5.0 cm should lead to denial. Regular follow-up is mandatory, with careful control of the blood pressure. In view of the relatively poor outcome of patients with aortic aneurysm after surgery, only the best risk subjects in whom coronary artery disease has been excluded may be considered for restricted certification. In applicants with a forme fruste of Marfan's syndrome and in whom the echocardiographic dimensions of the heart and great vessels remain within the normal range. Any valvular regurgitation, whether aortic or mitral, should be minimal before restricted certification may be considered subject to indefinite subsequent review.

PERIPHERAL VASCULAR DISEASE

Peripheral vascular disease powerfully predicts the presence of a generalized arteriopathy that is likely to involve the coronary and cerebral circulations. The discovery of absent (lower) limb pulses, with or without symptoms suggestive of intermittent claudication, should always provoke full cardiovascular review. In 84 consecutive patients with peripheral vascular disease but no cardiac symptoms followed for a mean of 66 months, more than two-thirds had significant coronary artery disease on angiography and their mean left ventricular ejection fraction was reduced at 44 per cent (Darbar et al. 1996). There were 23 events in the follow-up period. Dipyridamole thallium scintigraphy was a significant predictor of outcome. In general terms, the younger the age of onset, the worse the outcome; the presence of peripheral vascular disease following coronary artery surgery is associated with a significantly higher mortality. On account of the co-morbid risk of a coronary event associated with peripheral vascular disease all such applicants should at least undergo pharmacological stress thallium scintigraphy. If abnormal, certification should be denied unless a subsequent coronary angiogram satisfies the standard requirements for minor coronary artery disease (see above). Indefinite supervision is required, with likely limitation of the licence.

VENOUS THROMBOSIS

A number of factors predispose to deep venous thrombosis, with consequent risk of pulmonary embolism. This is covered in detail in Chapter 43.

Pulmonary embolism

Pulmonary embolism is an important complication of deep venous thrombosis and is now often investigated by spiral computed tomography (CT) scanning. This procedure has taken over from ventilation/perfusion (V/Q) scanning. Pulmonary angiography may be performed if the pulmonary artery pressure is also to be measured. It is essential to secure the diagnosis in view of the risk of recurrence although this is low in the absence of a risk factor.

Warfarin is the mainstay of treatment. At present, it disbars from any form of certification in Europe, due to the cumulative risk of haemorrhage. A new direct thrombin inhibitor, ximelagatran, is under trial. This does not require follow-up of the prothrombin time and may have a lower rate of haemorrhagic complication (see atrial fibrillation, p. 581).

Following pulmonary embolus the pulmonary artery pressure must be shown to be normal before a return to flying can be considered. Good Doppler signals may enable a non-invasive assessment of the tricuspid valve regurgitant velocity and thereby assessment of the pulmonary peak systolic pressure; if not, right heart catheterization will be required. As a period of six months is usually recommended for treatment with warfarin following such event, fitness cannot be restored during this time. Pulmonary hypertension (systolic pressure > 30 mmHg), whether primary or secondary, should disbar from all forms of certification to fly.

SYNCOPE

Syncope may be defined as transient loss of consciousness, usually associated with falling. The mechanism is global cerebral hypoperfusion due to a number of causes. As a rule recovery is spontaneous and complete, however, although recovery is usually rapid, full return of intellectual function may be delayed. Depending on cause, syncope may be abrupt and without warning, or there may be a prodrome (presyncope) of variable length with symptoms such as nausea, weakness, lightheadedness and visual disturbance. Retrograde amnesia occurs in some, particularly older, individuals. Recovery, although somewhat subjective, may be rapid (seconds/minutes) as in the case of an Adams–Stokes attack (i.e. transient complete atrioventricular block), or prolonged sometimes, in vasovagal syncope. If the attack is complicated by an anoxic epileptic seizure, then recovery will inevitably be delayed further (Brignole et al. 2001).

Differential diagnosis of syncope due to circulatory cause

- Neurocardiogenic syncope is triggered by a variety of circumstances, including nausea and gastrointestinal disturbance, and is associated with systemic hypotension and cerebral hypoperfusion. It may be associated with either bradycardia or tachycardia.
- Orthostatic hypotension may be caused by blood loss or impairment of autonomic regulation from a number of causes. It occurs in severe left (or right) ventricular dysfunction. It is a common transient experience in normotensive subjects on gaining the erect position.
- Structural heart disease exemplified by valvar aortic stenosis (or subaortic stenosis as in some forms of hypertrophic cardiomyopathy), if severe, is associated with syncope. More than one mechanism is involved.
- Cardiac arrhythmias including supraventricular and ventricular tachycardias and sino-atrial or atrioventricular conduction disorders may be complicated by syncope.
- The 'steal' syndromes in which there is competitive demand for cerebral perfusion are rarely seen in the pilot population.

Consciousness may also be impaired or lost due to hypoglycaemia, hypoxia, hyperventilation, somatization disorders and epilepsy.

Vasovagal (neurocardiogenic) syncope

Vasovagal (neurocardiogenic) syncope or the common faint was described over 200 years ago and is the mechanism of what used to be known, in classical literature, as the 'drawing-room swoon'. It is a common phenomenon – it has been suggested that between one-third and two-thirds of the population experience an attack at least once during their lifetime. The attacks are sporadic and often cluster; and the population is heterogeneous. It often presents in teenage years and then disappears, reappearing later in life sometimes as clusters of episodes. It contributes to at least 40 per cent of the syncopal events seen in the outpatient setting. It is difficult to manage partly because the triggering mechanisms, even after having been investigated extensively, are imperfectly understood (Fenton *et al.* 2000).

The regulation of the circulation involves a number of interacting reflexes. Initially baroreflex mechanisms are activated to counteract the effect of gravity on the venous blood pool. The renin–angiotensin–aldosterone axis is also involved, both interacting with the autonomic nervous system and influencing salt and water metabolism. Adequate blood pressure is needed to maintain the blood supply to the vital organs, including the brain, kidneys and gut. If it falls beyond a certain point cerebral auto-regulation fails and the subject loses consciousness. With an abrupt fall in blood pressure this occurs very rapidly – within five to ten seconds. Provided the pressure is restored rapidly (often brought about by the patient falling to the ground), recovery of consciousness ensues but, depending on the provocative circumstances, a minimum period of some 30 minutes is required for effective recovery. This can be prolonged considerably if there is recurrence of the syncopal episode, if the provocative circumstance is ongoing, e.g. in the case of nausea or vomiting, or if the period of hypotension was sufficiently prolonged for cerebral anoxia to provoke epileptic seizure. Twitching movements during the period of unconsciousness are common and should not be confused with epileptic seizure.

Maintenance of the systemic blood pressure requires adequate circulating blood volume, sufficient peripheral arteriolar tone in the 'resistance' vessels, proper regulation of the 'capacitance' vessels (which contain 70 per cent of the circulating blood volume), and regulation of the inotropic and chronotropic state of the heart. In vasovagal syncope these interacting mechanisms go awry but the causes are controversial and ill understood. All patients experience a profound fall in the blood pressure with ensuing impairment of consciousness; in some there is a profound bradycardia but in others there is a tachycardia. This paradox involves loss of regulation of venous tone (and return of circulating blood to the heart) and inadequate arteriolar tone.

The symptoms of vasovagal syncope include a prodromal syndrome of variable duration with light-headedness, weakness, a sensation of air hunger or hyperventilation, detachment from surroundings, palpitations, blurring of vision and field disturbance, nausea, dizziness and eventually syncope. Malignant syncope is characterized by little or no warning and injury may result. Another definition of the malignant form relates to the period of asystole during tilt testing. Depending on the circumstances, recovery may be prolonged by repeated episodes of hypotension followed by partial recovery of consciousness. Recovery invariably takes place but the symptoms can persist for hours. Patients with the condition have a normal life expectancy unless the incident causes hazard, e.g. when driving or flying.

Provocative factors in vasovagal syncope are several although some of the features may form part of the syndrome. Specifically, nausea, vomiting, a sensation of abdominal churning, diarrhoea, an awareness of warmth, heat or coldness, and sweatiness are common. Other input may come from fatigue, emotional disturbance or anxiety, circadian stress, dehydration, pain or visual stimuli, such as the sight of a needle. Sometimes cause and effect can be blurred. A glass of wine on an empty stomach in a susceptible individual may have the same effect. As up to one-third of aircrew may experience incapacitation at some time in their career, in 60 per cent of cases due to gastroenteritis, the likelihood of such an event in a susceptible individual is significant.

Investigation of vasovagal syncope is based on a characteristic history and a positive tilt test. All other investigations, such as resting, exercise and 24-hour (Holter) ECG and echocardiography, should be normal, as should the electroencephalogram (EEG) and brain CT/MRI scan. The head-up tilt test, in which the subject is raised from the supine position to an angle of 60 degrees for 45 minutes, is the investigation of choice. In the most severely affected individuals, the test is almost 100 per cent sensitive; in others, it is about 70 per cent sensitive with provocation with nitroglycerine. The false-positive rate is about 13 per cent, rising to 20 per cent with nitroglycerine. The reproducibility of the test is in the range of 70–80 per cent, but a negative test cannot be taken as an assumption that the diagnosis in incorrect or that the condition has improved.

The treatment of vasovagal syncope is unsatisfactory due partly to its sporadic appearance, often with long intervals between attacks. Drug therapy e.g. with beta-blocking agents, has to be taken continuously, and the results are disappointing. Few convincing trials have been carried out. Endocardial pacemaking is helpful in a few cases. Subjects with the syndrome have a normal life expectancy unless syncope causes some accident, such as falling under a vehicle, or occurs while driving a vehicle or flying as the single crew member in a light aircraft. This has been recorded in the UK. Intervention is for symptoms alone, as it has no effect on prognosis.

The certification of subjects with vasovagal syncope in the aviation environment is problematic, as it is a potential cause of sudden, total or subtle incapacitation. The Second European Workshop concluded that whereas a single syncopal episode would be likely to be followed by a recertification with certain safeguards (following a negative tilt test), 'a history of repetitive, or clustered attacks would be likely to disbar'. This was based on the unpredictability of the episodes, their tendency to cluster, their variable symptomatology and the undesirability of an aviator being incapacitated for an uncertain length of time. The aviation environment is one that is marked by fatigue due to disrupted sleep, circadian stress, at times warm temperatures and humidity in places that are visited. There is also a significant risk of gastroenteritis which may provoke an episode in a vulnerable individual. Malignant and recurrent vasovagal syncope should disbar (Sutton 1999).

Following a single episode of unexplained (but possibly vasovagal) syncope, full cardiological assessment is required together with neurological review. A demonstrable cause due to structural abnormality of the heart will disbar. Following an interval, arbitrarily six months, restricted certification may be permitted with full certification no sooner than five years provided there has been

no recurrence. Aircrew in whom the diagnosis has been made need to be counselled about the condition and told when attacks are likely to occur.

REFERENCES

ALLHAT Collaborative Research Group. Major outcomes in moderately hypercholesterolemic, hypertensive patients randomized to pravastatin vs usual care. *Journal of the American Medical Association* 2002: **288**: 2998–3007.

American College of Cardiology. 1st Bethesda Conference. Standards of fitness of aircrew. *American Journal of Cardiology* 1966; **18**: 630–36.

American College of Cardiology. 8th Bethesda Conference. Cardiovascular problems associated with aviation safety. *American Journal of Cardiology* 1975; **36**: 573–620.

Brignole M, Alboni P, Benditt D, *ct al.* Guidelines on management (diagnosis and treatment) of syncope. Task force on Syncope, European Society of Cardiology. *European Heart Journal* 2001; **22**: 1256–306.

Broustet, JP, Douard H, Oysel N, Rougier P, Koch M. What is the predictive value of exercise electrocardiography in the investigation of male aircrew aged 40-60 years old? *European Heart Journal* 1991; **13** (suppl. H): 59–69.

Brown KA. Prognostic value of thallium-201 myocardial perfusion imaging: a diagnostic tool comes of age. *Circulation* 1991; **83**: 363–81.

Bruce RA, Fisher LD. Exercise enhanced assessment of risk factors for coronary heart disease in healthy men. *Journal of Electrocardiology* 1987; **20** (suppl. 1): 162–6.

Bruschke AVG, Proudfit NL, Sones FM. Progress study of five hundred and ninety consecutive non-surgical cases of coronary artery disease followed 5–9 years. I. Arteriographic correlations. *Circulation* 1972; **47**: 114–53.

Bypass Angioplasty Revascularization Investigation (BARI). Comparison of coronary bypass surgery with angioplasty in patients with multi-vessel disease. *New England Journal of Medicine* 1996; **335**: 217–25.

CABRI. First-year results of CABRI (Coronary Angioplasty versus Bypass Revascularization Investigation). *Lancet* 1995; **346**: 1179–84.

Campbell RWF. Ventricular rhythm disturbances in the normal heart. *European Heart Journal* 1992; **13** (suppl. H): 139–43.

Cardiology Committee of the Royal College of Physicians of London. Report of the Working Party of the Cardiology Committee of the Royal College of Physicians of London. Cardiovascular fitness of airline pilots. *British Heart Journal* 1978; **40**: 335–50.

Chaitman BK, Davis KB, Dodge HT, *et al.* Should airline pilots be eligible to resume flight status after coronary artery bypass surgery? A CASS registry study. *Journal of the American College of Cardiologists* 1986; **8**: 1318–24.

Cohen M, Fuster V, Steele PM, *et al.* Coarctation of the aorta: long-term follow-up and prediction of outcome after surgical correction. *Circulation* 1989; **80**: 840–45.

Cullen SE, Celermajer DS, Franklin RC, *et al.* Prognostic significance of ventricular arrhythmias after repair of tetralogy of Fallot: a 12 year prospective study. *Journal of the American College of Cardiologists* 1994; **23** 1151–5.

Darbar D, Gillespie N, Main G, *et al*. Prediction of late cardiac events by dipyridamole thallium scintigraphy in patients with intermittent claudication and occult coronary artery disease. *American Journal of Cardiology* 1996; **78**: 736–40.

De Backer G, Ambrosioni E, Borch JK, *et al*. European guidelines on cardiovascular disease prevention in clinical practice. Third Joint Task Force of European and Other Societies on Cardiovascular Disease Prevention in Clinical Practice. *European Journal of Cardiovascular Prevention and Rehabilitation* 2003; **10**: S1–10.

Department of Trade and Industry. Trident 1 G-ARPI. Civil Aircraft Accident Report, 4-73. London: HMSO, 1973.

Downs JR, Clearfield M, Weis S, *et al*. Primary prevention of acute coronary events with lovastatin in men and women with average cholesterol levels: results of AFCAPS/TexCAPS. *Journal of the American Medical Association* 1998; **279**: 1615–22.

Doyle JT, Kannel WB, McNamarra PM, *et al*. Factors relating to suddenness of death from coronary disease: combined Albany–Framingham studies. *American Journal of Cardiology* 1976; **37**: 1073–8.

Dubach P, Froelicher VF, Klein J, Detrano R. Use of the exercise test to predict prognosis after coronary artery bypass grafting. *American Journal of Cardiology* 1989; **63**: 530–33.

European Atrial Fibrillation Consensus Conference. What is known, what is currently accepted, and what needs to be proven in atrial fibrillation? *European Heart Journal* 2003; **5** (suppl.): H1–55.

Evans SE, Cooke JNC. Cardiac effects of anthracycline treatment and their implications for aeromedical certification. *Aviation, Space, and Environmental Medicine* 2003; **74**: 1003–8.

Fenton A, Hammill SC, Rea R, *et al*. Vasovagal syncope. *Annals of Internal Medicine* 2000; **133**: 714–25.

Fitzsimmons PJ, McWhirter PD, Peterson DW, Kruyer WB. The natural history of Wolff–Parkinson–White syndrome in 228 military aviators: a long-term follow-up of 22 years. *American Heart Journal* 2001; **142**: 530–36.

Fleming HA. Cardiac sarcoidosis. In: James DG (ed.). *Sarcoidosis and the Granulomatous Disorders*, Vol. 73. New York: Marcel Decker, 1994; p. 323.

Gibbons RJ, Balady GJ, Beasley JW, *et al*. ACC/AHA guidelines for exercise testing: a report of the American College of Cardiology/American Heart Association Task Force on Practice Guidelines (Committee on Exercise Testing). *Journal of the American College of Cardiology* 1997; **30**: 260–315.

Hachamovitch R, Hayes S, Friedman JD, *et al*. Determinants of risk and its temporal variation in patients with normal stress myocardial perfusion scans: what is the warranty period of a normal scan? *Journal of the American College of Cardiologists* 2003; **41**: 1329–40.

Heart Protection Study Collaborative Group. MRC/BHF Heart Protection Study of cholesterol lowering with simvastatin in 20,536 high-risk individuals: a randomised placebo-controlled trial. *Lancet* 2002; **360**: 7–22.

Hickman JR, Tolan GD, Gray GW, Hull DH. Clinical aerospace cardiovascular and pulmonary medicine. In: DeHart RL (ed.). *Fundamentals of Aerospace Medicine*, 2nd edn. Baltimore: Williams & Wilkins, 1996; pp. 463–518.

Hilla RA, Dundara Y, Bakhaib A, Dicksona R Walleya T. Drug-eluting stents: an early systematic review to inform policy. *European Heart Journal* 2004; **25**: 902–19.

Hiss RG, Lamb LE. Electrocardiographic findings in 122,043 individuals. *Circulation* 1962; **25**: 947–83.

Imamura H, Nishiyama S, Nakanishi S, Seki A. Influence of residual antegrade coronary blood flow on the long term prognosis of medically treated patients with myocardial infarction and single vessel disease. *Japanese Heart Journal* 1997; **38**: 27–38.

International Civil Aviation Organization. International Standards and Recommended Practices (ISARPSs). Personnel Licensing. Annex 1 to the Convention on International Civil Aviation. Montreal: International Civil Aviation Organization, 2001.

Iskandrian AS, Chae SC, Heo J, *et al*. Independent and incremental prognostic value of exercise single photon computed tomographic (SPECT) thallium imaging in coronary artery disease. *Journal of the American College of Cardiologists* 1993; **22**: 665–70.

Joint Aviation Authorities. Joint Aviation Requirements FCL Part 3 Medical. Hooddorp: Joint Aviation Authorities, 1998.

Joy M. Cardiovascular fitness to fly and to drive: an interface between cardiology and some statutory fitness requirements. In: Julian DG, Camm AJ, Fox KM, Hall RJC, Poole-Wilson PA (eds). *Diseases of the Heart*. London: Baillière-Tindall, 1989; pp. 1574–606.

Joy M (ed.). The first European Workshop in Aviation Cardiology. *European Heart Journal* 1992; **13**: (suppl. H): 1–175.

Joy M. Vocational aspects of coronary artery disease. In: Weatherall DJ, Ledingham JGG, Worrell DA (eds). *Oxford Textbook of Medicine*, 3rd edn. Oxford: Oxford University Press, 1996; pp. 2356-62.

Joy M (ed.). The second European Workshop in Aviation Cardiology. *European Heart Journal* 1999; suppls. D: 1–D136.

Joy M. Certificatory aspects of the long QT syndrome (LQTS) in the UK: a 10 year perspective. *Aviation, Space, and Environmental Medicine* 2004; **75**; B92.

Joy M, Bennett G (eds). The first United Kingdom Workshop in Aviation Cardiology. *European Heart Journal* 1984; **5** (suppl. A): 1-164.

Joy M, Bennett G (eds). The second United Kingdom Workshop in Aviation Cardiology. *European Heart Journal* 1988; **9** (suppl. G): 1–179.

Joy M, Broustet J-P. Cardiovascular fitness to fly and drive: the interface between cardiology and statutory fitness requirements. In: Julian DG, Camm AJ, Fox KM, Hall RJC, Poole-Wilson PA (eds). *Diseases of the Heart*, 2nd edn. London: Baillière-Tindall, 1996; pp. 1517-33.

Joy M, Trump DW. Significance of minor ST-segment and T wave changes in the resting electrocardiogram of asymptomatic subjects. *British Heart Journal* 1981; **45**: 48–55.

Kannel WB, Feinleib M, Dawber TR. The unrecognised myocardial infarction: fourteen year follow up experience in the Framingham study. *Geriatrics* 1970; **25**: 75–87.

Kasper EK, Agema WRP, Hutchins GM, *et al*. The causes of dilated cardiomyopathy: a clinicopathologic review of 673 consecutive patients. *Journal of the American College of Cardiologists* 1996; **23**: 586–90.

Kwok Y, Kim C, Grady D, *et al*. Meta-analysis of exercise testing to detect coronary artery disease in women. *American Journal of Cardiology* 1999; **83**: 660–66.

Legrand V, Raskinet, B, Laarman G, *et al*. Diagnostic value of exercise electrocardiography and angina after coronary artery stenting. Benestent Study Group. *American Heart Journal* 1997; **133**: 240–48.

Long-Term Intervention with Pravastatin Group in Ischaemic Disease (LIPID) Study Group. Prevention of cardiovascular events and death with pravastatin in patients with coronary heart disease and a broad range of initial cholesterol levels. *New England Journal of Medicine* 1998; **339**: 1349–57.

Loop FD, Little VW, Cosgrove DM, *et al.* Influence of the mammary artery graft on ten year survival and other cardiac events. *New England Journal of Medicine* 1986; **314**: 1–6.

Mark DB, Shaw L, Howe FE, *et al.* Prognostic value of a treadmill exercise score in outpatients with suspected coronary artery disease. *New England Journal of Medicine* 1991; **325**: 849–53.

Marsalese DL, Moodie DS, Lytle BW, *et al.* Cystic medial necrosis of the aorta in patients without Marfan's syndrome: surgical outcome and long-term follow up. *Journal of the American College of Cardiologists* 1990; **16**: 68–73.

McHenry PL, O'Donnell J, Morris SN, Jordan JJ. The abnormal exercise electrocardiogram in apparently healthy men: a predictor of angina pectoris as an initial coronary event during long term follow up. *Circulation* 1984; **70**: 547–51.

McKenna WJ, Behr EB. Hypertrophic cardiomyopathy: management, risk stratification, and prevention of sudden death. *Heart* 2002; **87**: 169–76.

Mitchell SJ, Evans AD. Flight safety and medical incapacitation risk of airline pilots. *Aviation, Space, and Environmental Medicine* 2004; **75**: 260-68.

Morise AP. Are the American College of Cardiology/American Heart Association guidelines for exercise testing for suspected coronary artery disease correct? *Chest* 2000; **118**: 535–41.

Morris CD, Menashe VD. 25-year mortality after surgical repair of congenital heart defect in childhood: a population-based cohort study. *Journal of the American Medical Association* 1991; **266**: 3447–52.

Mukai S, Yao H, Miyamoto M, *et al.* The long-term follow up results of elective surgical treatment for abdominal aortic aneurysm. *Annals of Thoracic and Cardiovascular Surgery* 2002; **8**: 39–41.

Murphy JG, Gersh BJ, Warnes CA. The late survival after surgical repair of isolated ventricular septal defect (VSD). *Circulation* 1989; **80** (suppl. II): 1–490.

Murphy JG, Gersh BJ, Mair DD, *et al.* Long-term outcome in patients undergoing surgical repair of tetralogy of Fallot. *New England Journal of Medicine* 1993; **329**: 593–9.

O'Rourke RA, Brundage BA, Froelicher VF, *et al.* American College of Cardiology/American Heart Association expert consensus document on electron-beam computed tomography for the diagnosis and prognosis of coronary artery disease. *Journal of the American College of Cardiologists* 2000; **36**: 326–40.

Parker DJ. Long term morbidity and mortality after aortic and mitral valve replacement with tissue valves and certification to fly. *European Heart Journal* 1988; **9** (suppl. G): 153–7.

Patel CRK, Bhopal RS. *The Epidemic of Coronary Heart Disease in South Asian Populations: Causes and Consequences.* Birmingham: South Asian Health Foundation, 2003.

Pedersen TR. Randomised trial of cholesterol lowering in 4444 patients with coronary heart disease; the Scandinavian Simvastatin Survival Study. *Lancet* 1994; **344**: 1383–9.

Perier P, Stumpf J, Gotz C, *et al.* Valve repair for mitral regurgitation caused by isolated prolapse of the posterior leaflet. *Annals of Thoracic Surgery* 1997; **64**: 445–50.

Perrier EH, Doireau P, Carlioz R, *et al.* Typical Brugada-type EKG issued of an aeronautical population: epidemiological data, clinical and aero-medical concerns. *Aviation, Space, and Environmental Medicine* 2003; **74**: 390.

Petersen S, Peto V, Rayner M. *Coronary Heart Disease Statistics.* London: British Heart Foundation, 2003.

Pitt B, Waters D, Brown WV, *et al.* Aggressive lipid-lowering therapy compared with angioplasty in stable coronary artery disease. *New England Journal of Medicine* 1999; **341**: 70–76.

Pocock SJ, Henderson RA, Rickards AF, *et al.* Meta-analysis of randomized trials comparing coronary angioplasty with bypass surgery. *Lancet* 1995; **346**: 1184–9.

Postma A, Bink-Boelkens MT, Beaufort-Krol GC, *et al.* Late cardiotoxicity after treatment for a malignant bone tumour. *Medical and Pediatric Oncology* 1996; **26**: 230–37.

Pressler V, McNamara JJ. Aneurysm of the thoracic aorta: review of 260 cases. *Journal of Thoracic and Cardiovascular Surgery* 1985; **89**: 50–58.

Priori SG, Aliot E, Blomstrom-Lundqvist C. Task Force on Sudden Cardiac Death: the European Society of Cardiology. *European Heart Journal* 2001; **22**: 1374–450.

Priori SG, Schwartz CN, Napolitano C, *et al.* Risk stratification in the long QT syndrome. *New England Journal of Medicine* 2003; **348**: 1866–74.

Rabkin SW, Mathewson FAL, Tate RB. Natural history of left bundle branch block. *British Heart Journal* 1980; **43**: 164–9.

Rahimtoola SH. Choice of prosthetic heart valve for adult patients. *Journal of the American College of Cardiologists* 2003; **41**: 894–904.

Serruys PW, Unger F, Sousa JE, *et al.* Comparison of coronary-artery bypass surgery and stenting for the treatment of multi-vessel disease. *New England Journal of Medicine* 2001; **344**: 1117–24.

Sever PS, Dahlöf B, Poulter NP, *et al.* Prevention of coronary and stroke events with atorvostatin in hypertensive patients who have average or lower-than-average cholesterol concentrations, in the Anglo Scandinavian Cardiac Outcomes Trial – Lipid Lowering Arm (ASCOT-LLA): a multi-centre randomized controlled trial. *Lancet* 2003; **361**: 1149–58.

Steinherz LJ, Steinherz PG, Tan CTC. Cardiac failure and dysrhythmia 9–16 years after anthracycline therapy: a series of 15 patients. *Medical and Pediatric Oncology* 1995; **24**: 352–61.

Svennson LG, Crawford ES, Coselli JS, *et al.* Impact of cardiovascular operation on survival in the Marfan patient. *Circulation* 1989; **80**: 1233–42.

Sutton R. Vasovagal syncope: prevalence and presentation. *European Heart Journal* 1999; (suppls): D109–13.

Toff WD, Camm AJ. Ventricular pre-excitation and professional aircrew licensing. *European Heart Journal* 1992; **13** (suppl. H): 149–61.

Totaro P, Tulumello E, Fellini O, *et al.* Mitral valve repair for isolated prolapse of the anterior leaflet: an 11-year follow up. *European Journal of Cardiothoracic Surgery* 1999; **15**: 119–26.

Tunstall-Pedoe H. Risk of a coronary heart attack in the normal population and how it might be modified in flyers. *European Heart Journal* 1984; **5** (suppl. A): 43–9.

Verheugt FWA, Antman EM. Anticoagulation in cardiac disease: new data – new options. *European Heart Journal* 2004; **6** (suppl.): B1–B26.

Webb-Peploe MM. Obliterative and restrictive cardiomyopathies. *European Heart Journal* 1988; **9** (suppl. G): 159–67.

Webb-Peploe MM. Mitral leaflet prolapse: aspects of fitness to fly. *European Heart Journal* 1992; **13** (suppl. H): 117–29.

West of Scotland Coronary Prevention Study Group. Prevention of coronary heart disease with pravastatin in men with hypercholesterolaemia. *New England Journal of Medicine* 1995; **333**: 1301–7.

Wilde AAM, Antzelevitch C, Borggrefe M, *et al.* Proposed diagnostic criteria for the Brugada syndrome. *European Heart Journal* 2002; **23**: 1648–54.

Xhang L, Timothy KW, Vincent GM, *et al.* Spectrum of ST-T-wave patterns and repolarization parameters in congenital long QT syndrome: ECG finding identify genotypes. *Circulation* 2000; **102**: 2849–55.

Yap Y, Duong T, Bland M, *et al.* Left ventricular ejection fraction in the thrombolytic era remains a powerful predictor of long-term but not short-term all-cause, cardiac and arrhythmic mortality after myocardial infarction: a secondary meta-analysis of 2,828 patients. *Heart* 2000; **83**: 55–60.

Zarr SP, Pickard J, Besich WJ, Thompson BT, Kruyer WB. Normal coronary angiography versus luminal irregularity only: is there a difference? *Aviation, Space, and Environmental Medicine* 2004; **75**: B91–2.

APPENDIX 37.1 ILLUSTRATIVE ELECTROCARDIOGRAMS

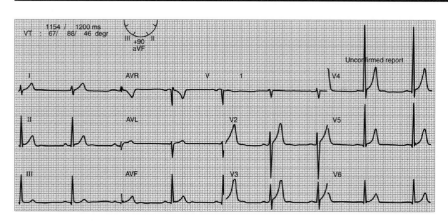

Figure A37.1 *Normal ECG of a 28-year-old pilot applying for class 1 status. The mean frontal axis is +90° (R and S waves are equal in S1). There is a sinus bradycardia, and the large voltages in the chest leads are normal in a slim individual.*

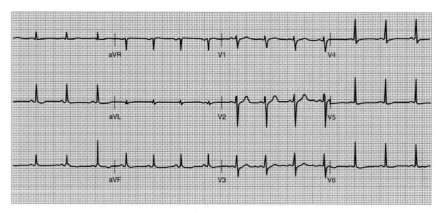

Figure A37.2 *ECG of a 29-year-old first officer, showing diffuse T-wave flattening. This is common in younger subjects and may be provoked by anxiety and/or hyperventilation. The exercise response will not be ischaemic, although sometimes it shows innocent repolarization anomalies. No restriction is needed.*

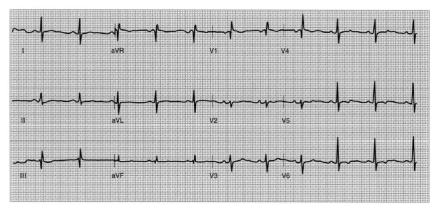

Figure A37.3 *ECG of a 34-year-old senior first officer, showing widespread T-wave notching. This is a normal variant, and the subject responded normally to exercise. Any doubt about the exercise response should require an echocardiogram to search for a possible muscle disorder and, in older subjects, myocardial scintigraphy. Incomplete right bundle branch block is also present.*

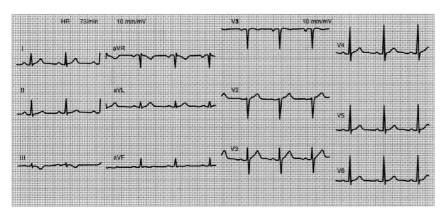

Figure A37.4 *ECG of a 44-year-old pilot. The ECG had been stable over many years, although both the T-wave inversion inferiorly and the QS in V1 were correctly reported as abnormal. The exercise ECG was normal, and the pilot was given unrestricted certification. As a new appearance, further investigation with thallium scanning or coronary angiography would be justified if the exercise response was doubtful. The inverted P wave in V1 may be explainable on the basis of mild hypertension.*

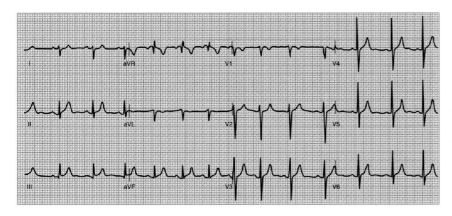

Figure A37.5 *ECG of a 30-year-old pilot, showing right axis deviation (S wave > R wave in S1). This is common in young tall subjects, but the additional slurring of the S wave in V1 raises the possibility of a secundum atrial septal defect. If small, it would be consistent with unrestricted certification.*

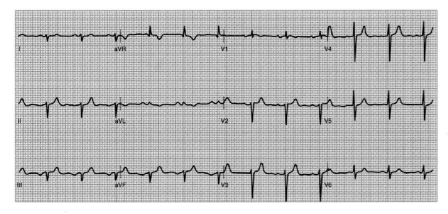

Figure A37.6 *ECG of a 45-year-old air traffic controller showing left axis deviation (S wave > R wave in S2). There is also clockwise rotation of the heart about its longitudinal axis with deep S waves in the left chest leads. This is seen as a variant of normal in young individuals and, in this case, had been present for many years. The exercise ECG was normal.*

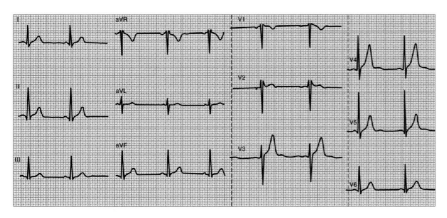

Figure A37.7 *ECG of a 41-year-old airline captain, showing incomplete (QRS duration < 120 ms) right bundle branch block (rSr' in V1, S wave in S1 and V6). This is most commonly a long-standing and normal variant. No investigation or restriction is necessary.*

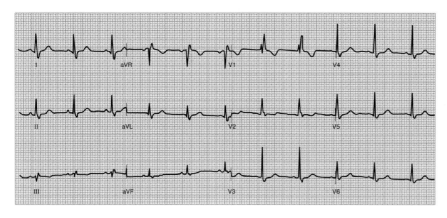

Figure A37.8   *ECG of a 54-year-old commercial pilot, showing complete right bundle branch block (slurred S waves in S1 and V6, RsR' in V1). As a new presentation, investigation is indicated (see text), but the condition is usually benign and long-term certification is to be expected (see page 583).*

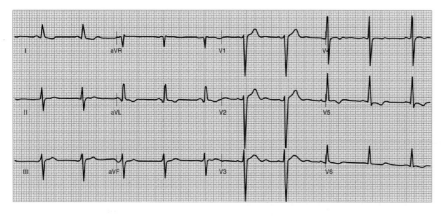

Figure A37.9   *ECG of a 51-year-old ex-military pilot, showing complete (QRS duration > 120 ms) left bundle branch block (absent q waves in S1, V5 and V6; RsR pattern in S1 and V6, with asymmetric T-wave inversion therein; poor r-wave progression in the chest leads). This pattern is less common than right bundle branch block in the pilot population and in the older pilot (> 45 years) carries an increased risk of adverse cardiac events (see page 583).*

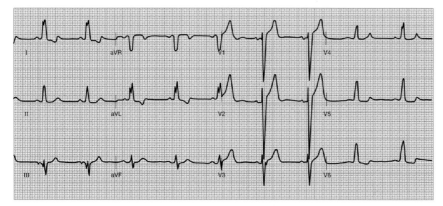

Figure A37.10   *ECG of a 61-year-old private pilot applicant with hypertension (178/98 mmHg). The T-wave inversion is the systolic overload pattern and the large voltages (on Sokolow's criteria) are suggestive of left ventricular hypertrophy. This carriers an increased risk of adverse outcome and demands full evaluation with vascular risk factor profiling (see page 569 – epidemiological considerations).*

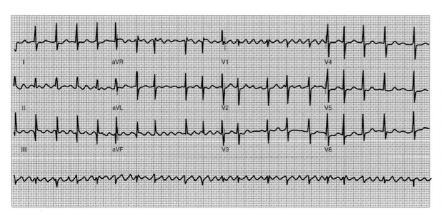

Figure A37.11   *ECG of a 48-year-old airline captain, showing (the less common) type 2 atrial flutter with regular flutter waves and variable atrioventricular (AV) conduction. The pilot was unaware of it. Due to the risk of one-to-one AV conduction, the condition is disbarring until the flutter circuit has been ablated.*

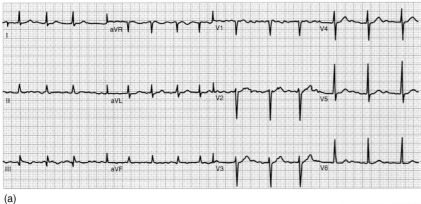

(a)

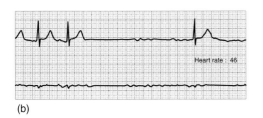

Heart rate : 46

(b)

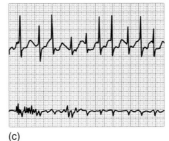

(c)

Figure A37.12 *ECG of a 49-year-old airline captain with atrial fibrillation. The rhythm is irregular and the baseline shows fibrillary waves (a); (b) Nocturnal pause on Holter monitoring (this should not exceed 3.5 s). Heart rate induced ST segment depression (c). A thallium scan was normal. The rhythm had been permanent for several years; as the heart was otherwise normal, restricted certification was permitted with regular follow-up.*

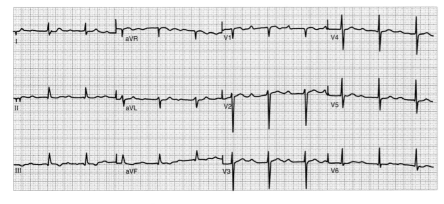

Figure A37.13 *ECG of a 34-year-old first officer with first-degree atrioventricular (AV) block. The PR interval is > 400 ms. Minor degrees of first-degree AV block (PR > 210 ms) are common and normally harmless provided the QRS duration is normal (< 90 ms). Even with this interval the condition appears to be benign although the P waves here are too wide (> 100 ms), suggesting left atrial overload. Exercise and Holter ECGs should be normal and the PR interval should shorten to < 180 ms with no decremental conduction on effort.*

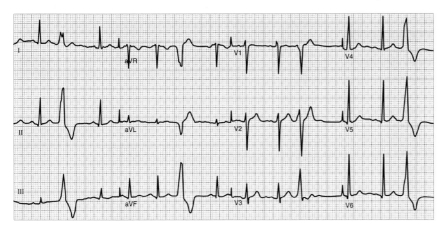

Figure A37.14 *ECG of a 44-year-old private pilot showing frequent right ventricular outflow tract premature contractions (left bundle branch block and right axis deviation). Provided they are suppressed by exercise, the echocardiogram is normal and no complex forms are seen (couplets or salvoes) on Holter monitoring, certification may be permitted, provided the subject is asymptomatic (see page 579).*

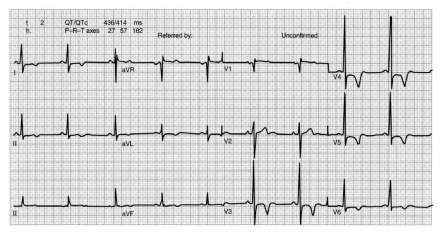

Figure A37.15 *ECG of a 56-year-old airline captain followed for many years with deep T wave inversion in V3–6. This is phenotypically a form of hypertrophic cardiomyopathy due to abnormality of the myosin C binding protein. Such individuals need to be restricted to multi-crew operation and be reviewed regularly with echocardiography, exercise ECG and Holter monitoring. Significant rhythm disturbance will disqualify.*

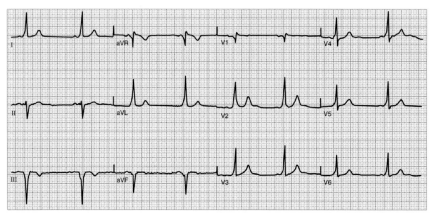

Figure A37.16 *ECG showing Wolff–Parkinson–White pattern in a 44-year-old asymptomatic private pilot applicant. There is a right posterior insertion of the Kent bundle accessory pathway. The PR interval is foreshortened (100 ms) and the slurred delta wave is seen in S1, aV1 and the chest leads. Subject to certain requirements class 2 and sometimes class 1 certification is achievable without restriction. If the syndrome is present (i.e. as atrioventricular re-entrant tachycardia) certification is possible only after ablation of the pathway (see page 582).*

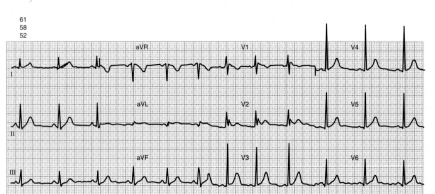

Figure A37.17 *ECG showing the Brugada pattern in a 46-year-old professional pilot. There is an abnormal ST segment drifting off the r′ in V1 and a convex upward segment ST in V2 with an RsR′ pattern. A sodium channelopathy is involved and the subject is at risk of sudden death. As prediction of outcome is unreliable all carriers of the gene involved, or Brugada phenotypes, should have restricted certification with denial for those who are symptomatic (see text).*

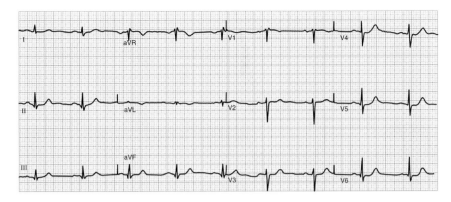

Figure A37.18 *ECG of a 61-year-old male private pilot with the long QT syndrome (LQTS). The corrected QT interval (QTc) is 455 ms (male normal < 440 ms). There are three different phenotypes LQTS (1, 2, 3), six different genotypes and some 200 mutations responsible for the sodium and potassium channelopathies involved. This is LQTS 1; although always asymptomatic, torsade de pointes type of ventricular tachycardia was recorded on Holter monitoring. Certification was denied (see page 584 – ion channelopathies).*

APPENDIX 37.2 ILLUSTRATIVE ANGIOGRAM AND ANGIOPLASTY

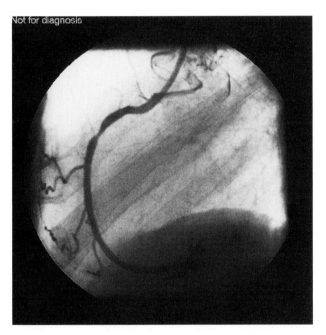

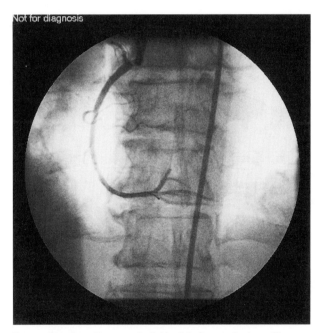

Figure A37.19 *Left anterior oblique image of the right coronary artery in a 54-year-old professional pilot with an 80% proximal stenosis. He presented with angina pectoris and responded abnormally to exercise. Six months after the intervention, the exercise ECG, echocardiogram and thallium scan were normal and restricted certification was permitted with annual follow-up.*

Figure A37.20 *The same individual during angioplasty. The index lesion has been dilated and is no longer visible. The guide wire can be seen in the posterior descending branch while the left ventricular branch appears blocked. Six months following the index intervention in the absence of symptoms when no abnormality had been demonstrated on exercise ECG, echocardiography or thallium scanning, restricted recertification was permitted subject to annual review.*

APPENDIX 37.3 ILLUSTRATIVE EXERCISE ELECTROCARDIOGRAM

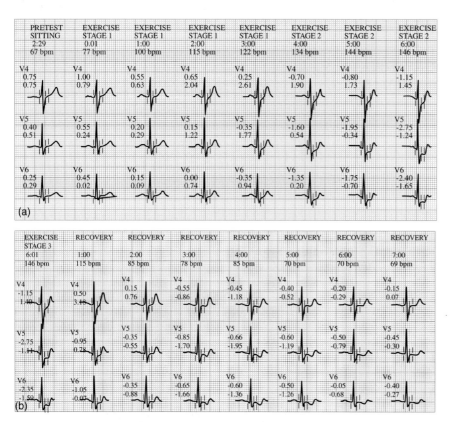

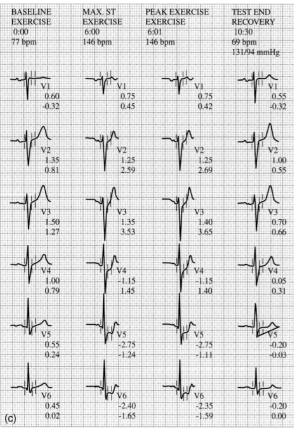

Figure A37.21 *Computer-synthesized exercise electrocardiographic summary of V4, 5, 6, (for simplicity) in a 59-year-old private pilot, who presented with a three-month history of chest pain on exertion during exercise (a) and recovery (b). The worst case deflections are seen in (c). It can be seen that although significant ST segment displacement is present at the end of exercise, the most significant hooked changes do not occur until the recovery period. The short walking time and prolonged recovery changes are of prognostic importance. The pilot had three-vessel coronary artery disease and subsequently underwent bypass grafting.*

38

Hypertension

ANTHONY J. BATCHELOR

INTRODUCTION

Hypertension is the most prevalent risk factor for arterial disease in the industrialized world (Wolf-Maier *et al.* 2003) and is a frequently encountered clinical problem in the aircrew population. One definition of hypertension can be considered as that level of blood pressure above which an excess morbidity and mortality is observed compared with a control population. However, it is now generally accepted that cardiovascular risk rises even across the range of pressures that traditionally have been regarded as falling within the 'normal' spectrum. Blood pressure is also seen to rise with age in industrialized populations in a manner not observed in people who have avoided the health hazards of Western civilization, and indeed it is likely that our evolutionary ancestors enjoyed substantially lower pressures than we do today. Moreover, blood pressure probably remained fairly static throughout the lifespan of primitive man, even if that life expectancy was often somewhat limited for other reasons. The same observations are likely to be true of other interacting risk factors for cardiovascular disease, with our early ancestors being lean in build, physically much more active, and with substantially lower serum lipid levels, no exposure to the smoking habit and no type 2 diabetes.

Against this background of multiple interrelated risk factors for cardiovascular disease, it can be seen that to separate out hypertension from other such adverse influences acting on the vascular system, and to consider blood pressure in isolation, is distinctly artificial. Furthermore, such an approach is likely to yield risk assessments of poor predictive power and with limited value for guiding clinical decision making.

MEASUREMENT OF BLOOD PRESSURE

Arterial systolic and diastolic blood pressures are continuously varying quantities, influenced by a host of extraneous factors. It is well recognized that stress and anxiety can elevate blood pressure, and the physician can be perceived as quite threatening in this context, particularly when occupational decisions are involved – leading to the so-called 'white-coat effect' or 'office effect'. Recent exercise and consumption of food, alcohol and caffeine can also affect blood pressure, as can the time of day, posture, ambient temperature and a host of other variables. Thus, the limitations of a single office blood pressure measurement can be readily appreciated, but equally it must be understood that most of the prognostic information concerning blood pressure has, until very recently, been related to data collected in precisely such a manner.

Attempts should be made to measure the blood pressure in controlled and standardized conditions. The patient should have avoided recent exercise, smoking, and caffeine or food consumption, and the blood pressure should be recorded on a number of occasions, with the subject seated in a comfortable ambient temperature and with the arm supported. Many errors of technique await the unwary, and it is not appropriate to delegate the collection of this critical risk data to the most junior members of the healthcare team alone, without the support of additional measurements made by the physician. It is important that the cuff is of adequate size for the arm: individuals whose biceps circumference exceeds 33 cm require a larger than standard cuff if overestimates of pressure are to be avoided. Other common sources of potential error include parallax problems in reading the column or dial, digit preference bias, excessively rapid cuff deflation, and uncertainty over which Korotkoff sounds correlate best with diastolic blood pressure – the disappearance of sounds (Korotkoff V) is now accepted as the most accurate correlation. Further errors may be introduced by poorly maintained equipment. Mercury-column sphygmomanometers are becoming increasingly uncommon in clinical practice and being replaced by aneroid or automated devices. The former require regular calibration, and only those automated instruments that have been validated by an appropriate authority and are maintained regularly should be relied upon.

Home blood pressure monitoring has become increasingly popular with the advent of modestly priced automated machines, but the accuracy and reliability of such instruments vary widely. Nevertheless, evidence that using validated home recorders can yield prognostically valuable information is emerging, and they may be a useful aid to risk assessments in aviators. Increasingly, however, the value of 24-hour ambulatory blood pressure recordings is being recognized, particularly where a white-coat effect is suspected, and this technique has particular application in the case of aircrew in whom the white-coat phenomenon is, to some degree, almost endemic. The method has the advantage of recording large numbers of measurements, which are taken with the subject removed from the clinical environment and which demonstrate not only the variability of blood pressure but also the effect of daily activities and the influence of sleep. Over the past decade, a number of studies have demonstrated the powerful prognostic value of this approach in assessing the risk of coronary events and stroke in relation to blood pressure (Staessen et al. 1989; Verdecchia et al. 1994). In addition, such studies have also shown that those subjects who lose the normal pattern of blood pressure fall, or 'dipping', during sleep carry a significant and additional level of risk (Verdecchia et al. 1994). Equally, however, while some data have indicated that white-coat hypertension may be relatively benign in the short term (Verdecchia et al. 1994), other studies have raised concerns over the longer-term risk of such subjects developing sustained hypertension (Bidlinger et al. 1996; Glen et al. 1996). It may be prudent to follow up individuals in this category with occasional 24-hour blood pressure profiles for a number of years, rather than discount the possibility of any future excess cardiovascular risk on the basis of one such recording.

With the increasing numbers of studies that have become available, it has been possible to recommend normal standards for ambulatory blood pressure and to start defining thresholds of risk. The British Hypertension Society has proposed that mean 24-hour values not exceeding 130/80 mmHg can be regarded as normal but that values in excess of 140/90 mmHg should be considered abnormal. The same guidelines suggest normal maximum mean values of 135/85 mmHg for daytime hours and 120/70 mmHg for night-time hours (O'Brien et al. 2000).

AEROMEDICAL CONCERNS

Hypertension is a major risk factor for coronary artery disease and stroke (MacMahon et al. 1990), with the level of systolic blood pressure appearing to have a more powerful risk predictive value than the diastolic pressure. It has been estimated that for each 10 mmHg rise in systolic pressure, there is an associated 30 per cent increase in coronary mortality risk (Prospective Studies Collaboration 2002), and this observation is clearly relevant to the professional aircrew population, in whom cardiovascular disorders are the most common single cause for loss of licence. Reassuringly, however, a large number of therapeutic trials have demonstrated that effective treatment of hypertension substantially, and relatively rapidly, reduces this excess risk (Collins et al. 1990). The effect of such treatment is greatest and realized most rapidly for stroke, but there is also good evidence for a reduction in coronary events of the order of at least 25 per cent with effective management of hypertension.

ASSESSMENT OF RISK

While significantly and persistently elevated blood pressure is a risk factor that warrants intervention in its own right, milder and borderline cases require consideration of other coexisting risks when planning management strategies. Whereas any one cardiovascular risk factor may have limited predictive power in isolation, additional factors such as hyperlipidaemia, smoking and diabetes substantially amplify each other when present in combination, and nor can age be ignored as a contributor to the risk equation. Long-term epidemiological studies, of which the ongoing Framingham Study (now into its third generation) is the best known, have provided the evidence base for constructing integrated risk formulae, and these in turn have been the basis for a number of risk-assessment charts and software calculators. Such aids permit a rapid and evidence-based estimate of total cardiovascular risk for individuals that not only has credibility with patients but also can guide informed management decision-making. Useful examples of such tools are the Joint British Societies

Coronary Risk Prediction Chart (which uses a traffic-light system) and the New Zealand Coronary Event Risk Chart. A number of software programs are available over the Internet, including a simple coronary and stroke risk calculator from the British Hypertension Society at www.bhsoc.org/. There is, however, some evidence to suggest that the Framingham data, which are frequently used to construct such guides, may somewhat overestimate cardiovascular event risk when applied to European populations (Brindle et al. 2003), and ideally risk-assessment tools would rely on epidemiological data collected from the population within which they are to be applied.

INVESTIGATION OF HYPERTENSION

Primary causes for hypertension are uncommon but, particularly in younger subjects, screening for renal disease (urinalysis, serum creatinine) and hyperaldosteronism (serum electrolytes) is prudent. Renal artery stenosis may be indicated by the presence of a renal bruit but is rare in younger subjects, and a full blood count will eliminate polycythaemia. In the absence of clues from the clinical history, routine screening for other causes such as phaeochromocytoma is rarely profitable, and careful examination of peripheral pulses should eliminate the unusual condition of aortic coarctation. A fasting survey of blood lipids and glucose aids the process of risk profiling, and evidence of end-organ changes should be positively looked for, including a clinical assessment of arterial compliance. The electrocardiogram (ECG) has somewhat limited specificity for identifying left ventricular hypertrophy, particularly in younger subjects. However, where such ECG indications coexist with elevated blood pressure, they should be regarded with concern and assessment of left ventricular mass by echocardiography undertaken if any doubt exists. Left ventricular hypertrophy demonstrated by the latter technique has been shown to have significant adverse prognostic implications for cardiovascular events in hypertensive subjects (Levy et al. 1990), and its presence would be a powerful indication for active pharmacological intervention in such cases.

MANAGEMENT OF HYPERTENSION

Pilots with raised blood pressure must first and foremost be regarded as patients who carry a significant cardiovascular risk factor, and it is primarily the healthcare considerations that should dictate their management. The current British Hypertension Society guidelines (BHS-IV) (Williams et al. 2004) recommend early intervention if the blood pressure is sustained above 160/100 mmHg or if levels in excess of 140/90 mmHg persist in the presence of cardiovascular complications, target-organ damage or diabetes, or in those cases where the total ten-year cardiovascular event risk is estimated to exceed 20 per cent. Individuals falling within these groups should be removed from all types of flying immediately and appropriate medical management initiated. For many aviators, however, it will be possible within these guidelines to observe those with more borderline initial blood pressures over a period of three to six months, while instituting lifestyle changes and introducing other risk-factor-reducing manoeuvres. The immediate discontinuation of smoking will have a profound effect on total risk in those who use cigarettes. Achieving an optimum body weight, reducing alcohol and salt intake, increasing fruit and vegetable consumption and taking regular aerobic exercise can all be expected to exert modest, but significant, favourable influences on blood pressure (Premier Collaborative Research Group 2003) and to have a positive influence on lipid status and glucose tolerance. Arguably, therefore, the flight surgeon's most useful consultations may be those held in the crew room, where informal interaction with aviators, health education and the active encouragement of a healthy lifestyle may help to avoid the future development of hypertension and arterial disease.

Drug treatment

Blood pressure thresholds for pharmacological intervention have tended to fall as the advantages of treatment have been comprehensively demonstrated by successive randomized controlled trials (Collins et al. 1990). At the same time, target levels for treated blood pressure have become more aggressive as the advantages of achieving lower levels have been documented (Hansson et al. 1998). The BHS-IV guidelines suggest targets for optimally treated blood pressure of less than 140/85 mmHg, or 135/80 mmHg in subjects with coexisting diabetes (Williams et al. 2004). Therapeutic endeavours in aviators should undoubtedly aim to match these figures. Multiple drug therapy is increasingly favoured as a means of achieving adequate blood pressure control without pushing single agents to their dose limits and increasing the risk of side effects. Most classes of modern antihypertensive agents are regarded as compatible with continued flying status, and it is also becoming increasingly clear that it is achieving the desired reduction in blood pressure, rather than the class of drug used, that is the critically important factor in influencing outcome in hypertensive patients. No apparent advantage was shown for any one class of agent in the uniquely large Antihypertensive and Lipid Lowering Therapy to Prevent Heart Attack Trial (ALLHAT Collaborative Research Group 2002), which compared a calcium channel-blocking drug and an angiotensin-converting enzyme (ACE) inhibitor with a thiazide diuretic.

Thiazide diuretics have a long history of use in the flying population and are certainly the initial therapy of choice, particularly for most older subjects. The dose–response curve does not favour pushing these drugs beyond a modest dose, and intakes in excess of bendroflumethiazide 2.5 mg daily, for example, are associated with minimal additional blood pressure-lowering advantage but risk being accompanied by increasing symptomatic and metabolic side effects. Provided this dose (or the equivalent of other thiazides) is not exceeded, side effects are uncommon and the metabolic impact is minimal. Aircrew with blood pressure that is controlled adequately with thiazides, with no other uncontrolled cardiovascular risk factors, and with no evidence of end-organ damage, are usually fit to return to unrestricted flying in military and civilian spheres.

ACE inhibitors are an alternative initial choice in younger aviators, are positively indicated in patients with type 2 diabetes, and have no adverse effects on serum lipids. Side effects, apart from an irritating cough, are uncommon. The cough tends to be dose-related, often not being seen if the dose remains modest (e.g. lisinopril $\leq$ 10 mg daily). An alternative approach is to switch to one of the angiotensin II type 1 receptor antagonists, which are considered to have even lower side-effect profiles and do not inhibit bradykinin metabolism, the mechanism held to be responsible for the cough with ACE inhibitors. Both agents can be combined usefully with a low-dose diuretic for amplified effect. Concerns that ACE inhibitors might have an adverse effect on G-tolerance have not been borne out by experience in either the US Air Force (Rhodes 2003) or the Royal Air Force (RAF), and the US Navy accepts these agents for unrestricted flying without G-tolerance testing.

Beta-blockers in low dosage can be effective but are less well tolerated by younger athletic individuals. Their potential for central effects, although usually minor, and their influence on cardiovascular homeostatic mechanisms are usually recognized by restricting their use in military aircrew to non-high-performance flying and multi-pilot operations. Long-acting cardioselective and hydrophilic agents such as atenolol are preferred; they should be limited to modest dosage (e.g. atenolol $\leq$ 50 mg daily). They may not be the best choice in overweight people, particularly in the face of glucose intolerance or adverse lipid profiles.

Calcium channel-blocking agents, which act by inducing arteriolar dilatation and reducing peripheral resistance, are associated with side effects such as flushing, mild headache and peripheral oedema in some subjects. Such effects are usually mild when longer-acting agents such as amlodipine are used, particularly if the dose is only moderate (e.g. amlodipine 5 mg daily). Because of their neutral influence on glucose metabolism and serum lipids, these drugs may be favoured in subjects with hyperlipidaemia or glucose intolerance.

Of the more commonly used modern agents, only alpha-blocking drugs and centrally acting antihypertensive drugs are contraindicated in the flight environment. The former can have unpredictable postural effects. Centrally acting antihypertensive drugs have yet to be been shown to have a benefit as first-line therapy, and the possibility of unwelcome central influences in the flight environment has not been excluded.

Follow-up

Although historically the first difficulty with managing raised blood pressure in the population has been the low rate of identification of subjects with hypertension, the second problem has been the low proportion of such individuals in whom adequate blood pressure control has subsequently been achieved with treatment (Mancia et al. 1997). Up to 40 per cent of treated hypertensive people have, in some studies, failed to achieve target blood pressures (Wolf-Maier et al. 2004). Regular follow-up of individuals with treated hypertension should be regarded as mandatory if adequate control is to be assured and maintained. Such reviews offer the opportunity for encouraging continued lifestyle changes and tight drug compliance, as well as allowing drug side effects to be enquired into and other cardiovascular risk factors to be reviewed. Repeated 24-hour ambulatory blood pressure profiles, performed at intervals, are a valuable means of confirming the improvement achieved and guiding treatment changes where necessary. Not only does this technique permit evaluation of control over the full 24-hour period, but also evidence exists to show that such measurements provide additional prognostic value for treated hypertensive people, with one study suggesting that 24-hour mean systolic pressures exceeding 135 mmHg are associated with a doubling of cardiovascular event risk compared with lower values (Clement et al. 2003). Additionally, there is some evidence that ambulatory 24-hour monitoring may assist not only in optimizing blood pressure control but also, in doing so with a drug regimen of reduced intensity and side-effect risk compared with a group monitored with office recordings alone (Staessen et al. 1997).

Subjects taking diuretics benefit from consuming a diet adequate in potassium and having their electrolytes, glucose and lipids rechecked four to six weeks after commencing therapy. Measuring serum creatinine levels in people on ACE inhibitors after one to two weeks of treatment should guard against the rare deterioration of renal function that might be seen with undiagnosed renal artery stenosis.

AEROMEDICAL DISPOSAL

Pilots with levels of blood pressure that, on repeated measurements, remain in excess of the current guidelines levels for early therapeutic intervention (BHS-IV 180/110 mmHg) must be removed promptly from flying duties and appropriate investigation and treatment instigated. For the majority of aviators in whom blood pressure is elevated to a less severe degree, but where it is still in excess of 150/90 mmHg, a judgement as to fitness for continued flying duties will be based on an assessment of the total risk factor profile and the presence or absence of any target-organ complications. Apart from aviators at the highest end of the risk profile, most will be fit to continue flying, perhaps with some limitation such as a multi-crew restriction, while further assessment is undertaken. However, aircrew should be grounded for a minimum of two weeks if drug therapy is commenced. Such an interval provides an opportunity for observation in order to ensure that no unacceptable or idiosyncratic side effects of therapy are encountered and, equally important, that adequate control of blood pressure is achieved. Most civil aircrew with uncomplicated hypertension, and without significant additional cardiovascular risk factors, will be fit to return to unrestricted flying status once blood pressure is controlled and stable. However, for military aircrew, rather more caution is needed. For the majority of military pilots without complications or additional risks, and who achieve adequate control with a low-dose diuretic or an ACE inhibitor, or a combination of the two, a return to unrestricted solo-pilot flying in the high-performance environment can be anticipated. Nevertheless, a monitored pressure-breathing test and a check of G-tolerance may be appropriate for those whose potential role could involve operating at high altitude (in excess of 40 000 feet) or in high-G environments, respectively. A similar approach is taken with hypertensive aviators using calcium-channel antagonists. Military aircrew requiring a beta-blocking agent would normally be restricted to the multi-crew environment and protected from regular exposure to levels of $+G_z$ exceeding 2.5.

CONCLUSION

The programme of regular occupational health assessments to which aircrew are exposed offers an excellent opportunity to provide an effective service in preventive medicine for this professional group. The identification and effective management of common cardiovascular risk factors, such as hypertension, provides a prime example of the potential benefits that such programmes bring to the aircrew population. By these means, the flight surgeon can exert a positive influence not only over the longer-term health and prognosis of their patients but, ultimately, also on flight safety, and can do so with the knowledge that the great majority of aviators with raised blood pressure will be manageable to modern standards of risk reduction while still being able to continue with full careers in their chosen profession.

REFERENCES

ALLHAT Collaborative Research Group. Major outcomes in high-risk hypertensive patients randomized to angiotensin-converting enzyme inhibitor or calcium channel blocker vs diuretic: the Antihypertensive and Lipid Lowering Therapy to Prevent Heart Attack Trial (ALLHAT). *Journal of the American Medical Association* 2002; **288**: 2981–97.

Bidlinger I, Burnier M, Bidlinger M, *et al.* Isolated office hypertension: a prehypertensive state? *Journal of Hypertension* 1996; **14**: 327–32.

Brindle P, Emberson J, Lampe F, *et al.* Predictive accuracy of the Framingham coronary risk score in British men: a prospective cohort study. *British Medical Journal* 2003; **327**: 1267–70.

Clement DL, De Buyzere ML, De Bacqer DA, *et al.* Prognostic value of ambulatory blood-pressure recordings in patients with treated hypertension. *New England Journal of Medicine* 2003; **348**: 2407–15.

Collins R, Peto R, MacMahon S, *et al.* Blood pressure, stroke, and coronary heart disease: part 2. *Lancet* 1990; **335**: 827–38.

Glen SK, Elliott HL, Curzio JL, *et al.* White-coat hypertension as a cause of cardiovascular dysfunction. *Lancet* 1996; **348**: 654–7.

Hansson L, Zanchetti A, Carruthers SG, *et al.* Effects of intensive blood-pressure lowering and low dose aspirin in patients with hypertension: principal results of the Hypertension Optimal Treatment (HOT) randomised trial. *Lancet* 1998; **351**: 1755–62.

Levy D, Garrison RJ, Savage DD, *et al.* Prognostic implications of echocardiographically determined left ventricular mass in the Framingham Heart Study. *New England Journal of Medicine* 1990; **322**: 1561–6.

MacMahon S, Peto R, Cutler J, *et al.* Blood pressure, stroke, and coronary heart disease: part 1. *Lancet* 1990; **335**: 765–74.

Mancia G, Sega R, Milesi C, *et al.* Blood-pressure control in the hypertensive population. *Lancet* 1997; **349**: 454–7.

O'Brien E, Coats A, Owens P, *et al.* Use and interpretation of ambulatory blood pressure monitoring: recommendations of the British Hypertension Society. *British Medical Journal* 2000; **320**: 1128–34.

Premier Collaborative Research Group. Effects of comprehensive lifestyle modification on blood pressure control (Premier Clinical Trial). *Journal of the American Medical Association* 2003; **289**: 2083–93.

Prospective Studies Collaboration. Age-specific relevance of usual blood pressure to vascular mortality: a meta-analysis of individual data for one million adults in 61 prospective studies. *Lancet* 2002; **360**: 1903–13.

Rhodes DB. Centrifuge testing of USAF aviators treated with lisinopril for hypertension. *Aviation, Space, and Environmental Medicine* 2003; **74**: 389.

Staessen J, Byttebier G, Buntinx F, *et al.* Antihypertensive treatment based on conventional or ambulatory blood pressure measurement. *Journal of the American Medical Association* 1997; **278**: 1065–72.

Staessen J A, Lutgarde T, Fagard R, *et al.* Predicting cardiovascular risk using conventional vs ambulatory blood pressure in older patients with systolic hypertension. *Journal of the American Medical Association* 1999; **282**: 539–46.

Verdecchia P, Porcellati C, Schillaci G, *et al.* Ambulatory blood pressure: an independent predictor of prognosis in essential hypertension. *Hypertension* 1994; **24**: 793–801.

Williams B, Poulter NR, Brown M J, *et al.* Guidelines for management of hypertension: report of the British Hypertension Society, 2004 – BHS IV. *Journal of Human Hypertension* 2004; **18**: 139–85.

Wolf-Maier K, Cooper RS, Banegas JR, *et al.* Hypertension prevalence and blood pressure levels in 6 European countries, Canada, and the United States. *Journal of the American Medical Association* 2003; **289**: 2363–9.

Wolf-Maier K, Cooper RS, Kramer H, *et al.* Hypertension treatment and control in five European countries, Canada, and the United States. *Hypertension* 2004; **43**: 10–17.

Yusuf S, Hawken S, Ounpuu S on behalf of the INTER HEART Study Investigators. Effect of potentially modifiable risk factors associated with myocardial infarction in 52 countries (the INTER HEART STUDY): case controlled study. *Lancet* 2004; **364**: 953–62.

39

Respiratory disease

GARY DAVIES

INTRODUCTION

Respiratory disease is the most common cause of emergency hospital attendance and the most common cause of morbidity and loss of productivity in the workplace, including the aviation industry. Consideration should be given not only to the disease itself but also to its natural history, treatment and possible sequelae. The potential for sudden incapacitation or the requirement for restrictions in the working environment (i.e. G force or pressure breathing) must be addressed when assessing fitness to return to work.

In this chapter, a distinction is made between trained aircrew, where considerable investment in time and money has been made, and initial applicants for aircrew training, where the potential uncertainty of the natural history of the disease may preclude acceptance.

The following diseases will be discussed. Although it is recognized that this is not an exhaustive list, it addresses the more common conditions that can present to the aviation medicine specialist:

- asthma
- sarcoidosis
- pneumothorax (spontaneous, traumatic)
- obstructive sleep apnoea
- chronic obstructive pulmonary disease (COPD)
- bullous lung disorders
- bronchiectasis
- mycobacterial diseases (tuberculosis (TB), atypical)
- interstitial lung disease (ILD)
- pulmonary thromboembolic disease
- pulmonary malignancies.

PASSENGER TRAVEL

It is commonly thought that modern passenger aircraft are pressurized in order to allow a normal sea-level environment. However, this is untrue and most are pressurized to cabin altitudes up to 2438 m (8000 feet), although this maximum may be breached in emergencies. At this cabin altitude, the partial pressure of oxygen will have dropped to the equivalent of breathing 15.1 per cent oxygen at sea level, and a healthy passenger will experience a fall in arterial oxygen tension (Pa_{O_2}) to 7.0–8.5 kPa (53–64 mmHg, arterial oxyhaemoglobin saturation (Sp_{O_2}) 85–91 per cent). This leads to concern that altitude exposure may exacerbate hypoxaemia in patients with lung disease, and particular caution seems justified in those who are hypoxaemic at sea level. Patients may experience mild to moderate hyperventilation (due to acute hypoxaemia) and a moderate tachycardia.

In such patients, the following assessment is recommended:

- History and examination with particular reference to cardiorespiratory disease, dyspnoea and previous flying experience.

- Spirometric tests.
- Measurement of O_2 saturation by pulse oximetry. Blood gas tensions are preferred if hypercapnia is known or suspected.

In those with resting oximetry between 92 and 95 per cent at sea level, hypoxic challenge testing is recommended. The hypoxic challenge test consists of breathing 15 per cent fraction of inspired oxygen (Fi_{O_2}) for 20 minutes with blood gas measurements being taken directly after.

The recommendations are as follows:

- Pa_{O_2} > 7.4 kPa (> 55 mmHg): oxygen not required.
- Pa_{O_2} 6.6–7.4 kPa (50–55 mmHg): borderline – walk test may be helpful.
- Pa_{O_2} < 6.6 kPa (< 50 mmHg): in-flight oxygen (2 l/min).

Often, the $P_{a_{O_2}}$ will be measured on 2 litres O_2 in order to ascertain whether a satisfactory improvement has occurred.

If the person's resting oximetry at sea level is less than 92 per cent, then supplementary oxygen will be required. If the person is on supplementary oxygen at sea level, then the flow rate will have to be increased during flight.

Patients are unable to use their own oxygen cylinders on the flight, and any oxygen that is required will have to be booked well in advance with the airline. Oxygen usually can be provided only in flow rates of 2 l/min or 4 l/min; therefore, if higher concentrations are required, the patient's fitness to fly should be put in doubt. In an extreme emergency, higher flow rates are possible. The price charged for supplying the oxygen in-flight varies between airline companies and can be an important factor in the overall cost of the flight.

At the end of each section in this chapter, passenger travel in patients with that particular respiratory disease will be discussed. These specific recommendations are a supplement to those stated above (British Thoracic Society Standards of Care Committee 2002).

ASTHMA

Introduction

Asthma is a chronic inflammatory disease confined to the airways of the lung and resulting in episodic airflow obstruction (Figure 39.1), which is reversible (spontaneously or as a result of treatment), and increased airway responsiveness to a variety of stimuli. Asthma is extremely common in many industrialized countries, with a prevalence of three to seven per cent. For reasons that are not well understood, the prevalence and severity of asthma

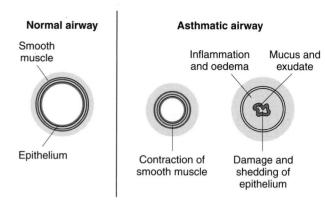

Figure 39.1 *Mechanism of airflow obstruction in asthma.*

appear to be increasing. Comparison of the prevalence of asthma in different parts of the world suggests that the high and increasing prevalence in the Western world is associated with urbanization and material prosperity.

Natural history

Over the past 15 years, research efforts by various clinicians and scientists have resulted in a paradigmatic shift in the way we view asthma. Rather than perceiving asthma as a disease consisting primarily of bronchospasm with resultant airway obstruction, we understand it to be an airway disorder resulting from a complex inflammatory process involving many cells, cytokines and other mediators.

Appreciation of the inflammatory nature of asthma has also led to recognition of the associated injury and damage to the airway wall – airway remodelling – which may lead to irreversible loss of function and be preventable by the early institution of anti-inflammatory treatment. Therefore, optimal medical management of asthma has been changed from regimens that relied almost exclusively on bronchodilators for control of symptoms to protocols emphasizing the importance of the use of anti-inflammatory agents.

Diagnosis

Diagnosing asthma can be difficult. The diagnosis is clinical, with no one diagnostic test. The symptoms of asthma can be associated with a number of other respiratory diseases, and so it is important to take a good history looking for the typical symptoms of wheeze, shortness of breath, cough (often only nocturnal) and specific triggers of symptoms. A family history of asthma or atopy may be helpful. The important indicators of asthma to look for are:

- intermittency
- variability

- nocturnal worsening of symptoms
- provocation of symptoms by specific triggers.

Lung-function testing and simple home peak-flow diaries are very important in the diagnosis of asthma. In these, the relevant features are:

- ≥ 20 per cent diurnal variation in peak expiratory flow (PEF) on three or more days within a two week period (home PEF diary) (use the formula $(best - worst)/best \times 100$)
- ≥ 15 per cent (or 200 ml, whichever is greater) improvement in forced expiratory volume in one minute (FEV$_1$) with either:
  - short acting beta-2 bronchodilator (e.g. 2.5 mg nebulized salbutamol) or
  - oral steroid trial (prednisolone 30 mg once daily for 14 days).

Lung-function testing also determines the degree of airflow obstruction (FEV$_1$/forced vital capacity (FVC)), the degree of air trapping (residual volume (RV)/total lung capacity (TLC)) and the degree of small-airways disease (maximum expiratory flow at 25 per cent of FVC (MEF$_{25}$) and maximum expiratory flow at 50 per cent of FVC (MEF$_{50}$)). Gas-transfer measurements will also allow assessment of any emphysema or pulmonary vascular disease.

Other tests may include:

- exercise testing (≥ 15 per cent decrease in FEV$_1$ after six minutes of exercise)
- exhaled nitric oxide (looking for airway inflammation)
- histamine or methacholine provocation test
- skin-prick testing and radioallergenosorbent (RAST) blood tests looking for specific allergens
- breath condensate (although this is still experimental at the time of writing, it will be in clinical use in the near future).

The differential diagnosis is large and it is important to also undertake chest X-ray (CXR), sputum testing for microscopy (including acid-fast bacilli (AFB) to exclude TB) and a detailed history looking for symptoms of bronchiectasis, COPD, ILD, bronchial tumour, foreign body, pulmonary emboli and hyperventilation.

Treatment

NON-PHARMACOLOGICAL TREATMENT

Allergen avoidance

Allergen avoidance can be useful in reducing the severity of existing disease. This can reduce both chronic disease and exacerbation rates. Avoidance of house dust mites by using bed-barrier covering, removing carpets and washing bed linen at high temperatures may reduce asthma symptoms.

Environmental factors

Smoking should be avoided completely. A patient with asthma who starts smoking in teenage years increases the risk of chronic asthma. Environmental pollutants may also play a role in asthma symptomatology. Workplace factors should also be investigated.

PHARMACOLOGICAL TREATMENT

The British Thoracic Society and the Scottish Intercollegiate Guidelines Network (SIGN) have reviewed their guidelines, which advocate a stepwise approach to treatment (Figure 39.2) (British Thoracic Society and Scottish Intercollegiate Guidelines Network 2003). This is a good guide to the treatment of asthma, the goal being to control symptoms on the lowest possible amount of inhaled steroids. The use of a long-acting beta-2 bronchodilators (LABA) with a lower dose of inhaled steroid is an important consideration, as is the use of leukotriene receptor antagonists, which looks very promising in a selected group of patients (especially exercise-induced asthma).

Aeromedical management problems

The major concern from an aviation medicine point of view is that of sudden incapacitation. This risk is likely to be exaggerated by the use of pressure-breathing masks and exposure to G forces. Unfortunately, there are few predictors of fatal or near-fatal asthma, except for a previous attack requiring hospitalization. The inclusion of newer treatments has led to better asthma control and, thus, reduced the likelihood of an asthma attack. It is also important to take into consideration any known precipitins and exposure avoided if possible.

From an operational point of view, there is a theoretical risk of an interaction between asthma and the prophylactic use of nerve agent pyridostigmine pretreatment (NAPP) tablets. This is because pyridostigmine could lead to cholinergic overstimulation, which may lead to bronchoconstriction. So far, there is no evidence that this is a clinical issue. In the military setting, there have been a large number of asthmatics given this drug prophylaxis without any reported problems. Research into this interaction and the possible use of long-acting anticholinergics is required.

Disposition

ENTRY TO PILOT TRAINING

Military

Candidates with a current or past history of confirmed asthma are permanently unfit for aircrew duties. Candidates who have had a single episode of wheeze in association with a respiratory tract infection should be

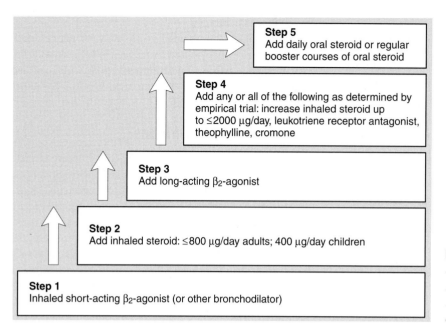

Figure 39.2 *Stepwise approach to asthma treatment. Adapted from draft British Thoracic Society and Scottish Intercollegiate Guidelines Network (SIGN) asthma guidelines.*

assessed formally for bronchial hyper-reactivity; if this is negative, they may be accepted as medically fit for aircrew selection.

Civilian

The following guidelines should be used in the assessment of candidates for commercial pilot training:

- There should be a minimum period of five years from the last acute attack, and no significant hospital admissions.
- Lung function tests should be acceptable: the FEV_1/FVC ratio should be greater than 70 per cent, with no appreciable drop after exercise.
- The asthma should be controlled on treatment with an inhaled steroid or cromoglycate, with or without an inhaled bronchodilator. Treatment with oral steroids should be disqualifying.
- There must be no bronchospasm (wheeze) on examination.
- There must be no bronchospasm with a mild respiratory infection (e.g. common cold).

For private flying, restrictions at selection may be less stringent:

- There should be a minimum period of two years since the last acute attack, and no significant hospital admissions.
- Lung function tests should be acceptable: the peak flow rate, a simple test that can be carried out by a general practitioner (GP), should be more than 80 per cent of the predicted normal.
- The asthma must be controlled well on treatment with an inhaled steroid or cromoglycate, with or without an

inhaled bronchodilator. Treatment with oral steroids is disqualifying.
- There must be no bronchospasm (wheeze) on examination.
- Bronchospasm with mild respiratory infection (e.g. common cold) should be controlled easily.

The above requirements should be confirmed by the prospective pilot's consultant physician.

TRAINED AIRCREW

The variability in both severity and prognosis of the disease demands that a specialist assessment is carried out in order to avoid unnecessary loss of trained aircrew. The aircrew member should be grounded while this assessment is taking place. The recommendation regarding return to flying duties will depend on the severity of the condition and drug treatment required.

Military

- Uncontrolled asthma: grounded.
- Persisting symptoms or requiring high-dose and/or multiple drug treatments: unfit solo flight, unfit pressure breathing.
- Asymptomatic on low-dose treatment: specialist review required, but may having flying restrictions lifted on specialist recommendation.
- Low-dose treatment category: should not necessarily be restricted to inhaled steroid only and may allow addition of LABA or leukotriene receptor antagonists on the recommendation of a specialist.
- Regular follow-up with formal lung-function testing is required.

Civilian

Existing commercial pilots who develop asthma require similar evaluation to that described above for entry to training. They may be restricted to multi-crew duties. Existing class private pilots who develop asthma require similar evaluation as for entry to training and may need a safety pilot limitation.

Passenger travel

Preventive and relieving inhalers should be carried in the hand luggage. Portable nebulizers may be used at the discretion of cabin crew. Some airlines can provide nebulizers for in-flight use, and patients should check with the carrier when booking. It is important to stress that spacers are as effective as nebulizers.

SARCOIDOSIS

Introduction

Sarcoidosis is a multisystem granulomatous disorder of unknown aetiology that typically affects young adults and is characterized by the presence of non-caseating granulomas in involved organs. The exact prevalence is not known for certain, due to the large numbers of asymptomatic people, but it is estimated to be in the region of 15 per 100 000 people. There is a significant difference in incidence between ethnic groups, with Afro–Caribbean people having about a three-fold higher incidence than white people. There is also heterogeneity of the illness, with Afro–Caribbean patients tending to have a more acute presentation and more severe disease than white people.

There has been substantial research into the cause of sarcoidosis, but as yet there is no definitive answer. The latest hypotheses involve a complex interaction between multiple genes and environmental factors or infection. At present, it is thought that there is no single causative antigen but that the disease results from chronic exposure to an antigen to which the individual is susceptible (Thomas and Hunninghake 2003). Another hypothesis suggests that the pattern of disease may, in part, be related to different underlying causes (Newman et al. 1997).

Clinical manifestations

Between 40 and 60 per cent of cases are asymptomatic and found incidentally, usually on a routine CXR. The most common presenting symptoms are respiratory (e.g. dry cough, dyspnoea, chest pain) or dermatological (e.g. erythema nodosum, sarcoid papules or plaques). Systemic symptoms (e.g. malaise, fatigue, night sweats, fever) may be present, but these are rarely the main presenting feature. Ophthalmologic (e.g. pain, visual change) and musculoskeletal (e.g. joint pains, myalgia) problems also occur. Rarely, there is neurological or cardiac involvement (see Chapter 37).

Lung involvement occurs in about 90 per cent of patients with sarcoidosis. CXR classically shows bilateral hilar lymphadenopathy (BHL). Staging of pulmonary sarcoidosis is based on the radiological stage of disease:

- Stage 1 – BHL (50 per cent): regression of BHL within one to three years occurs in about 75 per cent of patients. Around ten per cent develop chronic enlargement, which can persist for ten years or more.
- Stage 2 – BHL and pulmonary infiltrates (25 per cent): usually, the pulmonary infiltrates occur predominately in the upper zones. Two-thirds of patients undergo spontaneous resolution. Stage 2 patients usually have mild to moderate symptoms.
- Stage 3 – pulmonary infiltrates only: interstitial nodules commonly are present, predominately in the upper zones.
- Stage 4 – advanced pulmonary fibrosis.

Computed tomography (CT) scanning may show other associated features, including:

- beading of the fissures
- nodules
- bronchial wall thickening
- ground-glass opacification
- parenchymal masses or consolidation
- traction bronchiectasis.

Other pulmonary involvement includes endobronchial (40 per cent of stage 1, 70 per cent of stages 2 and 3), pleural sarcoid, superior vena cava obstruction (secondary to lymph-node compression) and pulmonary hypertension.

Investigations

Histology may show evidence of non-caseating granulomas, with exclusion of AFB. This can be from any available lesion (e.g. lymph node, cutaneous lesion) or transbronchial or endobronchial bronchoscopy biopsy.

Pulmonary function tests may show:

- restrictive pattern
- preserved flow rates
- reduced gas transfer factor.

Pulmonary function tests *may be normal*. Serial studies are useful for assessing treatment and progress.

Other investigations to support the diagnosis include:

- serum angiotensin-converting enzyme (ACE) level: raised in more than 75 per cent of untreated patients (NB: if the level is very high, consider lymphoma)

- bronchoalveolar lavage: lymphocytosis (increased numbers of activated T-cells)
- gallium scanning (uptake within the lung tissue)
- tuberculin skin test
- serum calcium.

Other tests may include electrocardiogram (ECG), echocardiogram, urinalysis, full blood count (FBC) and full neurological examination.

Treatment

Asymptomatic BHL rarely requires any treatment. Patients who are symptomatic or show signs of disease progression should be started on corticosteroid treatment. These drugs are usually given orally and continued for about 12 months, tailing off slowly. If an initial rapid benefit is required, then pulses of methylprednisolone can be given, with the added advantage of a lower maintenance dose of oral corticosteroids being required. All patients with organ dysfunction should be treated. Bone-density studies should be performed on people taking long-term corticosteroids.

Steroid-sparing agents can be used to minimize the amount of oral corticosteroid used in the long term. These include azathioprine, hydroxychloroquine and methotrexate.

Aeromedical management problems

The major concern is sudden incapacity due to arrhythmias and syncope secondary to the presence of cardiac sarcoid. Cardiological assessment is required for all patients with sarcoidosis. Pulmonary involvement may lead to symptoms that interfere with the individual's ability to perform their role and complete their mission. Steroid treatment itself has a variety of metabolic and central nervous system effects that may be hazardous to flying (see Chapter 51).

Disposition

ENTRY TO PILOT TRAINING

Because of the possibility of future cardiac involvement, candidates are considered unfit for aircrew training if sarcoidosis is present. This includes the presence of simple uncomplicated BHL. Candidates will be considered only following complete resolution and normal full evaluation by a specialist.

TRAINED AIRCREW

Military

The patient should be grounded on diagnosis until they have been investigated fully. To return to flying duties, the patient must show no evidence of active disease over a period of 12 months and have a full cardiac assessment (ECG, echocardiogram, Holter monitor, magnetic resonance imaging (MRI)) that is negative. Initially, they should return to multi-crew capacity, being upgraded to solo flying in a further year if the condition continues to be inactive.

Patients with chronic sarcoid or myocardial sarcoid or being treated with corticosteroids or immunosuppressants should be permanently unfit flying duties. Patients with isolated pulmonary fibrosis should be referred for specialist opinion and regular follow-up.

Civilian

Commercial flying is acceptable only if the patient is investigated fully with respect to the possibility of systemic involvement and then none is found. There must be no evidence of cardiac involvement. If lymphadenopathy is present, this should be limited to hilar lymphadenopathy only, and the applicant should be free of medication.

Passenger travel

Because of the risk of pulmonary fibrosis a hypoxic challenge test should be performed, and the results interpreted as per the previously stated recommendations (p. 612).

PNEUMOTHORAX

Introduction

A pneumothorax occurs when air enters the thoracic pleural space, the space between the visceral pleura and the parietal pleura. Air entering this space interrupts the usual negative intrathoracic pressure and causes a degree of lung collapse on that side. The degree of collapse is proportional to the size and duration of the leak. This can be either spontaneous or as the result of trauma.

Spontaneous pneumothorax

NATURAL HISTORY

Spontaneous pneumothorax is caused by a spontaneous rupture of the lung tissue leading to the escape of air into the pleural space. There is a bimodal distribution of incidence, with peaks occurring in young adults and in elderly people. The second peak is, however, becoming more diffuse and extending to an earlier age, as the age of patients with COPD decreases (Chen 2003).

In young adults, spontaneous pneumothorax is a consequence of a subpleural bleb rupturing. There is usually no underlying lung pathology. It occurs most commonly in tall, thin, fit men. Presentation can be with breathlessness or chest pain (usually pleuritic in nature). Often, symptoms are very minor.

In patients with underlying lung disease (usually in the older age group), i.e. secondary pneumothorax, the cause is usually due to rupture of a bulla. The most common cause of this is COPD. Presentation in this group tends to be with worsening breathlessness and chest pain. These patients tend to have a reduced respiratory reserve and can be significantly breathless, even with a small pneumothorax.

The major concern is a tension pneumothorax, which may occur when there is a flap valve at the site of the leak. This leads to a progressive increase in the size of the pneumothorax, which eventually becomes under pressure. The pressure causes cardiac compression and can lead to cardiorespiratory arrest. This requires immediate drainage and decompression.

Recurrence is a major problem. The recurrence rate, without definitive treatment, is approximately 30 per cent after the first episode, 50 per cent after a second episode and 80 per cent after a third episode (Cran and Rumball 1967). The vast majority occur within the first year, and the risk reduces dramatically with time after this. Risk of contralateral pneumothorax is about ten per cent.

INVESTIGATION

Tension pneumothorax should be treated immediately on clinical grounds, without further investigation. To confirm spontaneous pneumothorax, a CXR is the investigation of choice. A CT scan of the thorax may be required in cases where previous pleural adhesions may have occurred, e.g. previous pleurodesis.

Further investigation of aircrew should always include a routine CT thorax to exclude any underlying lung pathology. Full lung-function tests are also important in order to assess airways obstruction, increased RV and decreased gas transfer factor, which might suggest underlying emphysema.

TREATMENT

Initial treatment may not be required or should be with simple aspiration according to the British Thoracic Society guidelines (Henry *et al.* 2003). Occasionally, a chest drain may be required, usually in people with secondary pneumothorax.

In view of the increased risk of recurrence even after a single episode, it is recommended that aircrew undergo definitive treatment. Pleurectomy is the treatment of choice due to its low recurrence rate. This can be as an open operation or, more commonly, by a thoracoscopic approach. The latter has the advantages of being less inva-

sive and having a shorter recovery time (Baumann *et al.* 2001). Chemical pleurodesis is a further option but is not recommended in aircrew because of the higher failure rate (95–100 per cent versus 78–91 per cent) (Baumann *et al.* 2001).

AEROMEDICAL MANAGEMENT PROBLEMS

During flight, the chances of occurrence of a pneumothorax are increased. Increase in altitude (even cabin pressure) leads to expansion in the volume of air within the bullae, producing an increased risk of rupture. During pressure breathing, the higher pressure can lead to air trapping and increased risk of rupture. Fortunately, in-flight occurrence of pneumothoraces is rare, even with pressure breathing. The occurrence of a spontaneous pneumothorax during flight may result in incapacitation due to breathlessness and pain. Furthermore, during flight, the reduction in ambient pressure will cause a rapid increase in the percentage collapse (at 8000 feet, a pneumothorax will increase by about 30 per cent compared with at sea level).

DISPOSITION

Entry to pilot training

A spontaneous pneumothorax within two years and without definitive treatment is a bar to entry. Potential military aircrew should undergo pleurectomy, as discussed above. A single untreated pneumothorax more than two years previously is acceptable because of the small risk of recurrence after this time. Investigation for underlying lung pathology is recommended.

Trained aircrew

Military
Following successful pleurectomy after a single event, flying duties can resume after three months. If pleurectomy is not undertaken, then the patient should be grounded for 18 months. This is provided that this was a single episode. Repeat episodes, however, would require a pleurectomy for the aviator to continue with flying duties.

Investigation for underlying lung pathology is recommended.

Civilian
Full certification following a fully recovered single spontaneous pneumothorax may be acceptable after one year from the event, with full respiratory evaluation (pulmonary function testing, CT scanning) by a specialist.

Recertification in multi-pilot operations or under safety pilot conditions may be considered if the applicant recovers fully from a single spontaneous pneumothorax after six weeks, provided that pulmonary function testing and CT scanning show no underlying lung disease.

A recurrent spontaneous pneumothorax is disqualifying. Certification may be considered following surgical intervention with a satisfactory recovery.

PASSENGER TRAVEL

A patient with a current closed pneumothorax should not travel on commercial flights. The patient may be able to fly six weeks after a definitive surgical intervention and resolution of the pneumothorax. Careful medical assessment is required beforehand.

A patient who has not had surgery must have had a CXR confirming resolution, and at least six weeks must have elapsed following resolution before travel.

Traumatic pneumothorax

Trauma to the chest can cause a leak of air into the pleural space. This can be due to penetration through the chest wall, fractured rib(s) or blunt trauma to the lung tissue. The risk of recurrence after initial treatment is very small if no underlying lung pathology is present. No definitive treatment is required, and flying duties can resume three months after treatment.

BULLOUS LUNG DISEASES AND CYSTS

Introduction

Bullae are thin-walled airspaces greater than 1 cm in size. They may compress the surrounding lung tissue. They may be isolated in otherwise normal lungs or be part of generalized emphysema. Cysts may be caused by destruction of airspaces by respiratory disease.

Natural history

Isolated bullae in otherwise normal lungs in a young adult are usually stable and unlikely to progress. Presence of underlying lung disease suggests the likelihood of progression. The risk from bullae is associated with the risk of rupture and, therefore, pneumothorax. The other considerations are a ventilation/perfusion (V/Q) mismatch at the site of the bullae and potential compression of the surrounding normal lung.

Investigation

CT scanning and lung-function tests are the mainstay of investigation. CT scanning is important in order to assess the extent of bullae and to investigate any underlying lung disease. Lung-function testing is important in order to assess lung volumes and to investigate any airflow limitation. Radioactive assessment of ventilation and perfusion is also important in order to assess the degree of mismatch.

Treatment

Surgical treatment involves a bullectomy in patients with single bullae and otherwise normal lungs. There has been investigation into bronchoscopic reduction of emphysematous bullae with reasonable success. This is far less invasive but at the time of writing is still experimental.

Aeromedical management problems

The main hazard is bullous rupture and subsequent pneumothorax. The bullae may not communicate with the airway and, therefore, during decompression training may lead to an increase in size and pneumothorax (possibly tension pneumothorax, see earlier). Both rupture and pneumothorax would lead to sudden incapacitation.

Disposition

PILOT TRAINING

The presence of bullae makes the trainee unfit. Previous surgery for a single bulla with normal underlying lung can proceed following a full respiratory assessment.

TRAINED AIRCREW

An aviator with a single bulla but otherwise normal lungs must be grounded until definitive surgery has been performed. Multiple bullae or the presence of underlying lung disease are incompatible with flying.

OBSTRUCTIVE SLEEP APNOEA

Natural history

Obstructive sleep apnoea (OSA) is much more common than is widely thought. It typically affects middle-aged overweight men. OSA is characterized by:

- daytime somnolence
- snoring
- apnoeic attacks during sleep
- morning headaches
- perceived poor quality of sleep.

Collapse of the upper airway during sleep leads to recurrent periods of apnoea. These in turn lead to sudden arousals from sleep (usually not remembered by patient), poor-quality sleep as a consequence and daytime somnolence. Arousals from sleep are usually not recollected in the morning. Long-term effects include increased risk of cardiac events and nocturnal carbon dioxide retention.

Investigation

Clinically, an Epworth sleepiness score (out of 24) is of use. A sleep study (polysomnography) is the gold standard and will provide information on apnoeas and hypo-apnoeas as well as nocturnal oxygen desaturation and carbon dioxide retention. Overnight oximetry can detect the repetitive desaturations seen in severe OSA and may give a diagnosis in some patients. However, if the study is negative, full polysomnography is needed.

Treatment

Initial treatment of mild cases should involve addressing possible precipitating factors, such as obesity, excessive alcohol use, use of sedating drugs and cigarette smoking. Ear, nose and throat (ENT) problems and endocrine abnormalities, e.g. hypothyroidism, should also be corrected. For moderate to severe disease, and in people in whom simple measures have failed, the best treatment is with continuous positive airway pressure (CPAP). This can be provided nasally or via a full face mask. Intolerance of this treatment can occur, in which case a mandibular advancement device (or jaw advancement splint), tricyclic antidepressants or uvulopalatopharyngoplasty (removal of the tonsils, uvula and parts of the soft palate and pharyngeal folds) can be used, although the latter two are of minimal effectiveness.

Aeromedical management problems

The risk is that of incapacitation due to severe daytime somnolence. This may be either sudden, with onset of sleep, or chronic, with impairment of performance. Treatment corrects this and removes the risk of incapacitation.

Disposition

ENTRY TO PILOT TRAINING

A history of OSA should be disqualifying.

TRAINED AIRCREW

Grounding is required until a response to treatment and cure of daytime somnolence have been confirmed. Upon successful treatment, a return to unrestricted flying duties should be allowed. It is important to inform the aviator that they will need to contact the Driver and Vehicle Licensing Agency (DVLA) or equivalent driving (car or motorcycle) authority of the diagnosis.

Passenger travel

A doctor's letter is required outlining the medical diagnosis and stating that the CPAP machine should travel in the cabin as extra hand luggage. A patient with significant desaturation and intending to sleep during the flight should consider using their CPAP machine, although the majority of patients will not require CPAP during the flight. Battery-powered CPAP machines can be used during the flight but must be switched off before landing. Long-haul flights are best avoided. Patients should avoid drinking alcohol before and during the flight.

Patients with significant desaturation should use CPAP during sleep when visiting high-altitude destinations.

CHRONIC OBSTRUCTIVE PULMONARY DISEASE

Introduction

COPD is a disorder characterized by airflow limitation that is largely irreversible and progressive in nature. COPD encompasses chronic bronchitis and emphysema; the majority of patients have a combination of both. Chronic bronchitis is clinically a productive cough due to overproduction of bronchial secretions and without significant reversibility of airway obstruction. Emphysema is defined as enlarged airspaces distal to the terminal bronchiole, with destruction of airway walls without fibrosis. Other causes of emphysema are rare, e.g. alpha-1-anti-trypsin deficiency. The underlying cause in almost all cases is passive or active cigarette smoking. It has been found that there is a genetic susceptibility that may be used in the future to predict the chances of developing COPD. The mortality from COPD is rising worldwide.

Natural history

As COPD is a heterogeneous disease, there is a variable natural history. COPD patients tend to present late and often with an incorrect diagnosis of asthma. Symptoms consist of breathlessness, daily sputum production, cough and wheeze. Response to treatment is poor in comparison with asthma, with airflow obstruction being mainly irreversible in COPD. Recurrent respiratory infections are common. If smoking continues, the disease progression is relentless. Cessation of smoking at any stage will lead to a slowing of progression and is the *only* factor that has been shown to slow progression.

Pathogenesis

Risk factors for COPD include:

- smoking habit
- increasing age
- environmental pollution
- chronic childhood respiratory diseases and low birth weight.

Treatment

The treatment of COPD is difficult because of the usually fixed obstruction that is present.

The most important factor in the treatment of COPD is to stop smoking. This is the only intervention shown to reduce disease progression. Pulmonary rehabilitation programmes have been shown to be beneficial and should be undertaken if possible.

Pharmacological treatment involves the use of steroids and bronchodilators to reverse any reversible obstruction. The use of steroids is controversial, but a trial of oral steroids followed by inhaled steroids, if effective, should be considered. The use of new combination steroid and LABAs has been shown to be beneficial. Antimuscarinic bronchodilators are also used; tiotropium, a long-acting antimuscarinic bronchodilator, has been shown in trials to be of significant benefit. Oral theophyllines are also used, but much less so in recent years.

In patients with a significant emphysema element, bullectomy of any large bullae can improve lung function. This is usually performed by thoracotomy or mediastinoscopy. Bronchoscopic volume reduction has been tried, but this is still in its infancy and outcomes are awaited. Bronchoscopic methods involve the placement of one-way valves into the bronchi of a lobe, or subsegment of a lobe, that contains the bullae and allows deflation of the bullae.

Aeromedical management problems

Unlike asthma, COPD rarely causes sudden incapacitation, except when bullae are present, in which case the problems are those of a spontaneous pneumothorax. Patients with significant air trapping may experience problems with altitude (increase in volume of already trapped air) and with pressure breathing (an active increase in trapped air/pressure). This can lead to significant discomfort and compromise. Because of the nature of the disease, there is a greater rate of pulmonary infections, leading to reduction in operational efficiency and flying time.

In more advanced stages of COPD (usually passengers), the lower partial pressures of oxygen at altitude (discussed earlier), even in pressurized cockpits and aircraft, can lead to a significant reduction in the arterial oxygen saturation (SA_{O_2}). This reduction can lead to significant hypoxia. To overcome this, arterial blood gases and, if available, a fitness-to-fly test should be undertaken. A fitness-to-fly test involves arterial blood gas analysis while the patient breathes 15 per cent oxygen (simulation of cabin altitude). In a patient with significant reduction in P_{O_2}, 2 l/min of oxygen should be supplied for the journey. It is important that this is also assessed at the time to evaluate any CO_2 retention. It should be noted that cabin pressures and oxygen availability and cost vary between airlines.

Disposition

PILOT TRAINING

A diagnosis of COPD disqualifies pilot training. However, due to the nature of the disease, it would be very unusual in this group. A full specialist assessment is required in order to confirm the diagnosis.

TRAINED AIRCREW

In mild disease, with normal lung function and no CT evidence of bullae, unrestricted flying is allowed with regular respiratory follow-up. Strong advice to stop smoking should be given due to the disease progression.

Patients with moderate disease will require specialist assessment. They will be unfit fast-jet flying, but their suitability for other flying duties will depend on the amount of respiratory limitation.

Aircrew with frequent exacerbations, significantly decreased lung function ($FEV_1 < 50$ per cent predicted), presence of bullous disease or abnormalities of arterial blood gases are unfit any flying duties.

Passenger travel

Preventive and relieving inhalers should be carried in the hand luggage. Portable nebulizers may be used at the discretion of cabin crew. Some airlines can provide nebulizers for in-flight use, and patients should check with the carrier when booking. It is important to stress that spacers are as effective as nebulizers.

BRONCHIECTASIS

Introduction

Bronchiectasis is defined as a chronic dilation of one or more bronchi. Macroscopically, bronchiectatic lung reveals permanent dilation of subsegmental airways that are inflamed, tortuous and often partially or totally obstructed with secretions. The process also includes bronchioles, and at end stage there may be marked fibrosis of small airways. The overall appearance microscopically is of chronic inflammation in the bronchial wall, with inflammatory cells and mucus in the lumen. There is destruction of the elastin layer of the bronchial wall, with a variable amount of fibrosis. Causes are widespread, with the majority being idiopathic, post-infective (usually in childhood) or secondary to immunodeficiency. Cystic fibrosis is also a significant cause.

Natural history

There is often a history of childhood pulmonary infections or sinus/ENT problems. A cough is usually present, and symptoms of fatigue and breathlessness are common. Patients usually produce an increased amount of purulent sputum. The frequency of pulmonary infections increases with time if treatment is not instituted. Chronic rhinosinusitis is also often associated in adult life. Haemoptysis can be present, and worsening of constitutional symptoms also occurs. Examination classically shows finger-clubbing and crackles, usually at the bases.

Investigation

Abnormalities on plain CXR can be observed, but CXR can be normal in over 50 per cent of cases. Usually, a high-resolution CT scan is required in order to assess the extent of disease. Investigations of the underlying cause (immune deficiency, cystic fibrosis, connective tissue disease, ciliary dyskinesia, pulmonary aspergillosis) are very important and can indicate the course of treatment. Lung-function testing has a significant role in assessing small-airways disease. Sputum culture to culture infecting organisms is also important.

Treatment

If a treatable cause, e.g. hypogammaglobulinaemia or allergic bronchopulmonary aspergillosis, has been excluded, then the mainstay of treatment is sputum clearance. This usually involves the patient performing daily physiotherapy (postural drainage and/or breathing exercises) to expectorate as much of the sputum as possible. Recognizing pulmonary infective exacerbations and their prompt treatment with antibiotics is also very important. Infective exacerbations are defined by at least two of increased sputum volume, increased sputum colour and breathlessness.

In some patients, this management fails to prevent frequent infective exacerbations, thus causing morbidity and possibly disease progression. In these patients, prophylactic treatment is required. This usually involves either nebulized antibiotics or oral azithromycin, which requires only three doses a week. In severe disease, there may be the need for regular intravenous antibiotics.

Surgery for limited disease was used in the past, but this rarely leads to cure and is performed very infrequently nowadays.

Aeromedical management problems

Although this disease can be severe debilitating, resulting in significant loss of flying time, the risk of sudden incapacitation is small. The major feature is that of recurrent infective exacerbations. These can sometimes be controlled with prophylactic antibiotics, as stated above. Major haemoptysis is extremely rare and is insignificant as a cause of sudden incapacitation.

Disposition

PILOT TRAINING

A history of bronchiectasis is a bar to acceptance to pilot training. Patients with limited disease and who have had 'curative' surgery should be referred for specialist opinion but are unlikely to be fit for pilot training.

TRAINED AIRCREW

Patients with limited disease and who have minimal infective exacerbations and normal lung function should be fit for limited flying duties e.g. unfit fast jets, unfit solo flying. Those with more severe disease should be grounded permanently.

PULMONARY TUBERCULOSIS

Introduction

Pulmonary TB is a pneumonic infection caused by the organism *Mycobacterium tuberculosis*. TB is one of the most important diseases in the history of humanity and remains an extraordinary burden on human health today. The conquest of TB through the development of vaccines, drugs and diagnostics was a principal goal of biomedical research in the nineteenth and twentieth centuries. Despite the availability of curative chemotherapy for more than half a century, however, TB continues to cause an enormous amount of suffering, disability and mortality. It is still the leading cause of death from infectious disease worldwide.

Resurgence in the incidence of TB in the West has been caused by epidemics of human immunodeficiency virus (HIV)-related TB and multi-drug-resistant disease.

Natural history

After *M. tuberculosis* infection is acquired, the risk of developing disease depends on the host immunity. Tubercle bacilli are transmitted between people by aerosol particles (diameter < 1 μm), which remain airborne for long periods. Deposition of tubercle bacilli in the alveoli results in a series of protective responses by the cellular immune system that forestalls the development of disease in the majority of infected people. Alveolar macrophages ingest tubercle bacilli, which then multiply intracellularly and eventually cause cell lysis, with release of organisms. Additional alveolar macrophages engulf progeny bacilli, resulting in further intracellular growth and cell death. Over a period of weeks, as tubercle bacilli proliferate within macrophages and are released, infection spreads to regional lymph nodes, elsewhere in the lungs and systemically. The classic immunological response to infection with tubercle bacilli is the walling off of viable bacilli in granulomas. A calcified granuloma at the initial site of infection in the lung is referred to as a Ghon focus. For the majority of people acquiring a new tuberculous infection, the development of cell-mediated immunity to the organism is protective and holds the bacilli in check, although viability is usually maintained.

Clinical manifestations

Infection with TB is often asymptomatic. Pulmonary TB is usually a subacute respiratory infection with prominent constitutional symptoms. The most frequent symptoms of pulmonary TB are cough, fever, weight loss, night sweats and malaise. Cough in pulmonary TB is initially dry but often progresses to become productive of sputum and, in some instances, can cause haemoptysis. Occasionally, pleuritic pain is experienced, but this is usually with pleural involvement.

Presentation is usually late, with the patient being unwell for weeks or even months.

Investigations

Plain CXR may show the typical upper lobe infection, with cavitations. Consolidation or a pleural effusion may also be present. Enlarged hilar lymphadenopathy may be seen, but TB is a great mimic and can present in many ways, often suggesting other diseases.

Cutaneous tuberculin testing (Heaf or Mantoux) should be performed. Early-morning sputum tests on at least three consecutive days, looking for AFB, should be performed. If a pleural effusion is present, then pleural fluid should be examined for AFB. Often, bronchoscopic washing of the upper lobe is required if no sputum is available or the diagnosis is still suspected despite negative sputum microscopy. Sputum culture can take up to eight weeks but is essential for antibiotic sensitivity. Polymerase chain reaction (PCR) methods are also used extensively nowadays.

It is important to remember that if testing is negative but the diagnosis is still suspected, then continued investigation should proceed.

Treatment

Standard treatment of TB is with a combination of anti-tuberculous drugs. The usual regimen in the developed world, until sensitivities are known, is two months of isoniazid and rifampicin plus pyrazinamide ± ethambutol. Ethambutol is used especially if resistance is suspected. After the initial two months, depending on the sensitivities, drug treatment is reduced to isoniazid and rifampicin alone for a further four to seven months. The side effects of these drugs are extensive, the main significant effects being hepatitis and jaundice. Ethambutol may cause optic neuritis, which presents as colour-vision disturbance. For this reason, an ophthalmic opinion is suggested if ethambutol is to be used.

Aeromedical management problems

General illness caused by the disease and the intensity of the treatment is likely to mean that the patient is unable to fly. The risk of a spontaneous pneumothorax secondary to possible cavitations is also a concern.

Disposition

PILOT TRAINING

Candidates who have had previously fully treated TB and with no evidence of underlying lung disease and no evidence radiologically or on lung-function testing of residual lung damage are acceptable for pilot training.

TRAINED AIRCREW

An aviator with active disease and undergoing chemotherapy treatment should be grounded. Once they have completed the treatment and have been shown radiologically and on lung-function testing to have no residual lung damage, they may be upgraded to unrestricted flying duties.

Those who are taking prophylactic treatment should remain grounded for the length of the treatment.

Patients with evidence of residual lung damage or who are shown to have underlying lung pathology should be referred to a specialist for full radiological and lung-function assessment and judged on an individual basis.

Passenger travel

Patients with infectious TB must not travel by public air transportation until they are rendered non-infectious (three smear-negative sputum examinations on separate days).

ATYPICAL MYCOBACTERIAL DISEASE

Introduction

Atypical mycobacteria are ubiquitous in the environment and are low-grade pathogens. They include *Mycobacterium kanasii*, *M. xenopi*, *M. malmonoense* and *Mycobacterium intracellulare* complex (MAC), which is also known as MIAS due to the combination of organisms (*M. intracellulare*, *M. avium*, *M. scrofulaceum*). There are a number of other possible organisms, but these are a very rare cause of genuine infection. Exposure to them is unavoidable but does not constitute a threat to most people. Person-to-person spread is almost unheard of, with only one reported case. About five per cent of all mycobacterial pulmonary disease is caused by atypical mycobacteria. Usually, pre-existing lung disease (over 50 per cent having COPD) or an immunological defect is required before these organisms can cause genuine infection. Sometimes, the nature of the immunological defect is very hard to identify, but in the absence of pre-existing lung disease it should be sought by a specialist.

Clinical manifestations

The presentation is very similar to TB, with cough, sputum, fever, weight loss and increasing breathlessness. The symptoms tend to have an insidious onset, with a subacute or chronic illness picture, rather than an acute presentation. A significant proportion of patients (10–40 per cent) are asymptomatic.

Investigations

It is important to ascertain that the infection is genuine. It is impossible to distinguish TB from atypical infection on a chest X-ray. CT appearances have been described of a particular pattern of bronchiectasis that is associated with MAC, but this is still under investigation. Isolation and culture from sputum, bronchial lavage or lung biopsy are hindered by the same problems as TB (i.e. slow growth) and can require a number of different media and up to eight weeks to culture. This can be overcome on some occasions by the use of DNA probes and amplification techniques, but at present these are restricted to specialized reference laboratories.

Treatment

Rifampicin and ethambutol are the mainstays of treatment. This should be continued for between 15 and 24 months. The addition of one of isoniazid, clarithromycin, ciprofloxacin and streptomycin may be required, depending on sensitivities and progress of treatment. Lengthy treatment of many years' duration may be involved.

Aeromedical management problems

General illness secondary to the disease and the intensity of the treatment are likely to mean that the patient is unable to fly. The risk of a spontaneous pneumothorax secondary to possible cavitations is also a concern.

Disposition

PILOT TRAINING

The presence of active or previous atypical mycobacterial infection is a bar to acceptance to pilot training. This is not due to the disease itself but to the almost certain causative underlying lung disease or immunodeficiency.

TRAINED AIRCREW

The underlying lung disease or immunodeficiency, high recurrence rates and problems with inadequate treatment mean that the aviator should be permanently unfit flying duties.

INTERSTITIAL LUNG DISEASE

Introduction

ILD consists of a wide variety of lung disorders characterized by a diffuse parenchymal disease of the lung interstitium. The previous diagnosis of fibrosing alveolitis has now been superseded by a more encompassing classification (Figure 39.3). This classification includes information from radiology and histopathology.

Natural history

The presentation is usually breathlessness or an unsuspected abnormality on a chest X-ray. The natural history and treated course are critically dependent on the nature of the underlying disease process, which varies widely within this group of disorders. The diversity of this is beyond the scope of this chapter and should be investigated by a specialist.

Investigations

General investigations for presumed ILD should include the following:

- chest X-ray
- high-resolution CT thorax
- full lung-function testing, including transfer factor
- autoimmune screen, including extractable nuclear antibodies
- precipitins to known environmental factors, known to cause ILD.

Treatment

The mainstay of treatment of the lung disease is corticosteroids and immunosuppressants, but treatment of the underlying pathology or removal of exposure to a causative factor is also very important. The combination of these can be very complex and should be left to a specialist in this area. Lung transplantation may be required in end-stage disease.

Aeromedical management problems

Due to the nature of this group of diseases, they make flying duties impossible while the disease is active. Corticosteroids and immunosuppressants are associated with a number of problems of their own, such as increased risk of infection, neurological complications and blood dyscrasias, and are incompatible with flying duties. The

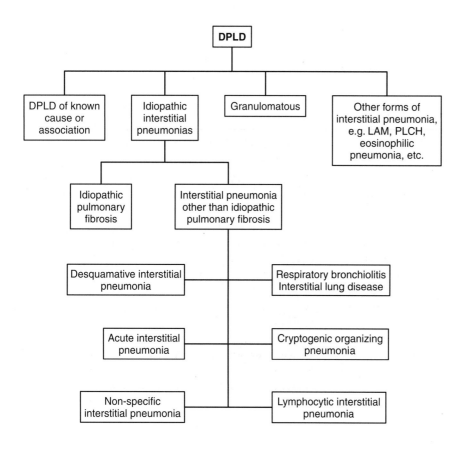

Figure 39.3 *Classification of interstitial lung disease. DPLD, diffuse parenchymal lung disease; LAM, lymphangioleiomyomatosis; PLCH, pulmonary Langerhans cell histiocytosis.*

other possible problem is that of hypoxia due to a reduced transfer factor. This may be present at sea level and should be picked up by investigation but may manifest only at altitude. Specific hypoxia tests can be performed at varying levels of P_{O_2} to assess this.

Disposition

PILOT TRAINING

A history of ILD is a bar to acceptance to pilot training.

TRAINED AIRCREW

The majority of diseases within this group are likely to lead to permanent grounding. There are some diseases within this group that, when treated, may enable a limited flying category, but this would require specialist recommendation. Referral to a specialized ILD unit is recommended.

Passenger travel

In ILD, a hypoxic challenge test consists of breathing 15 per cent $F_{I_{O_2}}$ is important in all but the most minor disease and if in any doubt should be performed. All those with a $Pa_{O_2} < 7.4$ kPa (< 55 mmHg) should be given supplementary oxygen.

PULMONARY THROMBOEMBOLIC DISEASE

Natural history

Pulmonary thromboembolic disease forms a large spectrum, from completely asymptomatic or a small amount of localized chest pain, through dyspnoea, to cardiorespiratory collapse and arrest. By definition, there is embolization from a clot within the vasculature, and so the causes are widespread but grouped grossly as due to:

- haemostasis, e.g. secondary to immobilization or tumour
- clotting disorder.

Embolization can occur before identification of the primary source. The most common source is from a deep vein thrombosis of the iliac or femoral veins.

Investigation

Investigation for pulmonary embolism is two-fold:

1. Investigation of the pulmonary embolus:

- Chest X-ray
  - may be normal
  - varying degrees of atelectasis, pleural effusion or hyperlucency
  - wedge-shaped infarct

- Arterial blood gases: hypoxia
- ECG
  - sinus tachycardia/atrial fibrillation
  - right bundle branch block
  - right ventricular strain pattern

- V/Q scan or computed tomography pulmonary angiogram (CTPA): probability of pulmonary embolism/definitive diagnosis

2. Investigation of the underlying primary source of the embolus:

- Doppler or venogram of iliac and femoral veins
- Bloods for clotting disorders (see Chapter 43)
- Search for possible underlying malignancy

Treatment

In severe cases, thrombolysis may be life-saving. In the vast majority of cases, initial treatment is subcutaneous low-molecular-weight heparin with oral warfarin. The subcutaneous low-molecular-weight heparin is continued until the international normalized ratio (INR) is greater than 2, at which point only warfarin is continued for six months.

Aeromedical management problems

A risk of recurrence is the main aeromedical problem. As stated previously, this could manifest as sudden incapacitation due to a large embolus or cause chest pain or dyspnoea, leading to a decrease in functional capacity. The other possible problem is that of hypoxia following a previous pulmonary embolism. This may be present at sea level and should be picked up by investigation but it may manifest only at altitude. Specific hypoxia tests can be performed at varying levels of P_{O_2} in order to assess this.

Disposition

PILOT TRAINING

Recurrent pulmonary embolism, a history of pulmonary embolism with no predisposing cause or a history of pulmonary embolism with an irreversible cause (e.g. clotting abnormality, malignancy) are disqualifying from pilot training. A history of a single pulmonary embolism with a reversible cause requires specialist assessment.

TRAINED AIRCREW

The aviator should be grounded for the length of investigation and treatment. Following treatment, and with a normal coagulation work-up and a defined cause found, flying duties can be resumed. Recurrent episodes or pulmonary embolisms with an irreversible cause mean permanent loss of flying.

Passenger travel

All patients with pulmonary thromboembolic disease when flying should avoid alcohol- and caffeine-containing drinks, take only short periods of sleep unless they can attain their normal sleeping position, and avoid the use sleeping pills. Pre-flight aspirin and graduating compression stockings may be recommended for those patients not on anticoagulant treatment.

PULMONARY MALIGNANCIES

Natural history

Pulmonary tumours can be benign or malignant, primary or secondary. Historically, lung cancer was more common in men than women, but this predominance is decreasing.

Primary malignant lung tumours can be classified histologically into small-cell (20 per cent) and non-small-cell (squamous cell 60 per cent, adenocarcinoma 10–15 per cent) tumours. They can present with cough, haemoptysis, chest pain, dyspnoea and systemic symptoms. Presentation is usually late in the disease. The major cause is cigarette smoking (a small proportion being due to passive smoking), with occupational exposure (asbestos, silicon, hydrocarbon fumes in coal-gas plants, arsenic, chromium, nickel, complex ethers) being the cause in a very small number.

Seeding of tumours to produce lung secondaries is common in a number of malignant tumours and can often be the presenting feature.

Prognosis is poor for malignant tumours if inoperable but depends on the histological type and the extent of the disease.

Investigation

Initial investigation is with chest X-ray. If a pulmonary malignancy is suspected, then the patient should be referred to a respiratory physician as soon as possible. In the UK, there is an organized pathway such that the patient can be investigated and treated as quickly as possible.

Investigation involves a high-resolution CT scan and bronchoscopy, with endobronchial biopsies if possible. Mediastinal lymph-node sampling can also be important in staging; this can be performed via a mediastinoscopy or less invasively via the bronchoscopic route.

Treatment

Management of lung cancer is based on several principles. It is important to establish whether the tumour is operable. If the disease is potentially curable by surgery, then the patient should be referred to a surgeon, regardless of the histology. Appropriate presurgical investigations are important.

A diagnosis of small-cell lung cancer is important, because these patients should be considered for multi-drug chemotherapy, with or without radiotherapy. Patients who are technically operable but refuse surgery or have other diseases that preclude operation (e.g. COPD, heart disease) should be considered for radical radiotherapy.

The evidence that anticancer treatment extends life expectancy in patients with inoperable disease is poor, with the possible exception of chemotherapy in some cases. However, both anticancer and medical treatments are required and are important for symptom palliation.

Local debulking of tumour for symptomatic relief can be performed bronchoscopically with electrocautery, cryotherapy or laser treatment.

Aeromedical management problems

Sudden incapacitation can occur from lung collapse or massive haemoptysis, but these are rare and mainly theoretical. More likely is general ill-health and malaise from systemic symptoms stopping the individual from flying. The risk of cerebral metastases and, therefore, seizures and loss of consciousness should also be taken into account. Endocrine abnormalities (including hypercalcaemia and hyponatraemia) may lead to confusion.

Disposition

PILOT TRAINING

A history of pulmonary malignancy is a bar to acceptance to pilot training. A history of a benign tumour would require extensive specialist assessment and individual recommendation.

TRAINED AIRCREW

Development of a pulmonary malignancy would lead to permanent grounding, even if operable, because of the risk of occult cerebral metastases. A history of a benign tumour would require extensive specialist assessment and individual recommendation.

REFERENCES

Baumann MH, Strange C, Heffner JE, *et al.* Management of spontaneous pneumothorax: an American College of Chest Physicians Delphi consensus statement. *Chest* 2001; **119**: 590–602.

British Thoracic Society and Scottish Intercollegiate Guidelines Network. British guideline on the management of asthma. *Thorax* 2003; **58** (suppl. 1): 1–94.

British Thoracic Society Standards of Care Committee. Managing passengers with respiratory disease planning air travel: British Thoracic Society recommendations. *Thorax* 2002; **57**: 289–304.

Chen J. Age at diagnosis of smoking-related disease. *Health Reports* 2003; **14**: 9–19.

Cran IR, Rumball CA. Survey of spontaneous pneumothoraces in the Royal Air Force. *Thorax* 1967; **22**: 462–5.

Henry M, Arnold T, Harvey J. BTS guidelines for the management of spontaneous pneumothorax. *Thorax* 2003; **58** (suppl. 2)ii: 39–52.

Newman LS, Rose CS, Maier LA. Sarcoidosis. *New England Journal of Medicine* 1997; **336**: 1224–34.

Thomas KW, Hunninghake GW. Sarcoidosis. *Journal of the American Medical Association* 2003; **289**: 3300–3.

40

Gastrointestinal disease

TREVOR LAUNDY

INTRODUCTION

Symptomatic gastrointestinal (GI) disease is common in the aviation environment and may cause acute incapacitation of crew or illness in passengers. Nevertheless, the occurrence of unheralded and catastrophic events is not the major concern that it is in the fields of neurological and cardiovascular disease. Acute GI illness, which frequently is self-resolving or relatively easily treated, is commonplace and often leads to no more than a temporary withdrawal from duty until treatment is completed and symptoms have settled. On the other hand, some of the chronic conditions affecting the GI tract are characterized by a poorly predictable relapsing and remitting course, which has significant implications for a flying career, particularly against backgrounds of major training investment, military fitness requirements and the dependence of employers on key personnel. Inflammatory bowel disease raises frequent problems in this regard but, conversely, improvements in the management of peptic ulcer disease have reduced its impact. Advances in endoscopic and radiological imaging, more accurate serological markers of disease, e.g. viral hepatitis and gluten enteropathy, and treatment advances in some areas have allowed more effective management of GI illness in the aviation community.

GASTRO-OESOPHAGEAL REFLUX DISEASE

Gastro-oesophageal reflux disease (GORD) is a common disorder in developed countries, with some surveys suggesting that up to 60 per cent of the adult population experience symptoms at some time. The cardinal symptoms are heartburn and regurgitation, often aggravated by postural change and relieved by antacids. There is commonly a history of preceding weight gain. When these are the only symptoms, a confident diagnosis of GORD can be made, but frequently there are other symptoms that raise the possibility of alternative diagnoses. In this situation, investigation is required, as it is when symptoms are particularly severe or there are alarm features such as dysphagia, weight loss, vomiting or GI bleeding. In the aviation setting, the exclusion of other diagnoses, including peptic ulcer disease, is a priority, and most patients will be referred for endoscopy. Some patients with symptomatic GORD have no abnormality on endoscopy, and subsequent investigation with oesophageal manometry or pH monitoring may be required. In practice, many aviators with GORD will have had the possibility of *Helicobacter pylori* infection raised; it may have been suggested by serological testing. Although this has no direct relevance to GORD, clarification of *Helicobacter* status with possible progression to eradication of a coincidental finding or resolution of iatrogenically induced concerns may justify endoscopy with near-patient biopsy urease testing and histological sampling.

Management of the condition involves a combination of lifestyle measures and acid neutralization or suppression. Weight reduction, smaller and more frequent meals, and sleeping with the head of the bed raised are all effective. Antacid/alginate drugs are usually the first-line choice of medication, but thereafter proton-pump inhibitors are commonly employed. All of these measures can be used to obtain symptomatic relief in aircrew. Restriction of aircrew status is rarely required, since in this population ulceration, bleeding and stricture are rare and the emphasis is on symptom and disease control. Surgical treatment occasionally may be indicated for young individuals with severe reflux requiring continuous therapy, for those who would rather avoid long-term drugs and for those with volume reflux. Interestingly, pressure breathing, negative G operations and positive G countermeasures rarely precipitate or aggravate reflux symptoms.

PEPTIC ULCER DISEASE

Peptic ulcer disease (Bebb *et al.* 2003) remains common in the community, although it now has less effect on aeromedical fitness than in the past. The prevalence of gastric and duodenal ulcer has decreased in developed countries over recent decades following a decrease in the prevalence of *H. pylori* as well as the introduction of highly effective acid-suppression drugs. Eradication of *H. pylori* heals ulcers and dramatically reduces relapse rates. Aspirin and non-steroidal anti-inflammatory drugs (NSAIDs) are independent causes of duodenal and, particularly, gastric ulceration. The prevalence and complication rates of peptic ulceration in the age group actively involved in aviation have reduced because of improvements in treatment. The diagnosis now rarely has a lasting effect on a flying career. Uncomplicated peptic ulcers typically cause epigastric pain related to eating and, frequently nausea, vomiting and weight loss, but they may be asymptomatic. Examination usually reveals epigastric tenderness as the only abnormality. The differential diagnosis often includes gastro-oesophageal reflux, gallstone disease, functional dyspepsia, gastric neoplasm, Crohn's disease and pancreatitis. Nevertheless, an unequivocal diagnosis of peptic ulceration can usually be made after upper-GI endoscopy and, when indicated, radiological imaging. The major aviation medicine concerns are the complications, of which bleeding and perforation are the most critical, although anaemia and gastric outflow obstruction are also significant. However, complications are now more a feature of disease in elderly people, where they are associated with aspirin and NSAID use. The combination of accurate and easily obtained diagnostic endoscopy with powerful acid-suppression treatment and effective *H. pylori* eradication strategies has revolutionized the outcome of diagnosed peptic ulcers. Cure is to be expected and can be confirmed by endoscopy, and most aviators can expect to return to unrestricted activity after treatment. Because bleeding and perforation may occur in patients with little or no dyspepsia, it might be thought that the management advances would not influence these emergencies, but in practice they are now less common in the younger population as a whole and have become rare in the aeromedical population.

When they do occur, a more delayed return to flying duties is to be expected.

INFLAMMATORY BOWEL DISEASE

Inflammatory bowel disease comprises collagenous colitis and lymphocytic colitis, together known as microscopic colitis, as well as the much more common ulcerative colitis and Crohn's disease. The latter two are of predominant importance in the aviation medicine context. Not only are they common diseases, but also their epidemiologies have particularly relevant features with high prevalences in the working age group and peak ages of onset in early adult life. They both have a relapsing and remitting course; this, together with variable response to treatment, causes difficulties for individuals, licensing authorities and employers. The high probability of relapse in the two conditions causes most employers and funders of training in the aviation world to categorize the conditions as disqualifying for recruits.

Ulcerative colitis

Ulcerative colitis is an inflammatory condition of unknown aetiology, which primarily affects the mucosa of the large bowel (Travis 2003). It always affects the rectum and extends proximally as it becomes more severe. There is undoubtedly a genetic susceptibility, demonstrated by a high incidence in first-degree relatives, but there is also evidence for environmental influences, with seasonal variations in presentation rates and a protective effect of smoking. Infection can cause relapses but does not appear to be the basic cause. Ulcerative colitis occurs worldwide but is more common in northern Europe and the USA than in southern Europe and the Far East. Studies in Scandinavia, the UK and the USA report an incidence of around 10 per 100 000 per year, with a prevalence of some ten times this figure. The classic presentation is with bloody diarrhoea, associated urgency of defecation and abdominal cramps. Onset is typically gradual, but there is wide variation in severity, ranging from a limited distal proctitis to an aggressive fulminant pancolitis. It has a relapsing and remitting course and is associated with a variety of extra-intestinal manifestations. Stool consistency, frequency and blood content are used to estimate severity, along with constitutional features (fatigue, anorexia, weight loss) and signs (anaemia, tachycardia, fever, abdominal tenderness).

The diagnosis is made by endoscopic observation of mucosal changes and their extent, combined with histological confirmation. At the time of first presentation, the differential diagnosis is usually between ulcerative colitis and infectious causes of bloody diarrhoea but it may also include Crohn's colitis (definitive distinction is occasionally not possible), radiation colitis, ischaemic colitis, microscopic colitis and drug-induced diarrhoea.

This brief clinical summary gives background to the aeromedical concerns with long-term fitness rather than the risk of acute incapacitation. Treatment is typically with oral and topical steroids in the acute phase and maintenance treatment with oral and topical 5-aminosalicylic acid (5-ASA), topical steroids and, possibly, oral steroids and azathioprine. Nevertheless, relapses are common and not predictable. Proctocolectomy may be indicated for severe or poorly controlled disease, steroid dependency or colitis complicated by dysplasia or cancer. Ileal-pouch construction is taking over from end-ileostomy as the procedure of choice, but there is a significant risk of major morbidity and a ten per cent risk of long-term failure, resulting in reversion to permanent ileostomy. Nevertheless, removal of the colon is essentially curative, and the introduction of ileal-pouch surgery has made it a more acceptable option for younger patients.

Familiarity with the spectrum of disease severity and progression is important in determining the aeromedical disposition. A limited distal proctitis may have no constitutional disturbance and only minor bowel symptoms and yet, occasionally, may be resistant to treatment and therefore troublesome. Conversely, an extensive colitis may produce major constitutional effects (or surprisingly little, in some younger patients), and the disturbed bowel habit may itself severely limit effective action in the air, even in aircraft with sanitary facilities. Moreover, even minor disturbances of bowel habit can be incompatible with long duty periods in small cockpits or ejection-seat aircraft. The risk of extension of distal disease can be assessed only after a period of follow-up.

An appreciation of the variability of the natural history and specialist assessment of individual cases is important for correct disposition. Patients newly diagnosed with ulcerative colitis should be grounded while the acute disease is treated, maintenance treatment established and some estimate made of disease extent and severity. Thereafter, a return to flying duties may be authorized, depending on the persons' response to, and tolerance of, maintenance treatment. Mild disease, limited in extent and controlled easily with oral or topical (enema or suppository) 5-ASA drugs may allow an early return to flying. Persisting severe and/or extensive disease, frequent relapse or a heavy therapeutic drug burden will prevent any return to flying. In all groups, endoscopic assessment is required. A few patients with initially aggressive disease achieve stable remission on maintenance regimens incorporating low-dose steroids (< 10 mg daily), azathioprine and 5-ASA preparations, and this may be compatible with limited aircrew duties. A return to some airborne duties may also be possible after proctocolectomy if general health is restored and good continence without undue urgency is achieved.

Crohn's disease

Crohn's disease (Jewell 2003) is an inflammatory disease that may affect any part of the GI tract, usually in a patchy fashion, involving only the large bowel in 30 per cent, only the small intestine in 40 per cent, and both the large and small intestines in 30 per cent. The distal ileum is the most common single site involved. Histologically, there is usually transmural inflammation. In contrast to the predominantly mucosal disease of active ulcerative colitis, there are frequent lymphoid aggregates, fewer neutrophils and crypt abscesses, and less goblet-cell depletion. Non-caseating granulomata are characteristic. The aetiology is unknown, but unlike ulcerative colitis it is more common in smokers. Crohn's disease occurs worldwide but appears to be most common in North America and Europe, where the incidence is reported to be around 4 per 100 000, with a prevalence of 60–80 per 100 000. Its apparent rarity in the developing world may be due, in part, to the diagnostic difficulties where intestinal tuberculosis is common. It begins most commonly in early adult life, follows a remitting relapsing pattern, and frequently is complicated by abscess and fistula formation, haemorrhage, perianal disease and obstructive symptoms.

The recurrence rate of Crohn's disease approaches 100 per cent at 10 years if endoscopic indications are taken into account, and 80 per cent of patients will require at least one surgical operation in the course of their disease. A subgroup of individuals with localized ileal resection and other characteristics such as youth and absence of perianal disease has a definably lower recurrence rate (Bernell et al. 2000). Nevertheless, many individuals with Crohn's disease have a degree of chronic ill health that makes a career in aviation untenable. In addition to local complications, nutritional deficiencies and anaemia are common, inflammatory markers are commonly raised, and remote manifestations affecting the skin, eyes, joints, back and liver are not rare. Treatment with corticosteroids is effective in active disease but is not indicated when patients are in remission. The 5-ASA preparation mesalazine may be beneficial in both active disease and the maintenance of remission. The strongest evidence for the latter is in relation to remission after ileal or ileocaecal resection. In patients with frequently relapsing disease and patients dependent on corticosteroids, the addition of azathioprine or 6-mercaptopurine may be of considerable benefit, with marked steroid-sparing effect. Crohn's disease can rarely be expected to be compatible with a return to full flying duties because of the unpredictable relapses and the symptoms and complications described above. With established remission over a significant time and absent endoscopic or haematological indicators of disease activity, a return to limited, selected aviation duties may be appropriate in trained personnel. The diagnosis can be regarded as disqualifying for recruitment to professional aviation activity.

IRRITABLE BOWEL SYNDROME

It is a frequent observation that in Western Europe and the USA, up to 50 per cent of patients referred to general gastroenterologists have no organic disease. Many of these are given a diagnostic label of irritable bowel syndrome (McCaughlin 2003). By contrast, in aviation medicine practice the diagnosis is rarely made, possibly due to an absence of healthcare-seeking behaviour in this population (Talley and Spiller 2002). Theories of causation have included motility disorders, heightened sensitivity to bowel distension and increased awareness of normal abdominal sensation; there is unlikely to be a single pathophysiology. For a 'syndrome' it is markedly heterogeneous: the Rome II criteria allow the diagnosis to be made in individuals who have frequent watery stools and in individuals who have infrequent, hard, pellet-like stools. While the pattern of symptoms is diverse, the common themes include abdominal pain, relief with defecation, fluctuating bowel habit, a feeling of incomplete evacuation and a sensation of abdominal bloating. By definition, the label is applied when there is no evidence of organic pathology. Well-established management guidelines exist for routine clinical practice, and for many individuals only limited investigation is required. In aviation medicine practice, the different epidemiology, together with occupational considerations, mean that a lower threshold for extensive investigation is often appropriate in patients presenting with non-specific bowel symptoms. If a conclusion of irritable bowel syndrome is reached, then the symptomatic burden may be incompatible with aircrew duties; in the absence of definable pathology or effective treatment, decisions on fitness must be made on empirical clinical grounds.

COELIAC DISEASE

Coeliac disease, or gluten enteropathy, is caused by an immunological reaction to the gluten content of cereals, mainly wheat, which causes morphological changes in the villous architecture of the proximal small intestine. Microscopic examination of specimens obtained by endoscopic small-intestinal biopsy reveals general flattening of the mucosa. The changes range from reduction in the normal villous height/crypt depth ratio to total absence of villi. The classic description of the disease in childhood, where it presents as malabsorption and growth failure, is not reproduced in adult life, where individuals can present with a wide range of symptoms. In an aviation medicine context, the most common presentations are with unexplained iron-deficiency anaemia, diarrhoea, abdominal bloating, non-specific abdominal symptoms, fatigue and general malaise. Less commonly, patients present with vitamin D or folate deficiency or dermatitis herpetiformis. The disease may mimic many other conditions or may be unmasked by acute intercurrent illness. There are associations with type I diabetes, autoimmune thyroid disease and osteopenia. In the long term, there is a predisposition to carcinoma of the oropharynx and oesophagus and small-bowel lymphoma. It is largely a disease of Caucasians; estimates of incidence vary widely between one per 100 and one per 2000, depending on the criteria used. Screening by antibody tests (tissue transglutaminase (tTG) is the antigen previously identified by anti-endomysial antibody) is 90 per cent sensitive and specific, but an associated immunoglobulin A (IgA) deficit may cause misleading results and it may be necessary to request immunoglobulin G (IgG) antibodies to gliadin or tTG specifically. Confirmation of the diagnosis depends on small-bowel biopsy and response to a gluten-free diet. Most cases enjoy a return to normal health when sources of gluten are excluded from the diet, although relapse is easily induced by dietary indiscretion or inadvertent consumption of gluten. The diagnosis in trained aircrew is compatible with an unrestricted flying category once symptoms have resolved and education is complete. However, the peripatetic lifestyle of most military and civil aircrew does make dietary compliance more difficult, and this is exacerbated by more prolonged military deployments during conflicts. Even in these circumstances, motivation in aviators is usually sufficient to ensure freedom from relapse. Regular follow-up is appropriate.

GASTROINTESTINAL INFECTIONS RELATED TO TRAVEL

Estimates of the number of people who cross international boundaries every year vary widely, but it is agreed by all that the number continues to increase after a temporary decline following the terrorist events of 11 September 2001. Notwithstanding these events, the majority of travellers do so by air, and for the general public the unit of distance between continents is hours' flight time by jet airliner. Thus, a large number of people are potentially exposed within a short period to enteropathogens of a different geographical location for which they are immunologically unprepared. Additionally, acute gastroenteritis has been long been recognized as one of the most common causes of incapacitation of flight crews; their peripatetic lifestyle undoubtedly adds to the baseline risk, although this may subsequently be reduced by frequent travel and development of immunity.

Travellers' diarrhoea is defined as three or more unformed stools each day during or after a journey, or any number of such stools accompanied by fever, cramping abdominal pain or vomiting. The major risk factors are destination and mode of travel. Travel between developed countries is of low risk, whereas travel from Europe or the USA to Asia, Africa or South America carries high risk. The aircrew member who uses transit hotel accommodation is at less risk than the backpacker who travels overland and eats in local facilities. Although disturbance of bowel habit may result from the changes in diet, routine and climate that are inevitable with travel and possibly from stress or anxiety in some flyers, most episodes of diarrhoea or vomiting in travellers result from intestinal infection.

The pattern of pathogens is related closely to the spectrum that is endemic in the destination country. Worldwide, the most common infectious agent isolated is enterotoxigenic *Escherichia coli* (ETEC), the highest rates being in Africa and Central America. *Shigella* infections are also relatively common in these areas. *Campylobacter* is identified more often in travellers to Asia, while *Giardia* is identified in parts of Eastern Europe. About ten per cent of infections are due to viruses, commonly the rotavirus and Norwalk viruses.

Individuals at high risk include those at the extremes of age, those with reduced stomach acidity (following gastric surgery, taking histamine H_2-receptor antagonists or proton-pump inhibitors) and those with immune deficiency. Travellers are advised to avoid uncooked foods, especially salads, to take care with drinking-water sources, including ice and ice-cream, and to avoid unpeeled fruit and vegetables. They should also be aware of the risks of ingesting water in swimming pools and even seawater in contaminated areas. Flight crews should be advised to choose different items from in-flight catering selections and restaurant menus, or even to eat at different restaurants. For people at high personal risk or those of critical mission importance, drug treatment for both prophylaxis and treatment may be indicated. Antibiotics, e.g. ciprofloxacin, are effective in shortening attacks, but at the expense of (minor) side effects (De Bruyn *et al.* 2000). For control of diarrhoea, loperamide is preferred, particularly in aircrew, for its lack of central nervous system effects.

LIVER DISEASE

Despite ongoing debate about the scientific merit of such policies, regular biochemical screening is still undertaken in many areas of the aviation industry, both for recruits and for trained personnel. Abnormalities of liver tests are common in this situation, and subsequent aeromedical disposal is a frequent cause of debate. Minor elevations of bilirubin ($< 70\,\mu mol/l$) occur in up to six per cent of the population and, in the absence of abnormalities of liver enzymes or evidence of haemolysis, may confidently be attributed to Gilbert's syndrome. This is commonly due to an abnormality of glucuronyl-transferase and the abnormality becomes more obvious with fasting or intercurrent infection. Patients and their medical advisors can be reassured that the condition is of no clinical significance. Isolated elevation of gamma-glucuronyl-transferase (GGT) is likely to result from enzyme induction, and ingestion of alcohol is a probable cause if the mixed corpuscular volume (MCV) is raised. If alkaline phosphatase (ALP) and GGT are both raised, then full investigation for cholestasis or hepatic infiltration is merited. Elevation of ALP alone is rarely hepatic in origin. If transaminase levels (alanine aminotransferase, ALT; aspartate aminotransferase, AST) are elevated significantly for any duration, then they require investigation. High levels (in the thousands) are seen in viral and drug-induced hepatitis, occasionally in cholangitis. The more common moderate elevations seen in asymptomatic populations will require exclusion of chronic viral hepatitis, disorders of iron and copper metabolism, and autoimmune hepatitis by appropriate blood tests. In the absence of a specific aetiology, liver ultrasound will commonly reveal increased parenchymal echogenicity, indicating fatty liver. Liver biopsy may be required if there is diagnostic doubt or a need to assess severity or progress of chronic liver disease but is not usually warranted with non-progressive, isolated, mild or moderate abnormalities of ALT or AST.

Hepatitis

Acute hepatitis A and E are enterically transmitted diseases with similar features, in that the clinical course is an acute self-limiting hepatitis that does not progress to chronic liver disease or a chronic carrier state. Although acute illness and convalescence may be disabling for several weeks, the importance of these conditions in the aeromedical context derives from the need to distinguish them from the causes of chronic hepatitis that have longer-lasting implications for aircrew fitness. The most common causes of chronic hepatitis are viral infections (hepatitis B and C), autoimmune hepatitis and drug reactions. Far less common are alpha-1-antitrypsin deficiency and Wilson's disease; haemochromatosis is discussed separately.

Worldwide, most patients with chronic hepatitis B are infected in childhood, although in some societies infection by the intravenous route is more common. The small percentage of patients who develop chronic disease after acute infection in adult life are usually men and commonly are immunocompromised. Chronic hepatitis B is sometimes asymptomatic, but general malaise, fatigue, arthralgia and right hypochondrial discomfort may proceed to hepatic decompensation or acute flare-ups of hepatitis. Later complications of cirrhosis, portal hypertension and hepatocellular carcinoma add to the aeromedical concerns.

Treatment with interferon-alfa and lamivudine is effective in some patients, but the side effects of the former and the treatment duration of the latter make them unsuitable for aircrew. As with other infectious diseases, real or perceived risks of infectivity will concern the employing authority in both military and public transport arenas. Modern assessment of antigen and antibody status, and their combinations, allows appropriate guidance to be offered.

Acute hepatitis C infection resolves completely (clearance of hepatitis C virus (HCV)-RNA from serum) in 15–40 per cent of those infected. The acute disease is often mild, and only 25 per cent of patients are icteric. Progression to chronic infection incurs the potential for development of cirrhosis, portal hypertension and hepatocellular carcinoma. In some parts of the world there is a high population prevalence, but in others the acquisition of infection is often associated with lifestyle practices, e.g. injecting drug use, or other health problems, e.g. haemodialysis. With antiviral treatment, e.g. pegylated interferon-alfa and ribavirin, viral clearance can be achieved in 30–56 per cent of patients with chronic hepatitis C (Brooks and Rosenberg 2002). Aircrew will require grounding during the initial treatment, mainly because of the potential side effects of interferon; after one month of treatment, if there are no adverse problems, then they can fly with a dual restriction. When HCV-polymerase chain reaction (PCR) is negative, they can return to unrestricted flying, subject to careful follow-up surveillance.

Autoimmune hepatitis

Autoimmune hepatitis (Ben-Ari and Czaja 2001) may be acute or, more commonly, chronic in presentation. It is associated with hyperglobulinaemia and other autoimmune disorders and, characteristically, with specific autoantibodies of three groups: (i) anti-nuclear antibodies (ANA) and smooth-muscle antibodies (SMA), (ii) anti-liver-kidney microsomal antibodies (anti-LKM), and (iii) anti-soluble liver antigen/liver pancreas antibody (anti-SLA/LP). The condition has a peak incidence in the age group 20–40 years and, therefore, is seen in the aviation environment. It affects women more commonly than men. Presentation ranges from insidious, with malaise, anorexia and fatigue, to fulminant, resembling acute viral or drug-induced hepatitis. Liver biopsy is needed to confirm the diagnosis (occasionally revealing it unexpectedly) and is used to monitor severity. The mainstay of treatment is immunosuppression with steroids and/or azathioprine.

Patients who can be stabilized on low-dose treatment (< 10 mg prednisolone daily, or azathioprine alone) may be fit for limited flying duties.

Other causes of hepatitis

Wilson's disease, an inherited disorder of copper metabolism, may present as hepatic, neurological or psychiatric disease. It is relevant to aviation medicine because it can present at any age, hepatic presentations are very varied and, rarely, the only feature may be an asymptomatic disturbance of serum aminotransferases in young men. Diagnosis is based on measurements of serum caeruloplasmin and urinary copper excretion, with liver biopsy often providing final confirmation. Life-long treatment with chelating agents is required. Side effects of treatment and concern about neuropsychiatric features of the condition usually preclude aviation activities. Alpha-1-antitrypsin deficiency is occasionally the cause of liver disease in young adults (Alpha-1 Association, www.alpha1.org/education/liver.asp). It is the most common genetic cause of liver disease in children, but in adults it more commonly manifests as emphysema. Delayed presentation of the liver disease as unexplained elevations of liver enzymes or cryptogenic cirrhosis may occur in the aviation population. The prognosis for this mode of presentation is relatively good, but in the absence of effective treatment (apart from transplantation) the aviation career implications are adverse.

Haemochromatosis

The classic description of haemochromatosis as a rare metabolic disease (bronze diabetes), has given way to an appreciation that this condition has a very common genetic basis, albeit with a low phenotypic penetrance. The development of complications comprising liver disease progressing to cirrhosis, cardiomyopathy, skin pigmentation, arthropathy and various endocrine disorders can be prevented by simple, cheap and safe treatment with venesection. The diagnosis can be made at an early stage. It is a disease of young adults, with men being affected at an earlier age than women because of the protective effect of iron loss related to reproductive function.

Haemochromatosis was recognized as a familial disorder in 1955 (Finch and Finch 1955). In 1996, the responsible gene (*HFE*) was isolated on chromosome 6p (Feder *et al.* 1996). Ninety per cent of cases of typical haemochromatosis are associated with homozygous substitution of tyrosine for cysteine (*C282Y*) at position 282 of the HFE protein. Another mutation at position 63 changes histidine to aspartic acid (*H63D*), but this appears to be associated with iron overload only in individuals who are compound heterozygotes for *C282Y* and *H63D*.

The disease may be defined in the aviation community following detection of minor abnormalities of liver function tests (LFTs) or, less commonly, during the assessment of impotence, arthralgia or general malaise. The diagnosis is made by elevations of transferrin saturation and raised ferritin levels. Confirmation with genotyping for *C282Y* and *H63D* is widely available, but these tests are positive in only 85 per cent of cases. Rarer abnormalities of the transferrin-receptor gene and ferroportin gene cause some cases, and there are presumed to be other, undefined, genetic polymorphisms. Although one in 300 of a Western population is homozygous for *C282Y*, only a minority of these individuals have iron overload. Some of this variation is known to be influenced by environmental factors, particularly alcohol and dietary overload, as well as blood loss, notably menstruation. Because of these factors, management of the disease should be based on clinical indicators. Early diagnosis is important, because the prognosis in patients detected before the onset of major organ damage and who receive treatment with regular phlebotomy approaches that of the normal population. Removal of excess iron is achieved by phlebotomy of 500 ml blood (200–250 mg iron) once or twice a week until serum ferritin is in the low normal range; this is then maintained by phlebotomy every few months.

It is now commonplace for trained aircrew to continue in unrestricted duties once treatment is stabilized. They are usually advised not to fly for 48 hours after having blood removed.

Alcohol and the liver and non–alcoholic steatohepatitis

Alcohol is the most common cause of liver injury in the Western world, and increasing consumption in young people suggests that death and disablement from alcoholic hepatitis and cirrhosis will continue to increase. Although the aviation community is generally health-conscious, the combination of youth, travel, work away from home, social opportunity, high disposable income and, in some circumstances, cultural pressures mean that alcoholic liver disease is not rare. Indeed, in the common circumstance of asymptomatic abnormalities of LFTs, alcohol is often the first suspected diagnosis. However, a proper index of suspicion for other causes of chronic hepatitis should be maintained, and haemochromatosis and non-alcoholic steatohepatitis (NASH) are common alternatives. NASH is now the most common cause of persistent isolated elevation of liver enzymes (usually ALT) without obvious other cause in the general population. It is relatively less common, but still frequent, in the aviation community. The concept was introduced in 1980 to define a condition that is histologically similar to alcoholic liver disease but in which alcohol per se is not implicated. NASH is associated with obesity, insulin resistance/type II diabetes, hyperlipidaemia and hypertension (the metabolic syndrome). The red blood cell (RBC) MCV is usually normal in NASH, in contrast to alcoholic liver disease, where it is frequently raised. In the long term, a proportion of people progress to cirrhosis and liver cancer, and it is probably responsible for the majority of so-called cryptogenic cirrhosis. Treatment advice that addresses the likely causative factors, i.e. weight reduction, lowering of serum lipids, exercise and medication to reduce insulin resistance, is especially appropriate in the context of aviation medicine.

GALLSTONES

Biliary colic is the only specific symptom of uncomplicated gallbladder disease. It occurs in less than ten per cent of individuals with gallstones. However, it manifests in an unpredictable fashion as sudden onset, incapacitating, severe epigastric or right hypochondrial pain lasting several hours, often associated with nausea and vomiting. This determines the aeromedical disposition facilitated by the availability and accuracy of ultrasound diagnosis. Asymptomatic large stones, discovered fortuitously, may be considered safe, but multiple small stones, particularly with a history of previous cholecystitis or biliary colic, have an unacceptable chance of producing incapacitation. In such cases, cholecystectomy will allow a return to full flying duties after recovery from surgery.

PANCREATITIS

Acute pancreatitis is commonly related to gallstones, alcohol use or congenital abnormalities of the gland and its ducts, but the list of other possible aetiologies is extensive. It is a serious illness, truly incapacitating in the acute phase, with a mortality approaching ten per cent. The likelihood of recurrence is related to the cause. Full recovery after an episode related to calculi in the biliary tree, and following cholecystectomy, may be compatible with a return to unrestricted aircrew duties. However, all other causes are likely to require a restriction to limited, multi-crew flying at best. Recurrent or chronic pancreatitis will usually lead to permanent grounding.

REFERENCES

Bebb J, James MW, Atherton J. Gastritis and peptic ulcer. *Medicine International* 2003; **Gastroenterology** (part 1): 15–18.

Ben-Ari Z, Czaja AJ. Autoimmune hepatitis and its variant syndromes. *Gut* 2001; **49**: 589–94.

Bernell O, Lapidus A, Hellers G. Risk factors for surgery and recurrence in 907 patients with primary ileocaecal Crohn's disease. *British Journal of Surgery* 2000; **87**: 1697–701.

Brooks CL, Rosenberg WM. Assessment and management of chronic hepatitis C infection. *Clinical Medicine* 2002; **2**: 302–6.

De Bruyn G, Hahn S, Borwick A. Antibiotic treatment for travellers diarrhoea. *Cochrane Database Systematic Review* 2000; **3**: CD002242.

Feder JN, Gnirke A, Thomas W, *et al.* A novel MHC class I-like gene is mutated in patients with hereditary haemochromatosis. *Nature Genetics* 1996; **13**: 399–408.

Finch SC, Finch CA. Idiopathic hemochromatosis, an iron storage disease. *Medicine* 1955; **34**: 381–430.

Jewell DP. Crohn's Disease. *Medicine International* 2003; **Gastroenterology** (part 2): 76–81.

McCaughlin J. Irritable bowel syndrome. *Medicine International* 2003; **Gastroenterology** (part 3): 88–90.

Talley NJ, Spiller R. Irritable bowel syndrome: a little understood organic bowel disease? *Lancet* 2002; **360**: 555–64.

Travis S. Ulcerative colitis. *Medicine International* 2003; **Gastroenterology** (part 2): 71–5.

41

Metabolic and endocrine disorders

RAYMOND V. JOHNSTON

DIABETES MELLITUS

Diabetes mellitus commonly affects approximately three per cent of the population (Bennettt *et al.* 1995). The prevalence increases with age. Data from the Oxford Community Diabetes study (Neil *et al.* 1987) are shown in Figure 41.1. The current terminology for the classification of diabetes mellitus is type 1, previously called insulin-dependent diabetes mellitus (IDDM), and type 2, formally known as non-insulin-dependent diabetes mellitus (NIDDM). This change in terminology is now used to reflect the greater use of insulin to improve control in NIDDM. These individuals are treated with insulin but are not truly insulin-dependent. Approximately 20 per cent of diabetic people are insulin-dependent and 80 per cent non-insulin-dependent.

Type 1 diabetes mellitus presents in the younger age group. The prevalence shows striking geographical variation. It is some 35 times more common in Finland than in Japan. Within the UK, the highest frequency is found in Scotland, where, as in several other countries, the incidence appears to have doubled within a decade. The basic problem in type 1 diabetes is insulin deficiency due to autoimmune destruction of the islet beta cells of the pancreas, which is determined partially by heredity. The genetic component of type 1, however, is less important than in type 2.

Type 2 diabetes mellitus is common. Its prevalence increases with age, inactivity and body weight. For example, in the USA, the prevalence is 4.3 per cent in white women aged between 45 and 54 years, rising to 8.9 per cent in those aged between 65 and 74 years. In type 2, raised fasting insulin levels are a response to fasting hyper-

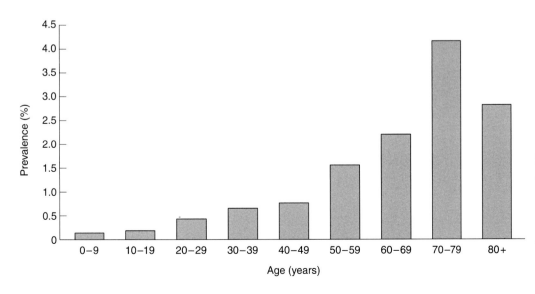

Figure 41.1 *Age-specific prevalence of diagnosed diabetes in the Oxford Community Diabetes Study (Neil et al. 1987). Reproduced with kind permission of Diabetes UK.*

glycaemia, but are inappropriately low for the abnormal blood glucose concentration. After eating a meal, the insulin response is poor, and so glucose concentrations go higher still and continue to stimulate further insulin secretion long after physiological insulin and glucose profiles have returned to basal levels.

Therapeutic options

DIET

The modern recommended diet for type 2 diabetes is free from refined carbohydrates but complex high-fibre carbohydrates are encouraged. It is low in fat and energy-restricted for obese people, but isocaloric with the existing diet for people of normal weight.

ORAL HYPOGLYCAEMIC AGENTS

If diet fails to control the diabetes, then the next therapeutic option is oral hypoglycaemic agents. The largest group of oral hypoglycaemic agents in clinical use are the sulphonylureas, but their use is best reserved for non-obese patients. The second major group are the biguanides, which are more appropriate for overweight patients. The main problem with sulphonylurea drugs is hypoglycaemia, which can be fairly prolonged with the long-acting preparation chlorpropamide. The prevalence of hypoglycaemia with sulphonylurea drugs in one study was approximately 20 per cent (Jennings *et al.* 1989). This is unacceptable in professional flying.

The only biguanide drug available is metformin since the withdrawal of phenformin some years ago due to the high incidence of lactic acidosis. Metformin has predominantly peripheral actions in lowering blood glucose and, to some extent, assists weight loss. The risks of lactic acidosis with metformin are minimal, but the drug should not be prescribed in the presence of hepatic or renal disease. An additional therapeutic option is the alpha-glycosidase inhibitors, e.g. acarbose, which inhibit digestion of glucose-containing polysaccharides from the gut. These may have a therapeutic role as an adjuvant to diet or oral hypoglycaemic therapy.

More recently, a new class of agents, the thiazolidine-diones (glitazones), has become available. These are interesting because they target the underlying problem in type 2 diabetes, i.e. insulin resistance, by enhancing insulin sensitivity. There is some evidence that this class of drug may have a beneficial effect on pancreatic beta-cell function, but this awaits confirmation by long-term well-controlled clinical trials. Until recently, the glitazones were licensed in Europe only for use in combination with sulfonylureas or metformin. These agents are now available for monotherapy, and long-term trials are awaited from the USA, where they have been used in this way for some time.

Control and complications

The reports of the Diabetes Control and Complications Trial research group (1993) in type 1 diabetes have shown that tight diabetic control may minimize the risk of microvascular disease and, possibly, the incidence of macrovascular complications. In type 2 diabetes, the UK Prospective Diabetes Study group (UKPDS 1998a) has shown that among patients allocated intensive blood-glucose control, there was a significant reduction in any diabetes-related endpoint, all-cause mortality and stroke. The effect was greatest in patients treated with metformin. The main parameter used in the assessment of quality of diabetic control is glycosylated haemoglobin. The percentage of glycosylated haemoglobin averaged over six to eight weeks is a useful measure of blood glucose control.

The phrase 'good metabolic control' encompasses other parameters in addition to glucose and haemoglobin A1 (HbA1) (Table 41.1). In order to achieve good metabolic

Table 41.1 *Targets for metabolic control*

Parameter	Unit	Good	Acceptable	Poor	Very poor
BMI	kg/m^2	< 25	25–27	> 27	–
HbA1 (normal 5.0–7.5)	%	< 7.5	7.5–8.8	> 8.8	> 10.0
HbA1c (normal 4.0–6.0)	%	< 6.0	6.0–7.0	> 7.0	> 8.0
Blood glucose:					
Fasting	mmol/l	< 6.7	< 8.01	> 10.0	–
Random	mmol/l	4.0–9.0	< 10.0	> 10.0	–
Total cholesterol	mmol/l	< 4.5	< 5.2	> 6.5	–
LDL cholesterol	mmol/l	< 2.5	< 3.0	> 3.5	–
HDL cholesterol	mmol/l	> 1.1	> 0.9	< 0.9	–
Triglyceride	mmol/l	< 1.7	< 2.0	> 2.2	–
Blood pressure	mmHg	< 130/80	< 145/95	> 160/95	–

BMI, body mass index; HbA1, haemoglobin A1; HbA1c, haemoglobin A1c; HDL, high-density lipoprotein; LDL, high-density lipoprotein.

control, it is important to set the patient realistic targets; the physician and other healthcare professionals should support the individual in the achievement of these goals with practical advice. The pilot population is particularly well motivated, and with appropriate guidance and under certain therapeutic and metabolic circumstances, may continue to fly.

Aeromedical implications of diabetes mellitus

The aim of medical certification is to reduce the medical component of human factors that may contribute to aircraft accidents to an acceptable level of risk. In the UK, the acceptable level of sudden or subtle incapacitation in professional pilots is one per cent per annum. Up to that figure, a professional pilot with a specific disease process that may cause incapacitation may return to flying in a multicrew situation. This approach is useful in diabetic pilots.

The risks in diabetic pilots may be divided into those intrinsic to diabetes mellitus itself and those that are iatrogenic due to therapeutic intervention in the disease process. The main risks intrinsic to the disease process are of cardiovascular disease, visual problems and nephropathy. The only significant iatrogenic complication with profound implications in aviation is hypoglycaemia. Having assessed the risk, how does one develop a certification policy? The simple approach would be to disqualify all diabetic pilots. However, a more scientific approach can be developed from a cautious literature review, which can then be applied to the diabetic population and audited over time. In this section, we summarize the literature and discuss the development of certification guidelines based on that literature.

CARDIOVASCULAR DISEASE

Premature vascular disease is one of the most common and serious complications of diabetes. The Whitehall Study showed that coronary heart disease mortality was approximately doubled for people with impaired glucose tolerance in a standard glucose tolerance test (Fuller et al. 1980). Data from a number of studies suggest that the risk of cardiovascular disease is two to four times higher in patients with diabetes compared with those without, and that the annual rate of fatal and non-fatal cardiovascular disease among patients with type 2 diabetes is 2.5 per cent (Entmacher et al. 1964). The risk of cardiovascular disease is high, even at the time of diagnosis, and is independent of the duration of diagnosed diabetes, because diabetes is present for approximately 7–12 years before formal diagnosis. Perhaps even before that time, patients would be classified as having impaired glucose tolerance, which is associated with an increased risk of cardiovascular disease (Fuller et al. 1980).

NEPHROPATHY

Kidney disease is a significant problem in the diabetic population. Nephropathy affects approximately 35 per cent of patients with type 1 diabetes and about five to ten per cent of patients with type 2 diabetes. Despite this lower prevalence, the impact of renal disease caused by type 2 diabetes is substantially greater, since type 2 is far more common, and cardiovascular complications are the major cause of death in these patients. The importance in identifying those at risk of developing nephropathy in potential or active aircrew lies in the findings that in type 1 patients with proteinuria, the relative mortality from cardiovascular disease is almost 40 times that of the general population. In patients without proteinuria, the relative cardiovascular mortality is only four times that of non-diabetic people (Borch-Johnson and Krenier 1987). Thus, the presence of nephropathy is a marker for cardiovascular disease. There is evidence that the presence of microalbuminuria (defined as urinary albumin excretion greater than 30 mg but less than 300 mg per 24 hours) may predict, with some accuracy, the development of diabetic nephropathy. There is also evidence that therapeutic intervention in type 1 diabetics with angiotensin-converting enzyme (ACE) inhibitors may halt this progression (Viberti et al. 1994). More recently, treatment with ACE inhibitors in patients with type 2 diabetes with microalbuminuria has been shown to reduce cardiovascular events by 25 per cent in both those with normal creatinine levels and in those with mild renal insufficiency (Mann et al. 2001). The Type 2 Diabetes, Hypertension, Cardiovascular Events and Ramipril (DIABHYCAR) study has shown, however, that the benefit of the ACE inhibitor ramipril in type 2 diabetes is dose-dependent (Marre et al. 2004). The measurement of microalbuminuria is a useful adjuvant to risk assessment in diabetic pilots.

VISUAL PROBLEMS

Approximately 80 per cent of flight information is accrued visually and, thus, any pathological process that interferes with visual function may result in human error and may contribute to an accident. Diabetes mellitus is known to affect all parts of the eye, e.g. cataract, retinal vein occlusion, ischaemic optic neuritis and cranial nerve palsies resulting in diplopia. Diabetic retinopathy, however, is a highly specific vascular complication of diabetes mellitus and is estimated to be the most frequent cause of new blindness among adults between the ages of 20 and 74 years. By 20 years after the first diagnosis, almost all insulin-dependent patients and more than 60 per cent of non-insulin-dependent patients have some degree of retinopathy (Klein et al. 1984). More than four-fifths of cases of blindness among type 1 diabetes patients and one-third of cases among type 2 diabetes patients are due to diabetic retinopathy. Many people forget that type 2 diabetes is not a benign disease, and it has been called a 'wolf in sheep's clothing'. The major determinants for the development of retinopathy are the quality of diabetic control and the duration of the diabetes.

HYPOGLYCAEMIA

Hypoglycaemia leads to a combination of neuroglycopenia and autonomic neural stimulation. This is characterized by faintness, tremor, sweating, hunger and coma. Any of these symptom complexes may degrade pilot performance. A study carried out in type 1 diabetes patients subjected to modest hypoglycaemia of 3.1 mmol/l showed a decrement in performance, which increased with the complexity of the task performed (Holmes et al. 1986). In this and other studies, researchers have shown that reaction times do not return to normal until some 20–30 minutes after euglycaemia has been restored. The implications in the aviation environment are self-evident.

Having accepted that hypoglycaemia is a significant concern in the aviation environment, it is vitally important for accurate risk assessment to have good data on the incidence of hypoglycaemia in both insulin- and non-insulin-dependent patients.

It is very difficult to assess the frequency of hypoglycaemia in insulin-treated diabetic populations because of the wide variation in severity and outcome. Another problem is the common occurrence of asymptomatic biochemical hypoglycaemia, which is evident only if blood glucose is measured frequently, and the failure to recognize or record many mild episodes, including those that occur during sleep. Severe hypoglycaemia, defined by the need for external assistance to resuscitate the patient, is a more robust and consistent measure for estimating frequency and is reliable even in retrospective reporting. Where a similar definition for severe hypoglycaemia has been applied, the lowest annual prevalence is nine per cent, but the average is approximately 20–30 per cent. Despite the difficulties in assessment, the frequency of mild hypoglycaemia in one good study was alarmingly high at 1.6 episodes per patient per week, i.e. approximately 83.6 episodes per patient per year (Praming et al. 1991).

Strict glycaemic control, usually from intensive insulin therapy, is recognized to be a risk factor for severe hypoglycaemia. In the Diabetes Control and Complications Trial, strict glycaemic control was associated with a three-fold increase in severe hypoglycaemia (Diabetes Control and Complications Trial Research Group 1993). The risk of severe hypoglycaemia increased continuously with lower monthly glycosylated haemoglobin values. Other risk factors for severe hypoglycaemia in the study were a longer duration of diabetes and a history of previous hypoglycaemia. Another worrying finding from this group was that no warning symptoms were experienced in 36 per cent of severe hypoglycaemic episodes that occurred while patients were awake. While loss of hypoglycaemic awareness is associated with strict diabetic control, it is also a complication acquired with increasing duration of diabetes, which may underline the emergence of age and duration of diabetes as risk factors for severe hypoglycaemia.

Type 2 diabetics can be managed on diet, diet and sulfonylureas, diet and biguanides, or diet and a combination of sulfonylurea and biguanide, and may be treated with insulin. In addition, the glitazones may be added to biguanide or metformin and, in this context, may cause hypoglycaemia, although this is not the case if used as monotherapy. The alpha-glycosidase inhibitors may potentiate the hypoglycaemic effect of a sulphonylurea. Severe hypoglycaemia associated with sulphonylureas is well documented, but the frequency of mild hypoglycaemia not requiring urgent hospital admission is more difficult to assess because symptoms are often brief and many patients treated with oral agents have poor knowledge of the symptoms of hypoglycaemia. Despite these difficulties, trials have recorded an incidence of symptomatic hypoglycaemia ranging from 1.9 to seven per cent per annum. The study by Jennings et al. (1989), as noted previously, found a prevalence of symptomatic hypoglycaemia of the order of 20 per cent when using direct questioning of the patients and the relatives. More recent data from the UK Prospective Diabetic Study (1998b) found the incidence of hypoglycaemia in type 2 diabetics on sulphonylureas to be ten per cent per annum overall, with that of major episodes being 1.5 per cent per annum. Since the withdrawal of phenformin in the early 1970s due to the incidence of metabolic acidosis, the only biguanide in use in the UK is metformin. Its mechanism of action does not involve the stimulation of insulin secretion and it does not cause hypoglycaemia. The incidence of metabolic acidosis is negligible but has been recorded as 0.04 cases per 1000 patient-years, with a mortality of 0.024 per 1000 patient-years (Berger 1985).

In summary, therefore, the sulphonylureas carry a risk of hypoglycaemia that lies outside the set limit of one per cent per annum proposed by the UK Civil Aviation Authority (CAA) and adopted by the European Joint Aviation Authorities (JAA). Metformin does not cause hypoglycaemia, and its risk of metabolic acidosis is acceptable in appropriately selected pilots.

Aeromedical disposal of civil pilots with diabetes mellitus

The prime determinant in declining certification to type 1 diabetic pilots and type 2 diabetic pilots on insulin is the unacceptable risk of hypoglycaemia. Other concerns in this group are the increase in coronary heart disease and the associated problems of retinopathy and nephropathy.

Since type 2 diabetes usually presents in the middle years, the majority of pilots with this type of diabetes are usually fully trained and may have a command. The airline is usually supportive of the pilot in this situation, as they do not wish to lose a trained individual. It is, thus, important that any aviation authority has a credible and sound certification policy to assess risk in this group.

Hypoglycaemia is not an issue in the risk assessment of pilots with diet-controlled diabetes, the main area of concern being the vascular complications. If a pilot with diet-controlled diabetes is to be returned to flying and their fitness status maintained, then it is vitally important that they are screened for coronary disease. The gold standard for diagnosing coronary artery disease is coronary angiography. However, this is not without risk, and it is not feasible to repeat on a regular basis. The resting electrocardiogram (ECG) alone lacks the sensitivity and specificity required in this group of higher-risk patients, and thus it is logical to use a non-invasive technique that will predict coronary artery disease at somewhat greater sensitivity than the resting tracing. The exercise ECG is a useful screening tool in this selected group of patients. It is not of value for widespread screening, as the prevalence of coronary artery disease in the otherwise healthy pilot population overall is low. If the exercise ECG is normal, then a diet-only-controlled diabetic pilot with good-quality control and no overt complications may return to flying, subject to an annual assessment with an exercise ECG and a satisfactory report from the treating diabetic physician. The alpha-glucosidase inhibitor acarbose is acceptable as an adjuvant to diet and will not affect decisions on certification.

A similar certification policy applies in this group to pilots whose diabetes is controlled by diet alone. However, those pilots treated with metformin tend to be overweight and do carry a small but acceptable risk of lactic acidosis and, thus, their overall risk is slightly greater than diet-only patients. Their assessment requires exemplary diabetic control and annual review, including an exercise ECG; if this is satisfactory, they may be returned to flying in the multi-crew situation. This approach is in line with the Scottish Intercollegiate Guidelines Network (SIGN) guidelines for the risk assessment of diabetic cardiovascular disease.

The incidence of hypoglycaemia in diabetics treated with the sulfonylureas does not meet the one per cent per annum level, as described previously, and thus these pilots are not acceptable for recertification in commercial operations. Pilots managed by metformin and a glitazone are not acceptable for certification, because hypoglycaemia is described as 'common' in the relevant drug data sheet. The situation with glitazones as monotherapy has not yet been clarified by the certification authorities, but in principle this approach would be acceptable in people intolerant of metformin.

Aeromedical disposal of military pilots with diabetes mellitus

Candidates with either diabetes mellitus or impaired glucose tolerance are unfit for selection for military service. Those who subsequently develop disorders of glucose metabolism are subjected to more stringent certification restriction than civil airline or private pilots. Impaired glucose tolerance does not disqualify trained personnel from aircrew duties, but frequent medical review is required because of the risk of progression to frank diabetes. Diabetes responsive to diet or biguanides is compatible with continued aircrew duties, but with a reduced medical category, unfit solo pilot/navigator and subject to regular medical review. Diabetes requiring insulin or sulfonylurea therapy renders the individual permanently unfit for aircrew duties.

Conclusion

The key to certification of this group of aircrew is to base policy on robust, good-quality scientific data which have been subjected to peer review. The aviation physician must liaise closely with the endocrinologist looking after the member of aircrew, so that the benefits of both disciplines can be consolidated, resulting in the fair and objective assessment of the pilot. Military operations make greater demands on the individual, both operationally and physiologically, and criteria for both initial flying training and subsequent possible return to aviation duties will be more stringent. All policies for medical certification of aircrew should be audited in the light of developments in world literature, and modified accordingly.

ENDOCRINE DISORDERS

The endocrine system is controlled by the hypothalamus, which is subject to regulatory influences from other parts of the brain, especially the limbic system. A number of releasing hormones from the hypothalamus cause stimulating hormones to be released from the anterior pituitary to act on specific end organs. The resulting hormone production from the end organs acts as a complex system of feedback to inhibit further production. In such a finely tuned homeostatic environment, any disturbance of secretion of the trophic hormone or of the end organ itself may result in clinical disease. In aircrew, the most important question the aviation specialist must ask is whether the disease or its treatment will affect performance. It is known that approximately 80 per cent of aviation accidents are due to human factors, and it is vitally important that the aviation physician is familiar with endocrine conditions that may cause sudden or subtle incapacitation and, thus, cause a problem in flight.

Anterior pituitary hypofunction

Hypopituitarism may be partial or complete and may result from either pituitary disease or hypothalamic disease resulting in a failure of the releasing hormone. Clinical manifestations vary depending on the extent and severity of the pituitary hormone deficiency. Thus, a patient may present in extremis with acute adrenal insufficiency or profound hypothyroidism, or with rather non-specific symptoms of fatigue or malaise, which could be labelled 'jet lag' or 'crew fatigue'.

AEROMEDICAL DISPOSAL

Hypopituitarism is treatable, and the patient should be able to perform normal activities as long as appropriate hormonal therapy is used consistently and properly. Once the appropriate regimen has been determined, with appropriate laboratory backup, the doses do not need to be changed, except for an increase in the glucocorticoid dose (which is generally doubled) during intermittent illness. Even after the proper regimen has been stabilized, lifelong follow-up by a specialist in endocrinology is required.

The implications for aviation are self-evident. In the military sphere, the requirement for instant transition to war, with all the adverse demands that makes, precludes these patients from service. In commercial aviation, the possibility of not having replacement drugs taken 'consistently and properly' and intermittent illness away from specialized help would preclude professional medical certification, as would concerns on the cardiovascular disease risk. Private pilots may be suitable for certification, endorsed with a safety pilot limitation, subject to satisfactory specialist reports and annual follow-up.

Anterior pituitary hyperfunction

Most syndromes of hyperfunction are due to pituitary tumours. The particular syndrome will depend on which cell type in the pituitary is involved.

ACROMEGALY

This diagnosis is made from the classic clinical features and confirmed by raised basal growth hormone levels on two or more occasions (> 5 mU/l). Growth hormone stimulates the production of insulin-like growth factor 1 (IGF-1), predominantly in the liver. IGF-1 can be used to assess disease activity, since, unlike growth hormone, the levels do not fluctuate throughout the day. Any pilot with a growth-hormone-

secreting tumour producing symptoms is unfit for flying duties. After treatment, the individual must be reviewed carefully to assess the efficacy of the treatment. Those with gross physical changes that do not regress are unlikely to be fit for professional or private certification. Specialist endocrinological and ophthalmic review would be required before any assessment by the aeromedical authority.

HYPERPROLACTINAEMIA

Prolactinomas are the most common functional pituitary adenomas and account for approximately 25 per cent of asymptomatic pituitary adenomas diagnosed at post mortem. The diagnosis is confirmed by raised prolactin levels. A prolactin level greater than 5000 mU/l suggests a prolactinoma, while a level below 2500 mU/l is more likely to be the result of compression of the pituitary stalk by an inactive adenoma. Any individual with an active pituitary tumour or an enlarged fossa is unfit. Many individuals on long-term treatment (except bromocriptine, because of its side effects) or post-curative surgery may be considered for certification after approximately three months. This will be subject to lifelong follow-up on an annual basis from endocrine and ophthalmic specialists. These individuals are unacceptable for military aircrew.

HYPERCORTISOLAEMIA

Cushing's disease, described by Harvey Cushing in 1932, is the term applied to Cushing's syndrome of pituitary origin. The signs and effects are those of excess cortisol production. Screening for Cushing's disease is performed most easily by measuring 24-hour urinary cortisol, increased levels above 280 mmol/day being diagnostic. If this is abnormal, then the dexamethasone suppression test is of value in differentiating between pituitary disease, primary adrenal disease and ectopic adrenocorticotropic hormone (ATCH) production by a tumour, e.g. small-cell bronchogenic carcinoma. Applicants for flying training with active Cushing's disease are unfit. After adequate treatment to suppress the cortisol excess, the patient may be reassessed at one year, with appropriate reports from the treating endocrinologist/neurosurgeon. They are not acceptable for military aircrew duties.

ANTIDIURETIC-HORMONE-DEFICIENCY DIABETES INSIPIDUS

The most marked symptoms are polydypsia and polyuria of greater than 3 l/day. The urine is of low osmolality (< 300 mosmol/kg). The long-acting vasopressin analogue desamino-D-arginine vasopressin (DDAVP) acts almost solely on the type I receptors in the renal tubule and is the mainstay of treatment. There is wide individual variation in the dose required to control symptoms. It is usually given by intranasal spray (5–40μg/day) as one to three doses daily. It can also be given orally in divided doses, and is used in a dose of 50–1200 μg/day. The sulphonylurea chlorpropamide enhances the renal response to antidiuretic hormone (ADH) and in the past was given in partial forms of diabetes insipidus, but it carries a risk of hypoglycaemia and, thus, is no longer used. Aeromedical certification should be on an individual basis, subject to satisfactory endocrinology reports and biochemistry. Military aircrew selection procedures are rather more stringent due to the role of the military pilot, and the need for long-term treatment will preclude selection.

Hypothyroidism

Isolated hypothyroidism beginning in adult life is almost always due to autoimmune thyroid disease or previously treated hyperthyroidism. It is a common condition, and one survey has indicated one per cent of the general population and four per cent of those over 60 years old are on long-term thyroxine (Parle *et al.* 1991). It is more common in females, with a 10–15 fold lower prevalence in males. Frank hypothyroidism requires a temporary unfit aeromedical assessment. Recertification should be possible once the individual is euthyroid on thyroxine. This should be subject to satisfactory endocrinology reports, and the follow-up should be indefinite. This policy is also acceptable in military aircrew.

Hyperthyroidism: thyrotoxicosis

Thyrotoxicosis is common, with a prevalence of one to two per cent in women and 0.1 per cent in men. The most common (70–80 per cent) cause is autoimmune thyroid disease (Grave's disease), although rarely it is due to a multinodular goitre or a single autonomously functioning solitary nodule ('toxic adenoma'). There are three forms of treatment for hyperthyroidism: medical, radioactive iodine and surgical. Only Grave's disease is 'cured' by anti-thyroid drugs, and even then approximately only 50 per cent of patients have a permanent remission. Remission occurs because the drugs notably reduce thyroid hormone synthesis by inhibiting thyroid peroxidase, but they also have an immunomodulatory effect. If the condition relapses, patients may be offered subtotal thyroidectomy. Patients over the age of 40 years are usually given radioactive iodine (^{131}I).

A thyrotoxic pilot is unfit for flying duties until stable euthyroidism has been established and a satisfactory report from the endocrinologist is received. If there have been eye signs, then an ophthalmic assessment is of value in order to establish that there is a good range of eye movement with no diplopia. Anti-thyroid drugs in the absence of side effects are not disqualifying.

Military aircrew may return to limited flying duties once euthyroid. It is possible to return to unrestricted flying after suitable surveillance, but only on the advice of an appropriate specialist. Long-term replacement therapy with thyroxine is compatible with unrestricted flying duties. Treatment with thyroid-suppressant therapy is compatible only with restricted flying duty. Providing the patient is euthyroid post radio-iodine therapy, unrestricted flying is permissible. All patients should remain under lifelong surveillance.

Addison's disease

After full investigation and stable maintenance treatment, an individual with Addison's disease may be considered for recertification in a multi-crew situation. It is unlikely that these individuals would be acceptable for military operations under normal circumstances, and the advice of a military aviation medical specialist should be sought.

Cushing's syndrome

Cushing's syndrome may be due to an adenoma or carcinoma of the adrenal cortex. Excessive alcohol use has also been associated with Cushing's syndrome. The aeromedical disposal needs to be highly individualized on the basis of the underlying lesion and the postoperative result.

Conn's syndrome (mineralocorticoid)

This is found in 0.5–3 per cent of the hypertensive population and presents with mild hypertension and hypokalaemia. It is associated with an adenoma (in approximately 80 per cent of cases) or hyperplasia of the zona glomerulosa of the adrenal glands due to enhanced sensitivity to angiotensin II (Stewart 1999). If an adenoma is demonstrated, the treatment is surgery. If bilateral hyperplasia is present, it is treated with the aldosterone antagonist spironolactone. If an adenoma is diagnosed and removed, this is curative and, thus, aeromedical recertification should not cause a problem, with regular follow-up. If the patient is on long-term spironolactone, amiloride or other medical treatment, then individual assessment is appropriate with full endocrinological reports. It is probable that recertification will be acceptable in a multi-crew situation.

Phaeochromocytoma

This is a rare tumour of the adrenal medulla. The incidence often quoted is 0.1 per cent of cases of hypertension.

Diagnosis is made by measurement of plasma adrenaline/noradrenaline or their many precursors or metabolites, vanillylmandelic acid (VMA), metanephrines and normetanephrines. The excretion may be paroxysmal and, thus, repeated sampling is mandatory. Tumours are localized by computed tomography (CT) or magnetic resonance imaging (MRI) of the abdomen or by scintigraphy.

If the tumour is removed completely, blood-pressure control is satisfactory, and there is no significant end-organ damage, then aeromedical certification should be possible on individual assessment. This may be multi-crew initially. Long-term follow-up is essential.

Calcium metabolism

HYPERCALCAEMIA

Hypercalcaemia may result from a wide range of causes, including vitamin D intoxication, sarcoidosis and malignancy. Endocrine disorders associated with hypercalcaemia are uncommon in aviation medical practice but are included here for the sake of completeness. Hyperparathyroidism is the most common of the parathyroid disorders, with a prevalence of about one in 1000 in the USA. Approximately 80 per cent of cases are associated with a single adenoma. The remaining cases have more than one adenoma or hyperplasia of all four glands. There may be associated multiple endocrine neoplasia. Secondary hyperparathyroidism occurs in chronic renal insufficiency and vitamin D deficiency when the parathyroid hormone (PTH) level rises in response to the hypocalcaemia. It can result in changes in bone mineralization. In some patients, long-standing hypersecretion (in secondary hyperparathyroidism) transforms to inappropriate autonomy and resultant hypercalcaemia. This is termed tertiary hyperparathyroidism, and the parathyroid glands show nodular hyperplasia.

HYPOCALCAEMIA

There are three main conditions that show hypocalcaemia and elevated phosphate in the presence of normal renal function. Idiopathic hypoparathyroidism presents in early adult life and is often associated with antibodies to parathyroid tissue. There may be other associated autoimmune disease, e.g. Addison's disease and autoimmune thyroiditis. Post-surgical hypoparathyroidism is the most common cause of hypocalcaemia, and the prevalence following thyroid or parathyroid surgery varies from 0.2 to two per cent. Pseudo-hypoparathyroidism is a rare condition thought to be due to a defect in the PTH receptor or to its coupling with adenylcyclase (Jüppner 1994). It is characterized by skeletal abnormality and mental deficiency and is unlikely to be encountered in aviation medicine practice.

The aeromedical certification of a member of aircrew with hypo- or hypercalcaemia depends on firstly making a temporarily unfit assessment until the cause is established and definitive management has been completed. The problems range from a well individual who has had a parathyroid adenoma successfully removed and is eucalcaemic and being followed up by their endocrinologist, who would be suitable for certification in all classes, to the individual who has hypercalcaemia secondary to carcinoma, and is not suitable for certification. The key to the certification process are good-quality data and close cooperation between the endocrinologist and the aviation physician.

Disturbances of lipid metabolism

AEROMEDICAL CONCERNS

The major concern with disturbances of lipid metabolism, whether primary or secondary, is accelerated atherogenesis and therefore a potential increase in the risk of sudden cardiovascular incapacity in the aviator.

LIPID METABOLISM

Lipids are not water-soluble and are transported in the blood in association with apoproteins as a lipoprotein complex. These lipoproteins are usually divided into five groups characterized by their ultracentrifugation densities. These are designated chylomicrons, very-low-density lipoproteins (VLDL), intermediate-density lipoproteins (IDL), low-density lipoproteins (LDL) and high-density lipoproteins (HDL). Apoproteins also play an important role in lipoprotein metabolism, by activation of enzymes and acting as receptor ligands.

In general terms, HDL and LDL are the major carriers of cholesterol, while triglycerides are carried on VLDL and chylomicrons. HDL cholesterol constitutes approximately 20–25 per cent of the total cholesterol. HDL lipoproteins are regarded as anti-atherogenic, whereas the major contributor to atherogenicity appears to be LDL. Lipoprotein(a) is a lipoprotein similar to LDL. Its apoprotein, protein(a), resembles plasminogen, and high levels are also proven to be atherogenic.

FAMILIAL HYPERCHOLESTEROLAEMIA

This is an inherited disorder of LDL receptors. In the homozygous condition there are virtually no effective receptors, whereas in the heterozygote only about 50 per cent of the receptors are active. It is characterized by high levels of both total and LDL cholesterol. Homozygotes will often have untreated levels of cholesterol of 15 mmol/l or greater, while those of heterozygotes may be around 8 mmol/l. Both groups are at risk of early coronary heart disease, events characteristically occurring in the second decade in homozygotes and in the fourth to fifth decades in heterozygotes.

Aeromedical disposal

A diagnosis of familial hypercholesterolaemia should lead to rejection of candidates for military aircrew training. For civil aviation certification, candidates are assessed on an individual basis. If they are on treatment, with well-controlled lipids and no evidence of cardiovascular disease, then they may be accepted without restriction. However, this will be subject to continued careful follow-up and assessment.

SECONDARY HYPERLIPIDAEMIA

Secondary hyperlipidaemias are common and are related to a variety of underlying disorders, the most common of which are obesity, diabetes mellitus, hypothyroidism, renal failure and nephrotic syndrome. Secondary hyperlipidaemias are also seen with excess alcohol ingestion, steroid or sex hormone therapy, and the use of thiazide or beta-blocker therapy.

The important implications for increased coronary risk with the secondary hyperlipidaemias in diabetes mellitus and renal disease are discussed more fully in Chapter 42. In aviation, the clinical problem is seen most frequently in obese people and in people who have an excessive intake of ethanol. Both are associated with a rise in triglycerides, but the fall in HDL is greater in obese people. The Framingham Study confirmed the increased coronary risk in both sexes with raised triglycerides and reduced HDL (Gordon et al. 1981).

Aeromedical disposal

Flying restrictions should be related to the cumulative risk factors. However, when lipid levels have been brought within acceptable limits, unrestricted flying may be possible subject to careful follow-up and a negative exercise ECG.

SCREENING

The arguments for lipid screening in aircrew were discussed at the first European Workshop in Aviation Cardiology (Keech and Sleight 1992).These have now been translated into appropriate programmes for both UK military aviators and the JAA. The military screens at initial entry and again at the age of 40 years. The JAA requires plasma lipids and serum cholesterol to be measured at the examination for first issue of a medical certificate and at the first examination after the age of 40 years.

TREATMENT OF HYPERLIPIDAEMIA IN AVIATORS

The rationale and supporting data for both primary and secondary prevention of coronary artery disease by treatment are presented in Chapter 37.

Causes of secondary hyperlipidaemia, such as those disorders listed above, should be excluded before initiation of therapy. First-line treatment should, where appropriate, be in terms of lifestyle management. Reduction in alcohol, cessation of smoking and increased exercise should be associated with commencement of a lipid-lowering diet. A lipid-lowering diet may result in a fall of up to 15 per cent in total cholesterol levels and often a marked decrease in triglycerides. An excellent example of an approach to dietary management may be found in Feher and Richmond (1991).

In those whose lipids remain sufficiently elevated to constitute an increased cardiovascular risk, drug therapy should be considered. In both civil and military aviation, hydroxymethylglutaryl coenzyme A (HMG-CoA) reductase inhibitors are the treatment of choice. The benefit of statin therapy in both primary and secondary prevention of cardiovascular morbidity is now well established (Jones 2003). In essence, a 20 per cent reduction in serum cholesterol reduces the relative cardiovascular risk by about a third. Standard therapeutic doses of HMG-CoA reductase inhibitors may be prescribed for aircrew and, in the absence of adverse side effects, are acceptable for unrestricted civil aviation certification and military flying.

REFERENCES

Bennett N, Dodd T, Flatley J, et al. Health Survey for England 1993. London: HMSO, 1995.

Berger W. Incidence of severe side-effects during therapy with sulphonylureas and biguanides. Hormone and Metabolic Research 1985; 17 (suppl. 15): 110–15.

Borch-Johnson K and Krenier S. Proteinuria: value as predictor of cardiovascular mortality in insulin dependent diabetes mellitus. British Medical Journal 1987; 294: 1651–4.

Cushing H. The basophil adenomas of the pituitary body and their clinical manifestations (pituitary basophilism). Bulletin of the Johns Hopkins Hospital 1932; 50: 137–95.

Diabetes Control and Complications Trial research group. The effect of intensive treatment of diabetes on the development and progression of long-term complications in insulin dependent diabetes mellitus. New England Journal of Medicine 1993; 329: 986–97.

Entmacher PS, Root HF, Marks MH. Longevity of diabetic patients in recent years. Diabetes 1964; 13: 373–82.

Feher MD, Richmond W. Why treat lipid disorders? In: Feher MD, Richmond W (eds). Lipids and Lipid Disorders. London: Wolfe, 1991; p. 61.

Fuller JH, Shipley MJ, Rose G, et al. Coronary heart disease risk and impaired glucose tolerance. Lancet 1980; i: 1373–6.

Gordon T, Kannel WB, Castelli WP, Dawber PR. Lipoproteins, cardiovascular disease and death. The Framingham study. Archives of Internal Medicine 1981; 141: 1128–31.

Holmes CS, Koepke KM, Thomson RG. Simple versus complex impairments at three blood glucose levels. Psychoneurology and Endocrinology 1986; 11: 353–7.

Jennings AM, Wilson RM, Ward JD. Symptomatic hypoglycaemia in NIDDM patients treated with oral hypoglycaemic agents. *Diabetes Care* 1989; **12**: 203–8.

Jones AF. The future of statin therapy. *Practical Cardiovascular Risk Management* 2003; **1**: 1, 5–8.

Jüppner H. Molecular cloning and characterization of a parathyroid hormone/parathyroid hormone receptor: a member of an ancient family of G protein-coupled receptors. *Current Opinion in Nephrology and Hypertension* 1994; **3**: 371–8.

Keech A, Sleight P. Lipid screening in aircrew: pros and cons. *European Heart Journal* 1992; **13**: 50–53.

Klein R, Klein BE, Moss SE, *et al*. The Wisconsin epidemiologic study of diabetic retinopathy. III. Prevalence and risk of diabetic retinopathy when age at diagnosis is 30 or more years. *Archives of Ophthalmology* 1984; **102**: 527–32.

Mann JFE, Gernstein HC, Pogue J, *et al*. Renal insufficiency as a predictor of cardiovascular outcomes and the impact of ramipril; the HOPE randomised trial. *Annals of Internal Medicine* 2001; **134**: 629–36.

Marre M, Lievre M, Chatellier G, *et al*. Effects of low dose ramipril on cardiovascular and renal outcomes in patients with type 2 diabetes and raised excretion of urinary albumin: randomised, double blind, placebo controlled trial (the DIABHYCAR study). *British Medical Journal* 2004; **328**: 495–9.

Neil HA, Gatling W, Mather HM, *et al*. The Oxford Community Diabetes Survey: evidence for an increase in prevalence of known diabetes in Great Britain. *Diabetes Medicine* 1987; **4**: 539–43.

Parle JV, Franklyn JA, Cross KW, *et al*. Prevalence and follow up of abnormal TSH concentrations in the elderly in the United Kingdom. *Clinical Endocrinology* 1991; **34**: 77–85.

Praming S, Thorstinsson B, Bendtson I, *et al*. Symptomatic hypoglycaemia in 411 type I diabetic patients. *Diabetes Medicine* 1991; **8**: 217–22.

Stewart PM. Mineralocorticoid hypertension. *Lancet* 1999; **353**: 1341–7.

UK Prospective Diabetes Study Group. Effect of intensive blood-glucose control with metformin on complications in overweight patients with type 2 diabetes (UKPDS 34). *Lancet* 1998a; **352**: 854–65.

UK Prospective Diabetes Study Group. Intensive blood-glucose control with sulphonylureas or insulin compared with conventional treatment and risk of complications in patients with type 2 diabetes. *Lancet* 1998b; **352**: 837–53.

Viberti GC, Mogensen CE, Groop L, *et al*. For the European Microalbuminuria Captoprin Study Group. The effect of captoprin on the progression to clinical proteinuria in patients with insulin dependent diabetes and microalbuminuria. *Journal of the American Medical Association* 1994; **271**: 275–9.

FURTHER READING

Scottish Intercollegiate Guidelines Network (SIGN). Management of diabetes. Clinical guideline no. 55. www.sign.ac.uk/guidelines/fulltext/55/index.html

UK Prospective Diabetic Study (UKPDS). www.dtu.ox.ac.uk/ukpds

42

Renal disease

DAVID J. RAINFORD

INTRODUCTION

Renal disease provides a considerable amount of work for physicians working within the sphere of aviation medicine. The spectrum is wide, ranging from the discovery of minor abnormalities in the urinary deposit at routine or selection medical through to the complex decision-making processes associated with returning those with chronic renal failure or renal replacement therapy back to work. This chapter will cover the majority of renal problems that will be encountered by the aviation physician and will discuss the principles underlying the medical certification process in the affected individual. For completeness, the common urological conditions will also be addressed.

RENAL RESPONSES TO THE FLYING ENVIRONMENT

An understanding of the physiological responses of the kidney to the flying environment is important in order to assist in distinguishing the physiological from the pathological. There are two important ways in which the kidney may respond to the flying environment: by changes in the handling of salt and water and by changes in the urinary deposit.

Salt and water

The handling of salt and water by the kidney in flight is modified both by changes in renal blood flow and by alterations in central blood volume. Positive radial acceleration ($+G_z$) causes a reduction in renal blood flow and a consequent fall in glomerular filtration rate (GFR). The associated antinatriuresis appears to be mediated by a decrease in filtered sodium load and enhanced tubular reabsorption (Epstein et al. 1974). The work of Park and colleagues (1994) in Korea demonstrated that high $+G_z$ ($+6\,G_z$ for 30 seconds) exposure in humans causes a significant reduction in plasma atrial natriuretic peptide concentration. It is likely, therefore, that the antinatriuresis of positive radial acceleration is mediated predominantly through the inhibition of atrial natriuretic peptide release as a response to an acute decrease in central blood volume.

In manned spaceflight, diuresis leads to a significant reduction in plasma volume. Work during long-term missions on board the space stations Salyut and Mir reviewed by Grigoriev and colleagues (1994) has helped to identify the mechanism. In essence, changes in atrial natriuretic peptide levels in the plasma are thought to contribute to the initiation of the natriuresis during spaceflight. There is also a fall in antidiuretic hormone (ADH) levels, which leads to an increased urinary flow. These acute changes are almost certainly a response to the redistribution of body fluids in weightlessness, with an increase in central blood volume, paralleling the results of head-out-of-water immersion experiments. In prolonged spaceflight, ADH levels rise, possibly due to altered sensitivity to the hormone, as is seen in head-down-tilt experiments (Sukhanov 1985). In flights of less than two weeks' duration, the reduction in plasma volume leads to increased plasma osmolality and increased sodium and chloride concentrations. In prolonged flight, normal homeostatic mechanisms appear to compensate.

Urinary deposit changes in response to flight

Changes in protein excretion during flight in response to $+G_z$ were first documented by Cromarty (1984) in an elegant study of urinalysis in fast-jet aircrew. Of 39 pilots studied, one-third ($n = 13$) showed at least a trace of protein in the urine after flight. It is likely that this is due to an increase of venous pressure within the kidney during $+G_z$ acceleration. Noddeland and colleagues (1986) found significant amounts of protein and hyaline casts in the urine of 17 of 20 pilots after centrifugation without anti-G suits. This was, however, not seen in a further group of 19 fighter pilots after air combat manoeuvre training with anti-G suits. Cromarty's study also showed the appearance of transient microscopic haematuria after flight in three of the 39 pilots studied.

Investigation of urinary deposit after spaceflight showed the presence of red cells, protein and protein casts, which disappeared during the recovery period (Popova *et al.* 1991). However, studies during spaceflight did not show significantly abnormal urinary deposit and, thus, it is suggested that the transient appearance of an abnormal urinary deposit is connected with the transfer from weightlessness to terrestrial gravitation (Gazenko *et al.* 1986).

HAEMATURIA

The complaint of frank haematuria leaves the physician in no doubt about management. The patient must be properly investigated and referred for specialist opinion. However, the finding of so-called 'reagent-strip haematuria' at routine medical examination raises a lot of questions. One thing is certain: it cannot be ignored. The modern reagent-strip test for haematuria is a reliable guide to the presence of abnormal numbers of red cells in the urine (Arm *et al.* 1986) and correlates very well with population studies that define an upper limit of normal of eight red blood cells (RBCs)/μl (8×10^9/l). Investigation should be full and include competent cystourethroscopy. Some cases will be found to be due to asymptomatic posterior urethritis/prostatitis and are treated easily. Carcinoma of the bladder, although uncommon before the age of 40 years, must be excluded. Most adults in whom the cause of the haematuria remains undiagnosed after full urological assessment have glomerular disease at renal biopsy. In examining fast-jet aircrew, it should be remembered that microscopic haematuria may occur following the application of $+G_z$ forces. Therefore, in order to avoid unnecessary investigation, it is probably wise to avoid urine testing within 24 hours of this kind of flying.

Aeromedical disposition

An initial applicant with haematuria should be investigated before the issue of a medical certificate for commercial flying and before acceptance for military training. Trained pilots who are found to have isolated microscopic haematuria in the course of their routine medical may be assessed fit while the investigations are carried out, but if frank haematuria has occurred, they should be made temporarily unfit because of the risk of recurrence and possible incapacitation due to clot colic or acute urinary retention. The presence of proteinuria in addition to microscopic haematuria (even a trace), or any suggestion of systemic disease or underlying disorder should also prompt immediate referral and a temporary unfit status.

After the exclusion of urological disease, the majority of cases will be found to have chronic glomerular disease. The discovery of chronic glomerular nephritis precludes entry to military flying training, but it may be permissible for training as a commercial pilot, provided that renal function is not significantly impaired. Candidates accepted for training with underlying glomerular disease must be warned of the potential danger of subsequent loss of licence should the disease progress. The discovery of glomerular disease in a trained pilot must be viewed differently. The most common causes of glomerular disease in patients presenting with microscopic haematuria are mesangial proliferative nephritis, usually of the immunoglobulin A (IgA) type, and thin membrane disease. In the presence of normal renal function, a normal blood pressure and the absence of proteinuria, IgA disease usually carries a good prognosis. Unrestricted medical certification is appropriate, subject to regular follow-up. Thin membrane disease is usually associated with a family history and is benign. Again, unrestricted medical certification may be allowed.

PROTEINURIA

Normal adults may excrete up to 150 mg of protein per 24 hours. The gold standard for the detection of proteinuria remains the laboratory quantification of the 24-hour excretion of protein. This is clearly an inappropriate method for screening purposes. Proteinuria thus is usually detected by urine reagent-strip analysis. A trace result occurs in response to as little as 50 mg of protein per litre, and a distinct colour change at the 1+ level at about 300 mg of protein per litre. Sensitivity of the reagent strip is of the order of 88 per cent and the specificity is 96 per cent. Trace results can be refined further by the simple expedient of repeat testing. If all strips show trace or less, then 90 per cent of patients tested will have a normal protein excretion. If any strip shows '+' or more, then abnormal protein excretion may be expected in greater than 80 per cent of cases and further investigation is warranted (Harrison *et al.* 1989).

Initially, the excretion of protein in the urine should be quantified either by analysis of a 24-hr urine collection, or measurement of the protein/creatinine ratio in a spot sample. Significant proteinuria is present if a 24-hour urine contains greater than 300 mg of protein, or if the protein/creatinine ratio on a spot urine is greater than 30. Significant proteinuria is nearly always a portent of underlying renal disease, and this is usually due to chronic glomerular nephritis. It may also be a sign of systemic disease affecting the kidney or of underlying malignancy causing a glomerular response. A full history and clinical examination therefore are essential.

Orthostatic proteinuria is present when protein is entirely absent from the urine in the recumbent position but appears in the upright posture. In general terms, this carries an excellent prognosis. The tendency of true orthostatic proteinuria is to resolution, with up to 50 per cent of patients remaining free from proteinuria in ten years. However, occasionally, early glomerular nephritis may have a postural element to protein excretion. Caution is advised, therefore, in making this diagnosis. The development of proteinuria in response to $+G_z$ in some aircrew is certainly benign, and this can be ignored. Urine testing should not be carried out within 24 hours of flight involving manoeuvres that subject the crew to repeated $+G_z$ stress. In general terms, proteinuria of less than 1 g daily in the presence of normal blood pressure, normal renal function and the absence of haematuria or systemic disease carries an excellent long-term prognosis.

Aeromedical disposition

An initial certificate of fitness to fly or acceptance for military flying training should not be issued until investigations are complete. Trained pilots and certificate holders with isolated mild proteinuria (< 1 g/day) may continue to fly while awaiting investigation. Where proteinuria exceeds 1 g/day, the aviator should be made temporarily unfit pending the results of investigations. Similarly, where the proteinuria is associated with haematuria, hypertension, renal impairment or signs of a systemic disorder, then the patient should be made temporarily unfit.

After full evaluation, aircrew with isolated proteinuria of less than 1 g/day may be allowed to return to full flying duties with no restrictions, provided that they are followed up carefully.

Patients with greater than 1 g/day of urinary protein excretion have an increased risk for the development of complications such as nephrotic syndrome, hypertension and renal failure. Single-pilot operations should not be allowed, in either commercial or military employment.

Flying with a co-pilot qualified on type is permissible, subject to regular follow-up. Stable proteinuria of greater than 1 g/day and with a normal plasma albumin may allow unrestricted private flying, although again subject to rigorous follow-up.

RENAL STONE DISEASE

Renal stone disease is common, affecting some two per cent of the adult population of the UK. The incidence is increasing, mainly because of changes in dietary habits. Stones occur approximately twice as frequently in males than in females, and a family history is often found. Development of renal stones may be more common in aircrew, possibly due to periods of relative dehydration in association with both the dry cabin environment and self-imposed reduction in fluid intake when flying. A study of active duty US army aviators recorded an incidence of almost double that of a control population (Clark 1990). Both the US and the Russian space programmes have identified an increased risk of stone formation in astronauts associated with the biochemical changes that result from microgravity adaptation and earth readaptation. The post-landing period is the most vulnerable time, when both hypercalciuria and hypocitraturia coexist (Jones and Whitson, in press).

The composition of renal stones varies in different continents and different ethnic groups. Uric acid and lower urinary tract stones are more common in the Middle East than in the western world, where idiopathic calcium oxalate stones in the upper urinary tract represent some 90 per cent of all occurrences. Idiopathic stone disease is defined as stone formation occurring when known causes, such as renal tubular acidosis, medullary sponge kidney, hypercalcaemia, hyperoxaluria and infection, have been excluded.

The concern of renal stone disease is that the development of acute renal colic may cause sudden incapacitation in flight. Aircrew who have suffered acute renal colic will readily testify that they would be concerned at their ability to control an aircraft during an attack.

Also of major consideration in the aviator is that renal stone disease is a disease of recurrence. The greatest incidence of recurrence is at two to three years after the first stone, but roughly half of the patients with a single stone episode will have suffered recurrence by five years and two-thirds by nine years; beyond 25 years, recurrence is almost 100 per cent. Recurrence, therefore, is likely during an aviator's flying career, and the passage of even one stone cannot be ignored. It is important, therefore, not only to investigate these patients thoroughly but also to institute effective measures to prevent recurrence where indicated and to establish close follow-up procedures.

Aeromedical disposition

All aircrew must be grounded at the first attack of renal colic or at the time of the discovery of renal calculi. They should be referred immediately for radiological investigation in order to exclude further stones and to ascertain urinary tract normality. A biochemical screen should be performed to exclude renal dysfunction, hypercalcaemia and hyperuricaemia. In the absence of any biochemical abnormality and the absence of further stones in the urinary tract, the patient is fit to return to full unrestricted flying. A metabolic assessment to exclude any underlying treatable urinary abnormality should be delayed until at least six weeks after passage of the stone, as a period of obstruction is often followed by a natriuresis and calciuresis, which will give a false impression of the presence of significant hypercalciuria.

In the presence of residual stones, aircrew must remain grounded until either they have passed the stone naturally or it has been removed. Virtually all residual stones can be dealt with by extracorporeal shock-wave lithotripsy (ESWL). This involves the minimum of trauma and the minimum of time on the ground.

Follow-up of aircrew following a stone episode is extremely important in view of the risk of recurrence. Following ESWL, recurrence may be as high as 30 per cent in the first year, and so surveillance is particularly important in this group. The principle is to detect any new stone formation early, so that it may be treated before constituting a hazard. Although ultrasound scanning is the most popular method of renal assessment for stones, radiographs are often preferred because they are capable of defining the small stones that may be missed by ultrasound. Occasionally, doubt exists as to the precise location of calcification in the renal area. If outside the collecting system, then there is very little risk and this can be determined effectively by the use of spiral computed tomography (CT). For aviators who have been shown to have urate stones, once clear on allopurinol therapy recurrence is uncommon and radiographic surveillance may be unnecessary. Although the majority of aircrew should be managed by simple surveillance, prophylactic treatment for patients with stone disease should be considered in those with frequent recurrence, those with a proven metabolic problem such as urate stones, and those with medullary sponge kidney. The single most effective form of therapy for prevention of further idiopathic stone formation is thiazide diuretics. Yendt and Cohanim (1978) showed that in people who took hydrochlorothiazide 50 mg twice daily on a regular basis, stone progression ceased in more than 90 per cent. Almost as effective and without the metabolic side effects of thiazides is the use of citrate supplements as a stone inhibitor. For aircrew, current practice is to use citrate in preference to thiazides in all frequent recurrent calcium stone formers who require prophylaxis, except in those with medullary sponge kidney, where thiazides remain the treatment of choice. Allopurinol should be used for those with proven urate lithiasis; often, only a small dose is required for effective prophylaxis. In frequent stone formers who do not respond effectively to thiazide or citrate prophylaxis, the addition of allopurinol will often reduce the recurrence rate. General advice about maintaining a good fluid intake and avoiding high oxalate intake should be given to all patients.

CHRONIC RENAL FAILURE

The concern of chronic renal failure is that its consequences may impair the ability to fly safely or lead to sudden incapacitation. This section will explore whether this concern is justified. If so, should all candidates with nephritis who apply be excluded? And should all existing aircrew found to have nephritis be grounded permanently? Decisions such as these have a profound impact on the careers and livelihoods of aircrew and must be taken only from the strength of evidence-based data.

The first and most important question to be answered is whether chronic renal failure per se leads to either sudden incapacitation or degradation in performance that might be a hazard to flight safety.

In the absence of nephrotic syndrome and its associated thrombotic potential, and in the absence of uncontrolled hypertension, chronic renal failure is insidious and symptoms are uncommon until creatinine clearance falls to about 20 ml/min. At much greater levels of function, there is impairment of vitamin D metabolism and haemopoiesis, but it is at about this level of creatinine clearance that retention of waste products may manifest with increasing acidosis, anaemia, problematic hypertension or acute gout. Therefore, with careful medical follow-up of patients with chronic renal impairment who are already trained, there is no reason to deny certification until their level of function falls to 20 ml/min. After this, the risk of sudden incapacitation or impairment of ability becomes too great and they should be grounded.

For those with chronic renal disease who wish to learn to fly, although they may be classified as fit at initial medical a serious warning needs to be given that they will not retain their certificate if their function falls below acceptable levels. This is vital to those who are contemplating flying as paid employment.

Whether pilots with chronic renal failure can return to flying following renal replacement therapy will depend on whether an annual risk of sudden incapacitation of less than one per cent can be achieved. From the risk-assessment point of view, the most important cause of mortality in the patient with any form of renal replacement therapy is cardiovascular disease. Cardiac disease due to atheroma, calcific aortic valves or cardiomyopathy accounts for more than 40 per cent of deaths on dialysis (Harnett *et al.* 1995). Patients on either haemodialysis or peritoneal dialysis have a cardiovascular mortality close to ten per cent per annum (Levy *et al.* 1998). These figures derive from a study of patients in the USA from a database of over 200 000 patients with end-stage renal disease (ESRD), and they are very similar to those recorded in the UK. Therefore, while on dialysis therapy, an acceptable cardiovascular mortality risk cannot be achieved. Patients on dialysis are therefore unfit certification to fly.

During the time on dialysis, and during the pre-dialysis period, multiple factors may have contributed to an increase in cardiovascular mortality risk. All of these factors are important, and evidence is amassing that early attention to these risk factors will improve prognosis. Data from both the European Dialysis and Transplant Association studies and the large US studies from Michigan show that after the first year, cardiovascular mortality falls significantly, although diabetes mellitus still remains a poor risk factor (Levy *et al.* 1998). Although the risk does not fall back to that of the general population, the risk in all except the people with diabetes falls below one per cent annual mortality. Age is a factor, and a one per cent per annum mortality is reached approximately 20 years earlier in transplant patient (Foley *et al.* 1998).

Whether the pilot can return to flying after transplantation depends, therefore, on individual risk analysis rather than a blanket decision to exclude all such patients. Using the evidence base, a protocol was developed. UK Civil Aviation Authority (CAA) aircrew have been assessed using the following guidelines:

- The first year after transplantation has the highest morbidity and mortality (including return to dialysis), and so all pilots should wait until one year post-transplant before assessment.
- Renal function must be stable and there must be no underlying systemic disorder that is likely to cause sudden change. Blood pressure must be within normal limits, although the use of approved hypotensive drugs may be acceptable.
- Any steroid dosage must be below 10 mg/day because of the unpredictable psychiatric effects of higher dosage. Levels of anti-rejection drugs such as ciclosporin must be within therapeutic limits in order to minimize side effects, as elevated levels of ciclosporin or its derivatives may cause tremor or even fits.
- Cardiovascular risk must be minimized by attention to smoking, lipids and glucose tolerance and assessed formally by a cardiologist.

The assessment of risk within this group of individuals, which has a high prevalence of coronary artery disease, may be achieved with the use of symptom-limited exercise stress ECG. Despite the limitations of exercise cardiography in asymptomatic individuals, the Seattle Heart Watch programme showed conclusively that people who had more than one positive test in the presence of vascular risk factors had an annual coronary event greater than five per cent (Bruce and Fisher 1987). By comparison, a normal stress test in the absence of vascular risk factors carried a risk of event of only 0.22 per cent. In the presence of vascular risk factors, a normal stress test carried a risk of event of 0.42 per cent. Despite incomplete sensitivity, this test does appear to allow identification of a group of people whose risk of event lies within the acceptable one per cent rule.

Using the above guidelines thus allows identification of those with an annual cardiovascular mortality risk of less than one per cent who can be allowed to fly. In the UK, half of those with chronic renal failure continue to fly; of those who have been transplanted, nearly 60 per cent have achieved some form of recertification.

In order to maintain validity of recertification, regular cardiovascular assessment in addition to renal assessment is a vital follow-up requirement. It must be remembered that these pilots may reach a cardiovascular mortality risk of greater than one per cent about 20 years earlier than their normal peers.

OTHER RENAL DISORDERS

Renal anomalies

Unilateral renal agenesis occurs in about one in 500 of the normal population. This may, therefore, be discovered from time to time as an incidental finding. It is of no clinical importance and, after documentation, may be ignored.

Horseshoe kidney occurs with about the same incidence as unilateral renal agenesis. These patients may be allowed to fly with no restrictions, but as there is an increased tendency to renal stone formation and urinary infection, any symptoms should be investigated rigorously and subsequent restrictions may need to be imposed.

Polycystic kidneys

Polycystic kidneys occur in about one in 1000 of the population. This is, therefore, one of the most common congenital renal disorders. In the adult type with which we are concerned, inheritance is autosomal dominant and so a family history is often obtained. Associated problems are cysts in other organs, and 5–16 per cent of affected people will have cerebral or abdominal arterial aneurysms. Ruptured intracranial aneurysms account for about six per cent of all deaths in people with this disorder.

The discovery of polycystic disease at initial medical examination will preclude acceptance for military aircrew training. Applicants for initial medical certification for commercial flying should also be rejected. The discovery of polycystic kidneys in trained aircrew requires a full renal assessment before decisions are made on fitness to continue flying. Complications include bleeding, urinary infections, renal calculi, hypertension and the development of chronic renal failure. Any decisions must, therefore, be made in the light of the presence or absence of these findings. The relatively high incidence of cerebral arterial aneurysms and the potential for subarachnoid haemorrhage should limit the pilot to multi-crew operations.

Post-nephrectomy

The removal of a traumatized or diseased kidney is no bar to a full flying career if the remaining kidney is normal and unaffected by disease. Long-term studies on US servicemen who had kidneys removed for trauma in the Second World War have shown no increase in morbidity or mortality.

Pelviureteric junction obstruction

Pelviureteric junction (PUJ) obstruction is a not uncommon cause of loin pain in young men. It is often of a colicky nature and follows a fluid load such as a few pints of beer. Radiologically, the renal pelvis is seen to be distended on intravenous urography, while the ureter below is not easily seen. Isotope studies will confirm either partial or complete blockage. Treatment is surgical, either by open pyeloplasty or by percutaneous techniques. Following repair, the patient is fit to return to full flying duties with no restrictions. Follow-up with isotope renography is essential, as occasionally the disorder is bilateral and both sides do not always manifest themselves simultaneously.

BENIGN PROSTATIC HYPERTROPHY

This is rarely a problem in pilots flying in the military because of the younger age spectrum, but it is a frequent problem in civil aviation, often as the pilot is coming towards the end of his career. Frequency of micturition and the risk of acute retention of urine are unacceptable, and intervention is required if the pilot is to fly both comfortably and in safety. Clearly, the definitive management that would present little problem with subsequent medical certification would be surgical. However, increasingly,

patients are loath to proceed to surgery without an adequate trial of medical treatment. Both alpha-adrenergic blockers and 5-alpha-reductase inhibitors have been shown to reduce symptoms and to delay or perhaps negate the need for surgery.

Alpha-adrenergic blockers are now in common use for the management of the symptoms of prostatism, but not all of these drugs have a margin of safety sufficient to allow control of an aircraft. As a group, they are proscribed for the management of hypertension in aircrew because as vasodilators they have risks of significant postural hypotension. The discovery of alpha-1a adrenoceptors in the prostate gland allowed the development of the selective alpha-1a adrenergic receptor antagonist tamsulosin, which is much safer than non-selective alpha-blockers. Tamsulosin is acceptable for use in aircrew providing that the usual period of grounding to assess side effects (as for the use of any new medication) is instituted and 24-hour ambulatory blood pressure recordings show no evidence of postural hypotension. It is wise to restrict these aircrew to multi-crew limitations, as there is a theoretical risk of postural hypotension if the aviator is relatively dehydrated in flight.

The 5-alpha-reductase inhibitors such as finasteride inhibit the production of dihydrotestosterone from testosterone and have been shown to effectively reduce prostatic volume. The side effects are mainly decreased libido and breast enlargement. Aircrew may, therefore, retain certification, but they should fly in a multi-crew role for a year to confirm prostatic volume reduction (and, therefore, minimal risk of acute urinary retention) before returning to unrestricted certification.

CARCINOMA OF THE BLADDER

Cancer of the bladder is the fourth most common cancer in men in the UK. It accounts for two per cent of all malignant disease. Fortunately, at diagnosis, 80 per cent of all bladder cancers are superficial, being non-invasive (Ta), invading only the lamina propria (T1) or appearing as carcinoma in situ (Tis). However, recurrence rates following initial treatment are high, at 50–70 per cent, and 10–30 per cent of these recurrences are invasive.

Provided that the cancer is non-invasive and the bladder is clear of tumour, then there is no requirement to restrict certification to fly. However, if the tumour is invasive, then restrictions will apply; each case must be assessed individually. Those aviators with local invasion possibly may be allowed to fly with another qualified pilot, whereas the presence of secondary deposits may merit permanent withdrawal of all certification.

The subject of urological malignancy is covered in more detail in Chapter 44.

REFERENCES

Arm JP, Peile EB, Rainford DJ, *et al*. Significance of dipstick haematuria. 1. Correlation with microscopy of the urine. *British Journal of Urology* 1986; **58**: 211–17.

Bruce RA, Fisher LD. Exercised enhancement of risk factors for coronary artery disease in healthy men. *Journal of Electrocardiology* 1987; **20** (suppl. 1): 162–6.

Clark JY. Renal calculi in army aviators. *Aviation, Space, and Environmental Medicine* 1990; **61**: 744–7.

Cromarty IJ. Microscopic haematuria in fast jet aircrew. MRCC project 042. London: Ministry of Defence, 1984.

Epstein M, Shubrooks SJ, Fishman LM, Duncan DC. Effects of positive acceleration ($+G_z$) on renal function and plasma renin in normal man. *Journal of Applied Physiology* 1974; **36**: 340–44.

Foley RN, Parfrey PS, Sarnak MJ. Clinical epidemiology of cardiovascular disease in chronic renal disease. *American Journal of Kidney Disease* 1998; **32** (suppl. 3): S112–19.

Gazenko OG, Grigoriev A, Natochin YV. Fluid–electrolyte balance and spaceflight. In: *Problems in Space Biology*, Vol. 54. Moscow: Nauka, 1986; pp. 1–238.

Grigoriev AI, Morukov BV, Vorobiev DV. Water and electrolyte studies during long-term missions onboard the space stations Salyut and Mir. *Clinical Investigation* 1994; **72**: 169-89.

Harnett JD, Kent GM, Foley RN, Parfrey PS. Cardiac function and haematocrit level. *American Journal of Kidney Disease* 1995; **25**: S3–7.

Harrison NA, Rainford DJ, Cullen SA, *et al*. Proteinuria: what value is the dipstick? *British Journal of Urology* 1989; **63**: 202–8.

Jones JA, Whitson PA. Renal and genitourinary concerns. In: Barratt M, Pool S (eds). *Principles of Clinical Medicine for Space Flight.* New York: Springer Verlag, in press.

Levy AS, Beto JA, Coronado BE, *et al*. Controlling the epidemic of cardiovascular disease in chronic renal disease: what do we know? What do we need to learn? Where do we go from here? National Kidney Foundation Task Force on Cardiovascular Disease. *American Journal of Kidney Disease* 1998; **32**: 853–906.

Noddeland H, Myhre K, Balldin U, Andersen H. Proteinuria in fighter pilots after high +Gz exposure. *Aviation, Space, and Environmental Medicine* 1986; **57**: 122–5.

Park JK, Seul KH, Park BO, *et al*. Effects of positive acceleration on atrial natriuretic peptide in humans. *Aviation, Space, and Environmental Medicine* 1994; **65**: 51–4.

Popova IA, Vetrova EG, Rustamyan LA. Evaluation of energy metabolism in cosmonauts. *Physiologist* 1991; **34**: S98–9.

Sukhanov YV. Study of human antidiuretic hormone in real and simulated space flights varying in duration. IBMP research report. Moscow: Institute for Biomedical Problems, 1985.

Yendt ER, Cohanim M. Prevention of calcium stones with thiazides. *Kidney International* 1978; **13**: 397–410.

43

Haematology

PAUL L.F. GIANGRANDE

INTRODUCTION

This chapter focuses on areas of general haematology that are of particular relevance to the practice of aviation medicine, as applied to both medical certification of flight crew as well as the transport of passengers in commercial aircraft. Several blood disorders, e.g. anaemia, can affect fitness to fly. At the same time, flight itself may lead to various problems, an important example of which is venous thromboembolism. This chapter covers a variety of non-malignant general haematological disorders. Malignant conditions such as the leukaemias are covered in Chapter 44. A list of normal haematological values is given in Appendix 43.1.

ANAEMIA

Haemoglobin in red blood cells (erythrocytes) is necessary for the uptake of oxygen in the lungs and its transport and transfer to peripheral tissues. The normal haemoglobin level is 13.5–17.5 g/dl for males and 11.5–15.5 g/dl for females. Anaemia is not in itself a diagnosis but may be a consequence of a wide variety of disorders, and it is important to determine the cause. Whatever the aetiology, cardiovascular reserve could be impaired, and this could pose a problem in an aircraft cabin with a pressure altitude of up to 8000 feet. Passengers with a haemoglobin level of 7.5 g/dl or more are not likely to experience problems with commercial air travel. However, the haemoglobin level alone cannot be relied on to decide whether a patient is fit to travel. A distinction must also be made between chronic and acute anaemia. Patients with long-standing anaemia, such as that associated with renal failure, often have good cardiovascular compensation and experience few problems with travel. By contrast, patients with anaemia of recent onset, such as after surgery, are more likely to experience problems. When assessing potential passengers for fitness to fly, it is also important to bear in mind that examination at rest may prove misleading; therefore, exercise tolerance should be assessed. As a general guideline, people who are able to walk about 50 m and to climb 10–12 stairs without symptoms should be able to fly without incident (Peffers 1978). Signs of haemodynamic instability precipitated by exertion include tachycardia or other arrhythmias, hypotension, chest pain and changes in the ST segment of the electrocardiogram (ECG). In addition to possible difficulties associated with the journey, travellers with anaemia should be advised of the possible hazards of blood transfusion in developing countries. This is particularly important for patients with chronic haematological conditions where periodic transfusion is required.

In the case of flight crew, there are no longer firm rules with regard to haemoglobin levels and medical certification. However, a finding of a haemoglobin level of 11 g/dl or less should prompt appropriate clinical enquiry and investigations. Final assessment will depend on the diagnosis and response to treatment.

Deficiencies of haematinics

Screening for deficiencies of haematinic agents such as iron, folic acid and vitamin B12 are normally included in the initial evaluation of a subject with anaemia. Iron deficiency is the most common cause of anaemia; the typical picture is a low haemoglobin associated with hypochromia (mean corpuscular haemoglobin (MCH) < 27 pg) and microcytosis (mean corpuscular volume (MCV)< 80 fL) of the red cells. The diagnosis can be confirmed by the finding of a low serum ferritin level. It is always important to establish the underlying cause of iron deficiency. It may simply reflect poor intake, e.g. in vegetarianism, or poor absorption, e.g. in coeliac disease, but the most common cause is chronic blood loss, e.g. menorrhagia, peptic ulcer or other gastrointestinal pathology.

Deficiency of folic acid or vitamin B12 may also cause anaemia. In this case, the red cells are unusually large (macrocytosis), with an MCV of 100 fL or more. Deficiency of folic acid is almost always the consequence of poor dietary intake, since this vitamin is plentiful in fresh fruit and vegetables. However, deficiency of folic acid may be a manifestation of malabsorption, and the possibility of coeliac disease needs to be considered in the differential diagnosis. Pernicious anaemia is an autoimmune condition characterized by chronic inflammatory gastritis associated with achlorhydria and the development of antibodies directed against intrinsic factor and/or gastric parietal cells. This results in malabsorption of vitamin B12 despite a normal dietary intake. Regular intramuscular injections, typically every three months, will restore normal haematopoiesis. The underlying gastritis is not corrected with this treatment, and there is a persisting long-term risk of the order of two to three of developing gastric cancer. It should also be borne in mind that there is also an association between pernicious anaemia and the subsequent development of other autoimmune disorders, in particular hypothyroidism. Severe vitamin B12 deficiency may be associated with both peripheral neuropathy and spinal cord demyelination, but this does not occur in association with folic acid deficiency.

Isolated macrocytosis associated with a normal haemoglobin level also merits documentation, as it may be an indicator of several conditions, including chronic liver disease, sustained high alcohol intake and hypothyroidism. It is a normal finding in pregnancy (Breedveld et al. 1981; Keenan 1989). Anaemia in association with thrombocytopenia and/or an abnormal leucocyte count deserves specialist investigation, and referral to a haematologist should be considered.

Haemolytic anaemias

The haemolytic anaemias can be defined as those forms of anaemia resulting from an increase in the rate of destruction of erythrocytes, which normally have a lifespan of around 120 days. Many of these are hereditary conditions. A classic example is hereditary spherocytosis, which is inherited as an autosomal dominant condition (Bolton-Maggs et al. 2004). Deficiency of a structural membrane protein, spectrin, results in premature destructions of the erythrocytes, leading to anaemia of variable degrees, which is often accompanied by mild jaundice and splenomegaly. Diagnosis is established easily by examination of the blood film and demonstration of reticulocytosis, but confirmatory tests include an osmotic fragility test and negative direct antiglobulin (Coombs') test. Splenectomy is beneficial in patients with significant anaemia, although this does result in increased susceptibility to certain bacterial infections (see below). Hereditary elliptocytosis is a similar condition, although any resulting anaemia is only slight and splenectomy is indicated only rarely.

Autoimmune haemolytic anaemia is caused by the destruction of erythrocytes by autoantibodies directed against red-cell antigens, resulting in anaemia of varying severity and often associated with mild splenomegaly (Pruss et al. 2003). It can develop at any age and both sexes are affected equally. It typically runs a chronic course, punctuated by intermittent remissions and relapses. Typical haematological findings include spherocytosis in the peripheral blood and a positive direct antiglobulin (Coombs') test. Treatment options include the use of steroids and immunosuppressive agents such as azathioprine or cyclophosphamide. Splenectomy may also be of value. Permanent remission is not common, and the requirement for continuous or intermittent therapy is likely to prejudice medical certification as flight crew.

Glucose-6-phosphate dehydrogenase (G6PD) deficiency deserves special mention because of the potential for development of severe and acute haemolytic anaemia in conditions when the erythrocytes are subjected to oxidative stress (Mehta et al. 2000). This form of haemolytic anaemia is inherited as a sex-linked condition and, thus, affects only males. It is by far the most common form of haemolytic anaemia. It is encountered particularly frequently in the Mediterranean, west Africa, the Middle East and South-East Asia. Although occasionally it is associated with persistent haemolytic anaemia and mild jaundice, most patients maintain a normal haemoglobin level. There will usually be no abnormality noted on routine laboratory screening. However, viral infections or other acute illnesses can precipitate rapid and sudden intravascular haemolysis associated with haemoglobinuria. Ingestion of broad (fava) beans and exposure to certain common drugs, including aspirin, quinine and penicillin, can have the same effect.

Sickle cell disease

Haemoglobinopathies are inherited disorders of haemoglobin resulting from synthesis of abnormal haemoglobin molecules. In general, these conditions are encountered in people originating from tropical areas, and it is believed that these conditions originally developed to confer protection against malaria. The gene frequency in people of Afro-Caribbean origin may be as high as five per cent. The gene is also found with a lower frequency among people of the Mediterranean, the Middle East and the Indian subcontinent. This condition is due to a single mutation in the beta-globin chain of the haemoglobin molecule: valine (V) is substituted for glutamic acid (E) at position 6. The abnormal haemoglobin is unstable and forms precipitates within the erythrocyte due to polymerization when deoxygenated.

It is of fundamental importance to distinguish between heterozygous carriers of this condition (sickle cell trait) from homozygous subjects. Sickle cell trait is a benign condition in which 20–40 per cent of the circulating haemoglobin is HbS and the rest is normal HbA. Heterozygotes have no clinical problems; indeed, the haemoglobin level is typically normal, and examination of the blood film shows no significant abnormality. In vitro tests show that sickling does not occur in sickle cell trait until the Po_2 falls to about 10 mmHg; thus, clinical problems will occur only in conditions of extreme hypoxia. Flight in pressurized commercial aircraft certainly poses no problems, and sickle cell trait is not a bar to a career in commercial civil aviation (Bendrick 1997). Similarly, sickle cell trait is no longer a bar to licensing of military aircrew in the UK and the USA. This was a controversial area in the past, and the previous policy of considering this to be a bar to certification of military aircrew was not reversed until the 1980s (Voge et al. 1991).

By contrast, homozygote subjects with sickle cell disease have a persistent anaemia, with a haemoglobin level typically in the range of 7–10 g/dl, and are prone to recurrent episodes of painful crises due to intramedullary necrosis following occlusion of small vessels (Claster and Vichinsky 2003). The most frequently involved areas are the knee, lumbosacral spine, elbow and femur, but the ribs, sternum, clavicles, calcaneus and facial bones may also be affected. Often there is no obvious precipitating cause, but it is recognized that infections, dehydration and exposure to cold or low levels of oxygen can provoke crises. Joint effusions are commonly seen when the knees or elbows are involved. Crises can be extremely painful, and opiate analgesics are usually needed. Extensive sickling within the lungs can be life-threatening. This can present initially with cough, fever and pleuritic chest pain; a chest radiograph will show extensive infiltration of either one or both lung fields. Other complications of homozygous sickle cell disease include episodes of painless haematuria, avascular necrosis of the hip, vaso-occlusive stroke, development of gallstones formed from aggregates of bilirubin, and development of intractable leg ulcers. Patients with sickle cell disease experience splenic infarction, leading to loss of immune function, and are, therefore, vulnerable to certain bacterial infections (see Splenectomy, p. 662). Repeated infarction within the hypertonic environment of the renal medulla often results in recurrent episodes of painless haematuria. Eventually, the ability to concentrate urine is impaired; therefore, patients are prone to dehydration.

It will be obvious from the above that a diagnosis of (homozygous) sickle cell disease is incompatible with medical certification as flight crew. With regard to passengers with sickle cell disease, data suggest that sickling crises and related problems in patients with homozygous sickle cell disease (HbSS) flying in pressurized commercial aircraft are extremely rare (Ware et al. 1998). There is, thus, reassuring evidence that permits a more relaxed attitude to flight in commercial aircraft. People with sickle cell disease should certainly be encouraged to drink plenty of water during the journey, as they are particularly prone to dehydration due to the impaired ability of the kidneys to concentrate urine. The risk of sickling with other variants, including combined haemoglobin sickle cell disease and haemoglobin S/beta-thalassaemia, is significantly higher. In such cases, it would be sensible to have oxygen available on board pressurized aircraft, although it is not necessary to use it on a prophylactic basis in flight. By contrast, there are several case reports describing the development of sickle cell crises in subjects with simple sickle cell trait in flight at altitude in unpressurized aircraft at altitudes above 8000 feet.

Thalassaemia

The thalassaemias are a group of haematological disorders in which a defect in the synthesis of one or more of the globin polypeptide chains is present, resulting in the formation of unstable aggregates of globin chains within erythrocyte precursors, which are destroyed prematurely. A full classification of the thalassaemias is beyond the scope of this chapter, but the principal division is that between disorders involving the alpha- and beta-chains of the haemoglobin molecule. The prevalence of the genes for thalassaemia is particularly high in Mediterranean countries (especially Greece, Italy, Cyprus and north Africa), the Middle East, the Indian subcontinent and South-East Asia. Carriers of beta-thalassaemia, the most common form in European countries, have no clinical problems, apart from a mild and persistent microcytic anaemia with a haemoglobin level typically in the range of 10–12 g/dl. The condition can, thus, be mistaken for iron-deficiency anaemia, but haemoglobin electrophoresis will permit the distinction through the demonstration of a mildly elevated level of haemoglobin A2. A diagnosis of heterozygosity (thalassaemia trait) is certainly not a barrier to medical certification for flight duties.

Beta-thalassaemia major is the homozygous form. This results in very severe anaemia, which becomes apparent three to six months after birth. This is accompanied by massive enlargement of the liver and spleen due to both excessive red-cell destruction and extramedullary erythropoiesis. Marked expansion of the bone marrow leads to thinning of the cortex in the bones, which can result in pathological fractures. Striking features in untreated children include prominence of the parietal and frontal bones and protrusion of the maxillary bones, leading to malocclusion of teeth and orthodontic problems. Somewhat paradoxically, many of the serious medical complications seen in thalassaemia actually result from treatment of the condition. A programme of regular transfusions to maintain a haemoglobin level of 10 g/dl will lead to regression of hepatosplenomegaly and skeletal changes. However, regular transfusion eventually results in iron overload and fibrosis in vital organs, which can lead to diabetes mellitus, cirrhosis and cardiac complications such as arrhythmias and congestive cardiac failure. The administration of iron-chelating agents such as desferrioxamine may postpone the onset of iron overload. A diagnosis of homozygous thalassaemia is clearly not compatible with medical certification as flight crew.

Polycythaemia

Polycythaemia is defined by an increase in the red-cell mass, resulting in a haemoglobin level of 17.5 g/dl or more in males and 15.5 g/dl or more in females. True polycythaemia rubra vera (PRV) is a myeloproliferative disease that can run a long clinical course but that transforms into myelofibrosis in about a third of cases (Stuart and Viera 2004). Acute myeloid leukaemia may also develop in about five per cent of patients. PRV typically develops in older people aged 50 years or older. Many of the clinical features are a consequence of hyperviscosity of the blood, hypermetabolism or hypervolaemia. Symptoms include headaches, dyspnoea, night sweats, pruritus, blurred vision and onset of gout. The typical facial appearance is plethoric with florid cyanosis. The diagnosis is based on the finding of an increased haematocrit associated with increased red-cell mass using radio-isotopic studies. A raised neutrophil and platelet count may also be observed. The haematocrit can be controlled effectively through regular venesection alone, although other treatment options include the use of alkylating agents (e.g. busulfan) or administration of phosphorus P-32. The median survival time is of the order of 10–16 years from diagnosis, regardless of the form of treatment used. Thrombosis and haemorrhage are common, and vascular accidents are a frequent cause of death. Increased viscosity of the blood, vascular stasis and high platelet counts may all contribute to the development of thrombosis. Vascular distension, infarcts of small vessels

and defective platelet function may promote haemorrhage. Although some discretion is allowed, a diagnosis of PRV is normally considered to be disqualifying from flying duties due to the potential for thromboembolic complications and unpredictable progression of the disorder.

BLEEDING DISORDERS

Haemorrhagic disorders may be congenital or acquired. Even in congenital cases, there is a wide spectrum of severity, as in the case of anaemia, and a diagnosis of a bleeding disorder does not necessarily preclude medical certification.

Thrombocytopenia

The normal range for the platelet count is $150-400 \times 10^9$/l, but when assessing the risk of the bleeding tendency it should be borne in mind that far more platelets are produced than are actually required to control bleeding. Easy bruising and persistent bleeding from cuts and scratches develop only when the platelet count falls below about 80×10^9/l. Serious internal bleeding, such as intracranial haemorrhage, may occur if the platelet count falls below 20×10^9/l. Many conditions result in thrombocytopenia, and the nature of the underlying disease and the trend in the count need to be considered when assessing a pilot for medical certification or a patient for suitability to travel. The risk of bleeding is not related only to the absolute platelet count: in autoimmune thrombocytopenia, there is a rapid turnover of young platelets, and serious bleeding is rarely a problem, even with very low counts.

As a general rule, a platelet count below 75×10^9/l should be considered the critical threshold for medical certification of pilots. However, it would be reasonable to permit a passenger to fly in a civil aircraft with a much lower threshold of 40×10^9/l. Patients with thrombocytopenia should not be given aspirin or similar non-steroidal drugs, as these will exacerbate the bleeding tendency through their inhibitory effect on platelet function. Paracetamol (acetaminophen) is a safe alternative analgesic. Patients who have undergone splenectomy for autoimmune thrombocytopenia will be permanently vulnerable to certain infections (see below).

There are various inherited forms of thrombocytopenia, and this may well be picked up as an incidental finding during a medical examination. Isolated thrombocytopenia is accompanied by a normal white cell count and haemoglobin level. Screening of other family members can help to prove the hereditary nature. There is often no clinical history suggestive of bleeding tendency, and an increased platelet size seems to compensate for the often modest reduction in the platelet count, to the extent that the bleeding time may be normal. Autoimmune thrombocytopenia (ITP) in childhood is a relatively common disorder, but complete remission is the most common outcome and the patient can be assured that relapse does not occur (Kuhne et al. 2001). For this reason, a history of an isolated episode of ITP years ago in childhood can be disregarded as being of no consequence for the purpose of medical certification of flight crew if the platelet count is normal. By contrast, ITP with onset in adult life typically has a chronic course (Provan and Newland 2003). Treatment options include steroids, infusion of intravenous immunoglobulin and splenectomy. Applicants with a history of chronic ITP who have undergone splenectomy and have stable platelet counts above the threshold of $75 \times 10^9/l$ may be considered for medical certification.

Haemophilia

Haemophilia A is a congenital disorder of coagulation characterized by a hereditary deficiency of factor VIII (Bolton-Maggs and Pasi 2003). Deficiency of factor IX results in an identical clinical condition known as haemophilia B (also known as Christmas disease). These are both sex-linked recessive disorders that almost exclusively affect only males. Severe haemophilia is defined by a coagulation factor level of less than one per cent; a level of one to five per cent is classed as moderately severe. The hallmark of severe haemophilia is recurrent and spontaneous bleeding into joints, principally the knees, elbows and ankles. Repeated bleeding into joints can result in disabling arthritis at an early age. Bleeding into muscles and soft tissues is also seen frequently, and there is also the potential for intracranial bleeding. About 10–15 per cent of patients with haemophilia A develop inhibitory antibodies to infused factor VVIII, which makes treatment more difficult. Mild cases of haemophilia may be picked up on routine screening before surgery. A factor VIII level of 30 per cent would represent a very mild case, with no problems whatsoever in day-to-day life and requiring treatment only in the setting of surgery or other invasive procedures. Although patients with severe haemophilia generally would not be regarded as suitable for medical certification as pilots, it must be emphasized that those with mild forms are not at increased risk of sudden incapacitation and medical certification should not necessarily be withheld.

By contrast, travel for a person with haemophilia as a passenger should present no significant problems. However, it should be borne in mind when assessing a patient for fitness to fly that a significant proportion of older patients have been exposed to hepatitis and/or human immunodeficiency virus (HIV) through their treatment with blood products. HIV-positive patients should not receive yellow fever, bacille Calmette-Guérin (BCG) or oral typhoid vaccines. People with haemophilia should carry an adequate quantity of coagulation factor concentrate for their stay abroad. The website of the World Federation of Hemophilia carries a database of specialist haemophilia centres around the world (www.wfh.org).

Von Willebrand disease

Von Willebrand disease (VWD) is a congenital bleeding disorder associated with a deficiency of von Willebrand factor (VWF) in the plasma, a protein that plays an essential role in the early phases of platelet adhesion and activation. VWD is now recognized to be the most common inherited bleeding disorder, with an estimated prevalence of at least one per 1000 in the general population. In contrast to haemophilia, it is transmitted in an autosomal dominant fashion, and so both sexes are affected.

The typical symptoms reflect the underlying defect in platelet function and include easy bruising and prolonged bleeding from cuts and scratches, epistaxis, menorrhagia and bleeding after dental extractions or surgery (Giangrande 2003). The severity of the bleeding tendency generally parallels the degree of deficiency of both factor VIII and VWF in the blood. Haemarthrosis is very unusual in VWD and tends to be seen only in patients with the severe form. A diagnosis of VWD does not necessarily preclude medical certification of flight crew if there is evidence that the phenotype is mild and there is no significant bleeding history, such that therapy is not required.

DEEP VEIN THROMBOSIS AND ANTICOAGULATION

The most common indication for anticoagulation is a deep vein thrombosis (DVT) in the veins of the leg. Pulmonary embolism has been estimated to occur in approximately one per cent of cases of DVT. The conventional approach to the treatment of venous thromboembolism involves anticoagulation with heparin and, subsequently, warfarin or a similar drug, such as acenocoumarol (nicoumalone). The primary purpose of anticoagulation is to prevent extension of the thrombosis; anticoagulation does not cause dissolution of the thrombus. In the case of an isolated distal venous thrombosis in the leg, warfarin treatment is continued for three months with a target international normalized ratio (INR) of 2.5 (Haemostasis and Thrombosis Task Force for the British Committee for Standards in Haematology 1998). If there is evidence of pulmonary embolism or the thrombosis extends proximally, then it is recommended that anticoagulation with warfarin be extended for a total of six months. Other conditions in which anticoagulation is indicated include atrial fibrillation, transient ischaemic attacks, peripheral arterial disease, ischaemic heart disease and following insertion of prosthetic heart valves. These conditions may themselves constitute an automatic bar to medical certification.

Anticoagulation is associated with a small but definite risk of bleeding complications, such as intracranial haemorrhage. In one review, the average annual frequencies of fatal, major and minor bleeding during warfarin therapy were 0.6 per cent, three per cent and 9.6 per cent, respectively (Landefeld and Beyth 1993). The risk of haemorrhagic complications, including intracranial bleeding, is particularly high in older subjects and in patients with an INR of greater than 4 (Heylek and Singer 1994; Rosand *et al.* 2004). Accordingly, the medical certificate must be suspended for the duration of anticoagulation with warfarin, because of the risk of potential incapacitation due to intracerebral or other haemorrhage.

Anticoagulation with warfarin does not pose any particular problems for passengers, but patients should ensure that they take adequate medication with them. If travelling on a long journey, perhaps with connecting flights, the tablets should be carried in the person's hand luggage. The risk of haemorrhagic complications is greatest in patients who are excessively anticoagulated with an INR greater than 5, and this emphasizes the need for continued laboratory control when away from home. If the patient is staying abroad for an extended period, arrangements should be made to have the usual periodic blood test to check the INR. Changes in diet, new medications and an increase in alcohol consumption may affect sensitivity to warfarin, and diarrhoea and vomiting may impair absorption of the drug. At the time of writing, a new class of oral anticoagulants is undergoing clinical trials, which may transform clinical practice in this area. Oral thrombin inhibitors such as ximelagatran appear to be as effective as warfarin but much safer in terms of risk of haemorrhagic complications while the patient is on therapy. These drugs are also given in fixed doses and do not require laboratory monitoring, and so it is possible that routine INR measurements may become obsolete in the not too distant future.

The long-term consequences of venous thromboembolism are not insignificant. Approximately 20 per cent of subjects will experience a recurrence of a DVT in the subsequent five years (Hansson *et al.* 2000). This raises the prospect of advising long-term anticoagulation, which inevitably will result in the loss of medical certification. Aspirin is an inhibitor of platelet function and is used in a number of conditions, quite apart from its use as a simple analgesic, including prevention of stroke. Consumption of aspirin per se is not incompatible with flying duties, although any underlying conditions are likely be contraindications. Aspirin has very little anti-thrombotic effect in the venous circulation and should not be used as an alternative to warfarin simply in order to avoid suspension of a medical certificate. There is often some perma-

nent damage to the valves in the veins, and this can lead to permanent circulatory problems, with persistent swelling of the limb or even chronic ulceration (post-phlebitic syndrome). Approximately 60 per cent of patients will develop post-phlebitic syndrome within two years, despite appropriate anticoagulant therapy, but the risk is reduced significantly by wearing compression hosiery on the affected leg for up to two years afterwards (Brandjes *et al.* 1987). A previous medical history of thrombosis will also preclude future prescription of hormone replacement therapy (HRT) or oestrogen-containing oral contraceptives for women and make it difficult to secure travel insurance in future because of the high risk of recurrence.

THROMBOPHILIA

A haematological abnormality may exist in an individual that predisposes to the development of venous thromboembolism (Bertina 2001). Such disorders include the relatively rare congenital (inherited) deficiencies of natural anticoagulants such as anti-thrombin, protein C or protein S. By far the most common genetic abnormality that predisposes to thrombosis is the factor V Leiden genotype, which is associated with resistance to activated protein C. The defect involves a single mutation in the factor V molecule (R506Q), which renders the molecule resistant to cleavage by protein C. This mutation is encountered in approximately four per cent of the European population, but it is very rare or even absent in other racial groups. It is associated with an approximately eight-fold increased risk of venous thrombosis, but there is a considerably higher risk in women taking oestrogen-containing oral contraceptives. Elevation of the plasma prothrombin level in association with a point mutation (nucleotide G20210A) in the prothrombin gene is another newly identified genetic risk factor for venous thrombosis. This is encountered in approximately two per cent of the Caucasian population and is associated with an approximately three-fold risk of thromboembolism. In addition to these inherited defects, the development of anti-phospholipid antibodies (lupus anticoagulant) is also associated with an increased risk of venous thromboembolism. Other acquired haematological disorders associated with an increased risk of thrombosis include myeloproliferative disorders such as polycythaemia and thrombocythaemia.

Screening for thrombophilia may be of value in selected individuals. Indications include thromboembolism at an unusually early age (under 40 years of age), recurrent thromboembolism, thrombosis at an unusual site or a strong family history. The full panel of tests can be done only once the subject has been off warfarin for at least one month. However, thrombophilic defects are increasingly being found in asymptomatic individuals as a result of family studies in relatives with a history of thrombosis. There is no justification for refusing medical certification in asymptomatic individuals with no personal history of thromboembolism, as the overall risk is still small in absolute terms. Even the identification of an underlying thrombophilic defect in a pilot who has experienced a single episode of venous thromboembolism does not, ipso facto, rule out certification once a course of warfarin therapy has been completed (Emonson 1997), although long-term warfarin therapy is likely to be recommended after further episodes.

AIR TRAVEL AND THROMBOSIS

It is now generally accepted that there is an association between any form of long-distance travel and venous thromboembolism, although the incidence is low and involves mainly passengers with additional risk factors for venous thromboembolism. However, the risk is not associated exclusively with air travel, and it has also been documented following long car, bus and train journeys. The alternative term of 'travellers' thrombosis' has been suggested as an alternative to the term 'economy-class syndrome'. It is possible to derive some general conclusions from published cases of venous thromboembolism associated with travel (Giangrande 2002). Thromboembolism is rarely observed after flights of less than five hours' duration and, typically, the flights are of 12 hours' duration or more. The risk rises with age: older people over the age of 50 years are more at risk, while those under the age of 40 years are less vulnerable. Symptoms of thromboembolism do not usually develop during or immediately after the flight but tend to appear within three days of arrival, when the patient may present far away from the airport, thus, the causal link may not be apparent immediately. Symptoms of thrombosis or pulmonary embolism have been reported up to two weeks after a long flight. Pulmonary embolism may be the first manifestation, without any symptoms in the lower limbs. Although most case reports and studies involve DVT in the lower limbs, there are also reports of cerebral venous thrombosis and arterial thrombosis associated with long flights.

The precise incidence of thromboembolism in relation to air travel is uncertain. A recent observational analysis from New Zealand, based on a review of 878 passengers who travelled extensively (at least ten hours within a six-week period; mean 39 hours) reported an incidence of venous thromboembolism of one per cent, including four cases of pulmonary embolism and five cases of DVT (Hughes et al. 2003). However, the incidence of latent asymptomatic thrombosis is likely to be even higher. A prospective study of long-haul air passengers over the age of 50 years reported that 12 of 116 (ten per cent) passen-

gers were found by ultrasound scanning to have asymptomatic DVT confined to the calf (Scurr et al. 2001).

The aetiology of venous thrombosis is usually multifactorial, with a combination of both constitutional and environmental factors responsible for causing a thrombosis in an individual at a given time (Rosendaal 1999). Stasis in the venous circulation of the lower limbs is undoubtedly the major factor in promoting the development of venous thromboembolism associated with travel. It has also been suggested that exposure to mild hypobaric hypoxia in pressurized aircraft may result in activation of the coagulation cascade, but data on this are conflicting (Bendz et al. 2000; Hodkinson et al. 2003). A number of other risk factors that predispose to venous thromboembolism are now also recognized, primarily through clinical experience in the setting of surgery (Table 43.1).

Table 43.1   *Factors predisposing to venous thromboembolism*

Age > 40 years, and especially > 65 years
Previous thrombotic episode, especially pulmonary embolism
Documented thrombophilic abnormality, e.g. anti-thrombin deficiency
Other haematological disorders (polycythaemia, thrombocythaemia)
Pregnancy and puerperium
Malignancy
Congestive heart failure, recent myocardial infarction
Recent surgery, especially lower-limb
Chronic venous insufficiency
Oestrogen therapy, e.g. oral contraceptive pill, HRT
Obesity
Prolonged recent immobility, e.g. after recent stroke
Dehydration (diarrhoea)

HRT, hormone replacement therapy.

The effect of age was highlighted in a study from Australia, which concluded that the annual risk of venous thromboembolism is increased by 12 per cent if one long-haul flight is undertaken annually (Kelman et al. 2003). Although the incidence of thromboembolism was less than one in 100 000 arriving passengers under the age of 40 years, it rose steadily to exceed 14 per 100 000 in those aged 75 years or older. It has been demonstrated that an inherited thrombophilic defect or use of an oral contraceptive pill increases the risk of thrombosis associated with air travel 16- and 14-fold, respectively (Martinelli et al. 2003).

A number of general measures may be taken in order to minimize the risk of thrombosis associated with long flights. Perhaps the most important step is to consider at the outset whether the patient is actually fit to fly in the first place. For example, it is probably wise to defer long-haul travel after recent major orthopaedic surgery. Passengers should be encouraged to carry out leg exercises from time to time while seated, e.g. flexion, extension and rotation of the ankles will help to promote circulation in the lower limbs. Hand luggage stowed under seats will also restrict movement. Passengers should also take advantage of stops on long-haul flights to get off the plane and walk around for a while. Adequate hydration should be ensured during the flight. It is not necessary to abstain from alcohol, but excessive consumption should be avoided, as this will both promote diuresis and discourage mobility. Similarly, the use of sedatives is best avoided. There is no value in screening passengers for thrombophilic defects before long-haul flights.

A number of randomized prospective studies have shown a clear benefit from the use of compression hosiery (flight socks) (Belcaro *et al.* 2002, 2003). These apply graduated pressure to the leg, which is maximal at the ankle, thus encouraging venous return. Quite apart from reducing the risk of thrombosis, compression hosiery help to prevent oedema of the legs and feet, which can itself cause discomfort after along flight. Aspirin has been advocated by some authors in the general prophylaxis of thrombosis associated with travel, but the beneficial effect is weak in absolute terms. It has been estimated that if the rate of travel-related DVT is 20 per 100 000 travellers, then 17 000 people would need to be treated with aspirin in order to prevent just one episode of DVT (Loke and Derry 2002). Furthermore, there is a potential for side effects, such as allergic reactions and gastrointestinal bleeding: 13 per cent of subjects taking aspirin in a study to evaluate its potential in preventing venous thrombosis associated with air travel reported mild gastrointestinal symptoms (Cesarone *et al.* 2002). In short, there is no firm evidence to support the indiscriminate use of aspirin as a routine prophylactic measure. The use of heparin may be considered in the relatively few passengers considered to be at particularly high risk of thrombosis, e.g. a patient flying home with their leg in plaster after a fracture.

BLOOD TRANSFUSION

Blood transfusion in many parts of the world still poses very real risks with regard to transmission of viral and other infections. Systematic screening of blood donations is not yet feasible in many developing countries, and needles may not even be sterilized properly before reuse. Infections that may be transmitted via transfusion of blood or plasma include HIV, hepatitis B and C, malaria, babesiosis, *Trypanosoma cruzi* (Chagas disease), brucellosis, syphilis, cytomegalovirus (CMV) and human T-cell lymphoma virus (HTLV-I). Patients with chronic disorders must be counselled about the possible risks in certain parts of the world if transfusion might be required. Patients sometimes enquire about the possibility of taking

blood from their home country with them abroad. This raises a number of technical and logistical problems, which are not easy to resolve, e.g. blood has to be stored at 4°C and has a limited shelf-life of up to six weeks. The international shipment of blood for transfusion is practical only when handled by agreement between two responsible organizations, such as national blood transfusion services. This mechanism is not feasible for the emergency needs of individual patients and should not be attempted by private individuals. In fact, emergency blood transfusion is required only rarely and is likely to be needed only in the setting of massive haemorrhage after trauma, gastrointestinal bleeding or obstetric emergencies. In developed countries, a decision to transfuse is far too often based solely on the haemoglobin level. In fact, the decision should be based on the clinical state and haemodynamic stability, e.g. pulse, blood pressure and respiratory rate, of the patient. It is by no means essential, for example, to transfuse a patient just because the haemoglobin has fallen to 8 g/dl. Even in the case of massive haemorrhage, resuscitation can often be achieved through the use of colloid or crystalloid plasma expanders instead of blood. Although it is not feasible to transport packs of blood abroad, plasma expanders may be transported much more readily, as they have a much longer shelf-life and do not require storage at 4°C. It might also be advisable in some cases to take sterile needles and other disposable equipment, such as giving sets.

Pilots are permitted to donate blood, but a period of 24 hours should elapse between donation and resuming normal duties because of the small risk of delayed fainting or other adverse reaction (12 hours in the case of air traffic controllers). The minimum recommended interval before duty for both aircrew and controllers after bone-marrow donation is 48 hours.

SPLENECTOMY

Splenectomy has already been referred to as a treatment option for some of the haematological disorders, including certain haemolytic anaemias and autoimmune thrombocytopenia, and some discussion of the hazards of splenectomy is therefore relevant. The most common reason for splenectomy is traumatic rupture following abdominal injury. The operation used to be carried out routinely in Hodgkin's lymphoma as part of the staging process before starting treatment. Patients with sickle cell disease are also effectively asplenic due to repeated infarction within the organ. Although splenectomy may control the underlying haematological condition, the patient will be left permanently vulnerable to certain infectious diseases (Conlon 1993; Mileno and Bia 1998). Asplenic individuals are particularly susceptible to encapsulated organisms such as

Streptococcus pneumoniae, Haemophilus influenzae and *Neisseria meningitidis.* Vaccination should be offered where possible, although the immunological response is better when the vaccine is given before elective splenectomy. Bacteraemia in asplenic individuals often has a fulminating course, leading rapidly to shock and coma, accompanied by disseminated intravascular coagulation. Patients should be treated with an antibiotic at the first sign of fever or respiratory illness, however trivial. Amoxicillin is preferred to penicillin V because of better absorption following oral administration and because it has a broader antibacterial spectrum that includes *H. influenzae.* Malaria in asplenic subjects is often fatal, and it is vital that asplenic subjects take appropriate prophylaxis where indicated. Although an applicant for medical certification may appear to be perfectly fit and healthy after splenectomy, the potential for medical complications should not be overlooked.

REFERENCES

Belcaro G, Cesarone MR, Shah SS, *et al.* Prevention of edema, flight microangiopathy and venous thrombosis in long flights with elastic stockings: a randomized trial. The LONFLIT 4 Concorde Edema-SSL Study. *Angiology* 2002; **53**: 635–45.

Belcaro G, Cesarone MR, Nicolaides AN, *et al.* Prevention of venous thrombosis with elastic stockings during long-haul flights: the LONFLIT 5 JAP study. *Clinical and Applied Thrombosis/Hemostasis* 2003; **9**: 197–201.

Bendrick GA. You're the flight surgeon: sickle cell trait and beta-thalassemia. *Aviation, Space, and Environmental Medicine* 1997; **68**: 244–5.

Bendz B, Rostrup M, Sevre K, *et al.* Association between hypobaric hypoxia and activation of coagulation in human beings. *Lancet* 2000; **356**: 1657–8.

Bertina RM. Genetic approach to thrombophilia. *Thrombosis and Haemostasis* 2001; **86**: 92–103.

Bolton-Maggs PH, Pasi JK. Haemophilias A and B. *Lancet* 2003; **351**: 1801–9.

Bolton-Maggs PH, Stevens RF, Dodd NJ, *et al.* General Haematology Task Force of the British Committee for Standards in Haematology. Guidelines for the diagnosis and management of hereditary spherocytosis. *British Journal of Haematology* 2004; **126**: 455–74.

Brandjes DP, Buller HR, Heijboer H, *et al.* Randomised trial of effect of compression stockings in patients with symptomatic proximal-vein thrombosis. *Lancet* 1997; **349**: 759–62.

Breedveld FC, Bieger R, van Wermeskerken RK. The clinical significance of macrocytosis. *Acta Medica Scandinavica* 1981; **209**: 319–22.

Cesarone MR, Belcaro G, Nicoliades AN, *et al.* Venous thrombosis from air travel: the LONFLIT 3 study – prevention with aspirin vs low-molecular-weight heparin in high-risk subjects: a randomised trial. *Angiology* 2002; **53**: 1–6.

Claster S, Vichinsky EP. Managing sickle cell disease. *British Medical Journal* 2003; **327**: 1151–5.

Conlon CP. The immunocompromised traveller. *British Medical Bulletin* 1993; **49**: 412–22.

Emonson DL. Activated protein C resistance as a 'new' cause of deep venous thrombosis in aviators. *Aviation, Space, and Environmental Medicine* 1997; **68**: 606–8.

Giangrande PLF Air travel and thrombosis. *British Journal of Haematology* 2002; **117**: 509–12.

Giangrande PLF. Von Willebrand disease. *Haematology Journal* 2003; **4** (suppl. 3): 168–74.

Haemostasis and Thrombosis Task Force for the British Committee for Standards in Haematology. Guidelines on oral anticoagulation: third edition. *British Journal of Haematology* 1998; **101**: 374–87.

Hansson PO, Sorbo J, Eriksson H. Recurrent venous thromboembolism after deep vein thrombosis. *Archives of Internal Medicine* 2000; **160**: 769–74.

Heylek EM, Singer DE. Risk factors for intracranial hemorrhage in outpatients taking warfarin. *Annals of Internal Medicine* 1994; **120**: 897–902.

Hodkinson PD, Hunt BJ, Parmar K, Ernsting J. Is mild normobaric hypoxia a risk factor for venous thromboembolism? *Journal of Thrombosis and Haemostasis* 2003; **1**: 2131–3.

Hughes RJ, Hopkins RJ, Hill S, *et al.* Frequency of venous thromboembolism in low to moderate risk long distance air travellers: the New Zealand Air Traveller's Thrombosis (NZATT) Study. *Lancet* 2003; **362**: 2039–44.

Keenan WF. Macrocytosis as an indicator of human disease. *Journal of the American Board Family Practice* 1989; **2**: 252–6.

Kelman CW, Kortt MA, Becker NG, *et al.* Deep vein thrombosis and air travel: record linkage study. *British Medical Journal* 2003; **327**: 1072–5.

Kuhne T, Imbach P, Bolton-Maggs PH, *et al.* Intercontinental Childhood ITP Study Group. Newly diagnosed idiopathic thrombocytopenic purpura in childhood: an observational study. *Lancet* 2001; **358**: 2122–5.

Landefeld CS, Beyth RJ. Anticoagulant-related bleeding: clinical epidemiology, prediction and prevention. *American Journal of Medicine* 1993; **95**: 315–28.

Loke YK, Derry S. Air travel and venous thrombosis: how much help might aspirin be? *Medscape General Medicine* 2002; **4**: 4.

Martinelli I, Taioli E, Battaglioli T, *et al.* Risk of venous thromboembolism after air travel: interaction with thrombophilia and oral contraceptives. *Archives of Internal Medicine* 2003; **163**: 2674–6.

Mehta A, Mason PJ, Vulliamy TJ. Glucose-6-phosphate dehydrogenase deficiency. *Bailliere's Best Practice and Research: Clinical Haematology* 2000; **13**: 21–38.

Mileno MD, Bia FJ. The compromised traveller. *Infectious Disease Clinics of North America* 1998; **12**: 369–412.

Peffers AS. Carriage of invalids by air. *Journal of the Royal College of Physicians of London* 1978; **12**: 136–42.

Provan D, Newland A. Idiopathic thrombocytopenic purpura in adults. *Journal of Pediatric Hematology/Oncology* 2003; **25** (suppl. 1): S34–8.

Pruss A, Salama A, Ahrens N, *et al.* Immune hemolysis-serological and clinical aspects. *Clinical and Experimental Medicine* 2003; **3**: 55–64.

Rosand J, Eckman MH, Knudsen KA, *et al.* The effect of warfarin and intensity of anticoagulation on outcome of intracerebral hemorrhage. *Archives of Internal Medicine* 2004; **164**: 880–84.

Rosendaal FR. Venous thrombosis: a multicausal disease. *Lancet* 1999; **353**: 1167–73.

Scurr JH, Machin SJ, Bailey-King S, *et al.* Frequency and prevention of symptomless deep-vein thrombosis in long-haul flights: a randomized trial. *Lancet* 2001; **357**: 1485–9.

Stuart BJ, Viera AJ. Polycythemia vera. *American Family Physician* 2004; **69**: 2139–44.

Voge VM, Rosado NR, Contiguglia JJ. Sickle cell anemia trait in the military aircrew population: a report from the Military Aviation Safety Subcommittee of the Aviation Safety Committee. *Aviation, Space, and Environmental Medicine* 1991; **62**: 1099–102.

Ware M, Tyghter D, Staniforth S, Serjeant G. Airline travel in sickle cell disease. *Lancet* 1998; **352**: 652.

APPENDIX: NORMAL HAEMATOLOGICAL VALUES

Parameter	Value
Haemoglobin	13.5–17.5 g/dl (males)
	11.50–15.5 g/dl (females)
MCV	80–95 fL
MCH	27–34 pg
WBC	$4.0–11.0 \times 10^9/l$
Neutrophils	$2.5–7.5 \times 10^9/l$
Lymphocytes	$1.5–3.5 \times 10^9/l$
Monocytes	$0.2–0.8 \times 10^9/l$
Eosinophils	$0.04–0.44 \times 10^9/l$
Platelets	$150–400 \times 10^9/l$
Serum ferritin	40–340 μg/l (males)
	14–150 μg/l (females)
Serum folate	3.0–15 μg/l
Red cell folate	160–640 μg/l
Serum vitamin B12	160–925 ng/l

Normal ranges for coagulation tests cannot be stated, as these vary according to the method and reagents used. The normal range for the laboratory that carried out the tests must, therefore, be consulted. MCH, mean content haemoglobin; MCV, mean corpuscular volume; WBC, white blood cells.

Malignant disease

SALLY EVANS

INTRODUCTION

The diagnosis of malignant disease has long-term implications for an individual's physical health and survival. For pilots and air traffic control officers (ATCOs), it also has implications for fitness to perform operational duties and represents a threat to their careers.

Licence holders often present early and with more localized disease than their peer groups. An awareness of their health, routine surveillance examinations, education and a professional responsibility to report symptoms of ill health may all contribute to this earlier presentation. This is countered somewhat by the tendency of tumours affecting young people to be biologically aggressive, and symptoms may be less likely to be attributed to a cancer than in an older person. There is no evidence that prognosis for any particular type of tumour in a pilot or ATCO is any different to that for the general population with the same condition.

Many studies have investigated the incidence of different types of cancer among pilots, but none has proven conclusively an occupational link. It remains to be determined whether the increased incidence of malignant melanoma demonstrated in a recent Icelandic study is linked directly to flying or more indirectly to occupation by increased exposure to the sun (Rafnsson et al. 2003).

After completing primary treatment, oncologists encourage their patients to return to work as soon as they feel well enough. Some patients even manage to continue working while receiving chemotherapy or radiotherapy. Because of the safety-critical role of licence holders, no professional pilot or ATCO should exercise the privileges of their licence while undergoing or recovering from primary treatment for malignant disease.

Palliative treatment given for the alleviation of symptoms rather than with the aim to be curative precludes future certification.

Once remission has been achieved, blood parameters have returned to normal values, and a full report including an estimated prognosis has been obtained from the oncologist, then an assessment of fitness for recertification can be undertaken. The assessment that has to be made is of the risk of incapacitation secondary to local or distant metastatic recurrence of the cancer. Most of the established staging systems are based on clinical and pathological evaluation, and there is increasing use of the TNM system, where T is tumour extent, N is extent of local lymph-node involvement and M is presence of distant metastatic spread.

International medical requirements for malignant disease

Annex 1 to the Convention on International Civil Aviation does not refer specifically to malignant disease. It states that for certification class 1, 2 and 3 'applicants with diseases of the blood and/or lymphatic system shall be assessed as unfit, unless adequately investigated and their conclusion is found unlikely to interfere with the safe exercise of their licence and rating privileges'. The *Manual of Civil Aviation*, published to amplify the standards of Annex 1, refers only briefly to acute and chronic leukaemias and lymphomas, stating that they require individual assessment.

Until the 1990s, it was rare for a licence holder with a history of malignant disease to be granted or regain a professional licence. An increasingly evidence-based approach to risk assessment, combined with greatly improved prognoses for a wide range of tumours, has permitted the development of a less cautious attitude without compromising flight safety.

Prevalence of malignant disease in professional licence holders

Most professional licence holders are male and between 20 and 60 years of age. The cancers that present in this population are representative of the types of malignant disease seen among the general population of working age. Cancer is the third most common reason for permanently withdrawing a pilot's medical certificate, ranking after cardiovascular disease and neuropsychiatric disorders. The prevalence of malignant disease within the professional pilot and ATCO population in the UK is shown in Figure 44.1. The four most common tumours – colorectal, lymphoid malignancies, melanoma, testicular tumours – make up over half the total numbers.

Primary treatment for malignant disease

SURGERY

Surgery may be the only primary treatment necessary, in which case the time to recertification depends on the postoperative recovery time, freedom from surgical complications and assessment of future risk of incapacitation from recurrence. Some examples of operations typically carried out on tumours discussed later in this chapter are shown in Table 44.1, together with the minimum postoperative time periods before recertification can be considered.

RADIOTHERAPY

Radiotherapy for malignant disease is usually given as an intensive course. It may be given with curative intent, such as that given to an isolated group of lymph nodes proven by biopsy to contain lymphoma. Alternatively, adjuvant radiotherapy may be used to reduce the risk of local recurrence, e.g. radiotherapy to abdominal lymph nodes following orchidectomy for seminoma of the testis.

Side effects such as skin erythema, diarrhoea and reduction in saliva production may occur as a result of tissue damage within the field of the radiation beam. More gen-

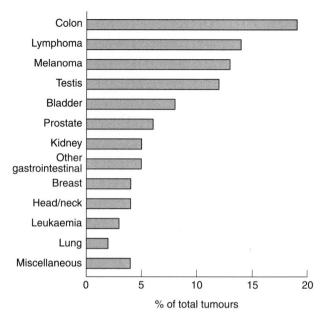

Figure 44.1 *Prevalence of malignant disease among professional pilots and air traffic control officers in the UK.*

Table 44.1 *Minimum time to recertification after various types of surgery*

Operation	Example	Minimum time to recertification (weeks)
Minor	Excision of naevus	1
Intermediate	Orchidectomy	3
Major	Hemicolectomy	8

eral sequelae, including fatigue and nausea, are very common, and the psychological effects of undergoing radiotherapy should not be underestimated. Prophylactic cranial irradiation can cause neurotoxicity and psychometric abnormalities. Small-vessel coronary artery disease may be a late effect if radiation has been directed to the left chest area, e.g. in Hodgkin's disease or left breast carcinoma, but clinical oncologists now take great care to exclude the heart from the radiation field whenever possible. Because non-specific side effects may occur in the post-treatment period, a minimum interval of four weeks should elapse before a return to operational duties can be considered.

CHEMOTHERAPY

Chemotherapeutic agents are toxic to dividing cells. They have a wide range of side effects as a result of the damage caused by their action on healthy cells, which inevitably occurs in addition to the intended toxic effect on malignant cells. These side effects may occur during treatment or may persist for many days, weeks or months after treatment has been completed (short-term effects). They may persist for longer than six months (long-term effects) or may present many months or years afterwards (delayed effects). Most chemotherapy protocols are complex and multifactorial, and there may be interactions between different types of therapy.

A minimum interval of two months should elapse before returning to flying after chemotherapy, subject to haematological indices remaining stable and within the normal range. Neutropenia is very common, and the risk of sepsis remains high for some time after completion of therapy. Enquiry should be undertaken to exclude any possible short-term sequelae that may be of potential flight-safety importance. Table 44.2 lists examples of systems that may be affected by common chemotherapeutic agents. Cardiotoxicity from anthracyclines, neuropathies from vinca alkaloids and hepatotoxicity from methotrexate may persist for a considerable length of time or remain permanently.

The assessment of future incapacitation risk should include the possibility of delayed side effects. Anthracycline cardiotoxicity is related to dose in the short term, but there is concern that long-term ventricular dysfunction and cardiac arrhythmias may not have a direct relationship to dose and may pose an increased risk of incapacitation to licence holders throughout their lives (Evans and Cooke 2003). Several drugs, including bleomycin and cyclophosphamide, may cause pulmonary fibrosis, and busulfan has been associated with lenticular changes.

As treatments have become more aggressive and efficacious, and a larger proportion of patients, including those treated as children, are surviving for longer, effectively being 'cured' of their cancer, an increased risk of developing a second malignancy is being seen. The anthracyclines, especially epirubicin, and etoposide are known to be leukaemogenic. The risks of a further malignancy are beginning to be quantified, and databases of 25-year survivors from Hodgkin's disease are now available (Swerdlow et al. 2000).

Considerable caution needs to be exercised with the introduction of new chemotherapeutic agents whose long-term side effects have not yet been evaluated fully. The potential long-term and delayed toxicities of all newly introduced treatment regimens require full appraisal, and clinical studies should confirm the absence of potentially incapacitating late sequelae before recertification can be considered.

As the periodic medical examination comprises a general physical assessment, tests of ophthalmic function and hearing, the majority of side effects should be detected routinely. Respiratory function tests and a thorough neurological examination can be included if the applicant is known to have received a drug that could have affected these systems. Specific cardiological investigations may be required if an anthracycline formed part of the chemotherapy protocol. Anthracyclines are used to treat a wide variety of malignancies, including those of the immune system, breast cancer, osteosarcoma and lung cancer.

Adjuvant hormone therapy

Steroids are preclusive for flying if given as adjuvant treatment for malignant disease. They can cause euphoria and subtle cognitive changes when given in large doses and usually are prescribed only for malignant disease to reduce inflammation around an active tumour. Tamoxifen, used for breast cancer, is acceptable, as is goserelin, a gonadorelin analogue used in the management of prostatic cancer. Bicalutamide, an anti-androgen, is also acceptable.

Serum tumour markers

The measurement of serum tumour markers is useful as a prognostic factor in colorectal, prostatic and ovarian cancers and, to a lesser extent, in breast cancer; in germ-cell

Table 44.2 *Examples of short-term side effects of chemotherapy of potential flight-safety importance*

System affected	Chemotherapeutic agent	Potential side effect
Cardiovascular	Anthracyclines	Arrhythmia, cardiomyopathy
	Cyclophosphamide	Myocarditis
	5-FU	Angina pectoris
Neurological	5-FU	Cerebellar syndrome
	Vinca alkaloids	Peripheral neuropathy
Auditory	Cisplatin	High-tone hearing loss
Renal	Cisplatin	Renal failure
Hepatic	Methotrexate	Hepatotoxicity
Immune	Cyclophosphamide	Suppression of antibody production
Psychological	Interferon	Depression

5-FU, 5-fluorouracil.

tumours of the testis, however, it is used only in staging. It is appropriate to request details of tumour markers for all these tumours before certification and at each review.

Psychological effects of cancer and its treatment

The psychological effects of the diagnosis of cancer and an individual's reaction to illness and to its treatment vary widely from one licence holder to another and from one month to the next in the same individual. This is often the first major illness experienced by a previously robustly fit individual, and it can have devastating effects on self-confidence and body image. Coupled with anxiety about future employment and financial security for themselves and their family, stress, anxiety, lability of mood, anger and depression are common. Stability of mood is essential before a pilot can be returned to flying duties or an ATCO to the operational environment.

Stem-cell transplantation

High-dose chemotherapy is used before autologous stem-cell rescue in a number of conditions, but especially for relapsed and refractory lymphoma. Following transplantation, recertification can be considered after a one- or two-year relapse-free interval. Graft-versus-host disease may complicate allogeneic transplants, and recertification can be considered only after a longer relapse-free period.

Central nervous system involvement

Malignant brain tumours are permanently disqualifying for certification. It may be possible to regain certification following removal of a benign tumour of the brain or spinal cord, once the risk of postoperative sequelae, including seizures, is sufficiently low.

Cerebral metastatic spread is disqualifying because of the unacceptably high risk of potentially incapacitating side effects from direct involvement of neural tissue or local inflammatory change. Common side effects include seizures, syncope, nausea and vomiting, paresis, cerebellar, motor or sensory disturbance, confusion, headache, cognitive dysfunction and personality change. Lung and breast cancers are frequently responsible for cerebral metastases, and melanoma and renal cell carcinomas also have a propensity to spread to the central nervous system. Both breast cancer and melanoma can result in the sudden presentation of a solitary brain metastasis after a 10–20-year disease-free interval.

Computed tomography (CT) and magnetic resonance imaging (MRI) of the brain can be used to detect cerebral metastases. These scans are becoming more useful as the resolution of the images continues to be refined. Positron-emission tomography (PET), when available, may also be useful.

CERTIFICATION AFTER TREATMENT FOR MALIGNANT DISEASE

Certification after treatment for malignant disease usually can be considered only if primary treatment (surgery, chemotherapy, radiotherapy) has been undertaken with curative intent and there is no residual clinical evidence of tumour. A few exceptions to this rule exist, including some lymphoid malignancies and early prostate cancer, for which no active treatment is indicated.

The aeromedical concern is whether recurrence or, in the exceptions mentioned above, progression of disease could present with symptoms that would jeopardize flight safety. As with other types of illness, it is the risk of sudden or subtle incapacitation that has to be assessed.

It is important to note that the certificatory assessments described in this chapter refer only to certification after primary treatment and do not apply after treatment for recurrence or relapse. For some tumours, certification after recurrence may be possible. However, survival after recurrence tends to be very much worse than after primary treatment, and the shorter the disease-free interval from the completion of treatment to recurrence, the worse the prognosis is likely to be.

The certification assessment method described uses published population survival rates, as data on recurrence are not available for most tumours. The use of survival rather than recurrence data tends to be 'fail-safe' in respect of incapacitation risk.

For each type of tumour, the survival figures vary according to the presenting features of the disease. The most important of these prognostic factors is usually the stage at presentation, but grade, tumour markers, site and biochemical parameters may also need to be considered. In addition, the age and gender of the individual may influence outcome. The certification assessment method takes into account survival data for homogeneous groups using the most important prognostic indicator or indicators. It is possible to vary the level of certification for an individual according to whether the prognostic factors that exist at presentation would weight the overall prognosis towards a substantially better or worse outcome.

As described in Chapter 36, the maximum acceptable annual risk of incapacitation for a pilot undertaking multi-crew operations is one per cent per annum. This is also the maximum permissible risk for an ATCO with a proximity endorsement. Unrestricted certification is possible only when the risk of incapacitation is substantially less than this.

Certification assessment method

There are three main factors to consider when assessing an individual's risk of recurrence of malignant disease in any one year. The first is the actual risk of recurrence, the second is the site of that recurrence, and the third is the risk of a recurrence at that site leading to incapacitation (Janvrin 1995).

The annual risk of incapacitation can be calculated as shown in Figure 44.2.

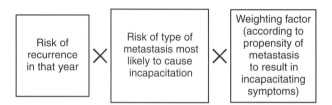

Figure 44.2 *Risk of incapacitation from recurrence of a tumour in any particular year.*

RISK OF RECURRENCE

The annual recurrence rate can be estimated from survival curves. Ideally, these should be disease-free survival curves, but for many tumours these are difficult to find and overall survival data will need to be used. However, as the prognosis after recurrence is often very poor, the overall survival and disease-free survival curves are usually very similar in shape, and the annual recurrence rate is similar to the annual mortality rate.

Overall survival figures do not allow for deaths from other causes. This is important for cancers that affect mainly older people. Figures quoted in published studies usually include patients over the age of 70 years, so they are often artificially poor for licence holders of working age. This is probably countered to some extent by the fact that individuals who develop tumours before the age of 40 years tend to have very aggressive disease. Also, survival figures will include cases where curative treatment has not been attempted.

Survival data are, by definition, historical data and represent the outcome from treatments given years ago. Improvement in survival from recently introduced treatment regimens will not be reflected in the certification assessment until published data can confirm the claims of increased efficacy of more modern treatment protocols.

These factors tend to push the certification assessment in the fail-safe direction and act to provide a regulatory safeguard.

SITE OF RECURRENCE

Each type of tumour has a propensity to recur at characteristic sites. However, it is often difficult to determine from the literature the risk of a first recurrence at a particular site. When these data do not exist, information may be obtained from post-mortems. Inevitably, post-mortem data include tissue that has become affected during the terminal phase of the disease, and sites that tend to become involved only in the late stages will be overrepresented.

Studies of malignant melanoma have shown that approximately a quarter of patients with evidence of cerebral metastases at post-mortem will have presented with a cerebral secondary as a first recurrence (Moseley *et al.* 1978). A broad assumption can be made that a similar proportion of patients with post-mortem brain involvement will be likely to present with a symptomatic cerebral metastasis.

WEIGHTING FACTOR

Each type of tumour tends to display a similar pattern of recurrence in specific organs, local to, or more distant from, the primary site. Studies that quantify the risk of presentation of recurrence with an incapacitating symptom are not widely available, as this is not the paramount concern of clinicians. The potential risk of incapacitation has, therefore, to be estimated for each likely location. The figure varies from five per cent for recurrence locally or in a regional lymph node basin to 100 per cent for sudden incapacitation from a cerebral metastasis. The possibility of subtle incapacitation also has to be considered, as many types of recurrence could result in a degradation of performance and, thus, affect the operational ability of a licence holder to some extent.

Table 44.3 shows the incapacitation risk weighting used to give a measure of the potential for sudden incapacitation from recurrence at various metastatic sites. The factor is deliberately weighted towards the upper level of expec-

Table 44.3 *Incapacitation risk weighting for recurrence at different metastatic sites*

Site	Incapacitation risk weighting (%)
Local	5
Lymph nodes	5
Liver	5
Lung	5
Bone	5
Bone marrow	20
Brain	100

tation in the interests of flight safety. It may be possible to assign a more accurate weighting factor that reflects the incapacitation risk from recurrence at different metastatic sites if quantitative data can be determined from relevant clinical studies.

Certification assessment for a theoretical tumour

In order to calculate the annual risk of incapacitation for an individual, the three parameters described above have to be determined. Figure 44.3 demonstrates the likelihood of survival for the five year period after completion of primary treatment for three stages of a theoretical tumour. The annual recurrence risk is the probability of developing a recurrence during each year and is calculated as shown in Table 44.4. As recurrence figures (in the form of disease-free survival rates) are often difficult to ascertain, overall survival figures usually have to be used. The number (or percentage) of survivors at the end of the year is divided by the total number (or percentage) alive at the start of the year in order to obtain the probability of surviving in any one-year period.

Using a theoretical example that three per cent of first recurrences will be a cerebral metastasis, with an incapacitation risk weighting of 100 per cent, the incapacitation risk for any year can be calculated by applying the formula described previously, i.e. recurrence risk × 3% × 100%, for each year.

Taking the annual recurrence risks for the theoretical tumour in Table 44.4, the annual risk of incapacitation for each stage of tumour is shown in Table 44.5.

For some malignancies, there is only a very small chance of cerebral spread and an alternative secondary site may present a greater risk of incapacitation. By knowing the likelihood of metastases affecting a particular site and applying the relevant incapacitation risk weighting, the annual incapacitation risk can be calculated.

As an incapacitation risk above 1 per cent per annum is incompatible with commercial flying, it is possible to determine the interval after primary treatment that should elapse before a licence holder can be given a certificate

Table 44.5 *Annual risk of incapacitation from recurrence of theoretical tumour*

Stage	Years since completion of primary treatment				
	1	2	3	4	5
I	0.15%	0.1%	0.07%	0.03%	0.03%
II	0.66%	0.57%	0.48%	0.28%	0.13%
III	1.5%	1.86%	1.1%	1.25%	0.86%

Assumes three per cent of recurrences will present as cerebral metastases.

Table 44.4 *Annual recurrence risk for three stages of theoretical tumour*

Stage	Years since completion of primary treatment				
	1	2	3	4	5
I	5/100 = 5%	3/95 = 3.2%	2/92 = 2.2%	1/90 = 1.1%	1/89 = 1.1%
II	22/100 = 22%	15/78 = 19.2%	10/63 = 15.9%	5/53 = 9.4%	2/48 = 4.2%
III	50/100 = 50%	31/50 = 62%	7/19 = 36.8%	5/12 = 41.7%	2/7 = 28.6%

Recurrence risk is stated as a probability and percentage for each year.

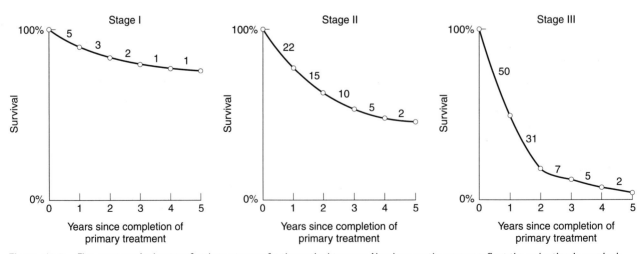

Figure 44.3 *Five-year survival curves for three stages of a theoretical tumour. Numbers on the curves reflect the reduction in survival percentage during each year.*

limited to multi-crew operations. A risk of incapacitation from tumour recurrence approaching 0.1 per cent per annum is normally required before unrestricted certification can be granted. This is demonstrated in Figure 44.4.

If prognostic factors are more favourable than those considered in the certification assessment, then it is reasonable to shift the transition point from no certification to multi-crew certification, or from multi-crew certification to unrestricted certification, to the left. Conversely, if prognostic factors are less favourable, then it is reasonable to wait for a longer period before relaxing the certificatory assessment. As the major prognostic factors will have been used in the assessment, this is likely to result in the reduction or addition of only a few months in either direction.

Similar bar charts can be created for any tumour if survival (or preferably recurrence) data are available, so that the annual recurrence rates can be calculated and the pattern of recurrence is known.

COLORECTAL CARCINOMA

Cancers of the lower gastrointestinal tract are the most common tumours seen in aircrew and the second most common malignancy seen in western societies. Survival data are usually based on whole-population studies. As the risk of colorectal carcinoma is much increased beyond the age of 60 years, it may not always be appropriate to use these data to predict prognosis in younger licence holders. As with other tumours, there is some evidence to suggest that they tend to be more aggressive in younger age groups, and this is likely to relate to genetic predisposition. Hereditary non-polyposis colorectal cancer is now known to be due to faults in the deoxyribonucleic acid (DNA) mismatch repair genes and may account for up to five per cent of all cases.

The most common site is the rectum (30 per cent), followed by the sigmoid colon (18 per cent) and the caecum

(13 per cent). Cancer of the rectum or rectosigmoid junction tends to have a slightly worse prognosis than colonic carcinoma, but the difference is sufficiently small to be of no relevance for certification.

The treatment of choice for tumour that has not spread beyond the bowel wall (Dukes' stage A or B) is curative resection. The overall rate of local or distant recurrence after surgery with curative intent is 33 per cent (Renehan *et al.* 2002). Adjuvant chemotherapy using 5-fluorouracil after surgery for Dukes' C colonic tumours, where nodal involvement has been demonstrated, has improved survival dramatically. Chemotherapy is also useful for Dukes' C rectal carcinoma and may be used in combination with preoperative radiotherapy. An alternative staging system is the TNM classification used by the American Joint Committee on Cancer (AJCC). In this system, stages T_{1-2} are equivalent to Dukes' stage A, T_{3-4} to Dukes' stage B and N_1 or more to Dukes' stage C.

The certification assessment chart for colorectal carcinoma has been created using the five-year cancer-specific survival figures for men of 90 per cent for stage A, 60 per cent for stage B and 40 per cent for stage C. Women have a slight survival advantage (McArdle *et al.* 2003). The risk of incapacitation from recurrence is low, as clinical follow-up surveillance is well established, and distant spread rarely presents symptomatically. This is reflected in the assessment, which permits early recertification, even after treatment for cancer with nodal involvement (Figure 44.5).

In addition to the stage of tumour at presentation, the grade and whether there is venous, lymphatic or perineural invasion influence the risk of local or distant relapse. The most common site of relapse is the liver, followed by local spread, pulmonary metastases and other abdominal sites. One per cent of all relapses affect cerebral tissue. Adverse prognostic factors include a short disease-free interval and the presence of multiple metastases. Distant metastatic spread is generally disqualifying. However, if recurrence can be demonstrated to be confined to a solitary metasta-

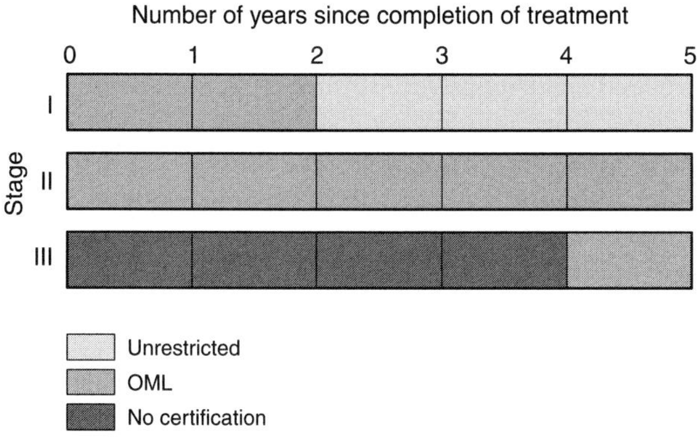

Figure 44.4 *Certification assessment during the first five years after treatment for a theoretical tumour. OML, operational multi-crew limitation.*

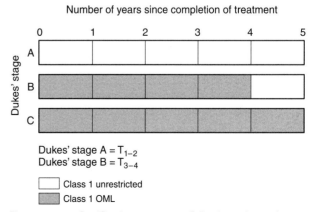

Dukes' stage A = T_{1-2}
Dukes' stage B = T_{3-4}

☐ Class 1 unrestricted
▨ Class 1 OML

Figure 44.5 *Certification assessment following colorectal cancer. OML, operational multi-crew limitation.*

sis in the liver or lung, and resection of the affected tissue is undertaken, then limited recertification may be reconsidered if the licence holder remains recurrence-free for three years post-surgery, as there appears to be a plateauing of survival after this period of time (Goldberg *et al.* 1998).

Carcinoembryonic antigen (CEA) levels may be useful as a marker of recurrence, but usually only if the levels were raised at presentation. If CEA levels are raised and a pulmonary metastasis is present, then no future certification is possible, as the prognosis is poor.

Long-term-follow up with regular CT scans and chest X-rays to look for hepatic and pulmonary metastases is essential for all licence holders, as even those with Dukes' stage A (T_{1-2}) disease have a distal relapse rate of approximately ten per cent (Gunderson *et al.* 2002).

LYMPHOID MALIGNANCY

The number of applicants for initial certification and recertification with a history of malignancy of the immune system has increased steadily during the past few years due to the increased efficacy of treatments available and consequent increase in survival. Lymphoid malignancies are a heterogeneous group of more than 25 conditions, with very different clinical features and widely varying management regimens. They have different patterns of relapse in terms of type, site and clinical presentation. The relapse-free, event-free and overall survival patterns follow completely different but quite characteristic time curves. The implications for aeromedical certification are, therefore, quite diverse.

The classification of lymphoid malignancies is complex. The World Health Organization (WHO) classification, based on the Revised European/American Lymphoma (REAL) classification, is now in widespread use. There are four broad groups: precursor cell lymphoma, B-cell neoplasms, T-cell and natural killer (NK) cell neoplasms, and Hodgkin's lymphoma. Excluding Hodgkin's disease, the peripheral B-cell neoplasms make up 85 per cent of all lymphoid malignancy seen in aviation medical practice. The most common are B-cell chronic lymphocytic leukaemia, follicular lymphoma and diffuse large B-cell lymphoma.

Hodgkin's lymphoma

The ten-year survival rates for stage I–IV Hodgkin's disease vary from 95 to 60 per cent. These figures have shown a steady improvement over the past 30 years and are continuing to improve. The risk of sudden incapacitation as a presentation of relapse of Hodgkin's disease is negligible.

As most cases are treated with an anthracycline, professional aircrew and controllers should undertake cardiological evaluation before certification. They will require lifelong follow-up because their risk of a second malignancy, either a solid tumour or leukaemia, following chemotherapy is raised (Swerdlow *et al.* 2000). Provided both oncology and cardiology reports are satisfactory, class 1 medical certification can be returned six months after completing treatment and the multi-crew limitation can be removed after two years of clinical remission. Hodgkin's lymphoma that is refractory to conventional therapy is sometimes treated with stem-cell transplantation. Certification is possible if remission is sustained for a minimum of 1 year after autologous transplantation and two or three years after allogeneic transplantation.

Other types of lymphoma

Lymphomas can be divided broadly into those that are aggressive but potentially curable and those that are indolent and inexorably progressive. The aggressive group has a survival curve that demonstrates a high mortality risk in the first year or two after diagnosis but once this time has elapsed the chance of relapse is very slim. The indolent group may stay in asymptomatic remission for long periods of time and pose the greater certificatory problem, as relapse, although inevitable, may be delayed for many years. Chemotherapy is often used to slow progression in this group, and certification can be considered even after one or more relapses. Cutaneous lymphomas are a very diverse group of conditions. The five-year survival ranges from 100 per cent to less than five per cent, depending on the individual condition, but most have a very good prognosis.

CERTIFICATION ASSESSMENT

All lymphoid malignancies have to be treated separately, as distinct entities, for certificatory purposes. For each type of lymphoid malignancy, published survival rates allow estimation of the likelihood of potential cure. They can be categorized into groups with similar prognoses (Table 44.6). Known prognostic factors at presentation, such as age, stage, lactate dehydrogenase level, number of extranodal sites involved and performance status, which is related to mobility impairment, have to be taken into account on a case-by-case basis. Performance status is scored according to the Eastern Co-operative Oncology Group scale, from 0 (fully active), to 1 (ambulatory) through to 4 (totally confined to bed).

Consideration also has to be given to the likelihood of central nervous system relapse and the time period to recertification must be weighted accordingly. An assessment of incapacitation risk can be undertaken when full clinical

Table 44.6 *Potential cure rates in patients with lymphoid malignancy*

Group	Potential cure (%)	Diagnosis
A	> 80	MZ MALT (stage I/II) DLBC (stage I/II) ALCL (stage I/II) Solitary plasmacytoma
B	50	Primary mediastinal lymphoma
C	30	DLBC (stage III/IV) ALCL (stage III/IV) including ALK negative MZ MALT (stage III/IV)
D	30	Burkitt's/Burkitt-like lymphoma Pre-B lymphoblastic lymphoma/leukaemia B-cell lymphoblastic lymphoma/leukaemia Multiple myeloma – BMT (csd)
E	10–20	Pre-T ALL Pre-T LBL Mantle cell lymphoma (two years symptom free)
F	< 10, moderately aggressive	Other peripheral T-cell and NK lymphoma/leukaemia Adult T-cell lymphoma (HTLV+) Mantle cell lymphoma Multiple myeloma (other) Subcutaneous panniculitis T-cell lymphoma
G	Considered incurable using current therapy, but indolent	Follicular lymphoma SLL B-cell CLL Lymphoplasmacytic lymphoma T-cell prolymphocytic leukaemia T-cell granular lymphocytic leukaemia Hairy cell leukaemia MZ B-cell lymphoma (nodal/splenic)
H	Miscellaneous group with a generally good prognosis	Primary cutaneous lymphoma

ALCL, anaplastic large cell lymphoma; ALK, anaplastic lymphoma kinase; BMT, bone marrow transplantation; CLL, chronic lymphocytic leukaemia; csd, compatible sibling donor; DLBC, diffuse large B-cell lymphoma; HTLV, human T-cell lymphoma/leukaemia virus 1; MALT, mucosa-associated lymphoid tissue; MZ, marginal zone lymphoma; NK, natural killer; Pre-T ALL, precursor T-cell lymphoblastic leukaemia; Pre-T LBL, precursor T-cell lymphoblastic lymphoma; SLL, small lymphocytic (B-cell) lymphoma.

details are known. Any central nervous system involvement would be permanently disqualifying for medical certification. Prerequisites for certification include a minimum period of time following completion of treatment in order to ensure that a sustained remission has been achieved and that there are no ongoing side effects from treatment and minimum levels for blood parameters, including haemoglobin, platelets and neutrophil count. A full oncology report should be obtained and a regular follow-up protocol established. Any reclassification as a result of transformation to a higher grade or restaging during treatment should be noted, as this may influence certification.

Relapse is suggested most frequently by the patient noticing a lump. It may present with general symptoms such as fatigue or localized symptoms such as direct pressure effects. Relapse is sometimes detected by blood testing for cytopenias or abnormal biochemistry, and scan results during restaging occasionally may highlight progressive disease. Symptomatic relapse is relatively uncommon, and sudden incapacitation is extremely rare. Potential short-term and long-term side effects of treatment also need to be considered.

Table 44.7 gives the minimum time to class 1 certification following completion of primary treatment. Certification is based on the likelihood of long-term relapse-free survival, acknowledging that if relapse occurs, then the symptoms are almost always insidious and detectable at an early stage by routine clinical follow-up. The malignancies in group D are weighted because of their propensity for central nervous system relapse. The cutaneous lymphomas in group H have to be assessed on an individual basis because of the heterogeneity of the group.

Table 44.7 *Minimum time to class 1 certification after lymphoid malignancy*

Group	Class 1 multi-crew	Class 1 unrestricted
A	3 months	3 months
B	6 months	2 years
C	1 year	2 years
D	2 years	3 years
E	2 years	3 years
F	5 years	10 years
G	3 months	1 year
H	6 weeks	6 weeks

Leukaemia

The myelogenous leukaemias are seen much less frequently than those of lymphoid origin in applicants for certification. This is due mainly to the poor prognosis of acute myeloblastic leukaemia and the fact that allogeneic bone-marrow transplant is currently the only potentially curative option for chronic myeloid leukaemia. After an appropriate period of remission, certificatory assessment can be undertaken using the same principles as described above for lymphoid malignancy.

CUTANEOUS MALIGNANT MELANOMA

The past few decades have seen an increase in the incidence of malignant melanoma in many parts of the world, and flight crew may be at particular risk. Whether this is because of lifestyle factors with enhanced opportunity for sun exposure, or whether it is related to ultraviolet irradiation in the cockpit, remains to be determined.

The prognosis of a primary malignant melanoma depends on the vertical thickness of the excised lesion, as first described by Clark *et al.* (1969) and subsequently confirmed by Breslow (1970), and whether there is lymph-node involvement or more distant spread (Breslow 1970).

Ulceration is now known to be associated with a poorer prognosis, and anatomical site also influences outcome. A lesion on the arm is more favourable than one on the trunk or leg; a lesion on the head or neck has the worst prognosis. Being male and over 50 years of age is also associated with a poorer prognosis, but the histological category is not of prognostic value.

Treatment is by surgical excision. Sentinel lymph-node mapping (identification of the lymph node to which the affected area of skin drains) and biopsy at the time of excision influences the decision to remove the complete lymph-node basin, but it has not been established whether this affects survival. The long-term benefits of immunotherapy and chemotherapy have yet to be proven, and trials are ongoing with vaccines containing melanoma-associated antigens to stimulate antibody production against the tumour.

Melanoma confined to the skin

Certification is possible only if there has been complete excision of the primary lesion with regular clinical examination for signs of local recurrence and regional and distant metastases. Clinical staging uses the TNM classification to describe the extent of disease. This method assesses tumour spread after primary excision and pathological staging, which takes into account microscopic evaluation of both the primary tumour and locoregional lymph nodes. A comparison of pathological and clinical staging, as described by the American Joint Committee on Cancer (AJCC), is shown in Table 44.8 (Balch *et al.* 2001).

If the primary tumour is ulcerated, then the prognosis has to be upstaged. For example, a T_2 tumour with ulceration has the prognosis of a T_3 tumour that is not ulcerated. A T_4 tumour with ulceration is equivalent in prognostic terms to a node-positive lesion.

The AJCC Melanoma Database consists of more than 30 000 patients, and complete prognostic factors are known for 17 600 of them. Survival data demonstrate a marked reduction in survival with higher stage and,

Table 44.8 *Comparison of staging classifications for malignant melanoma*

Pathological stage	Clinical stage	Tumour thickness (mm)	Nodes	Metastases
I	T1	≤ 1	No	No
	T2	1–2	No	No
II	T3	2–4	No	No
	T4	> 4	No	No
III	N1	Any	1	No
	N2	Any	2–3	No
	N3	Any	4+	No
IV	M	Any	Yes/no	Yes

importantly, a continued reduction in survival beyond ten years from primary treatment for stages I and II. This supports the clinical impression that recurrence of melanoma is notoriously difficult to predict, even many years after first presentation.

Assessment after excision of a primary cutaneous melanoma limited to skin or locoregional lymph nodes is shown in Figure 44.6. T_1 lesions have a good prognosis, and unrestricted certification is possible as soon as the wound has healed sufficiently to permit a return to operational duties.

Nodal involvement

Survival rates for microscopic lymph-node disease appear to be better than in cases where macroscopic disease has been demonstrated (Schuchter 2001). Microscopic disease may be detected on elective or selective lymph-node dissection or biopsy of the sentinel lymph node. Additionally, melanoma may be detected only in a lymph node by molecular diagnostic techniques such as immunohistological staining or reverse-transcriptase polymerase chain reaction (RT-PCR) to detect tyrosinase messenger ribonucleic acid (RNA).

Certification after macroscopic lymph-node involvement is more difficult than if only microscopic disease has been detected. The number of nodes affected – the N staging – also influences outcome. It may be reasonable to downstage by one stage, e.g. consider microscopic N_2 disease as N_1 or microscopic N_1 disease as T_4, if there are no lymph nodes affected on macroscopic examination in a similar way to the upstaging of disease if the primary lesion is ulcerated.

Metastatic disease

Metastatic disease beyond regional lymph nodes is incompatible with class 1 certification.

Local recurrence

The most common site of recurrence of a melanoma is in the scar from the original excision or in the surrounding skin. Five-year survival rates after local recurrence vary in the literature, from 60 per cent for in-scar recurrence (Cohn-Cedermark *et al.* 1997) to nine per cent for local skin (Balch *et al.* 2000). Recertification after local recur-

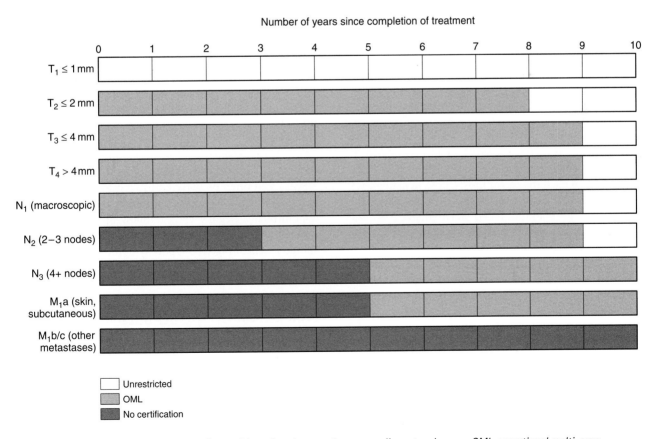

Figure 44.6   *Certification assessment after excision of a primary cutaneous malignant melanoma. OML, operational multi-crew limitation.*

rence has to be assessed, taking into account all of the known prognostic factors at the original presentation, as these continue to influence survival. The overall prognosis is similar for local recurrence, satellite disease and in-transit metastases, and these can be grouped together as 'regional stage III disease' and treated as such for certificatory purposes (Schuchter 2001).

Distant recurrence

The most common site of recurrence is local skin (40 per cent), followed by regional lymph nodes. Less common sites are the lungs (19 per cent), the brain (17 per cent) and the liver (six per cent) (Akslen et al. 1987). The incidence of cerebral metastases presenting as the first recurrence following treatment of a primary melanoma was found to be eight per cent in a large US and Australian series and was also exactly the same figure in a group of US Air Force personnel (Conrad et al. 1971). Cerebral spread often occurs alone, without evidence of regional lymph node spread or metastases to other sites, unlike spread to lung, liver or bone (Akslen et al. 1987). It is particularly important to identify latent cerebral spread in aircrew; as the resolution of the imaging techniques available continues to improve, MRI may become increasingly useful to detect asymptomatic cerebral secondaries.

GERM-CELL TUMOURS OF THE TESTIS

Testicular tumours are predominantly of germ-cell origin. There are two main types, seminoma and non-seminomatous germ-cell tumours (NSGCTs). They account for 15 per cent of aircrew seeking recertification following treatment for malignant disease. This is not surprising, as germ-cell tumours of the testis are the most common malignancy in males between the ages of 20 and 40 years. Since the introduction of platinum-based chemotherapy in the 1970s, over 95 per cent of patients can now expect to be cured (Dearnaley et al. 2001).

Germ-cell tumours arise from primitive germ cells, and more than 90 per cent arise in the testes. NSGCTs arising in other primary sites such as the mediastinum, and other types of testicular cancer, e.g. choriocarcinoma and embryonal carcinoma, tend to have a poorer prognosis and are not considered here.

A staging system based on disease site of origin, histology, tumour size and level of serum tumour markers has been developed by the International Germ Cell Cancer Collaborative Group (1997). The prognosis for seminoma and NSGCT is related to metastatic spread to secondary sites. The prognosis for NSGCT is also related to the level of serum tumour markers, alpha-fetoprotein (AFP),

human chorionic gonadotrophin (hCG) and lactate dehydrogenase (LDH) at presentation and to the extent of disease. If the AFP is raised, then the tumour cannot be a pure seminoma and is treated as a NSGCT.

Most licence holders present with early stage I disease confined to the testis. Standard treatment is orchidectomy, often combined with platinum-based chemotherapy if vascular invasion has occurred, for NSGCT, and radiotherapy to para-aortic lymph nodes for seminoma, which is a highly radiosensitive tumour. Even if salvage treatment for recurrence is subsequently required, the cure rate for stage I tumours approaches 100 per cent and unrestricted certification is, therefore, appropriate for this group.

Figure 44.7 shows the certification assessment following primary treatment for germ-cell tumours of the testis that have spread beyond the testis. In more extensive disease, the progression-free survival curves plateau two to four years after completion of treatment, irrespective of the initial stage, and most pilots will be able to achieve unrestricted certification once this time period has elapsed.

Even with metastatic disease, the prognosis in testicular cancer is good compared with that of other tumours. The organs most likely to be affected include the liver, lung, bone, brain and adrenal gland. Central nervous system relapse after chemotherapy for NSGCT is very rare and invariably occurs concomitantly with, or is preceded by, systemic metastases. For seminoma, the risk of cerebral relapse is negligible (Fosså et al. 1999). Seminoma with pulmonary metastases falls into the group with a good prognosis.

Survival rates for NSGCT and seminoma range from 92 and 86 per cent for good-prognosis tumours, to 80 and 72 per cent, respectively, for those with an intermediate prognosis, to less than 50 per cent for poor-prognosis NSGCT (International Germ Cell Cancer Collaborative Group 1997). The good-prognosis group accounts for three-quarters of all germ-cell tumours. Asymptomatic relapse in NSGCT can often be detected by elevated serum tumour markers, which are quantified routinely at oncology review appointments. Regular clinical follow-up, including chest radiography, is routine for all germ-cell tumours. Aircrew should be encouraged to report symptomatic relapse with pain or detection of a lump as soon as symptoms occur.

CARCINOMA OF THE BLADDER

Transitional cell carcinoma accounts for 90 per cent of all bladder cancers. Adenocarcinoma, squamous cell carcinoma and small-cell carcinoma are much less common. Bladder cancer is common among the general population but is seen relatively infrequently in licence holders. This is partly because it affects mainly men over the age of 60 years and partly because tobacco use is a major risk factor and a

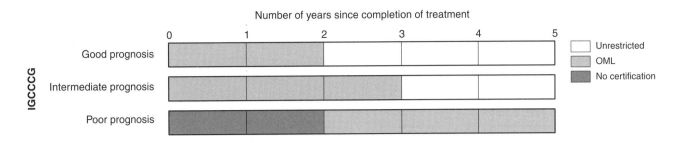

International Germ Cell Cancer Collaborative Group (IGCCCG) prognosis

Good prognosis =   All seminoma except non-pulmonary metastases
                        NSGCT: AFP < 1000 ng/ml
                                  hCG < 5000 IU/l
                                  LDH less than ×1.5 normal

Intermediate prognosis = Seminoma with non-pulmonary metastases
                          NSGCT: AFP < 10 000 ng/ml
                                    hCG < 50 000 IU/l
                                    LDH up to ×10 normal

Poor prognosis =   NSGCT   AFP > 10 000 ng/ml
                                  hCG > 50 000 IU/l
                                  LDH more than ×10 normal

Figure 44.7 *Certification assessment after treatment for a germ-cell tumour of the testis (other than stage I). AFP, alpha-fetoprotein; hCG, human chorionic gonadotrophin; LDH, lactate dehydrogenase; OML, operational multi-crew limitation.*

smaller proportion of licence holders smoke than in the general population.

Treatment of an early tumour is by transurethral resection followed by regular cystoscopic examination. More invasive tumours may require intravesical chemotherapy or immunotherapy with bacillus Calmette–Guérin (BCG) and possibly total cystectomy.

Following removal of an in situ carcinoma of the bladder, a licence holder may be given unrestricted class 1 certification. Lesions limited to the lamina propria (T_1) are also compatible with unrestricted class 1 certification, but 50 per cent are likely to progress and, thus, close surveillance is required (Borden *et al.* 2003). The prognosis is much poorer for tumours extending to muscle (T_2a and T_2b), and radical cystectomy is likely to be the treatment of choice. An operational multi-crew limitation (OML) limitation or unfit assessment may be appropriate in this circumstance. If there is microscopic or macroscopic extension beyond the bladder (T_3a or higher), then certification is unlikely to be possible.

ADENOCARCINOMA OF THE PROSTATE

The certification of licence holders with adenocarcinoma of the prostate is relatively straightforward compared with most other cancers. This is because progression of disease can, in the majority of cases, be tracked using the tumour marker prostate-specific antigen (PSA). The use of PSA as a screening tool is controversial, as less than a third of those with a raised PSA will have prostate cancer and up to 20 per cent of those with prostate cancer have a normal PSA. For disease monitoring, however, it is a useful indicator of activity and prognosis, and a raised PSA usually precedes clinical detection of progression by 6–12 months.

Prostate cancer is a disease of elderly men and is seen rarely before the age of 50 years. It is generally indolent, and watchful waiting is an acceptable management protocol for early, localized disease. Other treatments include surgical removal of affected tissue, radiotherapy (external beam or radioactive implants known as brachytherapy) and neoadjuvant hormone therapy, although even for high-grade tumours the treatment method has little influence on overall survival (So *et al.* 2003).

Nomograms are being used increasingly in clinical practice to predict outcome and are likely to be useful for aviation medical practice as they become more refined (Di Blasio *et al.* 2003). The main prognostic factors for recurrent disease are the pretreatment PSA, stage and Gleason score (determined by adding two gradings of biopsy tissue each scored from 1 to 5).

In aviation medicine, prostate cancer is of certificatory importance only if it extends beyond the prostatic capsule (stage T_3 or higher), the PSA trend is rising (especially when > 20 μg/l) and/or the Gleason score is 8–10. These factors relate to a higher probability of recurrence and a poorer prognosis. Certification is possible after treatment as long as the PSA remains suppressed and there is no evidence of nodal or bony spread on scanning. Even a pilot who has undergone radical prostatectomy with subsequent hormonal androgen suppression may be able to continue flying multi-crew operations with close surveillance if there is no evidence of active distant metastases.

CARCINOMA OF THE KIDNEY

Renal cell cancers comprise 90 per cent of all cancers affecting the kidney. Of renal cell cancers, three-quarters are clear-cell carcinomas and 10–15 per cent are papillary carcinomas. Collecting duct carcinoma, chromophobe and unclassified tumours are rare. Tumours arising from the renal pelvis are mainly transitional cell cancers and associated with a high risk of later bladder cancer.

Treatment is usually radical nephrectomy, often with postoperative cytokine-based immunotherapy. Partial nephrectomy is sometimes undertaken for small, localized tumours.

The most important prognostic factor is stage at diagnosis. T_1 tumours measure less than 7 cm and T_2 more than 7 cm; both are limited to the kidney. T_3 tumours do not extend beyond the Gerota fascia (they may involve the renal vein, vena cava or adrenal gland), but T_4 tumours do extend beyond this layer. Grade 1 tumours are associated with a relatively good prognosis, but any effect on general

mobility, as reflected by a performance score of more than zero, is associated with a poorer prognosis. These factors have been incorporated into the University of California, Los Angeles (UCLA) integrated staging system, as shown in Table 44.9 (Zisman *et al.* 2002).

Metastatic spread is detected in up to 50 per cent of patients at diagnosis. The most common sites are the lung (42 per cent) and bone (22 per cent), followed by the adrenal glands and brain (two per cent) (Janzen *et al.* 2003). Approximately half of T_3 tumours will recur, usually within two years of the original presentation. Cerebral metastases tend to be seen as a late manifestation of disease and invariably are associated with other metastases. The appearance of a late solitary cerebral metastasis more than ten years after treatment that seemed to have been curative is extremely rare, with only seven cases reported in the literature.

Certification after treatment for renal cell carcinoma is shown in Figure 44.8. The prognosis for tumours that have spread to nodes or more distantly, or have recurred after primary treatment, is poor. Fitness for certification has to be assessed on an individual basis but is unlikely to be possible for metastatic disease.

CARCINOMA OF THE BREAST

As the proportion of female licence holders is gradually increasing, there is likely to be an increase in prevalence of breast cancer within the aviation population with time. Male breast cancer and histological types other than invasive ductal, ductal carcinoma in situ or lobular carcinoma of the breast are rare and should be considered separately.

The most significant indicators of prognosis are tumour grade, stage as indicated by histological lymph-node involvement, and tumour size. The Nottingham Prognostic Index (NPI) (Haybittle *et al.* 1982) uses these factors to predict outcome on an individual basis by applying the following formula:

$$NPI = 0.2 \times size \text{ (in cm)} + stage \text{ (I–III)} + grade \text{ (1–3; good, moderate, poor)}$$

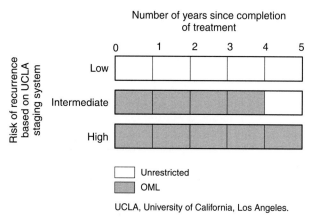

Figure 44.8 *Certification assessment after treatment for renal cell carcinoma. OML, operational multi-crew limitation.*

Table 44.9 *University of California, Los Angeles (UCLA) integrated staging system for N_0M_0 renal cell carcinoma*

Risk factor for recurrence	T stage	Grade	Performance status	5-year survival (%)
Low	1	1–2	0	91
Intermediate	1, 2 or 3	Any	Any	71–80
High	4 or 3	Any	1+	40–55

Performance status determined according to Eastern Co-operative Oncology Group criteria.

- Stage I: no lymph-node involvement.
- Stage II: lower axillary or internal mammary nodes positive.
- Stage III: apex or both axillary and mammary nodes positive.

The prognosis is, thus, assessed as good, intermediate or poor in terms of long-term survival (Table 44.10). Since it was first described, the NPI has been used to predict survival with tumours of less than 1 cm in size and in metastatic disease.

Table 44.10 *Fifteen-year survival for breast cancer using the Nottingham Prognostic Index (NPI) prognostic groups*

Prognosis	NPI	15-year survival (%)
Good	< 3.4	80
Moderate	3.4–5.4	42
Poor	> 5.4	13

Using this formula, the 15-year survival of the 'good' group is consistent with that of an age-matched female population (Galea *et al.* 1992) and, therefore, no certificatory restrictions need to be applied to licence holders with good-prognosis tumours. However, the prognosis for the other groups is considerably worse and notoriously difficult to estimate in an individual case. Recurrences continue to occur many years after primary treatment, and survival rates are influenced for many decades. Figure 44.9 shows the certification assessment after treatment for carcinoma of the breast.

Oestrogen receptor (ER) negativity appears to adversely influence survival, mainly in the first few years after diagnosis, but the effect is less marked with time.

Mastectomy or lumpectomy, with or without radiotherapy, is the mainstay of treatment. The use of adjuvant chemotherapy is determined by the extent of disease, menopausal and ER status. Postmenopausal ER-positive women may be given tamoxifen, which is compatible with certification. Other therapies, including aromatase inhibitors and hormone analogues, may be acceptable.

Genetic factors are likely to play an increasing role in both the therapy and the prognosis of breast cancer. Breast-cancer susceptibility is known to be increased in the presence of mutations of *BRCA1* and *BRCA2* genes. The expression of the human epidermal growth factor receptor-2 (HER-2) may influence prognosis and is used to provide a basis for therapeutic choices if an anthracycline is unacceptable.

In moderate- and poor-prognosis disease, the concern for aeromedical certification is the risk of a sudden incapacitation from covert metastatic disease. The most common sites involved are the liver, lung and bone. Cerebral metastases occur in 10–30 per cent of those with life-limiting disease, and there is some evidence to suggest that they may be more common in people with ER negativity. Because the course and prognosis of breast cancer are so variable, and there can be a long interval between primary treatment and the presentation of secondary spread, long-term oncology follow-up is important for certificatory purposes.

LUNG CANCER

Tumours of the lung are seen very rarely in aircrew. Although lung cancer is very common, it is seen mainly in elderly people, it is often not diagnosed before it has become inoperable, and the prognosis is very poor. This is especially true for small-cell lung cancer, which has a five-year survival of five per cent and for which there are limited treatment possibilities. It also has a high predilection for cerebral metastases (Janssen-Heijnen *et al.* 1998). Treatment often includes cranial irradiation as well as chemotherapy, and paraneoplastic syndromes may complicate the clinical situation. Future certification is unlikely to be possible with this condition.

Using the standard certification process described earlier in this chapter, it may be possible to recertificate a

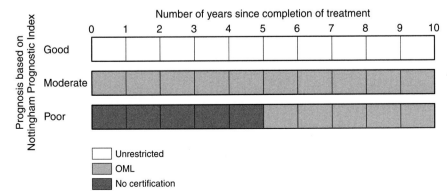

Figure 44.9 *Certification assessment after treatment for breast cancer. OML, operational multi-crew limitation.*

licence holder who has had a non-small-cell lung cancer (NSCLC) successfully resected and with no evidence of metastatic spread.

Figure 44.10 shows the certificatory possibilities following surgical treatment for the three most common types of NSCLC, adenocarcinoma, squamous cell carcinoma and large-cell (undifferentiated) carcinoma. Other types of NSCLC should be considered separately. Staging is based on the TNM classification (Mountain 1986). Stages I and II tend to be described as 'localized' tumours and have a much better prognosis than stage IIIA tumours. Five-year survival figures are 60 per cent, 58 per cent and 36 per cent, respectively, for patients under 40 years (Skarin *et al.* 2001) and 45 per cent, 25 per cent and 15 per cent for all ages (Mountain 1986). The prognosis for stage IIIB or IV is too poor to permit certification.

For resected stage I–IIIA disease, once a disease-free interval of five years has been reached, the future risk of recurrence is less than the risk of developing a second lung primary. The risk of late recurrence is not related to initial stage and has a much poorer outcome than a second primary.

CONCLUSION

Certificatory guidelines for fitness to fly after treatment for malignant disease have evolved during the past few years as more information has become available from clinical studies in respect of overall and disease-free survival rates from different types of cancer. This has allowed the more accurate estimation of future incapacitation risk from recurrence of disease or sequelae from treatment. Licence holders should be encouraged to report symptomatic recurrence as soon as they are aware of symptoms. Regular clinical follow-up and investigations to detect recurrence at the earliest possible stage, together with the use of modern imaging and biochemical techniques, facilitates certification with close surveillance.

The survival rates for many cancers, such as those of the immune system, are continuing to improve as more effective regimens are used. Treatment of many childhood cancers has shown particular improvement during the past few decades, and an increasing number of applicants for initial certification for professional flying or ATCO training declare a history of treatment for cancer as a child. The type of assessment described in this chapter enables consideration of these candidates who previously would not have been able to embark on a commercial career in aviation.

As the complexity of the human genome is starting to become unravelled, our understanding and knowledge of the development and progression of many cancers at the molecular genetic level is growing and may soon lead to the development of therapies targeted at a molecular level. Tumour markers are already in routine clinical use for some tumours, but new advances in molecular biology, such as the polymerase chain reaction (PCR), permit the detection of cells that it is not possible to identify using conventional microscopic techniques. In addition, molecular markers may, in the future, allow prognostic assessment on an individual basis. Attempts are being made to correlate markers of cell function with progression, likelihood of recurrence and survival.

Clinical trials of vaccination using autologous tumour cells are being undertaken for melanoma and colorectal carcinoma, and gene therapy using genetically modified viruses to selectively destroy cancer cells is also being tried. Whether these therapies will affect the long-term outcome has yet to be determined.

These certification guidelines will need to be reviewed constantly with the advent of effective new therapies and in the light of new outcome data. If more data can be obtained on the risk of incapacitation from recurrence and the type of presentation of relapse, then it may be possible to relax the certification assessments further. In the meantime, the outlook for licence holders with malignant disease remains hopeful, and the certification doctor has an important role to play in supporting the licence holder through the period of illness and back to fitness whenever possible.

REFERENCES

Akslen LA, Hove LM, Hartveit F. Metastatic distribution in malignant melanoma: a 30-year autopsy study. *Invasion and Metastasis* 1987; 7: 253–63.

Balch MB, Soong S-J, Smith T, *et al.* Long-term results of a prospective surgical trial comparing 2cm vs. 4cm excision margins for 740 patients with 1–4mm melanomas. *Annals of Surgical Oncology* 2000; 8: 101–8.

Balch CM, Buzaid AC, Soong S-J, *et al.* Final version of the American Joint Committee on Cancer staging system for cutaneous melanoma. *Journal of Clinical Oncology* 2001; 19: 3635–48.

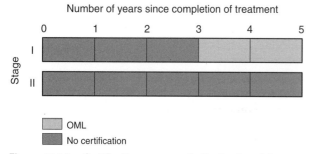

Figure 44.10 *Certification assessment after treatment for non-small-cell lung cancer. OML, operational multi-crew limitation.*

Borden LS, Clark PE, Craig Hall M. Bladder cancer. *Current Opinions in Oncology* 2003; **15**: 227–33.

Breslow A. Thickness, cross-sectional areas and depth of invasion in the prognosis of cutaneous melanoma. *Annals of surgery* 1970; **172**: 902–8.

Clark W, From L, Bernardino E, Mihm M. The histogenesis and biologic behavior of primary human malignant melanomas of the skin. *Cancer Research* 1969; **29**: 705–26.

Cohn-Cedermark G, Månsson-Brahme E, Rutqvist LE, *et al.* Outcomes of patients with local recurrence of cutaneous malignant melanoma. *Cancer* 1997; **80**: 1418–25.

Conrad FG, Rossing RG, Allen MF, Bales MR. Hazard rate of recurrence in patients with malignant melanoma. *Aerospace Medicine* 1971; **42**: 1219–25.

Dearnaley DP, Huddart RA, Horwich A. Managing testicular cancer. *British Medical Journal* 2001; **322**: 1583–8.

Di Blasio CJ, Rhee AC, Cho D, *et al.* Predicting clinical end points: treatment nomograms in prostate cancer. *Seminars in Oncology* 2003; **30**: 567–86.

Evans SA, Cooke JNC. Cardiac effects of anthracycline treatment and their implications for aeromedical certification. *Aviation, Space, and Environmental Medicine* 2003; **74**: 1003–8.

Fosså SD, Bokemeyer C, Gerl A, *et al.* Treatment outcome of patients with brain metastases from malignant germ cell tumours. *Cancer* 1999; **85**: 988–97.

Galea MH, Blamey RW, Elston CE, *et al.* The Nottingham Prognostic Index in primary breast cancer. *Breast Cancer Research and Treatment* 1992; **22**: 207–19.

Goldberg RM, Fleming TR, Tangen CM, *et al.* Surgery for recurrent colon cancer: strategies for identifying respectable recurrence and success rates after resection. *Annals of Internal Medicine* 1998; **129**: 27–35.

Gunderson LL, Sargent DJ, Tepper JE, *et al.* Impact of T and N substage on survival and disease relapse in adjuvant rectal cancer: a pooled analysis. *International Journal of Radiation, Oncology, Biology, Physics* 2002; **54**: 386–96.

Haybittle JL, Blamey RW, Elston CW, *et al.* A prognostic index in primary breast cancer. *British Journal of Cancer* 1982; **45**: 361–6.

International Civil Aviation Organization. Annex 1 to the Convention on International Civil Aviation 2001, 9th edn. Montreal: International Civil Aviation Organization, 2001.

International Germ Cell Cancer Collaborative Group. The International Germ Cell Consensus Classification: a prognostic factor-based staging system for metastatic germ cell cancer. *Journal of Clinical Oncology* 1997; **15**: 594–603.

Janssen-Heijnen MLG, Gatta G, Forman D, *et al.* Variation in survival of patients with lung cancer in Europe 1985–1989. *European Journal of Cancer* 1998; **34**: 2191–6.

Janvrin S. Aeromedical certification after treatment for malignant disease. Dissertation. London: Royal College of Physicians, Faculty of Occupational Medicine, 1995.

Janzen NK, Kim HL, Figlin RA, Belldegrun AS. Surveillance after radical or partial nephrectomy for localized renal cell carcinoma and management of recurrent disease. *Urology Clinics of North America* 2003; **30**: 843–52.

McArdle CS, McMillan DC, Hole DJ. Male gender adversely affects survival following surgery for colorectal cancer. *British Journal of Surgery* 2003; **90**: 711–15.

Moseley HS, Nizze A, Morton DL. Disseminated melanoma presenting as a catastrophic event. *Aviation, Space, and Environmental Medicine* 1978; **49**: 1342–6.

Mountain CF. A new international staging system for lung cancer. *Chest* 1986; **89**: 225–335.

Rafnsson V, Hrafnkelsson J, Tulinius H, *et al.* Risk factors for cutaneous malignant melanoma among aircrews and a random sample of the population. *Occupational and Environmental Medicine* 2003; **60**: 815–820.

Renehan AG, Egger M, Saunders MP, O'Dwyer ST. Impact on survival of intensive follow up after curative resection for colorectal cancer: systematic review and meta-analysis of randomised trials. *British Medical Journal* 2002; **324**: 813–16.

Schuchter LM. Review of the 2001 AJCC staging system for cutaneous malignant melanoma. *Current Oncology Reports* 2001; **3**: 332–7.

Skarin AT, Herbst RS, Leong TL, *et al.* Lung cancer in patients under 40. *Lung cancer* 2001; **32**: 255–64.

So A, Goldenberg SL, Gleave ME. Prostate specific antigen: an updated review. *Canadian Journal of Urology* 2003; **10**: 2040–50.

Swerdlow AJ, Barber JA, Hudson GV, *et al.* Risk of second malignancy after Hodgkin's disease in a collaborative British cohort; the relation to age at treatment. *Journal of Clinical Oncology* 2000; **18**: 498–509.

Zisman A, Pantuck AJ, Wieder J, *et al.* Risk group assessment and clinical outcome algorithm to predict the natural history of patients with surgically resected renal cell carcinoma. *Journal of Clinical Oncology* 2002; **20**: 4559–66.

FURTHER READING

Cancer Research UK. CancerStats reports. www.cancerresearchuk.org/statistics/cancerstats

Coleman MC. *Cancer Risk after Medical Treatment*, 1st edn. Oxford: Oxford University Press, 1991.

Crowther D, Sutcliffe SB, Bonadonna G. Hodgkin's disease in adults. In: Peckham M, Pineda HM, Veronesi U (eds). *Oxford Textbook of Oncology*, 1st edn. Oxford: Oxford University Press, 1995; pp. 1720–57.

Souhami RL, Tannock I, Hohenberger P, Horiot J-C (eds). *Oxford Textbook of Oncology*, 2nd edn, Oxford: Oxford University Press, 2002.

45

Neurological disease

ROBERT T.G. MERRY

INTRODUCTION

The prediction of future events in a disease requires a thorough knowledge of the natural history and epidemiology. Assessing flight-safety risk depends not only on this but also on the likelihood of the disease causing disability in flight, particularly if it is sudden and severe. The specific aircrew role of the individual is also important; different roles among aircrew, and whether solo or dual, in the event of incapacitation will cause different degrees of threat to flight safety. Also, the type of flying, whether military, professional civilian or private recreational flying, is associated with a different degree of risk and physical stress, so minimum standards of fitness will vary accordingly.

Unfortunately, reliable long-term epidemiological data for neurological diseases in a relatively young population are sparse, and inevitably decisions on flight safety in a particular individual may at times be overcautious. A decision on the fitness of an individual may also vary depending on whether they are an initial applicant for certification or a trained experienced member of aircrew, when continuation of flying in a more restricted role may be possible without compromising flight safety. Regardless of the restriction that is imposed, every member of a crew must be able to carry out all emergency procedures at all times.

Neurological diseases are a common cause of incapacitation, especially if they are unheralded, unpredictable, of sudden onset or have a high risk of recurrence. Unfortunately, many of the common neurological diseases such as stroke, epilepsy and migraine fit into this group and must be regarded as significant hazards to flight safety.

INJURY TO THE NERVOUS SYSTEM

Peripheral nerve injury

After recovery from a peripheral nerve injury, the assessment of an individual's ability to perform their particular role and all emergency procedures is performed most usefully by a qualified flying instructor, often with the aid of a simulator.

The rate of recovery from a peripheral nerve injury will depend on the severity or, in the case of surgical repair, how successful the anastomosis has been. Maximum achievable recovery may not be apparent in the early period after injury, and recovery may be gradual over a number of years. Although certain types of injury are known to be associated with a poor prognosis (e.g. avulsion of a nerve root from the spinal cord), most injuries are associated with a less certain prognosis and an adequate period should be allowed before a final decision on fitness is made. In cases of incomplete recovery, muscle tendon transfer may improve function and during recovery skilled physiotherapy is important.

Spinal cord injury

Compression of the spinal cord must be relieved as soon as possible in an attempt to reduce the degree of damage, but thereafter recovery is related to the severity of injury. Time must be allowed for recovery from acute spinal shock, but thereafter return of function depends on spontaneous recovery, although intensive physiotherapy and reduction of spasticity have a profound effect on the eventual outcome.

Head injury

Neurological complications of head injury include intracranial or intracerebral haemorrhage, focal neurological dysfunction, infection, epilepsy, cognitive dysfunction and damage to individual cranial nerves. After recovery from the acute phase, a decision on fitness to return to flying depends on full recovery of cognition, emotional stability, motor function, intact special senses and an acceptably low risk of epilepsy.

Any blunt head injury severe enough to cause disturbance of consciousness inevitably is associated with some degree of brain contusion, with a risk of permanent injury, and the more severe the contusion the higher the risk. Even a minor contusion can have profound temporary adverse effects on brain function, and in aircrew it is prudent to ground an individual until they have had sufficient time to recover (minimum period of four weeks) and are asymptomatic and free of signs of residual dysfunction or risk of the development of complications. In blunt head injury, the duration of unconsciousness is an indication of the severity of brain contusion, but this is difficult to assess in retrospect. However, the duration of post-traumatic amnesia (PTA) also correlates accurately with the severity of brain injury, and this period can be determined accurately by the patient and is retained permanently. Occasionally, if a head injury is followed by a period of natural sleep, or is associated with alcoholic amnesia or sedation, then the period of amnesia may be misleadingly prolonged, but provided allowance is made for these factors a reasonably good estimate of severity of injury to the brain can be made. Provided there are no other adverse factors and a full recovery has occurred, then a return to flying should be possible four to six weeks after a minor blunt head injury when the PTA is less than 30 minutes. If the head injury was more severe, then the period of grounding will be governed by the duration of PTA; if the PTA is longer than 24 hours, then the period of grounding should be for more than one year. A computed tomography (CT) head scan in the acute stage can also provide a guide to future complications, for if there is evidence of a haemorrhagic cerebral contusion, intracranial haemorrhage or haematoma, then the risk of permanent brain damage and epilepsy is increased.

Post-traumatic epilepsy

One of the most serious complications of a head injury is the development of epilepsy; the more severe the head injury, the higher the risk. The overall cumulative incidence of epilepsy is five per cent, but certain complications are associated with a higher incidence. Studies have shown that more than half of the cases of post-traumatic epilepsy (PTE) develop within one year, and 75 per cent within two years. In minor blunt head injuries the incidence returns to the risk of the general population by five years, but in severe head injuries associated with various complications the initial risk is much greater, and the incidence continues to increase for more than 20 years.

Jennett (1975) found that PTE was more likely if the head injury was complicated by a penetrating brain injury, depressed fracture of the skull with torn dura, focal neurological signs, intracranial haematoma or an early seizure. More recently, a large and prolonged follow-up study also showed that intracranial haemorrhage, particularly subdural haematoma with brain contusion, was associated with a significant risk, as were a fractured skull, PTA longer than 24 hours or age over 65 years (Annegers et al. 1998). CT scans were not available at the time of Jennett's study, and for only the past decade of the more recent study, but this showed that 34 subjects with evidence of brain contusion only on the scan did not develop PTE; another small study showed that it was those subjects whose scans showed evidence of intracerebral haemorrhage associated with an extracerebral haematoma who had the highest incidence of PTE (D'Alessandro et al. 1982). Table 45.1 gives a summary of the most important risk factors. The initial risk of the development of PTE can be calculated from the sum of the various risk factors, and thereafter the probable rate of diminution of risk can be estimated until an acceptable degree of risk of one per cent per annum for a return to dual flying is reached.

It has been shown that the electroencephalogram (EEG) was normal in 33 per cent of cases of PTE, and that when the EEG was abnormal the majority did not develop PTE. The EEG is, therefore, not useful in the prediction of PTE.

Table 45.1   *Complications of head injury associated with an increased risk of post-traumatic epilepsy*

Complication	Initial risk (%)
Penetrating brain injury	40
Depressed skull fracture with dural tear	30
Intracranial haemorrhage (subdural haematoma, intracranial haematoma)	35
Focal neurological signs	30
Early epileptic seizure	25
Late epileptic seizure	80
PTA > 24 h	13

PTA, post-traumatic amnesia.
Data from Jennett (1975).

Cranial nerve injury

OLFACTORY NERVE

Damage to the olfactory bulb fibres is a common complication of a blunt head injury and is usually permanent. Although anosmia might be considered a potential safety hazard, the ability to detect pungent or acrid fumes in the cockpit is preserved by intact nasal trigeminal perception, and so anosmia is not a contraindication to flying.

OPTIC NERVE AND VISUAL ACUITY

Visual acuity less than 6/18 in either eye results in loss of stereopsis and is below the standard required for military and professional pilots, but for private pilot certification monocular vision is not a contraindication.

OPHTHALMOPLEGIA CAUSING DOUBLE VISION

Double vision from any cause is incompatible with fitness to fly, and an individual must have recovered completely and have no significant risk of recurrence before resuming flying.

FACIAL PALSY

A severe facial palsy may impair the proper application and function of an oxygen mask in high-altitude military flying. An inability to close the eyelids may be a handicap in other aircrew roles, who may be exposed to dust or cold air, causing injury or excessive lacrimation.

HEARING LOSS

Unilateral severe deafness is incompatible with fitness for solo military pilots, but in other roles or types of flying adequate free-field hearing is often acceptable.

CEREBROVASCULAR DISEASE

The pathogenesis of stroke can be classified into ischaemic (85 per cent), haemorrhagic (14 per cent) and other (one per cent).

Ischaemic stroke

This type of stroke is due to either atherothromboembolism or lacunar infarcts of a perforating end artery. Transient cerebral ischaemic attacks (TIA) or cortical infarcts are often due to thromboembolism in a branch of a major cerebral artery. The embolus commonly arises from a thrombotic atherosclerotic plaque in a major cervical or cerebral artery, or from the heart, and is usually a symptom of more generalized atherosclerosis. Lacunar infarcts are due to a vasculopathy of small perforating cerebral end arteries, and although associated with atherosclerosis are particularly common in individuals with hypertension or diabetes and in heavy smokers.

Epidemiological studies of ischaemic stroke of both types in the general population show a poor prognosis. If an individual recovers from a first stroke or TIA, then the risk of recurrence is 11.8 per cent in the first year and five per cent per annum thereafter, so that after five years 30 per cent will have suffered another stroke or other vascular event such as a myocardial infarct; 25 per cent of these will be fatal (Sacco *et al.* 1982; Dennis *et al.* 1990; Bamford *et al.* 1987). These findings emphasize the fact that stroke is usually symptomatic of generalized atherosclerosis. Even in younger individuals who suffer a stroke, in those aged 45 years or above stroke is most commonly due to atherosclerosis, although in the group younger than 45 years the causes are more varied. In one study, atherosclerosis still accounted for 21.6 per cent, but other causes included cardioembolism (12.8 per cent), haematological disorder 8.1 (per cent), use of the contraceptive pill (11.5 per cent), dissection of major artery (ten per cent), other (16 per cent) and unknown 20 (per cent) (Lisovoski and Rousseau 1991).

Because ischaemic stroke in an individual over the age of 45 years is likely to be due to atherosclerotic thromboembolism, the prognosis is poor. The high risk of recurrence is incompatible with fitness to fly in any capacity and, therefore, should lead to grounding permanently. In ischaemic stroke in a person below the age of 45 years and in whom there is no evidence of atherosclerosis or other identifiable cause, then the prognosis is less certain and epidemiological data are scanty. It is acknowledged that in this circumstance the risk is lower, but even so the risk of recurrence is probably one to two per cent per annum, which is unacceptable.

There are, however, some causes of stroke that are known to be associated with a good prognosis. An example is a traumatic or spontaneous dissection of a major artery without evidence of constitutional arterial wall disease, e.g. Marfan syndrome. In this case, the recurrence risk is one per cent, and so if the person makes a full recovery from a stroke due to a dissection it is often possible to restore a restricted certificate; eventually, this restriction may be removed.

Cerebral haemorrhage

Stroke due to a spontaneous cerebral haemorrhage is often associated with hypertension, structural disease of a vessel or coagulation disorder. Because of the likely injury to the brain and the underlying predisposing condition, there is usually little chance of regaining fitness to fly.

SUBARACHNOID HAEMORRHAGE

The most common causes of spontaneous atraumatic sub-arachnoid haemorrhage are rupture of a berry aneurysm and arteriovenous malformation (AVM), although in ten per cent no cause is found – so-called perimesencephalic subarachnoid haemorrhage.

Berry aneurysm

A berry aneurysm is a saccular protrusion from an arterial vessel wall. They tend to occur at a branch of an intracerebral artery at various sites. They vary in diameter from a few millimetres to several centimetres. Because of the resulting weakness of the vessel, the wall tends to rupture. The risk of rupture has been estimated as one to two per cent per annum, although an international study has revealed considerable variability of risk, depending on size, site and whether there had been a previous subarachnoid haemorrhage (Wiebers 1998).

If an aneurysm is completely occluded, then there is no longer a risk of haemorrhage; in such cases, it is sometimes possible to permit a return to flying after a full recovery. This is particularly applicable to a single aneurysm on the vertebrobasilar artery, but an aneurysm arising on any of the major arteries above the tentorium cerebelli is associated with a risk of damage to the cerebral cortex, which may result in cognitive dysfunction, neuropsychiatric disorders or epilepsy. Supratentorial craniotomy for all causes is associated with an overall risk of epilepsy of 17 per cent (Foy *et al.* 1981), but the mean incidence of epilepsy after surgical clipping of a supratentorial aneurysm is 22 per cent, although the risk varies according to the site of the aneurysm (middle cerebral artery, 37 per cent; anterior cerebral artery, 21 per cent; posterior communicating artery, 13 per cent) (Cabral *et al.* 1976).

Because of this high incidence following surgery, the patient must be grounded for a certain period, the length of which will depend on the site of the aneurysm and the presence of any other complications (Table 45.2).

The development of the technique of endovascular embolization of intracranial aneurysms has resulted in a significant reduction in morbidity and mortality (Goddard *et al.* 2002), and possibly the incidence of epilepsy, where there is no evidence of other complications that might cause permanent brain injury. However, actual risk figures for different sites after longer follow-up are not available.

In 7–27 per cent of cases, no structural vascular disorder, whether intracranial or intraspinal, and no other systemic cause can be found to be the cause of the haemorrhage. These perimesencephalic subarachnoid haemorrhages are of unknown aetiology but are associated with a better prognosis. It is important to ensure that a small aneurysm has not been missed by angiography in the acute stage, although improved techniques in sophisticated neuroradiological centres have reduced the number of missed aneurysms significantly. Provided angiography has been performed at a good centre, and the individual was always in a good clinical state and not hypertensive, then the prognosis is good: there is a rebleed rate of four per cent in the first six months, but after six months this falls to 0.2–0.8 per cent per annum, and 80 per cent return to full employment and lead a normal life (Friedman 1991). In these circumstances, a return to flying may be possible after six months, but because of the slight residual risk the pilot should be restricted to dual for a few years.

Arteriovenous malformations

An intracranial AVM has a high risk of haemorrhage (two per cent per annum) and epilepsy. Treatment by surgical excision or embolization does not necessarily reduce the risk of epilepsy, unless the malformation was completely extradural, in which case complete eradication will allow a return to flying. Treatment of small intracerebral AVMs by stereotactic radiosurgery often will obliterate the malformation completely and, thus, remove the risk of future haemorrhage. However, although the residual risk of epilepsy in these cases is also thought to be reduced, currently longer follow-up is necessary before a more accurate degree of risk can be ascertained. At present, if there has not been the onset of de novo epilepsy two years after complete obliteration of a malformation by this technique, then it would be permissible to allow a return to restricted flying (dual only).

Table 45.2 *Intracranial aneurysm, risks of epilepsy after surgery, and disposal*

Site	Risk (%)	Ground	Restriction
Middle cerebral artery	37	6 years	Dual only, permanently
Anterior cerebral artery	21	3 years	Dual only, permanently
Posterior cerebral artery	13	2 years	Dual only for 10 years
Internal carotid bifurcation	5	6 months	Dual only for 2 years
Basilar artery	Nil	6 months	Nil

Data from Cabral *et al.* (1976).

Cavernous haemangioma (cavernoma)

A cavernous haemangioma is a malformation of capillaries that forms a local mass within the central nervous system. It has a tendency to repeated small localized haemorrhage, which results in deposition of haemosiderin locally and a characteristic appearance on magnetic resonance imaging (MRI) scan. Occasionally, a more severe haemorrhage may result in a local haematoma. Clinical symptoms depend on the situation of the cavernoma; if it lies in the brainstem, then the risk of sudden incapacitation from haemorrhage is much greater. The overall risk of haemorrhage has been calculated to be 0.7 per cent per annum. If the cavernoma occurs within the cerebral cortex, then there is a high risk of epilepsy; in a review of the literature and a retrospective case series, epilepsy occurred in 79 per cent (Moran et al. 1999). The true incidence of epilepsy awaits a prospective study of asymptomatic cavernomas; currently, however, in the knowledge that there is a risk of haemorrhage and that it is a structural abnormality that is potentially epileptogenic, an individual with such an abnormality should be permanently restricted (dual only) or in some cases grounded permanently.

NEURODEGENERATIVE DISEASES

Because these diseases are progressive, albeit at variable rates, their occurrence will usually be incompatible with continuing to fly, although some people with progressive neuromuscular diseases that present with little disability and progress slowly may be able to continue flying for a time while remaining under close supervision. Some cases of motor neurone disease, polyneuropathy or myopathy might be managed in this way, but there must be no suggestion or potential of cortical brain involvement that could lead to cognitive dysfunction. In such cases, fitness to fly will depend solely on the degree of physical handicap.

Dementias

Any neurodegenerative disease that can affect cognition is incompatible with fitness to fly. At the first suspicion of such an illness, an individual must be grounded while clinical assessment is being performed. Where there is any evidence of cognitive dysfunction, the person must remain grounded. A more definite diagnosis of any of the dementing illnesses, provided that depression or a treatable condition such as hypothyroidism or vitamin B12 deficiency has been excluded, must result in permanent loss of certification.

Parkinson's disease/parkinsonism

There are a number of neurodegenerative diseases of the brain that may present with signs of parkinsonism. Many of these diseases have a worse prognosis than idiopathic Parkinson's disease (IPD), with regard to the rate of progress and degree of disability. Certain clinical features and some investigations may help to distinguish between these diseases, but in a study comparing a clinical diagnosis of IPD made by neurologists and eventual pathological diagnosis at autopsy, the clinical diagnosis was found to be incorrect in 24 per cent of cases (Hughes et al. 1992). IPD is a progressive neurodegenerative disease of unknown aetiology due to degeneration of dopaminergic cells in the substantia nigra and locus coeruleus, leading to disturbance of function of the dopaminergic mesocorticolimbic neural pathways. Before clinical signs become apparent, 90 per cent of these dopaminergic cells will have died, and so clinical manifestation is a relatively late phase of the pathological process. F^{18}-dopa positron-emission tomography (PET) scanning of the brains of some asymptomatic relatives of people with familial Parkinson's disease have demonstrated characteristic abnormalities of dopamine function in the basal ganglia, and follow-up of these relatives has shown that they eventually develop clinical IPD. Those relatives who showed abnormalities of dopamine metabolism also showed evidence of cognitive dysfunction on psychological testing even in the preclinical phase, and in clinical IPD there is a high incidence of dysexecutive cognitive dysfunction characteristic of frontal lobe dysfunction apparent early in the clinical course, which does not correspond to the degree of physical disability (Lees and Smith 1983; Marsden 1994). In 10–20 per cent, this will lead on to dementia; in addition, depression occurs in a high proportion of cases. The motor disabilities of tremor and bradykinesia are also a serious potential safety hazard.

Previously, it has been considered safe to allow continuation of flying in a restricted capacity early in the illness, when the physical manifestations of the disease are minimal, provided the individual is kept under close clinical surveillance and undergoes frequent simulator assessment. However, in view of the above features of the illness, the variability of motor performance and the difficulty of detecting small but significant deterioration, it is probably best to withdraw all grades of certification permanently at the time of initial diagnosis.

TUMOURS

All intracerebral tumours are incompatible with fitness to fly because of the high risk of physical disability, high incidence of neuropsychiatric and cognitive disorder, and the risk of sudden incapacitation due to haemorrhage or epilepsy. Some tumours arising outside the nervous system, such as malignant melanoma, have a high propensity to metastasize to the brain and may present suddenly with a seizure, or cause rapid deterioration. Particular attention to this possibility must be made at follow-up after removal of a malignant melanoma, and consideration should be given to performing periodic brain scans.

Intracranial extracerebral tumours are often of a more benign nature but are often associated with a high risk of epilepsy. A common tumour of this type is a meningioma; although successful complete removal does diminish the risk of epilepsy, epilepsy persists in over half of those in whom it was a presenting symptom and also arises de novo in 22 per cent postoperatively. However, the risk of developing epilepsy diminishes with time; therefore, after two years, if epilepsy has not developed and there is no other significant residual handicap, then restricted certification may be granted, although unrestricted certification should never be restored.

If a benign extra-axial tumour arises below the tentorium cerebelli in the posterior fossa or spinal canal, then the probability of cerebral involvement is negligible and successful removal without significant neurological deficit may allow a return to flying, particularly if the histology suggests a low risk of recurrence. Even if the pathological features suggest a higher risk of recurrence, the person may be allowed to return to flying provided he or she is kept under close surveillance clinically and with the aid of regular MRI scans.

In intrinsic gliomas of a cerebellar hemisphere, the risk of epilepsy is nil and complete excision is easier to achieve surgically, with low risk of recurrence. In these cases, provided there is no significant neurological deficit, a return to flying may be allowed, although it would be prudent to keep the individual under periodic review.

In all cases, the decision on fitness to return to flying and whether a restriction is necessary will depend on the site and type of tumour, its likely natural history and whether there is any postoperative neurological deficit.

INFLAMMATORY DISEASES

Central nervous system

DEMYELINATION

This is the most common type of inflammation affecting the central nervous system. The various diseases due to demyelination are thought to be due to an autoimmune disorder, either following an acute infection or as a result of another, unknown cause. These diseases can be either monophasic or recurrent/progressive. At the time of the first clinical episode, it can be very difficult to distinguish between them. Acute disseminated encephalomyelitis is an acute illness that is usually triggered by an acute infection. It is monophasic and so it has a good prognosis, but often it is indistinguishable from the first clinical episode of multiple sclerosis (MS), which is a progressive disease, although the rate of progress and severity of disability are very variable. After a single clinical episode, an abnormal MRI scan can give guidance to the possibility of future relapse, which would then distinguish between a monophasic illness and MS. A scan showing areas of demyelination other than that causing the clinical syndrome is associated with a risk of recurrence of over 50 per cent within five years, whereas a scan that is otherwise normal has a risk of recurrence of less than ten per cent (Miller et al. 1989). These findings do not give guidance to the degree of disability in the future if MS develops, but an abnormal scan might suggest the need for closer surveillance over the next few years. After full clinical recovery from a first (possibly only) clinical episode, therefore, it is reasonable to allow a return to unrestricted flying. The need for future surveillance should be decided on each individual's clinical features.

A definite diagnosis of MS should result in an individual being kept under regular clinical review by a neurologist and restricted to flying dual. The risk of sudden incapacitation is less than five per cent lifetime, and so provided the person is in good physical condition (Kurtzke extended disability scale < 2.5) and has no cognitive dysfunction they may be allowed to continue flying with the above restriction.

OPTIC NEURITIS

If an aircrew member suffers an episode of optic neuritis but recovers visual acuity to an acceptable level and has no field defect or Uhthoff phenomenon, then they may be allowed to return to unrestricted flying. However, the risk of the subsequent development of MS is 50–60 per cent (Miller et al. 1988), and the closeness of follow-up will be determined in the same way as other first episodes of demyelination.

When confronted by an initial applicant for aircrew who has recovered from a single episode of presumed demyelination, their individual risk of the development of MS must be assessed and the applicant informed fully of the estimated risk of development of this disease and the possibility of premature restriction or loss of certification.

OTHER INFLAMMATORY DISEASES

Most of the other inflammatory diseases affecting the brain are not confined to the white matter and are associated with a greater risk of complications incompatible with fitness to fly.

Peripheral nervous system

PERIPHERAL NEUROPATHY

Acute post-infective demyelinating polyneuropathy (Guillain–Barré syndrome) is associated with a good outcome in the majority of cases, and there is a very low risk of recurrence. Any residual disability must be assessed with regard to flight safety along the lines mentioned earlier, but a full recovery should allow a return to unrestricted flying. The same applies to other inflammatory neuropathies with a good prognosis such as neuralgic amyotrophy, but chronic relapsing inflammatory demyelinating polyneuropathy is usually incompatible with fitness to fly. Other polyneuropathies, whether hereditary or acquired, may be allowed limited certification, depending on the degree of disability and likely natural history.

INFECTIONS

Human immunodeficiency virus infection

Neurological complications occur in 40 per cent of human immunodeficiency virus (HIV)-infected patients, most occurring when the individual has become immunocompromised (CD4 lymphocytes < 200/mm^3). Because of the very high incidence of cerebral involvement (acquired immunodeficiency syndrome (AIDS)–dementia complex) and opportunistic infections of the brain, a pilot in this clinical state should be grounded.

Meningitis

Aseptic viral meningitis is not associated with any significant sequelae, but pyogenic meningitis is associated with a slightly increased risk of seizures, particularly if seizures have occurred during the acute illness.

Viral encephalitis

Viral encephalitis is associated with a higher incidence of permanent brain damage, which may result in behavioural problems, cognitive dysfunction or epilepsy. Again, the risk of later epilepsy is increased if seizures occurred in the acute illness (Table 45.3).

The incidence of epilepsy after meningitis and encephalitis is highest in the first five years, but in cases with an initial high risk the incidence continues to rise slightly over many years (Annegers *et al.* 1988). For this reason, the period of grounding, or return to restricted flying, will depend on the type and severity of the acute illness and whether seizures occurred.

MYASTHENIA GRAVIS

Any evidence of significant muscular weakness at any time of the day is a bar to flying. An individual must be in good stable functional remission and off all treatment before being allowed to return to flying.

Ocular myasthenia that has remained confined to the eyes for more than two years and in which there are no antibodies to acetylcholine receptors is unlikely to become widespread, and therefore full remission off all treatment for at least three months will allow return to unrestricted flying. Any recurrence of symptoms means grounding while undergoing treatment.

PAROXYSMAL DISORDERS

Included among these disorders are some of the most common neurological conditions, such as migraine and epilepsy. Both of these disorders are latent, tend to recur with variable frequency, are unpredictable, and have no reliable biological markers for identification. Because they

Table 45.3 *Risk of seizures following intracranial infection*

Type	Seizure in acute illness	Seizure risk (%)		Ground	Restriction
		5 years	20 years		
Aseptic visual meningitis	0	No significant increased risk	2	6 months	Nil
Pyogenic meningitis	0		2.4	1 year	Nil
	+		13	2 years	Dual only, 5 years
Viral encephalitis	0		10	18 months	Dual only, 5 years
	+	10	22	3 years	Dual only, permanently
Cerebral abscess		Cumulative incidence 98%			Ground permanently

Data from Annegers *et al.* (1988).

are of sudden or rapid onset, they are potentially a serious safety hazard.

Migraine

Migraine is a common disorder. It is genetically determined, and so a predisposed individual will have a lifelong predisposition to attacks of variable frequency and severity. The highest incidence of clinical symptoms occurs during the reproductive phase of life. Population surveys have shown a prevalence of 15–20 per cent in females and eight to ten per cent in males. Attacks often occur in clusters and may remit for long periods, and so it is difficult to predict whether and when an attack might recur. Very rarely, attacks may follow a definite identifiable precipitant such as a specific dietary substance or may occur only while taking a particular medicine, usually the contraceptive pill. This so-called specific migraine should be viewed with scepticism, particularly as the diagnosis is based entirely on the personal history, and should be considered only if the individual remains completely free of attacks for a prolonged period after avoiding the suspected precipitant.

There are two clinical syndromes of migraine, migraine with an aura and migraine without an aura. The aura consists of a transient disturbance of brain function leading to a disturbance of vision, dysphasia or sensory or motor dysfunction of a limb, the most common being a visual disturbance. The aura often precedes the headache, so it may be the presenting symptom, and it can, therefore, be a serious safety hazard. The severity and rapidity of onset of headache, prostration from headache or severe vomiting, photophobia and occasional loss of consciousness are other symptoms that can be temporarily disabling. The severity of the headache and associated symptoms can be very variable and, if not accompanied by an aura, may be attributed to myriad other causes. In addition, an aura does not occur in every attack, so a person may suffer headache alone for many years before an aura occurs; therefore, it is not possible to be confident that an individual does not suffer from migraine with aura even after many years.

Recommended regulations for migraine are as follows:

RECRUITS OR INITIAL APPLICANTS

A past history of headache suggestive of migraine should exclude applicants for military aircrew, professional civilian pilots and air traffic controllers. Because it can be assumed that private pilots will be flying many fewer hours per annum, it is reasonable to be more lenient, so if attacks are infrequent (two or fewer per annum) and have not been accompanied by a severe aura, particularly visual, then they may be allowed unrestricted certification.

TRAINED PILOTS/AIRCREW

When migraine is diagnosed in an individual who is fully trained and holds unrestricted certification, they may be permitted to continue flying in a restricted capacity, unfit solo but fit dual, provided the attacks are infrequent. This restriction should be permanent. If attacks are very severe or frequent, then withdrawal of certification will be necessary.

TRAINED AIR TRAFFIC CONTROLLERS

Those with infrequent attacks should be made permanently unfit for solo controlling but may be allowed to continue controlling with a proximity restriction, although another appropriately qualified controller must be available in the immediate vicinity so that there is no possibility of delay in providing relief when necessary. Those who suffer frequent attacks are unfit controlling duties.

Transient global amnesia

Transient global amnesia (TGA) is a rare disorder of sudden onset which causes severe anterograde amnesia, accompanied by agitation and confusion, while retaining intact neurological function otherwise. The affected individual can perform familiar tasks during an attack, but the severe amnesia and agitation would be likely to be a safety hazard in flight.

The condition usually occurs in middle age, and is often precipitated by certain physical activities or psychological stress. The attack usually lasts for several hours before being followed by complete recovery, except that amnesia for the period of the attack persists permanently.

The aetiology is unknown but is probably a migrainous or vasospastic phenomenon in view of its benign natural history and absence of features associated with cerebrovascular disease.

It can be mimicked by a partial epileptic seizure, but these are usually of much shorter duration and show a high rate of recurrence within one year.

After an attack, a thorough clinical assessment, EEG and brain scan should be performed. If these reveal no abnormality and there has been no recurrence for more than a year, then the possibility of epilepsy is remote and a return to flying may be permitted. However, the recurrence rate has been shown to be at least three per cent per annum (Hodges 1991); because of this, a permanent restriction of unfit solo should apply to all forms of certification, including private pilot.

Trigeminal autonomic cephalgias

This is a group of disorders that includes cluster headache, which are characterized by severe paroxysmal unilateral headache accompanied by prominent autonomic features such as injection and watering of the eye and nasal congestion. Some of these disorders are chronic or require continuous prophylaxis, which would render the person unfit to fly. Others, such as cluster headache, are characterized by a periodicity of symptoms, often with long periods of remission. In these cases, the person should be unfit while symptoms persist, or while receiving treatment, but if he or she has been in complete remission and off treatment for three months, then a return to unrestricted flying may be permitted.

DISTURBANCE OF CONSCIOUSNESS

The most common causes of disturbance of consciousness among aircrew are syncope, cardiac arrhythmia or disease, and epilepsy. Two studies of drivers have shown that epilepsy is the most common medical condition to cause of accidents, presumably because the sudden onset allows no time to take appropriate avoiding action (Raffle 1983; Taylor 1983).

Syncope

Syncope can be difficult to distinguish from an epileptic seizure when it is complicated by an hypoxic convulsion. The occurrence of involuntary clonic or tonic movements, or urinary incontinence, during an attack does not necessarily mean that it was an epileptic seizure, although a severely bitten tongue does not usually occur with a secondary hypoxic convulsion, but is a common occurrence in an epileptic seizure. The diagnosis usually has to be made in retrospect and depends on the history, so a description from an eye witness is helpful. Features suggestive of syncope include a clear precipitant, build-up of typical prodromal symptoms (particularly visual), short duration and absence of prolonged postictal confusion. Even though a confident diagnosis of syncope sometimes can be made clinically when these typical symptoms are present, a careful clinical examination and electrocardiogram (ECG) should always be performed to exclude a cardiac conduction abnormality. In the event of a confident diagnosis of a single episode of syncope, with normal investigations, an immediate return to flying may be permissible. If there are recurrent typical syncopal episodes, then a tilt-table test may identify neurocardiological instability, and a decision on the need for a restriction on the certification (dual only) or permanent grounding will be made on an individual basis, but frequent syncope should result in permanent loss of certification.

Loss of consciousness of uncertain cause must undergo a more intensive cardiological and neurological assess-

ment. Neurological investigations that may be helpful are an EEG and brain scan. It can be difficult to distinguish in retrospect between syncope with a hypoxic convulsion and epilepsy. Apart from occasionally identifying a cardiac disorder, there are few useful biological markers. An epileptiform EEG may suggest that the cause was epileptic, but 0.5 per cent of the population show these features on an EEG, and prolonged follow-up has showed that only a small number develop epilepsy (Gregory *et al.* 1993). Conversely, only 50–70 per cent of epileptics show an abnormal interictal EEG, and so a normal EEG does not exclude the possibility of epilepsy. If doubt about the cause remains after thorough clinical assessment, then the individual must remain grounded for a minimum period of one year, and often longer, and should be allowed to return only to restricted flying (dual only).

Epilepsy

The occurrence of an epileptic seizure during flight is an extreme safety hazard, not only because of the sudden unheralded onset but also because the occurrence of a generalized seizure on a flight deck may result in disruption of the controls, or the onset of a partial seizure with automatism may not be immediately apparent to the co-pilot or other crew on the flight deck. In civilian flying the greatest hazard would be during takeoff or landing, but in military operations the hazard is high at all stages of the flight.

Epilepsy is, by definition, the occurrence of recurrent seizures. Because of the high safety risk, it is incompatible with fitness to fly, even in a restricted capacity. The occurrence of a single unprovoked seizure is associated with a risk of recurrence of 52–78 per cent over the next three years (Hopkins *et al.* 1988; Hart *et al.* 1990). Although most studies show a tendency for levelling out of the risk after a few years, there are very few follow-up studies over a longer period. Epidemiological studies suggest that a significant number of individuals who suffer a single seizure do not suffer a recurrence, but because of the high risk of recurrence and the difficulty of predicting individual risk, all aircrew who suffer a single unprovoked seizure must be grounded for a prolonged period. In military aircrew, this is permanent. In civilian flying, if there has been no recurrence after ten years and a consultant neurologist considers that there is no persisting increased risk of recurrence of seizures (assessment would include EEG and possibly MRI brain scan), then restricted certification may be granted.

Acute symptomatic seizures, such as those that occur immediately after a concussive head injury or acute metabolic disturbance such as renal failure, are not associated with an increased risk of epilepsy, and after full recovery the person may be able to regain certification. This may also apply to acute withdrawal seizures with alcoholism, but caution should be exercised in case the alcohol abuse unveiled a latent predisposition to epilepsy due to a past head injury or other illness or a mild underlying predisposition to primary generalized epilepsy.

Because of the serious potential hazard that epilepsy poses, every attempt is made to exclude anyone with a possible predisposition among initial applicants. A past history of seizures after the age of five years will exclude an applicant, unless there is a clear, well-documented history of one of the benign childhood epilepsy syndromes, which invariably remit in the second decade, e.g. benign rolandic epilepsy.

A past severe head injury, cerebral abscess or other infection or neurological condition associated with an increased risk will also disqualify. For many years, an EEG has been an obligatory part of the initial medical examination in an attempt to detect and exclude those who might have a latent predisposition to epilepsy. Disqualifying abnormalities include focal or generalized epileptiform spike or spike-wave activity at rest or during activating procedures, which must include photic stimulation at a range of frequencies. Non-epileptic equivalents such as 4–6-Hz spike and wave or 14-Hz positive spikes are acceptable. In a number of studies, unequivocal epileptiform activity has been found in 0.5 per cent, of which 59 per cent occurred only during photic stimulation (Gregory et al. 1993). It is known that half of those who show a photoconvulsive response have a predisposition to primary generalized epilepsy rather than a specific reflex photogenic epilepsy, but follow-up studies have shown only a slight increased risk of developing epilepsy (cumulative incidence of two to three per cent) – although the small number of subjects means that the confidence limits are wide. Subtle transient cognitive dysfunction has been demonstrated during asymptomatic epileptiform spike activity, which adds concern about individuals who show these abnormalities, but it is clear that the EEG is not a very efficient predictor of future epilepsy because of the high number of false positives, and that it will not predict symptomatic epilepsy. However, the low incidence of epilepsy in these clinical studies does not take into account the unusual environment of flying aircraft over long periods, particularly for people who are photosensitive being exposed to the intense flicker of rotating helicopter blades for prolonged periods, which may be a more powerful epileptogenic stimulus. It would, therefore, be wise to perform a screen EEG on candidates for helicopter aircrew, although the usefulness of performing an EEG on all applicants is more debatable.

It has been shown that 30 per cent of photosensitive subjects lose photosensitivity at a later age (Harding et al. 1997). Therefore, if a candidate shows only a photoconvulsive response on the initial EEG but suffers no seizures over the next five or more years, and shows no persisting photosensitivity on a repeat sleep-deprived EEG, then he or she may be granted full certification.

Suggested guidelines for management after loss of consciousness are as follows:

- *Single typical syncope with normal examination/ECG:* return to unrestricted flying after recovery.
- *Loss of consciousness of uncertain cause:* full cardiological and neurological assessment and investigations. Ground for minimum of one year, or longer according to clinical features until possibility of cardiac disease or epilepsy is unlikely. Restrict certification to dual only for longer period.
- *Recurrent typical syncope – infrequent:* permanent restriction on certification, dual only.
- *Recurrent typical syncope – frequent:* ground permanently.
- *Single epileptic seizure:*
  - Military aircrew: ground permanently.
  - Civilian professional or private: ground for minimum of ten years, after which may regain restricted certification.
- *Epilepsy:* permanently unfit.

Vertigo

Aircrew who suffer from vertigo are unfit to fly while they are symptomatic or after recovery if there is a significant risk of recurrence. In cases of doubt over prognosis, certain pilot and other aircrew roles may require a restriction to dual only; in pilots/navigators of high-performance military aircraft, a return to flying should be permitted only after full recovery, with no evidence of significant vestibular dysfunction on sophisticated testing.

Recurrent paroxysmal vestibular disorders such as periodic positional vertigo will require a permanent restriction to dual only, but a person with the more chronic benign positional vertigo should be grounded permanently unless cured completely by an Epley manoeuvre. In this case, there must be no recurrence of symptoms for at least six months; thereafter, the person should be fit dual only.

Neuralgia

The sudden onset, usually frequently recurrent, and extreme severity of the pain of trigeminal or other neuralgia is incompatible with fitness to fly. If an individual has been in remission, either spontaneously or following surgery, and has been off treatment for three months, then a return to flying is usually permitted.

Follow-up will depend on the estimated risk of relapse.

REFERENCES

Annegers JF, Hauser WA, Beghi E, *et al.* Risk of unprovoked seizures after encephalitis and meningitis. *Neurology* 1988; **38**: 1407–10.

Annegers JF, Hauser WA, Coan SP, Rocca PA. A population-based study of seizures after traumatic brain injuries. *New England Journal of Medicine* 1998; **338**: 20–24.

Bamford J, Sandercock P, Jones L, Warlow C. Natural history of lacunar infarction: the Oxford Community Stroke Project. *Stroke* 1987; **18**: 545–51.

Cabral RJ, King TT, Scott DF. Epilepsy after two different neurosurgical approaches to the treatment of ruptured intracranial aneurysm. *Journal of Neurology, Neurosurgery and Psychiatry* 1976; **39**: 1052–6.

D'Alessandro R, Tinuper P, Ferrara R, *et al.* CT scan prediction of late post-traumatic epilepsy. *Journal of Neurology, Neurosurgery and Psychiatry* 1982; **45**: 1153–5.

Dennis M, Bamford J, Sandercock P, Warlow C. Prognosis of TIA in the Oxford Community Stroke Project. *Stroke* 1990; **21**: 848–53.

Foy PM, Copeland GP, Shaw MDM. The incidence of post-operative seizures. *Acta Neurochirurgica* 1981; **55**: 253–64.

Friedman AH. Subarachnoid haemorrhage of unknown origin. In: Wilkins RH, Rengacharry SS (eds). *Neurosurgery Update 2.* New York: McGraw-Hall, 1991; pp. 73–7.

Goddard AJP, Annesley-Williams D, Gholkar A. Endovascular management of unruptured intracranial aneurysms: does outcome justify treatment? *Journal of Neurology, Neurosurgery and Psychiatry* 2002; **72**: 485–90.

Gregory RP, Oates TJ, Merry RTG. Electroencephalograph epileptiform abnormalities in candidates for aircrew training. *Electroencephalography and Clinical Neurophysiology* 1993; **86**: 75–7.

Harding GFA, Edson A, Jeavons PM. Persistence of photosensitivity. *Epilepsia* 1997; **38**: 663–9.

Hart YM, Sander JWAS, Johnson AL, Shorvon SD. National General Practice Study of Epilepsy: recurrence after first seizure. *Lancet* 1990; **336**: 1271–4.

Hodges JR. *Transient Global Amnesia.* London: WB Saunders, 1991.

Hopkins A, Garman A, Clarke C. The first seizure in adult life. *Lancet* 1988; **I**: 721–6.

Hughes AJ, Daniel SE, Kilford L, Lees AJ. Accuracy of clinical diagnosis of idiopathic Parkinson's disease: a clinico-pathological study of 100 cases. *Journal of Neurology, Neurosurgery and Psychiatry* 1992; **55**: 181–4.

Jennett B. *Epilepsy after Non-missile Head Injuries,* 2nd edn. London: Heinemann, 1975.

Lees AJ, Smith E. Cognitive deficits in the early stages of Parkinson's disease. *Brain* 1983; **106**: 257–70.

Lisovoski F, Rousseau P. Cerebral infarction in young people: a study of 148 patients. *Journal of Neurology, Neurosurgery and Psychiatry* 1991; **54**: 576–9.

Marsden CD. Parkinson's disease. *Journal of Neurology, Neurosurgery and Psychiatry* 1994; **57**: 672–81.

Moran NF, Fish DR, Kitchen N, *et al.* Supratentorial cavernous angiomas and epilepsy: a review of the literature and case series. *Journal of Neurology, Neurosurgery and Psychiatry* 1999; **66**: 561–8.

Miller DH, Ormerod IEC, McDonald WI, *et al.* Early risk of multiple sclerosis after optic neuritis. *Journal of Neurology, Neurosurgery and Psychiatry* 1988; **51**: 1561–71.

Miller DH, Ormerod IEC, Rudge P, *et al.* The early risk of multiple sclerosis following isolated acute syndromes of the brain stem and spinal cord. *Annals of Neurology* 1989; **26**: 635–9.

Raffle PAB. The HGV/PSV driver and loss of impairment of consciousness. In: Godwin-Austen EB, Espir MLE (eds). *Driving and Epilepsy and Other Causes of Impaired Consciousness.* London: Royal Society of Medicine; 1983: 35–9.

Sacco RL, Wolf PA, Kannel WB, McNamara PM. Survival and recurrence following stroke: the Framingham Study. *Stroke* 1982; **13**: 290–95.

Taylor JF. Epilepsy and other causes of collapse at the wheel. In: Godwin-Austen EB, Espir MLE (eds). *Driving and Epilepsy and Other Causes of Impaired Consciousness.* London: Royal Society of Medicine; 1983: 5–8.

Wiebers DO. International Study of Unruptured Intracranial Aneurysms Investigators. Unruptured intracranial aneurysms: risk of rupture and risks of surgical intervention. *New England Journal of Medicine* 1998; **339**: 1725–33.

46

Ophthalmology

ROBERT A.H. SCOTT AND PAUL WRIGHT

INTRODUCTION

Sight is the most important sense used in aviation. At least 80 per cent of all information acquired by pilots in flight is visual, from cockpit instruments and through the canopy. Over the past five to ten years, important advances have been made in cataract and corneal refractive surgery, contact lenses (CL) are gaining popularity among aircrew, and colour vision has become an important issue, with the onset of the electronic flight instrumentation systems (EFIS) used in modern aircraft.

With millions of pounds having to be spent to replace the loss of an experienced Royal Air Force (RAF) fast-jet pilot, any new ophthalmic interventions must be evaluated carefully to ensure that the risks are outweighed by the benefits of the procedure. In this chapter, we will describe and explain some of the visual characteristics of the eye relevant to aviation, and how to measure them, and discuss relevant ocular diseases in relation to the aviation environment.

VISUAL REQUIREMENTS FOR AVIATION

Aviators require two eyes that see distant and near objects clearly. The ocular muscle balance must be within normal limits, and colour vision must be normal. The visual fields must be full, and stereopsis must be present to the required standard.

Royal Air Force visual standards

The standards at selection for RAF aircrew are summarized in Table 46.1.

Poor vision in one eye

An individual with a single, or a single seeing, eye can fly an aircraft safely with certain restrictions. Uniocular subjects have a slightly reduced field of vision and no stereoscopic vision. The sensory loss and increased risk of complete visual incapacitation if the good eye is damaged pose a flight safety issue. An experienced private pilot is likely to be permitted to fly with a safety lookout if wearing appropriate eye protection, after a successful flight test. Professional pilots who become uniocular are restricted to fly as or with a qualified co-pilot. These restrictions appear to be adequate, as the US Federal Aviation Administration (FAA) reports no significant difference in accident rates between uniocular and binocular pilots.

REFRACTIVE ERROR IN AVIATION

Variation of refraction with age

The majority of neonates are hypermetropic. The magnitude increases until the age of eight years, when the refraction becomes relatively myopic until the end of the third decade, when refractive stability is attained. Increasing hypermetropia characterizes middle age as accommoda-

Table 46.1 Aircrew eyesight standards at selection

Branch	VA (uncorrected)	VA (corrected)	Near (33 cm)	Refraction range — Sph	Cyl	Muscle balance (max 'phoria)	Accommodation (minimum)	Convergence (cm)	CP
Pilot (includes UAS flying)	6/6 (RN/AAC 6/12)			Plano to +1.75 (RN/AAC −0.75 to +1.75)	+0.75	DV 6ESO to 8EXO 1 Hyperphoria	Age 17–20 9D Age 20–25 7D	To 10 cm or better	2
WSO	6/24	6/6	N5	−1.25 to +3.00		NV 6ESO to 16EXO 1 Hyperphoria			
ALM 1 (SAR)	6/9			−0.25 to +3.00					
ALM 2	6/24			−1.50 to +3.00	+1.25				
AEng	6/60			−2.00 to +3.00		No standard laid down	No standard laid down		4
WSOp									
WSOpL									

tion decreases. Myopia develops after the seventh decade due to the higher refractive index of the nucleosclerotic crystalline lens.

It is impossible to give an accurate prognosis of the progress of an individual's refractive error, as any individual will not necessarily adhere to the population norms. Myopes tend to demonstrate an earlier and more rapid myopic progression than hypermetropes. Care should be taken in assessing and accepting a young candidate for aviation training with low myopia, as the need for visual correction at an early age is likely.

Hypermetropia

In hypermetropia, light is focused behind the retina, making both distance and near objects blurred. When young, the eye can accommodate to compensate for this, but as the amplitude of accommodation declines with age, reading glasses are required at a younger age than normal and distance glasses will often be required later. Axial hypermetropia is the most common type; this occurs if the eye is short relative to its focal power. If the refractive power of a normal-sized eye is inadequate, then refractive hypermetropia occurs. Aphakia (no lens) is an extreme example of acquired refractive hypermetropia.

Hypermetropia can be divided into manifest and latent types. Manifest hypermetropia is the strongest convex lens correction accepted for clear distance vision. Latent hypermetropia is the remainder of the hypermetropia, masked by ciliary tone and involuntary accommodation. Latent hypermetropia is often significant in children, and cycloplegic refraction is necessary to measure it.

Hypermetropia that is overcome by accommodation is called facultative hypermetropia, while hypermetropia in excess of the amplitude of accommodation is called absolute hypermetropia. Hypermetropia is corrected with a convex (plus) lens.

Myopia

In a myopic eye, parallel rays of light are focused in front of the retina. Distant objects are blurred, but near objects are seen clearly, hence the synonyms 'near-sightedness' and 'short-sightedness'. This is often because the eye is abnormally long, i.e. axial myopia. In high myopia, there may be out-pouching of the posterior segment of the eye, known as posterior staphyloma.

The eye may be of normal length but the dioptric power may be increased, i.e. refractive or index myopia. Examples of acquired index myopia are keratoconus, in which the corneal refractive power is increased, and nucleosclerosis, in which the refractive power of the lens increases as the nucleus becomes denser.

Low myopia, the most common type, can be defined as less than −4.00 dioptres, moderate myopia as −4.00 to −7.75 dioptres, high myopia as −8.00 to −12.00 dioptres and extreme myopia as more than −12.00 dioptres. High and extreme myopia are associated with myopic macular degeneration and peripheral retinal degeneration, with a four per cent lifetime risk of retinal detachment.

Myopia is treated with concave (minus) lenses to correct the distance vision. Axial myopia most commonly becomes manifest in the early teens, progressing until the age of around 24 years. There is evidence that the reading associated with higher education induces progression of myopia. Aviators are usually selected under the age of 24 years and often develop low myopia by the time they have finished their flying training.

Figure 46.1 demonstrates emmetropia, hypermetropia and myopia.

Astigmatism

The refractive power of the astigmatic (literally, lacking a point) eye varies in different meridians. A point focus of light cannot be formed on the retina. There are several types of regular astigmatism, as follows:

- Compound hypermetropic astigmatism: rays in all meridians come to focus behind the retina.
- Simple hypermetropic astigmatism: rays in one meridian focus on the retina and the other focus lies behind the retina.
- Mixed astigmatism: one line focus lies in front of the retina and the other focuses behind the retina.
- Simple myopic astigmatism (Figure 46.2): one line focus lies on the retina and the other lies in front of the retina.

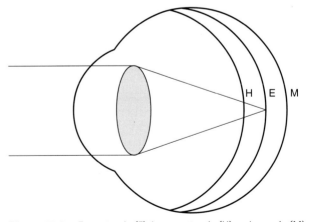

Figure 46.1 *Emmetropia (E), hypermetropia (H) and myopia (M). In emmetropia, parallel rays of light are focused on the retina. In hypermetropia, the eye is relatively short and the rays of light are focused behind the retina. In myopia, the eye is relatively too long and the rays of light are focused in front of the retina.*

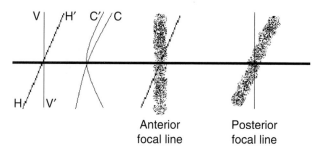

Anterior focal line

Posterior focal line

Figure 46.2 *Appearance of an image in simple myopic astigmatism. A cross with a vertical (VV') and horizontal (HH') limb is the object. Corneal astigmatism, in which the vertical diameter (C') is more curved than the horizontal diameter (C). The appearance of the image in simple myopic astigmatism is shown, where a focus in only one meridian is possible.*

- Compound myopic astigmatism: rays in all meridians come to a focus in front of the retina.

Astigmatism is corrected with a lens that is stronger in one meridian than the other. There are two types of astigmatic lenses, cylindrical and toric. Cylindrical lenses have one plain surface and form part of a cylinder. Thus, in one meridian the lens has no vergence power and is the axis of the cylinder at right-angles to this, i.e. the cylinder acts as a spherical lens. The total effect is the formation of a line image of a point object, the focal line that is projected parallel to the axis of the cylinder.

A toric lens can be thought of as a spherical lens with a cylindrical lens superimposed upon it. A toric lens may be defined numerically as a fraction, the spherical power being the numerator and the cylindrical power the denominator. For example, a toric lens with a power of +2.00 dioptres in one principle meridian and +4.00 dioptres in the other principle meridian can be regarded as a +2.00-dioptre sphere (DS) with a +2.00-dioptre cylinder (DC) superimposed. This is written as +2.00/+2.00 DC.

The cylindrical correction will be at an angle that is added to the prescription. If it is at 90 degrees, then the prescription is written as +2.00/+2.00 DC × 90 °

Anisometropia

When the refraction of the two eyes differs, the condition is know as anisometropia. Small degrees of anisometropia are commonplace and of no significance. Larger degrees in early childhood are a significant cause of refractive amblyopia. A disparity of more than 1 dioptre in a hypermetrope is enough to cause amblyopia of the more hypermetropic eye, because accommodation is a binocular function and the more hypermetropic eye remains out of focus. Myopes with anisometropia are less likely to develop amblyopia,

because both eyes have clear vision. However, when one eye is highly myopic, it usually becomes amblyopic. If anisometropia occurs in adulthood, it causes eye strain and diplopia, as the images from each eye are different sizes and are not resolved into one image by the brain.

Older people with nuclear sclerosis causing index myopia that affects one eye more than the other may not tolerate full spectacle correction of the more myopic eye, as they are not accustomed to coping with the anisometropia. Myopic patients who have been anisometropic for all their lives tolerate a higher degree of anisometropia and achieve binocular vision with more than 2 dioptres difference between the two eyes.

Presbyopia

The amplitude of accommodation declines steadily with age (Figure 46.3). This is related to sclerosis of the crystalline lens fibres and changes in the lens capsule that reduce spontaneous steeping of its surfaces on ciliary muscle contraction. The ciliary muscle itself may become less efficient with advancing age.

In infancy, the eye is capable of 14 dioptres of accommodation; by the age of 45 years, this has fallen to approximately 4 dioptres. There is an inexorable decline after that. In order to focus on an object at a reading distance of 25 cm, the emmetropic eye must accommodate by 4 dioptres. However, one-third of the available accommodation must be kept in reserve for comfortable near vision. A normal individual will begin to experience difficulty or discomfort with near vision at 25 cm when the accommodation has decayed to 6 dioptres between the ages of 40 and 45 years. Such individuals are presbyopic.

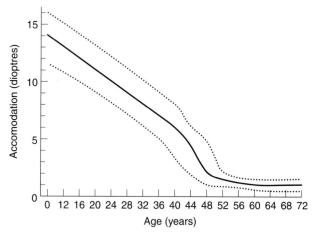

Figure 46.3 *Change in accommodation with age. The upper and lower lines represent the maximum and minimum accommodation, respectively. The middle line represents the mean. The figures are based on the observation of 4200 eyes and represent the greatest accommodative power of each individual.*

The onset of presbyopia occurs earlier with uncorrected hypermetropia than in emmetropia, because the individual with hypermetropia must accommodate more to achieve near vision.

MANAGEMENT OF REFRACTIVE ERRORS IN AIRCREW

Refractive correction in aircrew historically has been with corrective flying spectacles (CFS). Over the past 20 years, high-water-content soft CL have increasingly been introduced to RAF aircrew groups, and 53 per cent of aircrew who require refractive correction currently use these for flying.

Corrective flying spectacles

Aircrew who require refractive correction are not permitted to use their own civilian spectacles for flying duties. Defence-issue CFS are suitable for the working environment, in terms of both visual performance and robustness. A spare pair of CFS must be carried in an accessible place while flying in case of mechanical failure of the pair that is worn.

CFS are made to high specifications and are issued after a thorough eye examination by an approved optometrist. There are two CFS designs, both of which are an aviator shape in matt black-coated metal frames. One design is a general-purpose frame (9021A); the other has a wrap-around shape to the front for use with aircrew respirators and the AR5 hood (9013A). The low powers have CR39 acrylic lenses, while the higher powers have polycarbonate lenses in order to reduce the weight and thickness of the lenses. They all have anti-scratch and anti-reflection coatings. A full range of lenses is available in single-vision, multifocal and progressive forms. Half-eye reading designs are available for certain presbyopic aircrew who have good distance vision or who wear contact lenses (CL).

Multifocal lenses available to RAF aircrew include bifocal lenses, trifocal lenses and progressive power lenses. Executive bifocals, in which the whole lower portion of a lens is dedicated to near vision, are useful for people who perform a lot of reading. Invented by Benjamin Franklin, these were the first type of bifocal lens. D-segment bifocals have a small reading segment, allowing the greatest area of the lens to be devoted to distance vision. The D-segment bifocal is most popular with aircrew and allows a pilot to see the runway landing flare, in focus, out of the side of the distance portion of the lens. Trifocal lenses incorporate a further segment of intermediate power for mid-distance vision. These are often used when an individual has to read information from a computer screen or monitor.

Progressive power lenses are designed so the lens power changes gradually from top to bottom, with no visible interface between the distance and near portions. This leaves an area of peripheral distortion outside the transition zone of increasing power that reduces the field of view through the lenses. Such lenses are used with caution in aviators and are contraindicated for fast-jet aircrew.

CFS have been associated with significant problems in terms of comfort and safety. In one survey, flight safety incidents attributed to CFS were noted in five per cent of aircrew per year. The incidents were, for the most part, attributed to mechanical failure of the CFS and lens obscuration due to misting or sweat accumulation.

When prescribing a spectacle lens, the spherical and cylindrical components of the lens are specified in the following way. The power of the spherical lens is written, e.g. +2.50 DS or −4.25 DS, followed by the cylindrical component that specifies the cylindrical power and axis. The axis of the cylinder is marked on each trial frame according to a standard international convention. Thus, a cylinder of −2.50 dioptres placed with its axis vertically in the frame is written as $-2.50 \, DC \times 90\,°$. Astigmatic lens prescriptions may be transposed from a plus DS to a minus DS, and visa versa. This is often required when the examiner needs to compare the present refraction with a previous prescription. This can be accomplished in three steps, as follows:

1 The algebraic sum of DS and DC generates the new spherical power.
2 Change the sign of the cylinder retaining the numerical power.
3 Rotate the axis through 90 degrees.

For example:

$+5.50/-1.25 \times 125\,°$ becomes $+4.25/+1.25 \times 35\,°$
and $-1.75/+2.50 \times 20\,°$ becomes $+0.75/-2.50 \times 110\,°$

Aircrew contact lenses

CL (Figure 46.4) are the preferred option for visual correction across the whole spectrum of aircrew groups. Most aircrew contact-lens wearers wear daily disposable CL. These offer good visual performance, and they are hygienic and convenient. Daily disposable lenses are available in a wide range of spherical powers, but generally they are not used in astigmatism or dry eyes.

Different methods are used to stabilize CL orientation in order to correct astigmatism. Some are prism-ballasted, while others have thin zones that use the eyelid pressure on blinking to stabilize the lens. In addition to these, some lenses have the toric surface worked on the front surface and some have it on the back. These CL are non-disposable and must be cleaned and disinfected appropriately. In some people, several CL types are tried before a lens is found that sits at the correct orientation on the eye.

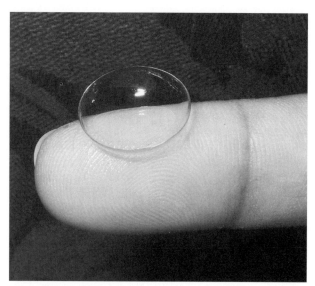

Figure 46.4 *Contact lens on finger. See also colour plate 46.4.*

Silicone hydrogel CL are made of low-water-content, highly oxygen-permeable material. They are used for excessively dry eyes and in eyes with high corneal oxygen demands. These CL can be used for 30-day extended wear, although this use has not been approved for general aircrew use. The lens type remains a useful option for problem cases.

Aircrew problems with CL are usually related to dehydration from individual or environmental factors. As a CL dehydrates, the surface deteriorates causing poor vision, reduced comfort and reduced oxygen transmission. Aircrew have a reduced blink rate, due to concentration on the tasks in the aircraft. The air-conditioning systems in large aircraft create a dry atmosphere that dehydrates individuals and their CL. If 'on-eye' dehydration is a problem, aircrew are advised to ensure adequate water intake, are made aware of the need to blink (at least once every four seconds), and may be given a written sheet detailing blinking exercises. Rewetting drops can also be used. If there is a problem with blocked meibomian glands, which results in a poor lipid layer and excessive tear evaporation, then the advice is to use hot compresses and lid massage. Lens movement is a problem that is reported occasionally; it has a number of causes. The usual reason is that the lens has dried due to reasons mentioned above and has, therefore, become uncomfortable and immobile, which initiates a strong 'squeeze-blink' reflex, which in turn can dislocate the lens. Sometimes, a toric lens is reported to rotate under high-g conditions; a blink usually corrects this.

Corneal hypoxia is seen occasionally, although usually only in cases where the lenses are persistently worn for too long or regularly left in overnight. The standard advice is to wear lenses for a maximum of 12 hours in a day for six days in a week and not to sleep in them. Chronic hypoxic changes include new vessels growing into the cornea from the limbus and corneal stromal swelling, which causes a change in refraction and topography. Acute hypoxia, which causes painful corneal oedema, is rare.

Microbial keratitis is a risk of soft CL use. Aircrew are made aware of the signs and symptoms of this and advised to seek immediate medical help if they suspect that they have such an infection.

Presbyopia is a problem as there are no truly successful soft bifocal CL. Some aircrew revert, unwillingly, to bifocals, although many pilots find that the cockpit instruments are far enough away and of large enough detail to manage without a reading correction. Reading glasses are reserved for use with maps, charts and checklists. A small number of rear crew, whose work is almost entirely visual display unit (VDU)-based, are successful with 'enhanced monovision' (a bifocal lens for the non-dominant eye and a distance vision lens for the dominant eye) or monovision (one eye distance, one eye near).

Refractive surgery

Radial keratotomy (RK) was the first large-volume surgical treatment for myopia. A series of corneal cuts are fashioned in a spoke-shaped pattern around the pupil, penetrating 85–95 per cent of the depth of the cornea. The incisions cause the perimeter of the cornea to bulge out, flattening the centre in order to correct myopia. Some of the problems associated with the technique were the result of the permanently weakened cornea and healing of the incisions, which caused regression of the myopic correction. The refraction changes during the day and at altitude after RK. These characteristics are not desirable in aviation, and RK has largely fallen out of favour as newer laser techniques have been developed.

The first laser corneal refractive surgery (CRS) for myopia, developed in the latter half of the 1980s, was photorefractive keratotomy (PRK). In this procedure, the anterior corneal surface is reshaped by photo-ablation using an ultraviolet excimer laser. The corneal epithelium is removed before treatment and grows back over the treated zone after four to six days (Figure 46.5).

Night vision abnormalities may occur after PRK, but these are minimized if a sufficient optical zone is reshaped. Corneal tissue healing after PRK may lead to haze and regression of the refractive correction over the first two to three months. This problem has been virtually abolished with improvements in laser technology and by restricting the use of PRK to lower orders of myopia (< −6.00). The integrity of the globe is unaffected by PRK and refractive stability is achieved within three to six months of surgery. No significant diurnal or altitude-related variations in refractive error or vision have been reported.

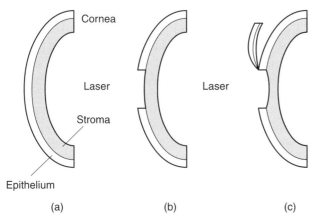

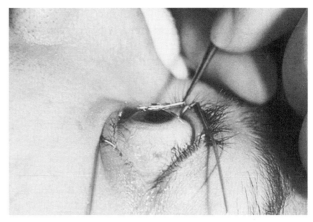

Figure 46.5 *Main types of corneal refractive surgical techniques. Diagrammatic representation of (a) normal cornea, (b) photorefractive keratotomy (PRK) and (c) laser in-situ keratomileusis (LASIK). The corneal epithelium must be removed before PRK but remains intact during LASIK.*

Figure 46.7 *Partial-thickness corneal laser in-situ keratomileusis (LASIK) flap before excimer laser treatment. See also colour plate 46.7.*

A variant of PRK, called laser epithelial keratomileusis (LASEK; not to be confused with LASIK – laser in-situ keratomileusis; see below), also displaces a flap of epithelium, which is replaced after the laser procedure and acts as a bandage (Figure 46.6). Recovery is faster and less painful than with standard PRK. The visual outcome is very similar to that of PRK and LASIK, but the pain and haze of PRK are minimized.

LASIK is the most popular refractive surgical technique at present. It provides a more predictable and safer method of correcting higher levels of myopia and low hypermetropia than PRK. It involves the cutting of a thin flap of corneal tissue and ablating the underlying stromal bed, before replacing the flap (Figure 46.7). Disruption of the epithelial layer is kept to a minimum, which avoids the aggressive healing response that leads to the formation of haze. Pain is minimized and the visual recovery is within one to two days.

Although LASIK provides a more predictable and safer method of correcting higher levels of myopia and low hypermetropia than PRK, it is about the same for the lower levels of myopia encountered in aircrew. Night-vision abnormalities, including a loss of contrast sensitivity with haloes and starbursts around light sources, can be a problem. Between one and three per cent of patients lose two or more lines of their best vision on a test chart after LASIK. The eye often becomes dry and requires lubricants for up to six months postoperatively. Occasionally, the corneal flap can become inflamed and melt or be displaced. Epithelial cells may grow under it, which need to be removed by lifting and scraping the flap clean. Corneal ectasia, in which the cornea thins and bulges out in a manner similar to keratoconus, can occur after LASIK for high myopia, where more tissue is removed, or if the procedure has been performed inappropriately on thin corneas. This complication distorts vision and may require a hard CL or even a corneal graft.

For myopia of less than −6.00 dioptres, over 90 per cent of patients will achieve 6/12 or better after both LASIK and PRK. Approximately 85 per cent of patients will achieve 6/6 or better. Aviators start with a low level of myopia and generally have excellent results from laser CRS. The glare and haze of PRK are roughly as debilitating as the haloes and starbursts of LASIK. Visual results and side effects are worse, as more myopia is corrected.

Wave-front aberrometry allows very accurate correction of not only the basic sphere and cylindrical errors that are corrected by spectacles but also the higher orders of ametropia responsible for poor night vision after CRS. It was conceived originally in order to correct higher orders of aberration in the atmosphere and to allow better resolution of the stars and planets in astronomy. Wave-front-guided surgery increases the proportion of patients who achieve excellent vision after treatment and is the most suitable for aircrew, as it reduces postoperative night-vision abnormalities.

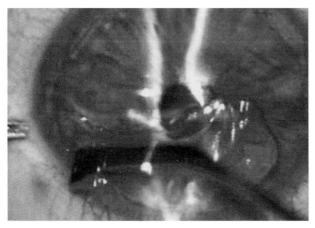

Figure 46.6 *Temporary removal of corneal epithelium during laser epithelial keratomileusis (LASEK). See also colour plate 46.6.*

Several surgical techniques are under investigation for the surgical reversal of presbyopia, but none have been proved to be safe and effective. Current approaches to correction of presbyopia include multifocal or accommodative intraocular lens (IOL) implantation, scleral expansion, laser presbyopia reversal and intrascleral segment surgery. If a patient is over the age of 45 years and has had full correction of a refractive error, then it is likely that some form of reading correction will be required. Reading glasses remain the most effective form of correction.

Other refractive techniques include implantable contact lenses (ICL), perspex lenses implanted inside the eye, similar to the intraocular lenses used in cataract surgery. These are capable of correcting individuals with high amounts of near- or far-sightedness beyond the range of LASIK (more than +6.00 dioptres of hyperopia and more than −15.00 dioptres myopia). The refractive correction is highly predictable, and the lens can be removed if required. The technique provides a high quality of vision.

Intrastromal corneal ring implants (INTACS™) are placed at the edge of the cornea, avoiding the line of sight. They are effective only for relatively low refractive errors and are useful in treating keratoconus (bulging cornea). They can be removed easily and safely if local deposits develop or glare makes vision uncomfortable. Occasionally, the cornea can be perforated during implantation, and they may cause astigmatism.

Diode lasers are low-powered lasers that gently heat spots near the edge of the cornea in order to correct hypermetropia and astigmatism. No tissue is removed. It avoids the line of sight, helping to preserve night vision. Generally this is a treatment for people over the age of 40 years. Laser thermal keratoplasty (LTK) is similar to diode laser and also avoids the visual axis. Less energy reaches the deeper layers than with a diode laser, and so there is a higher rate of regression of the treatment effect. As the laser system does not control the position of the eye, severe astigmatism can be induced if the eye moves suddenly or is treated off-target.

The US Air Force and US Navy experience of laser CRS is that PRK is safe in aircrew and allows a return to flying duties after three to six months once refractive stability have been proved. The procedure enhances flight performance in fast-jet pilots and does not cause a functionally significant loss of vision. Simulated cockpit studies after PRK found that although appreciation of low-contrast targets decreased, the operation did not decrease head-up display readability. The reduced contrast sensitivity did not appear to be clinically or operationally significant. Further treatment was required in 6–20 per cent of eyes in order to render them spectacle-independent. There are no data on the effects of LASIK on military aviation, and it is not sanctioned for use in US aircrew. PRK and LASEK are likely to be approved for UK military aircrew at the risk and expense of the individual, but satisfactory visual function must be demonstrated before a full flying category can be awarded.

If a civilian aviator has had successful refractive surgery, then class 1 certification will not normally be considered until one year after the operation. The preoperative refraction must not have exceeded ±5.00 dioptres. An ophthalmologist or optician must verify the preoperative refraction. An assessment by a Civil Aviation Authority (CAA) eye specialist is required before certification. Normally, class 2 certification will not be considered until one year after the operation. The preoperative refraction must not have exceeded +5.00 to −8.00 dioptres. An aircrew medical examiner (AME) report from an ophthalmologist about the surgery and its results is required, often with further special tests of vision, including contrast sensitivity and glare testing, in order to ensure that the vision is adequate for aviation.

OPHTHALMIC HISTORY AND EXAMINATION

Visual abnormalities and ophthalmic conditions are major causes of rejection from flying training, as stringent visual standards are set for aircrew entry. Prospective candidates are required to complete a detailed questionnaire relating to past ophthalmic disease, including the need for or use of refractive correction and any relevant family history.

Visual acuity

The uniocular distance visual acuities are assessed with a backlit Snellen chart at 6 m. The subject should attend with recently updated spectacles and a written copy of the current spectacle prescription. CL should not be worn for at least two weeks before the test. The visual acuity is recorded as the lowest line that is read correctly and completely. The test is first performed unaided and then repeated with spectacle correction. Common errors include facing the chart at the wrong distance and too much light in the chart causing glare and surface reflection; these affect the visual acuity. Occasionally, the candidate will memorize the letters before the test commences; therefore, a different chart face should be used for each eye. The occluded eye should not be pressed accidentally by the examiner or candidate, as this will change its shape and reduce its acuity. The subject should not be allowed to narrow the palpable fissures, as this minimizes the effects of a refractive error.

The uniocular and binocular near acuity are tested with the normal reading correction, using standard test types at 33 cm. If the visual acuity is normal at distance, then the reading correction is incorrect if N5 is not attained.

Testing for hypermetropia

It is important to identify any individuals who may be manifestly hypermetropic and who overcome their refractive error by accommodating to achieve a normal unaided visual acuity. These individuals will become presbyopic and then hyperopic towards middle age. Manifest hypermetropia can be diagnosed with a convex lens (usually +2.5D) and recording the visual acuity unaided and with the lens. An emmetropic individual who achieves 6/6 vision without correction will not be able to achieve that with a +2.5-dioptre lens. If they can read the line, then their manifest hypermetropia is at least +2.5 dioptres. The highest power of 'plus' lens through which the 6/6 Snellen line can be read quickly and correctly is the manifest hypermetropia. If the 6/6 Snellen line cannot be discerned, then the amount of 'plus' lens is reduced gradually until it can be read correctly. It is important to ensure that the subject does not try to remember or guess the Snellen letters and is given sufficient time to read the chart.

It is necessary sometimes to measure the total degree of hypermetropia by refraction using a topical cycloplegic. The most commonly used drug is cyclopentolate 1% (Mydrilate®), which acts by paralysing the ciliary muscle in order to abolish accommodation (cycloplegia) and the sphincter pupillae muscle in order to cause pupillary dilation (mydriasis).

Testing accommodation

If the unaided near acuity is reduced, then the accommodation may be quantified uniocularly and binocularly with and without correction using the RAF near-point rule. The drum with the near test-type is selected. The candidate places the shaped face piece of the rule on their cheekbones and holds the handle at the end of the rule. The drum is moved towards the subjective; the near point is when the N5 print becomes blurred.

When testing the uniocular accommodation, the right eye is made to focus on the last word of the N5 line and the left eye on the first word of that line. The amplitude of accommodation is measured in centimetres and is indicated by the end of the slide that carries the drum. Near correction should be worn during this test where appropriate. The accommodation is assessed for each eye separately and for both eyes together. Convergence weakness occurs when the near point of convergence is reduced.

Testing convergence

The line-and-dot test on the RAF near-point rule is used. The drum is moved towards the subject, who is instructed to declare when the single vertical line becomes double (not blurred). The distance, in centimetres, is the subjective convergence. One eye may be observed to hesitate, stop or diverge suddenly as the drum advances. This represents the point of objective convergence and is also measured in centimetres. Objective and subjective convergent measurements may differ in the same individual, who may not perceive the doubled vertical line. Subjective convergence should be measured initially; if this is unattainable, then the objective convergence should be measured and recorded.

Convergence weakness will often cause eyestrain (asthenopia). If this is problematic, then orthoptic exercises may greatly improve convergence and visual comfort. Symptomatic convergence weakness is often the result of ageing rather than significant pathology and is associated with presbyopia.

Stereopsis

Stereopsis is the ability to obtain an impression of depth by the superimposition of two images, one from each eye. Stereoscopic vision results from normal visual pathways that have developed optimally. Stereopsis may be perceived only by a subject possessing fully developed and integrated vision and eye-movement control.

The visual system reaches full maturity between the ages of seven and ten years. It may not realize its full stereoscopic potential due to ocular abnormalities, usually uncorrected refractive error or strabismus (squint). Subsequent stimulation to the visual system will have no significant effect in enhancing stereoscopic vision in a similar fashion to amblyopia. Psychological three-dimensional vision is depth perception independent of stereopsis gained by knowledge and experience of the known environment. It relies on the subject interpreting visual clues, including relative image size, light intensity, shadows and the movement of objects relative to each other (parallax). Stereopsis is a requirement for pilots and is desirable in all aircrew trades.

Stereopsis in aircrew is assessed with the *toatepast natuurwetenschep onderzoek* (TNO) random-dot stereogram stereo test. The TNO test insists of seven plates, each of which contains various shapes (squares, dots, crosses) created by random dots in complementary colours, which are viewed with red/green spectacles. The plates contain both visible features, which can be seen with and without spectacles, and hidden shapes, which are apparent only when the spectacles are worn and stereopsis is present. The first three plates enable the examiner to establish the presence of stereoscopic vision quickly; the other plates are used to determine its level. The TNO test provides a true measurement of stereopsis, as there are no monocular clues.

The Frisby test is a simpler test of stereovision that can be used for aircrew. It consists of three clear plastic plates, each containing four squares of small random shapes. One of the squares contains a hidden circle painted on the other side of the plate. The test does not require special spectacles, because the disparity is created by the thickness of the plate.

Testing ocular muscle balance

Normally, when the eyes are regarding a distant object, the visual axes are parallel. A state of ocular balance with image fusion without effort is termed orthophoria. Ocular imbalance results in varying degrees of squint or strabismus, in which the deviation can be manifest (tropia) or latent (phoria). Latent ocular misalignment, in which the ocular balance is maintained with effort, is phoric. When image fusion is absent and the eyes are misaligned, there is a manifest squint, or tropia. Diplopia (double vision) is rare in a congenital squint due to central cortical suppression of the image of one eye (strabismic amblyopia). If the manifest squint is associated with diplopia, then it is likely to be an acquired disorder of extraocular muscle function. Squints are assessed initially using the cover and alternate cover tests.

Cover/uncover test

The cover/uncover test is a monocular test designed to diagnose heterotropia. It should be performed for both near and distance vision. If the left eye shows a displacement of the corneal light reflex, then the examiner should cover the opposite right eye in search for any movement of that eye. A nasal movement to take up fixation indicates exotropia, a temporal movement esotropia, a downward movement hypertropia, and an upward movement hypotropia. If there is no movement of the left eye, then the test is repeated on the right eye. An eye may also fail to move on the cover/uncover test if there is eccentric fixation or if it is blind.

Alternate cover test

The alternate cover test is for heterophoria and is performed only if the cover/uncover test is normal. One eye is covered for about two seconds. The cover is then shifted quickly to the opposite eye. At this moment, the examiner notes any movement of the uncovered eye as it assumes fixation. If no movement occurs, the patient is orthophoric. A nasal movement indicates exophoria, a temporal movement esophoria and a downward movement hyperphoria. A person with heterophoria will, there-fore, have straight eyes, both before and after the alternate cover test has been performed, but during the test a deviation will be induced as a result of dissociation of the visual fusion mechanisms of the eyes.

Prism cover test

The prism and alternate cover test measures the total deviation (latent plus manifest) but does not separate heterotropia from heterophoria. Handheld prisms are placed in front of one eye, with the base of the prism placed in the direction that is opposite to the deviation. In a convergent squint, the prism is held base out. The alternate cover test is then performed; the endpoint is reached when the prism negates eye movement. The angle of deviation, in dioptres, is read from the strength of the prism. This test is the gold standard in the measurement of ocular deviations.

Maddox rod

The Maddox rod consists of a series of fused cylindrical red glass rods, which convert the appearance of a white spot of light into a red streak. The optical properties of the rods cause the streak of light to be at an angle of 90 degrees with the long axis of the rods. When the glass rods are held horizontally, the streak will be vertical, and visa versa.

The (red) rods are placed, by convention, in front of the right eye. This dissociates the two eyes, because the red streak seen by the right eye cannot be fused with the unaltered white spot seen by the left eye. The amount of dissociation is measured by the superimposition of the two images using prisms. The base of the prism is placed in the position opposite to the direction of the deviation. Both vertical and horizontal deviations can be measured in this fashion. When the white dot crosses to the right of the vertical line, there is an exophoria (Xophoria).

Maddox wing

The Maddox wing dissociates the two eyes for near fixation at 33 cm and measures the amount of heterophoria. The instrument is constructed in such a way that the right eye sees only a white vertical arrow and a red horizontal arrow and the left eye sees only a horizontal and a vertical row of numbers. The horizontal deviation is measured by asking the patient to which number the vertical arrow points. The vertical deviation is measured by asking the patient which number is intersected by the horizontal arrow. A cyclophoria (rotation) can be measured by asking the patient to move the horizontal arrow so that it is parallel with the horizontal row of numbers (Figure 46.8).

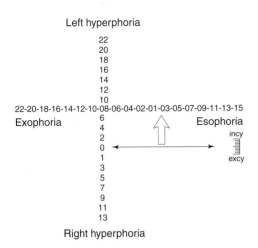

Left hyperphoria

22
20
18
16
14
12
10
22-20-18-16-14-12-10-08-06-04-02-01-03-05-07-09-11-13-15
Exophoria 6 Esophoria
4 incy
2
0
1 excy
3
5
7
9
11
13

Right hyperphoria

Figure 46.8 *Maddox wing test.*

Colour vision

In the past, very few colours were used in the cockpit, apart from red to signify stop and green to signify go. Today, colour is used in the cockpits of civil and military aircraft as well as air traffic control radar screens. There is a body of evidence that suggests that colour-defective pilots have significantly reduced target acquisition and lower reaction times to coloured visual stimuli than colour-normal people.

Three classes of cones with separate absorption spectra are responsible for colour vision in the human eye – blue, green and red. These are concentrated in the macular region and react to produce an electrical output in response to light of different hues. This output is modified in the retina, the visual pathway and the visual cortex in order to balance the relative input of colour information.

Colour deficiency may be congenital or acquired. Congenital red/green deficiency is a sex-linked characteristic and occurs in eight per cent of males and 0.4 per cent of females. Normal trichromats have normal amounts of all three cone types and normal colour vision. Anomalous trichromats are colour-weak and are slightly deficient in one of the cone types. Protanomaly is a deficiency in the red cone type (red-weak); it affects one per cent of males. Deuteranomaly is a slight deficiency in the green cone type (green-weak); it occurs in five to six per cent of males. Tritanomaly is a slight deficiency in the blue cone type (blue-yellow-weak); this occurs in 0.002–0.007 per cent of the population. Dichromats are completely colour-blind and have two cone types; protanopes lack the red cone (one per cent); deuteranopes lack the green cone (one per cent); and tritanopes, the rarest of congenital colour defectives (0.002–0.007 per cent), lack blue cones. Red-green deficiencies are all X-linked characteristics, blue-blue/yellow deficiency is an allelic characteristic with an equal sex ratio.

Acquired colour defects occur in 5–15 per cent of the population. They affect both sexes equally and typically cause a blue-yellow defect, although red-green discrimination may also be affected. They are associated with ageing, ocular disease, medications and drug ingestion. They may be insidious and precede any other visual loss. Drugs that commonly cause acquired colour vision deficits include oral contraceptives, oral diabetic agents, tetracyclines, antimalarial drugs, digoxin, ethanol, tobacco, sildenafil (Viagra®) and thiazide diuretics, several of which will commonly be used in aircrew. The use of sildenafil to boost sexual performance may have a particularly marked effect on blue/yellow colour discrimination and is associated with a bluish tinge visually. These effects have been reported in 30–50 per cent of users in a dose-dependent fashion; they last for one to six hours. An aviator who uses this drug must not fly for 24 hours after ingestion.

ELECTRONIC FLIGHT INSTRUMENTATION SYSTEMS

Electronic flight instrumentation systems (EFIS) allow colour-coded alphanumerical and analogue data for flight management and control. These are polychromatic data using more than eight colours, each of which can be displayed at different light intensities with graphics ranging from very small areas to entire backgrounds.

The conditions governing the use of colour have changed from previous cockpit designs, and the pilot observes these colour screens for long periods of time. The colour not only has safety connotations but also is used to save time when reading information; for example, the colour yellow is reserved for power information, while the colour magenta is used for track or trajectory processing. Cockpit control images may have several juxtaposed or superimposed colours. The intensity of contrast between a colour and a black background is no longer valid, as colour contrast against other colours is utilized.

The effects of EFIS displays maximize data presentation to colour-normal aviators by exploiting the increased sensitivity of blue-yellow colour discrimination. Colour-defective people have significant functional impairment when using EFIS. The effects of coloured visors and laser eye protection used in military aviation are not yet known.

MEASURING AND GRADING COLOUR PERCEPTION

At present, congenital red/green colour deficiency is tested in aircrew. A test for acquired defects may be required in the future. The tests used in British aviation are the Ishihara pseudo-isochromatic plate test for colour confusion in protanopes (confused greens and red) and deuteranopes (confused greens and purple). The standard 24-plate test is used under suitable lighting conditions. If the correct numbers are identified, then the individual is declared CP2 colour-normal and no further testing is performed.

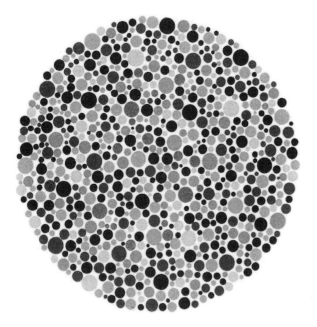

Figure 46.9 *Ishihara plate test card. The number '5' is read by red/green colour-normal people. See also colour plate 46.9.*

If the person fails the Ishihara plate test, the Holmes–Wright lantern (type A) test is the approved occupational colour-vision test for military aviators. It is also approved for European commercial pilots. The test requires an individual to tell the difference between red, green and white lights at different brightness and is a sensitive screen test for red-green colour deficiency. The lantern is used at 6 m in a darkened room; two lights, one above the other, are presented to the subject wearing normal spectacle correction. The colours are named and the test is repeated with various colour combinations. If no mistakes are made in the first run, then the individual passes and is declared CP3 colour-safe. If there is any red-green confusion, then the subject is automatically failed and is declared CP4 colour-unsafe. If there are any other mistakes in round one, then two extra runs are performed; if no mistakes are made in these, then the individual is passed as CP3. If there are any mistakes in the second or third run, other than red-green confusion, then the individual is dark-adapted for 20 minutes and a dark-adapted run is then performed. If the individual passes this run, then they are passed CP3. If there are any mistakes in the dark-adapted run, then the individual fails and is classed CP4 colour-unsafe.

CP1 is the situation in which an individual passes the Holmes–Wright lantern test in a light room with a device set on low brightness and is an entry standard for Royal Naval aviation. The colour vision grading system CP1–4 appears to be a political, rather than a functional, grading system. The Farnsworth lantern (Falant) test is a similar functional lantern test for aviation, though the Holmes–Wright lantern test has a superior correlation between other colour vision tests.

Visual fields

The visual field is an island of vision surrounded by a sea of darkness. It is not a flat plain but a three-dimensional structure. The outer aspect of the visual field extends approximately 60 degrees nasally, 90 degrees temporally, 50 degrees superiorly and 70 degrees inferiorly. The visual acuity is sharpest at the very top of the island and then declines progressively towards the periphery; the nasal slope is steeper than the temporal slope. The blind spot, where the optic nerve leaves the eye, is located temporally between 10 degrees and 20 degrees. A scotoma is either an absolute or relative defect in the visual field. An absolute scotoma represents total loss of vision. A relative scotoma is an area of partial visual loss within which some targets can and others cannot be seen. A scotoma may have sloping edges so that an absolute scotoma is surrounded by a relative scotoma. There is no set minimum visual field set for aviation, any visual field loss is assessed on an individual basis. Homonymous or bitemporal defects, whether hemianopic or quadrantanopic, are not accepted as safe (Figure 46.10).

Amsler grid

The Amsler grid is (Figure 46.11) used to test macular function and to detect central or paracentral scotomata by projecting a grid pattern on to the macula. The subject wears their usual reading correction and occludes one eye while the Amsler grid is held 33 cm in front of the open eye. The subject is asked what is in the centre of the page; failure to see the central dot indicates a central scotoma. The subject fixates on the central dot, or in the centre of the page if they cannot see the dot, and is asked whether all four corners of the diagram are visible or whether any of the boxes is missing. The subject is then asked whether all the lines are straight and continuous or whether some are distorted and broken. Any missing or distorted areas on the grid are outlined with a pencil. The procedure is repeated on the other eye. It is important to monitor any eye movement away from the central dot. A red Amsler grid may define more subtle defects.

OPHTHALMIC DISEASES COMMONLY ENCOUNTERED IN AVIATORS

Ocular adnexae

BLEPHARITIS

Chronic blepharitis is an inflammation of the eyelid margins. It is a very common external eye disorder. As well as

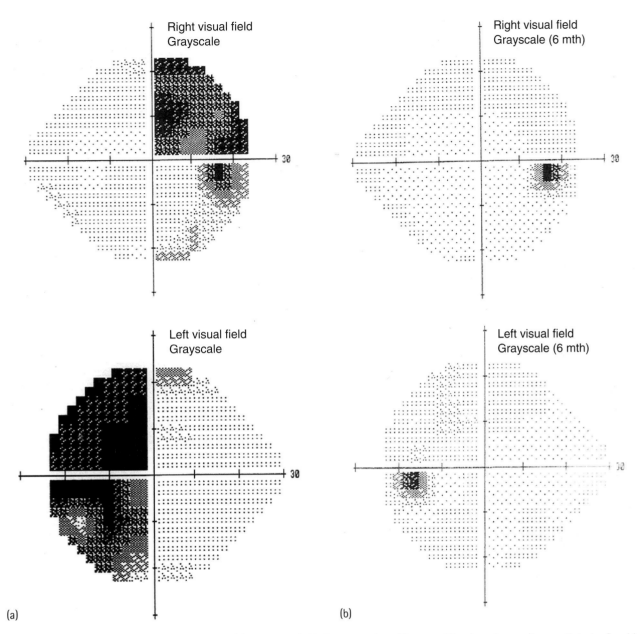

Figure 46.10 *Visual fields of a helicopter pilot. (a) This visual field, demonstrating a bitemporal hemianopia, was from a pilot who flew his own helicopter to the ophthalmic appointment to complain of vague visual disturbances. He had a pituitary prolactin-secreting adenoma diagnosed on magnetic resonance scanning and was treated successfully with cabergoline. Another pilot had to be dispatched to collect the helicopter and gave the individual a lift home. Post-treatment, the visual field returned to normal by six months. (b) The pilot was returned to full flying duties but subsequently always drove to follow-up appointments.*

causing annoying symptoms, it may interfere with the wearing of CL and aggravate the treatment of dry eyes. There are two main types of chronic blepharitis, anterior and posterior, but they are often mixed.

The symptoms include a foreign body sensation, mild photophobia and lid crusting. It is frequently worse in the mornings and characterized by remission and exacerbation. In anterior blepharitis (Figure 46.12), examination of the anterior lid margin demonstrates hyperaemia telangiectasia and scaling. In posterior blepharitis, there is lid thickening,

an excessively oily and foamy tear film, and a reddened posterior lid margin. The treatment of anterior blepharitis is with lid hygiene, using a cotton bud dipped in a cup of warm water that has been mixed with a few drops of baby shampoo or a pinch of sodium bicarbonate. The eyelids are scrubbed twice daily to remove the crusts. This will usually bring the disease under control. Artificial tears for the associated tear film instability will often be required.

If these simple measures do not work, then onward referral to an ophthalmic unit is recommended. Posterior

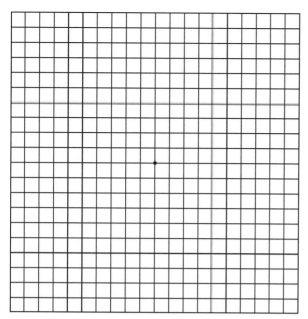

Figure 46.11 *Amsler grid test.*

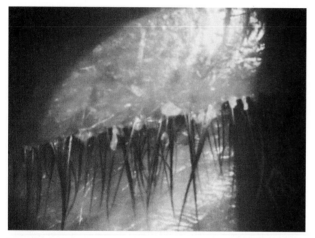

Figure 46.12 *Anterior blepharitis. See also colour plate 46.12.*

blepharitis (meibomitis) can be treated with systemic antibiotics (doxycycline 100 mg daily for at least one month). This is contraindicated in pregnant or lactating women and children under the age of 12 years, in which case erythromycin is substituted. Warm compresses are placed on the eyelids to melt solidified sebum.

CHALAZION (MEIBOMIAN CYST)

The meibomian glands lie within the lid tarsal plates and secrete lipid on to the eye surface. A chalazion (Figure 46.13) is a chronic inflammatory lesion caused by blockage of one of these gland orifices, with stagnation of the sebaceous secretion. They are painless roundish firm lesions in the tarsal plate. They may mechanically press on the

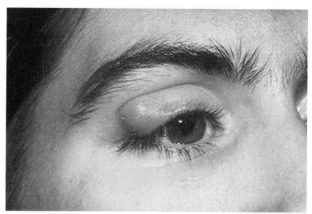

Figure 46.13 *Meibomian cyst (chalazion). See also colour plate 46.13.*

cornea, causing astigmatism and blurred vision. They are treated by incision or curettage, through the tarsal plate, under local anaesthesia.

EPIPHORA

Epiphora is excessive tearing and can be a cause of poor vision. It is caused by reflex overproduction of tears by corneal or conjunctival irritation, often due to irritation from misdirected eyelashes (trichiasis) or foreign bodies under the eyelid. Obstructive epiphora is caused by mechanical obstruction to tear drainage; the excessive watering is exacerbated by cold and windy atmosphere. The causes of the epiphora are usually managed with appropriate surgical manoeuvres. Occasionally, lacrimal pump failure causes epiphora secondary to lower lid laxity or weakness of the obicularis muscle, e.g. facial nerve palsy.

ORBITAL BLOW–OUT FRACTURE

A blow-out fracture of the orbit does not involve the orbital rim and is caused by a sudden increase in the orbital pressure by a striking object that is greater than 5 cm in diameter, such as a fist or a tennis ball. The fracture most frequently involves the orbital floor, although occasionally the medial orbital wall is also involved.

Signs of an acute blow-out fracture are ecchymosis, oedema and, occasionally, subcutaneous emphysema. The emphysema is worse on nose-blowing, and this should be discouraged. There is likely to be infraorbital nerve anaesthesia involving the lower-lid cheek side of the nose, upper teeth and gums, although this is usually transient. Enophthalmos, in which the eye sinks back into the socket, may occur later. Diplopia may be caused by mechanical entrapment of the inferior rectus muscle within the fracture or restriction of extraocular muscle movements due to haemorrhage and oedema.

Initial treatment is conservative, with prophylactic antibiotics if the fracture involves the maxillary sinus. The fracture needs to be confirmed with a computed tomography (CT) scan, and an orthoptic examination of the extraocular muscle balance should be made. Fractures involving more than half of the orbital floor, with entrapment of the orbital contents, and associated with persistent diplopia should be repaired within two weeks by placing a plate of synthetic material over the orbital floor. The diplopia is usually a restriction of up gaze, and an aviator's flight category will be determined by the results of surgery.

Ocular anterior segment

EPISCLERITIS

Episcleritis presents with mild uniocular discomfort, tenderness and watering of the eye. It is an idiopathic inflammation of the episcleral layer of the conjunctiva. It is a common, benign, recurrent but self-limiting disorder, which typically affects young adults. It is not associated with systemic disorders.

There are two types: simple and nodular. Simple episcleritis demonstrates sectorial or diffuse redness. In contrast, nodular episcleritis is localized to one area of the globe, forming a nodule with surrounding injection. Simple episcleritis usually resolves spontaneously within one to two weeks, but the nodular type may take longer to resolve. If discomfort is annoying, then topical steroids or topical non-steroidal anti-inflammatory drugs (NSAIDs) may be helpful. In the rare unresponsive recurrent cases, systemic flurbiprofen (100 mg three times daily) taken at the first symptom of recurrence may be successful in aborting the attack.

RECURRENT EROSION SYNDROME

This is a condition in which the corneal epithelial basement membrane complex is damaged by superficial corneal trauma, especially from a scratch. Its features are typically pain on waking, with lacrimation, photophobia and blurred vision. In mild cases, these symptoms resolve spontaneously within a few hours. It is recurrent and may cause problem for months or even years. After the initial episode has been treated with either pressure patching or debridement of the loose corneal epithelium, prophylactic ocular lubricants should be given using artificial tears four times daily and a simple lubricating ointment at night. Occasionally, further measures, such as bandage CL, antistromal puncture and phototherapeutic keratectomy, may be performed in order to cure the worst cases.

KERATOCONJUNCTIVITIS SICCA

Keratoconjunctivitis sicca, or dry eye, in aircrew is usually the result of meibomian gland dysfunction, which destabilizes the tear film. It may be secondary to autoimmune diseases, including Sjögren's syndrome, in which lacrimal salivary and salivary gland dysfunction are associated with rheumatoid arthritis and hypergammaglobulinaemia. The treatment is with topical ocular lubricants. If severe, temporary punctal occlusion may be performed using punctal plugs; occasionally, permanent punctal occlusion is indicated.

MICROBIAL KERATITIS

The only microbial pathogens that are able to produce corneal infection in the presence of an intact corneal epithelium are *Neisseria gonorrhoea*, *Corynebacterium diphtheriae*, *Listeria* spp. and *Haemophilus* spp. (Figure 46.14). Other bacteria are capable of producing keratitis only after loss of corneal epithelial integrity, especially associated with extended wear of soft CL and ocular surface disease such as post-herpetic corneal disease, trauma, bullous keratopathy, corneal exposure and dry eye. A bacterial corneal ulcer is associated with severe ocular pain and loss of vision in the affected eye. It is a sight-threatening condition that demands urgent identification and eradication of the causative organism. This is best performed with the patient hospitalized. A corneal scrape is taken for culture and sensitivity, and broad-spectrum topical antibiotics are administered intensively. Aviators may be susceptible to this condition, especially when wearing CL in hot and dry countries.

ADENOVIRAL KERATOCONJUNCTIVITIS

This highly contagious viral keratoconjunctivitis is common in the crowded conditions of military camps. It pres-

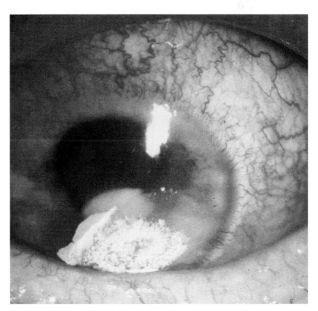

Figure 46.14 *Microbial keratitis in a wearer of soft contact lenses. The white precipitate is from the topical ofloxacin treatment. See also colour plate 46.14.*

ents with an acute onset of watering, redness, discomfort and photophobia. Both eyes are affected in approximately 60 per cent of cases. Examination demonstrates follicular conjunctivitis and lid oedema associated with a pre-auricular lymphadenopathy. In severe cases, subconjunctival haemorrhages chemosis and pseudo-membranes can develop.

Treatment is generally avoided unless the symptoms are severe, in which case topical steroids are instilled and spontaneous resolution occurs within two weeks. The patient must be isolated in order to avoid disease spread, which is often through shared towels. The cornea can also be affected with diffuse punctate epithelial keratitis, which resolves spontaneously, or focal white subepithelial opacities, which may persist for several months and may affect the visual axis. Topical steroids suppress corneal inflammation and improve vision, but they do not shorten the natural course of the disease and may need to be used for several months.

HERPETIC KERATITIS

Herpes simplex virus 1 predominantly causes infection above the waist (face, lips, eyes) and is usually acquired by coming into close contact with a person who has a cold sore or asymptomatic shedding of herpes labialus virus. Keratitis follows an attack of blepharoconjunctivitis and is characterized by a dendritic ulcer that stains with fluorescein dye (Figure 46.15). Treatment is initially with aciclovir 3% ointment five times daily for one week. Neurotrophic ulcers may occur after the primary infection. These are sterile ulcers with smooth margins in an area of stromal disease that persist despite antiviral therapy and are associated with stromal melting and corneal perforation.

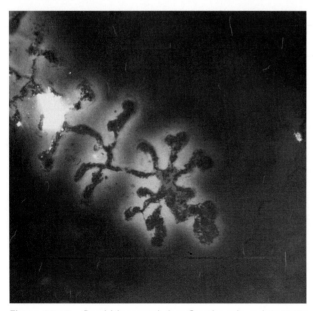

Figure 46.15 *Dendritic corneal ulcer. See also colour plate 46.15.*

Corneal stromal disease may occur with disciform keratitis, in which disc-shaped stromal oedema with an intact epithelium occurs. A mild iritis with localized granulomatous keratic precipitate is typical; the intraocular pressure may be raised. Necrotizing interstitial keratitis with multiple or diffuse whitish grey corneal stromal infiltrates may also occur, associated with corneal thinning and neovascularization. Treatment of disciform keratitis is with a combination of topical steroids and antiviral cover. This treatment is tapered slowly over several weeks. Occasionally, the patient will require continuous therapy.

KERATOCONUS

Keratoconus (conical cornea) (Figure 46.16) is a disorder in which the cornea thins and assumes an irregular conical shape. The hallmarks of keratoconus are paracentral stromal thinning, corneal protrusion and irregular astigmatism. The condition starts at around puberty and progresses slowly thereafter, although it may become stationary at any time. Both eyes are affected in about 85 per cent of cases, although the disease is asymmetrical. The aetiology of keratoconus is obscure. There is a hereditary component, as the offspring of keratoconic people have a ten per cent chance of being affected. Keratoconus is often associated with atopy and eczema. The wearing of hard CL and constant eye-rubbing have been proposed as predisposing factors.

The diagnosis is made using retinoscopy, keratometry, photokeratoscopy and slit-lamp biomicroscopy. Management is with spectacle correction in early cases, followed by hard CL to provide a regular refractive surface over the cone. When CL cannot be worn any more, a partial- or full-thickness penetrating keratoplasty is performed. Potential aircrew are screened for keratoconus. Early signs are seen in forme fruste keratoconus diagnosed in eyes that are otherwise refractively normal. A diagnosis of keratoconus or forme fruste keratoconus precludes an individual from aircrew selection, as there is a chance that the disease will progress and prevent the individual from completing a career in aviation.

UVEITIS

Uveitis is an inflammation of the uveal tract. It maybe subdivided into anterior uveitis, in which the iris and, occasionally, the anterior part of the ancillary body are inflamed, intermediate uveitis, in which the posterior part of the ciliary body is affected, posterior uveitis, in which the inflammation is located behind the posterior border of the ciliary body, and pan uveitis, in which the entire uveal tract is involved. Intermediate, posterior and pan uveitis are associated with progressive and severe visual loss. These diseases require systemic immunosuppression and usually will lead to a severely restricted flying category.

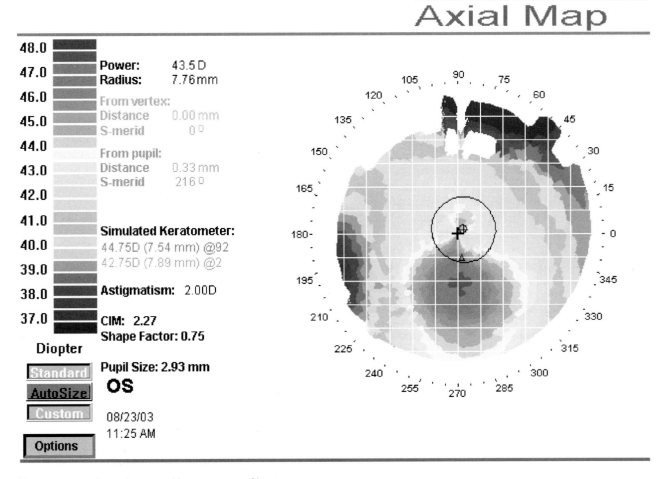

Axial Map

Power: 43.5 D
Radius: 7.76 mm

From vertex:
Distance   0.00 mm
S-merid   0 º

From pupil:
Distance   0.33 mm
S-merid   216 º

Simulated Keratometer:
44.75D (7.54 mm) @92
42.75D (7.89 mm) @2

Astigmatism: 2.00D

CIM: 2.27
Shape Factor: 0.75

Pupil Size: 2.93 mm
OS

08/23/03
11:25 AM

48.0
47.0
46.0
45.0
44.0
43.0
42.0
41.0
40.0
39.0
38.0
37.0
Diopter

Standard
AutoSize
Custom
Options

Figure 46.16 *Corneal topographic appearance of keratoconus.*

Anterior uveitis is the most common type, followed by intermediate posterior and pan uveitis. Anterior uveitis may be acute or chronic. The main symptoms of acute anterior uveitis are photophobia, pain, redness, decreased vision and lacrimation. In chronic anterior uveitis, the eye may be white and the symptoms minimal even in the presence of severe inflammation. The signs are a purplish reddish hue to the eye, associated with keratic precipitates, cellular deposits on the corneal epithelium. The anterior chamber has flare and cells, and the iris may be stuck to the lens by posterior synaechiae.

Anterior uveitis may be associated with arthritis and ankylosing spondylitis, especially in the presence of human leucocyte antigen HLA B27. Reiter's syndrome consists of a combination of non-specific urethritis, conjunctivitis and seronegative arthritis with iritis. The disease affects men more frequently than women. Approximately 75 per cent of patients are positive for HLA B27. The most common association is conjunctivitis, which follows the urethritis by approximately two weeks and precedes the onset of arthritis. This disease is rare in the general population but more common among the aircrew population, who will often be deployed to foreign countries and be exposed to sources of non-specific urethritis. The disease can also be triggered by gastroenteritis.

Treatment of anterior uveitis is with topical steroids and cycloplegia. Often, the disease is recurrent but intermittent. Commonsense should be employed when dealing with aircrew with recurrent anterior uveitis, and it is possible for people with this condition to attain a full flying career. They should not fly if the disease is active.

OCULAR HYPERTENSION AND GLAUCOMA

Aqueous humour is produced by active secretion from the ciliary body that lies behind the pupil. The aqueous humour passes through the pupil into the anterior chamber, where it drains under resistance through the trabecular meshwork that lies at the iridocorneal angle. Approximately ten per cent of the aqueous humour drains across the ciliary body and iris. The normal intraocular pressure (IOP) varies between 10 mmHg and 21 mmHg (mean 16 mmHg) and increases with age as the trabecular resistance increases.

Glaucoma is a term used to describe a collection of syndromes demonstrating a characteristic form of optic neuropathy, usually associated with a raised IOP. The many types of glaucoma can be classified as having either open iridocorneal angles or the angle-closure type, according to the manner by which aqueous outflow is impaired. The disorder may be primary or secondary, depending on the presence of associated factors contributing to the rise in intraocular pressure.

Ocular hypertension is diagnosed when an individual has a raised IOP without any clinical signs of glaucoma. Such individuals have an increased risk of developing glaucoma. Aircrew with intraocular hypertension require annual monitoring with visual field analysis and are likely to receive treatment if there are significant risk factors.

Primary open-angle glaucoma (POAG) has an insidious onset and is symptomatic only if the IOP is extremely high. It is a common disease, occurring in approximately one per cent of the population. If there is a positive family history of the disease in a first-degree relative, then the lifetime chance for developing POAG is ten per cent. Other associated factors include myopia, diabetes, increasing age

and ocular hypertension. A cupped optic disc is a cardinal sign of open-angle glaucoma. Visual fields are then performed, looking for the characteristic arcuate scotoma (Figure 46.17). Aircrew usually present with adult-type POAG in the latter stages of their flying careers.

When POAG is diagnosed, the initial treatment is medical, using topical ocular antihypertensives. If this fails, surgical treatments are used. The most common surgical intervention for POAG is a trabeculectomy, in which a guarded sclerostomy is fashioned to bypass the trabecular meshwork of the iridocorneal angle and allow aqueous to directly drain to the episcleral vessels at a lower pressure. The number of topical preparations for the treatment of POAG has increased over recent years. They act to suppress aqueous production by the ciliary body or increase uveoscleral outflow. The majority of aviators with glaucoma will continue to fly under medical surveillance, according to the nature of the glaucoma and the state of the visual fields. Specialist supervision of glaucoma patients is lifelong.

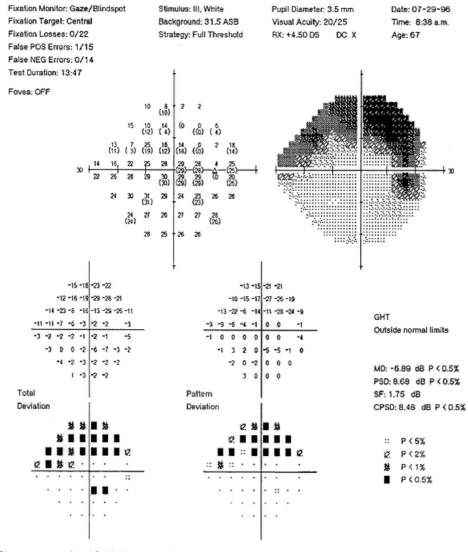

Figure 46.17 *Glaucomatous visual field, demonstrating an arcuate scotoma.*

CATARACTS

Cataracts are congenital or acquired opacities of the crystalline lens. They are classified according to their morphology, age of onset and causation. The vast majority of cataracts in the general population are age-related. In the younger aircrew population, cataracts are due more commonly to progression of congenital lens opacities or secondary to trauma, ocular inflammation, diabetes mellitus, steroid use or previous intraocular surgery. A cataract that does not cause visual symptoms need not impose limitations to flying in established aircrew but would be a bar to entry to flying training, as it might progress. The visual symptoms of cataracts include blurred and reduced visual acuity, reduced contrast sensitivity, significant glare that is worse when above the cloud canopy and at night, multiple uniocular images and progressive myopia.

The management of cataracts is surgical (Figure 46.18). The most common procedure is phacoemulsification with intraocular lens implant through a small (< 3 mm) corneal incision. The intraocular lenses are foldable and usually made of silicone or acrylic material. These are implanted into the capsular bag following the cataract extraction and focus light to the retina. A unifocal lens is used in aircrew. The lens is selected to give minimal postoperative refractive error with maximal distance vision. In prepresbyopic aircrew with unilateral cataracts, the unaffected lens accommodates for near vision, and no reading correction is required. Multifocal intraocular lenses are not recommended, as they reduce contrast sensitivity and increase glare. The intraocular lens selected for aircrew is designed to minimize visual aberrations that might cause glare.

Postoperative posterior lens-capsule opacification may occur in up to ten per cent of cases. Subjects complain of symptoms similar to those caused by the cataract. It is managed easily using an yttrium–aluminium–garnet (YAG) laser to make a hole in the opaque capsule over the visual axis in order to restore vision. There is sufficient remaining capsule to support the intraocular lens. The spe-

cific gravity of the intraocular lens is approximately the same as the fluids of the eye. This makes the effect of high G force and ejection negligible. No movement of an intraocular lens has ever been reported in pseudophakic ejectees. A full return to flying duties can be expected between 6 and 12 weeks after uncomplicated cataract surgery if the visual function is adequate.

Retinal disease

RETINAL DETACHMENT

In retinal detachment, fluid passes from the vitreous cavity under the retina, causing it to separate from its retinal pigment epithelium. The patient may notice flashes of light, floaters, a 'curtain' or shadow moving across the field of vision, and peripheral or central visual loss. On ophthalmoscopy, the retina will appear mobile, opaque and sometimes folded. In the aircrew population, trauma is the most common cause. Patients with an acute retinal detachment that threatens the macula should be operated on at the earliest opportunity in order to preserve the macular vision. Surgical repair is with either an external procedure, in which the retinal break is closed by indenting the sclera with a silicone explant, or a vitrectomy with internal tamponade with silicone oil or gas. The break is sealed in both cases by the creation of a chorioretinal scar using laser retinopexy or cryopexy.

Air travel is contraindicated in an eye with intraocular gas. If more than approximately 1 ml of the bubble remains, then it will expand at altitude, according to Boyle's law, causing an acute rise in IOP, which may be painful. Patients recovering from retinal-detachment surgery with intraocular gas and wishing to fly should do so only after being examined by their ophthalmologist. Silicone oil is also used as an intraocular tamponade agent; this will not expand at altitude. This allows air travel soon after the operation; the oil is removed at a later date. Visual recovery after retinal-detachment surgery depends on whether the macular has been affected and whether the visual field recovers after surgery.

CENTROSEROUS CHORIORETINOPATHY

Centroserous chorioretinopathy (CSC) is an idiopathic macular exudative disease that typically affects young to middle-aged men. The characteristic localized neurosensory detachment of the macular region is caused by leakage of fluid at the level of the retinal pigment epithelium that underlies the retina and normally removes fluid from the subretinal space. It presents with unilateral sudden-onset blurred vision associated with a greenish-brown positive scotoma, micropsia and metamorphopsia, with impaired dark adaptation. The diagnosis is made on careful clinical examination and confirmed by fluorescein

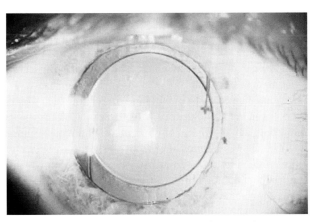

Figure 46.18 *Postoperative appearance of an eye after cataract surgery. The intraocular lens is visible in the centre of the eye.*

angiography, in which characteristic patterns of leakage are observed.

Approximately 80 per cent of eyes with CSC undergo spontaneous resolution of subretinal fluid, with a return to normal or near-normal visual acuity between six weeks and six months. Even if the visual acuity returns to normal, however, some degree of subjective visual impairment, such as micropsia, can persist. This seldom causes any significant disability. If there are recurrent and prolonged attacks, then progressive disturbance of the retinal pigment epithelium associated with permanent central visual loss can occur. Focal argon laser photocoagulation to the site of retinal pigment epithelial leakage reduces the length of time to resolution of the serous detachment, but it does not reduce the recurrence rate of CSC or prevent visual loss associated with chronic progressive retinal pigment epithelial changes. Aviators with CSC are often unfit aircrew duties while they have significant visual disturbances. They will often opt for laser treatment of the problem rather than wait for spontaneous resolution.

CENTRAL RETINAL VEIN OCCLUSION

Central retinal venous occlusion is associated with increasing age, systemic hypertension and blood dyscrasias. A subset of younger patients will develop central retinal vein occlusions, and the condition may be encountered in the aircrew population. It typically affects one eye of a healthy adult under the age of 40 years, and this probably represents a different disease process to that seen in older patients. It has been postulated that it may be caused by a congenital abnormality in the central retinal vein at the level of the lamina cribrosa, which gives rise to turbulent flow and thrombus formation.

Presentation is with visual impairment, which is characteristically worse in the mornings. Ophthalmoscopy during the acute stage demonstrates disc oedema and a moderate amount of retinal haemorrhage. Systemic causes of central retinal vein occlusions, including sarcoidosis and Behçet's disease, autoimmune collagen vascular diseases and anticardiolipin antibody syndrome. The prognosis is usually good if the retina does not become ischaemic. A poor outcome occurs occasionally, especially when ischaemia and exudative retinal detachment occur. If severe retinal ischaemia occurs, rubeosis iridis may develop, with associated secondary glaucoma. Pan-retinal argon laser photocoagulation is performed to prevent this.

Neurophthalmology

AMBLYOPIA AND SQUINT

Potential aircrew with a manifest squint and amblyopia will, for the most part, be screened out on selection. Amblyopia (lazy eye) is caused by suppression of central vision from suboptimal retinal stimulation during visual development in the first six to eight years of life. Amblyopia will occur in children with strabismus (strabismic amblyopia) or unequal refractive error (anisometropic amblyopia) or as a result of uniocular visual occlusion, often from cataracts, ptosis or eyelid tumours (stimulus deprivation amblyopia). Amblyopia is rarely bilateral, and the amount of reduced vision varies. Occasionally, individuals with mild forms of amblyopia will be fit for aircrew duties. The treatment of amblyopia is with adequate spectacle correction and patching of the good eye before visual maturation is completed at around seven years of age. After this, no treatment can improve the vision of the amblyopic eye.

Acquired squints may arise from extraocular muscle paralysis (III, IV and VI cranial nerve palsies) and will often cause diplopia. Systemic, intracranial, vascular and traumatic causes of these palsies should be excluded and treated if present. Where diplopia persists, prisms can be incorporated into the patient's glasses in order to give single vision. It is unlikely that a flying category will be awarded to a person with diplopia while looking straight ahead, even if it can be corrected with prisms. Occasionally, individuals with minimal diplopia in the far extremes of gaze and who do not require a great fusional effort to control it in the primary position may be awarded a flying category.

OPTIC NEUROPATHY

Optic neuropathy describes inflammatory or demyelinating disorders of the optic nerve. The most common type is retrobulbar neuritis, in which the optic nerve is inflamed behind the optic disc. It is associated with multiple sclerosis in approximately 75 per cent of women and 35 per cent of men over 15 years of age. Presentation is typically with an acute onset of monocular visual loss associated with periocular discomfort, which is made worse on moving the eye. There may also be frontal headache, with tenderness of the globe. Ophthalmoscopy is usually normal, although a few patients have papillitis. The visual acuity is markedly diminished, and colour vision is typically decreased, red targets having a washed-out appearance compared with those seen by the other eye. There is usually an afferent pupillary defect and electrodiagnostic tests of optic-nerve function are abnormal.

Seventy-five per cent of patients will recover their visual acuity over the ensuing four to six weeks. Colour vision and contrast sensitivity often remain abnormal. Optic atrophy may be observed after recovery. In the acute phase, intravenous and oral steroids may be used. Although the treatment does not improve the final visual outcome, it reduces the recovery period by approximately two weeks. An aviator with optic neuritis will regain a flying category only when the visual acuity, colour vision and visual fields have returned to satisfactory levels.

ABNORMAL PUPILLARY REACTIONS

Aircrew occasionally will present with abnormal pupils, usually complaining that one pupil is larger than the other. This is termed anisocoria and is either episodic or constant. Episodic anisocoria can be due to migrainous episodes, ocular inflammation or benign pupillary dilation, in which the papillary asymmetry may change. In the absence of any other medical abnormalities and normal pupillary light reactions, it is likely to be physiological anisocoria.

In constant anisocoria, with sluggish pupil reactions to light, and if iris trauma, pharmacological dilation and a third cranial nerve palsy have been excluded, then it is likely to be a Holmes–Adie pupil. This is caused by idiopathic denervation of the postganglionic parasympathetic nerve supply to the sphincter pupillae and ciliary muscles, occasionally following a viral illness. The affected pupil is typically large and irregular, with an absent or very slow light reflex. Constriction on accommodation is very slow and is associated with vermiform movements of the iris; re-dilation is also sluggish. It typically affects healthy young adults. It is unilateral in 80 per cent of cases. If there is a diminished Achilles tendon reflex, then it is termed Holmes–Adie syndrome. Patients with a Holmes–Adie pupil may have difficulty with glare and accommodation and can require a tint to their glasses as well as a reading correction, especially if both pupils are affected. Diagnosis is confirmed using 0.1% pilocarpine instilled to both eyes. The normal pupil will not constrict, as the concentration is too low to affect it, but the Holmes–Adie pupil constricts because of denervation hypersensitivity.

If there is constant anisocoria with good light reactions in both eyes, but which is greater in dim light, then Horner's syndrome should be suspected. This is due to congenital or acquired disruption of the sympathetic pathways innervating the eye and adnexal tissues. The lesion is usually unilateral and is characterized by mild ptosis as a result of a weakness of the sympathetically innervated component of the levator muscle, miosis from the unopposed action of the sphincter pupillae muscle, and apparent enophthalmos caused by the ptosis. There may be reduced ipsilateral facial sweating if the lesion is below the superior cervical ganglion and heterochromia iridis (different coloured irises) if the lesion is congenital. It is an important diagnosis to make, as it may be associated with tumours of the lung, carotid and aortic aneurysms, neck lesions (including malignant cervical lymph nodes), trauma or surgery, brainstem vascular disease, demyelination, syringomyelia and cluster headaches.

MIGRAINE

Migraine is characterized by recurrent attacks of headache that are widely variable in intensity frequency and duration and often with a familial tendency. The attacks are commonly unilateral and associated with anorexia, nausea and vomiting. Occasionally, they are preceded by neurological and mood disturbances.

People with classic migraines and retinal migraines will often present to ophthalmologists. A classic migraine is often associated with a visual aura, consisting of bright or dark spots, zigzag lines and scintillating scotomata as well as various visual field defects. After several minutes, the fortification spectrum expands, with an associated negative scotoma that progresses across the visual field and then breaks up. A headache is usually present and is similar to that found in common migraine. Retinal migraine is a rare variant, with acute transient unilateral visual loss identical to that seen in patients with amaurosis fugax. Cardiac and carotid artery disease must be excluded before making the diagnosis. Aircrew who suffer from attacks of migraine are unlikely to retain their full flying category because of the intermittent and unpredictable loss of visual function.

OPHTHALMIC DRUGS

Aircrew will usually be able to fly while using topical medications, as long as they do not affect their visual function. Allergy to the active component or the preservatives within the drops should be looked out for, and the drops changed as required. Cycloplegic drops, including atropine and cyclopentolate, will cause mydriasis and cycloplegia associated with abnormal glare and visual aberrations. Aircrew should not fly while using such drops. Mydriasis is also caused by alpha-sympathetic agonists such as phenylephrine and adrenaline (epinephrine); these drops should be avoided in aircrew. Miotic drops such as pilocarpine, used in glaucoma, cause a reduction of visual field due to pupillary constriction and should be avoided in aircrew. Topical beta-blockers are often used to treat glaucoma; systemic absorption may cause bradycardia and bronchoconstriction in susceptible individuals. Topical beta-blockers are contraindicated in patients with asthma or heart block. For the most part, they are tolerated well in aircrew.

Wearing of CL is usually discontinued when topical treatment is prescribed, as some drugs and preservatives in eye preparations accumulate in the CL and induce toxic reactions. When selecting a treatment for an aviator, the pharmacological vehicle should be considered. In general, drops and gels cause less visual disturbance than ointment, which blurs vision for up to half an hour after installation. It is prudent to tailor the medication to suit the needs of the aviator.

ACKNOWLEDGEMENTS

I would like to thank Ms Penny Shaw, Head of Optometry at OASC, RAF Cranwell, for her contribution on CFS and CL and Mrs Laura Walton for secretarial services.

FURTHER READING

Kanski JJ. *Clinical Ophthalmology*, 4th edn. Oxford: Butterworth Heinemann.

Tredici TJ, Ivan DJ. Ophthalmology in aerospace medicine. In: Dehart RL, Davis JR (eds). *Fundamentals of Aerospace Medicine*, 3rd edn. Philadelphia: Lippincott Williams & Wilkins, 2002; pp. 362–88.

Savant W, Dwarika D, Scott RAH, Stavrou P. Exudative retinal detachment following central retinal vein occlusion. *Eye* 2004; 18: 224–6.

Scott RA, Mushtaq B, Shaw P, Coker WJ. Survey of refractive correction in Royal Air Force aircrew. *Optometry in Practice* 2004; 5: 88–104.

Woodcock M, Good P, Scott RAH. A review of retinoid toxicity. *Investigative Ophthalmology and Visual Science* 2003; 44: 542.

47

Otorhinolaryngology

SALIYA CALDERA AND JOHN SKIPPER

INTRODUCTION

In order to understand the aviation medical aspects of otorhinolaryngology, it is important both to consider the normal physiological responses to the changes experienced in the flying environment and to appreciate how common conditions in ear, nose and throat (ENT) medicine impact on the ability of the aviator to perform his or her duties safely.

The problems associated with noise, spatial disorientation and motion sickness, although relevant to otolaryngological practice, are considered in Chapters 26, 28 and 29, respectively.

OTITIC BAROTRAUMA

One of the most common ENT problems encountered by the aviation medicine specialist is otitic barotrauma. This is defined as any damage to the ear that results from changes in pressure. The middle ear is enclosed within the petrous temporal bone and has as part of its lateral wall the tympanic membrane. Anteroinferiorly, the Eustachian tube extends from the middle ear to the lateral wall of the nasopharynx. In order to maintain maximum tympanic membrane compliance and, therefore, maximize hearing, the air pressure on either side of the tympanic membrane should be equal. The function of the Eustachian tube is to maintain this equality of air pressure around the tympanic membrane (Farmer 1985). In the normal state, absorption of gases from the middle ear through the mucous membrane results in a tendency towards negative pressure.

Changes in ambient atmospheric pressure affect the air pressure in the ear canal lateral to the tympanic membrane.

The Eustachian tube

In the resting state, the Eustachian tube remains closed. It is opened involuntarily by actions such as swallowing and yawning. The palatal muscles, principally the tensor veli palatini, attach to the tubal cartilage and on contraction pull on the tubal cartilage to facilitate opening of the lumen of the Eustachian tube. The other palatal muscles involved in this are the levator palatini, the salpingopharyngeus and the tensor tympani muscles. People with cleft palate often, even after apparently good repair, continue to have Eustachian tube dysfunction due to abnormalities in the pull of these muscles.

Within the aerospace environment, the gases within the tympanic cavity are subject to pressure changes, as described by Boyle's law. During ascent through the atmosphere, a given mass of gas will expand. Within the middle ear, this gaseous expansion initially pushes the tympanic membrane laterally. As the gas expands further, the Eustachian tube opens passively, followed by escape of air along the Eustachian tube into the nasopharynx.

During descent from altitude, increase in atmospheric pressure causes a decrease in the volume of the gas within the middle ear. This causes a relative negative pressure within the middle ear. The natural absorption of gases through the mucosal membrane of the middle ear also tends towards creating a negative pressure, and this is exacerbated during descent from altitude (King 1979).

In order to adjust this volume and pressure, the Eustachian tube must be opened. This requires an active process, such as swallowing, yawning or the Valsalva manoeuvre. If this active opening of the Eustachian tube does not occur, then increasing pressure differential around the Eustachian tube itself further prevents opening. If the negative pressure is not relieved by, for example, the Valsalva manoeuvre, then initially the tympanic membrane will medialize in order to absorb the pressure gradient. Further increasing the pressure gradient causes punctate haemorrhages on the tympanic membrane. Even further increases in the pressure gradient may cause serous exudate or haemorrhage into the middle ear from the middle-ear mucosa. Further pressure changes can cause rupture of the tympanic membrane.

Factors contributing to barotrauma

Anything that impedes the ability of the tympanic membrane or Eustachian tube to attempt to normalize pressure changes will predispose to barotrauma. Contributing factors include any condition that causes narrowing of the Eustachian tube lumen by oedema or that causes increased viscosity of mucus within the Eustachian tube.

The most common predisposing cause to Eustachian tube dysfunction is upper respiratory tract infection. Other common factors are allergy and rhinitis. As described earlier, the palatal muscles contribute to Eustachian tube opening, and any abnormalities of the palate may well be a predisposing factor in barotrauma. Also, anatomical obstruction of the Eustachian tube orifice by adenoidal hypertrophy or other nasopharyngeal masses will exacerbate the problem.

Scarring or tympanosclerosis of the tympanic membrane will limit the movement of the tympanic membrane and may be a contributing factor.

There have been many attempts to find a reliable test as a predictor of Eustachian tube dysfunction. So far, however, none has been successful. Even impedance tympanometry, which measures the mobility of the tympanic membrane in relation to pressure change within the external ear canal, has been found to be of little predictive value for barotrauma (Ashton and Watson 1999). Thus, the main predictors remain previous history of nasal or otologic disease and abnormal otoscopy.

Inner-ear barotrauma

The fluids of the inner ear are in close proximity to the middle ear cavity, separated by the oval and round windows. During a rise in atmospheric pressure, the round-window membrane bulges laterally in towards the tympanic cavity in order to offset some of the pressure changes. Further rises in pressure can result in rupture of this membrane or even rupture of the oval window. This

leads to the condition known as a perilymph fistula. This can produce sensorineural hearing loss, which can be sudden and severe, and also vertigo, which similarly can be sudden and incapacitating.

Alternobaric trauma

Alternobaric vertigo is a transient vestibular auditory dysfunction believed to occur as a result of elevated and probably asymmetric middle-ear pressure. Susceptibility towards vertigo results as a consequence of individual variations in the pressure required within the middle ear to passively open the Eustachian tube. Conditions that alter Eustachian tube patency, as described earlier, will contribute to the inability to passively open the Eustachian tube by rise in middle-ear pressure. Patients with such predisposing factors are more likely to experience alternobaric symptoms. It is thought that the mechanism of alternobaric vertigo is due to elevation of perilymph pressure due to medial bowing of the round-window membrane secondary to an increase in middle-ear pressure (Tjernström 1974).

Reversed ear: barotrauma of the external auditory meatus

If there is an obstruction at the external auditory meatal entrance, this will prevent an increase in pressure within the external canal. If there is increase in pressure within the middle ear through an open Eustachian tube, then this will cause bulging of the tympanic membrane laterally into the external canal. This can cause rupture of the tympanic membrane and haemorrhage of the external canal walls. In flying, the reversed ear is most often caused by a tight-fitting earplug.

Reversed ear is more common in diving than when flying, as in diving there is exposure to larger pressure differentials.

Delayed otitic barotrauma

Delayed otitic barotrauma is a clinical entity consisting of ear discomfort and hearing loss some hours after flight. This usually occurs after long flights, when breathing high oxygen concentrations. This results in a raised partial pressure of oxygen within the middle ear. Absorption of the oxygen through the mucous membrane of the middle ear over the following few hours results in significant negative pressure formation within the middle ear. This usually occurs during sleep, where there is the added insult of poor aeration of the middle-ear cleft due to a reduction in the rate of swallowing.

Management of otitic barotrauma

The main symptom of otic barotrauma is pain, and the immediate treatment is for pain relief with analgesics. The second mainstay of treatment involves attempts to ventilate the middle-ear cleft. Decongestants inserted topically into the nose are used in an attempt to reduce oedema of the Eustachian tube orifice mucosa.

Tympanic membrane perforations have a high frequency of infection due to the negative pressure in the middle ear, leading to debris being sucked into the cavity at the moment of perforation. Therefore, people with tympanic membrane perforations due to otic barotrauma should be prescribed prophylactic antibiotics.

The majority of cases of acute otic barotrauma will settle with such conservative measures. The majority of perforations due to otic barotrauma heal spontaneously.

With regard to further flying, the main cause of chronic otic barotrauma is either that the original predisposing factor is still persistent or that the oedema and bleeding caused by the original barotrauma have not recovered sufficiently. Therefore, it is important that sufficient time is given to recover from the episode of barotrauma before return to flying duties. It is difficult to give a precise length of time, as individuals vary and the degree of barotrauma varies. However, it would seem sensible that following barotrauma the tympanic membrane should look normal and Eustachian tube function should be demonstrated by auto-inflation during otoscopy before returning to flying duties.

Cases of recurrent or chronic barotrauma can be associated with nasal septal deviation, especially in the posterior bony nasal septum. In these cases, it may be possible to improve Eustachian tube function by septal surgery in order to correct the deformity of the nasal septum. In these cases, short-term ventilation tubes are sometimes inserted into the tympanic membrane in order to help aerate the middle ear while healing following surgery and return to normal functioning of the Eustachian tube occurs.

It is also technically possible to insert longer-term ventilation tubes into the tympanic membrane in order to prevent the pressure changes within the middle ear responsible for otic barotrauma. There are, however, significant side effects with long-term tubes, including a high association with perforations of the tympanic membrane, which has other consequences for aircrew, such as restrictions regarding getting water in the ears, which may prevent the person taking part in certain training drills.

If perilymph fistula is suspected, then the history and audiological findings of varying position-dependent hearing thresholds may be suggestive, but the definitive diagnosis of perilymph fistula is made by direct visualization of the fistula at exploratory operation (tympanotomy) (Goto *et al.* 2001). If perilymph fistula is diagnosed, then this can be closed by a tissue graft. Sufficient time for healing should be

given. Following such surgery, we would recommend full otological assessment and, if necessary, audiovestibular testing before considering return to flying duties.

Alternobaric vertigo is usually related to an underlying upper respiratory tract infection, and further flying should not be undertaken until normal Eustachian tube function can be demonstrated.

Delayed otic barotrauma is generally fairly mild in its symptomatology and is usually relieved by reintroducing air into the middle ear by gentle auto-inflation.

SINUS BAROTRAUMA

The sinuses are air spaces within the bones of the face that connect to the nasal cavity through narrow channels via the sinus ostia. The sinuses and the channels, together with the nasal cavities, are lined by respiratory mucosa consisting of pseudo-stratified columnar ciliated epithelium with numerous goblet cells. Mucus secreted by glands within the respiratory mucosa is cleared from the sinuses by ciliary activity towards the sinus ostia and in the nasal cavity towards the nasopharynx. For normal function, this drainage of the mucus is required, together with adequate ventilation of the sinuses. Any obstruction to this normal mucus flow, or to ventilation, may cause inflammation within the paranasal sinuses.

The air within the sinuses is subject to ambient pressure changes in a similar manner to the air within the middle-ear cleft. Unlike the middle ear, however, there is no voluntary control of the sinus ostium in the same way that there is voluntary control over the opening of the Eustachian tube.

During ascent, a decrease in ambient pressure leads to expansion of the gas within the sinus cavity. Generally, air passively vents from the sinus cavity through the sinus ostium and the channels leading to the nasal cavity. On descent, the relative negative pressure within the sinus is counteracted by passage of air from the nasal cavity into the sinus.

Obstruction of the sinus ostia or the channels leading into the nasal cavity, by mucosal oedema or some other obstruction such as polyp or neoplasm, can cause difficulties in such passage of air. Most often, sinus barotrauma occurs on descent; with obstructive lesions, however, such as polypoid changes to the sinus lining within the sinus, it is also possible to experience barotrauma during ascent.

During descent, the continued negative pressure within the sinus causes engorgement of the sinus mucosa, leading to rupture of the mucosal vessels, haematoma within the mucosa and sometimes frank haemorrhage within the sinus. Due to the circulatory patterns of mucous drainage within the sinuses, it is the frontal sinuses that are most commonly affected (Dickson and King 1956).

Predisposing factors to sinus barotrauma

The predisposing factors to sinus barotrauma most commonly involve upper respiratory tract infection or history of chronic inflammatory nasal disease, such as rhinitis or nasal polyps. Rarer causes include mucociliary disorders.

Management of sinus barotrauma

The main presenting feature is pain within the affected sinus. In some cases epistaxis occurs. Most cases of sinus barotrauma can be managed conservatively with topical nasal decongestion. This is to try to improve patency of the sinus ostium and the channels leading into the nose, in order to allow ventilation of the affected sinus and drainage. Prophylactic antibiotics can be used to prevent infection if there has been significant sinus barotrauma.

Once the symptoms of sinus barotrauma have resolved, and there is a healthy looking nasal cavity, it is possible for further flying duties to recommence.

Chronic or recurrent sinus barotrauma presents a more serious problem, as this condition rarely settles spontaneously and does not respond well to conservative management. The adaptation of endoscopic sinus surgery techniques to re-establish natural ventilation and drainage of the sinuses has made some improvement in the successful management of chronic sinus barotrauma (O'Reilly *et al.* 1996). The frontal sinus drainage pathway is a difficult area to access, and the surgery of this area has been improved by computer-assisted image-guided surgery. Reserving image-guided surgery for more severe cases has resulted in 100 per cent of aircrew returning to flying duties following this surgery over the past eight years in our unit.

Of course, it is important to ensure that there are no ongoing predisposing factors to the development of sinus obstruction. Following treatment of chronic sinus barotrauma, it is important that the ability of the sinus to withstand pressure changes is tested before further flying duties. This is usually assessed by decompression testing in hypobaric chambers.

HEARING LOSS

The two main types of hearing loss are conductive and sensorineural. Conductive hearing loss arises from any failure of transmission of sound waves through the external ear and middle ear, as far as the footplate of the stapes. Sensorineural hearing loss implies a defect in the central pathways of hearing from the cochlea through the cochlear nerve, brainstem and auditory cortex. The diagnosis is important in terms of aviation medicine, both in the man-agement of the condition and in the effect of the hearing loss within the aviation environment.

Sensorineural hearing loss

Sensorineural hearing depends on the integrated action of hair cells, stria vascularis cochlear neurones and the central neural network, all of which are dependent on continuous blood supply. Thus, various systemic disorders and local insults can impair sensorineural hearing.

PRESBYCUSIS

Presbycusis describes the bilateral symmetrical deterioration of hearing thresholds associated with ageing of the cellular elements of the cochlea. Typically, the loss is of the higher frequencies. Figure 47.1 shows the typical sloping pattern of hearing loss, which is worse in the higher frequencies, that occurs in presbycusis.

NOISE-INDUCED HEARING LOSS

Bilateral progressive hearing loss may also be caused by noise exposure. Excessive noise damages the hair cells of the organ of Corti. Noise-induced hearing loss may follow brief high-intensity exposure (acoustic trauma) or high-intensity exposure to noise over long periods of time. Typically, the hearing thresholds show a dip at 4 kHz (Figure 47.2).

Noise exposure is common in aviation. There are many sources, including transmission systems, propellers, jet flux, cabin-conditioning and cabin-pressurizing systems, hydraulic systems, communication equipment, sonic booms and armament discharge (Rood and James 1999).

OTOTOXIC DRUGS

Many agents are associated with cochlear toxicity, including antibiotics, especially aminoglycoside antibiotics, loop diuretics, anti-inflammatory medications, cancer chemotherapeutic drugs and haemolytic agents. Aminoglycosides are traditionally used by otolaryngologists as topical antibiotics in the ear, despite their potential ototoxic effects, but this practice is being evaluated.

VIRAL INFECTIONS

Many viral infections are associated with sensorineural hearing loss, including mumps, herpes zoster, Weil's disease, Epstein–Barr virus, cytomegalovirus and many adenoviruses and para-influenza viruses.

Other causes of sensorineural hearing loss include trauma, perilymph fistula, acoustic neuromas and Ménière's disease.

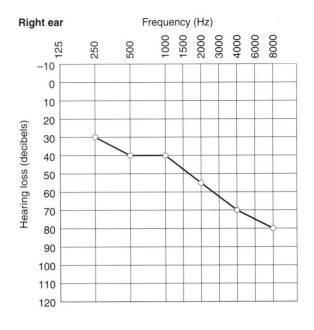

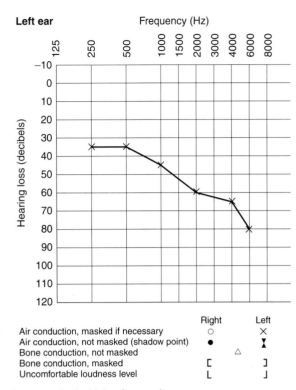

Figure 47.1   *Typical sloping pattern of hearing loss that occurs in presbycusis – worse in the higher frequencies.*

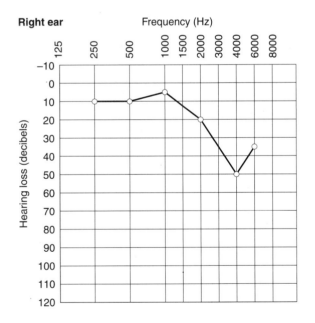

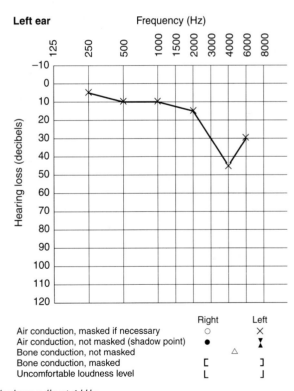

Figure 47.2   *In noise-induced hearing loss, typically the hearing thresholds show a dip at 4 kHz.*

Management and prognosis of sensorineural hearing loss are dependent on the underlying cause. Sensorineural losses that are severe enough can benefit from the use of hearing aids. If the underlying cause is due to noise exposure, then protection from further noise exposure is desirable, as it is believed that noise-induced hearing loss does not progress after exposure to noise ceases.

Hearing loss in the aerospace environment needs close assessment, due to the necessity for verbal communication within a noisy environment. Hearing loss can result in poor ability to understand radiocommunications in a cockpit environment. Ear defenders are designed to shield the ear from surrounding noise. The use of helmets with earmuffs, together with built-in transducers, produces good attenuation and allows some patients with significant hearing loss to function adequately within this environment.

Active noise reduction is a further technique used to attenuate surrounding noise while maintaining high signal intensity. This is achieved by sampling noise within the earshell of the headset with a small microphone. This noise is then inverted in phase and reintroduced into the shell, reducing the noise levels by destructive interference (Casali and Berger 1999). This has been shown to be an effective method of reducing noise levels at the ear of aircrew to acceptable levels. This reduction of noise improves speech discrimination, which is degraded by noise. This also helps people with sensorineural hearing loss due to other causes to maintain their ability to function within this environment.

Conductive hearing loss

Conductive hearing loss is often amenable to treatment, in contrast to many causes of sensorineural hearing loss.

Figure 47.3 shows an audiogram of conductive hearing loss, demonstrating the loss of air conduction thresholds with preservation of bone conduction thresholds. Treatments vary from simple to increasingly complicated, depending on the cause of the conductive hearing loss. In simple terms, there are five possible mechanical defects that contribute to conductive hearing loss:

- *Obstruction of the external ear canal:* this is caused most commonly by wax or debris due to otitis externa. Less common causes are foreign bodies within the ear canal and abnormalities of development. Rarer lesions in the ear canal include tumours.
- *Perforation of the ear drum:* depending on the size and position of the perforation, this can, to a lesser or greater extent, affect transmission of sound through the middle ear to the cochlea.
- *Discontinuity of the ossicular chain:* this can be caused by chronic infective processes, chronic inflammatory processes and trauma.
- *Fixation of the ossicular chain:* this can be secondary to infection or other inflammatory processes or otosclerosis, in which there is fixation of the footplate of the stapes within the oval window.
- *Eustachian tube abnormalities:* this leads to pressure changes within the middle ear cleft, which can lead to secretory otitis media or other chronic middle ear diseases.

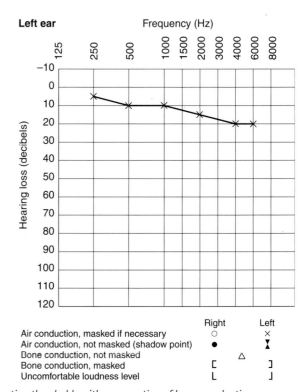

Figure 47.3 *Conductive hearing loss, demonstrating the loss of air-conduction thresholds with preservation of bone-conduction thresholds.*

MANAGEMENT OF CONDUCTIVE HEARING LOSS

Management of conductive hearing loss depends on the underlying condition. External ear canal obstruction is usually dealt with simply. Syringing the ears is essentially a safe technique when performed by appropriately trained personnel. In more difficult cases, the obstruction can be cleared with the use of an operating microscope.

Chronic otitis externa may require long-term medical or, rarely, surgical management.

Most perforations of the tympanic membrane will resolve spontaneously. Persistent defects in the tympanic membrane are normally repaired to prevent recurrent episodes of otitis media and possibly to improve hearing. This requires an operation known as a myringoplasty, which has a high success rate at closing the perforation (Kotecha *et al.* 1999). Following this type of surgery, we usually require that the patient does not fly until it is demonstrated that the tympanic membrane is healed and the Eustachian tube function has returned to normal.

Discontinuity of the ossicular chain and fixation of the ossicular chain require tympanotomy both for diagnosis and for surgical correction. It is possible sometimes to reconstruct the ossicular chain with prosthetic ossicles. In otosclerosis, the diagnosis is made at surgery; if there is fixation of the stapes footplate, then a stapedectomy can produce good improvement in hearing. The nature of the operation requires a fenestration to be made in the stapes footplate, which is then closed with the prosthesis and tissue graft. In aircrew, we would favour a stapedotomy fine fenestra technique with vein graft. There remains a risk of recurrent perilymph fistula. This risk is minimized by the use of vein graft to close the fenestration. The risk is greater for people exposed to rough pressure changes, such as fast-jet pilots (Thiringer and Arriaga 1998). In general, we would advise against such surgery in aircrew as long as reasonable speech discrimination is achieved through the headset.

Persistent secretory otitis media can be managed by myringotomy and aspiration of the effusion and insertion of ventilation tube into the tympanic membrane in order to allow aeration of the middle ear while improvement in Eustachian tube function is awaited.

Chronic middle-ear disease spreading from the middle ear into the mastoid segment may require mastoidectomy. The risk with this surgery is that there may be deterioration in hearing; there may also be some effect on vestibular function. Old-fashioned modified radical mastoidectomy procedures used to leave large mastoid cavities, which could result in the patient requiring frequent attention with discharge from the ear. However, new techniques such as small-cavity mastoidectomy, combined-approach tympanoplasty and mastoid-obliteration techniques have improved the outcome for patients requiring mastoidectomy (Black 1998). Following such surgery, careful con-

sideration must be given to the ability to perform flying duties. Individuals with a history of chronic middle-ear disease requiring such surgery can be at greater risk of problems in Eustachian tube function. Full assessment is required in the light of the type of flying duties required.

VERTIGO

Vertigo consists of an illusion of movement when the person believes, falsely, that he or she, or the environment, is moving.

Balance is obtained by use of sensory information from the eyes, proprioceptive receptors and vestibular labyrinth. This information is coordinated within the central nervous system, and there is subsequent motor output to the musculoskeletal system. Vertigo occurs when information from the vestibular sources conflicts with information from the other sensory systems. Vertigo is always a symptom of vestibular defect. The defect may lie within the peripheral labyrinth or within its central connections, the brainstem, cerebellum or temporal lobe cortex.

The causes of vertigo can be central, peripheral or due to external influences. External influences on the vestibular system include drugs, anaemia, hypoglycaemia, hypotension, viral infection, syphilis and middle-ear disease. The causes of central vertigo include multiple sclerosis, tumours, infarcts and cerebral abscesses. The main peripheral labyrinthine disorders include benign paroxysmal positional vertigo, sudden vestibular failure, Ménière's disease and vascular lesions.

Benign paroxysmal positional vertigo

This is the most common cause of vertigo. It is provoked by movements of the head. The vertigo lasts a few seconds. The cause is thought to be due to the detachment of calcium carbonate crystals from the otoconia within the posterior semicircular canal, which may be caused by injury, viral infection or ageing.

Particle-repositioning manoeuvres in order to try to expel the loose otoconia from the posterior semicircular canal have shown remarkable effectiveness (Epley 1992). Benign paroxysmal positional vertigo usually has a satisfactory outcome and, with resolution, most people will be fit to fly.

Sudden vestibular failure

This occurs when there is sudden hypofunction of one labyrinth. This generally causes severe vertigo, usually lasting over 24 hours, with gradual improvement over subsequent days. The common causes are head injury, viral infection, arterial occlusion and diabetic neuropathy. Presumed virally induced sudden vestibular failure is often called labyrinthitis.

Sudden vestibular failure usually improves as a result of central compensation. This central compensation is aided by the graded vestibular rehabilitation exercises involving head and eye movements, such as Cawthorne–Cooksey exercises (Dix 1979). Sudden vestibular failure usually recovers with good restoration of balance. Problems can still occur in situations where decompensation occurs, such as being tired, stressed or otherwise ill. Eventually, these problems seem to diminish and the patient may be fit for flying duties.

Ménière's disease

This is a disease of unknown aetiology consisting of a triad of symptoms of vertigo, hearing loss and tinnitus. There is usually also the associated symptom of fullness within the affected ear. The condition presents with exacerbations and remissions. The vertigo is usually severe, lasting for several hours. Associated with this, there is hearing loss and an increase in tinnitus. With resolution, the hearing may recover in between attacks. Over time, however, the hearing deteriorates and the hearing loss becomes perma-

nent. The audiometric pattern of hearing loss is typically loss of the lower frequency hearing (Figure 47.4).

Ménière's disease is thought to be a disorder of rise in pressure of the endolymph, probably because of an abnormality of the endolymphatic sac. Conservative treatment includes the use of bendrofluazide, a low-salt diet and betahistine. Surgical approaches to the management of Ménière's disease include endolymphatic-sac decompression and vestibular neuronectomy. Other treatments include chemical and surgical labyrinthectomies. The disease is a somewhat unpredictable condition. It may be possible for some patients with well-controlled symptoms to return to flying duties with a competent co-pilot (Gyot 1996; Johnson 1990). However, full assessment of vestibular function should be undertaken before returning to flying duties. Ménière's disease also affects hearing, and attention must be given to any hearing loss that occurs.

REFERENCES

Ashton DH, Watson LA. The use of tympanometry in predicting otitic barotrauma. *Aviation, Space, and Environmental Medicine* 1999; **61**: 763.

Black B. Mastoidectomy elimination; obliterate, reconstruct or ablate? *American Journal of Otology* 1998; **19**: 551–7.

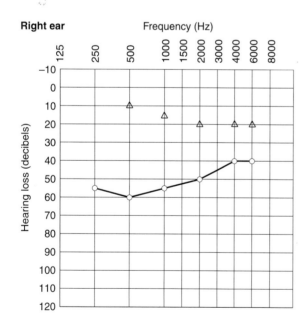

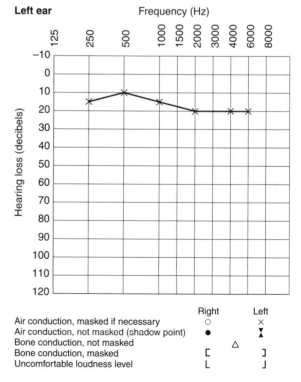

Figure 47.4 *Ménière's disease. The audiometric pattern of hearing loss is typically loss of lower-frequency hearing.*

Casali JG, Berger EH Technology advancements in hearing protection circa 1995: active noise reduction, frequency/amplitude-sensitivity, and uniform attenuation. *American Industrial Hygiene Association Journal* 1999; **57**: 175–85.

Dickson ED, King P. Results of treatment of otitic and sinus barotrauma. *Journal of Aviation Medicine* 1956; **27**: 92–9.

Dix MR. The rationale and technique of head exercises in the treatment of vertigo. *Acta Oto-Rhino-Laryngologica Belgica* 1979; **33**: 370–84.

Epley JM. The canalith repositioning procedure for treatment of benign paroxysmal positional vertigo. *Otolaryngology, Head and Neck Surgery* 1992; **107**: 399–404.

Farmer JC. Eustachian tube function: physiology and its role in otitis media. *Annals of Otology, Rhinology and Laryngology* 1985; **94** (suppl. 120): 1–6.

Goto F, Ogawa K, Kunihiro T, *et al.* Perilymph fistulas: 45 case analyses. *Auris, Nasus, Larynx* 2001; **28**: 29–33.

Gyot JP. Should a pilot suffering from Ménière's disease be grounded or lifted off to the moon? *Journal of Oto-Rhino-Laryngology* 1996; **58**: 304–5.

Johnson GP. Cases from the aerospace medicine residents teaching file. Case # 39. Ménière's disease. *Aviation, Space, and Environmental Medicine* 1990; **61**: 1160–62.

King PF. The Eustachian tube and its significance in flight. *Journal of Laryngology and Otology* 1979; **93**: 659–78.

Kotecha B, Fowler S, Topham J. Myringoplasty: a prospective audit study. *Clinical Otolaryngology* 1999; **24**: 126–9.

O'Reilly BJ, Lupa H, McRae A. The application of endoscopic sinus surgery to the treatment of recurrent sinus barotrauma. *Clinical Otolaryngology* 1996; **21**: 528–32.

Rood GM, James SH. Noise and communication. In: Ernsting JE, Nicholson AN, Rainford DJ (eds). *Aviation Medicine*, 3rd edn. London: Butterworth and Heinemann, 1999; pp. 489–521.

Thiringer JK, Arriaga MA. Stapedectomy in military aircrew. *Otolaryngology: Head and Neck Surgery* 1998; **118**: 9–14.

Tjernström O. Further studies on alternobaric vertigo. *Acta Otolaryngologica* 1974; **78**: 221–31.

48

Aviation psychiatry

GEOFFREY E. REID

INTRODUCTION

Although aviation psychiatry reflects the concerns of psychiatry as a whole, and almost any part of psychiatry has some relevance to aviation, it is the purpose of this chapter to concentrate on those aspects that are particularly significant to the occupational issues of aviation medicine. Psychiatric understanding and classification continue to develop at a rapid pace. This is not an appropriate place to provide a full lexicon of psychiatric syndromes as they are currently classified in either the *Diagnostic and Statistical Manual of Mental Disorders*, 4th edition (DSM-IV) or the *International Classification of Diseases*, 10th edition (ICD-10). This chapter provides a brief account of the current clinical situation in a number of diagnostic categories, with particular reference to the occupational aviation issues, and then discusses a number of specific aviation psychiatry topics. Those seeking a fuller account of psychiatric syndromes are referred to Gelder *et al.* (2000).

The scope of psychiatry is in a constant state of evolution. Although this is a truism for all medicine, the borders of psychiatry in particular may be expected to shift, as knowledge and understanding develop. Psychiatry deals rather more closely than other branches of medicine with issues that relate to our view of the intrinsic nature of humankind and the related moral and legal issues. In 1851, Samuel Cartwright described in the *New Orleans Medical and Surgical Journal* 'an unexplained tendency to run away in slaves', noting that the condition was 'practically confined to the Negro'. He called this disorder 'drapetomania'. Our contemporary understanding of such behaviour would, perhaps, take a different view of the context of the behaviour and the balance of social, psychological and bio-

logical factors involved. Disciplines that have relevance to psychiatry include anthropology, history, economics, sociology, psychology, ethnology, sociobiology and biology. All have their contribution to make to our understanding; each has their own particular virtues and limitations. In addition, human behaviour is influenced strongly by ideas, expectations, individual values and meanings. Those issues labelled as psychiatric disorder are but one part of this story. For those seeking a wider general understanding of human behaviour, a good starting point in the exploration of the human situation and human dilemmas will always be found in classic literature and drama.

It is important to distinguish between psychiatric symptoms and psychiatric syndromes. Mild anxiety symptoms, e.g. intrusive worrying thoughts, irritability, insomnia, physical and autonomic symptoms, are part of the common human experience from time to time, in response to stressful events, where they may be described as adjustment disorder. But they may also reflect the presence of one of the other disorders of anxiety (panic disorder with or without agoraphobia, social phobia, post-traumatic stress disorder (PTSD), generalized anxiety disorder, specific phobia) and may also occur in the context of another disorder. They may not necessarily be associated with the presence of any specific current external stressor. Symptoms are non-specific indicators that, as with medicine generally, should lead to a differential diagnosis.

It is also important to be clear on the difference between form and content. Although the content of a mental phenomenon may change in response to psychosocial and historical influences, the form remains a constant. Thus, the diagnosis of PTSD does not rely on the presence of specific thought content, but on the presence of a specific form of disturbance, with the characteristics of intrusive recollections, avoidance behaviour and chronic anxiety. The diagnosis rests on the identification of the form of the disorder, not on its specific content. In the past, delusionary experiences of outside influences, a symptom characteristic of schizophrenia, often had a religious content, but today they tend to feature television or computer images.

These distinctions are of major importance in an important feature of contemporary psychiatry: the development of systems for the classification of mental illnesses using operationalized criteria. There are two current systems: the ICD from the World Health Organization (WHO) and the DSM of the American Psychiatric Association. Although there are significant and important differences in detail, these systems are in broad agreement. ICD-10 was published in 1993 and DSM-IV in 1994. At the time of writing, DSM-V will be published shortly, followed by ICD-11. The aim of these classification systems has been to foster a common language for psychiatry, to operationalize definitions and to provide a lexicon of psychiatric syndromes independent of aetiological theory. However, all classifications of mental disorder are temporary and incomplete, improving as knowledge progresses. Psychiatric diagnosis still remains at descriptive syndrome level, the classifications describing symptom clusters rather than being based on aetiology. ICD-10 is in general use in the UK and is used throughout this chapter. UK psychiatrists also make extensive use of DSM-IV, reflecting the dynamic nature of developing knowledge and understanding; where appropriate, this is also referred to in this chapter.

Much hope still lies in the use of positron-emission tomography (PET) and single-photon-emission tomography (SPET) for investigating the pathophysiology of psychiatric disorders and the action of psychotropic drugs. Using these techniques, monoaminergic, cholinergic, opioid and benzodiazepine receptors, regional cerebral blood flow, and glucose and oxygen metabolism can be measured in the living brain. However, these techniques have not yet provided a diagnostic test for the major psychiatric disorders.

OCCUPATIONAL PSYCHIATRY

Any occupational health system runs the risk that it will become identified more closely with the needs of the employer rather than the employee. Mental health issues are readily stigmatized; the identification and management of significant mental health problems is essential to any safety critical task. The credibility of occupational mental health depends on the perception of their effectiveness.

A seven-year retrospective review of 214 US Air Force (USAF) active aircrew admitted to psychiatric facilities showed that 64.5 per cent had returned to flying within two years of admission (Flynn 1996). More than half (56.5

per cent) of this cohort had been referred for alcohol-related problems. However, the study does indicate a good short-term occupational recovery in USAF aircrew following psychiatric hospitalization.

CLINICAL PSYCHIATRIC SYNDROMES

Adjustment disorders

OCCUPATIONAL RISKS

* Need to avoid the unnecessary and inappropriate use of antidepressant medication.

CLINICAL FEATURES

These disorders are states of subjective distress and emotional disturbance arising in the course of adaptation to a significant life event or life change. They lie between normal behaviour and the major psychiatric morbidities and constitute subthreshold disorders. Precipitating events may include the disruption of an individual's social network (bereavement, separation) or a major developmental transition or crisis. The manifestations are variable and may include low mood, anxiety and worrying thoughts, a feeling of inability to cope, plan ahead or continue in the present situation, and conduct problems. They correspond to what is often understood by the term 'stress', but the precipitating situations are not of the severity associated with the development of acute stress disorder, acute PTSD, post-traumatic stress reaction or PTSD.

There are limitations to the construct of stress. Holmes and Rahe (1967) constructed a table weighting relative stressors, but this and other life-event scales have been shown to be inconsistent in their ability to link stress and illness. The vulnerability of the individual (e.g. ego strengths, support system, underlying personality disorders, the timing and combination of stress(es), the issue of control over the stressor, the desirability of the event) is an important modulating factor in the impact of the stressor on the individual.

MANAGEMENT

A problem-solving approach to management is helpful, the aim being to guide the patient in the use of such techniques rather than to solve the patient's problems for them. Pharmacological management has little role other than in short-term symptom relief, e.g. in the short-term relief of insomnia. This may, however, be of substantial benefit and should be considered. Nonetheless, the use of benzodiazepines may impair the habituation of anxiety and situational learning, and they have potential for dependence. The Royal College of Psychiatrists and the Royal College of

General Practitioners advise that benzodiazepines should not be prescribed for more than two weeks. The inappropriate use of antidepressants and other drugs should be avoided. Such medication is not compatible with flying duties.

OCCUPATIONAL DISPOSAL

Adjustment disorder usually has a good prognosis. Mild adjustment problems are probably compatible with the normal performance of routine flying duties, but aircrew with more severe or prolonged problems or involved in high-demand tasks should not fly until they have recovered. A case-by-case approach should be taken. Some aircrew may express concern that they have become a flight-safety hazard and request medical assistance in not flying. Such requests should be respected. A return to flying duties is generally to be expected.

Mood disorders

OCCUPATIONAL RISKS

- Boundaries between mood disorders and psychosocial distress (adjustment disorder).
- Use and safety of antidepressant medication.
- Risk of impaired performance of safety-critical tasks through poor performance and inattention.
- Cause of fear of flying.

CLINICAL FEATURES

Normal mood variation is related to sad or happy events. Depression and hypomania can be seen as extremes of these normal fluctuations in mood. However, clinical depression and mania are more than extremes of normal mood. They are syndromes in which, in addition to mood, there are disturbances in thought, psychomotor state, behaviour, motivation, physiology and psychosocial function.

Manic states often start as hypomania, characterized by heightened mood (euphoria), more and faster speech, quicker thought, brisker physical and mental activity levels, and more energy, together with a decreased need for sleep, irritability, perceptual acuity, paranoia, heightened sexuality and impulsivity. As the illness develops, it can progress to frank psychosis, with prominent paranoia and grandiose delusions. Mania can occur without any euphoric mood at all and may simply display an irritable quality. In fact, a common presentation of mania is a mixed episode, in which depressive mood predominates. These mixed states can be difficult to distinguish from pure agitated depression.

In depressive states mood is bleak, pessimistic and despairing. A deep sense of futility is often accompanied by the belief that the ability to experience pleasures is permanently gone. There is a slowing or decrease in almost all aspects of emotion and behaviour, including rate of thought and speech, energy, sexuality and the ability to experience pleasure. Basic physical activities are affected, such as eating, sleeping and grooming. Severity varies widely, ranging from mild physical and mental slowing to severe psychosis, with self-denigrating, profoundly negative delusions and hallucinations. Measurements of social behaviour and subjective state have shown that acute major depression is among the most disabling and distressing of medical disorders. The constant mental pain and the suicidal symptoms seriously affect the quality of life.

Unipolar depressive disorder is characterized by depressive episodes without any hypomanic or manic states. *Bipolar* disorder is characterized by manic or hypomanic states; the patient may be depressed, euthymic (normal in mood) or hypomanic/manic. Bipolar disorder differs from unipolar disorder by including manic states. Only one manic/hypomanic episode is required to diagnose bipolar rather than unipolar disorder. Bipolar disorder is conceptualized as a wide spectrum embracing all the milder forms of the disorder, ranging from cyclothymia and mild and brief hypomania, through hypomania, bipolar II disorder, and bipolar I disorder, to 'pure' mania.

There is an extended and continuing debate as to whether the depressive disorders are best thought of as comprising one or more distinct disorders. The dimensional view considers that there is one depressive disorder, varying essentially by severity. The binary view argues for two separate types, known previously as neurotic and endogenous depression. ICD-10 takes a dimensional view, describing depressive disorder as varying from mild to severe. DSM-IV has two principal 'stem' disorders, major depressive episode and dysthymia.

Biochemical understanding of depressive mechanisms has been associated predominantly with the monoamine neurotransmitters, noradrenaline (norepinephrine) and serotonin, with an occasional interest in the role of dopamine. It has been suggested that impaired function in these systems may exist before illness, producing a vulnerability to depressive illness when under stress. Such impaired function might have a genetic cause or be secondary to developmental events. Stressors may not only precipitate episodes but also increase such a pre-existent vulnerability, sensitizing individuals and making them more vulnerable to further episodes (kindling effect). The evidence for the involvement of serotonin in depressive illness is substantial, both from the antidepressant activity of highly selective serotonin-reuptake inhibitors (SSRIs) and from the results of neuroendocrine studies in depressed patients. It has been demonstrated that relapse of depressive illness can be produced by reducing the availability of serotonin in the brain. Similarly, depressive illness relapse can be produced by a reduction in the availability of nora-drenaline. More recently, a class of antidepressants known as serotonin- and noradrenaline-reuptake inhibitors (SNRIs) has appeared. All these drugs have proven antide-pressant activity, and the clinical choice of drug tends to depend on the side-effect profile.

It is essential that all patients thought to be suffering from any form of depressive disorder are assessed for the risk of suicide, employing direct questions on suicidal thoughts and intent and with a careful search for risk fac-tors (see Self-harm).

The development of a depressive illness is sometimes preceded by a period of symptomatology that may be indistinguishable from a generalized anxiety disorder, and aircrew may present during this time with flying-related anxiety. A psychiatric rule of thumb is that anyone pre-senting in middle age with anxiety symptoms, without a previous history of anxiety disorder and in the absence of a definite exceptional major stressor should be regarded as suffering from a depressive illness until proved otherwise. The aviation physician should also be aware of the 'smiling depressive' presenting with physical symptomatology, whose overt presentation may not suggest the presence of depressive illness but where further enquiry reveals the presence of significant depressed mood.

Most mood disorders have a course characterized by multiple recurrences; a minority manifest as a single episode or have a chronic course. In both bipolar disorder and unipolar depression, the time from the first to the sec-ond episode is, on average, much longer than that from the second to the third. This progressive shortening of cycles and free intervals then levels off.

Precipitating events play an important role in the onset of the first few episodes, but thereafter recurrence becomes more autonomous, with stressful events contributing less to the process. In bipolar illness, there is no difference in the quality of stressors precipitating depressive and manic episodes; the loss of a relative can induce either depression or hypomania. Single-episode bipolar disorders probably do not occur, and single-episode unipolar depression is observed in only 10–15 per cent of cases. A ten-year prospective study of 131 hospitalized bipolar patients found that most patients still had recurrences (Tohen *et al.* 1990). In a large representative study, unipolar depressive patients had strikingly lower recurrence rates than bipolar patients (Kessing *et al.* 1998).

MANAGEMENT

Clinical guidelines for the management of depression have been produced by the National Institute for Clinical Excellence (NICE 2004a). The ICD-10 classification of depression is used. Antidepressant medication is not rec-ommended for the initial treatment of mild depression. Guided self-help programmes based on cognitive-behav-ioural therapy (CBT), problem-solving therapy or brief CBT are recommended for mild/moderate depression. When antidepressant medication is required, SSRIs are recommended. For severe depression, a combination of an antidepressant and CBT is recommended. Antidepressants should be continued for at least six months following remission of depressive symptomatology, thereby greatly reducing the risk of relapse. Patients who have experienced two or more depressive episodes in the recent past are advised to continue antidepressant medication for two years. In view of the high recurrence rate, management must include the identification and resolution of any risk factors that are present.

Lithium and valproate are the drugs of first choice in the management of mania.

OCCUPATIONAL DISPOSAL

Aircrew with mood disorder are unfit to fly because of the cognitive difficulties, neurophysiological disturbances and the risk of suicide associated with the disorders. Following successful drug treatment and withdrawal of medication or completion of CBT, there should be a substantial moni-toring period of at least three months in order to guard against the risk of relapse before a return to flying. The high recurrence rate of mood disorders means that indi-vidual occupational psychiatrists may recommend a longer time off flying in the light of the particular history, experi-ence and conditions of employment. Patients requiring maintenance therapy are currently unfit to fly (but see Psychoactive medication and fitness to fly, p. 739). The very high recurrence rate with bipolar disorder together with the nature of the mood disorder itself makes a return to flying unlikely. The complex nature of mood disorders and the special requirements of aviation require that the decision regarding return to flying must be made by a psy-chiatrist with relevant occupational experience.

Self–harm, including attempted suicide and para–suicide

OCCUPATIONAL RISKS

- Risk of aircrew using aircraft to commit suicide.

CLINICAL FEATURES

Much self-harmful behaviour is impulsive and associated with psychosocial stressors. Sakinofsky *et al.* (1990) found that 46 per cent of 228 consecutive cases of deliberate self-harm or injury met DSM-III criteria for adjustment disor-der. There may be many motives, including even contradictory motives such as the hope of being rescued. Intentions may include attention-seeking or communica-tion of despair, appeal for help, tempting fate, a wish to escape, or a means for stress reduction. However, in about half of all suicides, a previous attempt is found in the person's history; prospectively, a history of previous attempts is one of the most powerful predictors of future non-fatal suicide attempts. Prospectively, suicide attempters have a high risk of committing suicide, and some 10–15 per cent eventually die through suicide. Suicide is a leading cause of premature death, especially among young adults. Sociodemographic risk factors associated with repetition are belonging to the age group of 25–49 years, being divorced, social isolation and unemployment. Psychosocial characteristics of repeaters include substance abuse, depression, hopelessness, powerlessness, personality disorders, unstable living conditions, living alone, criminal records, previous psychiatric treatment, and a history of stressful traumatic life events, including broken homes and family violence, especially physical and mental maltreatment by partners. Alcohol readily potentiates self-harmful behaviour through its disinhibiting effects. Fortunately, the use of aircraft to commit suicide is uncommon. A review of 1000 consecutive fatal aviation accidents (Cullen *et al.* 1997) found nine cases of alcohol intoxication and only three definite suicides not associated with intoxication. The risk factors associated with a high risk of suicide may be relatively uncommon within the aviation community.

MANAGEMENT

Self-harm is the subject of a clinical guideline from NICE (2004c).

OCCUPATIONAL DISPOSAL

All self-harmful behaviour must be taken seriously. Individuals with such behaviour should be unfit to fly until they have been assessed professionally, preferably by a psychiatrist with occupational experience.

Acute stress disorder

OCCUPATIONAL ISSUES

- Of military operational importance: combat stress reaction is a particular example of this disorder.
- Unable to function.

CLINICAL FEATURES

Acute stress disorder (ASD) is a transient reaction to exceptional physical or mental stress. The condition is polymorphic, but there is an initial stage of a 'daze', including narrowing of attention, inability to comprehend stimuli, and disorientation with subsequent anger, anxiety or low mood. In the military, the disturbance is managed in accord with the principles of proximity, immediacy and

expectancy (PIE). Affected personnel are managed in close proximity to their place of duty, as soon as possible after the onset of symptoms and with the expectation that they will return to their duties when recovered. Minimal formal psychiatric intervention is required. However, casualties with ASD are at risk of developing PTSD. Immediate intervention may reduce the long-term risk of PTSD. In a study during the Israel–Lebanon war, personnel managed by PIE had lower rates (40 per cent) of PTSD than personnel evacuated before management (70 per cent) (Solomon and Benbenishty 1986).

OCCUPATIONAL DISPOSAL

Military aircrew suffering from ASD have recovered, returned to duty and functioned effectively. However, such cases are at significant risk of developing PTSD and should be the subject of psychiatric review (see Operational aviation psychiatry, p. 739).

Post-traumatic stress disorder

OCCUPATIONAL RISKS

- Impaired performance of safety critical tasks through poor cognitive performance and inattention.

CLINICAL FEATURES

PTSD is a chronic, frequently disabling disorder that develops following exposure to a stressful event or situation of an exceptionally threatening or catastrophic nature. It is not a generic term for distress following an upsetting event, and it is not associated with 'normal' events such as divorce or a job loss. It is a common disorder in the general population, with estimated lifetime prevalence in the USA of 7.8 per cent (women 10.4 per cent, men five per cent) (Kessler *et al.* 1995). Its incidence and prevalence in military or civilian aircrew is unknown. Military personnel are, however, at particular risk for the disorder. The risk in the general US population of developing PTSD after a potentially traumatic event is 8.1 per cent in men and 20.4 per cent in women (Kessler *et al.* 1995).

There are three characteristic areas of symptomatology. The first consists of involuntary re-experiencing of the event, commonly as repetitive and intrusive images or other sensory impressions (e.g. smells), nightmares or flashbacks in which the event is re-experienced. Second, there is avoidance of any reminders of the event. Third, there are symptoms of chronic hyperarousal, such as hypervigilance, an exaggerated startle response, irritability, concentration difficulties and insomnia. Emotional numbing may be present, with the experience of an inability to have any feelings, a feeling of detachment from other people and amnesia for significant parts of the event. The disorder is often associated with depressive symptoms, conduct problems, substance misuse and marital disharmony; it may be through these associated features that the disorder is identified, the avoidance that is characteristic of the disorder often preventing its primary presentation.

The symptoms often develop immediately after an event (ASD, acute PTSD or post-traumatic stress reaction) but may be delayed. ASD is not a necessary precursor to PTSD.

Classic conditioning associates stimuli present at the time of a potentially traumatic event with anxiety and fear. Subsequently, stimuli (visual, auditory, olfactory, cognitive) resembling those that were present during the event trigger severe distress and avoidance. The disorder has been shown to be associated with hypothalamic–pituitary–adrenal (HPA) axis, neurochemical and hippocampal abnormalities. Sufferers show abnormally low levels of cortisol and may have an increased number of lymphocyte glucocorticoid receptors. The HPA axis produces large responses to further stressors. Several neurotransmitter systems may be dysregulated, and individuals with chronic PTSD may have smaller hippocampuses than controls. However, recent evidence suggests that the latter may be a vulnerability factor rather than a result of the precipitating experience.

Various vulnerability factors for PTSD have been identified (Ozer et al. 2003), including a previous personal or family history of anxiety or affective disorders, neuroticism, lower intelligence, female gender and a history of previous trauma. However, none of these is of sufficient predictive value to permit screening from high-risk occupations.

PTSD is only one of the many disorders that may be precipitated by a potentially traumatic event. Depressive disorders, specific phobias, adjustment disorders, neurological damage arising from injuries and psychotic disorder should all be considered. Comorbid diagnoses frequently exist.

PTSD is one of the differential diagnoses in fear of flying (p. 741).

MANAGEMENT

Clinical guidelines on the management of PTSD have been produced by NICE (2005).

The delivery of a brief, single-session psychological intervention shortly after the precipitating event ('debriefing') does not prevent the development of PTSD and should not be routine practice.

PTSD shows a substantial natural recovery rate, but in at least a third of individuals developing PTSD the disorder becomes chronic. However, many people settle within a short period of time, especially those with mild symptoms. In such cases, 'watchful waiting' with brief education, support and advice is an appropriate initial response. More severe PTSD symptomatology developing within the first three months of an event should be treated with trauma-

focused CBT. Chronic PTSD (after three months) should be similarly treated, with trauma-focused CBT or with eye-movement desensitization and reprocessing (EMDR). There are significant benefits from drug treatment with paroxetine, mirtazapine, amitriptyline and phenelzine. Only paroxetine has a current UK product licence for PTSD. However, drug treatment should not be used as the routine first-line treatment for PTSD in preference to CBT and is most useful as an adjunct therapy. Such drug treatment should be maintained for 12 months before gradual withdrawal.

The chances that PTSD will recover with appropriate treatment do not decrease with time elapsed from the precipitating event.

OCCUPATIONAL DISPOSAL

Aircrew diagnosed with PTSD should not fly. Following treatment and a good recovery, a return to flying can be expected. However, where the precipitating event involved flying, there may be a residual phobic anxiety for flying that may prevent a return to flying duties.

Agoraphobia with panic disorder

OCCUPATIONAL RISKS

- Severe and incapacitating form of anxiety.
- High risk of impaired performance of safety-critical tasks through poor cognitive performance and inattention.
- Cause of fear of flying.

CLINICAL FEATURES

Panic disorder draws its name from the god Pan. Pan was known for frightening animals and humans 'out of the blue'. The spontaneous 'out of the blue' and inappropriate character of panic attacks is the principal identifying characteristic of panic disorder and central to its recognition and diagnosis. Symptoms of panic attack include palpitations, pounding heart, tachycardia, sweating, trembling or shaking, shortness of breath or smothering, feeling of choking, chest pain or discomfort, nausea or abdominal distress, dizziness, unsteadiness, light-headedness, faintness, derealization or depersonalization, fear of losing control or going mad, fear of dying, paraesthesia, and chills or hot flushes. The disorder is distinct from situational or phobic anxiety.

Panic attacks are extremely frightening, and patients develop an anticipatory anxiety of having more attacks. A significant number of people with panic attacks go on to develop avoidance of situations that were associated with previous attacks. They particularly fear those situations where escape would be difficult or embarrassing, or where help might not be available. Most patients believe, mistakenly, that they will become incapacitated and incapable of taking care of themselves during a panic attack. Many go on to develop pervasive avoidance of a variety of situations. Factor analytical studies demonstrate that there is a cluster of situations associated with avoidance. These typically include public transportation (e.g. buses, trains, planes), riding in or driving a car, especially on heavily travelled roads, crowds (e.g. the cinema, a football match, large shopping centres), shopping (especially in supermarkets), particularly where one must stand in queues, and bridges, tunnels, elevators and other enclosed spaces (Burns and Thorpe 1977). Affected individuals fear situations where escape is difficult or impossible, e.g. airplanes, traffic jams on a bridge, dental appointments, etc. They do not fear the situation itself but rather reason that they will not be able to cope if the panic feelings occur while in that situation. There is a 'fear of the fear' (Goldstein and Chambless 1978).

In clinical samples, 75 per cent of patients who meet criteria for panic disorder also have associated significant agoraphobic avoidance. Some cognitive factors may differentiate those who develop agoraphobic avoidance. If patients believe the occurrence of a panic attack is evidence of a catastrophic medical problem such as a heart attack, then they are much more likely to develop agoraphobia (Thorpe and Burns 1983).

Agoraphobia may develop without a history of panic disorder. Current understanding is that these patients, although not meeting the full criteria for panic disorder, are otherwise very much like typical patients with panic disorder and agoraphobia, except that their anxiety attacks involve fewer symptoms. Some patients have only one or two symptoms, e.g. fear of loss of bladder or bowel control, tachycardia.

The dissociative experience of break-off (p. 742) can precipitate a panic attack and agoraphobic avoidance (fear of flying).

MANAGEMENT

Clinical guidelines for the management of panic disorder, with or without agoraphobia, have been produced by NICE (2004b). Psychological (CBT), pharmacological (SSRI) and combination treatments have been shown to be effective.

OCCUPATIONAL DISPOSAL

Panic disorder is one of the differential diagnoses of fear of flying (p. 742).

Obsessive–compulsive disorder

OCCUPATIONAL RISKS

- Impaired performance of safety-critical tasks through poor performance and inattention.

CLINICAL FEATURES

Obsessive–compulsive disorder (OCD) is a common, chronic, disabling disorder marked by obsessions and/or compulsions that are egodystonic. Obsessions are intrusive, repetitive thoughts that are unpleasant and produce anxiety but are recognized as being products of the person's own mind. Compulsions are repetitive goal-driven behaviours that have to be performed in order to prevent anxiety. Both are experienced as being irrational and are resisted, although resistance results in increasing anxiety. Resistance to the thoughts or behaviours diminishes with chronicity.

The differential diagnosis of OCD includes other anxiety disorders, schizophrenia, Tourette syndrome, autism, organic brain disease and anankastic personality disorder. Anankastic personality disorder is the lifelong presence of obsessional behavioural traits and ordered rigid, humourless and unspontaneous personality traits. Mild obsessional traits are not uncommon in professionals, including doctors and aircrew.

Genetic elements are present, with 35 per cent of first-degree relatives being affected and a higher monozygotic twin concordance rate.

MANAGEMENT

CBT and SSRI drugs are used. OCD is a chronic disorder. With treatment, significant improvement is seen in 20–30 per cent and moderate improvement in 40–50 per cent. Between 20 and 40 per cent become chronic.

OCCUPATIONAL DISPOSAL

A person with diagnosed OCD is unfit to fly. Fitness to return to flying must be assessed individually.

Personality disorder

OCCUPATIONAL RISKS

- Impaired performance of safety-critical tasks through poor performance and inattention.

CLINICAL FEATURES

Personality disorders are deeply ingrained and enduring behaviour patterns, manifesting themselves as inflexible responses to a broad range of personal and social situations (ICD-10). They are said to affect ten per cent of the general population. Medical practitioners should be aware of the great controversy surrounding this area of classification. They are divided into three clusters.

- *Cluster A:* paranoid, schizoid and schizotypal personality disorders.

- *Cluster B:* dissocial (antisocial), emotionally unstable (borderline) and histrionic personality disorders.
- *Cluster C:* anankastic (see above), anxious and dependent personality disorders.

OCCUPATIONAL DISPOSAL

An individual with a formal diagnosis of personality disorder would be unfit to fly.

Schizophrenia and other delusional disorders

OCCUPATIONAL RISKS

- Impaired performance of safety-critical tasks through poor performance and inattention.

CLINICAL FEATURES

The current definition of schizophrenia is a patchwork of features. Schizophrenia is characterized by delusions, hallucinations (thoughts being spoken aloud, voices arguing or discussing in the third person, or running a commentary on the patient's actions) and thought-alienation phenomena (thought withdrawal, insertion or broadcasting) deriving from abnormal mental processes. Genetic factors are the most important risk factor.

Schizoaffective disorder combines both schizophrenic and affective features.

Other delusional disorders are included within the schizophrenic spectrum and are characterized by a persistent delusional system but without the other features of schizophrenia.

Most patients with schizophrenia have a lifelong, remitting and relapsing course of illness, but there are no known ways of predicting this at initial onset. Schizoaffective disorder is considered to have a better prognosis than schizophrenia but a worse prognosis than affective disorder. Delusional disorders are often chronic.

OCCUPATIONAL DISPOSAL

An individual with a history of schizophrenia or other delusional disorder is unfit to fly.

Substance misuse

OCCUPATIONAL RISKS

- Impaired performance of safety-critical tasks through poor performance and inattention.

CLINICAL FEATURES

Humans have made use of psychotropic drugs since at least the Neolithic period – but generally not while flying. A

variety of disorders may be associated with the use of such substances, whether taken for recreational purposes or medically prescribed. They may be used harmfully, causing physical or mental damage, and they may cause the development of dependence syndrome and withdrawal states. Acute intoxication may result from the use of alcohol, opioids, cannabinoids, sedatives and hypnotics, cocaine, stimulants (including caffeine), hallucinogens, tobacco and volatile solvents. Delusional and schizophrenia-like symptoms may occur in association with or following psychoactive substance use or abuse. Psychoactive drugs reduce performance, disinhibit and impair judgement. The abuse of such substances while responsible for an aircraft cannot be compatible with air safety. A particular problem with lysergic acid diethylamide (LSD) is the phenomenon of flashbacks, in which the user experiences unpredictable recurrences of the original drug-induced state.

Acute intoxication due to the use of *alcohol* is characterized by disinhibition, argumentativeness, aggression, lability of mood, and impaired attention and judgement. When severe, it is accompanied by hypotension, hypothermia and depression of the gag reflex.

Acute intoxication due to *opioids* is characterized by apathy and sedation, disinhibition, psychomotor retardation, and impaired attention and judgement.

Acute intoxication due to *cannabinoids* is characterized by euphoria and disinhibition, anxiety or agitation, suspiciousness or paranoid ideation, temporal slowing, impaired judgement, impaired reaction time, auditory, visual or tactile illusions, and hallucinations with preserved orientation, depersonalization and derealization.

Acute intoxication due to *stimulants*, including caffeine is characterized by euphoria and a sensation of increased energy, hypervigilance, grandiose beliefs or actions, abusiveness or aggression, lability of mood, repetitive stereotyped behaviours, auditory, visual or tactile illusions, hallucinations (usually with intact orientation) and paranoid ideation.

Harmful use of psychoactive substances requires clear evidence of physical or psychological harm, including impaired judgement or dysfunctional behaviour.

Dependence syndrome develops after repeated substance use and includes a strong desire to take the drug, difficulties in controlling its use, persisting in its use despite harmful consequences, a higher priority given to drug use than to other activities, increased tolerance and sometimes a physical withdrawal state.

Withdrawal states are described with features characteristic of the particular drug, but typically including marked anxiety. People with alcohol withdrawal show tremor of the tongue, eyelids or outstretched hands, sweating, nausea, tachycardia, psychomotor agitation, headache, insomnia, transient visual, tactile or auditory hallucinations or illusions and grand mal convulsions.

Alcohol use

Alcohol is the world's favourite drug. The cause of both pleasure and destruction and therefore full of ambiguity, alcohol is a major contributor to disease, disability and premature mortality. The prevalence of alcohol problems varies markedly across different cultural and social settings. Certain environmental conditions appear to facilitate their development, while others seem to minimize them. The past 25 years have seen the development of an extensive literature on the effects of alcohol-control measures. In the UK, hazardous drinking is considered to start at 21 units/week for men and 16 units/week for women. In Canada, the upper limit for moderate drinking is estimated at 14 and 12 units/week, respectively. In the USA, the equivalent guidelines are 14 and 7 drinks per week.

OCCUPATIONAL RISKS

The effects of alcohol on performance are well identified. Euphoria is evident with blood alcohol concentration (BAC) of 25 mg%, lack of coordination occurs at 50–100 mg%, unsteadiness at 100–200 mg% and stupor at 200–400 mg%, with subsequent respiratory depression and death. Billings et al. (1972) demonstrated impairment of a pilot's ability to fly a single-engined, high-winged, piston aircraft down a glide slope with BACs from 40 mg% upwards. Alcohol reduces processing capacity, disrupting the ability to divide attention between competing tasks, the secondary task suffering more than the primary. The degree of impairment increases with the complexity or difficulty of the task. Moreover, the detrimental effects persist after the drug has been eliminated from the blood stream. Yesavage and Leirer (1986) demonstrated impaired performance on complex tasks in a simulator 14 hours after drinking enough alcohol to attain a BAC of 100 mg%. Other work has suggested individual differences in the susceptibility to impairment. Age or gender effects have not been demonstrated conclusively. An abnormality of vestibular function (positional alcohol nystagmus, PAN) has been demonstrated up to 34 hours after alcohol ingestion and, under the effects of +3 G, at up to 48 hours post-ingestion of only three units of alcohol (Oosterveld 1970). The symptoms of a hangover are worse when almost all ethanol and its metabolite acetaldehyde have been cleared, and peak blood ethanol or acetaldehyde levels are not related to the severity of hangover (Chapman 1970). It is thought that complex organic molecules such as polyphenols, higher alcohols including methanol, and histamine, collectively known as congeners, are the main causes of this phenomenon. Methanol is metabolized to formaldehyde and formic acid. The types of drink (brandy, red wine, rum, whisky) containing higher quantities of methanol are associated with more severe hangovers, the time course of methanol metabolism corresponded to the appearance of symptoms, and a small dose of ethanol ('hair of the dog', blocking the formation of formaldehyde and formic acid) may provide an effective treatment. Pathophysiological disturbances following alcohol ingestion include dehydration, metabolic acidosis, hypoglycaemia, disturbed prostaglandin synthesis, abnormal secretion of vasopressin, cortisol, aldosterone, renin and testosterone; cardiac output is increased, and vasodilation and tachycardia occur. Rehydration and anti-inflammatory analgesics are useful for the subjective discomforts, particularly if taken before bedtime (Bargiota and Corrall 1997). The bloody Mary, invented during the 'Roaring Twenties', is still said to be the ideal morning-after pick-me-up.

CLINICAL FEATURES

Excessive use of alcohol may exacerbate an existing psychiatric disorder. Individuals may drink as a result of psychiatric disorder. However, alcohol misuse itself is often the primary condition and the main cause of any psychological disturbance. Patients drinking excessively may present with depressive symptomatology, e.g. dysphoria, agitation, apathy, suicidal ideation, loss of libido, loss of appetite and weight loss. Although it induces sleep, alcohol also decreases both rapid-eye-movement (REM) sleep and slow-wave sleep. Rebound of REM sleep may follow withdrawal after regular use, with vivid dreams, nightmares and frequent awakenings. Alcohol, being metabolized rapidly, may result in rebound occurring early in the morning, giving rise to early-morning awakening. There may be diagnostic confusion with depressive disorders. Clinical experience has resulted in the advice that clinical treatment for a possible comorbid affective disorder should generally be withheld until the patient has been abstinent for four to six weeks.

The many physical consequences of excessive alcohol consumption include alcoholic liver disease, acute and chronic pancreatitis, gastritis, peptic ulcer, and cancers of the oral cavity, pharynx, oesophagus, liver, rectum and colon. Alcohol is an established risk factor for hypertension, and 30 per cent of 'essential' hypertension may be related to alcohol abuse. Gout, osteoporosis, avascular necrosis, gonadal atrophy, hypoglycaemia, and acute and chronic myopathy and cardiomyopathy are also associated.

The CAGE questionnaire (Ewing 1984) is a useful instrument for the identification and measurement of the harmful use of alcohol. The CAGE questionnaire asks four questions:

- Have you tried or felt you should *cut* down your drinking?
- Have you ever felt *annoyed* by criticisms about your drinking?
- Have you ever felt bad or *guilty* about your drinking?
- Have you had a drink first thing in the morning ('*eye*-opener') or before lunch to steady your nerves or get rid of a hangover?

Any single positive answer is significant. Two positive answers should raise serious suspicions of problem drinking.

Biological indicators include the gamma-glutamyltransferase (GGT). Raised GGT is one of the most sensitive tests for early liver disorder. Although the precise mechanism for its elevation is unknown, it is assumed to reflect enzyme induction. It can be elevated by factors other than alcohol, including other drugs (anticonvulsants, steroids, allopurinol), diabetes, and pancreatic, cardiac and renal disorders. Abnormalities of GGT begin to return to normal within two days of alcohol abstinence. A raised mixed corpuscular volume (MCV) is also common in excessive alcohol drinkers, and the combination of a raised MCV with raised GGT results in sensitivity of excessive alcohol consumption of 80 per cent. The MCV takes several weeks to begin to return to normal following abstention. The use of such biochemical and haematological measures is, however, not enough by itself to determine the presence of excessive alcohol use, and they should always be combined with the use of questionnaires, a full history and a clinical examination. Where diagnostic uncertainty exists, a trial of alcohol abstention will help to establish the role of alcohol.

MANAGEMENT

There is a positive relationship between per-capita alcohol consumption and alcohol misuse (Kendell 1979). Edwards *et al.* (1994) suggested a separation of alcohol dependence from the other alcohol-related physical, social and psychological problems, emphasizing that a mix of policies was necessary. Contextual policy aims to concentrate on specific hazardous situations, e.g. drinking-and-driving policy, where initiatives have been highly effective. In the field of aviation, Cook (1997a) has described two fundamental principles:

- Aircrew should not fly unless their BAC is 'zero', i.e. < 5 mg%.
- Post-alcohol impairment (PAI) suggests that aircrew should not fly until well after the BAC has reduced to zero.

Regulations reflect these principles either by imposing a legal limit for BAC or a safe interval between drinking and flying ('bottle-to-throttle time') or by prohibiting flying while 'under the influence' of alcohol. The US Federal Aviation Authority (FAA) imposes an eight-hour rule. The civil aviation regulations require that aircrew shall not consume alcohol less than eight hours before the specified reporting time for flight duty or the commencement of standby and shall not commence a flight duty period with a blood alcohol level in excess of 20 mg%. Cook (1997a) provides a full review of these issues.

There are three particular aspects of the management of alcohol misuse: withdrawal may need inpatient admission for detoxification; relapse prevention; and the management of any comorbid psychiatric disorder. Benzodiazepines are the main drug for the management of withdrawal; longer-acting drugs, e.g. diazepam, are preferred. Research into the duration and intensity of treatment aimed at relapse prevention continues to favour early recognition and brief, educative and motivational management. For more severely affected people, other treatments may be required.

Royal Air Force (RAF) aircrew identified as misusing alcohol are managed in accord with the RAF's alcohol policy, which integrates the medical and disciplinary aspects of alcohol misuse. Civil Aviation Authority (CAA) regulations state that alcohol dependence should be diagnosed if the individual's consumption regularly exceeds the 'amount culturally permitted'. Such an individual is to be assessed as medically unfit.

OCCUPATIONAL DISPOSAL

The return to flying duties of RAF aircrew is dependent upon compliance with the requirements of the policy, which applies to all RAF service personnel equally. Resumption of flying status under the CAA is permitted only after a course of treatment and complete abstention has been achieved, and only if the prognosis for continuing abstinence is good. Recertification at an earlier point for multi-pilot operations (class 1 operational multi-crew limitation, OML) or safety pilot restrictions (class 2 operational safety pilot limitation, OSL) may be considered providing that there is a minimum of four weeks' inpatient treatment, review by an approved psychiatric specialist, ongoing review including blood testing, and peer reports for a period of three years. Following discharge from inpatient treatment, there should be immediate review with the aeromedical section of the authority. Further review is undertaken at two, four, six and 12 weeks following discharge. If abstention is secure, then the pilot may be allowed to resume his or her flying role, but only in a multi-crew role. There is a requirement for continued attendance at Alcoholics Anonymous or an equivalent organization, and a peer on the same aircraft fleet is required to supervise and report to the relevant authority. Medical follow-up is continued at three-monthly intervals for a recommended period of three years. Multi-pilot or safety pilot restrictions may be reviewed after 18 months from recertification. Relapse may lead to permanent withdrawal of the aviation licence.

A full review of the issues of alcohol in aviation is provided by Cook (1997b).

Caffeinism

Aircrew consume prodigious quantities of coffee. The symptoms of caffeinism can include feelings of anxiety and nervousness, initial insomnia, restlessness, irritability, diuresis, tremulousness, palpitations and cardiac arrhythmias. Caffeinism can aggravate anxiety disorders.

Transsexualism

OCCUPATIONAL RISKS

The transition from one sexual identity to another is a process with considerable demands. Individuals are at risk of adjustment disorder.

CLINICAL FEATURES

Diagnostic criteria for gender identity disorder include a stated desire to be the other sex, a desire to live and be treated as the other sex, or the conviction that the person has the typical feelings and reactions of the other sex. The condition is not associated with chromosomal abnormalities or a physically intersexed condition. Findings from the Netherlands implicate the brain bed nucleus of the stria terminalis. In a series of six male transsexuals studied at post-mortem, the size of the nucleus was comparable to that of typical females and not males. It is believed that the nucleus size may be affected prenatally by sex-hormone levels. The behavioural phenomena of transsexualism are ancient. It has been recorded for centuries and in a broad range for cultures. Before recognition of transsexualism as a disorder deserving medical and psychiatric attention, many patients self-mutilated or committed suicide out of despair. The prevalence of gender-identity disorder in adults has been estimated at one in 10 000 males and one in 30 000 females.

MANAGEMENT

The Harry Benjamin International Gender Dysphoria Association (2001), the professional body dedicated to the study and treatment of transsexualism, has been setting an extensive series of requirements for evaluation and treatment of gender-identity disordered people. The purpose of these requirements is to ensure that transsexuals undergo comprehensive psychiatric evaluation and enter into an appropriate treatment programme. The programme includes, in addition to ongoing psychiatric or psychological monitoring, endocrine therapy and, depending on the outcome of a graduated trial period of cross-gender living, possibly sex reassignment surgical (SRS) procedures. The philosophy of treatment is to do reversible procedures before those that are irreversible. Thus, clothing change, name change and cross-gender role socialization should precede endocrine treatment. Genital surgical treatment for male patients includes penectomy, orchidectomy and creation of a neovagina. The neovagina may be created from penile skin, perhaps augmented by other skin, or

from a portion of large intestine. The cosmetic result is usually very good. Follow-up reports on operated transsexuals are generally quite favourable. Mate-Cole *et al.* (1990) reported on 40 male-to-female transsexuals undergoing surgery at Charing Cross Hospital, London. Patients were randomly assigned to two groups. Half of the patients were operated on in three months; the other half were kept on a waiting list for about two years. All patients completed a standardized assessment at acceptance for surgery and at the end of two years' follow-up. The group that received the earlier surgery showed significant improvement in a range of psychometric measures and maintained employment. The control group showed no improvement in psychological testing and deteriorated in employment.

OCCUPATIONAL DISPOSAL

The UK armed forces have a number of aircrew who have completed SRS successfully. On completion of the surgical procedure, they are fully fit to fly. Before completion of the procedures, they have been managed flexibly, being made unfit to fly as the developing circumstances required.

Eating disorders

OCCUPATIONAL ISSUES

Eating disorders may be associated with metabolic disturbances compromising physical health and placing aircrew at risk of incapacitation.

CLINICAL FEATURES

Anorexia nervosa and bulimia nervosa are protracted disorders that overlap in their clinical features.

MANAGEMENT

Clinical guidelines for the management of eating disorders have been produced by NICE (2004d).

OCCUPATIONAL DISPOSAL

The severity and impact of eating disorders vary widely. Aircrew developing an eating disorder must be the subject of individual assessment on fitness to fly.

SPECIFIC ISSUES IN AVIATION PSYCHIATRY

Selection to fly

Selection for flying training, selection for employment and fitness to fly once trained are separate issues requiring different criteria. RAF aircrew selection assesses both suitability for flying training and suitability for officer training. Use is made of psychometric aptitude tests, combined with an interview board for the assessment of personality factors. During the period between the two world wars, the RAF developed the sensorimotor apparatus 3 (SMA 3), requiring aircrew candidates to carry out coordinated movements of one arm and both legs while being distracted by visual or auditory stimuli that had to be cancelled using the other arm. Although this had been shown to provide a good indication of flying ability, the Air Ministry did not accept it. It was not until 1944 that the aircrew aptitude test battery, which included the SMA 3, was approved. Current psychometric tests, now computerized, continue to assess ability at complex sensorimotor tasks.

In 1971, a range of eight personality tests were trialled in RAF pilot selection. Of these, one, Eysenck's personality inventory (EPI), showed some promise. The RAF sample was found to be extraverted and with low scores on the neuroticism scale. Those more likely to succeed at flying training tended to have relatively lower neuroticism scores. These tests were subsequently trialled in army air corps candidates (Feggetter and Hammond 1976), achieving similar results, but not reaching statistical significance. Considerable interest was also shown in a Scandinavian psychometric test known as the defence mechanism test, purporting to identify abnormal psychological 'defence mechanisms'. Again, prospective studies did not demonstrate adequate validity and reliability (Cooper and Kline 1986; Kline 1987). The available evidence has not demonstrated adequate reliability and predictive value for such tests, and they are not routinely in service aircrew selection.

The use of psychological tests for selection for training or employment must always be evaluated adequately against specified criteria for reliability and predictive value.

The civil aviation requirements (JAR-FCL 3) for both class 1 and class 2 medical certificates state that the applicant shall have no established medical history or clinical diagnosis of any psychiatric disease or disability, condition or disorder, acute or chronic, congenital or acquired, that is likely to interfere with the safe exercise of the privileges of the licence. Any established condition including psychotic symptoms is disqualifying, and certification may be considered only if the original diagnosis can be shown to be inappropriate or inaccurate, or in the case of a single toxic episode. An established neurotic disorder disqualifies. An approved psychiatric specialist may consider certification after review and when all psychotropic medication has been stopped for at least three months. A single self-destructive act or repeated overt acts are disqualifying, certification being considered after full consideration of an individual case, and sometimes requiring psychological or psychiatric review. Alcohol, psychotropic drug or substance abuse, with or without dependency, is disqualifying. Certification may be considered after a period of two years' documented sobriety or freedom from drug use.

Fitness to fly

Normal behaviour in normal circumstances is associated with a significant risk of error. Errors may have disastrous consequences in the unforgiving environment of the air. Most psychiatric disorders, with their associated impairment of mental processes, increase this risk. There are only a few active psychiatric diagnoses that can be compatible with unrestricted flying. The issues have been considered above under the specific diagnoses.

Motivation to fly

There are considered to be two types of motivation: approach and avoidance. The social–cognitive theory of motivation considers that an individual's inclination to achieve specific goals depends on their feelings of self-efficacy. Self-efficacy is mediated by a person's beliefs or expectations about their ability to accomplish certain tasks successfully. Bandura (1997) postulates that these expectations determine whether a certain behaviour or performance will be attempted, the amount of effort the individual will contribute to the behaviour, and how long the behaviour will be sustained when obstacles are encountered. Bandura identifies four ways in which self-efficacy is learned and self-efficacy expectations are acquired: performance accomplishments, vicarious learning, verbal persuasion and physical/affective status. Behaviour, of course, is also a product of external controls and restraints, issues that are particularly pertinent in a military flying environment, where operational priorities and disciplinary controls ultimately may override individual motivation.

Flying has intrinsic rewards: the acquisition and performance of high-level skills, the social exclusiveness of the flying world, the social high esteem in which aircrew are held, and the high levels of physical health expected. The task itself has high levels of satisfaction in the successful performance of high-level sensorimotor skills, and there are emotional rewards, exemplified in the poem 'High Flight' ('Oh, I have slipped the surly bonds of earth/And danced the skies on laughter-silvered wings...'; Pilot Officer Gillespie Magee Jr, d. 11 December 1941).

Mastery and control are powerful reinforcers of behaviour. It is not unusual to hear aircrew describe having always wanted to fly. On direct questioning, many experienced aviators do describe their enjoyment of their sense of control in the air. There is also the sense of escape from more mundane concerns, a distancing from other, perhaps not so easily controllable issues. It is, for most, a highly enjoyable activity, and one that many of them relinquish reluctantly. However, other issues do intrude, and the factors motivating a young person may change when they are older. The motivation to fly is a dynamic drive, subject to change in the face of developmental and environmental factors. The cost–benefit ratio of a flying career may not have been assessed realistically, or new factors may change the assessment. A partner in a close relationship may, perhaps as a result of developmental or social changes, no longer be ready to accept the frequent absences from home commonly associated with the flying profession or the risks associated with military flying. An aviator's priorities and values may change and he or she may, for example, come to regret the associated absences from their family. These factors may result in the appearance of anxiety (usually non-clinical), a re-evaluation of the aviator's aims, a change in motivation to avoidance and a decision to leave flying. However, the person may find themselves unable to resolve conflicts between the domestic and other demands (perhaps financial) upon them and resolve their anxiety. An unresolved or unadmitted motivational issue is likely to confound attempts at treatment of any anxiety disorder that may develop, and it is important to evaluate the motivation to fly.

Psychoactive medication and fitness to fly

Any medication with significant psychoactive properties is not compatible with the performance of the safety-critical skills required for the flying environment. Recent years have seen controversy over the compatibility of antidepressant medication and flying. The advent of contemporary antidepressant drugs with fewer side effects has resulted in aircrew successfully recovering from depressive illness on medication that may have no demonstrable impairment of mental function. However, the contemporary drugs, although not having the profound general side effects of their tricyclic predecessors, do continue to have significant side effects, including the induction of hypomania and manic mood disorder. The potentially catastrophic nature of this precludes flying in the acute phase of treatment. Nonetheless, aircrew who have demonstrated long-term stability on maintenance treatment may become candidates for assessment by the regulatory authorities with a view to a return to limited flying duties.

The USAF has used stimulant drugs (amphetamines) to combat the effects of fatigue in aircrew. These were also used by astronauts during the Apollo spaceflights. A retrospective aircrew survey (Emonson and Vanderbeek 1995) suggested that over half the pilots who had used amphetamines considered them to have been beneficial or essential to operations, with very few reported problems. However, abusers of amphetamine are prone to accidents, because the drug produces excitation and grandiosity followed by excess fatigue and sleeplessness. A paranoid psychosis (amphetamine psychosis) may result from repeated moderate doses. Typical features of the psychosis include delusions of persecution, ideas of reference and feelings of omnipotence. The

inherent risks for misuse under operational pressures, the problems of accumulation of sleep debt and the capacity for catastrophic error would suggest that sleep-hygiene measures and the maintenance of an appropriate work–rest schedule are of greater long-term merit. It remains RAF policy to ensure adequate rest in aircrew through the use of a short-acting benzodiazepine with no residual effects (temazepam). The routine use of alcohol as a hypnotic is not to be recommended, in particular because of the development of tolerance. Similarly, care needs to be exercised in the use of temazepam, especially in high-stress environments. All anxiolytic medication has a high risk of the development of dependence, and its issue must be supervised closely.

RAF aircrew are not permitted to fly while taking any other psychoactive medication. In civil aviation, prescribed medication must be reviewed aeromedically before returning to flying duties (JAR-FCL 3.115). All other psychoactive substances are unacceptable.

Operational aviation psychiatry

Ethical issues and the pragmatic demands of operational imperatives particularly complicate psychiatric issues in wartime, where the occupational perspective can become paramount. The topic is perhaps best approached from the perspective of its history. Aviation psychiatry made its first appearance during the First World War, when J.L. Birley was put in charge of investigations into 'flying fatigue', only 13 years after Orville and Wilbur Wright's first successful powered, heavier-than-air flight on 17 December 1903. At first, the physical effects and demands of flight itself were thought to be the cause of the problems, but it was not long before it was realized that psychological factors were more important. The first textbook of aviation medicine was published in 1919. Oliver Gotch, physician at the RAF Central Hospital, stated: 'From the point of view of medical interest there is perhaps no more important subject than the study of the psychology of flying, in that the practical issues at stake are so great'. He considered that 'more cases of this nature than of any other present themselves in Air Force work'. In Birley's lecture 'The principles of medical science as applied to military aviation' to the Royal College of Physicians in 1920, he described the development of 'wind-up'. He considered that if unrecognized, this led to the affected individual becoming:

> ... irritable, unsociable, morose, losing his inspiring personality and adopting a black outlook on things in general. Although he feels tired, he is excitable and restless; unable to sit down to read or write, he must always be pottering about the aerodrome looking at the weather ... Sooner or later, he must give in.

'Wind-up' was recognized as an anxiety disorder. Its aetiology was held to lie in the gradual erosion, under the pressures of war, of those defence mechanisms developed by the individual to counter his or her natural instincts of self-preservation. Once developed fully, the individual's career as a war pilot was finished irrevocably. Treatment consisted of rest and recuperation; the results of mental therapy were disappointing. It was recognized that the disorder was 'dose-related'; through the introduction of 'short-shifts' the permanent wastage from this cause was reduced. Anderson (1919) reported that psychological disorder had developed in ten per cent of 600 pilots in squadrons under his care. Both Gotch and Birley emphasized the social consequences of the disorder. Gotch had described aeroneurosis developing in flying training and considered that it was infectious, commenting that 'one pupil who has given up flying [is] followed ... by 2 or 3 more in the same week'. He advised that once a pupil showed any signs of the disorder, they must be discharged from the air station as unfit for further flying. Birley stated that if individuals were allowed to remain once the disorder was definitely established, then 'the results might be disastrous' and 'could easily mar a squadron'.

Despite this recognition of the overwhelming importance of psychological stress in precipitating breakdown in aircrew, by the time of the Second World War the 'balance of opinion had been tilted back again by the physiological work done between the wars on oxygen lack and other factors specific to flying' (Reid 1979). The RAF medical training manuals of the time recognized that anxiety and depression would be common but implied that they would be observed chiefly in men who had been fatigued by a long period of operational duty. 'It soon became clear that many cases did not fit into this pattern' (Reid 1979) and the whole variety of anxiety disorders appeared.

During the Second World War, RAF bomber command casualties peaked in the winter of 1942–43, when heavy losses began to be sustained after the inception of daylight bombing operations. In the year ending February 1943, neuropsychiatrists saw 2919 cases of psychological disorder. Of these, 2200 were considered to have arisen mainly from flying duties (Symonds 1979). At that time, RAF bomber crews had no more than a ten per cent chance of surviving a full tour of 30 operations, and it was then that the phrase 'coffins or crackers' came into use. From that time onwards, the casualty rate receded.

A difficult issue during the Second World War was the management of men who had no previous history suggesting vulnerability to anxiety and who apparently had not been exposed to any special stress and yet who reported that they were 'unable to carry out their operational duties' (Reid 1979). It was thought that if such men were excused from operational duties but retained the privileges and prestige attached to flying status, then there was bound to be resentment among those who struggled successfully to control their own anxiety and fear and continued to face the perils of war. Balfour (1973), an under-secretary of

state for air, has described the perceived need for the category of 'lacking in moral fibre' (LMF). Poor morale was thought to be infectious, and speedy removal from the squadron was necessary, as perhaps also was dismissal from the service and enlistment in some other form of national service. The RAF medical branch was given the duty of stating whether there was medical reason for the man's behaviour. One in seven of the men referred for psychiatric assessment were determined to be not suffering from any psychiatric disorder but 'lacking in confidence' and referred to the executive.

Brandon (1996) has explored the issues of LMF. The first use of the term 'lacking in moral fibre' has been identified as being in 1940, in a letter outlining the procedures for identifying those 'whose conduct may cause them to forfeit the confidence of their Commanding Officer'. Men identified as showing evidence of physical or nervous illness were to be treated on the station. If the diagnosis was unclear, then they were to be transferred to not yet diagnosed neurosis (NYDN) centres, where a neuropsychiatric specialist was required to make the final diagnosis. If there was considered to be no evidence of psychiatric disorder, then the report eventually found its way to the secretary of state's office. Once confirmed, 'LMF' was stamped on the personal documents. Officers were cashiered, and non-commissioned officers (NCOs) were reduced to the lowest rank (aircraftsman, second class) and then either employed on menial duties or discharged. Once discharged, they were called up into the army or directed to work in the mines. There were criticisms of the policy at the time.

As noted above, the understanding of what constitutes a psychiatric case can be highly dependent on the context in which it occurs. In the combat situation, the population threshold for a diagnosable disorder shifts. Military aircrew receive extensive training in order to be able to perform their tasks under considerable pressure. Anxiety will be experienced by the majority of aircrew in a war environment. In war, it is the intent of both the ally and the foe to increase the stress continuously in pursuit of victory. A survey of 4500 US airmen with combat experience in 1944 showed that all but one per cent reported that they had experienced fear on at least some of their missions (Shaffer 1947). Gastrointestinal syndromes, low back pain, headaches, and exacerbations of pre-existing medical disorders are likely to be common. Despite this, the vast majority cope well and are considerably more resilient than might be expected. Reassurance and support from medical services in the field are appropriate, with the aim of maintaining the fighting force. Such reassurance should be credible, educative and specific, addressing both expressed and concealed fears (Kessel 1979). It should take into account the patient's assessment of the threat that they face. Fears that a more severe disturbance with loss of control may develop can be minimized by a simple explanation of the mechanisms involved in common anxiety symptoms, together with education on straightforward means of ameliorating their impact. Fears of more long-term problems, such as the development of PTSD, should be addressed. Again, such advice must be credible. Although it needs to be emphasized that the majority of individuals do not develop PTSD, it should not be denied that some individuals may develop problems. The means of avoiding such difficulties should be emphasized, including making use of peer support, supporting others and, perhaps most importantly, ensuring preparedness through training. It will be helpful to identify and address the common adjustment issues that may be experienced on the return home and to be able to identify the support that will be available post-operation. A supportive environment will do much to contain such difficulties and maintain morale. Traditionally, the medical officer can be a valuable source of informal personal support to the commander.

Aircrew developing an acute stress disorder or a severe adjustment disorder and who are no longer able to function should be managed as closely to their working environment as possible with regard to operational and medical conditions. They should be regarded as 'temporarily overwhelmed' and handled with the expectation that they will recover and return to their primary duties. They should not be isolated from their peers, who should be encouraged to visit as soon as is reasonable. Attention should be given to correcting risk factors (hydration, food, sleep, intercurrent illness), and they should be encouraged to talk. Explanation and reassurance should be given. Benzodiazepines and alcohol should be avoided in these circumstances, these drugs often having a disinhibiting effect. If sedation is necessary, a small dose of chlorpromazine (100 mg) can be given. The control of behaviour may require larger doses of chlorpromazine, this being preferred to haloperidol because of its sedative effect. Any persisting features suggestive of psychotic disorder should result in evacuation. The large majority of cases will be recovered within 72 hours and able to return to flying duty. Failure to recover fully should result in evacuation. Any doubts as to full recovery and fitness to return to flying duties should prompt a request for psychiatric assessment, preferably from a psychiatrist familiar with the requirements of the aviation environment. Other disorders that may be precipitated in such circumstances include brief reactive psychosis, self-mutilation, alcohol and other substance misuse, depression, catatonic reactions and dissociative reactions (e.g. amnesia, fugue states, conversion reactions).

Although it is hoped that in any future conflict, evacuated casualties would be accommodated within Service resources, the reduced availability of Service facilities may result in casualties, including aircrew, being cared for in the National Health Service (NHS). It is increasingly unusual in the general population for there to be any familiarity with service traditions and ways of life. Guidelines have been produced for civilian authorities on the psychiatric issues that might be encountered in the management of Service personnel (Brandon 1991). Casualties would have a strong service identity, strengthened by the common experience of combat. They would benefit from being kept together in the hospital and allowed to socialize together in appropriate facilities. Although opportunities for debriefing should be provided, helpers are advised not to probe too deeply but to limit intervention to dealing with war experiences and current problem-solving. Many casualties may express intense anger, guilt, resentment and derision. It will be helpful to have printed handouts available to casualties and their relatives, explaining the likely reactions. On arrival, casualties may still be suffering from acute stress disorder, showing fear, hyperarousal, and possibly hysterical symptoms such as amnesia or loss of motor or sensory function. There may be others who are withdrawn, apathetic or mute. Support, rest and reassurance are the appropriate initial steps, with minimal use of psychotropic drugs. Sedation should not be withheld, and benzodiazepines may be useful in these circumstances. However, some patients, particularly those troubled by flashbacks or nightmares, may find it easier to talk of their distress during the night, and over-sedation should be avoided. More detailed interventions should wait. Occasionally, an acute reactive psychosis may occur, requiring treatment with a major tranquillizer.

Fear of flying

Significant fear of flying is common in the general population, with a reported prevalence of 10–20 per cent (Agras et al. 1969; Fredrikson et al. 1996). Fear of flying is categorized as a simple phobia, but it is probably rather more complex than the present classification would suggest. In particular, fear of flying in experienced aircrew is thought to be a different issue from fear of flying in a novice or naive flyer.

Habituation is a decrease in the strength of a behavioural response that occurs when an initially novel eliciting stimulus is presented repeatedly. When an animal encounters a new stimulus, it first responds with a series of orienting reflexes. With repetition of the stimulus, if it is neither rewarding nor noxious, the animal reduces and ultimately suppresses its responses. Habituation is probably the most ubiquitous of all forms of learning. Through habituation, animals and humans learn to ignore stimuli that have lost novelty or meaning, thus freeing themselves to attend to stimuli that are important. An unusual sound in the presence of the family dog will make it respond by turning its head toward the sound. If the stimulus is given repeatedly and nothing either pleasant or unpleasant happens to the dog, it will soon cease to respond.

The process of habituation has been utilized in the therapeutic tactic known as systematic desensitization, used successfully in the treatment of specific phobias since the mid-1960s, and combining progressive relaxation and graduated exposure. The exposure component is thought to be responsible for the efficacy of systematic desensitization, while the decrease in autonomic arousal achieved by relaxation enhances habituation to the feared stimulus.

It is probable that habituation mechanisms function during an individual's early experiences of flying, resulting in the loss of anxiety. Habituation would be prevented by avoidance of flying, early adverse flying experiences or a high degree of initial arousal, giving rise to the symptom of fear of flying. There are likely to be a variety of aetiologies.

In vivo exposure is the most effective way of dealing with situational fear. Cognitive considerations have suggested that exposure is likely to be optimally effective when set up in a way that maximizes the extent to which patients are able to disconfirm their anxious cognitions. Exposure is now set up in a way that will maximize cognitive change.

Current management strategies for fear of flying in passengers utilize these principles, often incorporating educational measures to address the cognitive aspects. An international review of fear-of-flying programmes has been published (van Gerwen and Diekstra 2000). There are approximately 50 facilities with programmes for treating fear of flying in the western world. A flying phobia course is available for the UK Service population at the Department of Community Psychiatry, RAF Brize Norton.

In experienced fliers, habituation took place in training. The development of the symptom of fear of flying in this population should lead to a differential psychiatric diagnosis. Disorders to be considered would include adjustment disorder, acute stress disorder, PTSD, agoraphobia with panic disorder, agoraphobia without panic disorder and depressive illness. Management should be appropriate to the diagnosis (see individual diagnoses above). Motivational issues are important in resolving such disorders.

The dissociative phenomena of 'break-off' (see below) can precipitate a fear of flying.

Break-off

The phenomenon of break-off was first described by Clark and Graybiel (1957). They described 'sensations of separation from the ground, their environment, or from the aircraft while flying at high altitude in single seat jet aircraft'. In their survey, approximately one-third of the aircrew reported such feelings. Of these, two-thirds reported that the experience was pleasant and one-third expressed fear or anxiety in association with the phenomenon. The term 'break-off' derived from one of the aircrew who reported that he felt as if he had 'broken off from reality'. Sours

(1965) reported on the development of anxiety disorders and fear of flying in aircrew in association with the phenomenon. The phenomenon is an example of a dissociative state. Various similar experiences have been described, such as 'giant-hand' out-of-body experiences and the sensation of being 'balanced on a knife edge'. In the 'giant-hand' phenomenon, aircrew describe an experience of an inability to move the controls and 'as if a giant hand was thrusting the stick' (King 1962). The phenomena have been described in rotary-wing aircrew, and Durnford (1992) reported a prevalence of 16 per cent reporting an episode in a survey of 440 UK army air personnel. It may appear for the first time against a background of environmental and psychosocial stressors. Similar experiences have been described in other circumstances, e.g. in Inuit people ('kayak dizziness'), long-distance lorry drivers, snow-cat operators, and prisoners (Flinn 1965). Lyons and Simpson (1989), in a survey of 97 air personnel, reported that 15 had experienced the 'giant-hand' sensation. Durnford (1996) reported that 14 per cent of 299 US army rotary-wing aircrew members had experienced the 'giant hand'. The term 'break-off' is used in both the specific and generic senses.

UK military aircrew are made aware of the break-off phenomenon during their aviation medicine training. Civilian aircrew may not be aware of the phenomenon.

Aviation doctors need to be particularly aware of the phenomenon, which may be described by aircrew as developing a fear of heights.

Aircraft accidents

The idea that people carry within them the seeds of their own catastrophes is ancient (Connolly 1981) and has led to the concept of accident-proneness. Although in fact there is no evidence for there being accident-prone individuals, there is retrospective evidence of a temporary increase in the risk of accidental injury in association with clusters of life events, presumably in association with the development of adjustment issues.

Flying accidents are a cause of distress and illness. A retrospective study of 175 RAF aircrew members who had ejected suggested that 40 per cent had subsequent feelings of fear, anger, apprehension, disgust or altered motivation (Fowlie and Aveline 1985). The prevalence of PTSD in this group remains unknown. In the UK Kegworth air disaster, 79 per cent of 55 survivors (from a total of 79 survivors) met DSM-III-R criteria for psychiatric disorder; 50 per cent had PTSD (Gregg et al. 1996).

RAF medical policy requires the psychiatric assessment of aircrew following an accident before returning to flying duties. The station medical officer is required to take a full psychological history from anyone who has been involved in an aircraft accident before their return to duty. The station medical officer is assisted in the assessment by the use of screening instruments. This is a high-risk population in whom the use of screening instruments is justified. The RAF currently uses the Impact of Event Scale (Horowitz *et al.* 1979), with a score of 15 or more prompting psychiatric referral. A more recent version of the scale is the Impact of Event Scale – Revised (Weissman and Marmar 1997). Undue delay in returning to flying should be avoided; return to flying it should take place as soon as physical and psychiatric factors permit. RAF medical officers are required to take every opportunity to educate aircrew and the unit executive about the implications of stress-related conditions and the importance of their correct handling.

PTSD is not the only psychiatric syndrome that may be triggered by a potentially traumatic event. Differential diagnoses include depressive syndromes, specific phobias, adjustment disorders, personality change, neurological damage and psychotic syndromes. PTSD may exist comorbidly with any of these.

Lack of social support after a potentially traumatic event is associated with a greater risk of chronic PTSD (Ozer *et al.* 2003). The RAF has a long tradition of the 'aircrew wake', in which the squadron personnel gather in the bar and drink on a deceased colleague's bill, a tradition anecdotally acquired from the British cavalry. This has probable utility as a method of providing support to this particular population.

All aircrew should be provided with an assessment before returning to flying duties.

Psychiatric aeromedical evacuation

The earliest description of aeromedical psychiatric patients (US Army Air Corps, 1941) specified that psychiatric patients would not be transported by air except in great emergencies, and then only if there were sufficient attendants (Jones 1980). In 1944–45, 28 000 psychiatric patients were transported, 9000 being psychotic (Jones 1980). The experience showed that patients had to be properly classified and prepared, adequate equipment had to be available on board the aircraft, and properly trained personnel were essential. By 1970, the aeromedical transfer of psychiatric patients was a fairly standard procedure (Jones 1980).

Jones (1980) has emphasized that most psychiatric patients require only the good medical care and common courtesy needed by other ambulatory patients. However, from time to time, some psychiatric patients may behave either unpredictably or unacceptably, and some may not see themselves as ill. They may show resentment and anger. Such patients can be the cause of anxiety and anger both in the aircrew and in other patients and passengers. The fear of an unrestrained psychotic patient injuring others and perhaps endangering the whole aircraft is always an issue.

If reassured inadequately, then an aircraft captain may refuse to fly with such a patient on board.

The decision to move a psychiatric patient by air should be made carefully. The acutely ill psychiatric patient can be the cause of considerable anxiety in both relatives and medical staff, who may be unfamiliar with mental illness and motivated to move the patient quickly. However, flights can be delayed or diverted. It is highly desirable to ensure that the patient is stabilized before aeromedical evacuation.

Civilian airlines may require prior notification that a psychiatric patient is to be carried and have their own requirements. In the RAF, the movement of psychiatric patients by air is the responsibility of aeromedically trained registered mental nurses.

Assessment of the patient should pay particular attention to the risk of self-harm or violent uncontrolled behaviour. Pre-flight assessment should identify any self-harmful thoughts, and such a patient should be transported on a stretcher with sedation and restraint. The risk of self-harm is increased in single people, older people, alcohol-abusing people, people who live alone and people with a recent loss of someone close. Although women attempt suicide more often than men, men are more violent and successful in their suicidal behaviour. Violent behaviour might originate from a confusional state, psychosis or personality disorder. Any patient who has shown such behaviour before the flight should be evacuated on a stretcher, sedated and restrained.

Patients actively withdrawing from alcohol are unfit to travel except in an emergency. Early withdrawal symptoms include irritability, tremor, sleeplessness, poor appetite, an exaggerated startle response, agitation and restlessness; they may progress to delirium tremens and seizures.

Preparation of the patient for aeromedical evacuation is important. Flying is a cause of significant levels of anxiety in 20 per cent of the general population, and enquiry into previous flying experiences is essential. Flying can be associated with a number of unexpected sensations, including unusual noises, the expansion of gases in the abdomen and changes in middle-ear pressure. Moreover, there will be issues related to the new location that need to be addressed. A pre-flight briefing on these topics may identify possible problems and minimize others.

Although a restraint system is carried on board RAF aircraft roled for psychiatric aeromedical evacuation, its use is extremely unusual. Often, a stretcher flight harness together with the use of sedating medication provides sufficient restraint. The choice of medication must be made carefully. Psychoactive drugs that have not been used previously in the patient should be avoided. Drugs that oversedate will remove the patient's ability to care for themselves, requiring the attendant to be especially alert to the development of venous stasis with its risk of thrombophlebitis and the possibility of peripheral nerve palsies from prolonged maintenance of one position. The capacity of the patient to help themselves in the event of an emergency would be reduced. Patients nursed on a stretcher may develop expansion of trapped bowel gases, reducing respiratory tidal volume. Many of the drugs used in psychiatry (phenothiazines, tricyclic antidepressants and drugs used to counter the extrapyramidal side effects of the major tranquillizers) have anticholinergic effects. These may increase the risks of constipation, increased intestinal gases and acute urinary retention. Physostigmine 0.5–2 mg intramuscularly (IM) or intravenously (IV) will block anticholinergic effects and may be repeated every 30 minutes as necessary.

Chlorpromazine 50–200 mg IM is preferable to the less sedating drug haloperidol for pre-flight and flight sedation. It is preferable that any drugs given for the flight have been used on the patient before, such that the patient is familiar with their side effects, thus avoiding the risk of an idiosyncratic response in air. The most commonly used sedative drugs, however, are the benzodiazepines. Diazepam has a half-life of 20–50 hours; a dose of 5–10 mg orally should be given approximately one hour before the flight. Occasionally, these drugs may cause disinhibition.

Lithium carbonate is used widely in the management of manic–depressive disorder, recurrent depressive disorder and schizoaffective disorders. It is potentially toxic and must be maintained within narrowly defined plasma blood levels. Blood levels are, therefore, vulnerable to dehydration. Patients requiring lithium therapy preferably should be evacuated before it is commenced or the evacuation delayed until the patient has been stabilized on the drug. In-flight attention should be given to adequate fluid and electrolyte replacement. Indications of toxicity include confusion, clouding of consciousness, coma and fits.

Airshows and disaster planning

At the Ramstein Airshow, Germany, in August 1988, an aircraft of the Italian aerobatic display team crashed into the spectator enclosure, causing over 500 casualties. The risk of large numbers of casualties following such an accident is almost unequalled. In this particular accident, the Frecce Tricolori had just started their display when one aircraft struck the tail plane of another. This aircraft rolled out of control and hit the aircraft on its left. These two aircraft fell on to the airfield. One hit the ground immediately in front of the most densely packed area of the crowd before ploughing through the spectators. There was a fireball. Large pieces of the aircraft were hurled further into the crowd. Over the next 77 minutes, over 500 casualties were evacuated from the site using a 'scoop-and-run' concept.

Martin (1990) emphasizes the chaos and panic that ensued, the overwhelming numbers of casualties in widely dispersed groups, and the difficulties of applying concepts of triage in the presence of untrained helpers. Such a crowd is likely to have contained numbers of people, treated and untreated, suffering from major psychiatric disorders. A disaster will generate severely distressed people, people with acute stress disorders, people with acute exacerbation of pre-existing disorders, acute psychotic illness, and distraught parents and relatives of injured children and adults (Burkle 1996). Psychiatric casualties must be anticipated among the emergency services as well as among the survivors. Appropriate arrangements need to be made for the care of all these people and psychiatric services made available in sufficient numbers, preferably blended and co-located with the non-psychiatric caring agencies. The arrangements for the UK Royal International Air Tattoo include facilities for psychiatric care co-located with the acute medical and surgical facilities. The provision of debriefing is both unwarranted and impractical in the middle of a disaster, where the requirements of survival will take precedence, but there will be a requirement for support and emergency treatment. If not attended to, these issues are likely to impede the successful management of physically injured people.

Post-disaster, there is a risk of survivors developing PTSD, problems of grief among those bereaved by the disaster, and a risk of depressive disorder and other psychiatric illnesses. Lack of support in the aftermath of a disaster is associated with a greater risk of chronic PTSD (Ozer et al. 2003).

Conduct disorder in passengers

The UK CAA has reported on an analysis of disruptive passenger incidents reported from UK airlines in 2000–04. In the year to March 2004, there were 696 serious and significant incidents, against a background of 1.1 million passenger flights and about 110 million passengers. About one in every four million passengers was the cause of a serious disruptive incident. No case was reported in which disruptive passenger behaviour contributed to an aviation accident, although there were a number of incidents of violence against cabin crew. Similarly to previous years, 78 per cent of the incidents involved male passengers, People in the largest single age group, accounting for 35 per cent of the incidents, were in their thirties. About a third involved people travelling alone. Forty per cent of cases were of verbal abuse. Among the significant incidents, the most common misbehaviour was smoking in the toilet; violence was involved in 14 per cent of significant incidents. There were 28 serious incidents; many involved abuse of alcohol and varying degrees of violent, abusive or unacceptable behaviour.

In the majority of significant or serious incidents, a warning was delivered, which was thought to have been effective in 43 per cent of cases. In 20 cases, physical restraint was required. There were four occasions when the aircraft had to divert and seven when takeoff or taxi was aborted. In 80 incidents, the passengers were offloaded. Excessive consumption of alcohol (42 per cent of incidents) and smoking were the two main contributory factors, as in previous years.

Control of conduct disorder requires the training of cabin staff in de-escalation and restraint techniques. In 1998, British Airways was the first airline to introduce the 'yellow card', a warning card shown to abusive or disruptive passengers. The card spells out the legal position, the possibility of diversion and the consequent liabilities of the passenger.

REFERENCES

Agras WS, Sylvester D, Oliveau D. The epidemiology of common fears and phobias. *Comprehensive Psychiatry* 1969; **10**: 151–6.

Anderson HG. *Medical and Surgical Aspects of Aviation.* London: Oxford Medical Publications, 1919.

Balfour H. *Wings over Westminster.* London: Hutchinson, 1973.

Bandura A. *Self-Efficacy: The Exercise of Control.* New York: Freeman, 1997.

Bargiota A, Corrall RJM. Hangovers. *British Medical Journal* 1997; **314**: 2–3.

Billings CE, Wick RL, Gerke RJ, *et al.* The effects of alcohol on pilot performance during instrument flight. Federal Aviation Administration report no. FAA-AM-72-4. Washington, DC: Federal Aviation Administration, 1972.

Brandon S. The psychological aftermath of war. *British Medical Journal* 1991; **302**: 305–6.

Brandon S. LMF in Bomber Command 1939–45: diagnosis or denouncement? In: Freeman H, Berrios GE. *150 Years of British Psychiatry*, Vol. II. London: Athlone Press, 1996.

Burkle FM, Jr. Acute-phase mental health consequences of disasters: implications for triage and emergency medical services. *Annals of Emergency Medicine* 1996; **28**: 220–22.

Burns LE, Thorpe GL. The epidemiology of fears and phobias with particular reference to the national survey of agoraphobics. *Journal of International Medical Research* 1977; **5**: 1–7.

Chapman LF. Experimental induction of hangover. *Quarterly Journal of Studies of Alcohol Dependence* 1970; **5**: 67–85.

Clark B, Graybiel A. The break-off phenomenon: a feeling of separation from the earth experienced by pilots at high altitude. *Journal of Aviation Medicine* 1957; **28**: 121–6.

Connolly J. Accident proneness. *British Journal of Hospital Medicine* 1981; **26**: 470–81.

Cook CCH. Alcohol and aviation. *Addiction* 1997a; **92**: 539–55.

Cook CCH. Alcohol policy and aviation safety. *Addiction* 1997b; **92**: 793–804.

Cooper C, Kline P. An evaluation of the Defence Mechanism Test. *British Journal of Psychology* 1986; **77**: 19–31.

Cullen SA, Drysdale HC, Mayes RW. Role of medical factors in 1000 fatal aviation accidents: case note study. *British Medical Journal* 1997; **314**: 1592.

Durnford SJ. Disorientation and Flight Safety: A Survey of UK Army Aircrew. *AGARD Conference Proceedings* 1992; 532.

Durnford SJ. Spatial disorientation: a survey of US army rotary wing aircrew. US Army Aeromedical Research Laboratory report 96-16. Fort Rucker, AL: US Army Aeromedical Research Laboratory, 1996.

Edwards G, Anderson P, Babor TF, *et al. Alcohol Policy and the Public Good.* Oxford: Oxford University Press, 1994.

Emonson DL, Vanderbeek RD. The use of amphetamines in U.S. Air Force tactical operations during operation Desert Shield and Storm. *Aviation, Space, and Environmental Medicine* 1995; **66**: 260–63.

Ewing JA. Detecting alcoholism: the CAGE questionnaire. *Journal of the American Medical Association* 1984; **252**: 1905–7.

Feggetter SBG, Hammond DRF. The relationship between personality, flying aptitude and performance in rotary wing training. *Journal of Naval Science* 1976; **2**: 63–8.

Flinn DE. Functional states of altered awareness during flight. *Aerospace Medicine* 1965; **36**: 537–44.

Flynn CF, McGlohn S, Miles MPH. Occupational outcome in military aviators after psychiatric hospitalisation. *Aviation, Space, and Environmental Medicine* 1996; **67**: 8–13.

Fowlie DG, Aveline MO. The emotional consequences of ejection, rescue and rehabilitation in Royal Air Force aircrew. *British Journal of Psychiatry* 1985; **146**: 609–13.

Fredrikson M, Annas P, Fischer H, Wik G. Gender and age differences in the prevalence of specific fears and phobias. *Behaviour Research and Therapy* 1996; **34**: 33–9.

Gelder M, Lopez-Ibor JJ, Andreasen NC. *Oxford Textbook of Psychiatry.* Oxford: Oxford University Press, 2000.

Goldstein AJ, Chambless DL. A reanalysis of agoraphobia. *Behavioral Therapy* 1978; **9**: 47–59.

Gregg W, Medley L, Fowler-Dixon R, *et al.* Psychological consequences of the Kegworth air disaster. *British Journal of Psychiatry* 1996; **167**: 812–17.

Harry Benjamin International Gender Dysphoria Association. *Standards of Care*, 6th edn. Minneapolis: Harry Benjamin International Gender Dysphoria Association, 2001.

Holmes TH, Rahe RH. The social readjustment rating scale. *Journal of Psychosomatic Research* 1967; **11**: 213–18.

Horowitz MJ, Wilner N, Alvarez W. Impact of Event Scale: a measure of subjective stress. *Psychosomatic Medicine* 1979; **41**: 209–18.

Jones DR. Aeromedical transportation of psychiatric patients: historical review and present management. *Aviation, Space, and Environmental Medicine* 1980; **51**: 454–9.

Kendell RE. Alcoholism: a medical or political problem? *British Medical Journal* 1979; **1**: 367–71.

Kessel N. Hardiness and health: a prospective study. *Journal of Personal and Social Psychology* 1979; **42**: 168–77.

Kessing LV, Andersen PK, Mortensen PB, Bolwig TG. Recurrence in affective disorder. I. Case register study. *British Journal of Psychiatry* 1998; **172**: 23–8.

Kessler RC, Sonnega A, Bromet E, *et al.* Posttraumatic stress disorder in the National Comorbidity Survey. *Archives of General Psychiatry* 1995; **52**: 1048–60.

King PAH. A report of an incident of extreme spatial disorientation in flight. *Aeromedical Reports, Institute of Aviation Medicine, Royal Canadian Air Force, Toronto, Canada* 1962; **1**: 22–8.

Kline P. The scientific status of the DMT. *British Journal of Medical Psychology* 1987; **60**: 53–9.

Lyons TJ, Simpson CG. The giant hand phenomenon. *Aviation, Space, and Environmental Medicine* 1989; **60**: 64–6.

Martin TE. The Ramstein Airshow disaster. *Journal of the Royal Army Medical Corps* 1990; **136**: 19–26.

Mate-Cole C, Freschi M, Robin A. A controlled study of psychological and social change after surgical gender reassignment in selected male transsexuals. *British Journal of Psychiatry* 1990; **157**: 261–4.

NICE. *NICE Clinical Guideline 9: Eating Disorders.* London: National Institute for Clinical Excellence, 2004d.

NICE. *NICE Clinical Guideline 16: Self-harm.* London: National Institute for Clinical Excellence, 2004c.

NICE. *NICE Clinical Guideline 22: Anxiety.* London: National Institute for Clinical Excellence, 2004b.

NICE. *NICE Clinical Guideline 23: Depression.* London: National Institute for Clinical Excellence, 2004a.

NICE. *NICE Clinical Guideline 26: PTSD.* London: National Institute for Clinical Excellence, 2005.

Oosterveld WJ. Effect of gravity on positional alcohol nystagmus (PAN). *Aerospace Medicine* 1970; **41**: 557–60.

Ozer EJ, Best SR, Lipsey TL, *et al.* Predictors of posttraumatic stress disorder and symptoms in adults: a meta-analysis. *Psychological Bulletin* 2003; **129**: 52–73.

Reid DD. The historical background to wartime research in psychology and psychiatry in the Royal Air Force. In: Dearnley EJ, Warr PB (eds). *Aircrew Stress in Wartime Operations.* London: Academic Press, 1979.

Sakinofsky I, Roberts RS, Brown Y, *et al.* Problem resolution and repetition of para-suicide: a prospective study. *British Journal of Psychiatry* 1990; **156**: 395–9.

Shaffer L. Psychological studies of anxiety reaction to combat. USAAF Aviation Psychology report no. 14. Washington, DC: US Government Printing Office, 1947.

Solomon Z, Benbenishty R. The role of proximity, immediacy and expectancy in frontline treatment of combat stress reaction among Israelis in the Lebanon war. *American Journal of Psychiatry* 1986; **143**: 613–17.

Sours JA. The 'break-off phenomenon': a precipitant of anxiety in jet aviators. *Archives of General Psychiatry* 1965; **13**: 447–56.

Symonds CP. Clinical and statistical study of neurosis precipitated by flying duties. FPRC report 547. In: Dearnley EJ, Warr PB. *Aircrew Stress in Wartime Operations.* London: Academic Press, 1979.

Thorpe GL, Burns LE. *The agoraphobic syndrome.* New York: John Wiley & Sons, 1983.

Tohen M, Waternaux C, Tsuang MT. Outcome in mania: a 4-year prospective follow up of 75 patients utilizing survival analysis. *Archives of General Psychiatry* 1990; **47**: 1106–11.

Van Gerwen LJ, Diekstra RFW. Fear of flying treatment programs for passengers: an international review. *Aviation, Space, and Environmental Medicine* 2000; **71**: 430–37.

Weissman MM, Marmar CR. The Impact of Event Scale – revised. In: Wilson P, Keane TM (eds). *Assessing Psychological Trauma and PTSD.* New York: Guilford Press, 1997; pp. 399–411.

Yesavage JA, Leirer VO. Hangover effects on aircraft pilots 14 hours after alcohol ingestion: a preliminary report. *American Journal of Psychiatry* 1986; **143**: 1546–50.

49

Orthopaedics

IAN D. SARGEANT

INTRODUCTION

Aircrew may be expected to suffer from the full range of orthopaedic disorders seen in the general population of a similar age. In addition, their occupation may make them more vulnerable to certain types of back and neck injury. This chapter takes a systematic approach to those problems likely to be encountered in managing aircrew. The majority of patients suffering musculoskeletal symptoms will be managed successfully with analgesics and the passage of the time or the attention of physiotherapists, osteopaths or chiropractors. Orthopaedic surgeons might operate on the spine or limbs where there is reduced function due to congenital deformity or there is degenerative change, or to improve the expected outcome after trauma.

Muscle strength, range of joint movement and dexterity vary within the population, and there is a spectrum of performance that might be considered normal. These features, when considered in one person, also vary with age, training and practice.

DISABILITY

In order to understand the underlying principles of fitness assessment, it is important to understand the concept of disability and to appreciate its implications. Disability is defined variously and may be considered as the condition of suffering substantial long-term physical or mental impairment. The UK Disability Discrimination Act (DDA) 1995, Part I, gives statutory guidance on background information and matters that should be taken into account when determining questions relating to the definition of disability.

In the UK, employees of the armed forces and the police and people working on ships, hovercraft and aeroplanes were exempted from the provisions of the DDA 1995. However, the Disability Discrimination Act 1995 (Amendment) Regulations 2003, which came into force in the UK on 1 October 2004, gives these exempt groups protection under the act, although in the UK the armed forces are still exempt from the act (Department of Work and Pensions 2003).

An employer is discriminating against an employee or potential employee if the employer treats a disabled person less favourably than they treat or would treat others to whom that reason does not or would not apply, and there is no substantial justification for that decision that is relevant to the circumstances of the particular case. When performing medical assessments for potential and current aircrew employed in the UK, the provisions of the act should be remembered. Employees in other countries will be covered by regional variations in law.

A person suffering from a stiff little toe three years after a fracture will have a long-term restriction of joint movement, but if that person does not have substantial physical impairment in daily life then he or she is not disabled. A person suffering bilateral below-knee amputation might be considered to have substantial physical and long-term impairment, even if they are able to walk on artificial limbs without the help of sticks. With appropriate help, Douglas Bader was able to return to single-seat active combat flying during the Second World War. In the UK, an employer now has a duty to 'take such steps as it is reasonable' to reduce disadvantage to disabled workers that might be caused by 'provision, criterion or practice applied by or on behalf of an employer or any physical feature of premises occupied by the employer' (Department of Work and Pensions 2003).

For example, it is unlikely that to make major changes to a flight deck would be thought 'reasonable' modifications to be made by an employer to accommodate a pilot without the use of one arm, but it appears to be no longer justifiable in law to reject all aircrew applicants or remove the licence of qualified aircrew simply because they do not have a perfect health record. The applicant with the stiff little toe is likely to be fully fit for the tasks required or might need no more than minor reasonable adjustments, such as the provision of individually fitted shoes.

PRINCIPLES OF ASSESSING FITNESS

During assessment of the medical fitness of potential aircrew, the applicant should be functionally capable of sustained performance of the routine and emergency tasks required. There should be no underlying medical condition that is likely to cause current function to steadily and significantly deteriorate. If these conditions cannot be met, then there is substantial reason not to select the applicant.

The assessment of all musculoskeletal complaints can be made using the following broad headings (Magee 1992):

- *Mobility:* adequate joint mobility is required, allowing the pilot or member of aircrew to reach all areas of the working environment and perform an adequate lookout.
- *Strength:* the ability to demonstrate adequate and sustained limb strength without undue fatigability is required, allowing sustained force to be applied to controls in routine and emergency situations such as asymmetric engine failure or rapid operation of emergency escape systems.
- *Dexterity:* movements must be skilled and nimble and of adequate range and strength.
- *Tendency for sudden change in function:* the presence of conditions that might cause sudden and significant effects on physical performance, such as a tendency to shoulder dislocation or locking of the knee, must be assessed. If they are ongoing, untreated and likely to occur in the individual's working environment, and if the consequence of the occurrence would or could be serious, then the applicant is not fit to perform the task.
- *Pain:* the presence of conditions such as back and neck pain, which might cause gradually increasing and

painful distraction from the primary tasks, need assessment. Pain might also be referred to the limbs and provoked by flight duties where there may be no opportunity to gain relief by simple measures such as a change in position or stretching.

When assessing the medical fitness of current aircrew to return to flying before or after treatment, the above factors are similarly considered. The history of daily function is a valuable tool in assessing fitness for duties. The assessment of a person who might have returned to activities of daily living such as high-level recreational sport, prolonged driving of a motorcar, lifting, carrying, house maintenance and gardening can be relatively straightforward, with the successful performance of these tasks being an indicator of likely adequate function for duty. Aircrew who report symptoms provoked by their usual flight workload usually require management of the complaint. However, there is undoubtedly an incidence of unreported discomfort with symptoms among aircrew being treated and unknown to the employer, because of fear that reporting these symptoms might lead to a loss of flying category. The assessment of performance under normal flight conditions and emergency situations using a flight simulator can be valuable. If borderline restrictions in function cannot be improved, then it is often appropriate to allow aircrew to return to work with a co-pilot suitably qualified on aircraft type, or to restrict the duration of flights undertaken. A sympathetic, thorough and objective assessment of aircrew should reduce their fear of inappropriate restrictions on employment being imposed.

In the presence of a condition that might cause steady reduction in performance, regular monitoring of the condition and physical performance of the employee will allow his or her ongoing fitness for duty to be determined.

The overriding consideration is to determine the ability of aircrew to perform all duties safely. Appropriate and reasonable modifications to the workplace and regular assessment by the employer can allow prolonged and safe performance in the workplace by expensively trained and valuable aircrew, even in the presence of musculoskeletal symptoms.

ISSUES AFTER FRACTURE MANAGEMENT

The aims of treatment after fracture are to return the patient to maximum level of function as soon as possible (Ruedi and Murphy 2000). To achieve the best possible stable position of the fracture, implants such as screws, plates and intramedullary nails are often used. The implant is chosen aiming to give stability to the reduced fracture and to allow early movement of the muscles and joints close to the injury. The incidence of post-fracture arthritis is reduced by accurate reduction of intra-articular fractures, and the range of joint motion is improved by early movements of the joint and avoiding prolonged periods in plaster casts. The non-surgical treatment of fractures is frequently appropriate and effective for many fracture patterns.

Return to duties

The demonstration of a 'healed' fracture with adequate function of the affected area, no distracting discomfort and a satisfactory and relevant functional assessment should be the criteria used to confirm fitness to return to duties.

Removal of metalwork

After a patient returns to maximum function following a fracture, the issue of retained metalwork might be discussed. The historical practice of removing metalwork because it is there has good reasons to be avoided. Good reasons to remove the metalwork include reducing prominence and discomfort associated with the retained implant, or as part of the surgically assisted process of achieving fracture healing. There is a significant morbidity associated with metalwork removal, such as infection, painful scar, re-fracture of the bone through the screw holes, and damage to nerves or other soft tissue during the surgery. If a patient has returned to pain-free normal function, then removal of implants can only potentially reduce function. The long-term systemic effects of long-term retained metalwork appear to be insignificant.

The local mechanical effects or retained metalwork depend on the site and size of the implant. A retained single screw in the medial malleolus of the ankle will do very little to alter the mechanical properties of the tibia. Conversely, a short femoral nail might significantly alter the bending properties of the bone and the risk of future injury under load (Figure 49.1). Surgery to stiffen one or more segments of the spine following surgery for fracture or degenerative change will change the points at which axial loading and compression forces passing through the spine are concentrated.

The potential for a retained implant to cause increased risk of future injury varies with the patient and the size, type and site of the implant. Although the mechanical properties of the bone might be made more normal by removing the implant and the potentially increased risk of future fracture during a high-energy event reduced, the future event itself might be very unlikely. The risk associated with removal of metal work surgery should be balanced carefully against the risks associated with leaving metal in situ before the person submits themselves to surgery. The policy of insisting that pilots in the Royal Air Force (RAF) have lower-limb metalwork removed before returning to duty has been reviewed. If there is uncertainty about fitness to return to task or concern about unacceptable risk associated with retained metalwork, then the specialist opinion of an orthopaedic surgeon familiar with the issues should be sought.

Post-traumatic arthritis

Post-injury arthritis is usually associated with fractures that extend into a joint surface. It is likely that injury that

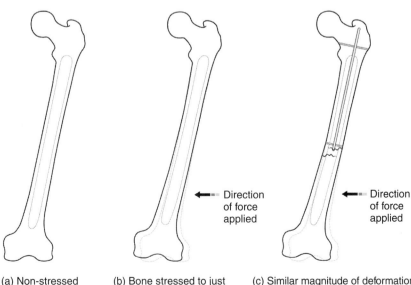

(a) Non-stressed bone

(b) Bone stressed to just within limit of fracture

(c) Similar magnitude of deformation Stiff segment due to metal rod Non-stiffened segment fractures

Figure 49.1   *Effect of force on a bone containing a metal rod.*

is going to provoke significant degenerative change will do so within two years or so of the cessation of treatment. The likelihood of arthritis developing is increased as the complexity of the fracture and the initial displacement increase. It is also associated with residual irregularity in the joint surface after treatment has been concluded. Some injuries, such as scaphoid fracture, hip dislocation and talar neck fracture, lead to risk of osteonecrosis. Scaphoid fracture is also associated with a significant non-union rate. The history of these conditions in an applicant for a strenuous type of job might reduce their period of unrestricted employment.

Residual long-bone deformity after fracture

Minor degrees of shortening after fracture of long bones may be tolerated well and the patient returned to high-level function. Following fracture to the humerus, significant healed fracture mal-alignment can be seen, with normal upper limb function due to the wide arc of movement of the shoulder possible in abduction, flexion and rotation. In other areas, residual angulation that cannot be compensated for by movement of an adjacent join in the plane of the deformity may be tolerated poorly. A history of mid-shaft forearm fracture and residual angulation will restrict pronation and supination.

UPPER LIMB

The function of the upper limb should be considered as a whole rather than by individual joints and areas. Areas of abnormal movement and stiffness in the upper limb can be compensated for readily in many patients. For instance, a patient with restriction of pronation of the wrist and forearm often adapts and compensates by abduction of the shoulder, thus bringing the palm of the hand towards the floor. This type of compensation manoeuvre would not be acceptable if the elbow had to be separated widely from the body and the applicant was to work in a confined environment. Minimal body–elbow separation not causing 'conflict' with other crew members or items of equipment could be acceptable.

Crushing or cutting injury to the digits of the hand is frequently associated with long-term stiffness and sensory abnormality. A normal thumb makes a major contribution to the hand function, and its dysfunction is not compensated for easily. Conversely, long-term sensory abnormality of the index finger provokes ready adaptation, with the majority of people using their middle and ring fingers and thumb for precision three-point fine pincer grip. As long as the index finger is not stiff, good function of the hand is likely.

Shoulder

Normal shoulder function depends on four joints – the sternoclavicular, acromioclavicular, glenohumeral and scapulothoracic joints – as well as the surrounding rotator cuff and other major muscles. These joints move in harmony to produce shoulder movement. Disorders of the shoulder such as arthritis, capsulitis, subacromial impingement and rotator cuff degeneration or tear cause certain patterns of symptoms and complaints. More than one of these conditions may be present and contributing to symptoms. The effect on function of untreated or residual symptoms and complaints can be considered, rather than discussing individual pathological conditions with overlapping symptoms and effect on limb function.

RANGE OF MOVEMENT

The shoulder has a large range of normal movement in flexion, abduction and rotation. Significant degrees of stiffness can be tolerated, with little effect on normal professional, daily, sporting and social activities. Stiffness in one of these joints, such as the glenohumeral joint, will still allow movement at the scapulothoracic joint that can be useful, even where the glenohumeral joint has been surgically fused. In the environment of the traditional cockpit, aircrew are expected to reach controls and switches in front, behind, to the side, above and below them. Significant stiffness in the shoulder has a profound effect upon reach – and much more effect than stiffness in the more peripheral limb joints. Consequently, shoulder stiffness can place major restrictions on the ability of pilots and aircrew to perform.

INSTABILITY

The advantages of mobility of the shoulder are balanced by the disadvantages of a relatively unstable joint. Dislocation of the shoulder can be associated with intrinsic soft-tissue laxity and can be habitual and multidirectional. Such a history in one shoulder suggests a tendency for the other shoulder to develop the condition in the future. Dislocation of the shoulder also often occurs for the first time after trauma. Dislocation is usually anterior. Re-dislocation after the first episode is common. The provocative position for anterior re-dislocation is with the shoulder elevated, extended and externally rotated, i.e. reaching above and behind the head. A history of untreated ongoing shoulder instability that might be provoked in the cockpit would be a major concern.

PAIN AND WEAKNESS

Significant shoulder pain reducing the pain-free arc of movement or shoulder weakness may have effects on active, uninhibited reach and, consequently, reduce the ability of aircrew to perform their duties. However, partial or full-thickness degenerative tears of the rotator cuff are not inevitably associated with loss of function. Rates of asymptomatic tear diagnosed with ultrasound ranging from 13 per cent in the age group 50–59 years to 51 per cent in the age group over 80 years have been reported (Tempelhof *et al.* 1999). It is important, therefore, to make clear functional assessments of patients when considering fitness for duty, rather than making an all-encompassing policy based purely on a diagnostic label.

Elbow, forearm and wrist

PAIN

The incidence of tennis elbow has been reported as affecting one to three per cent of the population between the ages of 40 and 60 years. Arthritis, epicondylitis, tenosynovitis, peripheral nerve compression and other 'degenerative' age-associated conditions tend to cause recurrent symptoms after first being experienced. The majority of symptoms can be managed successfully in the population and established aircrew without significant changes to their work practice. A history of these types of condition in the young adult is likely to have more profound implications on their long-term fitness for duties.

RANGE OF MOVEMENT

Pronation and supination of the forearm require a mobile radiocapitellar joint and proximal and distal radioulnar joints. Elbow movement essentially is otherwise a hinge-type mechanism. Other wrist movements depend on the radiocarpal joint and the mobility between the proximal and distal row of the carpals.

Conditions that cause stiffness of these areas will have less effect on reach when they affect a peripheral joint rather than a more proximal joint. Loss of the last few degrees of elbow extension might cause no more than minor embarrassment when stretching past a dining companion for the salt, and wrist stiffness may have little effect on reach at all. There may be no effect on the ability to perform cockpit tasks for a pilot.

The effect on the ability to access awkward areas and perform tasks is likely to be more affected by stiffness of peripheral joints. Minor loss of wrist dorsiflexion might result in functionally minor symptoms of pain under loaded dorsiflexion, such as when performing press-ups, but significant stiffness might impede the ability of aircrew or ground crew to access parts of the airplane and perform in-flight or ground-maintenance tasks.

Pronation and supination of the forearm have been discussed. An adequate range of movement without the use of exaggerated compensation manoeuvre is needed for function in tight working spaces.

Hand

Function of the hand is central to the traditional interface between human and machine (Burke *et al.* 1990). If techniques of adaptation and functional compensation for minor symptoms can be accepted higher in the limb, then they are less likely to be acceptable at this level. Assessment of the hand should ensure the ability to demonstrate adequate power grip, three-point pinch grip, key grip, rapid skilled precise movements and normal sensation. Performance below these levels is likely to need a thorough assessment of the ability to perform tasks safely and reliably.

LOWER LIMB

As with the upper limb, the effect of lower-limb pathology on function in the workplace as a whole needs assessment. Lower-limb dysfunction and symptoms can be referred from the spine or arise from local pathology. Early symptoms of osteoarthritis in the knee or the hip might cause little pain and no distraction during sitting. If the range of movement of the joint allows full performance in the work environment, then aircrew may continue to work safely.

Osteoarthritis may cause more severe symptoms of distracting ache, stiffness or episodic unpredictable short-lived severe pain. In these circumstances, fitness for primary task may be compromised.

Joint replacement

Knee and hip replacement are established surgical procedures with high rates of satisfaction from patients. After the surgical rehabilitation process has been completed, the functional outcome is often compatible with return to full flight-deck duties. A demonstrable ability to enter and leave the flight deck and perform all lower-limb flight tasks for an appropriate period should allow return to work. A discussion during questions at the British Medical Pilots Association meeting in 2004 revealed an audience member who had returned to light aircraft flying within two months of total knee replacement.

Primary total hip replacement is associated with postoperative dislocation in a small number (about one per cent) of cases. Most of the dislocations occur in the first three months following surgery. Dislocation is often associated with flexion and adduction of the hip. It would seem reasonable to allow at least three months for the hip to prove itself stable before allowing return to duties in possibly provocative positions. More recently, hip-resurfacing techniques and implants have been developed. Resurfacing achieves an intrinsically more stable joint because of the larger femoral head and acetabular radii. A stable range of movement approaching normal can be achieved. However, dislocations have been reported from some hospitals using this technique.

SPINE

The spine is a column of vertebrae and ligaments separated by discs with two synovial facet joints at each level. The column is supported by the paraspinal and abdominal muscles. Ageing is associated with the development of degenerative changes in the intervertebral discs at one or many levels. These changes are often asymptomatic and may be visible on magnetic resonance imaging (MRI) scans performed for unrelated reasons. The cause of back pain is likely to be associated with degenerative disc changes and secondary changes in many cases. These changes make the individual more likely to experience spontaneous or event-related pain. Secondary changes, such as disc-space narrowing, facet joint osteophytes and soft tissue hypertrophy, may narrow the nerve root canal, causing referred pain. Local back pain due to secondary tears of the annulus of the disc, facet joint degeneration and secondary inflammation occurs.

Other causes of pain such as spondylolysis and spondylolisthesis are often found in association with degenerative changes at the same or other levels. Surgery performed on these surgically treatable causes of back pain may give poor results due to the presence of other pain sources. It can be difficult to guarantee that the site of treatment is the source, or the only source, of pain.

Low back pain

Back pain is common in the population. Reported lifetime incidence of back pain is 49–69 per cent, with a point prevalence of 12–30 per cent. Other sources quote higher figures. In a cohort of previously asymptomatic individuals, 34 per cent of males and 37 per cent of females reported pain in the following year. A past history of back pain increases the chance of future back pain. If previous back pain is recognized, then there is a relative risk of 2.71 of future back pain. Higher incidence of back pain has been reported in certain groups of workers, such as truck drivers, heavy manual workers and nurses (Fairbank 2002). Factors that are thought to provoke back pain include vibration, posture and sudden maximal effort.

HELICOPTERS

Helicopter crew are exposed to vibration and may have to adopt uncomfortable postures for considerable periods. It is often not possible to relieve discomfort during flight with simple stretching manoeuvres. Vibration frequencies of between 2 and 16 Hz are recorded in helicopters. Exposures to vibration, smoking and driving have been linked to disc prolapse. In helicopter crew, backache is perceived as common, and the majority of sufferers rarely seek medical advice. Pain can be mild to moderate, appearing during or shortly after flight, without radiation and sited in the lumbar region or buttocks. It can also be more severe, radiate to the lower extremities with paraesthesia, and be longer-lasting after onset. A study in a mock-up of the UH-1H helicopter subjected pilots to two test periods of an hour each, one with vibration and one without. All experienced pain similar to the pain they reported in flight; the vibration made no difference to the pain. Other studies seem to suggest that the asymmetric posture adopted by pilots in helicopters contributes to the experience of back pain. It has been reported that chronic back pain is associated with the number of hours flown, developing after a career of 300–500 flight hours. It seems likely that the posture adopted by helicopter crew contributes to the incidence of back pain, and the vibration experienced may contribute to disc prolapse and referred pain. The symptoms may be short-lived regular provocation of symptoms from an underlying degenerative disc that may have otherwise been minimally symptomatic. It is unclear whether the environment in which crew work actually accelerates or provokes degenerative change.

Symptoms are likely to be reduced by further limitation of vibration in future helicopter designs and better working posture. For crew members who are distracted by back pain, adjustments to the seated position by the manufacture of relatively inexpensive lumbar supports can be effective. The natural progress of periods of exacerbation of symptoms is for them to usually improve. Physiotherapy aimed at improving posture and spinal-supporting muscle strength and coordination may give improvement of base-level symptoms and reduce frequency of exacerbations of pain.

Given the relative risk of recurrence of back pain in the general population, and the challenging environment of the helicopter, potential aircrew with a history of back pain or sciatica need to be assessed carefully before being accepted for training.

Although other aircraft types are less likely to submit the crew to vibration and asymmetric posture, G forces are still experienced by the crew, and back pain can be troublesome. Truck drivers have a higher incidence of back pain, even in the absence of G_z forces, which may be due to the adoption of prolonged symmetrical seated positions.

Cervical spine

As with the lumbar spine, degenerative change and symptoms of neck pain and, to a lesser extent, referred upper extremity symptoms are common in the population. A prevalence of seven or eight per cent has been reported in the general population. When considered by age, a prevalence of two per cent in the age group 15–24 years, and increasing to 40 per cent in the age group 55–64 years, has been reported. An uninhibited and adequate range of movement to perform flight tasks such as lookout is required. This required range of movement is likely to be greater in a single-seat aeroplane. As stated earlier, it is important to assess adequately a candidate for aircrew duties who has a history of neck pain before he or she is subjected to flight duties and stresses.

The potential for repeated exposure to G forces to cause degenerative change in the cervical spine was addressed by the Technology Watch (TW), which was established on the recommendation of the Aerospace Medical Panel of the former Advisory Group for Aerospace Research and Development, Working Group 17. The executive summary reported (Research and Technology Organisation 1999):

> This TW noted a very high rate of acute injury to soft tissues (muscles and ligaments) of the neck in fighter pilots that was a result of sustained G exposures. It also reported that in several pilot high-sustained G studies there were significantly greater incidences of degeneration of the cervical spine compared with low or no G exposed, age sex matched controls. Meta-analysis of 8 studies determined that there was a direct relationship between degenerative diseases of the spine and repeated exposures to sustained G. The statistical probability of this analysis was $P < 0.001$. The following hypothesis was developed. Acute injuries of neck muscles and ligaments commonly occur in fighter pilots. These injured soft tissues of the neck are less able to protect the cervical spine from reoccurring increased G generated external loads. Thus sub acute disc injuries occur that eventually lead to spinal degeneration and the development of osteophytes with vertebral strengthening. This G effect on the spine appears to be an acceleration of spinal degeneration that normally occurs with increasing age in low or

non-G controls. Thus it is hypothesised that both populations will eventually have similar levels of cervical spine degeneration after pilots are no longer exposed to sustained G.

EJECTION SEATS AND INJURY

The development of the ejector seat has made escape and survival from accidents in high-performance aircraft possible in flight conditions where otherwise there would have been death. There are three phases during an ejector seat being used when the pilot may be injured. Injured aircrew should be treated at the closest unit with experience and facility to treat severely injured patients. Particular patterns of injury associated with escape equipment can be assessed after initial life- and limb-saving treatment has been completed.

Seat acceleration

A high rate of onset of G force is associated with axial loading and flexion forces passing through the spine, which might result in fracture (Figure 49.2). Fractures are concentrated at the junctions between the mobile and less mobile sections of the spine, although they can occur at all levels. The cervicothoracic junction, thoracolumbar and lumbosacral areas are commonly affected. These injuries can be missed at initial assessment, particularly if there are other major injuries causing distracting pain. They can also be masked by the euphoria of a perceived 'escape without injury'. Displaced fractures of the vertebrae will usually be visible on plain X-ray films. In the presence of fracture, isotope bone scan is likely to be positive when performed after 48 hours and may show other unsuspected fractures. MRI scan is less invasive and will show minimally displaced fractures and trabecular fractures or 'bone bruise'. It will also allow the spinal ligaments and soft tissues to be assessed.

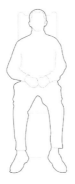 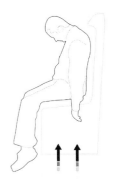 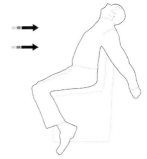

(a) Sitting in ejector seat   (b) Ejection vertical forces   (c) Wind flail forces   **Figure 49.2** *Ejection forces and injury.*

Wind flail injury

Aircrew ejecting at high airspeed will be subjected to rapid deceleration forces due to airflow. Mobile parts of the body may move in an uncontrolled manner past the usual range of movement and result in soft-tissue injury dislocation and fracture (Figure 49.2). The chance of wind flail injury to the legs and arms increases as the indicated airspeed at time of ejection increases. As well as the limbs being subjected to flail forces, the cervical spine can be submitted to multi-planar forces, including distraction pulling forces. These forces can result in severe soft-tissue ligamentous injury.

Injury on landing

The pattern of injury on landing depends on the rate of descent, the ability of the ejectee to perform parachute landing drills, and the type of surface. Axial loading forces passing through the foot, calcaneum, tibia, femur, pelvis and the axial spine can cause fracture at any site. As always in the presence of life-threatening injury or painful distracting injury, some of these injuries can be missed unless looked for specifically. If not identified, a potential treatment window that might improve long-term performance and function may be missed.

The particular forces that may be experienced by a person flying an aircraft equipped with an ejector seat mean that the issues of retained metalwork after fracture and the presence of joint replacements need to be considered in conjunction with the forces that might be experienced during and after ejection.

Management of the ejectee

The ejectee should be managed using standard protocols for the assessment and treatment of a severely injured patient. The specific issues of bony or ligamentous injury of the spine may be obvious with a severe injury, but occult and subtle injuries of the spine can be overlooked, particularly in the early euphoria of a successful ejection or if there are other, more severe distracting injuries. The treating team should have a high level of suspicion for spinal injury. The use of diagnostic aids such as MRI and isotope bone scanning is valuable in order to differentiate between minor soft-tissue sprain and more severe ligamentous injury or non-displaced fracture.

Return to ejection-seat flying

The decision to return to ejection-seat flying after ejection should be made after considering the functional performance of the pilot in general and the specific functional lim-itations that residual effect of injury might have after treatment has been completed. The prospect of returning to ejection-seat aircraft raises the issue of future ejection and the potential of increased risk of injury, especially to the spine. The conservative management of a minimally displaced anterior wedge fracture will usually give good functional outcome with minimal residual stiffness; in this circumstance, the increased risk of injury is slight and return to ejection-seat flight almost certain. If a more complex spinal fracture of two or more levels has been managed surgically with the insertion of rods and screws, then there will be a stiff segment of spine, even if the rods and screws are subsequently removed. Such a stiff segment will mean that the overall passive range of movement will be reduced. Future ejection causing passive flexion that might otherwise have been tolerated could now cause spinal injury and risk of neurological impairment. Other metalwork in limbs may change the tolerance to wind flail forces and landing forces.

CONGENITAL DEFORMITY

As with the previous discussions, the assessment of congenital deformity should be performed against functional criteria and with the potential for future deterioration of function in mind. Conditions that initially appear to be isolated and treated well often coexist with subtle or obvious hypoplasia of the remainder of the limb. For instance, treated club foot is often associated with a small calf, short leg and more subtle thigh hypoplasia. A well-treated club foot may allow all pilot duties to be performed but is likely to cause difficulty with other ground tasks and field craft skills that military pilots might perform.

OSTEOPOROSIS

The measurement of bone density is usually performed as a screening tool in the middle-aged to elderly person who has sustained fracture in order to exclude or treat reduced bone density. The relative risks of fracture, compared with the normal for age, in the femoral necks and the lumbar vertebrae are often given. Bone density below one standard deviation of the normal is considered osteopenic and below 2.5 considered osteoporotic. The history of bone-density studies being performed in a potential aircrew applicant should cause the result to be looked at carefully and the increased risk of fracture quantified. It is unusual for young people to undergo bone-density studies, and a spectrum of associated conditions that may be present and led to the decision to perform bone-density studies, such as previously treated pituitary hypoplasia, must be considered carefully.

REFERENCES

Burke FD, McGrouther DA, Smith PJ. *Principles of Hand Surgery*. Edinburgh: Churchill Livingstone, 1990.

Department for Work and Pensions. The Disability Discrimination Act 1995 (Amendment) Regulations. London: HMSO, 2003.

Fairbank CTJ. The thoracic and lumbar spine. In: Foy M, Fagg P (eds). *Medicolegal Reporting in Orthopaedic Trauma*. Edinburgh: Churchill Livingstone, 2002; pp. 383–92.

Magee DJ. *Orthopaedic Physical Assessment*. London: Saunders, 1992.

Research and Technology Organisation. Cervical spinal injury from repeated exposures to sustained acceleration. RTO Technical Report 4. RTO-TR-4 AC/323(HFM)TP/9. Neuilly-sur-Seine: Research and Technology Organisation, 1999.

Ruedi TP, Murphy WM. *AO Principles of Fracture Management*. Stuttgart: Thieme, 2000.

Tempelhof S, Rupp S, Seil R. Age-related prevelance of rotator cuff tears in asymptomatic shoulders. *Journal of Shoulder and Elbow Surgery* 1999; **8**: 296–9.

50

Clinical management of decompression illness

JANE RISDALL

INTRODUCTION

Decompression illness (DCI), encompassing both decompression sickness (DCS) and arterial gas embolism (AGE), is a potentially life-threatening condition encountered as a result of exposure to changes in barometric pressure. It can occur in astronauts and aviators as well as compressed-gas divers and caisson workers. DCI is a syndrome of numerous possible manifestations, thought to be initiated by the presence of bubbles of gas in the body tissues and circulation.

A reduction in environmental pressure may lead to bubble formation by two distinct mechanisms.

EVOLVED GAS DISEASE

Henry's law can be applied to describe the amount of dissolved gas held in tissues and blood. At sea level, both air and arterial blood contain approximately 0.8 atmospheres (80 kPa, 600 mmHg) of nitrogen, since the concentration of inert gas in arterial blood at equilibrium is approximately the same as in the gas mixture being breathed. During decompression (see Chapter 7), inert gas moves from the tissues into the blood, where it is carried to the lungs and exhaled. If this process occurs at a controlled rate, such that the inert gas tension in the tissues and blood does not achieve a sufficient level of supersaturation for bubbles to form, then decompression will proceed uneventfully. If the rate of decompression is such that the capacity of the tissues, circulation, heart and lungs is overwhelmed, then inert gas bubbles may start to form.

Humans are capable of tolerating a certain bubble load. Venous bubbles are efficiently filtered from the circulation by the lungs and numerous Doppler studies have demonstrated the presence of venous bubbles in otherwise asymptomatic subjects during subatmospheric exposures (Conkin et al. 1998). Bubbles may form in some tissues, such as adipose tissue, without causing overt symptoms: while in other tissues, such as the nervous system, the presence of even a small bubble load may result in tissue damage, symptoms and abnormal function. Pathological mechanisms for the deleterious effects of bubbles include disruption of tissue architecture, occlusion of the supporting microcirculation and the triggering of a range of injury cascades at the tissue–bubble interface.

Although the lungs provide an excellent bubble filter, their capacity is finite. Massive venous gas load may overwhelm this filter, resulting in venous bubbles transiting to the arterial circulation. Additionally, the presence of a right-to-left shunt may allow bubbles to bypass the pulmonary filter. Some 20–30 per cent of the normal adult population can be demonstrated to have a patent foramen ovale (PFO) (Hagen et al. 1984) and, although this relic of the fetal circulation normally results in no ill effects, it has the potential to promote arterialization of otherwise relatively harmless venous bubbles. The significance of a PFO to any individual aviator is currently uncertain.

ARTERIAL GAS EMBOLISM

The second method of bubble generation arises as the result of expansion of trapped gas (particularly in the lungs) as a consequence of Boyle's law. If gas from a ruptured lung enters the tissue planes it may present as subcutaneous emphysema or a pneumomediastinum. If it enters the pulmonary veins it will be carried to the left side of the heart and from there be distributed to the body as AGE. Two target organs that are particularly susceptible to AGE are the brain and the heart. A person who has sustained decompression pulmonary barotrauma should be assessed carefully for evidence of cardiac or neurological disturbance.

Pulmonary barotrauma due to lung overdistension has been considered a rare consequence of the loss of cabin pressure in flight (see Chapter 6), but it remains a real risk in experimental hypobaric chamber exposures. However, the advent of highly agile aircraft, capable of sustaining high $+G_z$ at high altitude and with life-support systems that deliver positive pressure breathing, have created the circumstances in which a sudden loss of cabin pressure during a $+G_z$ manoeuvre could occur while the aircrew's lungs were fully inflated. Additionally, performance of the anti-G straining manoeuvre will obstruct free flow of expanding gas from the lungs, further enhancing the risk of pulmonary barotrauma.

EBULLISM

Exposure to 63 000 feet introduces the additional hazard of ebullism. At this altitude, ambient pressure (47 mmHg, 6.25 kPa) equals the saturated vapour pressure of water at body temperature (37 °C) and spontaneous boiling and degassing of body fluids and tissues will occur (ebullism). Not only will water vapour continuously leave the body, resulting in rapid cooling, but also changes from the liquid to the gaseous phase in the tissues will produce gas cavities, and in certain animal species the body may rapidly increase in size. The changes are reversed on recompression as the gas phase reverts to liquid.

Most data available on ebullism are from animal studies (Billings 1973). These show that involvement of the cardiovascular system commences with the formation of bubbles in the low-pressure areas of the circulation (venous and capillary beds). The elastic walls of the arterial tree provide a degree of positive pressure protection. The bubbles can then occlude venous and pulmonary vessels and circulation ceases. Post-mortem findings generally demonstrate massive pulmonary damage with haemorrhage and atelectasis. However, if recompression is sufficiently rapid and pulmonary function re-established, the bubbles of ebullism revert to the liquid phase and recovery is possible.

Studies of ebullism in humans have been very limited, although successful short-term exposures to altitudes above 63 000 feet have been conducted using partial-pressure assemblies that increase intrapulmonary pressure and provide counter-pressure to certain areas of the body.

DIAGNOSIS OF DECOMPRESSION ILLNESS

There are no highly sensitive or specific diagnostic investigations for DCI, but it has been the practice in aviation medicine to regard any symptoms arising at altitude or simulated altitude, in the absence of hypoxia, as manifestations of DCI until proved otherwise. History and clinical examination are therefore key in assessing patients and establishing a diagnosis of DCI.

When suspected DCI occurs during flight, the opportunity for the clinician or flight surgeon to elicit a history may be very limited. Initially, examination of the patient may not be possible at all. Key facts to establish, therefore, are:

- nature of the symptoms being experienced
- evolution and severity of symptoms
- timing of onset of symptoms relative to exposure to altitude
- maximum altitude experienced
- rate of altitude exposure
- response of symptoms to oxygen
- response of symptoms to descent.

Onset of symptoms within five minutes or less of attaining altitude is suggestive of AGE, particularly if the decompression was rapid. Symptoms developing after five minutes at altitude are more likely to be due to evolved gas disease. Presenting symptoms can range from sudden loss of consciousness or sudden onset of chest pain, through shortness of breath, impaired level of consciousness, dizziness or paraesthesiae to joint pain or skin irritation.

PRESENTATION OF DECOMPRESSION ILLNESS

Since DCI can interfere with the function of a wide range of tissues, the potential number of manifestations is enormous. In the past, these have been grouped into 'syndromes' according to the anatomical site and presumed mechanism of disease. These have then been subdivided further according to the perceived severity, resulting in mild (Type 1) and serious (Type 2) decompression sickness (Elliott and Kindwall 1982). These terms are still used, but it is increasingly recognized that they are of limited value, because symptoms from the two groups may coexist or a 'Type 1' injury may progress to a 'Type 2'. A descriptive protocol focusing particularly on the evolution and manifestation of symptoms is preferred (Francis and Smith 1991).

Evolution

This term is used to describe the development of the symptoms before descent or recompression. DCI is frequently a dynamic condition, so this description may vary from one observation to the next. Typically, DCI presents initially as being *progressive*, as the patient becomes increasingly aware that something is wrong. If the symptomatology stabilizes, it may then be considered *static*. If there is improvement or even complete resolution without intervention (including descent or oxygen administration), then it may be described as *spontaneously improving* but if symptoms recur, the condition would be describe as *relapsing*.

Manifestations

There are a number of commonly occurring manifestations of DCI. Although each may present alone, combinations of symptoms are frequent and should always be actively sought and/or excluded.

PAIN

Limb pain is probably the most frequent manifestation of DCI. It describes a deep aching pain in a limb or joint, which may begin during ascent (decompression) or at altitude. In aviators, the lower limbs, particularly the knees, are most commonly involved. The pain usually begins gradually and is poorly localized. It may resolve spontaneously. Minor pain may migrate from joint to joint, a condition known as 'the niggles', or it may worsen, becoming localized to a particular joint and acquiring a dull, boring characteristic, frequently likened to toothache. The pain is seldom made worse by movement and often there are no objective signs on examination. Patients presenting with isolated limb pain must be examined fully to exclude any neurological deficit, as the pain may mask mild paraesthesiae, numbness or weakness. Limb pain DCI frequently resolves completely on descent to ground level.

Girdle or back pain often presents as a poorly localized aching or 'constricting' pain that originates in the mid to low back and often spreads, usually bilaterally, around the pelvis or abdomen in a girdle-like distribution. Occasionally, it may originate in the thoracic spine and spread around the chest or shoulder girdle. In the context of DCI, pain of this nature is associated with spinal cord involvement, and its presence may herald neurological deterioration.

NEUROLOGICAL

Involvement of the nervous system may range from the subtle, multifocal presentations of mild evolved gas disease to the dramatic catastrophic presentation of severe cerebral AGE. Both the central and peripheral nervous systems may be involved, giving a huge range of possible neurological manifestations. These can include alterations of higher functions (aberrant thought processes, altered affect, loss of memory, cognitive impairment), altered level of consciousness, seizure activity, impaired coordination, reduced strength or sensation in any distribution, presence of paraesthesiae, dysfunction of the special senses and loss of sphincter control.

The audiovestibular system may be damaged directly as a result of barotrauma or as a consequence of evolved gas disease affecting the cochlea, eighth nerve nuclei, cerebellar or cortical pathways. In individual cases it may be impossible to distinguish between these mechanisms or sites of injury by clinical examination alone. Consequently, audiovestibular DCI may describe any presentation that includes rotational vertigo, tinnitus, nystagmus or reduced auditory acuity after a provocative altitude exposure. Nausea and vomiting may accompany these symptoms but are insufficient in themselves to imply audiovestibular DCI.

CARDIOPULMONARY

Involvement of the lungs in DCI may be as a result of two distinct processes, namely decompression pulmonary barotrauma and the cardiopulmonary consequences of massive venous gas embolism. Cardiac involvement may also result from coronary artery AGE. Although the mechanisms involved are distinctly different, it may be difficult to distinguish between them in a clinical setting, because many of the symptoms and signs are shared. These include dyspnoea, tachypnoea, chest pain, cough, haemoptysis, cyanosis and, rarely, shock. Progression of symptoms at altitude may be due to either a tension pneumothorax or massive gas embolism of the lungs. The latter condition, often referred to as 'the chokes', presents initially with a sense of constriction around the lower chest and any attempt at deep inspiration is marked by an inspiratory 'catch'. This is accompanied by the development of retrosternal discomfort and paroxysmal coughing on inspiration. Breathlessness and cyanosis follow and shortly thereafter progress to collapse if the altitude exposure is maintained. Symptoms of respiratory DCI may persist for several hours after return to ground level and are thought to represent the reflex response of the pulmonary tissues to the venous gas load.

CUTANEOUS

Cutaneous manifestations often occur at altitude. They are usually transient and consist of itching, tingling ('the creeps') or formication. Occasionally, itching may be severe and accompanied by hyperaesthesia. More infrequently, erythematous, urticarial rashes or cyanotic mottling and marbling (cutis marmorata) are observed, usually in conjunction with other manifestations of DCI.

CONSTITUTIONAL

There are a number of non-specific symptoms that may be considered part of the constellation of DCI, including headache, malaise, fatigue, nausea, anorexia and anxiety. In a small proportion of people presenting with these symptoms, there is progression to diminished consciousness (primary collapse) without any other manifestations of DCI. Rapid recovery, often with an accompanying frontal headache, follows descent.

DIFFERENTIAL DIAGNOSIS

DCI may be mimicked by a variety of disorders, including intercurrent illness arising coincidentally with flight and conditions arising from the known environmental or psychological stresses of flight or simulated altitude exposure.

Intercurrent Illness

This should be rare in the well-screened aircrew population. Limb pains may arise for many reasons, including postural cramps and injury. Viral illnesses may manifest as constitutional symptoms evolving over the duration of longer exposures. More serious conditions, including ischaemic heart disease and cerebrovascular disease, may present for the first time during flight, provoking concerns of cardiopulmonary or serious neurological DCI. Descent in such cases will be required immediately and differentiation should present little difficulty once on the ground.

Environmental flight stresses

HYPOXIA

The clinical features of acute hypobaric hypoxia are summarized in Chapter 3. Almost all of the symptoms listed are equally applicable to an episode of DCI. The symptoms will be reversed rapidly by administration of an increased partial pressure of oxygen, but they will also respond favourably to recompression (descent) as the alveolar oxygen tension is raised.

GASTROINTESTINAL GAS DISTENSION

Free gas in the intestinal tract will expand as the ambient pressure is reduced (Boyle's law). If not vented adequately,

this can cause stretching of the visceral walls, with pain and reflex muscle contraction. In extreme cases, loss of consciousness can supervene. Significant abdominal pain due to gas expansion during ascent is uncommon at altitudes below 40 000 feet.

+G$_z$-RELATED ATELECTASIS

The aetiology of +G$_z$-related basal atelectasis is described in Chapter 8. The symptoms produced include inspiratory pain and retrosternal discomfort. In some individuals this will progress to paroxysmal coughing. The resemblance to cardiopulmonary DCI is clear. A detailed history, including the type of aircraft, flight profile and life-support equipment used, should help to make the distinction.

ALTERNOBARIC VERTIGO

In susceptible individuals rotational vertigo, nausea, vomiting and ataxia may occur if the pressure difference between the two middle ears exceeds a critical level (around 6 kPa, 45 mmHg). This is thought to be due to asymmetrical pressure stimulation of the vestibular apparatus. The problem occurs most commonly during ascent, but it has also been described during descent if a Valsalva or similar manoeuvre raises middle-ear pressure. If rotational vertigo occurs during ascent in the erect posture, the sensation of spinning will be towards the side with the poorest Eustachian tube function and, consequently, the highest middle-ear pressure (Ross 1976). Alternobaric vertigo is likely to occur at low altitudes, where the pressure changes are greater and generally below the threshold for DCI.

HYPERVENTILATION

Hyperventilation is not uncommon in conjunction with altitude exposure. It may be induced by a number of causes including anxiety, fear and unfamiliarity with breathing systems. It is usually easy to recognize by the rate and depth of respiration, development of paraesthesiae and light-headedness, and the history of the flight or altitude exposure. Confusing symptoms of recurrent loss of consciousness, tetany and acute apprehension with tachycardia persisting for some hours have been described but are very rare.

MANAGEMENT OF DECOMPRESSION ILLNESS

First aid

- Ensure the person is breathing 100 per cent oxygen, minimize activity and, if symptoms are severe, lie the person flat (not head-down).

- If the person is unconscious, put them in the recovery position if possible.
- Increase ambient pressure/descend to ground level as soon as is practicable.

In flight, a PAN call should be made, declaring a physiological emergency. In a simulated altitude exposure, appropriate assistance should be summoned to the chamber hall. The vast majority of cases will have resolved completely on return to ground level and many will improve spontaneously during descent to altitudes below 10 000 feet.

Management on the ground

Initial treatment on the ground should be directed towards stabilizing the patient along conventional trauma management guidelines, as dictated by the severity of symptoms. The response to first-aid treatment should be reviewed, a full history elicited and a thorough physical examination (including detailed neurological assessment) performed. If symptoms have resolved completely and no physical signs are detected, then the subject should be kept under observation, on 100 per cent oxygen, for two hours.

Dehydration almost invariably complicates DCI. All individuals should be rehydrated at the earliest opportunity with oral fluids, if conscious, or intravenous crystalloid solutions (not glucose-containing) if semiconscious or comatose.

If symptoms or signs are still present, consider hyperbaric recompression, with advice from a diving medicine specialist, plus adjunctive therapy as appropriate, particularly if recompression is not immediately available. In England, Wales and Northern Ireland, diving and hyperbaric medicine advice is provided by the Duty Diving Medical Officer at the Institute of Naval Medicine, available 24 hours a day (tel. 07831 151523). In Scotland, such advice is provided by the Aberdeen Royal Infirmary (tel. 01224 681818).

Role of hyperbaric recompression

Although first-aid measures will generally improve the subject's condition, recompression remains the definitive treatment for dysbaric disorders. This is effected initially by returning to ground level. However, persisting symptoms may be due to the continued presence of bubbles in the tissues or to a developing secondary injury (ischaemic damage, oedema, inflammation) as a result of trauma from evanescent bubbles. Further (hyperbaric) recompression will reduce the volume of any remaining gas bubbles in the tissues, reducing the pressure/stretch on tissues, restoring tissue architecture and improving blood flow. Bubble size

reduction is not linear but asymptotic and the biological effectiveness of the volume reduction will depend, in part, on bubble shape. A spherical bubble will reduce in all dimensions as its volume declines, whereas a cylindrical bubble, such as might occur inside a blood vessel, will experience a relatively greater reduction in length but may maintain a diameter sufficient to continue to impede blood flow for a similar decline in volume.

Administration of hyperbaric oxygen has several beneficial effects: it enhances the 'washout' of nitrogen from any remaining bubbles by increasing the diffusion gradients, it increases the blood oxygen content and, hence, oxygen delivery to injured tissues, it reduces endothelial dysfunction, and it lessens the consequences of reperfusion injury.

Recompression schedules

The diving medicine specialist will guide the choice of recompression table, but for altitude-induced DCI, compression to depths in excess of 18 m of seawater (msw) is unlikely to be required, since the inert gas burdens are low and recompression from point of injury to surface has already occurred.

ROYAL NAVY TREATMENT TABLE 61

Individuals with persisting pain-only or cutaneous symptoms can be treated using Royal Navy (RN) Treatment Table 61 (equivalent to US Navy (USN) Table 5), provided there are no neurological abnormalities in the history or on examination (Figure 50.1). The subject should start breathing oxygen on the surface and is then compressed to 18 msw (282 kPa, 2.8 ATA, 60 fsw, 2128 mmHg) over one

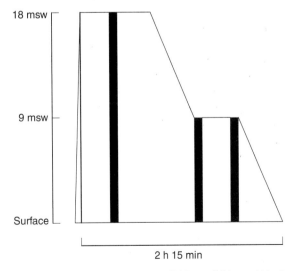

Figure 50.1 *Royal Navy Treatment Table 61. White and black areas represent oxygen-breathing and air breaks, respectively. See text for further details.*

or two minutes, stopping only if chamber occupants have difficulty clearing their ears. The time of treatment starts on reaching 18 msw. If the symptoms are relieved completely within ten minutes of starting treatment, subsequent decompression may proceed in accordance with RN Table 61. Otherwise, decompression should be conducted in accordance with RN Table 62 (USN Table 6) (Figure 50.2).

ROYAL NAVY TREATMENT TABLE 62

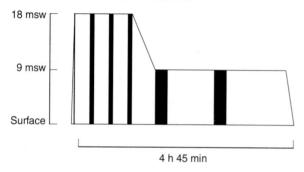

Figure 50.2 *Royal Navy Treatment Table 62. White and black areas represent oxygen-breathing and air breaks, respectively. See text for further details.*

This table is used for the majority of cases of DCI that do not meet the criteria for RN Table 61. Again, descent is to 18 msw on oxygen. If the symptoms have remained static or improved incompletely after three 20-minute periods on 100 per cent oxygen at 18 msw, the table may be extended by one, two or three further 20-minute oxygen-breathing periods, each separated by a five-minute air break, on the advice of the diving medicine specialist. The table may also be extended at 9 msw if symptoms recur during decompression. One or two one-hour oxygen-breathing periods, separated by 15-minute air breaks, may be added. In the event of incomplete relief of symptoms after a single hyperbaric recompression or if symptoms recur after leaving the chamber, it is thought to be beneficial to continue to treat daily with hyperbaric recompression until either there is no further improvement in the individual's symptomatology or complete resolution has occurred (Bennett and Moon 1990). Depending on the severity of the symptoms, retreatment may utilize a second RN Table 62 or follow RN Table 66 (USN Table 9) (Figure 50.3).

ROYAL NAVY TREATMENT TABLE 66

This table was developed specifically for the treatment of patients who require hyperbaric oxygen therapy. It limits the depth to 14 msw (242 kPa, 2.4 ATA, 45 fsw, 1824 mmHg), reducing the probability of oxygen toxicity with repeat exposures. It should not be used as a primary treatment for DCI.

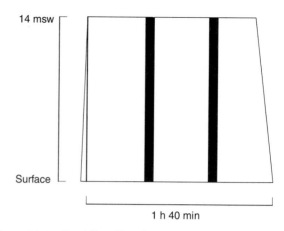

Figure 50.3 *Royal Navy Treatment Table 66. White and black areas represent oxygen-breathing and air breaks, respectively. See text for further details.*

Descent is to 14 msw on oxygen as quickly or as slowly as the subject's condition determines. Timing of treatment commences on reaching 14 msw and consists of three periods of 30 minutes breathing 100 per cent oxygen, separated by five-minute air breaks. Ascent is at a continuous rate of 1.4 msw per minute directly to surface.

Adjunctive measures

Although oxygen and recompression are the primary methods of treatment in DCI, hyperbaric recompression facilities are not always available immediately. Adjunctive therapies are recommended in order to optimize the patient's condition before transfer to more distant recompression facilities and to prevent or ameliorate secondary pathophysiological insults.

FLUIDS

The microcirculation is compromised in DCI, even in the absence of dehydration. This is thought to be the result of endothelial damage caused by circulating bubbles leading to plasma extravasation, platelet and leucocyte adhesion and platelet thrombi formation.

The efficacy of oral fluids in the treatment of DCI is not proven. However, fluids containing 60 mM sodium and 80–120 mM glucose have been used successfully for rehydration in other conditions (Cunha-Ferreira 1989). Provided the subject is not vomiting, an oral intake of 1–2 litres of fluid per hour is safe and tolerable. The gastric distension that occurs will stimulate gastric emptying, unless there is protein or a high concentration of glucose in the fluid ingested.

If significant symptoms are present, intravenous fluids are preferred, because:

- administration of oral fluids will interrupt breathing of 100 per cent oxygen
- most people have to sit up to swallow
- plasma volume can be replaced more rapidly with intravenous fluid administration
- oral fluids may increase the risk of vomiting and aspiration.

Isotonic intravenous fluids are preferred. Hypotonic solutions can induce osmolar gradients favouring entry of water into cells, possibly contributing to tissue oedema and glucose solutions should be avoided, since they may lead to worsening of neurological damage for similar reasons. The endpoint for fluid therapy should include a normal blood pressure, heart rate and haematocrit and a urine output of at least 1 ml/kg/h. Accurate fluid-balance recording is essential, since oliguria or anuria despite fluid administration may indicate persistent haemoconcentration or possible bladder dysfunction as a result of spinal cord damage. In either case, urinary catheterization is warranted.

The role of central nervous system (CNS) oedema in the outcome of neurological DCI has been debated. Circulating bubbles denude endothelial cells of surfactants, transiently increasing the permeability of the blood–brain barrier (BBB). Although this causes brain water to increase, this only appears to affect function if it is severe enough to cause a mass effect. The integrity of the BBB generally is restored within hours (Hills and James 1991). In contrast, brain function after gas embolism usually correlates well with blood flow, and consequently fluid load should be adequate in order to maintain cerebral perfusion. This is especially important after cerebral AGE, as cerebral autoregulation of blood flow is lost and cerebral perfusion passively follows systemic blood pressure.

LIDOCAINE

Lidocaine (lignocaine) is a cationic amide used therapeutically as a local anaesthetic and as a class Ib antiarrhythmic agent in ventricular tachyarrhythmias. At therapeutic (non-toxic) levels it has been shown to have the following CNS effects in animal models:

- preservation of neuroelectrical function
- reduction of infarct size
- preservation of brain blood flow
- reduction of brain oedema
- reduction of intracranial pressure.

Possible mechanisms for such cerebral protection include:

- reduction of sodium influx and neuronal depolarization in ischaemic cells
- reduction in cerebral metabolic demand for oxygen

- reduced release of glutamate and other ischaemia-related excitotoxins
- inhibition of leucocyte accumulation and migration.

Maturation of an ischaemic neurological lesion, and particularly ischaemic-reperfusion injury such as is seen in cerebral AGE, will take place over many hours and will involve activation of leucocytes, whose activities may be influenced by lidocaine. It follows that for optimal neuro-protection, lidocaine should be present in adequate concentrations for some time. Since plasma levels of this drug decline rapidly after a single bolus dose, a continuous infusion or repeated bolus doses will be required. With respect to dysbaric disease, there is sufficient evidence and a sufficiently low risk to justify expeditious use of lidocaine in cerebral AGE. Its use should be considered as an adjunct to first-aid oxygen therapy and hyperbaric recompression, but not as an alternative to recompression, unless the latter is unobtainable. The infusion should follow a conventional antiarrhythmic protocol, including electrocardiogram (ECG) monitoring, with a target plasma concentration in the lower half of the therapeutic range, and should be maintained for at least 24 and probably 48 hours.

There is less evidence to support the use of lidocaine in DCI other than AGE. However, there are anecdotal favourable case reports in the literature and the relevant neuroprotective spectrum of action would seem to favour its use in cases with significant neurological symptoms when there is likely to be a time delay in accessing hyperbaric recompression facilities.

ASPIRIN AND NON-STEROIDAL ANTI-INFLAMMATORY DRUGS

Bubbles induce platelet accumulation, adherence and thrombus formation. Consequently, a variety of antiplatelet agents, including aspirin, have been tried both prophylactically and therapeutically in DCI, but without significantly influencing outcome. There is class IIb evidence of benefit for the use of non-selective cyclo-oxygenase (COX) inhibitors in pain-only DCI, in that there appears to be a reduction in the number of recompressions required to achieve complete resolution of symptoms (Bennett et al. 2003). Operationally, the antiplatelet effects adversely affecting outcome in any subsequent trauma outweigh this benefit.

PREVENTION OF DECOMPRESSION ILLNESS

Most altitude exposures are planned to reduce the risk of DCI to a minimum. If DCI does occur, a detailed history of events surrounding the development of the symptoms is necessary to identify any predisposing factors that can be rectified or eliminated.

Risk factors

Exposure profile: the more rapid the rate of ascent and the longer and higher the exposure to altitude, the greater the risk of bubble formation and, hence, the greater the opportunity for DCI to occur.

Recent diving/hyperbaric exposure is likely to have increased the residual inert gas load, particularly if multiple dives have been performed over several days, predisposing to bubble formation during shorter exposures to lower altitudes than would otherwise be predicted.

The risk of DCI increases with increasing age, possibly reflecting alterations in tissue perfusion and inert gas washout. Areas of anatomical change, particularly tissue scarring, may have altered/reduced perfusion and be more susceptible to the effects of any bubble formation. This may also account for the observation that DCI symptoms often recur at sites previously affected (Case study 50.1). Equally, however, regions of reduced perfusion will also have an increased susceptibility to hypoxia at altitude.

Other potential risk factors that need to be considered include the following:

- Gender: females have a proportionally higher body fat content than males and thus are more susceptible to DCI for any given inert gas load.
- Poor aerobic fitness/obesity: increasing body fat content predisposes to DCI.
- Presence of a right-to-left shunt: increases the possibility of arterialization of venous gas emboli and may account for the presentation of symptoms after an otherwise non-provocative exposure.
- A single exposure is likely to generate bubble micronuclei, even if bubbles are not detectable. Repeat exposures will facilitate the development of bubbles around these nuclei and, hence, may predispose to symptoms (Case study 50.2).
- The circulatory turbulence induced by significant physical exertion before or during exposure may also generate micronuclei around which bubbles can form.

Strategies to reduce the risk of decompression illness

Standard schedules and procedures for altitude exposure should be followed, both in training and in operational flights. If operational circumstances force the use of less conservative schedules, then cognisance must be taken of the fact that in aviation DCI will occur when the subjects are on task, with the possibility of mission compromise (in the diving environment DCI usually occurs on return to surface).

Pre-exposure denitrogenation, by breathing 100 per cent oxygen, can be undertaken before provocative exposures or by subjects who know themselves to be susceptible to DCI. Including a period of exercise while oxygen is being breathed can further enhance the inert gas washout by increasing the cardiac output. However, the exercise should be at the beginning of the pre-oxygenation period and should be followed by resting oxygen breathing in order to allow the increased micronuclei generated to clear.

Staging the decompression, where possible, will also reduce the risk of DCI. This strategy, together with pre-oxygenation, is followed by National Aeronautics and Space Administration (NASA) astronauts before extra-vehicular activity (EVA) or spacewalk.

Adequate protection against hypoxia and adequate thermal protection will minimize the circulatory redistribution

---

CASE STUDY 50.1

A 32-year-old long-haul cabin-crew member suffered acute neurological decompression illness (DCI) after a weekend of scuba-diving. Symptoms resolved completely after recompression treatment following RN TT62 with three extensions at 18 m and five further daily treatments following RN TT66.

She was advised not to return to work until cleared to do so by her company medical officer and not to dive for six weeks.

Three weeks later, she flew long-haul as a passenger and during the flight developed paraesthesiae, impaired coordination, fatigue and malaise, which resolved spontaneously over the subsequent 24 hours. She reported no problems on the return flight.

At the six-week diving-clinic review, she had minimal evidence of impaired coordination, which was unchanged following a further RN TT66. In conjunction with her company medical officer, the decision was made to refer her for contrast echocardiography, which revealed a patent foramen ovale (PFO). After successful endovascular closure, she was referred for aviation medical assessment in order to determine her fitness to return to flying duties.

She underwent a two-hour hypobaric chamber 'flight' and on a separate occasion a 12-second rapid decompression from 8000 to 25 000 feet without any recurrence of symptoms and was made fit to return to flying.

CASE STUDY 50.2

A 30-year-old C130 pilot, with 2000 hours' experience, was flying as co-pilot on a sortie that included planned decompressions from 18 000 to 24 000 feet. The crew all went on to oxygen at 8000 feet and the first decompression run was conducted uneventfully. During the second run at 24 000 feet, the co-pilot developed paraesthesiae in both hands, which resolved spontaneously, and a dull ache over his lower back with an abnormal sensation in the overlying skin. These symptoms resolved on recompression to 18 000 feet and the third run was undertaken without any untoward events.

On landing, he reported well. Two and a half hours later, he developed pain in both knees, girdle pain at T12, headache, profound fatigue and a sensation of dizziness on standing.

He was referred for hyperbaric recompression and transferred to the chamber by road, on oxygen. Examination at the chamber was unremarkable, but a diagnosis of joint pain and probable neurological decompression illness (DCI) was made from the history.

Recompression following RN TT62 with three extensions at 18 m resulted in complete resolution of his symptoms. Unfortunately, he experienced a mild relapse of symptoms the following day and required three further daily treatments following RN TT66 until no further symptomatic improvement could be demonstrated.

After discussion at aviation medical review, he declined any further clinical investigations. He was restricted to an altitude of 18 000 feet and UK-based flights only for three months. At his second review, having had no further problems, his altitude restriction was lifted but his geographical restriction was retained. During this period, he was selected for and successfully completed his Captain's course. He had no further problems, and at his third review all restrictions were lifted. Should he experience another episode of DCI at altitude he will require clinical investigation.

---

that may compromise inert gas washout from particular tissues.

Where specific correctable factors are identified in an individual, correction is performed and subsequent controlled altitude exposures reveal no evidence of problems, return to full flying duties with a reduced DCI risk is possible (Case study 50.1). For aviators in whom correctable factors are not identified, aeromedical disposal and return to flying have to be managed on an individual basis (Case study 50.2).

FLYING AFTER DIVING AND AIR TRANSPORT OF THE DIVING CASUALTY

A diver at surface with an inert gas load from recent diving is at increased risk of DCI when exposed to the reduced pressure of a commercial aircraft cabin or unpressurized helicopter. In 1982, the UK Diving Medical Advisory Committee (DMAC) convened a workshop to examine the matter of flying commercial offshore divers back to shore. This group recommended a pre-flight surface interval for both nitrogen- and helium-based diving before ascent to cabin altitudes of 2000 feet and 8000 feet (610 m, 2438 m). They later revised the times conservatively before ascent to 8000 feet (Diving Medical Advisory Committee 2000). A workshop was also convened in 1989 by the Undersea and Hyperbaric Medical Society to address this issue for recreational divers. This workshop suggested a delay of 12

hours after less than two hours of no-stop diving in the preceding 48 hours, a 24-hour delay for multi-day or unlimited diving, and a 48-hour delay after decompression dives (Sheffield 1989). More stringent rules should apply to divers who have been treated successfully for DCI, in order to avoid the risk of precipitating recurrent symptoms. Where a diver has been treated but has residual symptoms, or a casualty with DCI needs to be transported by air, then advice should be obtained from the diving medicine specialist managing the case, but this will usually include the requirement to transport on oxygen and maintain the lowest practicable cabin altitude for the duration of the flight.

REFERENCES

Bennett PB, Moon RE. *Diving Accident Management*. Bethesda, MD: Undersea and Hyperbaric Medical Society, 1990.

Bennett MH, Mitchell SJ, Dominguez A. Adjunctive treatment of decompression illness with a non-steroidal anti-inflammatory drug (tenoxicam) reduces compression requirement. *Undersea and Hyperbaric Medicine* 2003; **30**: 195–205.

Billings CE. Barometric pressure. In: Parker JF, West VR (eds). *Bioastronautics Data Book*. Washington, DC: US Government Printing Office, 1973; pp. 35–63.

Conkin J, Powell MR, Foster PP, Waligora JM. Information about venous gas emboli improves prediction of hypobaric decompression sickness. *Aviation, Space, and Environmental Medicine* 1998; **69**: 8–16.

Cunha-Ferreira RMC. Optimising oral rehydration solution composition for the children of Europe. *Acta Paediatrica Scandinavica* 1989; **364** (suppl.): 31–9.

Diving Medical Advisory Committee. Recommendations for flying after diving. DMAC 07. London: Diving Medical Advisory Committee, 2000.

Elliott DH, Kindwall EP. Manifestations of the decompression disorders. In: Bennett PB, Elliott DH (eds). *The Physiology and Medicine of Diving*, 3rd edn. London: Ballière Tindall, 1982; pp. 461–72.

Francis TJR, Smith DH. Describing decompression illness. Presented at the 42nd Undersea and Hyperbaric Medical Society Workshop, Alverstoke, Gosport, UK, 9–10 October 1991.

Hagen PT, Scholz DG, Edwards WD. Incidence and size of patent foramen ovale during the first 10 decades of life: an autopsy study of 965 normal hearts. *Mayo Clinic Proceedings* 1984; **59**: 17–20.

Hills BA, James PB. Microbubble damage to the blood-brain barrier: relevance to decompression sickness. *Undersea Biomedical Research* 1991; **18**: 111–16.

Ross HE. The direction of apparent movement during transient pressure vertigo. *Undersea Biomedical Research* 1976; **3**: 311–14.

Sheffield PJ. Flying after diving. 77(FLYDIV)12/1/89. Bethesda, MD: Undersea and Hyperbaric Medical Society, 1989.

51

Medication and aircrew

ANTHONY J. BATCHELOR

INTRODUCTION

The explosive development in pharmacological science and technology over the past 30 years has led to the introduction of chemotherapeutic agents with ever greater clinical effectiveness but substantially more benign side-effect profiles than many of their antecedents. Such dramatic advances have had major implications for the medical management of aircrew with a variety of health concerns, with the result that many clinical conditions can now be treated effectively to modern evidence-based standards in pilots, while still permitting a continued useful flying career prospect for these individuals.

In discussing the selection of therapeutic agents that may be used safely in the aviation environment, there is an understandable temptation merely to draw up a list or formulary of acceptable drugs together with indications of any flying limitations that might be appropriate to impose with their use. Indeed, some useful guidelines have been published that adopt such an approach (Silberman 2003). However, such a method has significant limitations. Not only is it challenging to produce a formulary that is both comprehensive and up-to-date, but also such a list takes no account of the details of the patient's underlying condition or comorbidity. For the purposes of this discussion, therefore, such a simplistic approach needs to be modified so that due regard can be given to the circumstances of the individual patient, the natural history of the disorder for which he or she is being treated, and the response to that treatment. Furthermore, it must be flexible enough to take account of the rapid evolution in therapeutics that is taking place in many fields. It is, therefore, more useful to consider a few basic principles rather than to lay down an extensive and rigid framework of rules that are, inevitably destined to be outdated rapidly, and then to examine these in the context of some common clinical scenarios.

PRINCIPLES

The management of most acute conditions requiring short-term drug therapy will naturally require a break from the demands of a profession characterized by the daily need to maintain vigilance and rapid response times in a complex task environment. Thus, short courses of antibiotics, anti-inflammatory drugs and analgesics will usually be in response to symptoms that are accompanied, appropriately, by a brief period of grounding. A return to flying will be dependent on resolution of the underlying condition, by which time drug treatment will have been completed or possible side effects (e.g. from a continuing course of antibiotics) will have become evident.

However, the introduction of longer-term drug treatment for any condition in the aviator brings a range of possible concerns into focus. The potential for adverse career implications to be associated with the need for chronic therapy requires that due concern should be given, without ever prejudicing the most effective and evidence-based management of the patient, to ensuring that an adequate and legitimate indication exists for the introduction of such treatment. Furthermore, long-term therapy introduced for any reason not only must be shown to be effective in achieving the desired results in the short term, but also needs to be effectively monitored in the long term.

There is an obligation to ensure that there are no class side effects of the agent that would be unacceptable in the flying environment, the focus being particularly on those influences that might produce subtle impairments of psychomotor function, vigilance or disturbances of the special senses. The possibility of individual idiosyncratic drug responses must also be borne in mind and, for these reasons, it is appropriate to insist on a period of grounding at the start of treatment. This would normally be for a minimum of two weeks, until the treatment is shown not only to be producing the desired effect but also to be free from any undesirable side effects. As in any clinical situation, compatibility with other treatments is a consideration when introducing new drug treatment, and the necessity for a simple drug regimen in professional aviators cannot be overemphasized.

Ideally, a once-daily scheme of drug administration should be the aim, as compliance inevitably tends to be compromised by the irregular work pattern of aircrew. Complex regimens that demand the ingestion of chemotherapeutic agents at intervals more frequent than every 12 hours will rarely be adhered to in a profession where constantly changing work patterns are further challenged by the possibility of repeated time zone changes. There is also much to be said for limiting the dose of drugs to the lowest compatible with producing the desired response rather than increasing the dose of any single agent to the limit and risking side effects; in many situations, the introduction of a multi-drug approach may be appropriate. The modern management of hypertension is an excellent example of such a principle, but this is not unique. Naturally, situations where the sudden withdrawal of a drug could be dangerous (because of either rebound effects or rapid relapse of disease) should be avoided in aviators.

Finally, a cautious approach should be taken with the use of newly released drugs in the treatment of aircrew. Conservative management strategies using agents with well-proven track records are usually preferable until experience is gained in the general, non-pilot, population.

GENERAL PROBLEMS

Few drugs have been tested thoroughly in the aviation environment, and studies attempting to eliminate adverse effects on psychomotor performance, or to identify interactions with the physiological challenges of the flight environment, would be prohibitively costly if extended to all new therapeutic agents. However, the undesirable effects of modern drugs are explored more vigorously in the litigious environment of today than in years past, so that most modern agents have been studied extensively before marketing. Nevertheless, drugs that appear to be entirely satisfactory on the ground may still be associated with unexpected side effects in aircrew; such side effects can be extremely subtle, so decrements of performance can easily go unrecognized.

SPECIFIC PROBLEMS OF DRUG THERAPY

Antihypertensive agents

Drugs of this class are prescribed very commonly in the community. They have potential influences on flying performance, which need further consideration. They are discussed in detail in Chapter 38.

Lipid-lowering drugs

Hyperlipidaemia is a common cardiovascular risk factor. The number of prescriptions for 3-hydroxy-3-methylglutaryl coenzyme A (HMG-CoA) reductase inhibitors (statins) has been increasing exponentially in recent years, fuelled by the ever more robust evidence for the effectiveness of this class of cholesterol-lowering agents in both secondary and primary prevention of vascular disease. In the UK there are now two statins available for purchase without prescription, and when these drugs were first introduced, the possibility of subtle psychological side effects was a distinct concern. However, as trial evidence accumulated, it became clear that the excess of violent deaths among those taking active treatment in the earlier reports represented a statistical blip that was not supported by the many subsequent trials. Nevertheless, an influence on sleep patterns and memory was evident in some studies, raising questions as to the potential for these agents to impact on performance in the complex flying environment, where sleep/wake cycles were frequently challenging. Despite these concerns, however, the large accumulated experience has shown the statins to be a remarkably safe group of agents, and formal testing of vigilance and cognitive function on simulated flying tasks has been reassuring (Gibellato et al. 2001). In the absence of other contraindications, pilots may be allowed to fly without restriction while taking statins (see Chapter 41).

Diabetes mellitus and hypoglycaemic agents

The frequent incidence of hypoglycaemia, with its rapidly evolving and profound effects on central nervous function, renders insulin-treated diabetes mellitus entirely incompatible with professional flying. This observation extends to private flying in all but a few countries, where highly selected cases, subject to strict monitoring, are permitted to fly under tightly controlled conditions. Of the oral agents used in the management of type 2 diabetes, the alpha-glucosidase inhibitor acarbose is free from systemic effects, as it acts on the small intestine to regulate glucose absorption. For people who can tolerate the gastrointestinal side effects, this agent may be used in the flying environment without restriction. The biguanide metformin is the usual drug of first choice when diet and lifestyle modification fail to provide adequate glycaemic control and has the advantage of being free of significant risk of induced hypoglycaemia. This drug is, therefore, regarded as acceptable for professional flying in the multi-crew environment. The same advantages do not extend to the sulphonylurea group of agents, all of which – even the short-acting varieties – are associated with a significant risk of hypoglycaemia. The thiazolidinediones are, theoretically, an attractive second line of therapy for the aviator, but concerns that they might induce hypoglycaemia when used in the usual combination with metformin have yet to be resolved. The use of these drugs is discussed in detail in Chapter 41.

H1–antihistamines

The management of common allergic conditions in aircrew was substantially enhanced over 20 years ago by the introduction of antihistamines that were free from sedative effects. However, experience has shown that although some drugs may initially appear to be entirely safe, despite being tested to ensure lack of side effects relevant to the flight environment, unexpected and undesirable side effects can still become apparent, even after many years of use. The H1-antihistamine terfenadine is an excellent example of this phenomenon. This drug was used widely in the aviation medicine community from the early 1980s because of its effectiveness as an antihistamine, while being free of detectable hypnotic or sedative qualities. However, the drug has since been withdrawn because it is associated with a risk of precipitating episodes of life-threatening ventricular arrhythmias. This risk is now understood to be mediated by an influence on the rapid component of the delayed rectifier potassium current of myocardial cells, resulting in a prolongation of the QT interval on the electrocardiograph (ECG) and an enhanced risk of ventricular tachycardia, classically of the torsades de pointes variety (Simons 2004). While this risk is small, it is amplified by concurrent administration of other agents that compete for, or inhibit, the hepatic cytochrome P450-dependent metabolic pathway, including common macrolide antibiotics, some antifungal agents and even grapefruit juice. This phenomenon is not a class effect, but neither is it confined to terfenadine (astemizole has similar effects), and few of the H1-antihistamines are now considered entirely safe for use in the aviation environment. The exceptions that are currently accepted are loratadine,

des-loratidine and, possibly, fexofenadine (Nicholson *et al.* 2000).

Anticoagulants

Even in the most encouraging series, serious complication rates of less than two per cent per annum have been documented infrequently in patients taking oral anticoagulants. Furthermore, the risk of the underlying disease for which anticoagulation is indicated has to be considered, rendering the achievement of aeromedically acceptable total event rates in such cases even more challenging. Using the example of warfarin taken by subjects with mechanical prosthetic heart valves, the risks of thromboembolism and valve failure have to be added to the haemorrhage risk before the true event risk of the clinical situation can be appreciated. In one large follow-up study involving 6475 patient-years, the serious haemorrhage rate for such subjects was 2.7 per cent per annum, while the rate of cerebral embolism in the same group was 0.7 per cent (Cannegieter *et al.* 1995). Such studies have helped to define the optimal level of anticoagulation, expressed as international normalized ratio (INR), in order to achieve the ideal balance between the risks of haemorrhage and thrombosis, but an extensive review also acknowledges that the quality of anticoagulant monitoring and control can further influence this risk (Schulman 2003). Tighter control of the INR range in any individual will reduce the serious haemorrhage risk, and there are indications that this may be achievable with near-patient testing using portable INR-meters. Progress in this area may allow a re-examination of aeromedical certification and anticoagulant use in the future, but the dramatic nature of the possible complications dictate that caution is required, and currently the combination must be regarded as incompatible with flying status.

Antiarrhythmic agents

The management of cardiac dysrhythmias is discussed in detail in Chapter 37. The classes of drugs that can be considered as suitable in this situation for use in pilots are limited. Beta-blockers and sotalol may be acceptable for restricted flying under specific circumstances in pilots with paroxysmal atrial fibrillation, but few other drugs will normally be considered permissible. The pro-arrhythmic potential of many drugs, such as the class 1c agents, will rarely be acceptable for professional flying, and the ophthalmic side effects of amiodarone preclude most pilots using this otherwise effective drug from being considered for certification. Furthermore, the failure of a large follow-up study to demonstrate a survival advantage for people in whom sinus rhythm is maintained with drug therapy has weakened the clinical indications for such drugs (Wyse *et al.* 2002), and increasing emphasis is being directed on the rapid developments in intracardiac electrophysiological ablation techniques.

Anticonvulsants

Epilepsy, for self-evident reasons, is disqualifying for flying. However, anticonvulsant drugs are also used in the management of conditions other than epilepsy, particularly in neuralgic pain syndromes. The nature of these disorders makes it unlikely that they would be considered compatible with flying in most cases, but even if the condition is managed successfully with anticonvulsant agents, the risk of relapse and central effects from these drugs makes a return to flying inappropriate.

Psychotropic drugs

Currently, no drugs of this class are acceptable for professional flying. However, a vigorous debate is taking place in the aviation medicine community concerning the use of selective serotonin reuptake inhibitors (SSRIs) for the treatment of mild recurrent depression. Not only is this a common disorder in the general population, but anonymous surveys have suggested that a substantial proportion of pilots with the condition either avoid declaring and treating recurrent episodes or take SSRIs without informing the regulatory authority. It has been argued that appropriately monitored treatment for aircrew with depression, without automatic denial of certification, might be a considerably safer alternative to undeclared and unmonitored drug use or continued flying in pilots with untreated relapses (Jones and Ireland 2004).

Immunosuppressants

Many clinical conditions requiring therapy with immunosuppressant drugs will be incompatible with flying in their own right. However, the use of such agents in low doses to control conditions that have little capacity to challenge the functional performance of the aviator may be encountered, and each will require to be assessed on its merits. Psoriasis, uncomplicated by functionally significant arthropathy and controlled with low doses of an agent such as methotrexate might be one example, as would be chronic active hepatitis controlled on low-dose steroids (not exceeding prednisolone 10 mg daily) in symptom-free subjects with normal hepatic function. Freedom from drug-related side effects, control of the underlying disease process and close monitoring would be requirements in all cases. Conditions that could be associated with the sudden onset of symptoms if relapse occurred (e.g. temporal arteritis) would need to be excluded.

Antimalarial prophylaxis

The professional activities of many civil and military pilots take them to parts of the world where chemoprophylaxis against malaria is required. While the selection of agent will be guided by the local pattern of drug resistance, not all potential choices are compatible with flying duties, and caution is needed. Chloroquine and proguanil, while far from being free from side effects, have long been the mainstay of chemoprophylaxis in aviators and have proved remarkably safe. However, with the emergence of ever more chloroquine-resistant strains of malaria, the use of other agents is increasingly required. Doxycycline is a useful drug and is free of class effects that would preclude its use in pilots. Encouraging data have also been published on the combination of atavoquine and proguanil suggesting it is free from adverse influences on psychomotor performance (Paul *et al.* 2003). This drug combination also has the advantage of requiring an interval of only 24 hours following ingestion of the first dose before useful protection is achieved, particularly valuable in situations requiring sudden unexpected travel to malarial areas. Mefloquine has proved to be a valuable agent for prophylaxis in some areas of chloroquine resistance. However, while some uncontrolled studies have produced conflicting results, there is enough documented evidence of significant neuropsychiatric side effects from this agent, with an incidence reported as 11.8 per cent overall and disabling in 0.7 per cent in one study (Barrett *et al.* 1996), to render the drug unacceptable for use by aviators. The problems of malaria treatment and prophylaxis are covered in more detail in Chapter 55.

Treatment of erectile dysfunction

The professional pilot population contains large numbers of middle-aged men in whom concerns over failing erectile function are not uncommon. The management of such cases requires identification and treatment of underlying conditions such as diabetes and peripheral vascular disease, together with the addressing of psychological problems. Indeed, in older pilots, it has been suggested that coronary artery disease should be positively excluded in those presenting with erectile difficulties, given the known association with vascular disease in this group (Grossman *et al.* 2004). In recent years, the availability of treatment with phosphodiesterase inhibitors has provided an effective solution for increasing numbers of patients suffering with such symptoms, and aircrew suffering erectile problems naturally are anxious to have access to such therapy.

The primary action of these agents is to inhibit the breakdown of cyclic guanosine monophosphate (cGMP), produced under the influence of nitric oxide released in the corpora cavernosa. This in turn is responsible for vascular smooth-muscle relaxation via its influence on intracellular calcium levels. Of the more commonly reported side effects of this expanding class of drugs, headache, rhinitis and disturbances of colour vision all have potential relevance in the aviation medicine sphere; fortunately, these are relatively short-lived and usually mild. Avoiding flying for a period of 12 hours after using drugs of this class should be advised and should avoid any aeromedical risk.

Prostatism and alpha-blocking agents

Another relatively common affliction of the mature male population, and to which pilots are certainly not immune, is benign prostatic hypertrophy. For those in whom surgery is not indicated, alpha-blocking agents have proved moderately effective in controlling the urinary symptoms in the short to medium term. However, for the same reasons that this class of drugs is not acceptable in pilots with hypertension, most alpha-blockers used for this indication are not compatible with professional flying status. The risk of orthostatic hypotension that is common with these agents does, however, appear to be a rare accompaniment of the prostate-selective drug tamsulosin (De Mey et al. 1998). Therefore, provided an adequate period of observation with lying and standing blood pressure estimations on the ground confirms the absence of any significant postural blood pressure drop in subjects taking this agent, it may be possible to consider a return to professional flying in a multi-crew environment (see Chapter 42).

OTHER POTENTIAL PITFALLS

Over-the-counter drugs

An increasing range of drugs is becoming available for purchase without prescription, more so in some countries than others. The potential aeromedical risks of taking agents so readily available to the public are unlikely to be appreciated by many and yet may be very real. Commonly available analgesic combinations, for example, frequently include codeine, an opioid with significant central effects. The need for aircrew to adopt a cautious approach to self-medication, and for them to be educated to seek appropriate advice before self-treatment, cannot be overemphasized. Even prescribed drugs call for a similar approach before a return to flying if the health practitioner involved has no experience of the requirements for private or professional flying.

Complementary medicines

There is a widespread conception among the non-medical public that complementary and herbal medicines are 'natural' and, therefore, safe from concerns over unwanted side effects. Many such preparations, however, contain pharmacologically active ingredients with the potential to produce unwanted effects and may also have the potential for significant interactions with prescribed medication.

Drug compliance and time zones

Compliance with prescribed drug regimens is an inevitable issue with aircrew, who lead irregular lives with ever-changing duty times. Wherever possible, once-daily medication should be provided. On long-haul operations involving transmeridian flights, medication should be taken according to base time where possible. Such advice is equally relevant for airline passengers with conditions such as epilepsy or diabetes, which require critical control of drug timing, and should be maintained until they reach their destination.

CONCLUSION

The aviator needs to be aware of his or her responsibility to seek advice from authoritative sources whenever the initiation of drug therapy is contemplated. Furthermore, rather like the professional athlete, he or she needs to reflect very carefully before taking any agent that might have active pharmacological properties, no matter how innocuous the substance may appear. With appropriate precautions and advice, however, it is gratifying to acknowledge that many of the advances of modern medicine are now available for inclusion in the healthcare of professional pilots without compromise to their continued active flying careers.

REFERENCES

Barrett PJ, Emmins PD, Clarke PD, Bradley DJ. Comparison of adverse effects associated with the use of mefloquine and combination of chloroquine and proguanil as antimalarial prophylaxis: postal and telephone survey of travellers. British Medical Journal 1996; 313: 525–8.

Cannegieter SC, Rosendaal FER, Wintzen AR, et al. Optimal oral anticoagulant therapy in patients with mechanical heart valves. New England Journal of Medicine 1995; 333: 11–17.

De Mey C, Michel MC, McEwen J, Moreland T. A double-blind comparison of terazosin and tamsulosin on their different effects on ambulatory blood pressure and nocturnal othostatic stress testing. *European Urology* 1998; 33: 481–8.

Gibellato MG, Moore JL, Selby K, *et al*. Effects of lovastatin and pravastatin on cognitive function in military aircrew. *Aviation, Space, and Environmental Medicine* 2001; 72: 805–12.

Grossman A, Barenboim E, Azaria B, *et al*. Oral drug therapy for erectile dysfunction: overview and aeromedical implications. *Aviation, Space, and Environmental Medicine* 2004; 75: 997–1000.

Jones DR, Ireland RR. Aeromedical regulation of aviators using selective serotonin reuptake inhibitors for depressive disorders. *Aviation, Space, and Environmental Medicine* 2004; 75: 461–70.

Nicholson AN, Stone BM, Turner C, Mills SL. Antihistamines and aircrew: usefulness of fexofenadine. *Aviation, Space, and Environmental Medicine* 2000; 71: 2–6.

Paul MA, McCarthy AE, Gibson N, *et al*. The impact of Malarone and primaquine on psychomotor performance. *Aviation, Space, and Environmental Medicine* 2003; 74: 738–45.

Schulman S. Care of patients receiving long-term anticoagulant therapy. *New England Journal of Medicine* 2003; 349: 675–83.

Silberman WS. Medications in civil aviation: what is acceptable and what is not? *Aviation, Space, and Environmental Medicine* 2003; 74: 85–6.

Simons FER. Advances in H1-antihistamines. *New England Journal of Medicine* 2004; 351: 2203–17.

Wyse DG, Waldo AL, DiMarco JP, *et al*. A comparison of rate control and rhythm control in patients with atrial fibrillation. *New England Journal of Medicine* 2002; 347: 1825–33.

FURTHER READING

Ediger E, Benson A, Danese D, *et al*. Medication for military aircrew: current use, issues, and strategies for expanded options. NATO/RTO technical report 14. Neuilly-sur-Seine: RTO/NATO, 2001.

52

Aviator fatigue and relevant fatigue countermeasures

JOHN A. CALDWELL

BACKGROUND

Pilot fatigue from long duty periods, unpredictable work hours, circadian disruptions and sleep restriction has become a significant risk factor in modern civilian and military aviation operations (Neville et al. 1994; Samel et al. 1995). This is due in part to the fact that an escalation in the demand for aviation services has occurred in tandem with large-scale corporate and military workforce reductions. As a result, the present contingent of pilots faces serious fatigue-related difficulties associated with increased time pressure, greater workloads and heightened scheduling demands. While the full impact of this situation is presently unclear, accident statistics, aviator surveys and expert opinions indicate that aircrew fatigue is a significant problem that poses a serious threat to flight safety.

Statistics

A US National Transportation Safety Board (NTSB; 1994) study of major domestic air-carrier accidents from 1978 through 1990 concluded that extended duty/wakefulness periods are associated with more errors overall and significantly more procedural and tactical decision errors in commercial flights. Kirsch (1996) calculated that fatigue may be responsible for four to seven per cent of civil aviation mishaps, although there are recent indications that this may be an underestimation. Statistics compiled by the US Air Force Safety Center suggest that 7.8 per cent of the reportable class A Air Force mishaps over the past 30 years have been, at least to some extent, attributable to fatigue (Luna 2003).

Survey data

Survey data indicate that tired pilots are having an adverse effect on flight safety. Petrie and Dawson (1997) reported that international commercial aircrews consider fatigue-related sleepiness and lethargy, cognitive slowness, concentration difficulties and irritability to be serious concerns in long-haul flight operations. Bourgeois-Bougrine et al. (2003) found that short-haul (domestic) pilots frequently complained of schedule-related sleep deprivation. Among regional airline pilots and corporate/executive pilots (who typically engage in shorter-duration flights), fatigue has been identified as a moderate to serious safety concern, and approximately three-quarters of survey respondents from these groups admitted to having actually nodded off during a flight as a result of excessive fatigue (Co et al. 1999; Rosekind et al. 2000). Within the military, Caldwell and Gilreath (2002) reported that US Army helicopter pilots and crews frequently blamed inadequate sleep and/or insufficient sleep quality for impaired on-the-job alertness; like their commercial counterparts, they indicated that fatigue in general was a significant problem. K.G. Cornum (personal communication, 1994) reported that during Operation Desert Storm, Air Force F-15 pilots routinely experienced significant alertness impairments from the circadian disruptions and sleep deprivation produced by around-the-clock task demands and minimal recovery periods.

Expert consensus

In light of such evidence, it is little wonder that sleep and fatigue experts have voiced strong opinions regarding the need to acknowledge fully the impact of fatigue on air safety and to systematically implement scientifically sound fatigue countermeasures. It has been noted that 'fatigue (sleepiness, tiredness) is the largest identifiable and preventable cause of accidents in transport operations (between 15 and 20% of all accidents), surpassing that of alcohol- or drug-related incidents in all modes' and that 'official statistics often underestimate this contribution' (Akerstedt 2000). Thus, it is clear that aviator fatigue cannot be ignored. However, it is equally clear that the performance and alertness of pilots and crews can be enhanced by applying the scientific knowledge of fatigue, sleep, shift work and circadian physiology that has been gained over the past 40 years but that has not been transitioned effectively into operational practices (Dinges *et al.* 1996).

ALERTNESS-MANAGEMENT TECHNIQUES

Scheduling demands and human physiology are at the centre of fatigue-related problems in aviation. Humans simply were not designed to cope effectively with the multiple flight legs, long duty hours, limited time off, early report times, less-than-optimal sleeping conditions, rotating and non-standard work shifts and jet lag that have become the hallmarks of today's flight operations. Whether conducting short-haul commercial flights, long-range transoceanic operations or around-the-clock military missions, a well-planned, science-based alertness-management strategy is critical for countering the acute sleep loss/sleep debt, the sustained periods of wakefulness, and the circadian factors that are primary contributors to fatigue-related flight mishaps (Rosekind *et al.* 1996). The strategies summarized below will contribute to improved safety, performance and productivity in a variety of operational contexts. Unfortunately, there is no one-size-fits-all solution to pilot fatigue. However, a comprehensive programme that takes into account human physiological makeup, unique mission characteristics and the specific requirements of available alertness-management techniques can optimize safety in operational contexts.

Alertness-management strategies can be classified broadly into two major categories: non-pharmacological and pharmacological. Generally speaking, it is best to utilize the non-pharmacological approaches until there is evidence that uncontrollable operational factors are rendering these techniques ineffective or unfeasible. Once this occurs, pharmacological strategies can be implemented without hesitation, provided that such options are allowed under current regulatory guidance and there is sufficient medical oversight to ensure proper dispensing and administration of approved medications.

Non-pharmacological strategies

The most palatable measures for the prevention or remedy of operator sleepiness/fatigue often are those of a non-pharmacological nature. These measures generally are viewed as benign and natural ways of improving on-the-job alertness, since they do not require 'medical' intervention. Non-pharmacological strategies generally include administrative/regulatory approaches (education, schedules, work-hour restrictions) and behavioural interventions (breaks and/or naps), but some environmental countermeasures (bright lights) occasionally are included as well. In the context of the present discussion, only the non-pharmacological techniques backed up by some degree of scientific validation will be emphasized.

EDUCATION

Studies have demonstrated that sleep restrictions of as little as one to two hours per day rapidly compromise vigilance and performance in subsequent duty periods (Belenky *et al.* 2003; Van Dongen *et al.* 2003). Thus, it is critical that aviation personnel be educated about the dangers of fatigue and the importance of acquiring adequate sleep. Ultimately, the pilots themselves and the staff scheduling the pilots' duty periods must be convinced that quality off-duty sleep is the best possible anti-fatigue strategy. Aircrews should be taught that (i) fatigue is a physiological problem that cannot be overcome by motivation, training or willpower; (ii) people cannot reliably judge their own level of fatigue-related impairment; (iii) there are wide individual differences in fatigue susceptibility, which cannot be predicted reliably; and (iv) there is no one-size-fits-all 'magic bullet' (other than adequate sleep) that can counter fatigue for every person in every situation. In addition, they should be advised that (i) adequate off-duty sleep is the key to optimal on-the-job alertness; (ii) an average of eight hours of sleep per day, either in a consolidated block or in a series of naps, is the goal, even during long trips or on rotating schedules; and (iii) the 'good sleep habits' summarized in Table 52.1 are essential for maximizing sleep quantity and quality (Caldwell and Caldwell 2003).

ON-BOARD SLEEP

For some commercial and military flight operations, in-flight, out-of-cockpit sleep is permitted when an augmented crew (at least three pilots) is on board, and on-board rest facilities are available (in the USA, augmented crews are mandated for commercial long-haul flights of more than 12 hours' duration). This provision offers pilots an opportunity to partially attenuate the increased homeostatic sleep drive that occurs due to the longer duty period between takeoffs and landings on long-

Table 52.1 *Good sleep habits*

- Stick to a consistent wakeup and bedtime every day of the week when possible
- Use the bedroom only for sleep and sex
- Resolve daily dilemmas outside of the sleep area
- Engage in a consistent getting-ready-for-bed routine as often as possible
- Establish an aerobic exercise routine and stick to it
- Create a quiet and comfortable sleep environment whenever possible
- Use a sleep mask to block out environmental light
- Minimize disturbing environmental noises with a fan or earplugs
- Don't consume caffeine within four hours of bedtime
- Don't use alcohol as a sleep aid, because it disrupts the normal sleep process
- Don't take naps during the day if you are having difficulties sleeping at night*
- Don't smoke cigarettes immediately before bed

*This does not apply to strategic naps used specifically to compensate for insufficient consolidated sleep.

duration flights (Rosekind *et al.* 2000). On transoceanic flights, one of the pilots in a three-person crew and two of the pilots comprising a four-person crew can leave the cockpit during the cruise segment of the flight in order to gain some in-flight sleep while another pilot or pilots fly the aircraft. In some military operations, a modified strategy may be implemented in multi-crew aircraft. For instance, in the case of the B-2 bomber, in which the maximum crew complement is only two, one of the pilots may sleep in a cot located behind the seats during low-workload flight phases while the other pilot maintains control of the aircraft. Such in-flight sleep is an absolutely essential tool for B-2 missions, which often remain aloft for 44 continuous hours. Clearly, on-board crew sleep is an important aviation fatigue countermeasure in any situation, military or civilian, involving flights of longer than 10–12 hours' duration. Although the quality of on-board sleep may not equal that which would be obtained in a normal home setting (Rosekind *et al.* 2000), it is nevertheless profoundly beneficial in comparison with an extended period of continuous wakefulness.

COCKPIT NAPS

A strategy related to on-board crew rest is the cockpit nap in which one pilot actually sleeps in his or her cockpit seat, rather than moving to another part of the aircraft, while the other pilot assumes command of the flight deck. National Aeronautics and Space Administration (NASA) studies on commercial pilots have shown that cockpit naps averaging approximately 30 minutes in duration are both safe and effective (Rosekind *et al.* 1995). As a result, many

international airlines, including those of the UK but not of the USA, currently take advantage of cockpit napping in order to promote or maintain flight-crew alertness on long flights. Specific cockpit-napping procedures vary as a function of the airline and the governing organization, the crew complement on board, and other factors, but on British carriers a nap duration of 30 minutes, followed by a recovery period of 20 minutes, is recommended (for circumstances in which napping is permitted).[1] In some military operations (US and others), cockpit naps are used in multi-crew aircraft as long as another alert pilot is at the controls. Although cockpit napping is not as beneficial as on-board sleep in a designated out-of-cockpit facility, it is nonetheless an effective strategy for partially attenuating the increased sleepiness that accompanies extended periods of continuous wakefulness.

CONTROLLED REST BREAKS

The liberal distribution of rest breaks is recommended as a method to provide short-term relief from boredom and fatigue, especially during long, tedious and repetitive tasks (Rosa 1995). Pilots often use some type of rest-break strategy (chatting, standing up, walking around, etc.) in order to sustain alertness during lengthy flights. Although controlled studies of the efficacy of this countermeasure in aviation contexts are scarce, Neri *et al.* (2002) reported that Boeing 747 pilots who were offered brief hourly breaks during a six-hour simulated night flight showed significant post-break reductions in slow eye movements, theta-band electroencephalogram (EEG) activity, unintended sleep episodes and subjective sleepiness for up to 15–25 minutes. Benefits were particularly noticeable near the time of the circadian trough. Along similar lines, Caldwell *et al.* (2003a) found that simply assuming a more upright posture, as opposed to remaining seated, reduced the amount of slow-wave EEG activity and enhanced performance on a ten-minute vigilance task during the later part of a 28-hour sleep-deprivation cycle. Although no information was provided on how long alertness was improved following this manipulation, it is certainly possible that posture-related benefits contributed to the positive effects of rest breaks found earlier by Neri *et al.* (2002). Thus, simply walking off the flight deck for a few minutes each hour during long-duration flights can provide at least a brief respite from operator fatigue.

---

[1]The 20-minute recovery period is designed to give the pilot time to recover from any sleep-inertia (post-nap grogginess) that may be present on awakening. Sleep inertia is a common experience when awakening from sleep. The magnitude of sleep inertia is thought to be a function of the amount of prior wakefulness, the depth of sleep that was obtained and, possibly, the time of day at which the sleep period occurred. However, most scientists agree that sufficient recovery in most cases occurs within 20–30 minutes.

PROPER CREW WORK–REST SCHEDULING

One method for improving aircrew sleep and alertness is to devise and implement crew schedules that consider the realities of the homeostatic and circadian sleep/alertness mechanisms. However, both airline-pilot schedulers and military-pilot schedulers traditionally have minimized or ignored these factors and have focused instead on time-on-task restrictions in order to reduce boredom effects, etc. Complex regulations limiting the number of hours that pilots can work and fly have been implemented throughout the world, and these regulations have been valuable. Goode (2003) showed that longer continuous duty periods are associated with an increase in accident risk (pilots working 13 or more hours were five times more likely to be involved in a mishap). Thus, it is important to regulate aircrew duty periods. However, flight-time limits alone have not protected aircrews adequately from the dangers of fatigue. Although this prescriptive approach is attractive to managers and schedulers because it is relatively easy to establish and monitor, it fails to account for the complex physiological factors that underlie human performance, such as the quality and quantity of pre-duty sleep, the duration of continuous wakefulness, circadian peaks and troughs, disturbances to the body's internal clock, and a variety of other important factors. It is difficult to integrate fully such complexities into flight schedules, which are often driven by passenger demands and/or mission deadlines. However, this difficulty is being mitigated to some extent by the development of computerized scheduling tools such as the Fatigue Avoidance Scheduling Tool (FAST) (Hursh et al. 2004) and the System for Aircrew Fatigue Evaluation (SAFE) (Belyavin and Spencer 2004). These software tools predict alertness decrements and optimal sleep times based on factors such as the amount of continuous wakefulness, the circadian phase and the quality of recovery sleep. Armed with this information, schedulers can devise work/rest options that minimize crew fatigue and maximize operational efficiency and safety. Although computerized scheduling aids have not been validated fully across a wide range of aviation settings, they are being used in some operational contexts with great success.

MELATONIN AS A CHRONOBIOTIC

In aviation operations involving rapid schedule changes, the administration of melatonin may help to overcome jet lag and shift lag. There is a substantial amount of research to indicate that appropriate administration of this hormone can improve circadian adaptation to new time schedules (Arendt et al. 1995). There is also evidence that melatonin possesses weak hypnotic or 'soporific' properties that may facilitate out-of-phase sleep (Sack et al. 1998; Wirz-Justice and Armstrong 1996). One strategy for using melatonin to adjust to eastward transitions of eight or more hours is to ingest 5 mg at 1800–1900 local time on the day of departure and subsequently to ingest 5 mg melatonin at 2200–2300 for four nights after arriving in the new time zone.[2] A strategy for adjusting to westward transitions is to avoid pre-departure melatonin but to take 5 mg melatonin at 2300 local bedtime for four nights after arriving at the destination (Arendt and Deacon 1997). However, in both cases, users must be cautioned that melatonin-related sleepiness could interfere with the performance of complex tasks if these tasks occur shortly after the administration time. In the USA, melatonin is not considered a drug and is available widely both to commercial pilots and to military aviators. Generally speaking, US civil aviators can use it with few restrictions, but it has not been authorized for military use. In the UK, procurement of melatonin is more difficult, since it is considered a drug rather than a food supplement. British civil aviators and military aircrews are not authorized to self-administer this substance. Melatonin's primary drawback is that it can produce negative effects on alertness and performance if its administration is not timed properly, and most potential users likely possess insufficient knowledge about circadian rhythms and/or endogenous melatonin secretion to make the best decisions in this regard. Caldwell (2000) has concluded that 'currently, melatonin use is unacceptable for aviators'.

BRIGHT LIGHT AS A CIRCADIAN RESYNCHRONIZER

As an alternative to melatonin, some studies have shown that properly timed bright light can facilitate circadian resynchronization after schedule changes (Daan and Lewy 1984; Gander et al. 1989; Samel and Wegmann 1997). However, at present, there remains debate over the optimal levels of light exposure and whether personnel are able to readily determine the appropriate times at which bright light exposures should occur. Lewy et al. (1988) discuss the use of both melatonin and light in order to adjust circadian rhythms, and this detailed reference should be consulted in an effort to maximize the success of using either strategy. The difficulties in appropriate timing of both methods suggest that perhaps the safest self-administered strategy for jet-lagged pilots seeking to adjust to new schedules is simply to take advantage of naps and local time cues when possible (Waterhouse et al. 1997). Natural light exposure is most readily useable by westward travellers after transitions of up to eight hours; in this situation, it is reasonably clear that sunlight in the evening will promote adjustment to the new time zone. For eastward transitions, the proper timing of light exposure is far more complex, and incorrect timing can prolong the adaptation period (Waterhouse et

---

[2]Note that this eastward adaptation strategy cannot be used by pilots flying an aircraft during west–east flights because the soporific properties of melatonin will likely impair alertness and performance.

al. 1997). For pilots, who are likely suffering from shift lag as well as jet lag, the best strategy may be simply to avoid light exposure (or minimize it with very dark glasses) before a period of daytime sleep. Also, it should be noted that since aviation personnel often remain in the new time zone or on the new work shift only temporarily, attempts at adaptation may not be beneficial.

Pharmacological strategies

As noted previously, adequate daily sleep is the primary key to optimum alertness in the aviation environment. Educational efforts, good sleep hygiene, on-board bunk rest and cockpit naps are focused on preventing sleep deprivation in operational contexts. Well-designed crew schedules ensure that sleep opportunities occur at favourable points in the circadian cycle, and both melatonin and bright-light therapy help to attenuate bodyclock disruptions known to impair or prevent adequate pre-mission or recovery sleep. The comprehensive application of all of these strategies will solve a large percentage of the fatigue-related problems in aviation. However, in situations where the non-pharmacological approaches are either not feasible or not sufficient, as is sometimes the case in military or emergency operations, pharmacological fatigue countermeasures should be considered.

Medication-based options are useful for (i) optimizing sleep opportunities when such opportunities are available but difficult to utilize and (ii) sustaining alertness in the face of unavoidable sleep deprivation. In aviation settings, where there is a high degree of medical oversight, such drug-based avenues are both safe and effective. Both the US military and the Royal Air Force (RAF) have approved the use of certain hypnotics to optimize the sleep of their aircrew. In the US military, although not in the RAF, the use of stimulants for aircrew has also been authorized. The present discussion will include information on the compounds that are currently authorized under US Air Force policy for preventing or mitigating severe fatigue in specific operational contexts.[3]

SLEEP-PROMOTING COMPOUNDS

Sleep is often difficult to obtain in operational contexts, even in situations where efforts have been made to ensure the existence of adequate sleep opportunities. There are a number of reasons for this, but generally speaking the difficulties are due to the fact that (i) the sleep environment is less than optimal (too noisy, too hot, uncomfortable), (ii) the state of the individual is incompatible with the ability to sleep (too much excitement, apprehension, anxiety) or (iii) the sleep opportunity occurs at a time that is not biologically conducive to rapid sleep onset and/or sufficient sleep maintenance due to shift lag or jet lag. For such circumstances, the US Air Force and the US Army have approved the limited use of temazepam, zolpidem and zaleplon. These hypnotics can optimize the quality of crew rest in circumstances where sleep is possible but difficult to obtain. The choice of which compound is best for each circumstance must take several factors into account, including time of day, half-life of the compound, length of the sleep period, and the probability of an earlier-than-expected awakening. However, appropriate hypnotic therapy is clearly a valuable adjunct to the non-pharmacological strategies discussed previously.

Temazepam

Temazepam (15–30 mg) may be the best choice for optimizing eight-hour sleep periods that are out of phase with the body's circadian cycle because, under these circumstances, sleep is often easy to initiate but difficult to maintain due to the circadian rise in alertness. Personnel who work at night often fall asleep easily after the work shift, since sleep pressure is high from the previous night of wakefulness. However, once the day progresses, they are frequently plagued by late-morning or noontime awakenings that result from circadian-based alerting cues. The day sleep of night workers is typically two or more hours shorter per day than their typical night sleep (Costa 1997; Tilley *et al.* 1982). For these individuals, the long half-life of temazepam is desirable because the problem usually is one of sleep maintenance rather than sleep initiation. Temazepam, particularly in the 30-mg dose and in the 20-mg soft gel formulation, has been shown to objectively and subjectively improve daytime sleep (Muller *et al.* 1987); as a result, temazepam has been found to improve night-time performance (Porcu *et al.* 1997). A recent study of US Army pilots who were working and flying at night in a simulated shift-work environment verified that night-time performance, vigilance and alertness were enhanced significantly as a function of temazepam-induced improvements in daytime sleep (Caldwell *et al.* 2003b). Thus, short-term temazepam therapy can be extremely valuable to pilots rotating from day to night schedules. It is important to note that in the UK and several other countries, temazepam is now available only in tablets of 10-mg and 20-mg formulation, the gel capsules having been withdrawn because of intravenous drug abuse. Temazepam is also a good choice for temporarily augmenting the nighttime sleep of personnel who are deployed westward across as many as 9–11 time zones (Nicholson 1990; Stone and Turner 1997). Upon arrival at their destination, these individuals will likely be able to fall asleep quickly, since their local bedtime in the new time zone is much later than the one established by their circadian clock (from the origina-

---

[3]Although numerous other potentially useful medications are currently on the market, and many new ones being developed, a complete review of these compounds is beyond the scope of this chapter.

tion time zone); however, they may be unable to sleep throughout the night. While awaiting adjustment to the new time zone, temazepam can support adequate sleep maintenance despite conflicting circadian signals, and the obvious benefit will be less performance-degrading sleep restriction.

Zolpidem

Zolpidem (5–10 mg) may be the optimal choice for sleep periods of less than eight hours or sleep periods that could be shortened unexpectedly due to operational need. This drug is especially useful for promoting short- to moderate-length sleep durations (four to seven hours) when sleep opportunities occur at the 'wrong' circadian times. Daytime naps fall into this category because, like daytime sleep in general, these naps are difficult to maintain (Costa 1997; Lavie 1986; Tilley et al. 1982). Furthermore, unless the naps are placed early in the morning or shortly after noon, they can be extremely difficult to initiate (Gillberg 1984). Zolpidem is a good choice for facilitating such naps, because its relatively short half-life of 2.5 hours promotes rapid sleep onset with minimal post-nap hangover. A US Army study demonstrated that zolpidem-induced prophylactic naps enhanced the subsequent (post-nap) alertness and performance of sleep-deprived pilots during the last portion of a 38-hour period of continuous wakefulness without producing troublesome hangover effects (Caldwell and Caldwell 1998). Thus, zolpidem is useful for shift-work environments and sustained operations. Zolpidem is also helpful for promoting the sleep of personnel who have travelled eastward across three to nine time zones (Suhner et al. 2001). Unlike westward travellers, who experience sleep-maintenance difficulties, eastward-bound personnel will likely suffer from sleep-initiation problems. Zolpidem can help these personnel by rapidly initiating sleep and maintaining sleep until normal circadian factors take over. Since the drug's half-life is short, hangover effects will be minimized. As with temazepam, the zolpidem-enhanced sleep will not alleviate the symptoms of jet lag completely, but it will attenuate the sleep restriction and sleep disturbances that can degrade subsequent alertness and performance.

Zaleplon

Zaleplon (5–10 mg) may be the best choice for initiating very short naps (one to two hours) or for initiating early sleep onset in personnel who are trying to sleep earlier than usual in preparation for a very early start time the next morning. With regard to facilitating early report times, zaleplon or zolpidem may be used, but both compounds are important for the same reason. Since it is typically difficult for people to initiate sleep two to four hours before their usual bedtimes (Akerstedt 2003; Lavie 1986), requirements to be at the flight line in the pre-dawn hours often lead to two to three hours of sleep restriction. Since this amount of sleep truncation has been shown to significantly impair both alertness and performance (Belenky et al. 2003; Roehrs et al. 2003; Van Dongen et al. 2003), it is understandable that short-haul pilots often attribute a large part of their fatigue-related problems to such early duty schedules (Bourgeois-Bougrine et al. 2003). Zaleplon can help in this situation by hastening sleep-initiation (Chagan and Cicero 1999), thus extending the overall sleep period, and its ultra-short half-life of one hour is unlikely to pose hazards in terms of residual drug effects. Paul et al. (2004) suggest that zaleplon can be used safely to support sleep periods as short as three hours, since a study of 10 mg zaleplon revealed minimal drowsiness three to five hours post-dose. Thus, zaleplon (10 mg) is a good hypnotic for promoting early-to-bed sleep periods and short naps (of two to four hours) that would otherwise be difficult to initiate and maintain. In addition, as was the case with zolpidem, zaleplon can be considered useful for the treatment of sleep-onset insomnia in eastward travellers who are experiencing mild cases of jet lag. For instance, those who have transitioned eastward only three to four time zones can use this short-acting drug to initiate and maintain what the body believes to be an early sleep period.

General precautions for hypnotic therapy

Sleep-promoting compounds can be extremely useful for overcoming sleep problems in operational contexts. However, like all medications, there are both benefits and risks that should be considered by the prescribing flight surgeon and the individual pilot receiving treatment. Although temazepam, zolpidem and zaleplon are recognized widely as being safe and effective, personnel should be cautioned about potential side effects and instructed to bring any that occur to the attention of the unit flight surgeon. Potential problems may include performance-impairing hangover effects, dizziness and amnesia associated with premature awakenings (before the drug is metabolized fully), and/or various idiosyncratic effects (Balter and Uhlenhuth 1992; Menkes 2000; Nicholson 1990; Roth and Roehrs 1991). The appearance of side effects may necessitate discontinuation of therapy, the use of an alternative compound, or the modification of dosing strategies (Nicholson 1990). Hypnotics should not be used by personnel who are on call and may be awakened for immediate duty. Operational use of hypnotics should be preceded by a test dose given under medical supervision. When using hypnotics to aid in advancing or delaying circadian rhythms in response to time-zone shifts, caution is advised because of the many complexities associated with properly resynchronizing internal rhythms (Nicholson 1990; Stone and Turner 1997; Waterhouse et al. 1987). All of these cautions should be weighed against the fact that in many cases, the administration of hypnotics is the only practical means by which severe sleep deprivation (and the consequent negative effects of fatigue) can be prevented. Thus, while there are potential drawbacks associated with the use of these medications, the payoff can be far more significant.

ALERTNESS-ENHANCING COMPOUNDS

For situations in which, despite the best intentions, adequate sleep opportunities are simply non-existent, stimulants or alertness-enhancing drugs represent a viable option for temporarily staving off the deleterious effects of fatigue. Unavoidable manpower constraints, hostile environmental circumstances, extremely high workloads and/or unexpected enemy attacks may all require a postponement of sleep until a break in the operational tempo permits rest and recuperation. Although stimulants should not be viewed as a substitute for proper staffing or adequate work/rest cycles, they can be life-saving in circumstances in which sleep deprivation is unavoidable (Cornum et al. 1997). Stimulants have the advantages of being effective and easy to use. Because their feasibility is not dependent upon environmental manipulations or scheduling modifications, their usefulness, especially for short-term applications, is significant (e.g. see Kenegy et al. 2004). These advantages explain why pharmacological compounds such as amphetamines have been used extensively to overcome unavoidable sleep deprivation in several past military conflicts.

Although stimulants other than caffeine currently are not authorized for civilian or military use in the UK, caffeine, modafinil and dextro-amphetamine are approved for certain aviation operations by the US Air Force, and caffeine and dextro-amphetamine are approved for limited use by the US Army and the US Navy. Each of these compounds is discussed briefly below.

Caffeine

Caffeine is a good choice for situations in which medical oversight of drug administration is not available. Caffeine is already in widespread use, is not a prescription drug and generally is viewed as quite safe. It is readily available in many forms, including tablets, gums, candies, beverages and foods. An eight-ounce cup of drip-brewed coffee contains an average of 135 mg of caffeine, an eight-ounce cup of brewed tea contains approximately 50 mg of caffeine, and a 12-ounce cola drink contains an average of 44 mg caffeine. An eight-ounce cup of Starbucks™ (Starbucks Short®) contains 250 mg of caffeine (Schardt and Schmidt 1996). Research has shown that the effects of caffeine are variable, depending on the dose administered, the task measured and the level of tolerance (James 1998; Lieberman et al. 1987; Yeomans et al. 2002). Side effects can include increased heart rate, nervousness, anxiety, restlessness, nausea, increased frequency of urination and reductions in fine motor control (Serafin 1996). In general, caffeine improves reaction time and cognitive performance, elevates mood, and reduces sleepiness in fatigued subjects (Committee on Military Nutrition Research 2002;

Lieberman et al. 1987; Penetar et al. 1993). Studies have shown that 600-mg doses of caffeine can temporarily restore the performance and alertness of sleep-deprived personnel kept awake for over 50 continuous hours (Wesensten et al. 2002). For shorter periods of sleep loss (less than 24 hours), 150–300-mg bolus doses of caffeine are beneficial (Penetar et al. 1993). However, despite these and other positive findings, wholesale dependence on caffeine to mitigate the effects of sleep deprivation in the operational environment is controversial, since the effects of caffeine tolerance have not been studied adequately (Wyatt et al. 2004). Although a recent report suggested that doses of 200–800 mg of caffeine should be considered a first-line remedy for the drowsiness associated with insufficient sleep in operational military settings (Committee on Military Nutrition Research 2002), Rogers and Dernoncourt (1998) concluded that many of the effects of caffeine result more from the alleviation of caffeine withdrawal in habitual users than from a true performance-enhancing action. At present, further research on the tolerance issue is required for the following reasons: (i) over 80 per cent of adults in the USA daily consume behaviourally active doses of caffeine, (ii) tolerance to the subjective effects of caffeine has been shown to occur within four days of chronic dosing, and (iii) tolerance to the sleep-disrupting effects of caffeine has been observed after seven days of consistent caffeine administration at 1200 mg/day (Griffiths and Mumford 1995). Together, these facts suggest the possibility that the already widespread use of caffeine may diminish its effectiveness as a wake-promoting agent in severely fatigued individuals. Nonetheless, the generally positive impact of caffeine on alertness, combined with its safety and availability, make it a good starting point for the pharmacologically based management of aviation fatigue. Although there is some indication that caffeine's short half-life of only four to six hours may make it undesirable for situations in which a long-term boost is needed, this same quality may make caffeine optimal for situations in which there is the possibility that an unexpected sleep opportunity may arise shortly after the dose administration time.

Modafinil

The prescription drug modafinil (100–200 mg) may be a better choice for sustaining alertness and performance in operational contexts, as long as sufficient medical oversight is available to supervise its use. Although doses in the range of 200–800 mg have been observed to increase anxiety, insomnia, headaches, palpitations, blood pressure and pulse rate (Buguet et al. 2003), the frequency of side effects is low. There appears to be little or no drug tolerance with modafinil, even after weeks of continuous use, and the abuse liability is limited (Cephalon 1998). Furthermore, modafinil exerts only a small adverse effect on recovery sleep, even when given fairly close to the time of sleep onset

(Buguet *et al.* 1995). Thus, it may be optimal for sustained operations in which there is a possibility that an unexpected sleep opportunity could arise. Modafinil exerts a wide array of positive effects on alertness and performance. Lagarde and Batejat (1995) found that 200-mg doses every eight hours reduced episodes of micro-sleeps and maintained more normal (i.e. rested) mental states and performance levels than placebo for 44 hours of continuous wakefulness (but not the full 60 hours of sleep deprivation). Wesensten *et al.* (2002) found that 200–400-mg doses of modafinil effectively countered performance and alertness decrements in volunteers kept awake for over 48 hours. Caldwell *et al.* (2000a) found that 200 mg of modafinil every four hours maintained the simulator flight performance of pilots at near-well-rested levels despite 40 hours of continuous wakefulness, but there were complaints of nausea and vertigo, likely due to the high dosage used. A more recent study with Air Force F-117 pilots indicated that three 100-mg doses of modafinil (administered every five hours) sustained flight performance within 27 per cent of baseline levels during the latter part of a 37-hour period of continuous wakefulness. Performance under the no-treatment condition degraded by over 82 per cent (Caldwell *et al.* 2004). Similar beneficial effects were seen on measures of alertness and cognitive performance. Furthermore, the lower dose produced these positive effects without causing the side effects noted in the earlier study (Lagarde and Batejat 1995). Due to these and other positive results, modafinil is gaining popularity as a way to enhance the alertness of sleepy personnel, largely because it is considered safer and less addictive than compounds such as the amphetamines. Modafinil also produces less cardiovascular stimulation than amphetamine and, despite its half-life of approximately 12–15 hours (Medical Economics 2003a; Robertson and Hillriegel 2003), the drug's impact on sleep architecture is minimal. However, it should be kept in mind that modafinil has not been tested thoroughly in real-world operational environments, its efficacy for the long-term sustainment of wakefulness (i.e. beyond 40 hours) in sleep-deprived subjects has not been well established, and work with clinical populations suggests that modafinil is less effective than amphetamine (Mitler and Aldrich 2000). Nevertheless, modafinil has already received limited approval for use in certain long-range US Air Force bomber missions, and ongoing flight-performance research will likely pave the way for wider reliance on this compound as an effective fatigue countermeasure, at least for military aviation applications.

Amphetamine

Dextro-amphetamine (5–10 mg) has been researched for many years, and several studies have provided evidence that this compound is effective for maintaining alertness and performance in sleep-deprived people in a variety of settings. Although dextro-amphetamine can produce side effects such as palpitations, tachycardia, elevated blood pressure, restlessness, euphoria and dryness of the mouth (Medical Economics 2003b), the properly controlled administration of this compound remains a viable (and fairly routine) strategy for the sustainment of combat performance in select military aviation operations where sleep is difficult or impossible to obtain. The US Navy's *Performance Maintenance Guide* (US Naval Strike and Air Warfare Center 2000) and the US Army's *Leader's Guide for Crew Endurance* (Comperatore *et al.* 1996) both discuss the use of dextro-amphetamine for the sustainment of aviator performance in continuous flight operations. The US Air Force has authorized the use of dextro-amphetamine in certain types of lengthy (12 or more hours) single-seat and dual-seat flight missions. In comparison with caffeine, dextro-amphetamine appears to offer a more consistent and prolonged alerting effect (Weiss and Laties 1962). In comparison with modafinil, studies suggest that amphetamine is either more efficacious (Mitler and Aldrich 2000) or, at least in the case of 40-hour sleep-deprivation periods, equivalent (Caldwell 2001; Pigeau *et al.* 1995; Wesensten *et al.* 2004). In terms of the efficacy of amphetamine as a fatigue countermeasure, Newhouse *et al.* (1992) studied dextro-amphetamine (5, 10 or 20 mg) in people deprived of sleep for over 48 hours and found that 20 mg dextro-amphetamine (administered after 41 hours of continuous wakefulness) produced marked improvements in addition/subtraction (lasting for over ten hours), a gradual improvement in logical-reasoning (significant between 5.5 and 7.5 hours post-dose), a long-lasting improvement in the speed of responding during the choice reaction-time task (lasting for ten hours), and an increase in alertness (lasting for seven hours). It was noted that the drug did not impair judgement. The 10-mg dose exerted fewer and shorter-lasting effects, whereas the 5-mg dose was ineffective. Two flight-simulation studies involving US Army pilots indicated that repeated 10-mg doses of dextro-amphetamine (given at midnight, 0400 and 0800) maintained flight performance and alertness nearly at well-rested levels throughout 40 continuous hours of wakefulness (Caldwell *et al.* 1995, 1997). Benefits were especially noticeable between 0300 and 1100, when fatigue-related problems were most severe. In a later study, ten pilots completed a series of one-hour sorties in a especially-instrumented UH-60 helicopter during 40 hours of sleep deprivation. The results revealed that 10-mg doses of dextro-amphetamine sustained performance nearly as well under actual in-flight conditions as in the laboratory (Caldwell and Caldwell 1997). A follow-on simulator investigation extended these findings by showing that with additional amphetamine dosing, pilot performance and alertness could be sustained for over 58 continuous hours of wakefulness (two nights of sleep loss) (Caldwell *et al.* 2000b). Reports from the field indicate that dextro-amphetamine has been used successfully in a number of combat situations, such as Vietnam (Cornum *et al.* 1995), the 1986 Air Force strike on Libya (Senechal 1988) and Operation Desert Shield/Storm (Cornum *et al.* 1997). Emonson and Vanderbeek (1995) found that US Air Force pilots who were administered dextro-amphetamine during Operation Desert Shield/Storm were better able to maintain acceptable performance during continuous and sustained missions, and that the medication contributed to both safety and effectiveness. To date, no major side effects or other problems have been reported from the medical use of dextro-amphetamine in military settings. In light of these and other findings, dextro-amphetamine doses of 10–20 mg (not to exceed 60 mg/day) are recommended for situations in which heavily fatigued military pilots simply must complete the mission despite dangerous levels of sleep deprivation.

General precautions for stimulant therapy

Alertness-enhancing compounds can be extremely useful for temporarily mitigating the impact of sustained wakefulness in operational contexts where sleep opportunities are severely limited. However, there are both benefits and risks associated with the use of these compounds that deserve consideration from the prescribing flight surgeon and the individual pilot before use. Although caffeine, modafinil and dextro-amphetamine are recognized widely as being safe and effective when used under proper medical supervision, personnel should be cautioned about potential side effects, which may include irregular heartbeats, accelerated heart rate, elevated blood pressure, dry mouth, diarrhoea, constipation, loss of appetite, restlessness, dizziness, light-headedness, tremor, headaches nausea and reduced libido (Medical Economics 2003a,b). Furthermore, pilots and flight surgeons considering the use or administration of dextro-amphetamine should remain cognizant of the risks associated with abuse and dependence. Also, it should be noted that people taking amphetamine have experienced psychotic episodes on rare occasions; however, this typically occurs when recommended dose levels are exceeded or the drug is injected rather than taken orally (Kosman and Unna 1968; Poole and Brabbins 1996; Segal and Kuczenski 1997). If any difficulties occur during the course of treatment with caffeine, modafinil or dextro-amphetamine, alertness-enhancement therapy may need to be discontinued altogether, the specific compound may need to be changed, or the dosage may need to be modified. It should be noted that the potential difficulties associated with the use of stimulants must be weighed against the fact that these medications are often the only practical means available to preserve the performance of severely sleep-deprived pilots. Although stimulants should never be used as a replacement for sound work/rest scheduling, they can make the difference between life and death when, despite everyone's best efforts, significant sleep loss is simply unavoidable. It is well known that personnel cannot otherwise overcome severe fatigue even when they are highly motivated to do so.

SUMMARY

As technological advancements, customer demands and mission-related pressures continue to escalate, pilots and crews will increasingly face the risks posed by fatigue in aviation operations. However, with appropriate planning, one or more of the previously mentioned non-pharmacological or pharmacological alertness-management strategies can contribute significantly to pilot effectiveness and flight safety, even under the most daunting circumstances. With proper training and education, crews, schedulers and leaders can improve crew work/rest schedules and effectively utilize on-board rest opportunities, cockpit napping, controlled rest breaks and other techniques to optimize alertness on the flight deck. In exceptionally demanding circumstances, where administrative, behavioural and environmental strategies prove insufficient, pharmacological agents can be used to reliably enhance operational performance by optimizing available sleep opportunities and/or by temporarily countering the deleterious effects of unavoidable sleep deprivation.

REFERENCES

Akerstedt T. Consensus statement: fatigue and accidents in transport operations. *Journal of Sleep Research* 2000; **9**: 395.

Akerstedt T. Shift work and disturbed sleep/wakefulness. *Occupational Medicine* 2003; **53**: 89–94.

Arendt J, Deacon S. Treatment of circadian rhythm disorders: melatonin. *Chronobiology International* 1997; **14**: 185–204.

Arendt J, Deacon S, English J, Hampton S, Morgan L. Melatonin and adjustment to phase shift. *Journal of Sleep Research* 1995; **4** (suppl. 2): 74–9.

Balter MB, Uhlenhuth EH. New epidemiologic findings about insomnia and its treatment. *Journal of Clinical Psychiatry* 1992; **53** (suppl.): 34–9.

Belenky G, Wesensten NJ, Thorne DR, *et al.* Patterns of performance degradation and restoration during sleep restriction and subsequent recovery: a sleep dose–response study. *Journal of Sleep Research* 2003; **12**: 1–12.

Belyavin AJ, Spencer MB. Modeling performance and alertness: the QinetiQ approach. *Aviation, Space, and Environmental Medicine* 2004; **75** (suppl.): A93–103.

Bourgeois-Bougrine S, Carbon P, Gounelle C, Mollard R, Coblentz A. Perceived fatigue for short- and long-haul flights: a survey of 739 airline pilots. *Aviation, Space, and Environmental Medicine* 2003; **74**: 1072–7.

Buguet A, Montmayeur A, Pigeau R, Naitoh P. Modafinil, d-amphetamine and placebo during 64 hours of sustained mental work. II. Effects on two night of recovery sleep. *Journal of Sleep Research* 1995; **4**: 229-1.

Buguet A, Moroz DE, Radomski MW. Modafinil: medical considerations for use in sustained operations. *Aviation, Space, and Environmental Medicine* 2003; **74**: 659-63.

Caldwell JA. Efficacy of stimulants for fatigue management: the effects of Provigil and Dexedrine on sleep-deprived aviators. *Transportation Research* 2001; **4** (part F): 19-37.

Caldwell JA, Caldwell JL. An in-flight investigation of the efficacy of dextroamphetamine for sustaining helicopter pilot performance. *Aviation, Space, and Environmental Medicine* 1997; **68**: 1073-80.

Caldwell JA, Caldwell JL. Comparison of the effects of zolpidem-induced prophylactic nap to placebo naps and forced rest periods in prolonged work schedules. *Sleep* 1998; **21**: 79-90.

Caldwell JA, Caldwell JL. *Fatigue in Aviation: A Guide to Staying Awake at the Stick*. Burlington, VT: Ashgate Publishing Company, 2003.

Caldwell JA, Caldwell JL, Crowley JS. Sustaining female helicopter pilot performance with Dexedrine during sustained operations. *International Journal of Aviation Psychology* 1997; **7**: 15-36.

Caldwell JA, Caldwell JL, Crowley JS, Jones HD. Sustaining helicopter pilot performance with Dexedrine during periods of sleep deprivation. *Aviation, Space, and Environmental Medicine* 1995; **66**: 659-63.

Caldwell JA, Caldwell JL, Smith JK, Brown DL. Modafinil's effects on simulator performance and mood in pilots during 37 h without sleep. *Aviation, Space, and Environmental Medicine* 2004; **75**: 777-84.

Caldwell JA, Caldwell JL, Smythe N, Hall KK. A double-blind, placebo-controlled investigation of the efficacy of modafinil for sustaining the alertness and performance of aviators: a helicopter simulator study. *Psychopharmacology* 2000a; **150**: 272-82.

Caldwell JA, Gilreath SR. A survey of aircrew fatigue in a sample of U.S. Army aviation personnel. *Aviation, Space, and Environmental Medicine* 2002; **73**: 472-80.

Caldwell JA, Prazinko BF, Caldwell JL. Body posture affects electroencephalographic activity and psychomotor vigilance task performance in sleep deprived subjects. *Clinical Neurophysiology* 2003a; **114**: 23-31.

Caldwell JA, Smythe NK, Leduc PA, Caldwell JL. Efficacy of dextroamphetamine for maintaining aviator performance during 64 hours of sustained wakefulness: a simulator study. *Aviation, Space, and Environmental Medicine* 2000b; **71**: 7-18.

Caldwell JL. The use of melatonin: an information paper. *Aviation, Space, and Environmental Medicine* 2000; **71**: 238-44.

Caldwell JL, Prazinko BF, Rowe T, *et al*. Improving daytime sleep with temazepam as a countermeasure for shift lag. *Aviation, Space, and Environmental Medicine* 2003b; **74**: 153-63.

Cephalon. *Clinical Investigator's Brochure*. Frazer, PA: Cephalon, 1998.

Chagan L, Cicero LA. Zaleplon: a possible advance in the treatment of insomnia. *Pharmacy and Therapeutics* 1999; **24**: 590-99.

Co EL, Gregory KB, Johnson JM, Rosekind MR. Crew factors in flight operations XI: a survey of fatigue factors in regional airline operations. Report no. NASA/TM-1999-208799. Moffett Field, CA: NASA AMES Research Center, 1999.

Committee on Military Nutrition Research. *Caffeine for the Sustainment of Mental Task Performance: Formulations for Military Operations*. Washington, DC: National Academy Press, 2002.

Comperatore CA, Caldwell JA, Caldwell JL. *Leader's Guide to Crew Endurance*. Fort Rucker, AL: US Army Aeromedical Research Laboratory and US Army Safety Center, 1996.

Cornum KG, Cornum R, Storm WF. Use of psychostimulants in extended flight operations: a Desert Shield experience. In: *Advisory Group for Aerospace Research and Development. Neurological limitations of aircraft operations: human performance implications. Conference proceedings no. 579*. Nuilley-sur-Seine: NATO Advisory Group for Aerospace Research and Development, 1995; pp. 371-4.

Cornum RC, Caldwell JA, Cornum K. Stimulant use in extended flight operations. *Airpower* 1997; **11**: 53-8.

Costa G. The problem: shiftwork. *Chronobiology International* 1997; **14**: 89-98.

Daan S, Lewy AJ. Scheduled exposure to daylight: a potential strategy to reduce 'jet lag' following transmeridian flight. *Psychopharmacology Bulletin* 1984; **20**: 566-8.

Dinges DF, Graeber RC, Rosekind MR, Samel A, Wegmann HM. Principles and guidelines for duty and rest scheduling in commercial aviation. NASA/TM report no. 110404. Moffett Field, CA: NASA Ames Research Center, 1996.

Emonson DL, Vanderbeek RD. The use of amphetamines in U.S. Air Force tactical operations during Desert Shield and Storm. *Aviation, Space, and Environmental Medicine* 1995; **66**: 260-63.

Gander PH, Myhre G, Graeber RC, Anderson HT, Lauber JK. Adjustment of sleep and the circadian temperature rhythm after flights across nine time zones. *Aviation, Space, and Environmental Medicine* 1989; **60**: 733-43.

Gillberg M. The effects of two alternative timings of a one-hour nap on early morning performance. *Biological Psychology* 1984; **19**: 45-54.

Goode JH. Are pilots at risk of accidents due to fatigue? *Journal of Safety Research* 2003; **34**: 309-13.

Griffiths RR, Mumford GK. Caffeine: a drug of abuse? In: Bloom FE, Kupfer DJ (eds). *Psychopharmacology: The Fourth Generation of Progress*. New York: Raven Press, 1995; pp. 1699-713.

Hursh SR, Redmond DP, Johnson ML, *et al*. Fatigue models for applied research in warfighting. *Aviation, Space, and Environmental Medicine* 2004; **75** (suppl.): A44-53.

James JE. Acute and chronic effects of caffeine on performance, mood, headache, and sleep. *Neuropsychobiology* 1998; **38**: 32-41.

Kenagy DN, Bird CT, Webber CM, Fischer JR. Dextroamphetamine use during B-2 combat missions. *Aviation, Space, and Environmental Medicine* 2004; **75**: 381-6.

Kirsch AD. Report on the statistical methods employed by the U.S. Federal Aviation Administration in its cost/benefit analysis of the proposed 'Flight Crewmember Duty Period Limitations, Flight Time Limitations And Rest Requirements'. In: *Federal Aviation Administration. Comments of the Air Transport Association of American to FAA notice 95-18, FAA Docket No. 28081*, Appendix D. Washington, DC: Federal Aviation Administration, 1996; pp. 1-36.

Kosman ME, Unna KR. Effects of chronic administration of the amphetamines and other stimulants on behavior. Clinical Pharmacology and Therapeutics 1968; **9**: 240-54.

Lagarde DP, Batejat DM. Disrupted sleep-wake rhythm and performance: advantages of modafinil. *Military Psychology* 1995; **7**: 165-91.

Lavie P. Ultrashort sleep-waking schedule. III. 'Gates' and 'forbidden zones' for sleep. *Electroencephalography and Clinical Neurophysiology* 1986; **63**: 414–25.

Lewy AJ, Bauer VK, Ahmed S, *et al*. The human phase response curve (PRC) to melatonin is about 12 hours out of phase with the PRC to light. *Chronobiology International* 1998; **15**: 71–83.

Lieberman HR, Wurtman RJ, Emde GG, Roberts C, Coviella ILG. The effects of low doses of caffeine on human performance and mood. *Psychopharmacology* 1987; **92**: 308–12.

Luna T. Fatigue in context: USAF mishap experience. *Aviation, Space, and Environmental Medicine* 2003; **74**: 388.

Medical Economics. *Physicians' Desk Reference: Modafinil*. Montvale, NJ: Medical Economics Co., Inc., 2003a.

Medical Economics. *Physicians' Desk Reference: Dexedrine (Brand of Dextroamphetamine Sulfate)*. Montvale, NJ: Medical Economics Co., Inc., 2003b.

Menkes DB. Hypnosedatives and anxiolytics. In: Dukes MNG, Aronson JK (eds). *Meyler's Side Effects of Drugs*, 14th edn. Amsterdam: Elsevier Science, 2000; pp. 121–38.

Mitler MM, Aldrich MS. Stimulants: efficacy and adverse effects. In: Kryger MH, Roth T, Dement WC (eds). *Principles and Practice of Sleep Medicine*. Philadelphia: W.B. Saunders, 2000; pp. 429–40.

Muller FO, Dyk MV, Hundt HKL, *et al*. Pharmacokinetics of temazepam after day-time and night-time oral administration. *European Journal of Clinical Pharmacology* 1987; **33**: 211–14.

National Transportation Safety Board. A review of flightcrew-involved, major accidents of U.S. air carriers, 1978 through 1990. NTSB safety study. Report no. SS-94-01.Washington, DC: National Transportation Safety Board, 1994.

Neri DF, Oyung RL, Colletti LM, *et al*. Controlled breaks as a fatigue countermeasure on the flight deck. *Aviation, Space, and Environmental Medicine* 2002; **73**: 654–64.

Neville HJ, Bisson RU, French J, Boll PA, Storm WF. Subjective fatigue of C-141 aircrews during Operation Desert Storm. *Human Factors* 1994; **36**: 339–49.

Newhouse PA, Penetar DM, Fertig JB, *et al*. Stimulant drug effects on performance and behavior after prolonged sleep deprivation: a comparison of amphetamine, nicotine, and deprenyl. *Military Psychology* 1992; **4**: 207–33.

Nicholson AN. Hypnotics and occupational medicine. *Journal of Occupational Medicine* 1990; **32**: 335–41.

Paul MA, Gray G, MacLellan M, Pigeau RA. Sleep-inducing pharmaceuticals: a comparison of melatonin, zaleplon, zopiclone, and temazepam. *Aviation, Space, and Environmental Medicine* 2004; **75**: 512–19.

Penetar DM, McCann U, Thorne DR, *et al*. Caffeine reversal of sleep deprivation effects on alertness and mood. *Psychopharmacology* 1993; **112**: 359–65.

Petrie KJ, Dawson AG. Symptoms of fatigue and coping strategies in international pilots. *International Journal of Aviation Psychology* 1997; **7**: 251–8.

Pigeau RA, Naitoh P, Buguet A, *et al*. Modafinil, d-amphetamine and placebo during 64 hours of sustained mental work. I. Effects on mood, fatigue, cognitive performance and body temperature. *Journal of Sleep Research* 1995; **4**: 212–28.

Poole R, Brabbins C. Drug induced psychosis. *British Journal of Psychiatry* 1996; **168**: 135–8.

Porcu S, Bellatreccia A, Ferrara M, Casagrande M. Performance, ability to stay awake, and tendency to fall asleep during the night after a diurnal sleep with temazepam or placebo. *Sleep* 1997; **20**: 535–41.

Robertson P, Hillriegel ET. Clinical pharmacokinetic profile of modafinil. *Clinical Pharmacokinetics* 2003; **42**: 123–37.

Roehrs T, Burduvali E, Bonohoom A, Drake C, Roth T. Ethanol and sleep loss: a 'dose' comparison of impairing effects. *Sleep* 2003; **26**: 981–5.

Rogers PJ, Dernoncourt C. Regular caffeine consumption: a balance of adverse and beneficial effects for mood and psychomotor performance. *Pharmacology, Biochemistry, and Behavior* 1998; **59**: 1039–45.

Rosa RR. Extended workshifts and excessive fatigue. *Journal of Sleep Research* 1995; **4** (suppl. 2): 51–6.

Rosekind MR, Gregory KB, Miller DL, *et al*. Crew fatigue factors in the Guantanamo Bay Aviation Accident. *Sleep Research* 1996; **25**: 571.

Rosekind MR, Gregory KB, Co EL, Miller DL, Dinges DF. Crew factors in flight operations XII: a survey of sleep quantity and quality in on-board crew rest facilities. Report no. 2000-209611. Moffett Field, CA: NASA, 2000.

Rosekind MR, Smith RM, Miller DL, *et al*. Alertness management: strategic naps in operational settings. *Journal of Sleep Research* 1995; **4** (suppl. 2): 62–6.

Roth T, Roehrs T. A review of the safety profiles of benzodiazepine hypnotics. *Journal of Clinical Psychiatry* 1991; **52** (suppl.): 38–47.

Sack RL, Lewy AJ, Hughes RJ. Use of melatonin for sleep and circadian rhythm disorders. *Annals of Medicine* 1998; **30**: 115–21.

Samel A, Wegmann HM. Bright light: a countermeasure for jet lag? *Chronobiology International* 1997; **14**: 173–83.

Samel A, Wegmann HM, Vejvoda M. Jet lag and sleepiness in aircrew. *Journal of Sleep Research* 1995; **4** (suppl. 2): 30–36.

Schardt D, Schmidt S. Caffeine: the inside scoop. *Nutrition Action Healthletter* 1996; December.

Segal DS, Kuczenski R. An escalating dose 'binge' model of amphetamine psychosis: behavioral and neurochemical characteristics. *Journal of Neuroscience* 1997; **17**: 2551–66.

Senechal PK. Flight surgeon support of combat operations at RAF Upper Heyford. *Aviation, Space, and Environmental Medicine* 1988; **59**: 776–7.

Serafin WE. Drugs used in the treatment of asthma. In: Hardman JG, Limbird LE, Molinoff PB, Ruddon RW, Gilman AG (eds). *Goodman and Gilman's The Pharmacological Basis of Therapeutics*. New York: McGraw Hill, 1996; pp. 659–82.

Stone BM, Turner C. Promoting sleep in shiftworkers and intercontinental travelers. *Chronobiology International* 1997; **14**: 133–43.

Suhner A, Schlagenhauf P, Hofer I, *et al*. Effectiveness and tolerability of melatonin and zolpidem for the alleviation of jet lag. *Aviation, Space, and Environmental Medicine* 2001; **72**: 638–46.

Tilley AJ, Wilkinson RT, Warren PSG, Watson B, Drud M. The sleep and performance of shift workers. *Human Factors* 1982; **24**: 629–41.

US Naval Strike and Air Warfare Center. Performance maintenance during continuous flight operations: a guide for flight surgeons. Report no. NAVMED-P-6410. Pensacola, FL: US Naval Strike and Air Warfare Center, 2000.

Van Dongen HPA, Maislin G, Mullington JM, Dinges DF. The cumulative cost of additional wakefulness: dose–response effects on neurobehavioral functions and sleep physiology from chronic sleep restriction and total sleep deprivation. *Sleep* 2003; **26**: 117–26.

Waterhouse J, Reilly T, Atkinson G. Jet lag. *Lancet* 1997; **350**: 1611–16.

Weiss B, Laties VG. Enhancement of human performance by caffeine and the amphetamines. *Pharmacology Review* 1962; **14**: 1–36.

Wesensten NH, Balkin TJ, Thorne DR, *et al*. Caffeine, dextroamphetamine, and modafinil during 85 hours of sleep deprivation. I. Performance and alertness effects. *Aviation, Space, and Environmental Medicine* 2004; **75**: B108.

Wesensten NH, Belenky G, Kautz MA, *et al*. Maintaining alertness and performance during sleep deprivation: modafinil versus caffeine. *Psychopharmacology* 2002; **159**: 238–47.

Wirz-Justice A, Armstrong SM. Melatonin. Nature's soporific? *Journal of Sleep Research* 1996; **5**: 137–41.

Wyatt JK, Cajochen C, Ritz-De Cecco A, Czeisler CA, Dijk D. Low-dose repeated caffeine administration for circadian-phase-dependent performance degradation during extended wakefulness. *Sleep* 2004; **27**: 374–81.

Yeomans MR, Ripley T, Davies LH, Rusted JM, Rogers PJ. Effects of caffeine on performance and mood depend on the level of caffeine abstinence. *Psychopharmacology* 2002; **164**: 241–9.

53

The ageing pilot

JOHN COOKE

INTRODUCTION

Since the first powered and controlled flights were made by the Wright brothers, there has been immense worldwide development of all forms of aviation, which has brought with it an inevitable increase in the number of older pilots. In 1991, the Federal Aviation Administration (FAA) found that nearly 50 per cent of all civilian pilots in the USA were over 40 years of age. At the same time, significant demographic changes have begun to affect those same advanced nations in which most of the world's aviation industry is based. In these nations, the increasing expectation of life is causing some governmental re-examination of national retirement ages and also some encouragement for the extension of professional careers. However, in aviation, air safety must take precedence over any other consideration. The problems of these ageing pilots may best be considered by assessing the risks associated with ageing, their management, and the present and future place of age limitations of licensing.

AGE AS A RISK FACTOR

Ageing is a major factor in the aetiology of many pathological conditions. Population statistics show that after about the age of 35 years, increasing age is associated with increasing mortality. A large number of influences affect expectation of life, including gender, family history, ethnic and environmental factors, and the nature of employment. In relation to the latter of these, Booze (1989) showed in a study of general aviation pilots that their overall mortality and their liability to coronary artery disease (CAD) was less than that of their contemporaries in the general population. This seemed not unexpected in a population selected by initial medical examination and followed by regular medical revalidations. Nevertheless, professional pilots in the USA raised the question as to whether the perceived stresses of their work could cause adverse effects on health and longevity. To answer this, the FAA sponsored a study that compared the mortality and survival rates of retired American Airlines pilots with that of the white male population (Besco et al. 1995). The results were conclusive: retired pilots had very significantly better survival after the age of 60 years. Thus, it would seem that age may be a lesser single risk in pilots than in the general population. However, the ageing pilot remains a problem, and it is important to consider the effect of ageing on the more important systems that relate to the fitness of a pilot to fly. Those systems are:

- the cardiovascular system
- the special senses
- the psychological and mental processes
- other systems.

AGE AND CARDIOVASCULAR DISEASE

Sudden incapacity of a pilot due to a cardiovascular cause remains an important concern of both licensing authorities and the general public. A number of published studies have shown that there is a clear relationship between increasing age and an increasing risk of cardiovascular events. Tunstall-Pedoe (1992) reviewed these data in regard to the medical certification of pilots. He based his well-known one per cent rule on the statistical expectation that between the ages of 60 and 64 years, British males have a one per cent per year likelihood of death due to a cardiovascular event. It was partially on this hypothesis that the Joint Aviation Authorities (JAA) framed its age limit rules for airline pilots. The results of a personal retrospective study of CAA medical documents relating age to the diagnosis of CAD in 174 professional pilots in the UK showed that over 70 per cent of the total cases were aged over 50 years and the incidence increased after that age. All of these cases were male, which might confirm the gender advantage of women, if it were not that over the period of study only about seven per cent of professional pilots in the UK were female.

Cullen (2002) has published good autopsy evidence of the increased CAD found in older pilots. He reported the results of the examination of coronary arteries of 1188 pilots killed in aircraft accidents. His results showed a clear-cut progression of increasing CAD with age in both the frequency and the severity of the condition. In pilots between the ages of 56 and 60 years, over 70 per cent showed a significant degree of CAD. However, only in a very small percentage of cases did it appear that CAD was a contributory or main cause of the fatal accident.

Stroke is the other cardiovascular condition that is related clearly to age. Its main causal factor of hypertension is also more frequent in later life. However, as blood pressure is monitored at every medical examination for revalidation, the incidence of stroke is very low in pilots. Another common cardiac problem tending to appear in later age is atrial fibrillation. Medical records at the CAA show that of professional pilots diagnosed with this arrhythmia, 66 per cent were aged over 50 years at the date of first diagnosis. In addition, there is good evidence that the statistical chance of an incapacitating thromboembolism due to atrial fibrillation increases sharply after the age of 60 years.

Management of age-related cardiovascular problems

The single most important principle in the management of ageing pilots is the avoidance of any additional associated risk. In cardiovascular disease, the three classic risk factors are smoking, hyperlipidaemia and hypertension. Of these, smoking is the single entirely avoidable risk. Nevertheless, evidence obtained from the medical examination application forms at the CAA has shown that at the end of the twentieth century, nearly ten per cent of British professional pilots still smoked. This finding is not unique to the UK, and this is despite the non-smoking policy in aircraft imposed by many airlines. Hypertension is eminently treatable and, for this reason, was until recently the main focus of attention in preventive measures. Since the introduction of new drugs with very few significant side effects, such as the angiotensin antagonists, the results look extremely promising in the reduction of risk of cardiovascular events. The problem of raised blood lipids is receiving increasing attention, and the desirable 'normal' levels have been lowered. At the same time, effective treatment has been developed in the form of the statin group of drugs. For effective prophylaxis, there is a need for blood lipid measurements to be made in symptomless individuals. Some of the licensing authorities, such as the JAA, have already instituted such tests, and this policy is also carried out by some airlines and some air forces. The publicity about the dangers of hyperlipidaemia has also meant that more people are getting these tests carried out on a voluntary basis.

AGEING AND THE SPECIAL SENSES

Presbyopia is a virtually universal complaint that accompanies increasing age. Although the age of onset is quite variable, the problem of accommodation for near and intermediate vision will at some stage require the use of visual aids, despite the reluctance of some pilots to accept that fact. The use of such devices poses no problem for the vast majority of commercial and private pilots, it but can impose definite limitations on the military pilot of high-speed jet aircraft. More serious age-related ophthalmic conditions include cataract, glaucoma and macular degeneration. Of these, cataract and glaucoma are both treatable, and successful treatment may allow the maintenance of fitness to fly. Macular degeneration is not treatable effectively and is a disqualifying disability.

Deafness has an obvious association with increasing age. This may arise from a number of causes. It may be related to cumulative damage caused by noise, by conductive deafness and otosclerosis, and by the causes of perceptive deafness. Except when deafness causes difficulty in understanding speech, the problem can usually be overcome simply by increasing the gain to a satisfactorily fitting headset. Much more complex are problems involving vertigo, but in a few cases recovery will be possible as result of specialist advice and in treatment.

AGEING AND PSYCHOLOGICAL AND MENTAL PROCESSES

There is a great deal of experimental evidence to show that ageing is associated with a general decline in mental ability. In relation to aviation, these researches have been concentrated mainly on the psychometric approach and the assessment of older pilots in simulators. Some studies have claimed to show a slow progressive decrement of cognitive processes in pilots with increasing age (Tsang 1992). However, this is very far from a universal finding, particularly since there seems little supporting evidence that in reality the performance of the ageing pilot is significantly degraded (Hardy and Parasuraman 1997), and there is certainly little evidence of increased liability to accident. It might appear that the skill and judgement resulting from long experience can offset a minor decrement of performance.

The characteristic changes in behaviour due to ageing may consist of some increase in rigidity of outlook and habit. These changes are easily recognized by younger colleagues, their seniors generally being unaware of them. On occasions, this can result in personality problems on the flight deck. It is also clear that difficulty may arise for some older pilots when asked to undertake new tasks or to convert to new aircraft. Pelegrib *et al.* (1995) showed that 16 per cent of pilots over the age of 49 years failed a conversion course for the Airbus A320. Such problems usually show up in simulator training and in-flight checks and may lead to licensing problems. Overt psychiatric illness in the ageing pilot may arise as an exacerbation of an existing problem that has not been severe enough to be recognized previously. This is particularly true of the affective group of disorders. Neuroses may also become a disability, usually as a result of cumulative stress, particularly in domestic affairs. If mental decline of a significant degree due to ageing occurs, then it is often characterized by difficulties involving short-term memory, not of a severe nature but adding to the disability in learning new procedures and technology. On the positive side, there does not seem to be any direct relationship between ageing and the abuse of alcohol or drugs.

The only effective management in order to avoid the risks of these conditions is an acceptance by colleagues of the necessity for observation and reporting of abnormal behaviour. The consequent requisite action by the competent authorities will need the aid of consultant psychiatric advice.

AGEING EFFECTS ON OTHER SYSTEMS

'After 60 everything hurts.' The truth of this saying lies in the cumulative orthopaedic disabilities that affect many individuals by the age of 60 years. Backache and spinal problems seem to be common in transport pilots, possibly because of the long hours that they spend sitting on the flight deck. Military pilots may suffer spinal injuries due to ejection. Osteoarthritis of large joints can be a particular problem both in access to cockpits and in the use of controls. Prognosis in relation to flying will, of course, depend on the results of the requisite treatment. Old age can bring problems in the function of other systems, particularly the genitourinary and alimentary tracts. Except when there are serious causes present, these symptoms are rarely disabling.

AGE LIMITATIONS

Set ages for retirement are a standard feature of the social and employment organization of all the developed nations. Age limits for professional pilots generally are the responsibility of national licensing authorities and employers. Their purpose is two-fold: to reduce any risk to aviation safety that might be caused by the physical or mental deterioration of the ageing pilot and to enable employers to offer a progressive career in aviation. These age limits are a continuing subject of heated debate. In the case of professional pilots, the International Civil Aviation Organization (ICAO) made a recommendation in 1978 that the age limit should be 60 years of age. However, it soon became apparent that the degree of compliance with the '60-year rule' was subject to very considerable national variation. Because of this, in 1996 ICAO made a survey by a questionnaire of national practices that called for information of each nation's present policy and of any changes that the nation might propose for the future. A total of 70 nations responded. The survey confirmed the wide differences in attitude: 49 nations, importantly including the USA, which is the world's largest airline operator, conformed to the age limit of 60 years for airline transport pilots; in contrast, 13 nations, including three major operators, imposed no age limit for airline pilots but relied on other measures, such as increased medical and operational scrutiny. Additionally, the majority of nations imposed no age limit on commercial pilots other than those flying airline passenger operations. On the aspect of proposals for changing the regulations, a large number of nations seemed to favour some relaxation of the rule.

Meanwhile, the JAA regulations were being agreed by 37 nations. These allowed airline pilots between the ages of 60 and 65 years to continue flying airline passenger operations, but only in multi-pilot crews where the other pilot was under the age of 60 years. With regard to small aircraft and other general aviation operations, no restriction other than a compulsory exercise electrocardiogram (ECG) at the age of 65 years was required. In the USA, there have been continuing efforts by the political supporters of the airline pilots to introduce bills into Congress that would allow relaxation of the 'age 60 rule'. At the time of writing, it appears likely that ICAO will undertake a new review of national attitudes to this age limit.

Employers are free to impose their own age limits for their pilots. The larger airlines do this by fixing retirement ages from the company as part of the processes that allow promotion and company pensions. In Europe, most of these retirement ages have been between 55 and 60 years. This is shown in Figure 53.1, where the residual numbers of professional pilots in the UK fall dramatically after the age of 60 years.

AGEING OF PRIVATE AND SPORT PILOTS

There are many more older private pilots than professional pilots. In the UK, there are 1628 licensed pilots over 70 years of age, of whom 178 are more than 80 years old (Figure 53.2). The large majority of nations impose no age limits on private and sport pilots, the latter of which includes micro-light, motor-glider, glider and private balloon pilots. This general attitude is based on the statistical evidence from air accident investigations, which shows that the majority of accidents involving this group of pilots are due to human error. Such pilots have much less experience them professionals and fly much less frequently, and their aircraft are usually much less equipped with avionics. They are particularly vulnerable to bad weather conditions. Other factors are that they usually fly as single pilots, and the majority of their aircraft have a single engine. There is also the possible effect of their lesser medical standards, and there is a debate as to whether these contribute to any significant degree to the causal factors of fatal accidents. As might be expected with an older age group, about 3.5 per cent of fatal accidents may have been caused partly or fully by physical incapacity. The majority of these were shown by Cullen (2002) to be due to cardiovascular causes in accordance with his other data of the correlation of CAD with ageing.

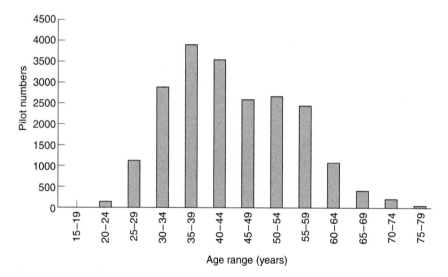

Figure 53.1   *Age distribution of UK professional pilots, 2003.*

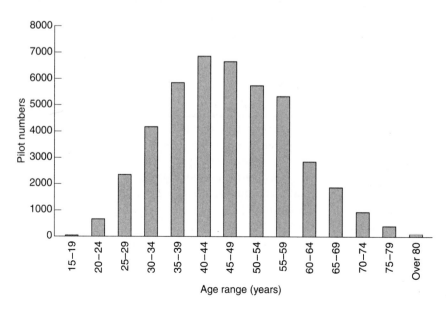

Figure 53.2   *Age distribution of UK private pilots, 2003.*

MILITARY AVIATION

Only in recent years have any age limits needed consideration in service aviation. Fast-jet and other combat aircraft remain the province of the young pilot, or at least those of no more than middle age. However, there has been recognition that transport and communication aircraft tasks remain within the ability of the older pilot, as they do in civil aviation. Although career structure and retirement ages in military aviation will vary with national requirements, it is unlikely that many military pilots will continue after the age of 55 years.

DISCUSSION AND CONCLUSIONS

We must accept that it is not possible to eliminate all risk in aviation. Machine failure has been reduced to a very low level by the enormous improvements in design, manufacture and maintenance. Human factors in the broadest terms are now the cause of the majority of accidents. The reduction of these human causes of failure remains a continuing target. It is important to examine the degree to which ageing contributes to these accidents and how much regulation is justified.

The human factors that affect performance include errors of judgement, lack of skill or attention, and fatigue. These are mainly responsible for accidents, and theoretically they might be made worse by the slow general decline in mental ability and cognitive processes that have been shown to occur as part of the ageing process. This would imply that older pilots would have a higher accident rate than their juniors. An overview of aviation accidents confirms that there are very few airline accidents and significantly more general aviation accidents, and that private and sport aviation has the highest accident rate of all (Bennett 1984). In general, private pilots are older than pilots in the other groups, but there are a lot more important factors in the causes of their accidents. An FAA study examining the ages of pilots involved in accidents found that in both commercial general aviation and private flying, the highest accident rate was in the youngest pilots (Kay et al. 1994). With increasing experience, the accident rate fell to a lower steady level, which did not appear to increase significantly after the age of 60 years. The same study has been made on FAA class 1 airline pilots. Although the accident rate was much lower than that found in the other groups, the pattern of the relationship to age of the pilots was the same up to the age of 60 years, when they had to retire from airline operations. On this evidence, it would seem that ageing confers little increased risk in the field of human factors.

The other important aspect of human failure is the possibility of sudden incapacity due to physical or mental causes. While a number of instances of incapacitation of a pilot due to physical causes are reported every year and may be more frequent in older pilots, the largest proportion of these are gastrointestinal upsets. Acute incapacity due to CAD is comparatively rare, even in old private pilots. Most of the fatal accidents attributed to mental causes have involved a suicidal tendency, where ageing is not contributory. The greatest concern has always been the possibility of collapse or subtle incapacity due to a cardiovascular event. Here, there is clearly some increased risk, as shown by the relationship to age of such events in private pilots. Some degree of risk continues in commercial aviation where there are single-pilot operations, such as air taxis and flying instruction. In many countries, no age limits apply to these pilots. There is an obvious anomaly, whereby airline pilots may retire from multi-crew duties to become single pilots in general aviation. In the UK, the CAA recognized this problem in 1994 and decided to submit professional pilots to increased medical surveillance in the form of an exercise stress ECG at the age of 70 years. Two results were noted: many fewer pilots applied for revalidation at that age, and 20 per cent of those who submitted to the test showed clearly abnormal exercise ECGs, which required further investigation. Subsequently, the JAA have decided that such a test should be applied to commercial pilots at the age of 65 years. In airline operations, the main safeguard is the presence of two pilots. There was one fatal airline accident in the UK in 1972 in which the captain suffered a coronary occlusion that contributed to or caused a loss of control that was not retrieved by the co-pilot. As a result, there has been greatly increased emphasis on crew training to recognize incapacity and for the unaffected pilot to take over control without delay (Chapman 1984). This policy has been successful: every year, collected international statistics have recorded a few incidents of pilot incapacitation due to CAD without danger to passengers. There has been no fatal accident due to the physical incapacity of a pilot in a British airliner since that in 1972. In summary, it appears that age contributes a continuing small increase of risk for single-pilot operations, but the risk is virtually negated in airline operations by the thorough training of two pilot crews.

Given these data, it might seem difficult to produce a convincing argument for the imposition of age limits on pilots, provide that they have adequate surveillance in the form of their medical examinations for revalidation. Furthermore, there is an argument that setting the age limit as low as 60 years for airline pilots may be eliminating individuals of great skill and experience before there is any likelihood of deterioration. But despite all this evidence and experience, it seems certain that age limits will be continued. Partly, this is undoubtedly due to public concern and anxiety about air travel, which is generally greater than for other forms of public transport, despite the statistical evidence that flying as a passenger is safe. There is also the background of both national and employment retirement ages, which, in the view of the public, mark a boundary that divides working life from the concept of the ageing pensioner. It is also difficult to provide any fair alternative for age limits. Many airline pilots are very happy to retire by the time they reach 60 years of age. It seems inevitable that those who wish to continue will necessarily have to come under some restriction of licensing and increased surveillance. Nevertheless, the number of professional pilots older than 60 years and licensed by the CAA has more than doubled since 1998. The new review by ICAO will certainly cause further discussion and reflection on these problems, but while there may be some further relaxation of the 'age 60 rule', it seems certain that some age limits will remain for airline pilots.

As regards the increased risk of private and sport flying and single-pilot commercial operations, there is not likely to be any change in policy. The pragmatic view will continue that any fatal accident that might be attributed to an ageing pilot will not be a major incident or kill more than a few people. Finally, the authorities are well aware that any attempt to impose age limits on private or sport pilots would be met by furious resistance. There would be no political advantage to be gained.

What of the future? Excepting some cataclysm, it seems likely that in the short term, the development and expansion of aviation will continue and the number of ageing pilots will increase. This will result from continuing demographic changes in developed nations spreading to other nations as they advance. The process is likely to be enhanced by future advances in medicine both in public health and in new prophylactic treatments that extend life. Serious debate about the necessary policies has only just begun, and it will certainly need to continue.

REFERENCES

Bennett G. Aviation accident risk and aircrew licensing. *European Heart Journal* 1984; **5** (suppl. A): 9–13.

Besco RO, Sangal SP, Nesthuis TE. A longevity and survival analysis for a cohort of retired airline pilots. Final report. Washington, DC: Federal Aviation Administration Office of Aviation Medicine, 1995.

Booze CF. Sudden in-flight incapacitation in general aviation. *Aviation, Space, and Environmental Medicine* 1989; **60**: 332–5.

Chapman PJC. The consequences of in-flight incapacitation in civil aviation. *Aviation, Space, and Environmental Medicine* 1984; **55**: 497–500.

Cullen SA. The contribution of pathology to the investigation of fatal aviation accidents. Thesis for the degree of Doctor of Medicine. Liverpool: University of Liverpool, 2002.

Hardy DJ, Parasuraman R. Cognition and flight performance in older pilots. *Journal of Experimental Psychology* 1997; **3**: 313–48.

Kay EJ, Hillmsn DJ, Hyland DT, *et al*. Age 60 rule research: consolidated database experiments. Final report. Washington, DC: Federal Aviation Administration Office of Aviation Medicine, 1994.

Pelegrib C, Maho V, Amalberti R. Pilot age and training performance. In: *Proceedings of the 21st Conference of the European Association for Aviation Psychology*. Brookfield, VT: Avebury Aviation, 1995.

Tsang PS. Reappraisal of ageing and pilot performance. *International Journal of Aviation Psychology* 1992; **2**: 193–212.

Tunstall-Pedoe H. Cardiovascular risk and risk factors in the context of aircrew certification. *European Heart Journal* 1992; **13** (suppl. H): 16–20.

FURTHER READING

Cooke JNC. The ageing pilot: is increased scrutiny justified? *European Heart Journal* 1999; **1** (suppl. D): 48–52.

Hyland DT, Kay EJ, Deimler JD, Gurman EB. Age 60 rule research. Part II. Airline pilot age and performance: a review of the scientific literature. Washington, DC: Federal Aviation Administration Office of Aviation Medicine, 1994.

54

Commercial passenger fitness to fly

MICHAEL BAGSHAW

PASSENGER HEALTH

Introduction

Flying as a passenger should be no problem for the fit, healthy, mobile individual. For the passenger with certain pre-existing conditions, however, the cabin environment may exacerbate their underlying problems. Although many problems relate to the physiological effects of hypoxia and expansion of trapped gases, it should be remembered that the complex airport environment can be stressful and challenging to the passenger, leading to problems before even getting airborne.

Whereas passengers with medical needs require medical clearance to travel from the airline, passengers with disabilities do not. Disabled passengers do need to notify the requirement for special needs, such as wheelchair assistance or assignment of seats with lifting armrests, and this should be done at the time of booking.

An in-flight medical emergency initially will be dealt with by the cabin crew, who may make use of the on-board emergency medical kit. In some cases, advice will be taken from a ground-based medical professional utilizing radio- or satellite communication. This may involve transmission of digitized medical data or might simply involve speech communication. A medical professional travelling as a passenger who offers assistance to the crew is known as a 'good Samaritan'. The outcome may involve an unscheduled diversion and landing at the nearest suitable airport, or the aircraft may return to the airport of origin or continue on to the planned destination, depending on the circumstances.

This chapter covers the principles supporting the decision-making process regarding passenger fitness to fly and details the international guidelines. Specific detailed guidance for individual diseases may be found in the clinical section of this book.

Pre-flight assessment and medical clearance

The objectives of medical clearance are to provide advice to passengers and their medical attendants on fitness to fly and to prevent delays and diversions of the flight as a result of deterioration in the passenger's wellbeing. It depends on self-declaration by the passenger and on the attending physician having an awareness of the flight environment and how this might affect the patient's condition.

Most major airlines provide services for those passengers who require extra help, and most have a medical advisor to assess the fitness for travel of those with medical needs. Individual airlines work with their own guidelines, but these are generally based on those published by the Aerospace Medical Association (2003) on fitness for travel.

The International Air Transport Association (IATA) publishes a recommended Medical Information Form (MEDIF) for use by member airlines, which is available from airlines' reservations departments or websites. The MEDIF should be completed by the passenger's medical attendant and passed to the airline or travel agent at the time of booking to ensure timely medical clearance.

Medical clearance is required when:

- fitness to travel is in doubt as a result of recent illness, hospitalization, injury, surgery or instability of an acute or chronic medical condition;
- special services are required, e.g. oxygen, stretcher or authority to carry or use accompanying medical equipment such as a ventilator or a nebulizer.

Medical clearance is not required for carriage of an invalid passenger outside these categories, although special needs, such as a wheelchair, must be reported to the airline at the time of booking. Cabin-crew members are unable to provide individual special assistance to invalid passengers beyond the provision of normal in-flight service. Passengers who are unable to look after their own personal needs (e.g. toileting, feeding) during flight will be asked to travel with an accompanying adult who can assist.

It is vital that passengers remember to carry with them any essential medication and not pack it in their checked-in hold baggage.

Deterioration on holiday or on a business trip of a previously stable condition, such as asthma, diabetes or epilepsy, or accidental trauma can often give rise to the need for medical clearance for the return journey. A stretcher may be required, together with medical support, and this can incur considerable cost. It is important for all travellers to have adequate travel insurance that includes provision for the use of a specialist repatriation company to provide the necessary medical support.

Assessment criteria

In determining the passenger's fitness to fly, a basic knowledge of aviation physiology and physics can be applied. Any trapped gas will expand in volume by up to 30 per cent during flight, and consideration must be given to the effects of the relative hypoxia encountered at a cabin altitude of up to 8000 feet above mean sea level. The altitude of the destination airport may also need to be taken into account in deciding the fitness of an individual to undertake a particular journey.

The passenger's exercise tolerance can provide a useful guide on fitness to fly. If they are unable to walk a distance greater than about 50 m without developing dyspnoea, then there is a risk that the passenger will be unable to tolerate the relative hypoxia of the pressurized cabin. More specific guidance can be gained from knowledge of the passenger's baseline sea-level blood gas levels and haemoglobin concentration.

Table 54.1 shows the guidelines recommended by one international carrier. This list is not exhaustive, and it should be remembered that individual cases might require individual assessment by the attending physician.

The prolonged period of immobility associated with long haul-flying can be a risk for people predisposed to develop deep venous thrombosis (DVT). Pre-existing risk factors include:

- blood disorders and clotting factor abnormalities
- cardiovascular disease
- malignancy
- major surgery
- lower limb/abdominal trauma
- DVT history
- pregnancy
- oestrogen therapy, including oral contraception and hormone replacement therapy
- age over 40 years
- immobilization
- pathological body fluid depletion
- smoking
- obesity
- varicose veins.

Although many airlines promote lower limb exercise via their in-flight magazine and videos, and encourage mobility within the cabin, those passengers known to be vulnerable to DVT should seek guidance from their attending physician on the use of compression stockings and/or anticoagulants. There is currently no evidence that flying, per se, is a risk factor for the development of DVT, but people at high risk should avoid any form of prolonged immobilization. The issue of DVT and air travel is covered in greater detail in Chapter 43.

CONSIDERATIONS OF PHYSICAL DISABILITY OR IMMOBILITY

In addition to the reduction in ambient pressure and the relative hypoxia, it is important to consider the physical constraints of the passenger cabin. A passenger with a disability must not impede the free egress of the cabin occupants in case of emergency evacuation.

There is limited leg space in an economy-class seat, and a passenger with an above-knee leg plaster or an ankylosed knee or hip may simply not fit in the available space. The long period of immobility in an uncomfortable position must be taken into account, and it is imperative to ensure adequate pain control for the duration of the journey, particularly following surgery or trauma.

Even in premier-class cabins, with more available legroom, there are limits to space. To avoid impeding emergency egress, immobilized or disabled passengers cannot be seated adjacent to emergency exits, despite the availability of increased legroom at many of these positions. Similarly, a plastered leg cannot be stretched into the aisle, because of the conflict with safety regulations.

Table 54.1 *Guidelines for medical clearance*

Category	Do not accept	Remarks
Cardiovascular disorders	Uncomplicated myocardial infarction within 7 days	Myocardial infarction less than 21 days requires MEDIF assessment
	Uncontrolled heart failure	
	Open heart surgery within 10 days	This includes CABG and valve surgery
		MEDIF assessment required up to 21 days post-operative
		Transpositions, ASD/VSD, transplants, etc. will require discussion with airline medical advisor
	Angioplasty: no stenting, 3 days: with stenting, 5 days	
Circulatory disorders	Active thrombophlebitis of lower limbs	
	Bleeding/clotting conditions	Recently commenced anticoagulation therapy requires assessment
	Blood disorders	
	Haemoglobin less than 7.5 g/dl	MEDIF assessment required for Hb less than 10 g/dl
	History of sickling crisis within 10 days	
Respiratory disorders	Pneumothorax that is not fully inflated, or within 14 days after full inflation	
	Major chest surgery within 10 days	MEDIF assessment required up to 21 days post-surgery
	If breathless after walking 50 m on ground or on continuous oxygen therapy on ground	Consider mobility and all aspects of total journey
Gastrointestinal disorders	General surgery within 10 days	Laparoscopic investigation may travel after 24 h if all gas absorbed; laparoscopic surgery requires MEDIF up to 10 days
	Gastrointestinal tract bleeding within 24 h	MEDIF required up to 10 days
CNS disorders	Stroke, including subarachnoid haemorrhage, within 3 days	Consider mobility/oxygenation aspects
		MEDIF up to 10 days
	Generalized seizures within 24 h	Petit mal or minor twitching – common sense prevails
	Brain surgery within 10 days	Cranium must be free from air
ENT disorders	Otitis media and sinusitis	
	Middle-ear surgery within 10 days	
	Tonsilectomy within 1 week	
	Wired jaw, unless escorted and with wire cutters	If fitted with self-quick-release wiring, may be acceptable without escort
Eye disorders	Penetrating eye injury/intraocular surgery within 1 week	If gas in globe, total absorption necessary – may be up to 6 weeks, specialist check necessary
Acute psychiatric disorders	Unless escorted with appropriate medication carried by escort, competent to administer such	MEDIF required. Medical, nursing or highly competent companion/relative escort
Pregnancy	After end of 36th week for single uncomplicated	Passenger advised to carry medical certificate
	After end of 32nd week for multiple uncomplicated	
Neonates	Within 48 h of birth	Accept after 48 h if no complications present
Infectious disease	If in infectious stage	As defined by the American Public Health Association
Terminal illness	Until individual case assessed by airline medical advisor	Individual case assessment
Decompression	Symptomatic cases (bends, staggers, etc.) within 10 days	May need diving or aviation physician advice
Scuba diving	Within 24 h	
Fractures in plaster	Within 48 h unless splint bivalved	Extent site and type of plaster may allow relaxation of guidelines. Exercise caution with fibre-glass casts
Burns	Consult airline medical advisor	

ASD, atrial septal defect; CABG, coronary artery bypass graft; CNS, central nervous system; ENT, ear, nose and throat; MEDIF, International Air Transport Association (IATA) Medical Information Form; VSD, ventricular septal defect.

There is limited space in aircraft toilet compartments. If assistance is necessary, a travelling companion is required.

The complexities of the airport environment should not be underestimated and must be considered during the assessment of fitness to fly. The formalities of check-in and departure procedures are demanding and can be stressful, and this can be compounded by illness and disability, language difficulties and jet lag.

The operational effect of the use of equipment such as wheelchairs, ambulances and stretchers must be taken into account, and the possibility of aircraft delays or diversion to another airport must be considered. It may be necessary to change aircraft and transit between terminals during the course of a long journey, and landside medical facilities will not be available to a transiting passenger.

There is often a long distance between the check-in desk and the boarding gate. Not all flights depart from or arrive at jetties, and it may be necessary to climb up or down stairs and board transfer coaches. Passengers should specify the level of assistance required when booking facilities such as wheelchairs.

SCHEDULED OXYGEN

In addition to the main gaseous system, all commercial aircraft carry an emergency oxygen supply for use in the event of failure of the pressurization system or during emergencies such as fire or smoke in the cabin. The passenger supply is delivered through dropdown masks from chemical generators or an emergency reservoir, and the crew supply from oxygen bottles located strategically within the cabin. The dropdown masks are released automatically en masse (the so-called 'rubber jungle') in the event of the cabin altitude exceeding a predetermined level of between 10 and 14 000 feet. This passenger emergency supply has a limited duration if provided by chemical generators, usually in the region of ten minutes. The flow rate is between 4 and 8 litres (normal temperature and pressure, NTP)/min and is continuous once the supply is triggered by the passenger pulling on the connecting tube. Oxygen supplied from an emergency reservoir is delivered to the cabin via a ring main. In some aircraft, it is possible to plug a mask into this ring main to provide supplementary oxygen for a passenger.

Sufficient first-aid oxygen bottles are carried to allow the delivery of oxygen to a passenger in case of a medical emergency in-flight, at a rate of 2 or 4 litres (NTP)/min. This cannot be used to provide a premeditated supply for a passenger requiring it continuously throughout a journey, however, since it would then not be available for emergency use.

If a passenger has a condition requiring continuous ('scheduled') oxygen for a journey, then they must pre-notify the airline at the time of booking the ticket. Most airlines make a charge to contribute to the cost of its provision.

Normally, it is not possible for a passenger to supply their oxygen. Oxygen bottles, regulators and masks must meet minimum safety standards set by the regulatory authorities, and the oxygen must be of aviation quality, which is a higher specification than medical quality with respect to water content. For further information regarding therapeutic oxygen for airline passengers, see the websites http://www.medaire.com and http://www.airsep.com.

IN-FLIGHT MEDICAL EMERGENCIES

An in-flight medical emergency is defined as a medical occurrence requiring the assistance of the cabin crew. It may or may not involve the use of medical equipment or drugs and may or may not involve a request for assistance from a medical professional travelling as a passenger on the flight. It can be something as simple as a headache or a vasovagal episode or something major, such as a myocardial infarction or impending childbirth.

The incidence is comparatively low, although the media impact of an event can be significant. One major international airline reported 3022 incidents occurring in more than 34 million passengers carried in one year. The breakdown of these incidents into generalized causes is shown in Table 54.2 (Bagshaw 1996; Bagshaw and Byrne 1999).

The top six in-flight emergency medical conditions reported by the same airline are shown in Table 54.3 (Bagshaw 1996; Bagshaw and Byrne 1999). Any acute medical condition occurring during the course of a flight can be alarming for the passenger and crew because of the remoteness of the environment. The cabin crew receive training in advanced first aid, basic life support and the use of the emergency medical equipment carried on board the

Table 54.2 *In-flight incidents reported in one year by a major airline*

Type of medical incident	%
Gastrointestinal system	22.3
Cardiovascular system	21.8
Musculoskeletal system/skin	13.4
Central nervous system	15.5
Respiratory system	10.2
Urogenital system	3.3
Metabolic system	2.5
Otorhinolaryngology (ENT)	1.4
Miscellaneous	9.6

Total 3022 incidents in 34 million passengers

Table 54.3 *Six most common in-flight medical incidents reported in one year by a major airline*

Type of medical incident	%
Fainting	14.9
Diarrhoea	11.5
Head injury	6.3
Vomiting	6.1
Collapse	5.4
Asthma	4.9

Total 3022 incidents in 34 million passengers

aircraft. Many airlines give training in excess of the regulatory requirement, particularly when an extended range of medical equipment is carried.

GOOD SAMARITANS

Although the crew members are trained to handle common medical emergencies, in serious cases they may request assistance from a medical professional travelling as a passenger. Such assisting professionals are referred to as 'good Samaritans'. Cabin-crew members attempt to establish the bona fide medical professionals offering to assist, but much has to be taken on trust.

The international nature of air travel can lead to complications in terms of professional qualification and certification, specialist knowledge and professional liability. An aircraft in flight is subject to the laws of the state in which it is registered, although when not moving under its own power, i.e. when it is stationary at the airport, it is subject to the local law. In some countries, e.g. France, it is a statutory requirement for a medical professional to offer assistance to a sick or injured person, whereas in other states, e.g. the UK and the USA, no such law exists.

Some countries, e.g. the USA, have enacted a Good Samaritan Law, whereby an assisting professional delivering emergency medical care within the bounds of his or her competence is not liable for prosecution for negligence. In the UK, the major medical defence insurance companies provide indemnity for their members acting as good Samaritans.

Some airlines provide full indemnity for medical professionals assisting in response to a request from the crew, whereas other airlines take the view that a professional relationship is established between the sick passenger and the good Samaritan and any liability lies within that relationship. At the time of writing, there has been no case of successful action against a good Samaritan providing assistance on board an aircraft.

Recognition by the airline of the assistance given by the good Samaritan is complicated by the special nature of the relationship between the professional, the patient and the airline. Indemnity, whether provided by the airline or the professional's defence organization, depends on the fact that a good Samaritan act is performed.

If a professional fee is claimed or offered, then the relationship moves away from being that of a good Samaritan act to one of a professional interaction with an acceptance of clinical responsibility. This implies that the professional is suitably trained, qualified and experienced to diagnose, treat and follow up the particular case, and the good Samaritan indemnity provision no longer applies.

Follow-up of the passenger after disembarkation is frequently difficult, because the sick passenger is no longer in the care of the airline and becomes the responsibility of the receiving hospital or medical practitioner.

AIRCRAFT MEDICAL DIVERSION

Responsibility for the conduct of the flight rests with the aircraft captain, who makes the final decision as to whether an immediate unscheduled landing or diversion is required for the wellbeing of a sick passenger. The captain has to take into account operational factors and the medical condition of the sick passenger.

In practice, it is rarely possible to land immediately; even if a suitable airport is in the vicinity, the aircraft has to descend from cruising altitude, possibly jettison fuel to reduce to landing weight, and then fly the approach procedure to land.

Consideration has to be given to the availability of appropriate medical facilities, and in many cases it is of greater benefit for the sick passenger to continue to the scheduled destination, where the advantage of appropriate facilities will outweigh the risks of continuing the flight.

Operational factors to be considered include the suitability of an airport to receive the particular aircraft type. The runway must be of sufficient length and load-bearing capacity, the terminal must be able to accommodate the number of passengers on the flight, and if the crew go out of duty time there must be sufficient hotel accommodation to allow an overnight stay of crew and passengers.

The cost to the airline may be substantial, including the effects of aircraft and crew unavailability for the next scheduled sector, as well as the direct airport and fuel costs of the diversion. In making the decision as to whether to divert, the captain will take advice from all sources. If a good Samaritan is assisting, then he or she has an important role to play, perhaps in radio consultation with the airline medical advisor.

TELEMEDICINE

Many airlines use an air-to-ground link that allows the captain and/or the good Samaritan to confer with the airline medical adviser regarding the diagnosis, treatment and prognosis for the sick passenger. The airline operations department is also involved in the decision-making process. Some airlines maintain a worldwide database of medical facilities available at or near the major airports; others subscribe to a third-party provider giving access to immediate medical advice and assistance with arranging emergency medical care for the sick passenger at the diversion airport.

The link from the aircraft is made using radio-telephone voice or data link (very high frequency (VHF) aircraft communications and reporting system (ACARS)), high-frequency (HF) radio-communication or a satellite communication system (Satcom). Satcom is installed in newer long-range aircraft and is gradually replacing HF as the industry norm for long-range communication. The advantage of Satcom is that it is unaffected by terrain, topography or atmospheric conditions and allows good transmission of voice and data from over any point on the globe. Digitization and telephone transmission of physiological parameters is a well-established practice, particularly in remote areas of the world. An aircraft cabin at 37 000 feet can be considered a remote location in terms of availability of medical support, and the digital technology used in Satcom is similar to that used in modern ground-to-ground communication. The advent of Satcom has enabled the development of air-to-ground transmission to assist in diagnosis. Pulse oximetry and electrocardiography (ECG) are examples of data that can assist the medical advisor to give appropriate advice to the aircraft captain, although the cost–benefit analysis of installing such equipment and training crew in its use has to be weighed very carefully.

AIRCRAFT EMERGENCY MEDICAL EQUIPMENT

National regulatory authorities stipulate the minimum scale and standard of all equipment to be carried on aircraft operating under their jurisdiction, which includes emergency medical equipment. These standards stipulate the minimum requirement, although in practice many airlines carry considerably more equipment.

Tables 54.4 and 54.5 give the minimum standard of equipment mandated by the Federal Aviation Administration (FAA) to be carried by aircraft registered in the USA, while Table 54.6 gives the standard determined by the Joint Aviation Authorities (JAA) for aircraft registered in European states.

In determining the type and quantity of equipment and drugs to include in the medical kits, the airline must fulfil the statutory requirements laid down by the regulatory authority. Other factors to be considered are as follows:

- *The route structure and stage lengths flown:* nations vary in their regulations on what might be imported and exported, particularly in terms of drugs. For example, it is illegal to import morphine derivatives into the USA, even if locked securely in a medical kit.
- *Passenger expectations:* premier-class business passengers from the developed world expect a higher standard of care and medical provision than passengers travelling on a relatively inexpensive package holiday flight.
- *Training of cabin crew:* the crew must have a knowledge and understanding of the kit contents, for use by themselves or in assisting a good Samaritan. They must be proficient in first aid, resuscitation and basic life support.
- *Differences in medical cultures:* ideally, the kit contents should be familiar to any good Samaritan, irrespective of nationality or training. Some authorities require information and drug names to be given in more than one language.
- *Equipment and drugs appropriate for likely medical emergencies:* it is important to audit the incidence and outcome of in-flight medical emergencies and maintain a review of the kit content. This review should also take into account changes in medical practice.
- *Space and weight:* the medical equipment must be accessible but stowed securely. Some airlines divide the equipment and drugs between basic first-aid kits that are readily accessible on the catering trolleys and a more comprehensive emergency medical kit that is sealed and stowed with other emergency equipment. Space and weight are always at a premium within the cabin, and the medical kits must be as light and compact as possible.
- *Shelf-life and replenishment:* a tracking system for each kit must be in place to ensure that contents have not exceeded their designated shelf-life. Similarly, after use of a kit, there has to be a procedure for replenishment. In practice, the aircraft can depart if the kit contents meet the statutory minimum, even though drugs or equipment have been used from the non-statutory part of the kit. Many airlines subcontract the tracking and replenishment to a specialist medical supply company.

RESUSCITATION EQUIPMENT

Although basic cardiopulmonary resuscitation (CPR) techniques are an essential part of cabin-crew training, the outcome of an in-flight cardiac event may be improved if

Table 54.4 *Federal Aviation Regulations Part 121: first-aid and emergency medical kits*

First-aid kits

Approved first-aid kits required by B121.309 must meet the following specifications and requirements:

(1) Each first-aid kit must be dust- and moisture-proof, and contain only materials that either meet Federal Specification GG-K-291a, as revised, or are approved.
(2) Required first-aid kits must be distributed as evenly as practicable throughout the aircraft and be readily accessible to the cabin flight attendants
(3) The minimum number of first-aid kits required as set forth in the table below:

No. of passenger seats	No. of first aid kits
0–50	1
51–150	2
151–250	3
More than 250	4

(4) Except as provided in paragraph (5), each first-aid kit must contain at least the following or other approved contents:

Contents of first-aid kits	Quantity
Adhesive bandage compresses, 10-inch	16
Antiseptic swabs	20
Ammonia inhalants	16
Bandage compresses, 4-inch	8
Triangular bandage compresses, 10-inch	5
Burn compound, 1/8-ounce or an equivalent of other burn remedy	6
Arm splint, non-inflatable	1
Leg splint, non-inflatable	1
Roller bandage, 4-inch	4
Adhesive tape, 1-inch standard roll	2
Bandage scissors	1

(5) Arm and leg splints that do not fit within a first-aid kit may be stowed in a readily accessible location that is as near as practicable to the kit.

Emergency medical kits

The approved emergency medical kit required by B121.309 for passenger flights must meet the following specifications and requirements:

(1) Approved emergency medical equipment shall be stored securely so as to keep it free from dust, moisture, and damaging temperatures.
(2) One approved emergency medical kit shall be provided for each aircraft during each passenger flight and shall be located so as to be readily accessible to crew members.
(3) The approved emergency medical kit must contain, as a minimum, the following appropriately maintained contents in the specified quantities.

Contents of emergency medical kits	Quantity
Sphygmomanometer	1
Stethoscope	1
Airways, oropharyngeal (three sizes)	3
Syringes (sizes necessary to administer required drugs)	4
Needles (sizes necessary to administer required drugs)	6
50% Dextrose injection 50 ml	1
Epinephrine (adrenaline) 1: 1000, single dose ampoule or equivalent	2
Diphenhydramine HCl injection, single dose ampoule or equivalent	2
Nitroglycerine tablets	10
Basic instructions for use of the drugs in the kit	11

appropriate resuscitation equipment is available. This can range from a simple mouth-to-mouth face guard, to a resuscitation bag and mask and airway, to an endotracheal tube and laryngoscope, to an automatic external defibrillator (AED).

The decision on the scale of equipment to be carried has to take account of the same parameters used in determining the content of the emergency medical kits (see Table 54.4). In addition, a cost–benefit analysis has to balance the cost of acquisition, maintenance and training against the probability of need and the expectation of the travelling public.

The European Resuscitation Committee and the American Heart Association endorse the concept of early defibrillation as the standard of care for a cardiac event, both in and out of the hospital setting. However, the protocol includes early transfer to an intensive care facility for continuing monitoring and treatment, which is not always possible in the flight environment.

Despite this inability to complete the resuscitation chain, it is becoming increasingly common for commercial aircraft to be equipped with AEDs and for the cabin crew to be trained in their use. This has been mandated in the USA by the FAA (see Table 54.5). Experience of those airlines that carry AEDs indicates that there may be benefits to the airline operation as well as to the passenger. Some types of AED have a cardiac monitoring facility, and this can be of benefit in reaching the decision on whether to

Table 54.5 *US Aviation Medical Assistance Act (1998)*

Rule issued by Federal Aviation Administration (FAA), April 2001

US aircraft weighing more than 7500 lb and having at least one flight attendant must carry an automated external defibrillator (AED) and enhanced medical kit (EMK) on all domestic and international flights within 3 years

The following items will be added to each EMK
- Oral antihistamine
- Non-narcotic analgesic
- Aspirin
- Atropine
- Bronchodilator inhaler
- Lidocaine and saline
- IV administration kit with connectors
- CPR masks

An EMK is already equipped with
- Sphygmomanometer (measures blood pressure)
- Stethoscope
- Three sizes of oral airways (breathing tubes)
- Syringes
- Needles
- 50% dextrose injection (for hypoglycemia or insulin shock)
- Epinephrine (adrenaline) (for asthma or acute allergic reactions)
- Diphenhydramine (for allergic reactions)
- Nitroglycerin tablets (for cardiac-related pain)
- Basic instructions on the use of the drugs
- Latex gloves

All crew members will receive initial training on the EMK and on the location, function, and intended operation of an AED. Flight attendants will receive initial and recurrent training in CPR and on the use of AEDs. Medical personnel are frequently onboard and can assist fellow passengers during an in-flight medical event. In addition, a 'Good Samaritan' provision in the aviation medical assistance act of 1998 limits the liability of air carriers and non-employee passengers unless the assistance is grossly negligent or willful misconduct is evident

CPR, cardiopulmonary resuscitation.

Table 54.6 *European Joint Aviation requirements (JAR-OPS 1, sub-part L)*

First-aid kits

The following should be included in the first-aid kits:
- Bandages (unspecified)
- Burns dressings (unspecified)
- Wound dressings, large and small
- Adhesive tape, safety pins and scissors
- Small adhesive dressings
- Antiseptic wound cleaner
- Adhesive wound closures
- Adhesive tape
- Disposable resuscitation aid
- Simple analgesic (e.g. paracetamol)
- Antiemetic (e.g. cinnarizine)
- Nasal decongestant
- First-aid handbook
- Splints, suitable for upper and lower limbs
- Gastrointestinal antacid
- Anti-diarrhoeal medication (e.g. loperamide)
- Ground/air visual signal code for use by survivors
- Disposable gloves

A list of contents in at least two languages (English and one other). This should include information on the effects and side effects of drugs carried

Note: An eye irrigator, while not required to be carried in the first-aid kit, should, where possible, be available for use on the ground

In addition, for aeroplanes with more than nine passenger seats installed, an **Emergency medical kit** must be carried

The following should be included in the emergency medical kit:
- Sphygmomanometer – non-mercury
- Stethoscope
- Syringes and needles
- Oropharyngeal airways (two sizes)
- Tourniquet
- Coronary vasodilator (e.g. nitroglycerine)
- Anti-spasmodic (e.g. hyoscine)
- Epinephrine (adrenaline) 1:1000
- Adrenocortical steroid (e.g. hydrocortisone)
- Major analgesic (e.g. nalbuphine)
- Diuretic (e.g. furosemide)
- Antihistamine (e.g. diphenhydramine hydrochloride)
- Sedative/anticonvulsant (e.g. diazepam)
- Medication for hypoglycemia (e.g. hypertonic glucose)
- Antiemetic (e.g. metoclopramide)
- Atropine
- Digoxin
- Uterine contractant (e.g. ergometrine/oxytocin)
- Disposable gloves
- Bronchial dilator, including an injectable form
- Needle disposal box
- Antispasmodic drug
- Catheter

A list of contents in at least two languages (English and one other). This should include information on the effects and side effects of drugs carried

divert. For example, there is no point in initiating a diversion if the monitor shows asystole or if it suggests that the chest pain is unlikely to be cardiac in origin.

Lives have been saved by the use of AEDs on aircraft and diversions have been avoided, so it could be argued that the cost–benefit analysis is weighted in favour of carrying AEDs as part of the aircraft medical equipment. Nonetheless, it is important that unrealistic expectations are not raised. An aircraft cabin is not an intensive care unit, and the AED forms only a part of the first-aid and resuscitation equipment.

Many airlines have in place a procedure for the follow-up of crew members involved in a distressing event such as a serious medical emergency. This can be valuable in avoiding long-term post-traumatic stress disorder and also in reinforcing the training that the crew member has already undergone.

CONCLUSION

The passenger cabin of a commercial airliner is designed to carry the maximum number of passengers in safety and comfort, within the constraints of cost effectiveness. It is incompatible with providing the facilities of an ambulance, an emergency room, an intensive care unit, a delivery suite or a mortuary.

The ease and accessibility of air travel to a population of changing demographics inevitably means that there are those who wish to fly who may not cope with the hostile physical environment of the airport or the hostile physiological environment of the pressurized passenger cabin. It is important for medical professionals to be aware of the relevant factors and for unrealistic public expectations to be avoided.

Most airlines have a medical advisor who may be consulted before flight to discuss the implications for a particular passenger. Such pre-flight notification can prevent the development of an in-flight medical emergency that is hazardous to the passenger concerned, inconvenient to fellow passengers, and expensive for the airline.

For a person with a disability but not an acute medical problem, pre-flight notification of special needs and assistance will reduce the stress of the journey and enhance the standard of service delivered by the airline.

The importance of adequate medical insurance coverage for all travellers cannot be overemphasized. Finally, as is normal practice in commercial aviation, there is a continuing audit of activity and an ongoing risk–benefit analysis. The industry is under constant evolution and is now truly global in its activity. Application of basic physics and physiology, and an understanding of how this may affect underlying pathology, will minimize the medical risks to the travelling public (Aerospace Medical Association 2003; British Medical Association 2004).

REFERENCES

Aerospace Medical Association. Medical guidelines for airline travel, 2nd edn. *Aviation, Space, and Environmental Medicine* 2003; **74**: II: A1–19.

Bagshaw M. Telemedicine in British Airways. *Journal of Telemedicine and Telecare* 1996; **2**: 36–8.

Bagshaw M, Byrne NJ. La sante des passagers. *Urgence Pratique* 1999; **36**: 37–43.

British Medical Association. *The Impact of Flying on Passenger Health: A Guide for Healthcare Professionals.* London: British Medical Association, 2004. Available on www.bma.org.uk

55

International travel and disease

ANDREW D. GREEN

INTRODUCTION

People who travel overseas expect to get ill with infectious diseases. This is often treated as a source of amusement, as witnessed by the numerous eponyms for travel-associated gastrointestinal disease and jokes about the safety of drinking water. Folklore does have its foundations in fact, and there is good evidence that, for a variety of reasons, the traveller is more likely to be ill than someone who has remained at home. However, clinics treating individuals with infectious diseases acquired abroad often focus on patient management and forget that there may be broader public-health matters to consider. By definition, the patient has travelled, and for the majority this will have been on a commercial passenger aircraft with many other people. The patient may well have acquired the illness overseas, but he or she might also have been infected during flight or transmitted the infection to others.

This chapter examines the relationship between air travel and infectious diseases. A series of issues are discussed, and practical solutions are offered for each. The aim is not to convert the aviation medicine specialist into an expert infectious diseases practitioner, but rather to provide a practical and pragmatic approach to common problems.

SCALE OF THE PROBLEM

Commercial air travel has seen dramatic growth in passenger numbers in recent years. The advent of low-cost carriers and the latest generation of wide-body aircraft mean that travel will become even more accessible and affordable in the future. It is estimated that in excess of 1000 million people flew on commercial aircraft in 2003, and many of these crossed international borders. Holidaymakers are visiting ever more distant locations. Many choose to immerse themselves fully in local culture, sampling local food and indulging in behaviour normal for that society (World Tourism Organization 2003). The proportion of travellers who seek health advice before travel is small, and in some groups is less than ten per cent (D.J. Bradley, Malaria Reference Laboratory, personal communication, 2004).

The risk of a traveller developing an infectious disease varies with each individual. Factors include the reason for travel (e.g. business or pleasure), type of travel (e.g. luxury or backpacker), occupation (e.g. medical aid worker or pilot) and destination (e.g. Western Europe or West Africa). Part of the attraction of travel is the opportunity to sample different cultures, and although some business people have little control over their choice of food for many others the chance to sample local cuisine is a major reason for travel. Pre-travel advice in the travel clinic for those who seek guidance is, therefore, usually a balance between what is desirable and what is achievable.

As a result, illness in travellers remains common, despite the best efforts of medical experts. Detailed incidence data are not easily obtained, but most studies suggest that on average 30 per cent of all people who spend two weeks or more overseas develop some sort of illness either during travel or within two weeks of return. For 'high-risk' travel in 'high-risk' destinations, the incidence may be as high as 80 per cent (Cossar *et al.* 1990). Surveillance data from patients with infectious diseases in England and Wales confirm that a significant proportion are ill directly as a result of travel (National Travel Health Network and Centre 2004). A simple calculation suggests that very large numbers suffer from travel-related illness – perhaps a third or more of all passengers on some passenger aircraft.

The key questions for the aviation medicine practitioner are:

- If some passengers on *every* flight are ill, what threat do they pose to other passengers and crew?
- What precautions should be taken for *every* flight to limit spread of disease?
- How can individuals who might have an infectious disease be identified?
- How can risks be minimized when someone falls ill in flight?
- What can alert authorities to the possibility that infectious diseases have been transmitted in flight?

DEFINITIONS

Lazy terminology leads easily to confusion, and this field is no exception.

An *infectious disease* is defined as a clinical pathological process caused by a biological agent or the effects of its products. Some microorganisms multiply themselves within the host to cause invasive disease, while others produce proteins or lipopolysaccharides called *toxins*, which may lead to disease in the absence of the organism itself.

Only living organisms may be *infected*, since infection implies a disease process. Inanimate objects such as aircraft where microorganisms are found are *colonized* or *contaminated*.

Many infectious diseases have an *incubation period*. This is the period from the time of exposure to a microorganism until the development of typical clinical disease. The period may vary from hours to months for different conditions. Some diseases produce non-specific symptoms and signs during the incubation period, which is termed the *prodromal* illness.

An infectious disease that can pass directly from person to person is *transmissible*. Many infectious diseases are *non-transmissible*. Differentiation is important, as individual patient management and public-health control measures differ. In the aviation medicine context, it is transmissible infectious disease that is of greatest concern.

EVIDENCE BASE

Despite the large numbers of aircraft passengers travelling each year, there are very few reports of illness attributable to flight. A number of factors contribute to underreporting of disease, as follows:

- *Passenger expectations:* illness following foreign travel is common, and passengers may attribute disease to their visit rather than the flight.
- *Patient behaviour:* few individuals with common diseases are recorded by national disease-reporting systems. Most people self-medicate, and those that do seek medical help rarely submit specimens for laboratory examination. In the UK, it has been estimated that each laboratory-confirmed case of gastrointestinal infection represents nearly 150 other cases in the community (Wheeler *et al.* 1999).
- *Incubation periods:* unless a disease has an incubation period of less than the time of flight, then transmission during flight is unlikely to be recognized easily. Passengers who have been infected may not develop symptoms until several days later, by which time they will have been dispersed widely.
- *Lack of systematic surveillance:* proactive disease surveillance is labour-intensive and costly and needs specifically defined aims. For airline operators, this would require systematic detailed follow-up of every passenger for symptoms of illness, which is impractical outside of research studies. Passive surveillance relies on routine disease notification, with alerts being generated if any association with aircraft is suggested. It is being introduced within Europe, allowing cross-border identification and follow-up of individuals who may have contracted illness during flight.

ROUTES OF TRANSMISSION

The ways in which diseases spread are many and varied. Some travellers need to be made aware of some of the more unusual routes of transmission. For example, pot-holing in Mexico is associated with a fungal infection caused by *Histoplasma* species, white-water rafting in Jamaica is associated with leptospirosis as a result of bacteria entering minor abrasions, and eating giant land snails can lead to eosinophilic meningitis due to a parasitic infection by *Angiostrongylus* species. However, even the most adventurous airline operators are unlikely to offer any of the above as in-flight entertainment, and it is sensible to focus on those diseases that might be associated with spread in the aircraft cabin environment.

With few exceptions, person-to-person transmission of disease occurs from people who are *symptomatic*. This has important implications for passenger aircraft:

- Asymptomatic individuals uncommonly transmit infections to others.
- Identification of symptomatic individuals will allow targeting of resources in order to reduce disease transmission.
- Infection-control precautions can be tailored to the symptoms of the individual, e.g. respiratory precautions for a coughing patient.
- Exclusion of symptomatic people from aircraft will further reduce the risks of in-flight disease transmission.
- Patients who require aeromedical evacuation may be at higher risk of transmitting disease, and this risk may vary according to diagnosis and symptoms.
- Passengers who have been incubating disease may become symptomatic for the first time during flight.

Respiratory infection

Infection by the respiratory route is most commonly by droplets. These are particles greater than $10\,\mu$m in diameter that fall to the ground rapidly after being generated. The majority of patients with respiratory symptoms such as coughs and sneezes produce droplets containing microorganisms that can directly infect the upper respiratory tracts of other people. For practical purposes, these are relatively easy to contain by the use of physical barrier methods, such as simple masks and ventilator filters, around the airways of patients and medical attendants. However, droplets may be expelled with force, so that other mucous membranes such as conjunctivae may require protection. Environmental contamination is common in the immediate area of a symptomatic individual, and hands are easily colonized; organisms are then passed readily to the mouth or mucous membranes of the patient or another person.

In contrast, smaller particles measuring less than $10\,\mu$m in diameter remain in the air and are termed aerosols. They behave more like gases and are able to penetrate as far as the alveoli, together with any organisms they contain. Higher levels of respiratory protection are required to contain spread. Aerosol transmission is much less common than droplet spread.

Examples of diseases spread by the respiratory route include the following:

- *Legionella pneumophila* aerosol inhalation of environmental organisms; no person-to-person spread.
- *Mycobacterium tuberculosis*: person-to-person droplet spread.
- Varicella (chickenpox): highly transmissible person-to-person by droplets and aerosols.

Evidence for transmission of respiratory diseases on aircraft is scanty. Reports of respiratory symptoms such as drying of mucous membranes or cough following extended flights are common and are usually related to environmental conditions. These are relatively easy to enumerate by subjective questionnaire surveys, since many individuals on each flight report similar symptoms. In contrast, the nature of infectious disease makes a transmission event irregular and unpredictable, and large-scale prospective studies would be required to provide an accurate estimate of risk.

There are few reports of incidents, and these generally have been identified through a series of unusual circumstances, such as the following:

- Influenza A transmitted during an internal flight in Alaska. An index case with symptoms boarded an aircraft, which then was delayed on the runway for four hours with the air-conditioning turned off. All passengers and crew were able to be followed up as they stayed in the same small town for 24 hours post-flight and were easy to identify when a large number presented ill simultaneously (Moser *et al.* 1979).
- Flu-like illness transmitted during an internal flight in Australia. A group of miners flew for three hours to a remote mine, where 20 developed illness over the following week. The nature of the closed community allowed recognition of the incident and enabled the association with the flight to be established (Marsden 2003).
- *Mycobacterium tuberculosis*. A series of incidents in the mid-1990s were investigated by the Centers for Disease Control in the USA. The US strategy for control of tuberculosis relies on identification of newly infected people by skin testing, and this allowed detailed investigation of six reported incidents of patients with symptomatic tuberculosis flying on aircraft. In only one case was there evidence of transmission. Six individuals on a Boeing 747 during a long-haul flight were infected, but these were only those passengers with extended close contact with the symptomatic index case (Kenyon *et al.* 1996).
- Severe acute respiratory syndrome (SARS). In 2003, the World Health Organization (WHO) declared a global emergency following the appearance of a new respiratory infection, subsequently identified as due to a novel coronavirus. Although the disease was largely confined to China and South-East Asia, outbreaks did occur elsewhere, most notably in Canada. During the early stages of the epidemic, a number of patients flew between countries, and in three flights transmission to other passengers was subsequently confirmed. The risk of transmission correlated with the extent of symptoms in the index cases; one sick individual infected 22 passengers and crew, while another flight

carrying four confirmed cases infected only one other passenger. Transmission occurred only to those in close contact with cases and was not documented from any patients who flew with asymptomatic disease or during disease incubation (Olsen *et al.* 2003).

In the absence of compelling evidence of disease transmission based on outbreak reports, research has focused on the theoretical mechanisms for spread of microorganisms. Direct measurement of pathogenic viruses and bacteria in the aircraft environment requires both a full complement of passengers and for some of them to be symptomatic and shedding microorganisms. Such studies are technically difficult, rely on the presence of individuals with disease, and almost certainly are unethical. Instead, surrogate markers of transmission have been investigated. These include measurement of total bacterial counts in air, as is common practice in operating-theatre sampling. This is, in reality, largely only an indicator of organisms present on skin scales – bacterial numbers increase when people shed skin scales, typically when they move about. Measurements in flight have shown highest numbers of bacteria during embarkation and disembarkation and during level flight, when passengers are most frequently in movement (Dechow *et al.* 1997). The total number of bacteria present in air during quiet periods is no different than that found in equivalent locations on the ground, such as buses and public meeting areas. No increase in numbers has been demonstrated with recirculation of cabin air (Wick and Irvine 1995).

High-efficiency particulate air (HEPA) filters are now fitted to air-conditioning systems of most new passenger aircraft. Despite the absence of data implicating recycled air as a risk, it is perceived to be of commercial benefit by addressing the theoretical mode of disease transmission. Filter manufacturers regularly examine filters for their physical integrity and the presence of viruses and bacteria when they are changed at routine service intervals, but pathogens have not been found to date (K. Bull, PALL Industries, personal communication, 2003).

Patterns of air movement have been studied in various aircraft types. In commercial airliners, this has been used to determine optimum levels of comfort without creation of draughts or temperature loss, which vary with both the type of aircraft and its configuration. In military aircraft, this has been extended to predict theoretical transmission of infection. One study showed that up to ten per cent of bacteria released into the rear of a C130 aircraft were detectable on the flight deck (Clayton *et al.* 1976). The US Air Force has assessed airflow patterns in all of its aircraft used for aeromedical evacuation and advised that only those with front-to-rear air flows should be used for potentially infectious patients, in order to reduce the risk to aircrew (United States Air Force Transportation Command 2003).

International guidelines for control of respiratory infection on aircraft have been produced for both tuberculosis and SARS. The WHO guidance on tuberculosis stresses the importance of pre-flight identification of open cases of disease and preventing their travel, advises on contact-tracing procedures following the inadvertent transportation of a case on a long-haul flight, and emphasizes the low risk to those not in the immediate proximity. However, the guidance also recommends that HEPA filters are fitted to all commercial passenger aircraft, despite acknowledging that there is no evidence base for this advice (World Health Organization 1999). It is interesting to note that the guidelines would not have prevented any of the incidents that provoked the initial report, since each of the cases failed to declare their illness before flight.

Guidance for SARS has been produced by the Centers for Disease Control, which had concerns about transmission during international flights, and Health Canada, which focused on internal movements. As with tuberculosis, the emphasis is on identification of symptomatic individuals before flight and delaying travel until they are symptom-free. Personal hygiene for all individuals on all flights is highlighted and the importance of hand-washing stressed. Should a passenger develop symptoms during flight, then basic source isolation (if practical) is advised, with a face-mask for the individual rather than all other passengers. Contact details are collected from everyone on the flight, but enhanced surveillance measures are undertaken only for those people in close contact with the case. No further action is recommended for flights when asymptomatic individuals have travelled but later found to have developed disease (Centers for Disease Control 2004; Health Canada 2003).

In summary:

- Transmission of respiratory infection on aircraft is rarely reported.
- Spread is by direct contact with a symptomatic individual.
- Ideally, individuals with symptoms suggesting respiratory infection should not be carried.
- If a passenger develops symptoms during flight, then basic source-isolation precautions should be adopted, as far as is practical.
- Only those passengers and crew in close contact with a symptomatic individual are at risk of acquiring infection.
- There is no evidence of transmission through recirculation of aircraft cabin air.

Gastrointestinal infection

Most gastrointestinal infections are transmitted by the faecal–oral route. Organisms enter the mouth, either in food/water or on the hands. They originate from the gut of humans and animals and may multiply in the environment under favourable conditions. These simple facts underlie the basic principles of gastrointestinal disease control, which aim to interrupt this cycle of infection. In the aviation medicine field, this includes control measures such as water purity, food safety, catering practices, sanitation and personal hygiene. It also explains why intuitively sensible measures such as disposable cutlery and plates are of little practical use: eating from sterile plates is meaningless if the food served has been prepared poorly and the passengers' hands are covered with faecal organisms.

Examples of diseases spread by the faecal–oral route include the following:

- *Campylobacter* species: animal gut origin, direct contamination of foodstuffs without environmental multiplication.
- *Salmonella* species: animal gut origin, direct contamination of foodstuffs with significant further multiplication in the environment.
- *Shigella* species: human gut origin, spread primarily person-to-person by contamination of environment and hands.

In the aircraft cabin, the principal sources of infection are likely to be the food and water consumed and other passengers with disease. Catering practices and water management are dealt with more fully in Chapter 34.

Incidents of food poisoning on aircraft are reported infrequently, with fewer than 50 incidents recorded (Tauxe *et al.* 1987). In part, this is due to poor recognition and reporting, but it also reflects the high standards now adopted by airline operators. The improved international surveillance systems developed in recent years have helped identify some incidents that previously would have passed unnoticed, but the absence of flight-related cases of illness against the large background number of travellers suggests that aircraft catering is now well regulated. In many of the incidents reported, the implicated foodstuff was ingested pre-flight, with symptoms developing during flight 24–48 hours later after an incubation period (Green *et al.* 1995). In contrast, for a food-poisoning incident resulting from food ingested in flight, the incubation period for illness must be short enough for symptoms to appear before landing. Very few conditions have an incubation period shorter than even the longest long-haul flights.

The greatest threat to passengers of infective gastrointestinal disease is from other passengers. Many are likely to have contracted an infective condition before flight, and some will be unwell when they travel. In common with other infections, people without symptoms are unlikely to pose a threat to others. In contrast, the infecting dose of many organisms, most notably *Shigella* species and the enteric viruses, may be extremely small, such that minimal environmental contamination may lead to disease spread in the absence of high standards of personal hygiene.

Despite the estimates of numbers of passengers with disease, actual incidents of acute illness during flight or faecal contamination of toilets or seating are rarely reported (N. Byrne, British Airways Health Services, personal communication, 2004). Cabin crew are trained in dealing with handling vomit and faeces, and contaminated areas are cordoned off from passengers. There have been no reported transmissions of disease from any such incidents. In contrast, there are well-documented incidents on buses and coaches where an index case has been sick and produced a significant number of secondary cases related to direct contact with, and droplet spread of, vomit.

Gastrointestinal disease on military operations is common, and the nature of field conditions means that person-to-person spread of highly transmissible agents is the usual cause. Although most individuals will suffer a benign self-limiting illness, a proportion may be affected more severely and require medical care. Some of these might require aeromedical evacuation for their clinical condition or for operational reasons. Such individuals will usually be symptomatic, and there will need to be a careful assessment of the need for immediate evacuation against infective risks to other passengers and crew. Infection-control precautions in flight should reduce but cannot eliminate the risk of transmission. In one medical repatriation of a seriously ill casualty with norovirus infection, the patient infected medical attendants during flight and ground personnel who handled faecally-contaminated equipment post-flight (Brown *et al.* 2002).

In summary:

- food poisoning on aircraft is difficult to recognize but probably is rare;
- faecal–oral spread of infection is most likely to result from a symptomatic passenger;
- risk of infection to all passengers and crew may be reduced by high standards of personal hygiene.

Blood–borne infection

Infections spread by the blood-borne route are difficult to acquire. Casual contact does not transmit infection, and there is a requirement for blood from an infective individual to come into contact with either broken skin or mucous membranes. Some infections are preventable by immunization, but many others are not. Risk-reduction measures are therefore generic and focus on treating all blood exposures in the same way. Although it is possible for some blood-borne infections to be spread by the droplet route, e.g. following a haematemesis, this is largely theoretical and there is little evidence that this is an important means of spread.

Examples of disease spread by the blood-borne route include the following:

- Hepatitis B: highly infective with high viral load individuals; vaccine-preventable.
- Human immunodeficiency virus (HIV): 100-fold less infective than hepatitis B; no vaccine, but in some circumstances antiviral drugs may reduce transmission post-exposure.
- Viral haemorrhagic fevers, such as Ebola and Lassa fevers: despite the common perception of high transmissibility of these diseases, these are in fact transmitted in a very similar way to hepatitis B and are of similar infectivity.

There are no reports of blood-borne virus transmissions on aircraft. However, every passenger should be considered a potential carrier of any virus, and policies for managing at-risk exposures of crew and other passengers considered. This is particularly important during aeromedical evacuations, when blood spills and sharps injuries are most likely. Policies should also be in place for all other flights: many passengers have insulin-dependent diabetes and carry needles and syringes, which sometimes are discarded in refuse, while immigration controls mean that to avoid arrest many intravenous drug users hide their needles before disembarkation. Both of these actions have resulted in injuries to personnel cleaning aircraft.

Education and personal protective measures should form the cornerstone of risk reduction. Cabin crew should be trained to recognize and respect the significance of blood and blood-stained bodily fluids. Physical protection, including gloves and aprons should be available, along with material to contain and collect spills; this would normally include a coagulant such as cellulose powder, a scraper to collect the spill, and a plastic bag for disposal. Chemical disinfectants may damage aircraft alloys, and few such disinfectants are safe to use in this environment. Furthermore, they have minimal effect in the presence of organic material such as blood and offer no real advantages over physical cleaning. The simple kits described above can also be used for clearing other bodily fluids. Basic personal hygiene with emphasis on hand-washing is critical. Incidents involving blood contact should be reported to occupational health as soon as is practical, so that the exposure may be documented on the crew member's health record and further action taken if necessary. This might include post-exposure immunization for hepatitis B or anti-retroviral drugs for HIV, according to the risk assessment of the incident.

Passengers with viral haemorrhagic fevers have, occasionally, flown on commercial aircraft. Affected individuals have always been in the early stages of illness before haemorrhagic symptoms have been manifest, and as a result there have been no high-risk exposures on the aircraft. In 2000, six cases of Lassa fever were imported by air into Europe. Of over 500 people in 'normal' close contact with the patients, including passengers on the aircraft, none was infected. The only secondary case was in a junior doctor who was heavily contaminated in the mouth and eyes after examining one patient before the diagnosis had been established.

In contrast to the asymptomatic passenger, the planned aeromedical evacuation of a patient known or suspected to have a viral haemorrhagic fever would need to be circumspect. Such patients will have established diseases and might be likely to develop bleeding problems. Although the risk of aerosolization is low, the spillage of significant volumes of infective blood in a closed environment such as an aircraft would be considered a significant hazard. A careful reappraisal of the need to move the patient is required; should this still be considered necessary, a detailed plan of containment must be drawn up, including coverage of the following issues:

- Rationale for containment: protection of medical attendants, other passengers, crew and airframe.
- Diagnosis and condition of patient: likelihood of blood exposure.
- Surveillance of personnel post-evacuation: all involved or only those in contact with bodily fluids?
- Immediate protocols for exposure of staff to blood or sharps injury.
- Collection of patient from destination site, delivery to aircraft, and delivery to receiving hospital after evacuation.
- Clinical-waste management during flight, and subsequent disposal.
- International health regulations, politics and publicity.
- Education and training of medical personnel and aviators.

In practice, this means long and complex planning, i.e. it is not something to be attempted as an emergency evacuation. Although such diseases are rare, the increasing numbers of travellers to remote locations and the operational deployment of military forces to areas endemic for viral haemorrhagic fevers mean that such plans are prudent.

Various solutions have been proposed. Few aeromedical organizations can maintain dedicated aircraft for potentially highly infective patients. Measures are, therefore, generally aimed to protect both personnel and maintain integrity of the airframe. Examples include the use of a conventional road ambulance within the hold of a transport aircraft, the use of a specially modified road ambulance with HEPA-filtered air, and the covering of a transport aircraft floor with plastic sheeting with use of individual protective equipment by medical attendants. The Royal Air Force (RAF) has evacuated three patients with Lassa fever from Sierra Leone using a purpose-built air-transportable patient isolator; the patient is managed within a HEPA-filtered sealed environment, which fully contains any blood spills.

In summary:

- Blood-borne infections are not transmitted easily in the normal aircraft environment.
- Blood exposure is most likely during aeromedical evacuation.
- Spill kits should be available on all passenger aircraft, and cabin crew should be trained in their use.
- Occupational health services must expect to deal with personnel who have been exposed to blood or blood-stained bodily fluids.
- Viral haemorrhagic fevers behave like any other blood-borne infection – there is significant risk only when patients are symptomatic and bleeding.
- Evacuation of patients with known or suspected viral haemorrhagic fevers can be undertaken but requires detailed planning and resourcing.

AEROMEDICAL EVACUATION OF INFECTIOUS PATIENTS

Any 'normal' passenger may have been exposed to an infectious agent and at embarkation be symptomatic or asymptomatic. Those without symptoms may be incubating disease, have a prodromal illness, have mild or subclinical infection, or be recovering from their acute illness. For some infections, an extended healthy carrier state may develop post-infection. As discussed above, only those individuals with symptoms pose any infective risk to other passengers or crew.

Patients who are being aeromedically evacuated will have been exposed to the same risks as any other traveller. However, they pose a greater risk of transmitting an infection for a number of reasons:

- Infectious disease may be the diagnosis leading to repatriation.
- They may have been hospitalized and acquired a healthcare-associated infection.
- Their clinical condition may require the use of supportive medical techniques such as assisted ventilation, vascular access and renal support, each with associated hazards to medical personnel.
- Aeromedical flights often carry multiple patients. Transmission of infectious agents between susceptible individuals with predisposing factors is common in any environment, but particularly when staff are working under pressure in difficult surroundings.
- Aeromedical patients usually will be repatriated to a medical facility. The consequences of introducing a novel infectious agent into a hospital environment may be serious.
- Clinical waste is generated in flight.

A prudent approach is to try to identify those patients who might prove to be an infective hazard. Although this would be impractical for routine commercial passenger flights, it can be achieved for aeromedical evacuation, since an expert medical assessment is required for every patient. Such a policy also embraces current international guidance on diseases such as SARS.

The aim of the initial screen is to find those patients who have symptoms that might prove hazardous to other passengers and crew if an infective agent is involved. It does not attempt to accurately identify underlying diagnosis or even confirm an infective aetiology; in practice, the risk is related to the symptom rather than the agent involved. The screen should be sensitive rather than specific and should identify every patient with any potentially transmissible infective condition.

A series of simple questions can be added to the initial aeromedical assessment. These might include asking about specific symptoms such as:

- cough
- vomiting or diarrhoea
- bleeding
- rash
- fever.

There is no need to accurately define each of these terms, as might be the case in other medical contexts. Any patient with a suspect symptom is referred for an aeromedical opinion, such that more detailed assessment of the relevant feature can be made. This will allow judgement as to the likelihood of a transmissible infectious agent being involved. If doubts exist, then infectious diseases specialist advice should be sought.

For patients who are assessed, there may be a number of possible outcomes:

- The symptom does not indicate that an infectious agent is involved and no special precautions are required (e.g. rash due to drug allergy).
- An infectious agent may be involved, and special precautions may be required in flight (e.g. patient with jaundice).
- An infectious agent may be involved, and the patient should not be aeromedically evacuated (e.g. patient with profuse vomiting).

The decision to delay aeromedical evacuation would normally take into account the patient's clinical condition, the risks of transmission as assessed, and the operational circumstances such as standards of medical care on site or military context. In most cases, it is prudent to delay evacuation until the symptoms have resolved. Should the need dictate, individuals who are possibly infective could still be moved but with specialist infection-control precautions and enhanced surveillance of other passengers and medical attendants.

The decision and mode of repatriation may also be influenced by the following:

- Numbers of patients affected: with large groups of patients, it may be impractical to move; with smaller numbers of patients, patients with similar symptoms may be nursed as a cohort and evacuated together.
- Specialist medical staff: potentially infective patients ideally should have dedicated medical attendants. In some circumstances, this might not be possible and repatriation might be delayed.
- Diagnosis: a credible suspected diagnosis of a viral haemorrhagic fever would dictate the use of a specialist evacuation technique.

As an adjunct to all aeromedical evacuations, specific data collection and surveillance are desirable. Information regarding the numbers and types of infection developed by patients post-aeromedical evacuation and detailed occupational health records allow periodic evaluation of the efficacy of control measures in place.

MALARIA

Malaria is a parasitic infection of blood transmitted by the bite of the female anopheline mosquito. Over 400 million people are infected annually worldwide. *Plasmodium falciparum*, *P. malariae* and *P. ovale* are true tropical diseases found only in equatorial regions, while *P. vivax* can be transmitted in temperate areas during summer months. In the UK, over 2000 cases are imported each year, most in travellers who have returned recently from endemic areas. The vast majority of cases occur in people who have taken either no or inappropriate chemoprophylaxis.

Deaths from malaria occur regularly; in non-immune populations, this is frequently the result of delayed or missed diagnosis. The disease may be deceptively innocuous, even with high levels of parasitaemia, and terminal decline may occur within hours.

Malaria-carrying mosquitoes may, occasionally, be carried on aircraft, and rare reports of 'airport malaria' result from disease transmission in non-endemic countries. Such introductions are unimportant from the public-health perspective; more problematic is the importation of a human reservoir that might act as a focus for transmission by endogenous *Anopheles* species (Zucker 1996). The aim of disinsection processes, as described in Chapter 34, is to prevent the accidental introduction of insect vectors into a receptive area and is concerned particularly with the vectors of yellow fever and dengue.

The principles of malaria prevention are simple. The risk of acquiring disease can be reduced by a series of pre-cautions; importantly, however, the risk cannot be eliminated entirely. The key points are as follows:

- Awareness: travellers must be educated regarding:
  - mode of malaria transmission – by mosquito bite
  - symptoms – any illness, especially non-specific 'flu-like
  - actions to take if disease is suspected – seek immediate medical advice.
- Bite avoidance: measures to reduce the number of potentially infective bites include:
  - repellents – diethyltoluamide (DEET) or citronella-containing preparations are available widely and effective
  - bed-nets – impregnated with an insecticide such as permethrin and used appropriately
  - knockdown insecticides – for use in confined areas
  - clothing covering wrists and ankles after dusk – preferably impregnated with insecticide
  - window screens on rooms.
- Chemoprophylaxis: drugs should be:
  - appropriate for area of travel – up-to-date advice is required
  - suitable for individual – different drugs may be contraindicated for different people
  - taken – even the best drugs are ineffective if they do not enter the body
  - started before exposure and continued for an appropriate time after return.
- Diagnosis: since no precaution will be entirely effective, malaria must be considered as a diagnosis in any individual who has been in an endemic area. Although most cases present within a few weeks of return, a small proportion will not become ill until a year or more later.

Aviation issues

The incidence of malaria in aviators is difficult to assess, as cases are rarely reported by occupational group. For commercial pilots, it has been argued that their risks are lower than for other travellers, as they generally stay overnight for short periods in good-standard accommodation in large cities, where malaria transmission is relatively low. Work looking prospectively at commercial pilots suggest that malaria is uncommon in those staying for short periods and that chemoprophylaxis might not be required for this group (Byrne and Behrens 2004). In other groups, this will not be true, and the risks will be the same as for other comparable travellers.

Bite prevention

Most discussion about malaria and aviation deals with choice of chemoprophylaxis. It must be emphasized that this forms only one part of the approach to malaria prevention: bite-reduction measures are of equal or greater importance. When the UK deployed a large military force to West Africa in May 2000, over 200 cases of malaria resulted. The first six cases were in aircrew who had taken appropriate chemoprophylaxis; they had deployed in field conditions without impregnated uniforms or bed-nets and not been trained in the same bite-prevention techniques as their infantry counterparts (Tuck *et al.* 2003). A number of countries are now using flying suits impregnated with insecticide. These suits are technically difficult to produce without compromising the flame-retardant properties of the material. They would be useful in reducing malaria incidence only if aircrew were night-flying or sleeping in their flying suits.

Chemoprophylaxis regimens and self-treatment

The use of drugs to prevent an infectious disease is not unique but is practised widely only for malaria. Adverse events to drugs when used for therapy may be acceptable to clinicians and patients, since the underlying condition requires treatment and relatively few patients are involved. In contrast, the same drugs are required to be almost entirely free of adverse events when used for disease prevention in otherwise healthy individuals, despite the use of lower doses than for therapy.

There is a perception by some individuals that malaria is mild and that precautions are not always needed. The relative rarity of the disease in non-endemic areas means that knowledge there is scanty; in contrast, the frequent repeated infections in semi-immune adults in endemic areas lead to its trivialization. In the latter situation, it is often forgotten that the adults are the survivors and that up to 30 per cent of their peers will have died from malaria in childhood.

Maps of malaria distribution are often misleading, as they generally indicate geographical areas where the disease is found, rather than intensity of transmission. For example, malaria is transmitted in equatorial regions around the world. However, the infective bite rates in West Africa are ten times higher than for East Africa and 100 times higher than for South America or South-East Asia. It is easy for travellers to convince themselves that their neglect of malaria advice on visits to malarious areas of low transmission enables them to ignore similar advice in future when travelling to far riskier environments.

Finally, there is an interesting aspect of traveller psychology. People often compare malaria chemoprophylaxis regimens when meeting others on their travels and may decide to follow the advice of the individual taking the least intrusive protocol. Often, this means stopping effective chemoprophylaxis, and deaths have been recorded as a direct result.

These factors all combine to help explain poor compliance with malaria chemoprophylaxis. Aviators as a group are generally well educated and very concerned about their health. Despite this, their compliance with recommended prophylaxis is extremely poor and in one study was less than four per cent (Dunlop 1991).

The drugs advised for travellers are usually based on the guidance of national expert groups. There is, therefore, no international consensus, since not only do opinions differ but also licensing, manufacture, costing and distribution of preparations vary markedly. Consistent advice within countries is important, and every effort should be made to ensure that the latest guidance is available widely to both health professionals and travelling populations. Examples of information sources are given at the end of this chapter.

Not all chemoprophylactic drugs are recognized as safe to use in aircrew. There has been some debate regarding the suitability of mefloquine in aviators, with research focused on trying to establish the true incidence of psychomotor impairment when the drug is used in low doses (Schlagenhof *et al.* 1997). Few national bodies recommend the use of mefloquine in aircrew, and this is unlikely to change, even if research fails to demonstrate an effect on simulated flight performance studies. A low-incidence event cannot be detected easily in the laboratory when small numbers of subjects are examined and usually appears during post-marketing surveillance after introduction of a new product to a large population. The known effects on motor coordination of the high doses of mefloquine used during malaria therapy mean that any use in aviators is unlikely to be approved.

The advent of sensitive and specific rapid diagnostic kit technology that can be used by non-laboratory personnel has allowed new strategies to be developed. In the past, some travellers opted to treat themselves for suspected malaria, but this often resulted in overuse of therapeutic drugs, as many mild illnesses were treated mistakenly. Accurate diagnosis combined with effective oral therapies such as atovaquone/proguanil and co-artemether (artemether with lumefantrine) means that early treatment of infection has become a practical option.

A number of approaches to chemoprophylaxis in aircrew have been suggested:

- No antimalarials:

  - practised effectively by many non-compliant aircrew
  - appropriate for selected destinations and accommodation
  - requires educated aircrew who report sickness early and are either treated or repatriated urgently.

- Rapid diagnostic kits:

  - use if not taking prophylaxis, or for all travellers;
  - education and hands-on training required *before* travel
  - best for groups, so that sick individual does not test him- or herself
  - needs appropriate therapeutic drugs included as part of protocol
  - first-aid measure – individuals should seek expert advice as soon as practical.

- Tailored advice for each trip:

  - consistent with advice for other travellers
  - impractical for aircrew flying repeatedly to malaria areas
  - difficult to provide individual advice to many aviators.

- Continuous prophylaxis:

  - assumes unpredictable work patterns and regular flying to malaria areas
  - suitable for some selected groups, e.g. military transport crews on defined tour of duty
  - compliance likely to be very poor
  - concerns about long-term tolerability for drugs taken over many years.

- Cluster tours of duty:

  - work pattern adjusted to allow all flying into malaria areas to be grouped together over a period of weeks or months
  - chemoprophylaxis taken only when required – not taken throughout remainder of year for other duties
  - no evidence base of improved compliance
  - requires sympathetic and motivated employers
  - difficult to implement for military aviators.

The choice of drugs used for chemoprophylaxis will vary according to the type of travel and the destination, and will usually follow national guidance, as described above. There are particular aviation issues with each of the commonly used drugs:

CHLOROQUINE

- Much experience – considered safe in aircrew.
- Once-weekly dose – one week before first exposure until four weeks after last exposure.
- Has been used continuously for up to 30 years in some individuals.
- No evidence of cumulative eye toxicity when used in malaria-prophylaxis doses.
- Parasite resistance now widespread – limited utility.

PROGUANIL

- Much experience – considered safe in aircrew.
- Rarely used alone – usually in combination with chloroquine.
- Daily dose – one week before first exposure until four weeks after last exposure.
- Considered safe for long-term use.
- Parasite resistance now widespread – limited utility.

MEFLOQUINE

- Very effective antimalarial agent.
- Not generally accepted as safe to use in aircrew.
- Adverse events uncommon in prophylactic doses.
- Once-weekly dose – one week before first exposure (three weeks advised in some countries) until four weeks after last exposure.
- Parasite resistance uncommon – effective in sub-Saharan Africa.
- Long-term use safe, although licence limits use to one year in some countries.
- Suitable for use in aircrew who are not in control of aircraft and in ground-support personnel.

DOXYCYCLINE

- Effective antimalarial – similar level of protection as mefloquine.
- Considered safe in aircrew.
- Adverse events not common.
- Daily dose – one week before first exposure until four weeks after last exposure.
- Short half-life means rigorous compliance is essential in order to maintain protection.
- Parasite resistance uncommon – effective in sub-Saharan Africa.

ATOVAQUONE/PROGUANIL

- Effective antimalarial – similar level of protection as mefloquine.
- Considered safe in aircrew (Paul *et al.* 2003).
- Adverse events not common.
- Daily dose – two days before first exposure until seven days after last exposure.
- Parasite resistance uncommon – effective in sub-Saharan Africa.

The addition of atovaquone/proguanil to the available drugs for chemoprophylaxis has significant potential benefits for aviators. The drug combination is safe to use in flying crew and has a pharmacokinetic profile and mode of action that allows it to be taken for a much shorter time before and after exposure. This means that good compliance is much more likely. There is also the possibility of starting the drug around the time of first exposure, meaning that it could be suitable for both passengers and crew on aircraft that make unscheduled diversions to high-transmission areas.

REFERENCES

Brown D, Gray J, Green AD, et al. Outbreak of acute gastroenteritis associated with Norwalk-like viruses among British military personnel – Afghanistan, May 2002. *Morbidity and Mortality Weekly Report* 2002; **51**: 477–9.

Centers for Disease Control. *Guidance on Air Medical Transport for SARS patients.* Atlanta, GA: Centers for Disease Control, 2004.

Clayton AJ, O'Connell DC, Gaunt RA, et al. Study of the microbiological environment within long and medium range Canadian Forces aircraft. *Aviation, Space, and Environmental Medicine* 1976; **47**: 471–82.

Cossar JH, Reid D, Fallon RJ, et al. A cumulative review of studies on travellers, their experience of illness and the implication of these findings. *Journal of Infection* 1990; **21**: 27–42.

Dechow M, Sohn H, Steinhanses J. Concentrations of selected contaminants in cabin air of Airbus aircraft. *Chemosphere* 1997; **35**: 21–31.

Dunlop J. Malaria prophylaxis in flying staff: compliance with advice. In: Steffen R. (ed.). *Abstracts of the Second International Conference on Travel Medicine.* Atlanta, GA: International Society of Travel Medicine, 1991.

Green AD, Connor MP, Elphinstone LH. Food poisoning on Royal Air Force aircraft 1990–4. In: Dupont H. (ed.). *Abstracts of the 4th International Conference on Travel Medicine.* Stone Mountain, GA: International Society of Travel Medicine, 1995.

Health Canada. *Infection Control Guidance for Air Flight Cabin Crew Staff.* Ottawa: Health Canada, 2003.

Kenyon TA, Valway SE, Ihle WW, et al. Transmission of multi-drug resistant *Mycobacterium tuberculosis* during a long airborne flight. *New England Journal of Medicine* 1996; **334**: 933–8.

Marsden AG. Influenza outbreak related to air travel. *Medical Journal of Australia* 2003; **179**: 172–3.

Moser MR, Bender TR, Margolis GR, et al. An outbreak of influenza aboard a commercial airliner. *American Journal of Epidemiology* 1979; **110**: 1–6.

National Travel Health Network and Centre. Illness in England, Wales and Northern Ireland associated with foreign travel: a baseline report to 2002. London: Health Protection Agency, 2004.

Olsen SJ, Chang H, Cheung T, et al. Transmission of the severe acute respiratory syndrome on aircraft. *New England Journal of Medicine* 2003; **349**: 2416–22.

Paul MA, McCarthy AE, Gibson N, et al. The impact of Malarone and primaquine on psychomotor performance. *Aviation, Space, and Environmental Medicine* 2003; **74**: 738–45.

Schlagenhof P, Lobel H, Steffen R, et al. Tolerance of mefloquine by SwissAir trainee pilots. *American Journal of Tropical Medicine and Hygiene* 1997; **56**: 235–40.

Tauxe RV, Tormey MP, Masola L, et al. Salmonellosis outbreak on transatlantic flights: foodborne illness on aircraft 1947–84. *American Journal of Epidemiology* 1987; **125**: 150–57.

Tuck JJ, Green AD, Roberts KI. A malaria outbreak following a British military deployment to Sierra Leone. *Journal of Infection* 2003; **47**: 225–30.

United States Air Force Transportation Command. Interim policy on movement regulation of aeromedical evacuation of bioterrorism and Centers for Disease Control Critical List Agent casualties. Washington, DC: United States Air Force Transportation Command, 2003.

Wheeler JG, Sethi D, Cowden JM, et al. Study of infectious intestinal disease in England: rates in the community presenting to general practice and reported to national surveillance. *British Medical Journal* 1999; **319**: 1046–50.

Wick RL, Irvine LA. The microbiological composition of airline cabin air. *Aviation, Space, and Environmental Medicine* 1995; **66**: 220–24.

World Health Organization. *Tuberculosis and Air Travel: Guidelines for Prevention and Control.* Geneva: World Health Organization, 1999.

World Tourism Organization. *World Tourism in 2002: Better than Expected.* Madrid: World Tourism Organization, 2003.

Zucker J. Changing patterns of autochthonous malaria transmission in the United States: a review of recent outbreaks. *Emerging Infectious Diseases* 1996; **2**: 37–43.

FURTHER READING

Bradley DJ, Bannister B, on behalf of the Health Protection Agency Advisory Committee on Malaria Prevention for UK Travellers. Guidelines for malaria prevention in travellers from the United Kingdom for 2003. *Communicable Diseases and Public Health* 2003; **6**: 180–99.

Byrne NJ, Behrens RH. Airline crews' risk for malaria on layovers in urban sub-Saharan Africa: risk assessment and appropriate prevention policy. *Journal of Travel Medicine* 2004; **11**: 359–61.

Lockie C, Walker E, Calvert L. *Travel Medicine and Migrant Health.* London: Churchill Livingstone, 2000.

USEFUL WEBSITES

Centers for Disease Control and Prevention: Travelers' Health. www.cdc.gov/travel

Health Protection Agency. www.hpa.org.uk

Health Protection Scotland. www.fitfortravel.scot.nhs.uk

National Travel Health Network and Centre. www.nathnac.org

World Health Organization. International travel and health. www.who.int/ith/en

56

Aeromedical evacuation: medical aspects

WILLIAM J. COKER

INTRODUCTION

Aeromedical evacuation (AE) is defined as the movement of patients by air because other methods either involve an unacceptable delay in treatment or are not practicable. This includes both emergency AE to reduce mortality and morbidity and routine AE, where surface means of evacuation are non-existent or not practical. Patients for AE can be stable, stabilized or unstable. Stable patients require minimal treatment in flight but will often require careful observation because the demands of the flight environment may impose physiological stresses, which may cause their condition to deteriorate. Stabilized patients will have received initial treatment but will be moved for urgent treatment elsewhere. They will require careful observation and treatment in flight, but they will usually have a stabilized airway, any haemorrhage will be controlled, fluid replacement may be in progress, and any fractures will be stabilized. They will have a higher risk of medical decompensation than patients who are stable. Unstable patients are moved by air only when they cannot be treated before flight. They require a full medical team with resuscitation and airway-management skills. They usually have a life-threatening condition, and the purpose of the AE is to bring them as quickly as possible to a well-equipped treatment facility.

HISTORY

The history of AE is nearly as old as powered flight itself (evacuation of patients by balloon during the siege of Paris in 1870 is not supported by contemporary records). A French medical officer, Eugene Chassaing, adapted military aircraft for use as air ambulances during the First World War. However, AE was not used to any great extent in this conflict. Between the two world wars, Great Britain, France and the USA all used modified aircraft to transport patients. The Second World War saw a rapid expansion in casualty transportation by air and, with this, specific training of flight personnel for the specific purpose of medical escort duties. The Vietnam War demonstrated the suitability of the helicopter for the rapid removal of injured troops close to the point of wounding. No soldier in Vietnam was more than 35 minutes away from a medical facility because of this 'scoop-and-run' system. This rapid transfer to specialist medical care almost certainly contributed towards the lower mortality rate of wounded casualties in Vietnam compared with earlier conflicts.

Since the 1980s, the helicopter evacuation of civilian casualties from road-traffic accidents and for inter-hospital transfer of critically ill patients has become a common feature of everyday life. An example is the London-based Helicopter Emergency Medical Service (HEMS), which was established in 1990. This was originally set up as an exercise to define the role of helicopter-based pre-hospital care in the UK. Military AE has also continued to evacuate serving personnel from conflicts where, although the numbers of casualties are small by the standards of previous wars, casualties often need to be evacuated over long distances because there is little holding capacity in the forward areas. The casualties are, therefore, stabilized rather than stable. In the Iraq war of 2003, the Royal Air Force (RAF) aeromedically evacuated more than 2000 casualties. The growth of civilian air travel in this period has also led to the increased use of jet aircraft to aeromedically evacuate travellers from both popular and remote locations around the world.

GENERAL PRINCIPLES

Table 56.1 shows the different types of AE in civilian and military situations. From the emergency evacuation of a battlefield casualty by a military helicopter manned by a military medical assistant to the planned AE of a holiday-maker with a stable fracture in a civilian airliner with a nurse escort, there is a whole range of AE activity. There are, however, a number of fundamental principles that should be remembered when AE is proposed for any patient, as follows:

- AE should offer a clear advantage to the patient. This will often be obvious when more sophisticated medical care is required urgently, but sometimes the advantage of AE has to be weighed against the benefits of maintaining medical care on the ground and the potential complications of AE.
- AE is not a therapeutic procedure, although, like many therapeutic procedures, it does have its own side effects and complications.
- Although there are no absolute contraindications to AE, some conditions place a heavy load on the AE escort team and can be anticipated to cause difficulty. The AE of these patients needs careful planning and preparation.
- It is better to anticipate problems and prepare for them before flight than to be surprised by them at 30 000 feet in the back of a dark, noisy, vibrating aircraft. Assume 'Murphy's law' applies, i.e. if anything can go wrong, it will. Therefore, prepare for it!

- Patients should be reassessed regularly throughout the AE process. This must often take place in less than ideal circumstances.
- Time spent checking and preparing AE equipment before flight is never wasted.
- The type of aircraft and the composition of the escort team will be determined by the number and clinical condition of the casualties and the distance they need to be moved.
- AE is straightforward, as long as you remember that humans were designed for living on, or very near, the surface of the Earth.

CATEGORIZATION OF PATIENTS

The purpose of categorizing patients for AE is to give medical, nursing and movements staff a simple and standardized means of assessing the degree of urgency; the appropriate in-flight equipment and personnel required; and the space requirements for each patient. For strategic AE, the RAF has codes for priority, clinical dependency and classification (see Table 56.2).

CHOICE OF AIRCRAFT

There are many factors that determine the type of aircraft used for any particular AE. Only some of these factors will be medical. The distance the patient is required to move and the type and length of the nearest landing strip or runway will limit the choice of aircraft. In turn, the number of patients and the complexity of the care they require will also determine the type of aircraft. Sophisticated medical equipment, consumable supplies, oxygen cylinders and

Table 56.1 *Types of aeromedical evacuation (AE)*

Military	Civilian
Forward AE: helicopter evacuation from point of wounding to emergency medical/surgical treatment	*Emergency helicopter service:* transport of critically ill patients from scene of accident to nearest appropriate hospital
SAR: search-and-rescue helicopter – RN, RAF, Coastguard	*Helicopter AE:* inter-hospital transfers within the UK
Tactical AE: theatre-wide plan for AE comprising a coordinated chain to deliver casualties from an intra-theatre facility to a hub airfield, from which strategic AE can return them to the UK; can use either rotary- or fixed-wing aircraft	*Fixed-wing AE:* conventional scheduled flights in passenger aircraft with either sitting patients or stretcher patients; or
Strategic AE: transfer of patients from an operational theatre to the UK; in peacetime, this is carried out globally year-round; due to the distances involved, fixed-wing aircraft are generally used	*Dedicated AE:* flight using pressurized jet aircraft or single-/multi-engine non-pressurized aircraft

RAF, Royal Air Force; RN, Royal Navy; SAR, search and rescue.

Table 56.2 *Categorization of patients for aeromedical evacuation (AE)*

Priority

This category allows more urgent patients to be evacuated before less urgent patients if aircraft space is limited.

Priority	Explanation
1: urgent	Patient for whom AE is necessary to save life or limb, or to avoid serious permanent disability; normally returned to the UK within 24 h
2: priority	Patient who requires specialized treatment not available locally and who will suffer pain and disability unless evacuated with the least possible delay; normally returned to the UK within 48 h
3: routine	Patient whose immediate treatment can be undertaken locally, but who would benefit from further treatment in the UK; normally returned within 3–4 days, but could wait up to 7 days

Dependency

This category gives an indication of the level of medical care required during AE.

Dependency	Explanation
1: high	Patient who requires intensive medical and nursing care in flight; may be ventilated and require intracranial pressure monitoring, central venous pressure or cardiac monitoring
2: medium	Patient who, although not requiring intensive support, requires frequent monitoring and whose condition may deteriorate in flight; may require oxygen and multiple IV infusions and have drains and catheters in situ
3: low	Patient whose condition is stable and is not expected to deteriorate in flight; requires nursing care and may need regular medical therapy while in flight
4: minimal	Patient who does not require nursing or medical care in flight, but who may need help with mobility or with bodily functions

Classification

This category defines the patient's need for space on the aircraft and gives an indication of the patient's mobility in the event of an aircraft emergency. It also describes the degree of supervision required by psychiatric patients.

Class	Explanation
1A: severely disturbed psychiatric patients	Disturbed patient who will require very close supervision in flight; may also require sedation and even physical restraint
1B: psychiatric patients of intermediate severity	Patient who is not disturbed before flight but who may react badly to flight and require sedation; needs close supervision
1C: mildly disturbed psychiatric patients	Patient who is stable, cooperative and has proved reliable under pre-flight observation is at low risk of requiring sedation during flight
2A: immobile stretcher patients	Patient who is unable to move without aid and who, in an aircraft emergency, would require assistance to leave the aircraft
2B: mobile stretcher patients	Patient who requires a stretcher while in flight but who, in an emergency, could leave the aircraft without help
3A: sitting patients	Patient who, in an emergency, would require help to leave the aircraft
3B: sitting patients	Patient who, in an emergency, could leave the aircraft unassisted
4: walking patients	Patient who requires no nursing care and is able to travel unattended; may require assistance with their baggage

batteries to power the equipment take up a considerable amount of room and weight. The electrical equipment must also be checked to make sure it does not interfere with the operation of the aircraft.

Stretcher access to the aircraft can also be critical. A retractable ramp is ideal for stretcher loading, but not all aircraft used for AE will have this facility. Although some nations have the luxury of dedicated aircraft for AE, most, particularly in war, will rely on opportunistic aircraft. These will fly out to the theatre of operations loaded with personnel, material etc., and then be reconfigured to carry AE patients back home on the return trip. This requires the AE team to reconfigure the aircraft, depending on the number and type of patients.

The pressurization of the aircraft cabin is an important factor in AE. All modern jet aircraft are pressurized to a cabin altitude of 6000–8000 ft. Although most medical conditions are unaffected by decreased pressure, several conditions would be critically compromised by this altitude, e.g. decompression sickness or air in the cranium. To request a cabin altitude of sea level places a large limitation in terms of fuel and speed on the operation of the aircraft. The cabin altitude will be sufficient to cause a degree of hypoxia in some patients, particularly those with cardiovascular and respiratory disorders. Oxygen should be considered as potentially necessary in all AE patients, especially those requiring intensive treatment. Most aircraft used opportunistically for AE will not carry medical oxygen, and this will have to be carried in large, heavy cylinders.

If patients require intensive care during flight, then it is essential that the team has room to operate around the patient. This can become a problem when patients are carried in tiers, when the space between patients for most military AE configurations will be as little as 53 cm. If procedures need to be carried out, then such patients will need to be removed from the stretcher tier. Aircraft used in civilian practice for single patients may also have limited space. The C-21 Lear Jet is highly effective for AE, requiring little runway for takeoff and having a good range and speed. However, cabin space is extremely limited, with little headroom and difficult stretcher access.

The C-130 Hercules is the workhorse for a great deal of AE. Its versatility in takeoff and landing, with its large capacity, make it very useful in evacuating large numbers of patients from remote locations. However, its noise level is between 95 and 100 dB, and auscultation is impossible under these circumstances. Aircraft used in the strategic AE role, such as the Lockheed TriStar, are far more comfortable, are quieter and have better temperature control than the C-130, but they could not operate under the same conditions as the versatile Hercules. The C-17 Globemaster has a huge capacity and can land on almost any semi-improved airfield. Access is easy, both to the aircraft and to the stretcher patients when they are accommodated on the stanchions. Noise and lighting are excellent, and climate control is good. It has been modified to supply piped oxygen to patients and has already been extremely useful in the AE role.

GENERAL MEDICAL CONSIDERATIONS

Gas expansion

At the highest cabin altitude expected during flight in a pressurized aircraft (8000 feet), gas will increase in volume by approximately 30 per cent. Gas trapped in body cavities can cause pain on expansion; this is most likely to happen in the ears, sinuses, gastrointestinal tract and, rarely, the teeth. Such pain may be difficult to determine in comatose or disoriented patients. Examination of the tympanic membrane or abdomen may be necessary if the patient shows increased irritability or agitation on ascent or descent.

Hypoxia

The decrease in barometric pressure mentioned above will cause a corresponding fall in the partial pressure of oxygen in the inspired air. The barometric pressure at 8000 feet will be 565 mmHg, with an arterial oxygen pressure (Pa_{O_2}) of about 55 mmHg. If this is plotted on the oxyhaemoglobin dissociation curve, the blood oxygen saturation is 90 per cent. Although healthy travellers can compensate for this degree of hypoxaemia, in patients with pre-existing cardiac or pulmonary disease or anaemia, who already have a lowered arterial oxygen pressure, this fall may be enough to bring them to the steep part of the oxygen dissociation curve. This may cause very low arterial oxygen saturation, resulting in functional impairment. Oxygen may, therefore, be required in patients with certain medical conditions, even though they appear well oxygenated before flight.

Vibration

Vibration is common in all forms of transport, particularly in military transport aircraft and most helicopters. It may interfere with patient assessment and physiological monitoring, as well as having an effect on the patient per se. Vibration increases metabolic rate, equivalent to that seen in gentle exercise. It can also cause hyperventilation and induce motion sickness, fatigue and irritability. To reduce the effects of vibration, patients should be secured comfortably and adequate padding should be provided.

Temperature control

Temperature decreases with increasing altitude at a rate of 2 °C for every 1000 feet up to 35 000 feet. Aircraft collecting patients from a desert environment and flying back to a temperate climate at 35 000 feet may subject patients to a considerable variation in cabin temperature. Sick patients may also be in metabolic overdrive and may have lost their thermoregulatory mechanisms. The AE team should, therefore, monitor cabin temperature changes and assess the effect of these changes on their patients.

Noise

Noise, or 'unwanted sound', is another characteristic of helicopters and military aircraft. It interferes with communication between the AE team and their patients, and it can cause fatigue in both staff and patients. Communication must continue using other methods. These will include close observation and visual alarm systems. Auscultation will be impossible, even with specially designed stethoscopes. Hearing protection should be worn by staff and patients in aircraft such as the C-130 Hercules. Disposable ear plugs or ear defenders should be available for patients, while staff should be provided with a headset to attenuate noise and facilitate communication between AE team members and aircrew.

Airsickness

This is a variety of motion sickness and is characterized by nausea, vomiting, pallor and cold sweating. It is a normal response to unfamiliar motion and will, therefore, disappear as personnel become adapted to the aircraft movement. Patients, however, may suffer, particularly if the aircraft is subject to turbulence during AE. If this is anticipated, or if a patient has a previous history of airsickness, then an antiemetic can be given before takeoff. Transdermal hyoscine is effective but will cause drowsiness. Medication is unlikely to help once symptoms have occurred. Vomiting due to airsickness should be avoided in patients who have recently had any form of abdominal surgery, because of the increased tension this could put on suture lines.

Fear of flying

A significant fear of flying is experienced by up to 15 per cent of the population, with a proportion of this group being handicapped socially and in their working lives by this phobia. In the aeromedical situation, this could aggravate a patient's condition, making them more vulnerable to the effects of vibration and airsickness. AE staff should be aware of the frequency of this condition and should offer reassurance and, if necessary and appropriate clinically, mild sedation to those affected. Patients may express anxieties to staff on the AE team about flying, or they may betray signs of anxiety such as hyperventilation, pallor and cold sweating, especially during periods of turbulence.

Medication and time zones

On strategic AE flights the aircraft may transit through several different time zones. For medication that has been started before the flight, it is easiest if this is given according to the time at the point of departure. This should be communicated to the staff taking over the patient at the end of the flight. The time and time zone pertaining to the medication given should be annotated clearly on the drug card. For patients with type 1 diabetes, it should be remembered that when travelling east, the travel day will be shortened; if more than two hours are lost, then it may be necessary to take fewer units of intermediate- or long-acting insulin. When travelling west, the travel day will be extended; if it is extended by more than two hours, then it may be necessary to supplement with additional injections of soluble insulin or an increased dose of intermediate-acting insulin. On long flights, the use of short-acting soluble insulin using a pen device is most convenient. This allows insulin to be given with each meal for the duration of the flight.

Organization of aeromedical evacuation

When AE is requested, physician-to-physician referral is always to the patient's advantage. Whereas contact across time zones, even with mobile telephones, does not always allow for this personal contact, the receiving hospital should always have notice of the patient's arrival. After the request has been made by the referring medical practitioner, the patient should be assessed for AE. This will involve categorization and should be carried out by a medical practitioner with experience in aviation medicine. Liaison with the AE team should also take place, in order to enable the team to arrive with the appropriate equipment and medical support. Ground transport to the receiving hospital from the airhead must always be arranged; usually, the AE team will deliver patients to the receiving hospital. The patients' records, including notes written during the flight and details of any drugs given, should accompany the patients to the receiving hospital.

Before the flight, the AE team leader will discuss any specific points with the aircraft captain, e.g. a request for an altitude limitation. The stowage of equipment or disposition of stretchers will be discussed either with the load master or the senior cabin steward. AE in peacetime is relatively straightforward, but in the operational setting it requires considerable coordination of aircraft movements, the careful disposition and composition of the AE teams, and the support of receiving hospitals.

CLINICAL CONSIDERATIONS

Neurological problems

All patients with head injury need careful assessment, both before and during AE. The Glasgow Coma Scale (GCS) will give some degree of objective uniformity, the important factor being any change during AE. Unconscious patients with head injury need a secure airway and supplemental oxygen to maintain maximal oxygenation and prevent any degree of cerebral hypoxia. Intravenous access should be in place so that mannitol or dexamethasone can be given for cerebral oedema, or anticonvulsants can be administered acutely if indicated. If the patient is conscious, then anti-emetics should be considered, as retching and vomiting must be avoided to prevent the accompanying rise of intracranial pressure. However, most anti-emetics will cause drowsiness and thus affect the GCS.

Free air within the cranial cavity is hazardous in flight. It may arise from a recent craniotomy, a penetrating wound of the head or a cerebrospinal fluid (CSF) leak from the ears or nose, suggesting a basal skull fracture. The danger is that the air will expand with increasing altitude and compress vital structures. This may progress to herniation of brain tissue, either in the temporal lobe or tonsillar region, both of which can cause death. CSF leakage may occur more rapidly with increasing altitude. On descent, air and bacteria could be forced back into the cranium. The presence of air in the cranium can be determined by a lateral skull X-ray or computed tomography (CT) scan. Ideally, patients should not fly within seven days of a craniotomy; if a patient with air in the cranium does have to fly, then the cabin pressure must be kept the same as that at the originating airfield. This advice also applies to patients with CSF leak.

Patients who have suffered a cerebrovascular event, such as cerebral thrombosis or haemorrhage, already have an impaired cerebral circulation, and any further cause of cerebral hypoxia must be avoided. Ideally, the neurological condition should be stable before flight. If they require AE before this occurs, they will need supplemental oxygen during flight. Blood pressure and pulse rate should be controlled with medication if required.

Patients with space-occupying lesions (SOL) are safe to fly, although the stresses of flight, particularly hypoxia, will make the risk of seizures more likely in those already disposed to seizures because of their SOL. Seizures in flight should be controlled with intravenous and oral therapy and the patient should be observed for any signs of increasing intracranial pressure.

The AE of patients who have had a recent subarachnoid haemorrhage (SAH) is always problematic. Following an SAH, 25 per cent of patients will die within 24 hours and a further 25 per cent will die within the first month. As the first week is the time of maximum rebleeding, the aneurysm should be clipped as soon as possible. As the risk of surgery is high if the patient is unconscious, it is probably reasonable to fly a stable, conscious patient who has had a SAH if this is necessary in order to obtain access to a neurosurgical facility.

Patients with idiopathic epilepsy are safe to fly if they are stable, either on or off medication. However, patients with uncontrolled or poorly controlled epilepsy are at risk, due to the lowering of the convulsive threshold by hypoxia. If they are aeromedically evacuated for other conditions, they should be on an optimum treatment regimen, and strict compliance with medication times should be observed. If convulsive episodes occur during flight, then parenteral therapy should be available (although not paraldehyde). Good airway management and oxygen are essential in this situation.

Cardiovascular conditions

Hypoxia is the biggest threat to patients with heart disease during AE. Patients with poor cardiac reserve may not tolerate the decreased oxygen saturation that results from the reduced cabin pressure and may deteriorate clinically. The AE of a patient who has had a myocardial infarction (MI) should be delayed until their condition is stable and there are no complications such as cardiac failure or dysrhythmias. The absence of complications is a more important factor than the time after MI. However, it has been shown that the majority of complications in flight occur within the first 14 days following MI, and it would seem sensible to delay AE until 14 days post-MI if possible.

Well-controlled angina is compatible with flying. If the patient can walk 80 m on the flat or manage an average flight of stairs, then it is unlikely that they will develop problems in flight. Unstable angina is a relative contraindication to flying; the risk of hypoxia and the catecholamine release produced by the stress and excitement of flight may well provoke a cardiac dysrhythmia. Similarly, uncontrolled cardiac failure is also a relative contraindication to AE, and every attempt should be made to control failure before AE is undertaken. All patients with cardiac disease should be given supplemental oxygen during AE and should have pulse oximetry to ensure their oxygen saturation remains greater than 95 per cent. Cardiac monitoring should be carried out if there is even a small risk of rhythm disturbance. The AE of any patient with significant heart disease will require a full team that is able to resuscitate, defibrillate, pace and ventilate, as necessary. All equipment used in RAF aeromedical flights is compatible with the aircraft avionic systems, but it is standard procedure to alert the aircrew if defibrillation or synchronized cardioversion is due to be carried out.

Respiratory disease

Patients with well-controlled respiratory disease at sea level may deteriorate in flight due to the fall in the partial pressure of oxygen in the inspired cabin air. If a patient exhibits respiratory symptoms on the ground, then these will certainly worsen at cabin altitude. Equations to predict the arterial oxygen tension at altitude in normocapnoeic patients with chronic airways obstruction have been derived. These require measurement of the arterial oxygen tension at ground level; if the resultant arterial oxygen tension at altitude is unacceptably low (< 6.5 kPa), then varying oxygen concentrations can be administered on the ground until a satisfactory predicted result for the appropriate altitude is obtained. Alternatively, the altitude can be adjusted to maintain a satisfactory oxygen tension. It should also be remembered that the use of 100 per cent oxygen will worsen patients with chronic obstructive pulmonary disease (COPD), who depend on a hypoxic drive for ventilation. Other factors that can cause deterioration in a patient with COPD are pulmonary embolism, spontaneous pneumothorax and acute pulmonary infection. Gastric distension, due to the expansion of swallowed air at altitude, can restrict diaphragmatic movement and thereby reduce vital capacity. Pulse oximetry should be used in flight to monitor all patients with COPD; patients should also be observed for signs of dyspnoea, tachycardia, restlessness and distress. The AE of a patient with unstable COPD should be undertaken only by a team that has the expertise and facilities to carry out endotracheal intubation and mechanical ventilation.

Stable bronchial asthma should not present any problems in flight. Treatment with inhalers can be continued, although a spacer attachment is probably more effective than an inhaler alone. Unstable asthma should be controlled before AE. Asthmatic patients deteriorating in flight and unresponsive to medical treatment will require mechanical ventilation.

The AE of patients with respiratory failure requires a full intensive care team. The condition will inevitably be worsened by the cabin altitude induced hypoxia. Respiratory failure caused by adult respiratory distress syndrome (ARDS), in addition to increasing the inspired oxygen concentration, may require a combination of positive-pressure ventilation and positive end expiratory pressure.

An untreated pneumothorax is a contraindication to AE and must be corrected before flight. Unless this is done, there is a risk that the pneumothorax will expand in flight and a tension pneumothorax develop. Following successful drainage of a pneumothorax, it is advisable to wait for two weeks and then check radiologically that the lung remains inflated. Patients can be aeromedically evacuated with a chest drain in situ; this should be fitted with a Heimlich valve. A chest X-ray should be taken before AE to check that the tube is sited properly and is working satisfactorily. Patients with persistent bronchopleural fistulae can also fly with a functioning drain and Heimlich valve.

Patients with pleural effusions should have these drained and the aetiology determined before flight. A chest X-ray should be taken before AE to ensure that fluid has not re-accumulated or that a pneumothorax has not occurred during thoracocentesis.

Haematological conditions

Severe anaemia (< 7 g/dl) will accentuate the problems of hypoxia and is a relative contraindication to AE, although this judgement must take into account the chronicity and cause of the anaemia as well as the presence of any other condition. Patients with chronic anaemia are more tolerant of their condition, for any given level of haemoglobin (Hb), than those patients with an acute cause for their anaemia. Conditions such as myocardial ischaemia will be aggravated by anaemia, and careful pre-flight blood transfusion will be necessary in these situations. The aim of transfusion should be to raise the Hb above 10 g/dl.

Sickle cell crises can be precipitated by hypoxia in subjects with sickle cell haemoglobin C disease and sickle cell beta-thalassaemia. These individuals should receive oxygen during AE. They should also be well hydrated before and during flight. Patients with sickle cell trait present no problems in aircraft pressurized to normal cabin altitudes (6000–8000 m).

Gastrointestinal conditions

Air within the gastrointestinal tract or free within the peritoneum are the main concerns, as this will increase in volume with altitude. The gastrointestinal tract normally contains a small amount of air, although expansion of this rarely causes problems, as the excess volume can be vented by belching or flatulence. Trapped gas in an ileus, hernia or volvulus can expand and produce pain or even compromise the circulation of blood in the bowel. Patients with an ileostomy or colostomy should be warned about the increased volume of gas at altitude, which will increase faecal output, as patients will need to change bags more frequently than when on the ground.

Following abdominal surgery, the expansion of gas can cause added tension on suture lines, which could lead to breakdown or bleeding. Following gastrointestinal haemorrhage, distension has been associated with an increase risk of rebleeding. Ideally, patients should not be aeromedically evacuated until at least seven days after surgery. If AE must be carried out before this, then it should be undertaken after discussion with the surgical team. A nasogastric tube should be inserted before flight and suction should be available. A height restriction should also be considered. For AE after damage control surgery, some surgical authorities would advise a mass closure technique with retention sutures, rather than the standard layered abdominal closure. This allows for peritoneal expansion and further inspection and assessment at the receiving hospital.

Following colonoscopy involving multiple biopsies or polypectomy, flight should be delayed for at least 24 hours due to the residual gas in the large bowel and the increased risk of bleeding from the biopsy/polypectomy sites. After laparoscopic abdominal procedures, residual carbon dioxide gas is absorbed rapidly and is not a complicating factor. Laparoscopic procedures are less associated with ileus than are open procedures, and the timing of AE of these patients should be discussed with the surgical team; usually, AE can take place earlier following laparoscopic procedures than open procedures.

Orthopaedic considerations

All casts used for splinting fractured limbs should be split (bivalved) before AE. This is because the material of the cast, whether Plaster of Paris or fibreglass, may contain air pockets that will increase in volume during flight, thereby compressing limbs, with resulting damage to nerve or vascular structures. Additionally, pockets of air could be trapped beneath the cast and expand. There is also the possibility that soft tissue will expand in flight, this often being related to the original injury. An alternative procedure to splitting the cast is to apply a back-slab splint before flight. Splitting casts or applying a back-slab carries the added advantage of allowing access to any wounds during flight in order to check for bleeding or tension. The use of pneumatic splints in AE is not recommended, as air would have to be released from these splints to allow for gas expansion at altitude. Likewise, free-weight traction should not be used in AE, due to the adverse effects of movement, turbulence and G forces on these systems.

The risk of fat embolism in all patients with multiple or serious long-bone fractures should be remembered. The usually insidious onset of dyspnoea, distress, confusion or convulsions in patients with fractures makes this a possible diagnosis. Such patients will require oxygen and may require intubation and ventilatory support. Pulmonary embolism from a venous origin is also possible, although its onset is more sudden and it generally occurs later than fat embolism.

As a general principle, the optimum time to transport a patient with a fracture is when the fracture is stabilized. This will prevent pain, bleeding and further tissue damage, and reduce the chance of fat embolism. For minor fractures, transport can take place when the swelling has diminished after two to three days; for major fractures, it will ideally be after the immune response period (approximately seven days). Haemoglobin, platelet count and clotting factors should all be normal. Consideration should be given to the need for prophylaxis against venous thrombosis; this will be essential for some fractures, e.g. fractures of the pelvis. Stabilization of the fracture should be maintained during transport by fixation or splinting. Patients who have had spinal surgery should be checked for air in the spinal canal, as this can increase in volume with altitude and cause further neurological damage.

Ophthalmic patients

The AE of patients with ophthalmic conditions will depend on the severity of the condition and the availability of skilled ophthalmic help. In the military situation, eight to ten per cent of all combat injuries involve the eye, and a significant proportion of these injuries will be complicated and severe, involving the threat of loss of vision. Statistically, open eye injuries do better when ophthalmic care is not delayed, but in these battlefield injuries such help will not be available immediately. Consequently, AE may provide the only possibility of saving sight in this group.

The concern is that trapped air may cause a problem at altitude, although if air is present in the eye as a result of a penetrating laceration, then small amounts would not be expected to be a significant problem in an open eye. The risk assessment has to be made between the possibility of an expanding bubble of trapped air causing additional ocular damage and the advantage of getting the patient to more definitive care as quickly as possible.

Rupture of the globe of the eye is a relatively common combat-related injury and needs urgent AE. During AE these patients should be transported in the reclining position, with the head elevated and face up. The eye should be covered, but no pressure should be applied to the globe. All extraocular movements should be minimized.

Ophthalmological procedures for retinal detachment involve the intraocular injection of one of several gases to temporarily increase intraocular pressure. Guidelines have been published regarding air travel following such intraocular surgery. This is different from the situation where air is introduced into an eye by a penetrating wound. The advice is that until the intraocular bubble has decreased to less than 30 per cent of the vitreous, flight is contraindicated. All ophthalmic patients for AE should be secured firmly in their seats and offered anti-emetics if airsickness is a problem; retching and vomiting should be avoided in order to prevent the associated rise in intraocular pressure.

Patients with infectious disease

Patients with infectious disease can be aeromedically evacuated because of the infectious condition per se, or they may be evacuated because of a non-infectious condition that is complicated by infection, or they may have an infection unrelated to the condition requiring AE. In the latter cases, the infection may not be diagnosed until AE is complete. The type of AE required by a patient with a known infectious condition will depend on the severity of the condition and its mode of transmission. Most patients with infectious disease can be evacuated on commercial passenger aircraft, provided routine infection control measures are taken. For reasons of economy, cabin air is recirculated; to maintain air quality, high-efficiency particulate air (HEPA) filters are installed in the air-circulation systems. These will filter out aerosolized contaminants, including droplet nuclei carrying virus and bacterial particles.

One of the most important concerns relating to AE and infectious disease is awareness of the possibility that any AE patient may have an infectious condition. Table 56.3 is used as a checklist on all RAF AE flights in order to consider this possibility.

There may be circumstances when it is necessary to evacuate a patient with a severe and highly infectious disease from an endemic to a non-endemic area. It should be stressed that this will be undertaken only in exceptional circumstances, but it can be done using an air-transportable patient isolator (ATI). This is a totally enclosed unit comprising a sealed plastic envelope enclosing a stretcher system, which can be moved and adjusted in the horizontal plane. Sealed access points allow medical and nursing staff to care for the patient. If necessary, a patient can be ventilated while in the ATI. The RAF has three patient isolators. Although used rarely, they are exercised regularly by both military and civilian personnel as a cooperative venture.

Biological and chemical casualties

In the event of casualties being contaminated by chemical or biological material, either occupationally as a result of an accident or as the result of war or terrorist activity, then the first priority is the decontamination of the casualty before AE. Unless decontamination is complete, AE will present a risk to aircrew and clinical staff. Once decontamination is complete, further precautions will depend on the agent itself and the patient's condition. A patient contaminated with certain biological agents could be moved in the ATI described above, although resource limitations would make this impractical for the large-scale AE of biological casualties.

Psychiatric conditions

The most important element concerning the AE of psychiatric patients is the careful assessment of each patient. This has to be carried out by an individual with training in psychiatry and acquainted with the practice of AE. The major concern is that a psychiatric patient will harm themselves or others within the confines of an aircraft, with the possibility of serious interruption to the flight or even danger to the whole aircraft. Sometimes pressure will be exerted on the AE team to move a psychiatric patient quickly because he or she is seen as potentially troublesome. Wherever possible, psychiatric patients should be stabilized before AE. Careful pre-flight assessment will indicate those rare patients where violent behaviour or self-harm is likely and where physical restraint during flight may be necessary.

A patient's psychiatric medication should be continued during flight, but it is generally unwise to start a patient for AE on new drugs immediately before or during flight. It is also preferable to stabilize a patient on a drug before AE, in order to avoid the problems of under- or overdosage. It is important to avoid oversedation, as this will reduce the patient's ability to look after themselves in an emergency and could even cause life-threatening respiratory depression. Heavy sedation will also predispose to deep vein thrombosis and barotrauma. Many drugs used in psychiatry have anticholinergic side effects, which will increase the likelihood of urinary retention, constipation, increased bowel gas and dry mouth; these conditions can be further aggravated on a long flight. The selective serotonin reuptake inhibitors (SSRIs) cause fewer anticholin-

Table 56.3 *Checklist for possible infectious illness in aeromedically evacuated patients*

Pyrexia
- Oral temperature $\geq$ 38.9 °C

Diarrhoea
- Diarrhoea possibly due to an infective agent

Abnormal bleeding
- Any bleeding from gums or mucus membranes?
- Any report of petechial haemorrhage from mouth and palate?
- Any presence of conjunctival injection?
- History of blood in stools or vomit?

Lymphadenopathy
- Any report of tender or painful lymph nodes?
- Any unusual coloured, enlarged or discharging lymph nodes?

Skin
- Any report of petechial or purpuric rash on skin?
- Any report of 'pox'-like skin lesion or rash?
- Any indication of jaundice?
- Presence of infective or discharging wounds?

Respiratory
- Rapid progression to severe symptoms over a period of less than three days?
- Any report of cough *and* fever, particularly if in combination with any of haemoptysis, purpuric skin rash or lymphadenopathy?

Exposure
- Any history of close contact with individuals known to have an infectious disease?
- Exposure to sewage, bodily fluids or animals before illness?
- History of insect bites?

ergic side effects than tricyclic antidepressants, but they are less sedating, which may be a disadvantage in this situation.

Anxiety is a common symptom before and during flight in 15–20 per cent of the population. It is, therefore, important to brief psychiatric patients before flight to forewarn them about particular noises in flight and of some of the physiological disturbances they may experience. If they are on no other sedating medication, then they may benefit from an anxiolytic such as diazepam, taken in a dose of 5–10 mg orally one hour before flight.

If a stable psychiatric patient, or a non-psychiatric patient, becomes acutely agitated or violent during AE, then they may require psychotropic medication. Ideally, this should have a quick calming effect with minimal risk of oversedation. Drugs such as haloperidol, lorazepam and diphenhydramine are ideal in this situation. If haloperidol is used during AE, benztropine should also be carried to counteract any extrapyramidal or dystonic symptoms that may occur. Alternatively, haloperidol could be given with diphenhydramine. If physical restraint is necessary during AE, then a sufficient number of people to provide adequate restraint must be available, both to restrain and to protect the patient from damage. Medication can be given by syringe and the patient subsequently restrained. This restraint may be provided by a stretcher and harness fit or can, if necessary, use four-point Velcro™ restraints.

Pregnancy, air travel and aeromedical evacuation

A cabin altitude of up to 8000 feet poses no threat to a normal pregnancy. At this altitude, the maternal haemoglobin remains 90 per cent saturated, even though the maternal Pa_{O_2} falls to 65 mmHg. The fetal Pa_{O_2} remains virtually unchanged due to the increased oxygen-carrying properties of fetal haemoglobin and the Bohr effect. Passengers in early pregnancy should be aware of the increased risk of vomiting due to motion sickness, while those in the third trimester of pregnancy should guard against sudden unexpected movement due to turbulence, as even relatively minor trauma could result in abruption. Pregnancy increases the risk of deep vein thrombosis due to compression of the inferior vena cava by the gravid uterus. The level of fibrinogen and other coagulation factors are also increased in pregnancy. This situation can be exacerbated by long periods of immobility, sitting in a relatively cramped position with the legs dependent, the so called 'economy-class syndrome'. This can be helped by compression stockings, comfortable non-restrictive clothing, and regular exercises and/or movement around the aircraft cabin wherever possible, preferably every hour. Pregnant passengers should also consider the destination to which

they are flying. Factors such as the need for malaria prophylaxis, endemic disease patterns and the medical care available in the event of a complication in their pregnancy should all be taken into account. Neonates should not fly for the first 48 hours of life, as not all alveoli will have expanded and there will be some ventilation/perfusion inequality. In these cases, the already low arterial oxygen pressure could be worsened by increasing altitude.

Emergencies in pregnant passengers are rarely caused by flying or the cabin environment. When they do occur during flight, the medical response is limited by the facilities available. The modern airliner is not an ideal delivery suite, and it is for this reason that long-distance air travel should not be undertaken after the thirty-fifth week of a normal singleton pregnancy. Women with an otherwise uncomplicated twin pregnancy should avoid long-haul flights after the twenty-seventh week of pregnancy. Women with a history of vaginal bleeding in pregnancy, preterm delivery, cervical incompetence or increased uterine activity should be advised to avoid long-haul flights at any stage of the pregnancy, especially if these involve long flights over water. The onset of labour during a commercial flight is an indication to divert to the nearest large airport for hospital delivery.

As far as the AE of pregnant patients is concerned, all those with reduced oxygen-carrying capacity should have this corrected before flight wherever possible. Patients with conditions such as intrauterine growth retardation, postmaturity, pre-eclampsia and placental infarction should have supplemental oxygen during flight. Active bleeding in the first trimester of pregnancy is generally a contraindication for AE. However, when an ectopic pregnancy has been excluded and if the bleeding is relatively light, i.e. less than a menstrual period, and with no abdominal cramping, then AE can be considered if medical facilities are not available locally. All such patients should have an intravenous cannula in situ, the haemoglobin should be greater than 12 g/dl before AE and an obstetric team should accompany the patient. The patient should be haemodynamically stable before flight. If the bleeding becomes severe during flight, then an emergency diversion should be considered. Patients being treated non-surgically for ectopic pregnancy, e.g. with methotrexate, should not be transported by elective AE until serum beta-human chorionic gonadotrophin (HCG) levels are undetectable.

Vaginal bleeding in the third trimester of pregnancy, due to abruptio placenta or placenta praevia, is potentially life-threatening and is a relative contraindication to AE. However, in some locations, AE by helicopter over a short distance may give these patients the best chance of survival if local facilities are lacking or non-existent. Severe pre-eclampsia is a contraindication to AE, although patients with this condition can be aeromedically evacuated if the condition is stabilized. This will require antihypertensive medication and appropriate anti-seizure medication. Seizures due to eclampsia in a patient already in the air and receiving treatment for raised blood pressure are best treated with intravenous diazepam, although an infant born within an hour or two of this treatment will show signs of respiratory depression. Patients with premature rupture of membranes are liable to go into premature labour and, therefore, AE should be delayed for 12 hours. If after this time labour has not started, then AE can be considered. However, tocolytic therapy should be available in flight, as should trained personnel able to undertake vaginal delivery if this becomes necessary.

If there is no local facility for delivery and delivery is likely during AE, then ideally an obstetric team should accompany the patient. If at all possible, delivery should be avoided in flight. As with all other forms of AE, a risk assessment should be carried out in each individual case, balancing the outcome using available local facilities against the risk of complications in flight. If the decision to undertake AE is made, then everything should be done to stabilize the patient's condition before AE.

CONCLUSION

AE can now provide high-quality medical care in the air. Given the appropriately trained nursing and medical staff and the right equipment, there are few patients who cannot be moved electively, and even stabilized patients can be moved large distances, given the right conditions. Effective AE has changed the way in which military operations are conducted. In civilian practice, patients, however seriously injured or unwell, can be returned home from anywhere in the world. For further detailed information on AE, the reader is advised to consult the texts mentioned below.

FURTHER READING

Aerospace Medical Association Medical Guidelines Task Force. Medical guidelines for airline travel. *Aviation, Space, and Environmental Medicine* 2003; **74** (5 suppl.): A1–19.

AGARD. Aeromedical support issues in contingency operations. AGARD conference proceedings 599. Neuilly-sur-Seine: AGARD/NATO, 1998.

Cox GR, Peterson J, Bouchel L, Delmas JJ. Safety of commercial air travel following myocardial infarction. *Aviation, Space, and Environmental Medicine* 1996; **67**: 976–82.

Davies GRW, Degotardi PR. Inflight medical facilities. *Aviation, Space, and Environmental Medicine* 1982; **53**: 694–700.

DeHart RL, Davis JR. *Fundamentals of Aerospace Medicine*, 3rd edn. Philadelphia: Lippincott Williams & Wilkins, 2002.

Gong H. Air travel and oxygen therapy in cardiopulmonary patients. *Chest* 1992; **101**:1104–13.

Harding RM, Mills FJ. *Aviation Medicine*, 3rd edn. London: BMJ Books, 1993.

Hays MB. Physicians and airline medical emergencies. *Aviation, Space, and Environmental Medicine* 1977; **48**: 468–70.

Holleran RS. *Air and Surface Patient Transport, Principles and Practice*, 3rd edn. St Louis, MO: Mosby, 2003.

Hopkirk JAC, Denison DM. Aerospace medicine. In: Weatherall DJ, Ledingham JGG, Warrell DA (eds). *Oxford Textbook of Medicine*, 3rd edn, Vol. 1. Oxford: Oxford University Press, 1996; p. 1202.

Hurd WW, Jernigan JG. *Aeromedical Evacuation, Management of Acute and Stabilized Patients*. New York: Springer, 2003.

Johnston RV. Clinical aviation medicine: safe travel by air. *Clinical Medicine* 2001; **1**: 385–8.

Morton NS, Pollack MM, Wallace PGM. *Stabilization and Transport of the Critically Ill*. New York: Churchill Livingstone, 1997.

Neel S. Army aeromedical evacuation procedures in Vietnam: implications for rural America. *Journal of the American Medical Association* 1968; **204**: 99–103.

Rayman RB, Hastings JD, Kruyer WB, Levy RA. *Clinical Aviation Medicine*, 3rd edn. New York: Castle Connolly Graduate Medical Publishing, 2000.

Skjenna OW, Evans JF, Moore MS, *et al.* Helping patients travel by air. *Canadian Medical Association Journal* 1991; **144**: 287–93.

57

Aeromedical transfer of the critically ill patient

NEIL MCGUIRE

INTRODUCTION

In this chapter, the focus will be on patients who are critically ill and who have been categorized dependency 1 or 2 by North Atlantic Treaty Organization (NATO) definitions, as defined in Chapter 56. These two chapters are complementary and should be read in conjunction.

Trunkey (1983) provided a model of the timescales related to casualty death following trauma (Figure 57.1). Using this model, it is clear that in order to make any impact on mortality, high-standard medical care needs to be provided at an early stage. If this approach is adopted, then the support for early resuscitation and life- and limb-

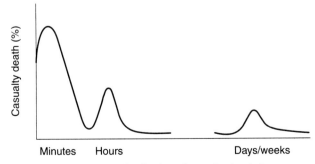

Figure 57.1 *Trimodal distribution of casualty death. From Trunkey (1983).*

saving surgery requires critical-care provision to complete the chain.

Once critical care is commenced, the requirement to evacuate the critically ill patient with all of the attendant care is established. This may be in the circumstances of primary, delayed primary (after a number of hours usually with inadequate resources) or secondary transfer. This chapter is, therefore, directed mainly at delayed primary or secondary transfer of critically ill patients by air, but the principles of transfer do not have truly fixed boundaries.

For critical-care transfers in particular, the initial premise is that they should never be undertaken lightly. In all circumstances, only appropriately trained personnel should be used. They should have equipment that can deliver care to the same standard that is offered in the fixed hospital environment (see below). It must be remembered that the journey begins as soon as the patient leaves a secure environment (piped gas supplies, mains power, immediate assistance) and ends only when a secure environment is regained.

TEAM COMPOSITION

The medical personnel should be trained in anaesthesia and intensive care and must maintain their currency outside missions by working in those areas. Nursing personnel should be critical-care-trained and in some organizations are also nurse anaesthetists. Single-patient missions are based on a full team and may be supplemented by additional personnel as required.

EQUIPMENT

Critical-care provision requires the application of modern medicine at the highest level to succeed. Delivering this care requires a considerable amount of extremely costly and complex support equipment (Figure 57.2). Traditionally, this type of equipment has been heavy, bulky and entirely dependent on fixed facilities with constant power supplies. In the transfer environment, there are considerable difficulties presented by this type of equipment. The aviation environment imposes further constraints, as discussed in Chapter 56. Many of the features of equipment used in the transfer environment require similar characteristics of robustness, reliability and the ability to use multiple power supplies. It is of interest that the most common cause of critical incidents during transfer is power failure (Thames Valley Critical Care Network, working party transfer surveys, unpublished data, 2003, 2004).

Ventilators

The use of continuous positive airways pressure (CPAP), intermittent positive-pressure ventilation (IPPV), positive end-expiratory pressure (PEEP), and alteration of the inspiratory to expiratory ratio are all employed in the ventilatory support of the critically ill. Ventilators used for transfer must be able to emulate all of the modes used in a fixed intensive care unit (ICU) facility if appropriate care is to be provided. They must have low power consumption, be able to use a variety of power supplies and be able to function with low oxygen consumption, preferably without using oxygen as a driving gas.

Monitors

Monitors must be able to monitor all parameters required to ensure continuity of care. They must also support proactive care and be sensitive enough to track the changes to make this possible. More modern equipment is multi-role and may have accessories such as defibrillators and external pacemakers. Likewise, the ability to perform investigations such as 12-lead electrocardiography (ECG), is necessary. These have marked advantages in terms of weight and space-saving. Monitors must meet at least minimal standards set by professional bodies, but for most patients these requirements should be exceeded in the hostile air environment.

Pacemakers

Temporary transvenous pacemakers are usually life-vital and as such must have high reliability with extended battery life. The indication of battery depletion must be timely and the brief act of changing the battery must not interrupt function.

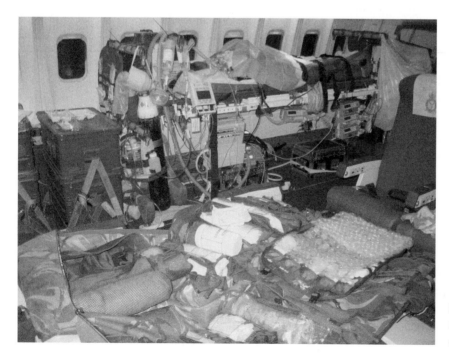

Figure 57.2 *Example of equipment required to support the critically ill patient during aeromedical transfer.*

Syringe pumps and volumetric pumps

In a critically ill patient, syringe and volumetric pumps may be life-vital equipment, particularly if they are delivering drugs that directly support the circulation. Again, these items of equipment must be able to emulate those within the fixed hospital environment closely enough to provide full support.

Suction apparatus

Suction apparatus must be fully portable, have high flow capability and be able to collect fluid waste in a manner that protects staff and be safely disposable.

Blood analysis

The ability to perform blood gas, electrolyte, glucose, lactate and other blood analyses is at the heart of critical care. Assessment of arterial oxygen, carbon dioxide, bicarbonate pH, glucose and potassium should be carried out at least every hour during transfer as a routine. This should also be undertaken if any changes are made to ventilation, including change of ventilator, or if the patient's clinical condition changes. Portable machines capable of this analysis are therefore essential.

Peripheral nerve stimulators

The ability to assess neuromuscular junction function is essential when using neuromuscular junction-blocking drugs. This allows for more exact control and helps to avoid the physiological consequences of under- or overdosage.

Disposable equipment

There is also a requirement for a considerable array of disposable equipment to support the patient directly and indirectly via machines. The use of this type of equipment has simplified the care of the patient from an infection-control perspective and aids in the rapid replenishment of supplies. It has, however caused equal difficulties of continuity of supply when operating in isolated locations and issues of disposal of waste generated in the confines of the transfer environment.

CRITICAL ILLNESS

To understand the need for complex support for critically ill patients, it is necessary to appreciate some of the underlying processes in critical illness. Definitions of terms and processes associated with critical illness are described below.

Systemic inflammatory response syndrome (SIRS) is a clinical syndrome occurring due to certain pathological processes (pancreatitis, trauma, burns) characterized by two or more of the following: temperature over 38 °C or under 36 °C, heart rate over 90 beats/min, respiratory rate over 20 breaths/min or alveolar carbon dioxide tension (Pa_{CO_2}) less than 4.3 kPa (32 mmHg), and white cell count over 12 000 cells/mm^3 or less than 4000 cells/mm^3, or greater than ten per cent immature (band) forms (American College of Chest Physicians/Society of Critical Care Medicine 1992). This is to distinguish it from the response occurring due to infection that is referred to as 'sepsis'.

Severe sepsis is associated with organ dysfunction, hypoperfusion and/or hypotension. This may lead to lactic acidosis and oliguria as part of a spectrum of abnormalities. In septic shock, these elements are present despite resuscitation and require further levels of support. In this instance, multiple organ dysfunction syndrome can occur and lead to eventual multiple organ failure (MOF). The mortality associated with sepsis syndrome and MOF is in excess of 50 per cent.

Disseminated intravascular coagulation (DIC) is a disorder of coagulation caused by massive uncontrolled activation of the coagulation mechanism. It is so severe that the anticoagulation mechanism is overwhelmed. DIC usually presents with haemorrhage, but thrombosis or a mixture of both may be seen. Underlying the condition is thrombosis occurring at the microcirculatory level.

EFFECT OF ALTITUDE

In addition to the reduction in oxygen tension with increasing altitude, there are other influences on gas exchange. There are similarities between anaesthesia and treatments used in the critical-care setting. During anaesthesia, the use of analgesic and sedative drugs interferes with gas exchange, as does IPPV. A moderate increase in the inspired oxygen concentration usually attenuates the effect on arterial oxygen tension, but the situation is more complicated in critically ill patients.

The additional factors in critically ill patients are usually due to a combination of hypoventilation, impaired diffusion, ventilation perfusion mismatching, physiological shunt and abnormalities in oxygen delivery and utilization. The influence of each will vary according to the pathophysiological process occurring in any given patient at any time during the different phases of their illness.

Impaired diffusion following acute lung injury (ALI) results from inflammatory processes such as those seen in

SIRS. There is thickening of the alveolar membranes and an increase in interstitial lung water from non-cardiogenic pulmonary oedema. Changes in pulmonary blood flow also occur, which may be due to abnormal responses to hypoxia within the pulmonary vasculature or a reflection of the general state of the circulation (see below). There are also problems related to oxygen delivery and utilization, which in turn are aggravated by changes in body temperature, pH and acid–base balance.

Air in the cerebrospinal fluid (CSF), or air in general, expanding within the skull can raise intracranial pressure. This is of particular significance when the normal compensatory mechanisms for finely adjusting the intracranial pressure are compromised. Normally, autoregulatory mechanisms adjust blood flow when there are changes in arterial carbon dioxide, arterial blood pressure and central venous pressure. CSF production and absorption are also controlled closely. In the case of serious head injury or a patient with a large space-occupying lesion, some or all of these mechanisms may be disrupted globally or regionally in the brain. A sudden increase in volume caused by the presence of air may lead to acute cardiovascular instability or even precipitate further neurological damage.

Air-containing cavities within the lung, bullae, post-surgery or air leaks from trauma can all lead to pneumothorax. Expanding air in the pleura or pericardium may lead to the conversion of a simple pneumothorax or pneumopericardium to a tension pneumothorax or pneumopericardium, both of which are life-threatening. Expansion of mediastinal air may also lead to air tracking into the pleura and the formation of pneumothoraces and/or pneumopericardium.

Patients who are post-trauma, post-surgery, on certain drugs or critically ill from whatever cause are likely to have impaired gastric motility. Delayed gastric emptying will result in raised gastric volume and may lead to nausea, vomiting, regurgitation and electrolyte disturbances. Passive regurgitation in the unconscious critically ill patient will lead to pulmonary aspiration and the risk of chemical pneumonitis and pulmonary sepsis. Acute gastric dilation is also a serious complication and adds impaired respiratory function to the list of problems.

Surgery in the peritoneal cavity initially leaves residual air trapped after closure. If this expands, then it may cause pain. In large amounts, it may lead to a rise in intra-abdominal pressure and a degree of intra-abdominal hypertension. Air or other gases within the lumen of the bowel also expand, giving rise to pain and discomfort and put anastomotic suture lines at risk. Ileus or deranged bowel motility, common in acute phases of critical illness and during the course of critical illness, may also lead to raised intra-abdominal pressure and intra-abdominal hypertension de novo. Expanding gas will exacerbate this problem.

Intra-abdominal hypertension interferes with intra-abdominal organ function as well as respiratory and cardiovascular function. Renal function may be impaired, with a rise in creatinine and urea. The kidneys are particularly at risk in critical illness, and the additional insult of intra-abdominal hypertension may precipitate renal failure. The liver is also vulnerable, and deranged hepatic function may occur.

Critically ill patients from diving accidents who have been treated inadequately or divers who have had other problems requiring air evacuation are at risk of nitrogen-bubble formation and the attendant cardiovascular, respiratory, neurological and locomotor complications (see Chapter 50).

RESPIRATORY SYSTEM

If the airway is compromised, intubation should be undertaken under controlled circumstances. This should be with the appropriate drugs, preferably either by the team taking over the care of the patient or in their presence. During induction maintaining stability is difficult and requires experience if marked, and even life-threatening, physiological changes are to be avoided. This includes complete preparation before induction, pre-oxygenation, precautions against gastro-oesophageal reflux and the correct therapeutic agents in the correct dosage. There must be provision for resuscitation should complications occur. Induction agents such as midazolam or etomidate, alone or in combination, are usually used. Analgesics such as alfentanil and fentanyl and antiarrhythmics such as lidocaine may be useful adjuncts. Non-depolarizing neuromuscular blocking agents such as rocuronium, atracurium and pancuronium are the drugs of preference, depending on the circumstances. The depolarizing neuromuscular blocking agent suxamethonium should normally be avoided in the critically ill, due to its effects on the intracellular to extracellular potassium ratio. Following the procedure, the patient should be established on ventilation, arterial blood gases checked (see below) and a chest X-ray performed. Patients who have been burned around the airway require particular attention, as oedema, although not present initially, may develop quickly and preclude subsequent access.

In a patient who is already intubated, the endotracheal tube should be checked and a chest X-ray performed to determine the tube position. Endotracheal tube cuff pressures should be checked and monitored during flight. The previous recommendation of filling the cuff with saline is no longer supported (Dirven 2002). The chest X-ray will also serve to aid in the assessment of the current state of the lung fields and the presence of any other pathology. The absence of a visible pneumothorax on X-ray does not preclude the diagnosis, and in the case of reasonable suspicion a tube thoracostomy should be performed.

Tube thoracostomies that have been placed for drainage of air, blood or fluids should remain in situ. They should be on free drainage, not be clamped at any stage and remain dependent. If possible, systems that do not require fluid to function and have non-return systems should be used. The use of the Heimlich-type valve incorporated in the system or certain types of emergency chest drainage systems, as used in acute trauma, may be problematic. These are prone to blockage and can give rise to tension pneumothorax, which may be difficult to detect initially or distinguish from other causes of sudden deterioration. Emergency drainage bags, often used with these devices, are usually open-vented and are prone to spill, presenting a biohazard.

During transfers the presence of an endotracheal tube may cause respiratory and cardiovascular effects. The usual approach is to increase sedation and add neuromuscular blockade to the patient's therapeutic regimen. This manoeuvre, however, may mask the inadequacy of inferior transfer ventilators and is often to the patient's detriment. If the patient is in the recovery phase of critical illness and is being weaned from ventilatory support, then it is important not to compromise that recovery. There are a number of possible solutions to this problem:

- The use of tracheostomy may be considered, but it is important to remember that this is not without risk. The patient should not be transferred until the risk of immediate post-procedure haemorrhage has passed (at least 24 hours) and a tract has begun to form. If a newly provided tracheostomy is displaced, particularly if it was performed for upper-airway obstruction, then regaining control of the airway may be impossible in the transfer situation. Even with the upper airway clear, patients have died during attempts to provide an airway in the controlled environment of an ICU. In the case of an established tracheostomy, this requires the same checks as for an endotracheal tube.
- The use of ICU-level ventilation also serves to attenuate the effects of intubation. It should be provided for all critical-care patients who require ventilation. In the initial 'scoop-and-run' following trauma, or acute collapse from other reasons, it may be acceptable to use low-specification ventilators. Similarly, in the immediate recovery phase from surgery or head injury without pulmonary complications, it may also be acceptable. Within a short time, however, these initial events may be followed by pulmonary compromise from dependent atelectasis, secretions, pulmonary sepsis and ALI. In this situation, ventilation becomes a more complex issue and should not be approached as if the patient has normal lungs and is simply being ventilated for routine surgery.

In these circumstances, the use of high-specification ventilators that provide the basic ICU facilities of PEEP, pressure control, inverse inspiration/expiration ratios, compensate for changes in compliance and have appropriate alarms and back-up systems, are essential. Transfer ventilation should emulate, or be of a higher standard than, that which the patient was receiving in the transferring hospital. When a patient is transferred from one ventilator to another, they should be stabilized for a period of time and arterial blood gases checked to ensure there has been no deterioration. This should occur regardless of the similarity of settings.

CARDIOVASCULAR SYSTEM

In the critically ill patient, fluid balance must be finely tuned to compensate for the effects of continuing fluid loss, IPPV and PEEP, oxygenation, renal impairment (see below) and cardiovascular performance. It is important to understand that replacing losses and restricting fluids are not always mutually exclusive, because baseline maintenance requirements and insensible losses, which often are overlooked, also have to be considered.

Inotropic sympathomimetics such as adrenaline (epinephrine), dopexamine, dobutamine and dopamine may already be in use to treat the patient. In addition, vascular support may be augmented by vasoconstrictive sympathomimetics such as noradrenaline (norepinephrine) and terlipressin. These drugs may be considered life-vital components of care, as any sudden interruption in their administration may result in severe instability or cardiac arrest. Other drugs are considered below.

To attenuate the effects of flight, the circulation must be optimally filled and supported. Some patients, such as those with major trauma or burns, may require additional fluids to ensure that they have been filled adequately. To ensure that changes related to fluid balance may be dealt with and appropriate drugs given, adequate access to the circulation must be available. For continued resuscitation, large-bore cannulae are required. Vasoactive drugs require administration via the central venous route, and this must also be available. This also provides for monitoring of central venous pressure to aid cardiovascular monitoring.

Patients with SIRS affecting the circulation will also require optimal filling but may need increases in support from inotropic or vasoconstrictive drugs as transfer begins. Patients with spinal-cord injury are discussed below. If the potential for instability is suspected, then drugs to support the circulation should be prepared in advance and be available immediately with adequate central venous access.

Impaired myocardial contractility occurs in critically ill patients due to the effects of changes in acid–base balance, electrolyte disturbance and the inflammatory substances released in SIRS. Arrhythmias compound these effects and may be caused by the same factors. Addressing the issues by monitoring and correcting acid–base balance, arterial blood gases and electrolytes, particularly potassium and magnesium, will do much to attenuate these problems.

Following myocardial infarction, the myocardium may be extremely irritable and prone to arrhythmias, which may precipitate cardiac arrest. Cardiac failure and cardiogenic shock may also occur. It is unwise to attempt to subject these patients to a secondary aeromedical transfer until these issues have been treated adequately and in any event not within the first 48 hours. It is also possible that the patient may not have received what is regarded as adequate treatment for their initial infarction, and angina may be a feature.

Angina in this circumstance, or unstable angina occurring without evidence of preceding infarction, should lead to the patient being regarded as critically ill, and he or she should be attended by a critical-care transfer team as the risk of deterioration is high. The worst-case scenario of acute arrhythmia and cardiac arrest can be managed safely only with appropriately trained individuals and equipment. If the patient survives, then he or she will not necessarily wake or maintain ventilation adequately and will need critical-care support.

The situation may be complicated further by the preparation to move the patient, which may lead to increased intrinsic sympathomimetic activity and, thus, mask the effects of inadequate filling and vagal influences. In some instances, this may lead to unwanted tachycardia and hypertension. In other patients, the opposite occurs, with acute vagal stimulation from, e.g. moving the patient's head when they are intubated. Finally, the adjuvant therapy with sedation, analgesia or neuromuscular blockade that is given customarily to reduce the effects of transfer may precipitate bradycardia and acute vasodilation in the cardiovascularly compromised patient.

GASTROINTESTINAL TRACT

Support of the gastrointestinal tract is achieved by initial drainage, early feeding, optimizing fluid balance, gas exchange and improving perfusion generally. The placement of a nasogastric drainage tube is normally a requirement for aeromedical transfers of critically ill patients, and there are few exceptions. Decompressing the stomach of gas and fluid reduces the potential effects discussed above. Feeding should be stopped a number of hours before transfer, in order to reduce the likelihood of reflux. The use of prokinetic drugs such as metoclopramide or erythromycin may be considered. Nasogastric or orogastric tubes should be aspirated and then placed on free drainage, while

remaining dependent. As drainage bags expand, they should be decompressed regularly.

In order to reduce the incidence of upper-gastrointestinal tract haemorrhage over the period of cessation of feeding, or in patients who are not fed, H_2-receptor-blocking drugs such as ranitidine or proton-pump inhibitors such as omeprazole should be used. For long transfers, feeding may be recommenced at the discretion of the attending physician. The choice and volume of food depend on the individual patient's requirement.

If there has been intra-abdominal surgery and/or bowel surgery without sufficient time to allow anastomoses to heal and ileus to settle, then sea-level cabin altitude should be requested. If there is ileus from medical causes, with a risk of perforation or acute uncontrollable haemorrhage, then transfer should be delayed until this has resolved, by either therapeutic or surgical means.

HEPATIC FUNCTION

Hepatic dysfunction may be primary, due to ingestion of drugs, or as a result of viral hepatitis. In the critically ill patient, changes in blood flow, the presence of toxins and drugs in the circulation, and the direct effects of infective agents compromise hepatic function. Also, increased intra-abdominal pressure (intra-abdominal compartment syndrome) due to ileus or haematoma may compromise hepatic function indirectly by impairing perfusion.

Impaired hepatocyte function increases the potential for coagulopathy and for altered metabolism of drugs. In practice, mildly deranged hepatic function is of little significance during transfer. However, in the case of acute hepatic failure, even short-distance ground transfer may be extremely hazardous due to the circulatory and neurological effects associated with the condition. Transfer by air to enable the patient to receive hepatic transplantation may be justified and the attendant risk accepted.

In the last instance, issues such as management of blood glucose, circulatory maintenance, coagulation and management of neurological status need to be addressed. Patients with cerebral oedema are particularly at risk and should have intracranial pressure measurement. As with all transfers, the ability to treat must accompany the ability to monitor.

RENAL FUNCTION

Reduced blood flow to and within the kidney occurs in critically ill patients. It is caused by systemic hypotension and the effects of sepsis. Intrinsic renal damage may result and be aggravated by hypoxia and the nephrotoxic effects of drugs. Usually there is a combination of factors, and they may result in impaired renal function and even renal failure.

Impaired renal function may also be due to existing renal disease, which may or may not have been identified previously. The goal in critically ill patients is to maintain function or, where it is impaired or lost, to replace it. In the modern critical-care environment, acute renal failure is not an individual cause of mortality, and renal replacement is available routinely.

Patients who are treated inadequately may be subject to changes in electrolytes during the flight, which will compromise their safety. If this occurs, then there is a limited response available and the patient may suffer irreversible cardiac dysfunction. Temporizing treatments with sodium bicarbonate, calcium salts, glucose and insulin or ion-exchange resins have a limited role and allow the patient to survive a short journey, but they are not recommended except in extreme circumstances.

Renal replacement is provided to control fluid balance, acid–base balance and electrolytes. In the air-transfer environment, provision of support has been to the level only of addressing fluid balance (Stevens *et al.* 1986). The ability to control acid–base balance and electrolytes requires sophisticated equipment, which, given the nature of weight-activated controls, will not function correctly in the air. It is usually bulky, requires mains power and uses large quantities of fluid in the process. For this reason, patients who have the physiobiochemical derangements associated with renal impairment require renal replacement before transfer, with a period of stabilization post-treatment. Even if the measured parameters are acceptable, treatment in the immediate period before transfer is advisable in patients who are known to be reliant on this therapy. If this is not available locally, then renal support must be provided by the aeromedical team before the patient is moved, in order to ensure optimization.

Urinary catheters need to be checked to ensure that there is free drainage. Urine output should be measured hourly, as in the ICU.

CENTRAL NERVOUS SYSTEM

The major goals in the management of cerebral injury are the avoidance of hypoxia, the normalization of arterial carbon dioxide and the maintenance of cerebral perfusion pressure. Cerebral perfusion pressure is dependent on the mean arterial blood pressure, the central venous pressure and the intracranial pressure. The aim is to reduce the incidence of preventable secondary brain injury.

Head injury may lead to altered level of consciousness and is quantified by assessing the Glasgow coma scale (GCS). Restless uncooperative patients are difficult to manage. They may be a danger to themselves and may even

present a hazard to the aircraft. It is tempting to sedate such patients to manage them, but this is often considered without regard for the underlying pathology or the consequences of reducing the level of consciousness further.

If the level of consciousness is reduced sufficiently, then it is associated with hypoventilation. Hypoventilation will lead initially to hypercarbia and then to hypoxia. Hypercarbia leads to an increase in intracranial pressure, which may be critical for the already injured brain. Hypoxia will also lead to further neurological injury. It is essential that the airway be maintained and that ventilation is controlled in order to avoid this.

Patients with a GCS of 8 or less should be intubated and ventilated (care for the cervical spine should also be practised routinely where trauma has occurred) (Association of Anaesthetists of Great Britain and Northern Ireland 1996). This will require the correct use of drugs to induce anaesthesia. Vasodilation caused by induction agents may lead to hypotension and cerebral hypoperfusion. Conversely, intubation may lead to a marked sympathetic stimulation and a marked increase in intracranial pressure.

The lower cervical spine and the junction between the thoracic spine and the lumbar spine are the most common sites of injury. Spinal fractures and dislocations lead to disturbances of not only sensory and motor but also autonomic function.

Injuries to the cervical and upper thoracic region may lead to cardiovascular instability due to loss of cardio-accelerator nerve output and vascular tone. Below T5, sympathetic innervation of the myocardium is preserved. Ventilation and bronchomotor tone are also affected. These effects are much greater than is normally appreciated (Table 57.1). Ileus, urinary retention, gastric ulceration and haemorrhage may also occur in the early period. These patients have a markedly increased risk of deep venous thrombosis. Later post-injury, general nutrition issues and pressure areas are a problem.

Injury of the thoracic spine due to trauma is likely to be complicated by other thoracic injury, including pulmonary contusion, as discussed above. This adds to the problems of secretion retention and the potential to develop pulmonary sepsis. Adequate, preferably closed-system, suction apparatus is essential in order to reduce the effects of bronchial plugging, which can lead to rapid desaturation. However, it must also be remembered that patients with unopposed vagal influence due to high spinal-cord injury may be prone to profound bradycardia or even asystole when subjected to endobronchial suctioning.

BURNS AND TRAUMA

Patients who have been injured due to burns or trauma may, in addition to their original injury, develop a SIRS

Table 57.1   *Effects of spinal-cord dysfunction*

Location	Cardiovascular effects	Bronchial tone effects	Ventilation effects
High cervical	Bradycardia, hypotension	Variable tone, potential for bronchospasm	Failure of ventilation, requires immediate intervention
Mid-cervical	Bradycardia, hypotension	Variable tone, potential for bronchospasm	Paradoxical ventilation, reduced functional residual capacity, inability to cough
Low cervical	Bradycardia, hypotension	Variable tone, potential for bronchospasm	Hypoventilation, sputum retention, deterioration of ventilation likely after initial period
Upper thoracic	Bradycardia, hypotension		Loss of intercostals, peripheral diaphragm, hypoventilation, cough reduced, sputum retention
Lower thoracic	Hypotension		Loss of abdominal-wall tone, reduced cough

picture. It is unpredictable who will develop this complication, which may carry a genetic predisposition. Some patients who have received what might be considered a relatively minor injury may be affected, whereas others who are severely injured may not.

Following limb trauma, care must be taken to exclude compartment syndromes and any required fasciotomies should be undertaken pre-transfer. Fractures need to be stabilized adequately, preferably with a rigid fixation device. This is particularly important if there is any question of vascular compromise. In the case of serious pelvic fracture, where there is risk of further haemorrhage, external fixation is also essential.

TEMPERATURE

Control of temperature is important in the critically ill patient. During sedation and with the use of neuro-muscular blockade, normal temperature-control mechanisms are disrupted. This is accentuated by critical illness, where normal metabolic processes are compromised. In these circumstances, the patient tends to become hypothermic (core temperature below 35 °C). This is aggravated by other temperature losses, such as those occurring during ventilation, the administration of intravenous fluids, from evaporation from fluid loss in haemorrhage post-trauma or burns, and exposure to the environment.

Hypothermia interferes with normal metabolic processes, including the metabolism of drugs, and it can delay elimination of drugs. This is probably of less significance in the context of aeromedical evacuation. Hypothermia affects cardiovascular function; when severe, this leads to life-threatening arrhythmias. It also interferes with clotting mechanisms. The latter is of particular significance in aeromedical evacuation required during the acute phase of post-trauma, where haemorrhage continues

and further resuscitation is required. It may mean the difference between survival and exsanguination.

THERAPEUTICS

Transfer critical care requires, at a minimum, drugs reflecting the therapeutic regimen on which the patient is established before transfer. This will normally include, at the very basic level, analgesia, sedation and often neuro-muscular blockade. Some of the issues of neuromuscular blockade have been discussed above. Others, including the precipitation or aggravation of critical-care neuropathy, are too complex for the purposes of this discussion.

As a general principle, the patients should remain on an established regimen if they are stable and are suitable for transfer. Apart from the drugs that maintain analgesia, sedation and muscle relaxation, there may be others supporting the patient. These drugs may be life-vital as well as generally supportive and must be continued. If drugs are changed just before transfer, then there may be serious consequences, such as severe cardiovascular instability. Drugs should, therefore, be added only to facilitate transfer, and any changes to drugs should be studied over a period of time to judge properly the therapeutic effects of those changes.

In addition to the drugs mentioned already, the critically ill patient requires other therapeutic agents such as antimicrobials, anticoagulants, antiarrhythmics and drugs to aid in the prevention of gastrointestinal haemorrhage (H_2-receptor-blocking drugs, proton-pump inhibitors). These drugs may all be at therapeutic levels before transfer, but during a prolonged transfer further administration will be required.

This approach sometimes means that patients may be on a therapeutic regimen that is not normally used by the transfer team, but the similarity of the drug effects may be read across and the patient can be maintained safely on the drugs from the transferring facility. If this is the situation, then uplifting adequate supplies to cover the transfer should be undertaken.

TRANSFER

When all of the above have been considered, and any potential for optimization has been exploited, the patient is ready to be transferred. This begins with transfer on to the portable equipment before the movement of the patient is actually contemplated. Once this has been successful and a period of observation has passed, in order to ensure that no adverse effects have occurred, the patient may be moved.

The selection of team members is potentially different for each phase of the transfer. Short transfers by rotary-wing aircraft or by road to fixed-wing aircraft can be achieved by the minimum of a critical-care aeromedical physician and a critical-care aeromedical nurse. For longer, fixed-wing flights, technical support and additional logistic personnel should be included.

SUMMARY

Moving the patient requires many skills, including currency in critical-care practice and transfer medicine. It takes a high level of expertise and experience accompanied by constant vigilance and the ability to function in the potentially harsh environment of the aircraft. It can be accomplished safely only by properly trained medical and nursing personnel, with the correct equipment and supported by appropriate technical and logistic support. Even if all these conditions are satisfied, there remains the potential for adverse events when dealing with critically ill patients.

REFERENCES

American College of Chest Physicians/Society of Critical Care Medicine. Consensus conference: definitions for sepsis and organ failure and guidelines for the use of innovative therapies in sepsis. *Critical Care Medicine* 1992; **20**: 864–74.

Association of Anaesthetists of Great Britain and Northern Ireland. *Recommendations for the Transfer of Patients with Acute Head Injuries to Neurosurgical Units.* London: Association of Anaesthetists of Great Britain and Northern Ireland, 1996.

Dirven PJA. Minimal sealing pressures of endotracheal tube cuffs filled with saline in a model of the airway. Presented at AIRMED 2002 World Congress, 17–20 September 2002. Interlaken, Switzerland.

Stevens PE, Bloodworth LL, Rainford DJ. High altitude haemofiltration. *British Medical Journal (Clinical Research Edition)* 1986; **292**: 1354.

Trunkey DD. Trauma. *Scientific American* 1983; **249**: 20–27.

Appendix: units of measurements

Table A1 *General physical units and useful equivalents*

Quantity	Symbol	SI unit	Other units	Abbreviations	Useful equivalents	Notes
Acceleration:						
Linear	a	metre per second squared		m/s^2	$3.281\ ft/s^2$	1
			foot per second squared	ft/s^2	$0.305\ m/s^2$	
			inch per second squared	in/s^2	$0.025\ m/s^2$	
Angular	α	radian per second squared		rad/s^2	$57.296°/s^2$	
			Degree per second squared	$°/s^2$	$0.01745\ rad/s^2$	
Angle:						
Plane	$\alpha, \beta, \gamma,$ etc.	radian		rad	$0.001\ rad$	2,3
			milliradian	mrad	$1.745 \times 10^{-2}\ rad$	
			degree	°	$2.909 \times 10^{-4}\ rad$	
			minute of arc	′	$4.898 \times 10^{-6}\ rad$	
			second of arc	″		
Solid	Ω	steradian		sr		2
Area	A or S	square metre		m^2	$10.76\ feet^2$	
			square kilometre	km^2	$1.0 \times 10^6\ m^2$	
			square centimetre	cm^2	$1.0 \times 10^{-4}\ m^2$	
			square millimetre	mm^2	$1.0 \times 10^{-6}\ m^2$	
			square hectometre (hectare)	ha	$1.0 \times 10^4\ m^2$	
			square inch	in^2	$6.452\ cm^2$	
			square foot	ft^2	$0.0929\ m^2$, $929.03\ cm^2$	
			square yard	yd^2	$0.836\ m^2$	
			acre		$4047\ m^2$	
			square mile	$mile^2$	$2.59\ km^2$	
Density	ρ	kilogram per cubic metre		kg/m^3		
			gram per cubic centimetre	g/cm^3	$1.0 \times 10^{-3}\ kg/m^3$	
			pound mass per cubic inch	lb/in^3	$2.768 \times 10^4\ kg/m^3$	
			pound mass per cubic foot	lb/in^3	$16.018\ kg/m^3$	
Electric current	I	ampere		A	$1 \times$ coulomb/s	
Energy, work, amount of heat		joule (J) (newton metre)		$J = N.m$	$0.738\ ft\ lbf$,	4
			foot pound force	ft lbf	$9.478 \times 10^{-4}\ BTU$,	
					$0.239ca1$	
			British Thermal Unit	BTU	$1.356\ J$	
			kilowatt hour	kWh	$1055.06\ J$.	
			kilocalorie	kcal	$3.6 \times 10^6\ J$	
			calorie	cal	$4185.5\ J$	
			horsepower hour	hph	$4.185\ J$	
			foot poundal	ft pdl	$2.684 \times 10^6\ J$	
			erg	erg	$0.042\ J$	
					$1.0 \times 10^{-7}\ J$	

Table A1 *(Continued.)*

Quantity	Symbol	SI unit	Other units	Abbreviations	Useful equivalents	Notes
Force	F	newton (N)		N = kg.m/s²	0.245 lbf	5
			kilogram force (kilopond)	kgf (kp)	9.807 N	
			pound force	lbf (Lb)	4.448 N	
			ounce force	ozf	0.278 N	
			poundal	pdl	0.138N	
			dyne	dyn	1.0×10^{-5} N	
			pond	p	9.807×10^{-3} N	
Frequency	f	Hertz (Hz) (events per second)		Hz	2π rad/s, 6.283 rad/s	
			cycles per second	cps	1 Hz	
	ω		radians per second	rad/s	0.1592 Hz	
Heat, production	H	watt		W = J/s		
Heat, transfer						
Convective	C					
Conductive	K					
Evaporative	E	watt (W)		W = J/s		
Radiant	R					
Illumination		lumen per square metre (lux (lx))		lx = lm/m² = cd/sr/m²		6
			lumen per square foot	lm/ft²	10.764 lx	
			foot-candle	ft-candle	10.764 lx	
Length	L	metre		m	3.281 feet	7
			kilometre	km	1.0×10^{3} m, 0.621 mile	
			centimetre	cm	1.0×10^{-2} m, 0.594 in	
			millimetre	mm	1.0×10^{-3} m	
			micrometre	μm	1.0×10^{-6} m	
			nanometre	nm	1.0×10^{-9} m	
			inch	in	2.54 cm	
			foot	ft	0.305 m	
			yard	yd	0.914 m	
			mile: statute	mile	1.609 km	
			nautical (UK)	nm (UK)	1.853km, 1.152 mile	
			nautical (Int)	nm (Int)	1.852km	
Luminance (surface brightness)		candelas per square metre		cd/m²		
			candelas per square foot	cd/ft²	10.764 cd/m²	
			foot-Lambert	ft L	3.426 cd/m²	
Luminous flux		lumen		cd/sr		8
Luminous intensity		candela		cd		7

Table A1 *(Continued.)*

Quantity	Symbol	SI unit	Other units	Abbreviations	Useful equivalents	Notes
Mass	m	kilogram		kg	2.205 lb	7
			gram	g	1.0×10^{-3} kg	
			ounce	oz	28.35 g	
			pound	lb	0.454kg	
			ton (imperial)	ton	1016.05 kg	
			tonne (metric ton)	t	1.0×10^3 kg	
Matter	n	mole		mol		7,9
Moment of inertia			kilogram metre squared	kg m²		
			pound foot squared	lb ft²	0.04214 kg m²	
			slug foot squared	slug ft²	1.356 kg m²	
Moment of force (torque)			newton metre	Nm		
			pound force foot	lbf ft	1.356 Nm	
Pressure	p	pascal (Pa) (newton per square metre)		Pa = N/m²	0.021 lbf/ft²	
			kilopascal	kPa	1000 Pa, 7.501 mm Hg (Torr)	
			micropascal	μPa	1.0×10^{-6} Pa	
			bar	b	1.0×10^5 pa, 14.504 lbf/in²	
			millibar	mbar	1.0×10^2 Pa, 1.0×10^{-3} b	
			millimetre of water	mm H₂O	9.807 Pa	
			centimetre of water	cm H₂O	98.067 Pa	
			inch of water	in H₂O	249.081 Pa, 1.868 mmHg (Torr)	
			millimetre of mercury	mmHg (Torr)	133.322 Pa, 0.133 kPa, 0.019 lbf/in²	
			pound force per square foot	lbf/ft²	47.88 Pa, 0.359 mmHg (Torr)	
			pound force per square inch	lbf/in² (psi)	6894.74 Pa,68.948 mbar, 51.715 mmHg (Torr)	
			atmosphere (standard)	atm	101.325 kPa, 1013.25 mbar, 760.00 mmHg (Torr), 14.696 lbf/in² (psi)	
Power (work rate)	P	watt (W)		W = J/s	0.738 ft lbf/s, 0.102 kgf m/s	10
			kilogram force metre per second	kgf m/s	9.807 W	
			foot pound force per second	ft lbf/s	1.356 W	
			horsepower	hp	745.7 W, 550.0 feet lbf/s	
			kilocalorie per hour	kcal/h	1.16 W	

Table A1   (Continued.)

Quantity	Symbol	SI unit	Other units	Abbreviations	Useful equivalents	Notes
Radiation:						
Quantity	D	gray (Gy)	radiation absorbed dose	Gy = J/kg, rad	100.0 rad, 0.01 Gy	
Dose equivalent		sievert (Sv)	roentgen equivalent, man	Sv = J/kg, rem	100.0 rem, 0.01 Sv	
Relative humidity	rh			%		
Revolution (frequency of rotation)		n(r)	units per minute	n/min = (rpm)		
Skin wettedness	w			%		
Sound:						
Pressure	p	pascal (Pa) (newton per square metre)	dynes per square centimetre (microbar)	Pa = N/m², dyn/cm² (μbar)		
Pressure level	Lp		decibel	dB		11
Specific heat	c	joule per kilogram per degree Celsius		J/(kg.°C)		
Temperature	T	kelvin		K	°C + 273.15, (5/9) (°F + 459.67)	7
			degree Celsius	°C	K − 273.15, (5/9) (°F − 32)	
			degree Fahrenheit	°F	(9/5)°C + 32, (9/5) K − 459.67	
Thermal:						
Conductance	C			W/(m².°C)		
Conductivity	k or λ	watt per metre per kelvin		W/(m.K)		
Insulation	I		tog, clo	°C.m²/W	0.1°C.m²/W, 0.645 clo, 1.55 tog	
Resistance	R			°C.m²/W		
Storage	S	watt (W)		W = J/s		
Time	t	second	minute, hour, day	s, min, h, d	60 s, 360 s, 8460 s	7

Torque – see Moment of force

Table A1 (Continued.)

Quantity	Symbol	SI unit	Other units	Abbreviations	Useful equivalents	Notes
Velocity: Linear	v	metre per second		m/s	3.281 ft/s	
			kilometre per hour	km/h	0.278 m/s, 0.621 mph	
			feet per minute	ft/min	0.005 m/s	
			feet per second	ft/s	0.305 m/s	
			mile per hour	mph	0.447 m/s, 1.609 km/h, 1.46 ft/s	
			nautical mile (UK) per hour	kt	0.515 m/s, 1.853 km/h	
Angular	ω	radian per second		rad/s	57.296°/s	
			degree per second	°/s	0.01745 rad/s	
			revolutions per minute	rpm	6°/s, 0.1047 rad/s	
Volume	V	cubic metre		m³	2.832×10^{-2} feet³	
			cubic centimetre	cm³ (cc)	1.0×10^{-6} m³	
			cubic decimetre	dm³	1.0×10^{-3} m³ 1000 cm³ = 1000 ml	
			litre	L (dm³)	0.035 feet³, 1000 cm³, 61.025 in³	
			millilitre	ml (cm)	1.0×10^{-6} m³	
			cubic inch	in³	16.387 cm³, 0.016 L	
			cubic foot	ft³	28.317 L	
			pint	pint	0.568 L	
			gallon (UK)	gal (UK)	4.546 L	
			gallon (US)	gal (US)	3.785 L	
Volume flow	V	cubic metre per second		m³/s	1.0×10^{-3} m³/s	12
			litres per second	L/s	1.667×10^{-3} m³/s, 0.035 ft³/min	
			litres per minute	L/min	28.317 L/min	
			cubic foot per minute	ft³/min		
			gallon per hour	gal/h	4.546 L/h	

1. Standard acceleration due to gravity (gn) = 9.80665 m/s² = 32.174 ft/s².
2. Supplementary base unit of the SI.
3. A complete circle subtends an angle of 2π rad.
4. The joule is the energy expended in the application of a force of 1 newton through a distance of 1 metre.
5. The newton is the force required to accelerate a mass of 1 kilogram at 1 metre per second per second.
6. The lux is the illumination of a surface at an intensity of 1 lumen per square metre.
7. Base unit of the SI.
8. The lumen is the luminous flux emitted within a solid angle of 1 steradian by a point source having a luminous intensity of 1 candela.
9. One mole of an atomic, molecular or ionic substance is the amount of the substance that contains 6.023×10^{23} atoms, molecules or ions.
10. The watt is the power which in one second gives rise to an energy of 1 joule.
11. The decibel (dB) is a logarithmic measure of relative intensity, and dB = $20 \log_{10}$ (P measured/P reference). In the measurement of sound, P reference is a sound pressure of 2.0×10^{-5} Pa = 2.0×10^{-4} μbar = 20 μPa.
12. 1 lb air at 760 mmHg (Torr) and 20°C occupies 13.3 ft³ or 376.6 L. 1 ft³ air at 760 mmHg (Torr) and 20°C weighs 0.075 lbf or 34.0 g.

Table A2   *Derivation of SI units*

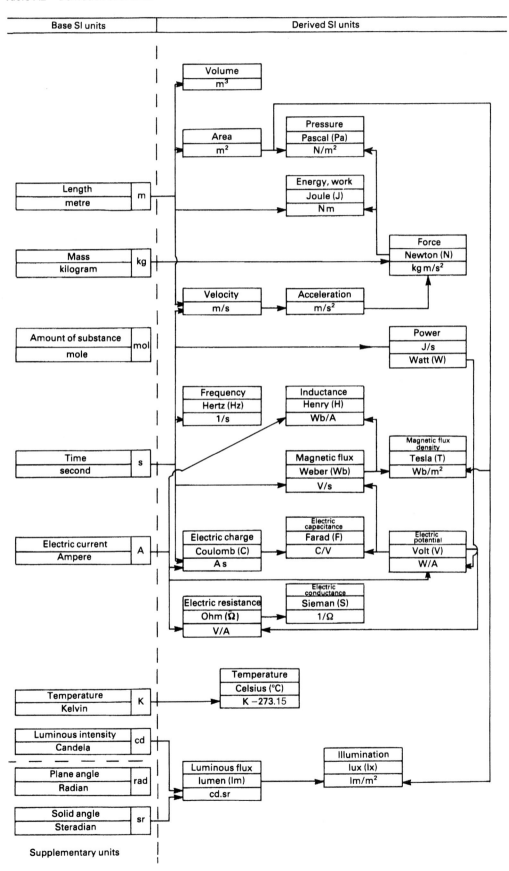

Table A3 *Conversion table for units of pressure*

To/From	kPa	Pa (N/m²)	b	mbar	atm	mmHg (Torr)	in Hg	cm H₂O	in H₂O	lbf/ft²	lbf/in²
kPa	1	1000	0.01	10	9.872×10^{-3}	7.501	0.295	10.197	4.014	20.885	0.145
Pa (N/m²)	0.001	1	1×10^{-5}	0.01	9.872×10^{-6}	7.501×10^{-3}	2.953×10^{-4}	0.01	4.014×10^{-3}	0.021	1.45×10^{-4}
b	100	1×10^{5}	1	1000	0.987	750.062	29.53	1019.71	401.436	2088.543	14.504
mbar	0.1	100	0.001	1	9.87×10^{-4}	0.75	0.029	1.02	0.401	2.088	0.014
atm	101.325	1.013×10^{5}	1.013	1013.25	1	760	29.92	1033.26	406.78	2116.216	14.696
mm Hg (Torr)	0.133	133.322	1.333×10^{-3}	1.333	1.316×10^{-3}	1	0.039	1.359	0.535	2.784	0.019
in Hg	3.386	3386.4	0.034	33.864	0.033	25.4	1	34.531	13.595	70.726	0.491
cm H₂O	0.098	98.067	9.806×10^{-4}	0.981	9.679×10^{-4}	0.735	0.029	1	0.394	2.048	0.014
in H₂O	0.249	249.081	2.491×10^{-3}	2.491	2.458×10^{-3}	1.868	0.074	2.54	1	5.202	0.036
lbf/ft²	0.048	47.88	4.788×10^{-4}	0.479	4.725×10^{-4}	0.359	0.014	0.488	0.192	1	6.94×10^{-3}
lbf/in²	6.895	6894.74	0.069	68.948	0.068	51.715	2.036	70.376	27.707	144	1

Table A4 *Conversion table for units of energy*

To/from	J(N/m)	ft/bf	BTU	kWh	kilocal	cal	hph
J(N/m)	1	0.738	9.471×10^{-4}	2.778×10^{-7}	2.387×10^{-4}	0.239	3.777×10^{-7}
ftlbf	1.356	1	1.284×10^{-3}	3.766×10^{-7}	3.236×10^{-4}	0.324	5.12×10^{-7}
BTU	1055.06	778.768	1	2.933×10^{-4}	0.252	251.2	3.987×10^{-4}
kWh	3.6×10^{6}	2.655×10^{-6}	3409.52	1	859.184	8.592×10^{5}	1.36
kilocal	4185.5	3090.4	3.968	1.164×10^{-3}	1	1000	1.581×10^{-3}
cal	4.185	3.09	3.968×10^{-3}	1.164×10^{-6}	0.001	1	1.581×10^{-6}
hph	2.684×10^{6}	1.952×10^{6}	2507.9	0.735	632.61	6.326×10^{5}	1

Table A5 *Respiratory symbology*

	Symbol	Definition
Quantitative variables:	F	Fractional concentration of gas
	f	Respiratory frequency
	P	Pressure in general
	Q	Blood volume in general
	$\dot{Q}$	Blood volume per unit time (flow)
	R	Respiratory exchange ratio
	S	Saturation
	t	Temperature
	V	Gas volume in general
	$\dot{V}$	Gas volume per unit time (flow)
	$\dot{v}$	Instantaneous gas flow per unit time
Qualifying terms (subscripts):		
Gas phase	A	Alveolar
	B	Barometric
	D	Dead space
	E	Expired
	$\bar{E}$	Mixed expired*
	ET	End-tidal
	I	Inspired
	T	Tidal
Blood phase	a	Arterial
	c	Capillary
	V	Venous
General	ATPD	Ambient temperature and pressure, dry
	ATPS	Ambient temperature and pressure, saturated with water
	BTPS	Body temperature (37°C) and ambient pressure, saturated with water
	STPD	Standard temperature (0°C) and pressure (760 mmHg), dry
	NTP	Normal temperature (15°C) and pressure (760 mmHg)

*NB: A bar over any symbol indicates a mean value.

Table A6   *Thermal symbology*

	Symbol	Definition
Quantitative variables:	A	Area
	I	Thermal insulation
	p	Pressure in general
	T	Temperature
Qualifying terms (subscripts):		
Physical	a	Air
	b	Body
	c	Convective
	cl	Clothing
	db	Drybulb
	dp	Dew point
	e	Evaporative
	eff	Effective
	g	Globe
	k	Conductive
	n	Natural (vs ventilated)
	o	Operative
	r	Radiant
	v	Ventilated
	w	Water (vapour)
	wb	Wet bulb
Physiological	a	Arterial
	ac	Auditory canal
	b	Body
	bl	Blood
	bs	Bodysurface
	co	Core
	gi	Gastrointestinal
	lb	Lean body
	oe	Oesophageal
	re	Rectal
	sk	Skin
	tr	Tracheal
	ty	Tympanic

Table A7   *Vibration/biodynamics symbology*

	Symbol	Definition
Quantitative variables:	g	Gravitational constant
	G	Gravitoinertial force
	s	Displacement
	v	Velocity
	a	Acceleration
	c	Coefficient of damping
	c_c	Coefficient for critical damping
	ζ	Damping factor (c/c_c)
	m	Mass
	k	Stiffness
	f	Frequency
	f_n	Undamped natural frequency
	Ω	Angular frequency
Qualifying terms:	x	Antero-posterior
(directional subscripts with	y	Lateral
respect to body)	z	Cranio-caudal
	ϕ	Rotation about x axis (roll)
	θ	Rotation about y axis (pitch)
	ψ	Rotation about z axis (yaw)

Index